4TH EDITION

MOLECULAR BIOTECHNOLOGY

Principles and Applications of Recombinant DNA

Bernard R. Glick and Jack J. Pasternak

Department of Biology, University of Waterloo
Waterloo, Ontario, Canada

Cheryl L. Patten

Biology Department, University of New Brunswick
Fredericton, New Brunswick, Canada

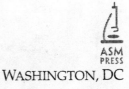

ASM
PRESS

WASHINGTON, DC

Address editorial correspondence to ASM Press, 1752 N St. NW, Washington, DC 20036-2904, USA

Send orders to ASM Press, P.O. Box 605, Herndon, VA 20172, USA
Phone: (800) 546-2416 or (703) 661-1593
Fax: (703) 661-1501
E-mail: books@asmusa.org
Online: estore.asm.org

Library of Congress Cataloging-in-Publication Data

Glick, Bernard R.
 Molecular biotechnology : principles and applications of recombinant DNA / Bernard R. Glick, Jack J. Pasternak, and Cheryl L. Patten. — 4th ed.
 p. ; cm.
 Includes bibliographical references and index.
 ISBN 978-1-55581-498-4 (hardcover)
 1. Biotechnology. 2. Genetic engineering. 3. Molecular biology. I. Pasternak, Jack J. II. Patten, Cheryl L. III. Title.
 [DNLM: 1. Biotechnology. 2. Genetic Engineering. 3. Molecular Biology. TP 248.2 G559m 2010]
 TP248.2.G58 2010
 660.6′5—dc22

 2009026838

10 9 8 7 6 5 4 3 2 1

Cover and interior design: Susan Brown Schmidler
Cover illustration: Terese Winslow

In memory of Lili Pasternak (1938–2008),
an extraordinary human being

This page intentionally left blank

Contents

PART II
MOLECULAR BIOTECHNOLOGY OF MICROBIAL SYSTEMS 331

PART III
MOLECULAR BIOTECHNOLOGY OF EUKARYOTIC SYSTEMS 723

PART IV
MOLECULAR BIOTECHNOLOGY AND SOCIETY 895

Preface

SINCE THE EARLY 1970S, when recombinant DNA technology was first developed, there has been a veritable explosion of knowledge in the biological sciences. Since that time, with the advent of PCR, chemical DNA synthesis, DNA sequencing, monoclonal antibodies, directed mutagenesis, genomics, proteomics, and metabolomics, our understanding of and ability to manipulate the biological world have grown exponentially. When the first edition of *Molecular Biotechnology: Principles and Applications of Recombinant DNA* was published in 1994, nearly all of the transgenic organisms that were produced included only a single introduced gene. Just 15 years later, it is not uncommon for researchers to engineer organisms by modifying both the activity and the regulation of existing genes while at the same time introducing entire new pathways. In 1994, only a handful of products produced by this new technology were available in the marketplace. Today, molecular biotechnology has given us several hundred new therapeutic agents, with many more in the pipeline, as well as dozens of transgenic plants. The use of DNA has become a cornerstone of modern forensics, paternity testing, and ancestry determination. Several new recombinant vaccines have been developed, with many more on the horizon. The list goes on and on. Molecular biotechnology really has lived up to its promise, to all of the original hype. It has been estimated that worldwide there are currently several thousand biotechnology companies employing tens of thousands of scientists. When the exciting science being done at universities, government labs, and research institutes around the world is factored in, the rate of change and of discovery in the biological sciences is astounding. This fourth edition of *Molecular Biotechnology*, building upon the fundamentals that were established in the previous three editions, endeavors to provide readers with a window on some of the major developments in this growing field in the past several years. Of necessity, we have had to be highly selective in the material that is included in this edition. Moreover, the window that we are looking through is moving. This notwithstanding, we both expect and look forward to the commercialization of many of these discoveries as well as to the development of new approaches, insights, and discoveries.

BERNARD R. GLICK
JACK J. PASTERNAK
CHERYL L. PATTEN

This page intentionally left blank

Preface to the First Edition

MOLECULAR BIOTECHNOLOGY EMERGED as a new research field that arose as a result of the fusion in the late 1970s of recombinant DNA technology and traditional industrial microbiology. Whether one goes to the movies to see *Jurassic Park* with its ingenious but scientifically untenable plot of cloning dinosaurs, reads in the newspaper about the commercialization of a new "biotech" tomato that has an extended shelf life, or hears one of the critics of molecular biotechnology talking about the possibility of dire consequences from genetic engineering, there is a significant public awareness about recombinant DNA technology. In this book, we introduce and explain what molecular biotechnology actually is as a scientific discipline, how the research in the area is conducted, and how this technology may realistically impact on our lives in the future.

We have written *Molecular Biotechnology: Principles and Applications of Recombinant DNA* to serve as a text for courses in biotechnology, recombinant DNA technology, and genetic engineering or for any course introducing both the principles and the applications of contemporary molecular biology methods. The book is based on the biotechnology course we have offered for the past 12 years to advanced undergraduate and graduate students from the biological and engineering sciences at the University of Waterloo. We have written this text for students who have an understanding of basic ideas from biochemistry, molecular genetics, and microbiology. We are aware that it is unlikely that students will have had all of these courses before taking a course on biotechnology. Thus, we have tried to develop the topics in this text by explaining their broader biological context before delving into molecular details.

This text emphasizes how recombinant DNA technology can be used to create various useful products. We have, wherever possible, used experimental results and actual methodological strategies to illustrate basic concepts, and we have tried to capture the flavor and feel of how molecular biotechnology operates as a scientific venture. The examples that we have selected—from a vast and rapidly growing literature—were chosen as case studies that not only illustrate particular points but also provide the reader with a solid basis for understanding current research in specialized areas of molecular biotechnology. Nevertheless, we expect that some of our examples will be out of date by the time the book is published, because molecular biotechnology is such a rapidly changing discipline.

For the ease of the day-to-day practitioners, scientific disciplines often develop specialized terms and nomenclature. We have tried to minimize the use of technical jargon and, in many instances, have deliberately used a simple phrase to describe a phenomenon or process that might otherwise have been expressed more succinctly with technical jargon. In any field of study, synonymous terms that describe the same phenomenon exist. In molecular biotechnology, for example, recombinant DNA technology, gene cloning, and genetic engineering, in a broad sense, have the same meaning. When an important term or concept appears for the first time in this text, it is followed in parentheses with a synonym or equivalent expression. An extensive glossary can be found at the end of the book to help the reader with the terminology of molecular biotechnology.

Each chapter opens with an outline of topics and concludes with a detailed summary and list of review questions to sharpen students' critical thinking skills. All of the key ideas in the book are carefully illustrated by the more than 200 full-color diagrams in the pedagogical belief that a picture is indeed worth a thousand words. After introducing molecular biotechnology as a scientific and economic venture in Chapter 1, the next five chapters (2 to 6) deal with the methodologies of molecular biotechnology. The chapters of Part I act as a stepping-stone for the remainder of the book. Chapters 7 to 12 in Part II present examples of microbial molecular biotechnology covering such topics as the production of metabolites, vaccines, therapeutics, diagnostics, bioremediation, biomass utilization, bacterial fertilizers, and microbial pesticides. Chapter 13 describes some of the key components of large-scale fermentation processes using genetically engineered (recombinant) microorganisms. In Part III, we deal with the molecular biotechnology of plants and animals (Chapters 14 and 15). The isolation of human disease-causing genes by using recombinant DNA technology and how, although it is in its early stages, genetic manipulation is being currently contemplated for the treatment of human diseases are presented in Chapters 16 and 17. The book concludes with coverage of the regulation of molecular biotechnology and patents in Part IV.

A brief mention should be made about the reference sections that follow each chapter. Within many of the chapters we have relied upon the published work of various researchers. In all cases, although not cited directly in the body of a chapter, the original published articles are noted in the reference section of the appropriate chapter. In some cases, we have taken "pedagogic license" and either extracted or reformulated data from the original publications. Clearly, we are responsible for any distortions or misrepresentations from these simplifications, although we hope that none has occurred. The reference sections also contain other sources that we used in a general way, which might, if consulted, bring the readers closer to a particular subject.

Acknowledgments

We express our appreciation to the following people who reviewed various parts of the manuscript as it was being developed. The comments of these expert scientists and teachers helped us immeasurably: Arthur I. Aronson, Purdue University; Ronald M. Atlas, University of Louisville; Fred Ausubel, Massachusetts General Hospital; David R. Benson, University of Connecticut; Jean E. Brenchley, Pennsylvania State University; A. M. Chakrabarty, University of Illinois at Chicago; Stan Gelvin, Purdue

University; Janet H. Glaser, University of Illinois at Urbana-Champaign; David Gwynne, Cambridge NeuroScience; George D. Hegeman, Indiana University; James B. Kaper, University of Maryland at Baltimore; Donald R. Lightfoot, Eastern Washington University at Cheney and Spokane; Cynthia Moore, Washington University; William E. Newton, Virginia Polytechnic University; Danton H. O'Day, University of Toronto in Mississauga; Richard D. Palmiter, University of Washington; David H. Persing, Mayo Clinic; William S. Reznikoff, University of Wisconsin; Campbell W. Robinson, University of Waterloo; Marc Siegel, University of Waterloo; Aaron J. Shatkin, Center for Advanced Biotechnology and Medicine at Rutgers University; Jim Schwartz, Genentech; Daniel C. Stein, University of Maryland at College Park; Dean A. Stetler, University of Kansas; and Robert T. Vinopal, University of Connecticut.

The following professionals at ASM Press worked on the book and deserve our thanks: Susan Birch, senior production editor; Ruth Siegal, developmental editor; Jodi Simpson, copy editor; Susan Schmidler, designer and art director; Peg Markow at Ruttle, Shaw & Wetherill, Inc., senior project manager; and Network Graphics, illustrators. Finally we are indebted to Patrick Fitzgerald, Director of ASM Press, who, in all possible ways, helped transform our original efforts into an acceptable final form. His encouragement as a persistent and friendly "torturer" was deeply appreciated.

BERNARD R. GLICK
JACK J. PASTERNAK

This page intentionally left blank

I FUNDAMENTALS OF MOLECULAR BIOTECHNOLOGY

MOLECULAR BIOTECHNOLOGY is an exciting scientific discipline that is based on the ability of researchers to transfer specific units of genetic information from one organism to another. This conveyance of a gene or genes relies on the techniques of genetic engineering (recombinant DNA technology). The objective of recombinant DNA technology is often to create a useful product or a commercial process. In part I, the concept of molecular biotechnology, some fundamentals of molecular biology, and recombinant DNA procedures are presented. Essential molecular biotechnology laboratory techniques, including chemical synthesis of genes, the polymerase chain reaction (PCR), and DNA sequencing, are discussed. Developments in sequencing technologies have led to the sequencing of the entire genomes of many organisms, and this has enabled researchers to begin to understand organisms from their sequences and to identify novel genes with potentially useful functions. In addition to isolation (cloning) of genes, it is important that these genes function properly in a host organism. To this end, strategies for optimizing the expression of a cloned gene in either prokaryotic or eukaryotic cells are reviewed. Finally, procedures for modifying cloned genes by the introduction of specific nucleotide changes (in vitro mutagenesis) to enhance the properties of the target proteins are examined. Together, the chapters in part I provide the conceptual and technical underpinnings for understanding the applications of molecular biotechnology that are described in the ensuing chapters.

This page intentionally left blank

The Development of Molecular Biotechnology

The Emergence of Molecular Biotechnology

LONG BEFORE WE KNEW THAT MICROORGANISMS EXISTED or that genes were the units of inheritance, humans looked to the natural world to develop methods to increase food production, preserve food, and heal the sick. Our ancestors discovered that grains could be preserved through fermentation into beer; that storing horse saddles in a warm, damp corner of the stable resulted in the growth of a saddle mold that could heal infected saddle sores; and that intentional exposure to a "contagion" could somehow provide protection from an infectious disease on subsequent exposure. Since the discovery of the microscopic world in the 17th century, microorganisms have been employed in the development of numerous useful processes and products. Many of these are found in our households and backyards. Lactic acid bacteria are used to prepare yogurt and probiotics, insecticide-producing bacteria are sprayed on many of the plants from which the vegetables in our refrigerator were harvested, nitrogen-fixing bacteria are added to the soil used for cultivation of legumes, the enzymatic stain removers in laundry detergent came from a microorganism, and antibiotics derived from common soil microbes are used to treat infectious diseases. These are just a few examples of traditional biotechnologies that have improved our lives. Up to the early 1970s, however, traditional biotechnology was not a well-recognized scientific discipline, and research in this area was centered in departments of chemical engineering and occasionally in specialized microbiology programs.

In a broad sense, biotechnology is concerned with the production of commercial products generated by the metabolic action of microorganisms. More formally, biotechnology may be defined as "the application of scientific and engineering principles to the processing of material by biological agents to provide goods and services." The term "biotechnology" was first used in 1917 by a Hungarian engineer, Karl Ereky, to describe an integrated process for the large-scale production of pigs by using sugar beets as the source of food. According to Ereky, biotechnology was "all lines of work by which products are produced from raw materials with the aid of living

3

FIGURE 1.1 Principal steps of a bioengineered biotechnology process. Parenthetically, Karl Ereky's scheme entailed using inexpensive sugar beets (raw material) to feed pigs (biotransformation) for the production of pork (downstream processing).

things." This fairly precise definition was more or less ignored. For a number of years, the term biotechnology was used to describe two very different engineering disciplines. On one hand, it referred to industrial fermentation. On the other, it was used for the study of efficiency in the workplace—what is now called ergonomics. This ambiguity ended in 1961 when the Swedish microbiologist Carl Göran Hedén recommended that the title of a scientific journal dedicated to publishing research in the fields of applied microbiology and industrial fermentation be changed from the *Journal of Microbiological and Biochemical Engineering and Technology* to *Biotechnology and Bioengineering*. From that time on, biotechnology has clearly and irrevocably been associated with the study of "the industrial production of goods and services by processes using biological organisms, systems, and processes," and it has been firmly grounded in expertise in microbiology, biochemistry, and chemical engineering.

An industrial biotechnology process that uses microorganisms for producing a commercial product typically has three key stages (Fig. 1.1):

1. Upstream processing: preparation of the microorganism and the raw materials required for the microorganism to grow and produce the desired product
2. Fermentation and transformation: growth (fermentation) of the target microorganism in a large bioreactor (usually >100 liters) with the consequent production (biotransformation) of a desired compound, which can be, for example, an antibiotic, an amino acid, or a protein
3. Downstream processing: purification of the desired compound from either the cell medium or the cell mass

Biotechnology research is dedicated to maximizing the overall efficiency of each of these steps and to finding microorganisms that make products that are useful in the preparation of foods, food supplements, and drugs. During the 1960s and 1970s, this research focused on upstream processing, bioreactor design, and downstream processing. These studies led to enhanced bioinstrumentation for monitoring and controlling the fermentation process and to efficient large-scale growth facilities that increased the yields of various products.

The biotransformation component of the overall process was the most difficult phase to manipulate. Commodity production by naturally occurring microbial strains on a large scale was often considerably less than optimal. Initial efforts to enhance product yields focused on creating variants (mutants) by using chemical mutagens or ultraviolet radiation to induce changes in the genetic constitution of existing strains. However, the level of improvement that could be achieved in this way was usually limited biologically. If a mutated strain, for example, synthesized too much of a compound, other metabolic functions often were impaired, thereby causing the strain's growth during large-scale fermentation to be less than desired. Despite this constraint, the traditional "induced mutagenesis and selection" strategies of strain improvement were extremely successful for a number of processes, such as the production of antibiotics.

The traditional genetic improvement regimens were tedious, time-consuming, and costly because of the large numbers of colonies that had to be selected, screened, and tested. Moreover, the best result that could be expected with this approach was the improvement of an existing inherited property of a strain rather than the expansion of its genetic capabilities.

Despite these limitations, by the late 1970s, effective processes for the mass production of a wide range of commercial products had been perfected.

Today, we have acquired sufficient knowledge of the biochemistry, genetics, and molecular biology of microorganisms to accelerate the development of useful and improved biological products and processes and to create new products that would not otherwise occur. Distinct from traditional biotechnology, the modern methods require knowledge of and manipulation of genes, the functional units of inheritance, and the discipline that is concerned with the manipulation of genes for the purpose of producing useful goods and services using living organisms is known as molecular biotechnology. The pivotal development that enabled this technology was the establishment of techniques to isolate genes and to transfer them from one organism to another. This technology is known as recombinant deoxyribonucleic acid (DNA) technology, and it began as a lunchtime conversation between two scientists working in different fields who met at a scientific conference in 1973. In his laboratory at Stanford University in California, Stanley Cohen had been developing methods to transfer plasmids, small circular DNA molecules, into bacterial cells. Meanwhile, Herbert Boyer of the University of California at San Francisco was working with enzymes that cut DNA at specific nucleotide sequences. Over lunch at a scientific meeting, they reasoned that Boyer's enzyme could be used to splice a specific segment of DNA into a plasmid and then the recombinant plasmid could be introduced into a host bacterium using Cohen's method.

Recombinant DNA Technology

It was clear to Cohen and Boyer and others that recombinant DNA technology had far-reaching possibilities. As Cohen noted at the time, "It may be possible to introduce in *E. coli*, genes specifying metabolic or synthetic functions such as photosynthesis or antibiotic production indigenous to other biological classes." The first commercial product produced using recombinant DNA technology was human insulin, which is used in the treatment of diabetes. The DNA sequence that encodes human insulin was synthesized, a remarkable feat in itself at the time, and was transplanted into a plasmid that could be maintained in the common bacterium *Escherichia coli*. The bacterial host cells acted as biological factories for the production of the two peptide chains of human insulin, which, after being combined, could be purified and used to treat diabetics who were allergic to the commercially available porcine (pig) insulin. In the previous decade, this achievement would have seemed absolutely impossible. By today's standards, however, this type of genetic engineering is considered commonplace.

The nature of biotechnology was changed forever by the development of recombinant DNA technology. With these techniques, the maximization of the biotransformation phase of a biotechnology process was achieved more directly. Genetic engineering provided the means to create, rather than merely isolate, highly productive strains. Not long after the production of the first commercial preparation of recombinant human insulin, bacteria and then eukaryotic cells were used for the production of insulin, interferon, growth hormone, viral antigens, and a variety of other therapeutic proteins. Recombinant DNA technology could also be used to facilitate the biological production of large amounts of useful low-molecular-weight compounds and macromolecules that occur naturally in minuscule quantities. Plants and animals became targets to act as natural bioreactors for

producing new or altered gene products that could never have been created either by mutagenesis and selection or by crossbreeding. Molecular biotechnology has become the standard method for developing living systems with novel functions and capabilities for the synthesis of important commercial products.

Most new scientific disciplines do not arise entirely on their own. They are often formed by the amalgamation of knowledge from different areas of research. For molecular biotechnology, the biotechnology component was perfected by industrial microbiologists and chemical engineers, whereas the recombinant DNA technology portion owes much to discoveries in molecular biology, bacterial genetics, and nucleic acid enzymology (Table 1.1). In a broad sense, molecular biotechnology draws on knowledge from a diverse set of fundamental scientific disciplines to create commercial products that are useful in a wide range of applications (Fig. 1.2).

The Cohen and Boyer strategy for gene cloning was an experiment "heard round the world." Once their concept was made public, many other researchers immediately appreciated the power of being able to clone genes. Consequently, scientists created a large variety of experimental protocols that made identifying, isolating, characterizing, and utilizing genes more efficient and relatively easy. These technological developments have had an enormous impact on generating new knowledge in practically all biological disciplines, including animal behavior, developmental biology, molecular evolution, cell biology, and human genetics. Indeed, the emergence of the field of genomics was dependent on the ability to clone large fragments of DNA into plasmids in preparation for sequence determination.

Commercialization of Molecular Biotechnology

The potential of recombinant DNA technology reached the public with a frenzy of excitement, and many people became rich on its promise. Indeed,

FIGURE 1.2 Many scientific disciplines contribute to molecular biotechnology, which generates a wide range of commercial products.

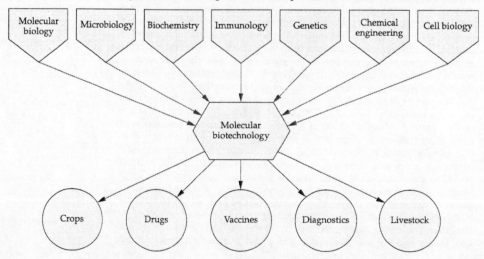

TABLE 1.1 Selected developments in the history of molecular biotechnology

Date	Event
1917	Karl Ereky coins the term "biotechnology"
1940	A. Jost coins the term "genetic engineering"
1943	Penicillin is produced on an industrial scale
1944	Avery, MacLeod, and McCarty demonstrate that DNA is the genetic material
1953	Watson and Crick determine the structure of DNA
1961	The journal *Biotechnology and Bioengineering* is established
1961–1966	Entire genetic code is deciphered
1970	First restriction endonuclease is isolated
1972	Khorana and coworkers synthesize an entire tRNA gene
1973	Boyer and Cohen establish recombinant DNA technology
1975	Kohler and Milstein describe the production of monoclonal antibodies
1976	First guidelines for the conduct of recombinant DNA research are issued
1976	Techniques are developed to determine the sequence of DNA
1978	Genentech produces human insulin in *E. coli*
1980	U.S. Supreme Court rules in the case of Diamond *v.* Chakrabarty that genetically manipulated microorganisms can be patented
1981	First commercial, automated DNA synthesizers are sold
1981	First monoclonal antibody-based diagnostic kit is approved for use in the United States
1982	First animal vaccine produced by recombinant DNA methodologies is approved for use in Europe
1983	Engineered Ti plasmids are used to transform plants
1988	U.S. patent is granted for a genetically engineered mouse susceptible to cancer
1988	PCR method is published
1990	Approval is granted in the United States for a trial of human somatic cell gene therapy
1990	Human Genome Project is officially initiated
1990	Recombinant chymosin is used for cheese making in the United States
1994–1995	Detailed genetic and physical maps of human chromosomes are published
1994	FDA announces that genetically engineered tomatoes are as safe as conventionally bred tomatoes
1995	First genome sequence of a cellular organism, the bacterium *Haemophilus influenzae*, is completed
1996	First recombinant protein, erythropoietin, exceeds $1 billion in annual sales
1996	Complete DNA sequence of all the chromosomes of a eukaryotic organism, the yeast *Saccharomyces cerevisiae*, is determined
1996	Commercial planting of genetically modified crops begins
1997	Nuclear cloning of a mammal (a sheep) with a differentiated cell nucleus is accomplished
1998	FDA approves first antisense drug
1999	FDA approves recombinant fusion protein (diphtheria toxin–interleukin-2) for cutaneous T-cell lymphoma
2000	*Arabidopsis* genome is sequenced
2000	Monoclonal antibodies exceed $2 billion in annual sales
2000	Development of "golden rice" (provitamin-A-producing rice) is announced
2000	Over $33 billion is invested in U.S. biotechnology companies
2001	Human genome is sequenced
2002	Complete human gene microarrays (gene chips) become commercially available
2002	FDA approves first nucleic acid test system to screen whole blood from donors for HIV and HCV
2004	Large-scale sequencing of the Sargasso Sea metagenome begins
2005	NCBI announces that there are 100 gigabases of nucleotides in the GenBank sequence database
2006	Recombinant cancer vaccine becomes available to protect against cervical cancer
2008	Two-billionth acre of genetically engineered crops is planted
2009	FDA approves first drug produced in a genetically engineered animal (a goat)

FDA, Food and Drug Administration; HCV, hepatitis C virus; HIV, human immunodeficiency virus; NCBI, National Center for Biotechnology Information; PCR, polymerase chain reaction; tRNA, transfer ribonucleic acid.

within 20 minutes of the start of trading on the New York Stock Exchange on 14 October 1980, the price of shares in Genentech, the company, founded by Cohen and Boyer with chemist and entrepreneur Robert Swanson, that produced recombinant human insulin, went from $35 to $89. This was the fastest increase in the value of any initial public offering in the history of the market. It was predicted that some genetically engineered microorganisms would replace chemical fertilizers and others would eat up oil spills, plants with inherited resistance to a variety of pests and exceptional nutritional content would be created, and livestock would have faster growing times, more efficient feed utilization, and meat with low fat content. Many were convinced that as long as a biological characteristic was genetically determined by one or a few genes, organisms with novel genetic constitutions could be readily created. Today we see that, despite the commercial hype that dominated reality in the beginning, this infatuation with recombinant DNA technology was not totally unfounded. A number of the more sensible versions of the initial claims, although trimmed in scope, have become realities.

In the 25 years since the commercial production of recombinant human insulin, more than 200 new drugs produced by recombinant DNA technology have been used to treat over 300 million people for diseases such as cancer, multiple sclerosis, cystic fibrosis, and strokes and to provide protection against infectious diseases. Over 400 new drugs are in the process of being tested in human trials to treat Alzheimer disease and heart disease (to name only two). Similarly, many new molecular biotechnology products for enhancing crop and livestock yields, decreasing pesticide use, and improving industrial processes, such as the manufacture of pulp and paper, food, energy, and textiles, have been created and are being marketed.

The impact on agriculture has been tremendous. According to the Food and Agriculture Organization of the United Nations, yield improvements of all major crops have decreased due to poor agricultural management practices, decreased acreage of arable land, and increased reliance on fertilizers and pesticides that diminish soil quality. To produce more food on less land, 13 million farmers in 25 countries are now planting genetically engineered crops on 300 million acres of land. These crops are predominantly corn, cotton, canola, and soybeans that are resistant to herbicides and insects. Over the last 10 years in the United States, genetically engineered crops contributed to $44 million in economic gains due to increased yields and lower production costs. The global market value of genetically modified crops is currently $7.5 billion. Small resource-poor farmers are among the beneficiaries of agricultural biotechnology. In a comparative study of small cotton farms in South Africa, it was found that the yield of cotton from plants that were genetically engineered to produce a bacterial insecticide was on average about 70% greater than those from non-genetically modified plants over three seasons. Higher yields and reduced pesticide and labor costs translated into doubled revenues despite the slightly higher costs of the transgenic seeds. Similarly, in India, farmers who planted genetically modified cotton increased their yields by 31% in 2008 while decreasing insecticide use by 39%. This resulted in an 88% increase in profits for small farmers.

The ultimate objective of all biotechnology research is the development of commercial products. Consequently, molecular biotechnology is driven, to a great extent, by economics. Not only does financial investment currently sustain molecular biotechnology, but clearly the expectation of finan-

MILESTONE

Construction of Biologically Functional Bacterial Plasmids In Vitro

S. N. COHEN, A. C. Y. CHANG, H. W. BOYER, and R. B. HELLING

Proc. Natl. Acad. Sci. USA 70:3240–3244, 1973

The landmark study of Cohen et al. established the foundation for recombinant DNA technology by showing how genetic information from different sources could be joined to create a novel, replicatable genetic structure. In this instance, the new genetic entities were derived from bacterial autonomously replicating extrachromosomal DNA structures called plasmids. In a previous study, Cohen and Chang (*Proc. Natl. Acad. Sci. USA* 70:1293–1297, 1973) produced a small plasmid from a large naturally occurring plasmid by shearing the larger plasmid into smaller random pieces and introducing the mixture of pieces into a host cell, the bacterium *E. coli*. By chance, one of the fragments that was about 1/10 the size of the original plasmid was perpetuated as a functional plasmid. To overcome the randomness of this approach and to make the genetic manipulation of plasmids more manageable, Cohen and his coworkers decided to use an enzyme (restriction endonuclease) that cuts a DNA molecule at a specific site and produces a short extension at each end. The extensions of the cut ends of a restriction endonuclease-treated DNA molecule can combine with the extensions of another DNA molecule that has been cleaved with the same restriction endonuclease.

Consequently, when DNA molecules from different sources are treated with the same restriction endonuclease and mixed together, new DNA combinations that never existed before can be formed. In this way, Cohen et al. not only introduced a gene from one plasmid into another plasmid, but also demonstrated that the introduced gene was biologically active. To their credit, these authors fully appreciated that their strategy was "potentially useful for insertion of specific sequences from prokaryotic or eukaryotic chromosomes or extrachromosomal DNA into independently replicating bacterial plasmids." In other words, any gene from any organism could theoretically be cloned into a plasmid, which, after introduction into a host cell, would be maintained indefinitely and, perhaps, produce the protein encoded by the cloned gene. By demonstrating the feasibility of gene cloning, Cohen et al. provided the experimental basis for recombinant DNA technology; established that plasmids could act as vehicles (vectors) for maintaining cloned genes; motivated others to pursue research in this area that rapidly led to the development of more sophisticated vectors and gene-cloning strategies; engendered concerns about the safety and ethics of this kind of research that, in turn, was responsible for the establishment of official guidelines and governmental agencies for conducting and regulating recombinant DNA research, respectively; and contributed to the formation of the molecular biotechnology industry.

cial gain was responsible for the considerable interest and excitement during the initial stages of its development. By nightfall on 14 October 1980, the principal shareholders of Genentech stock were worth millions of dollars. The unprecedented enthusiastic public response to Genentech encouraged others to follow. Between 1980 and 1983, about 200 small biotechnology companies were founded in the United States with the help of tax incentives and funding from both stock market speculation and private investment. Like Herbert Boyer, who was first a research scientist at the University of California at San Francisco and then a vice president of Genentech, university professors started many of the early companies.

Much of the commercial development of molecular biotechnology has been centered in the United States. By 1985, there were over 400 biotechnology companies, including many with names that contained variants of the word "gene" to emphasize their expertise in gene cloning: Biogen, Amgen, Calgene, Engenics, Genex, and Cangene. Today, there are about 1,500 biotechnology companies in the United States, 3,000 in Europe, and more than 8,000 worldwide, most in the health care sector. All large multinational chemical and pharmaceutical companies, including Monsanto, Du Pont, Pfizer, Eli Lilly, GlaxoSmithKline, Merck, Novartis, and Hoffmann-LaRoche, to name but a few, have made significant research commitments to molecular biotechnology. During the rapid proliferation of the biotechnology business in the 1980s, small companies were absorbed

by larger ones, strategic mergers took place, and joint ventures were undertaken. For example, in 1991, 60% of Genentech was sold to Hoffmann-LaRoche for $2.1 billion. Also, inevitably, for various reasons, there were a number of bankruptcies. This state of flux is a characteristic feature of the biotechnology industry.

The annual earnings of the biotechnology industry have increased from about $6 million in 1986 to more than $70 billion in 2003. Worldwide, the biotechnology industry employs about 180,000 people. Since the 1980s, new, independent molecular biotechnology companies have usually been specialized and have tended to stress the use of one particular aspect of recombinant DNA technology. The extent of this specialization is often reflected in their names. For example, after the formation of companies dedicated to the cloning of commercially important genes—Biogen, Amgen, Genzyme, Genentech, and so on—several U.S. molecular biotechnology companies, including ImmunoGen, Immunomedics, and MedImmune, were formed to produce genetically engineered antibodies for treating infectious diseases, cancer, and other disorders in humans. Currently, the roster of biotechnology companies is extensive and includes those focused on cardiovascular disorders, tissue engineering, cell replacement, drug delivery, vaccines, gene therapy, antisense drugs, microarray detection systems, diagnostics, genomics, proteomics, and agricultural biotechnology.

Concerns and Consequences

While many people appreciate the potential of molecular biotechnology to solve important problems in agriculture, medicine, and industry, they recognize the need to be cautious about its widespread application. Indeed, one of the first scientific responses to this new technology was a voluntary moratorium on certain experiments that were thought to be potentially hazardous. This research ban was self-imposed by a group of molecular biologists, including Cohen and Boyer. They were concerned that combining genes from two different organisms might accidentally create a novel organism with undesirable and dangerous properties. Within a few years, however, these apprehensions were allayed as scientists gained laboratory experience with this technology and safety guidelines were formulated for recombinant DNA research. The temporary cessation of some recombinant DNA research projects did not dampen the enthusiasm for genetic engineering. In fact, the new technology continued to receive unprecedented attention from both the public and the scientific community.

Molecular biotechnology can contribute benefits to humanity. It can:

- Provide opportunities to accurately diagnose, prevent, or cure a wide range of infectious and genetic diseases
- Significantly increase crop yields by creating plants that are resistant to insect predation, fungal and viral diseases, and environmental stresses, such as short-term drought and excessive heat, and at the same time reduce applications of hazardous agrichemicals
- Develop microorganisms that will produce chemicals, antibiotics, polymers, amino acids, enzymes, and various food additives that are important for food production and other industries
- Develop livestock and other animals that have genetically enhanced attributes

- Facilitate the removal of pollutants and waste materials from the environment

Although it is exciting and important to emphasize the positive aspects of new advances, there are also social concerns and consequences that must be addressed. The following are some examples.

- Will some genetically engineered organisms be harmful either to other organisms or to the environment?
- Will the development and use of genetically engineered organisms reduce natural genetic diversity?
- Should humans be genetically engineered?
- Will new diagnostic procedures undermine individual privacy?
- Will financial support for molecular biotechnology constrain the development of other important technologies?
- Will the emphasis on commercial success mean that the benefits of molecular biotechnology will be available only to wealthy nations?
- Will agricultural molecular biotechnology undermine traditional farming practices?

FIGURE 1.3 *The Farm,* by Alexis Rockman. According to the artist, "The Farm explores the iconography of agriculture. The Farm is set on a wide-angled field with all its usual trappings—animals, fruits, and vegetables. The situation, however familiar, is far from predictable. A disproportionately enormous and savage cow has an overabundance of teats. The pig is a human organ factory. And the chicken, which boasts three pairs of wings and no feathers, is ready for basting. The fruit fly, the workhorse of many a genetic study, is present as is a mouse with a human ear cartilage projecting from its back....Past, present, and future states are threaded together here with barbed wire, woven baskets and DNA....The Farm shows how the bodies of these animals have been—and may one day be—transformed to suit our aesthetic, medical, gastronomic needs." © Alexis Rockman, 2000. Reprinted with the permission of the artist.

- Will medical therapies based on molecular biotechnology supersede equally effective traditional treatments?
- Will the quest for patents inhibit the free exchange of ideas among research scientists?

These and many other issues have been considered by government commissions, discussed extensively at conferences, and thoughtfully debated and analyzed by individuals in both popular and academic publications. On this basis, rules and regulations have been formulated, guidelines have been established, and policies have been created. There has been active and extensive participation by both scientists and the general public in deciding how molecular biotechnology should proceed, although some controversies still remain.

Molecular biotechnology, with much fuss and fanfare, became a comprehensive scientific and commercial venture in a remarkably short time. Many scientific and business publications are now devoted to the subject, and graduate and undergraduate programs and courses are available at universities throughout the world to teach it. Even artists have depicted their perception of molecular biotechnology (Fig. 1.3). It could be debated whether the early promise of biotechnology has been fulfilled in the way that was predicted in a 1987 document published by the U.S. Office of Technology Assessment, which declared that molecular biotechnology is "a new scientific revolution that could change the lives and futures of . . . citizens as dramatically as did the Industrial Revolution two centuries ago and the computer revolution today. The ability to manipulate genetic material to achieve specified outcomes in living organisms . . . promises major changes in many aspects of modern life." It does, however, offer solutions to some serious global problems, including the spread of infectious diseases, the burden of waste accumulation, and food shortages. The potential of molecular biotechnology to solve some of these imminent problems is the subject of this book.

SUMMARY

In 1973, Stanley Cohen, Herbert Boyer, and their coworkers devised a method for transferring genetic information (genes) from one organism to another. This procedure, which became known as recombinant DNA technology, enabled researchers to isolate specific genes and to perpetuate them in host organisms. Recombinant DNA technology has been beneficial to many different areas of study. However, its impact on biotechnology has been extraordinary.

Biotechnology, for the most part, uses microorganisms on a large scale for the production of commercially important products. Before the advent of recombinant DNA technology, the most effective way of increasing the productivity of an organism was to induce mutations and then use selection procedures to identify organisms with superior traits. This process was not foolproof; it was time-consuming, labor-intensive, and costly; and only a small set of traits could be enhanced in this way. Recombinant DNA technology, however, provided a rapid, efficient, and powerful means for creating microorganisms with specific genetic attributes. Moreover, the tools of recombinant DNA technology enable not only microorganisms, but also plants and animals, to be genetically engineered. Combining recombinant DNA technology with biotechnology created a dynamic and exciting discipline called molecular biotechnology.

From its beginning, molecular biotechnology captured the imagination of the public. Many small companies dedicated to gene cloning (recombinant DNA technology) were established with funding from private investors. Although these biotechnology companies took somewhat longer than expected to bring their products to the marketplace, a large number of recombinant DNA-based products are currently available, and many more are expected soon.

Because of its broad impact, molecular biotechnology has been scrutinized carefully for its potential effects on society. Some of the concerns that have been raised are its safety, its possible negative effects on the environment, and the private or public ownership of genetically engineered organisms.

REFERENCES

Anonymous. 1987. *New Developments in Biotechnology—Background Paper: Public Perceptions of Biotechnology.* Office of Technology Assessment, U.S. Congress, U.S. Government Printing Office, Washington, DC.

Bud, R. 1991. Biotechnology in the twentieth century. *Soc. Stud. Sci.* 21:415–457.

Bud, R. 1993. *The Uses of Life: a History of Biotechnology.* Cambridge University Press, Cambridge, United Kingdom.

Busch, L., W. B. Lacy, J. Burkhardt, and L. R. Lacy. 1992. *Plants, Power, and Profit: Social, Economic and Ethical Consequences of the New Biotechnologies.*

Blackwell Publishers, Cambridge, MA.

Cohen, S. N., and A. C. Chang. 1973. Recircularization and autonomous replication of a sheared R-factor DNA segment in *Escherichia coli* transformants. *Proc. Natl. Acad. Sci. USA* 70:1293–1297.

Cohen, S. N., A. C. Y. Chang, H. W. Boyer, and R. B. Helling. 1973. Construction of biologically functional bacterial plasmids in vitro. *Proc. Natl. Acad. Sci. USA* 70:3240–3244.

Davis, B. D. (ed.). 1991. *The Genetic Revolution: Scientific Prospects and Public Perceptions.* Johns Hopkins University Press, Baltimore, MD.

Grace, E. S. 1997. *Biotechnology Unzipped: Promises & Realities.* Trifolium Press, Inc., Toronto, Canada.

Morse, S., R. Bennett, and Y. Ismael. 2004. Why *Bt* cotton pays for small-scale producers in South Africa. *Nat. Biotechnol.* 22:379–380.

Robbins-Roth, C. 2000. *From Alchemy to IPO: the Business of Biotechnology.* Perseus Publishing, Cambridge, MA.

Van Beuzekom, B., and A. Arundel. 2006. *OECD Biotechnology Statistics 2006.* OECD Publishing, Paris, France.

REVIEW QUESTIONS

1. What is biotechnology?

2. Distinguish between traditional biotechnology and molecular biotechnology.

3. Describe the basic steps of a bioengineered biotechnology process.

4. What are the shortcomings of the "mutation and selection" method for developing enhanced organisms for commercial purposes?

5. Why was the work reported by Cohen and Boyer and their coworkers in 1973 considered important?

6. How did recombinant DNA technology enable the production of human insulin?

7. What are some of the problems that molecular biotechnology has the potential to solve?

8. Discuss the statement "molecular biotechnology is a diverse science."

9. Discuss some of the social concerns that have been raised about molecular biotechnology.

10. Go to http://www.nytimes.com, http://news.yahoo.com, or an equivalent news website and conduct a search with the word "biotechnology." Describe and discuss three recent biotechnology news stories.

DNA, RNA, and Protein Synthesis

THE INFORMATION ENCODED IN GENETIC MATERIAL is responsible for establishing and maintaining the cellular and biochemical functions of an organism. In most organisms, the genetic material is a long double-stranded DNA polymer. The sequence of units (deoxyribonucleotides) of one DNA strand is complementary to the deoxyribonucleotides of the other strand. This complementarity enables new DNA molecules to be synthesized with the same linear order of deoxyribonucleotides in each strand as an original DNA molecule. The process of DNA synthesis is called replication. A specific order of deoxyribonucleotides determines the information content of an individual genetic element (gene). Some genes encode proteins, and others encode only ribonucleic acid (RNA) molecules. The protein-coding genes (structural genes) are decoded by two successive major cellular processes: RNA synthesis (transcription) and protein synthesis (translation). First, a messenger RNA (mRNA) molecule is synthesized from a structural gene using one of the two DNA strands as a template. Second, an individual mRNA molecule interacts with other components, including ribosomes, transfer RNAs (tRNAs), and enzymes, to produce a protein molecule. A protein consists of a precise sequence of amino acids, which is essential for its activity.

Although the deoxyribonucleotide sequences are different in genes encoding different functions, and for genes encoding similar functions in different organisms, the chemical compositions are the same. This enables molecular biotechnologists to transfer genes among a variety of organisms to create beneficial products. To understand how this is accomplished, it is helpful to know about the structure of DNA, replication, transcription, and translation.

Structure of DNA

The chemistry of DNA has been studied since 1868. By the 1940s, it was known that DNA is made up of individual units called nucleotides that are linked to each other to form long chains. A nucleotide consists of an organic base (base), a five-carbon sugar (pentose), and a phosphate group (Fig.

A

B

FIGURE 2.1 Chemical structures of the components of DNA. **(A)** A representative nucleotide. The term "base" denotes any of the four bases (adenine, guanine, cytosine, and thymine) that are found in DNA. The deoxyribose sugar is enclosed by dashed lines. The numbers with primes mark the carbon atoms of the deoxyribose moiety. **(B)** The bases of DNA. The circled nitrogen atom is the site of attachment of the base to the 1′ carbon atom of the deoxyribose moiety.

2.1A). The sugar of DNA is 2′-deoxyribose because it does not have a hydroxyl (OH) group on the 2′ carbon; rather, it has a hydroxyl group only on the 3′ carbon of the sugar moiety. By contrast, in mRNA, the five-carbon sugar ribose has hydroxyl groups at both the 2′ and 3′ carbons of the pentose ring. In both DNA and RNA, the phosphate group and base are attached to the 5′ carbon and 1′ carbon atoms of the sugar moiety, respectively. In DNA, there are four kinds of bases: adenine (A), guanine (G), cytosine (C), and thymine (T) (Fig. 2.1B). The nucleotide subunits of DNA are joined by phosphodiester bonds, with the phosphate group of the 5′ carbon of one nucleotide linked to the 3′ OH group of the deoxyribose of the adjacent nucleotide (Fig. 2.2). A polynucleotide strand has a 3′ OH group at one end (the 3′ end) and a 5′ phosphate group at the other (the 5′ end).

5′ end

$$O=P-O-CH_2$$

Adenine

Phosphodiester
linkage

Thymine

Guanine

Cytosine

3′ end

FIGURE 2.2 Chemical structure of a single strand of DNA.

FIGURE 2.3 A rod–ribbon model of double-helical DNA. The rods represent the complementary base pairs, and the ribbons represent the deoxyribose–phosphate backbones.

In 1953, James Watson and Francis Crick, using X-ray diffraction analysis of crystallized DNA, discovered that DNA consists of two long chains (strands) that form a double-stranded helix (Fig. 2.3). The two polynucleotide chains of DNA are held together by hydrogen bonds between the bases of the opposite strands. Base pairing occurs only between specific, complementary bases (Fig. 2.4). A pairs only with T, and G pairs only with C. The A·T base pairs are held together by two hydrogen bonds, and the G·C base pairs are held together by three. The number of complementary base pairs is often used to characterize the length of a double-stranded DNA molecule. For DNA molecules with thousands or millions of base pairs, the designations are kilobase pairs and megabase pairs, respectively. For example, the DNA of human chromosome 1 is one double-stranded helix that has about 263 megabase pairs (Mb).

The A·T and G·C base pairs lie within the interior of the molecule, and the 5′-to-3′-linked phosphate and deoxyribose components form the backbone of each strand (Fig. 2.4). The two strands of a duplex DNA molecule run in opposite directions to each other (antiparallel chains). One chain is oriented in a 3′-to-5′ direction, and the other is oriented in a 5′-to-3′ direction. Because of the base-pairing requirements, when one strand of DNA has, for example, the base sequence 5′-TAGGCAT-3′, the complementary strand must be 3′-ATCCGTA-5′. In this case, the double-stranded form would be $_{3'-ATCCGTA-5'}^{5'-TAGGCAT-3'}$. By convention, when DNA is drawn on a horizontal plane, the 5′ end of the upper strand is on the left.

Genetic material has two major functions. It encodes the information for the production of proteins, and it is reproduced (replicated) with a high degree of accuracy to pass the encoded information to new cells. The Watson–Crick model of DNA fully meets these important requirements. First, because of base complementarity, each preexisting DNA strand can act as a template for the production of a new complementary strand.

FIGURE 2.4 Chemical structure of double-stranded DNA.

FIGURE 2.5 DNA replication. **(A)** The incoming nucleotide is a deoxyribonucleoside triphosphate that is directed by DNA polymerase to pair with the complementary base of the template strand. (*continued*)

Consequently, after one round of replication, two daughter molecules are produced, with each having the same sequence of nucleotide pairs as the original DNA molecule. Second, the sequence of nucleotides of a gene provides the code for the production of a protein. The linear order of amino acids in a protein is determined by the linear sequence of deoxyribonucleotides in a gene.

DNA Replication

As predicted by the Watson–Crick model of DNA, each strand of an existing DNA molecule acts as a template for the production of a new strand, and the sequence of nucleotides of the synthesized (growing) strand is determined by base complementarity. During replication, the

FIGURE 2.5 (*continued*) **(B)** The α phosphate of the incoming nucleotide forms a phosphodiester bond with the 3′ hydroxyl group of the growing strand. The next incoming nucleotide of the growing strand that is complementary to the nucleotide of the template strand is positioned by DNA polymerase.

phosphate group of each incoming nucleotide is enzymatically joined by a phosphodiester linkage to the 3′ OH group of the last nucleotide that was incorporated in the growing strand (Fig. 2.5A). The nucleotides that are used for DNA replication are triphosphate deoxyribonucleotides that have three consecutive phosphate groups attached to the 5′ carbon of the deoxyribose sugar moiety. The phosphate that is attached to the 5′ carbon is designated the α phosphate, the next phosphate is the β phosphate, and the third one is the γ phosphate (Fig. 2.6). During the replication process, the β and γ phosphates are cleaved off as a unit, and the α phosphate is linked to the 3′ OH group of the previously incorporated nucleotide (Fig. 2.5B). The DNA synthesis machinery of prokaryotes and eukaryotes includes a large number of different proteins. Of these, DNA polymerases are responsible for binding deoxyribonucleotides, fitting the correct nucleotide into place

MILESTONE

A Structure for Deoxyribose Nucleic Acid
J. D. WATSON AND F. H. C. CRICK
Nature 171:737–738, 1953

The elucidation of the structure of the genetic material (DNA) was undoubtedly one of the most important scientific breakthroughs of the 20th century. James Watson and Francis Crick, who, with Maurice Wilkins, were awarded the Nobel Prize in physiology or medicine in 1962 for this work, suggested "a structure for the salt of deoxyribonucleic acid (D. N. A.). This structure has novel features which are of considerable biological interest....This structure has two helical chains each coiled around the same axis....Both chains follow right handed helices, but . . . the sequences of the atoms in the two chains run in opposite directions.... The novel feature of the structure is the manner in which the two chains are held together by the purine and pyrimidine bases....They are joined in pairs, a single base from one chain being hydrogen bonded to a single base from the other chain....One of the pair must be a purine and the other a pyrimidine for bonding to occur....If adenine forms one member of a pair, on either chain, then...the other member must be a thymine; similarly for guanine and cytosine. The sequence of bases on a single chain does not appear to be restricted in any way....It has not escaped our notice that the specific pairing we have postulated immediately suggests a possible copying mechanism for the genetic material." In another article a few months later (*Nature* 171:964–967, 1953), Watson and Crick discussed more implications for their model. "The phosphate-sugar backbone of our model is completely regular but any sequence of the pairs of bases can fit into the structure. It follows that in a long molecule many different permutations are possible, and it therefore seems likely that the precise sequence of bases is the code which carries the genetic information....Our model suggests possible explanations for a number of other phenomena. For example, spontaneous mutations may be due to a base occasionally in one of its less likely tautomeric forms. Again, the pairing between homologous chromosomes at meiosis may depend on pairing between specific bases."

Within a decade of the demonstration of the double-helical nature of DNA with its complementary base pairs, the molecular aspects of DNA replication were known, the cellular processes that are responsible for both decoding and regulating the synthesis of gene products were understood, and many of the kinds of changes that lead to altered gene products were recognized. From the time of its publication to the present, the scientific impact of the Watson–Crick discovery has been pervasive and, for the most part, inestimable. As one small example, recombinant DNA technology would not exist without knowledge of the structure of DNA.

according to the base-pairing requirement of the template strand, and forming the phosphodiester linkage.

In bacteria, DNA replication is initiated at a specific region of the (usually circular) chromosome called the origin of replication (or origin) and, in *Escherichia coli*, proceeds at the rate of about 1,000 nucleotides per second. In eukaryotes, a chromosome has many different sites of initiation of replication. Because of these multiple origins of replication, part of the eukaryotic replication process includes enzymatically joining (ligating) segments of newly synthesized DNA together with phosphodiester bonds. Furthermore, in eukaryotes, a special replication enzyme called telomerase is used for the completion of the linear ends (telomeres) of each chromosome.

Decoding Genetic Information: RNA and Protein

The vast majority of genes encode information for the production of protein chains. Proteins are essential polymers that are involved in almost all biological functions. They catalyze chemical reactions; transport molecules within cells; escort molecules between cells; control membrane permeability; give support to cells, organs, and body structures; cause movement; provide protection against infectious agents and toxins; and regulate the differential production of other gene products. A protein chain consists of

FIGURE 2.6 Structure of a deoxyribonucleoside triphosphate. The phosphate units are designated α, β, and γ. The α phosphate is directly attached to the 5' carbon of the deoxyribose sugar. During DNA synthesis, the α phosphate participates in the formation of the phosphodiester bond, and the β and γ phosphate groups are released as a unit (pyrophosphate).

a specific sequence of units called amino acids. All amino acids have the same basic chemical structure. There is a central carbon atom (the α carbon) that has a hydrogen (H), a carboxyl group (COO^-), an amino group (NH_3^+), and an R group attached to it (Fig. 2.7A). An R group can be any 1 of 20 different side chains (groups) that make up the 20 different amino acids found in proteins. When R, for example, is a methyl group (CH_3), then the amino acid is alanine. The amino acids of proteins are designated by either a three- or a one-letter notation (see the table following chapter 23). For example, alanine is abbreviated Ala or A. In a protein, each amino acid is linked to an adjacent amino acid by a peptide bond that joins the carboxyl group of one amino acid to the amino group of the adjacent one (Fig. 2.7B). The first amino acid of a protein has a free amino group (N terminus), and the last amino acid in the polypeptide chain has a free carboxyl group (C terminus).

Proteins range in length from about 40 to more than 1,000 amino acid residues. A protein folds into a particular shape (configuration, or conformation) depending on the locations of specific amino acid residues and the overall amino acid composition. Individual amino acids have different characteristics that are determined by the properties of their side chains, and these influence the folding of the protein into a particular three-dimensional shape. The shape of a protein in turn helps to determine its function. Also, many functional proteins consist of two or more polypeptide chains. In some cases, multiples of the same polypeptide chain are required for an active protein molecule (homomeric protein). In other instances, a set of different protein chains (subunits) assembles to form a functional protein (heteromeric protein). Finally, large protein complexes that are made up of many different subunits often perform important cellular functions.

The decoding of genetic information is carried out through intermediary RNA molecules that are transcribed from discrete regions of the DNA. RNA molecules are linear polynucleotide chains that differ from DNA in two important respects. First, the sugar moiety of the nucleotides of RNA is ribose, which has hydroxyl groups on both the 2' and 3' carbons of the sugar. Second, instead of thymine, the base uracil (U) is found in RNA. Most RNA molecules are single stranded, although often there are segments of nucleotides within a single chain that are complementary to each other and form double-stranded regions (intrastrand pairing) (Fig. 2.8). The base pairing within a single RNA strand is the same as the base

FIGURE 2.7 Generalized structures of an amino acid and a peptide bond. **(A)** An amino acid. The R represents the location of the side chain. **(B)** A peptide bond. The peptide bond is encircled, and R1 and R2 represent different side chains.

Peptide bond

pairing between complementary sequences of DNA, except that uracil pairs with adenine. Base pairing can occur between two RNA molecules if they contain complementary sequences of base pairs.

The major kinds of RNA molecules that are essential for the decoding of genetic information are mRNA, ribosomal RNA (rRNA), and tRNA. The production of RNA from DNA is called transcription. In most prokaryotes, a single RNA polymerase is responsible for the transcription of all types of RNA. In eukaryotic organisms, mRNA, rRNA, and tRNA are each transcribed by a different RNA polymerase.

In many of its features, transcription resembles replication. Briefly, one strand of the DNA of a specific region acts as a template for the synthesis of a polymer of ribonucleotides. RNA polymerase sequentially joins, via 3'-5' phosphodiester linkages, ribonucleotides that are complementary to the nucleotides of the template DNA strand (Fig. 2.9). As transcription proceeds, the newly synthesized RNA is released from the DNA and the DNA helix re-forms. Since only specific segments of DNA molecules are transcribed, sets of short stretches of base pairs within the DNA are required to ensure that transcription is initiated at the correct nucleotide and that it terminates at a specific nucleotide. The sequences that control the initiation of transcription usually precede the coding sequence, and the termination signal sequences follow it. The DNA segment that precedes a gene is called the 5'-flanking or upstream region, and the one following a gene is the

FIGURE 2.8 Secondary structure of an RNA molecule. The lines represent hydrogen bonding between complementary base pairs. The ribose–phosphate backbone is omitted.

FIGURE 2.9 Schematic representation of transcription. The arrow indicates the direction of transcription.

3'-flanking or downstream region. To initiate transcription, RNA polymerase binds to a specific sequence of nucleotides upstream of the coding sequence known as the promoter. Similarly, a specific sequence of nucleotides downstream of the coding sequence, known as the transcriptional terminator, signals RNA polymerase to stop RNA synthesis.

From a molecular perspective, a gene is a specific nucleotide sequence that is transcribed into RNA. Structural genes, which make up the vast majority of transcribed DNA sequences, encode proteins; however, the initial transcription product of a structural gene is an mRNA. In prokaryotes, a contiguous DNA segment forms a structural gene (the coding region). Prokaryotic transcription entails the binding of RNA polymerase to a promoter region, the initiation of transcription at a nucleotide upstream of the structural gene, and the cessation of transcription at a termination sequence that lies downstream from the coding region (Fig. 2.10). In eukaryotic organisms, a structural gene usually consists of several coding regions (exons) that are separated by noncoding regions (introns, or intervening sequences). After RNA polymerase has bound to the promoter and the entire eukaryotic structural gene is transcribed, the introns are removed from the primary transcript, and the exons, in the correct order, are linked (spliced) together to form a functional mRNA (Fig. 2.11 and 2.12). In general, exons tend to be 150 to 300 bases in length, and introns can vary from as few as 40 to over 10,000 bases. A small number of eukaryotic structural genes lack introns,

FIGURE 2.10 Schematic representation of a prokaryotic structural gene. The promoter region (p), the site of initiation and direction of transcription (the right-angled arrow), and the termination sequence for RNA polymerase (t) are depicted. A prokaryotic structural gene is transcribed into mRNA and then directly into protein.

DNA

FIGURE 2.11 Schematic representation of a eukaryotic structural gene. The promoter region (p), the site of initiation and direction of transcription (the right-angled arrow), and the termination sequence for RNA polymerase (t) are depicted. The numbers 1 to 5 mark the exons of the structural gene, and the letters a to d mark the introns. The primary transcript is polyadenylated at the 3' end and capped with a modified guanine (G) nucleotide at the 5' end. Processing of the primary transcript removes the introns. The functional RNA is translated into protein.

and in some instances, the introns in a primary transcript may be legitimately removed in more than one way in a process known as alternate splicing. For example, in one kind of tissue, all the exons of the primary transcript may be spliced together to form a functional mRNA, whereas in another tissue, the initial transcript may undergo a different pattern of exon splicing, with an exon being skipped during the process of intron removal and a novel functional mRNA being produced. The exon-skipping mechanism generates different gene products in different tissues from the same

FIGURE 2.12 Splicing of a eukaryotic primary RNA transcript. The bracketing arrows mark the sites that are spliced together after the removal of the intervening RNA regions. In this example, introns a and b are spliced out of the primary transcript, and exons 1, 2, and 3 are spliced together to form a functional mRNA.

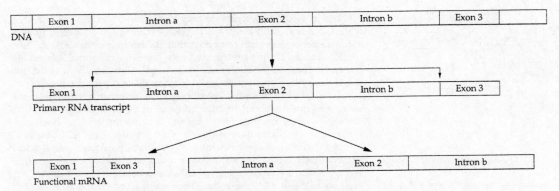

FIGURE 2.13 Alternative splicing of a eukaryotic primary RNA transcript. The bracketing arrows mark the sites that are spliced together after the removal of the intervening RNA region. In this example, exon 2, flanked by introns a and b, is spliced out of the primary transcript, and exons 1 and 3 are spliced together to form a functional mRNA transcript.

structural gene (Fig. 2.13). For example, in *Drosophila*, the fruit fly that is commonly used in genetic studies, two different mRNAs are produced from the *doublesex (dsx)* gene as a consequence of alternate splicing of the exons contained in the gene (Fig. 2.14). One form is produced exclusively in female flies and the other only in male flies, and each encodes a protein that has a different activity. The protein produced in female flies prevents the development of some male-specific characteristics, including male genitalia, and conversely, the protein produced in male flies prevents the development of female-specific traits.

Most (>90%) of the RNA in a metabolically active cell is rRNA found in ribosomes. Although there can be hundreds to thousands of different

FIGURE 2.14 Alternative splicing of the *doublesex (dsx)* primary transcript produces two different mRNAs in the fruit fly *Drosophila melanogaster*. The first three exons are spliced together in both male and female flies; however, in male flies, exon 4 is skipped, resulting in the splicing of exon 3 to exons 5 and 6. In female flies, exon 3 is spliced to exon 4, which contains a signal for the addition of a poly(A) tail (pA), resulting in a shortened mRNA. The numbered boxes indicate exons, while the red and blue lines indicate intron sequences that are spliced out of the primary transcript in female and male flies, respectively. Adapted from Maniatis and Tasic, *Nature* **418**:236–243, 2002.

FIGURE 2.15 Conformation of a charged tRNA. The amino acid is attached to the 3′ end of the tRNA, and the location of the anticodon region is enclosed by dashed lines.

mRNAs in a cell, they represent only about 3 to 5% of the cellular RNA, while tRNA represents about 4%. The rRNA combines with specific proteins to form ribonucleoprotein complexes that make up the large and small ribosomal subunits. During protein synthesis, one large ribosomal subunit and one small ribosomal subunit combine to form a ribosome. Both of the ribosomal subunits of eukaryotes are larger than those of prokaryotes.

In addition to thousands of ribosomes, a cell that is actively synthesizing proteins has about 60 different types of tRNA molecules. The tRNA molecules range in length from about 75 to 93 nucleotides. Because of intrastrand complementary segments of nucleotides, each tRNA molecule forms a folded, L-shaped structure (Fig. 2.15). A particular amino acid is enzymatically linked by its carboxyl end to the 3′ end of a specific tRNA. For example, the enzyme arginyl-tRNA synthetase adds the amino acid arginine to the tRNAArg molecule. There is at least one tRNA for each of the 20 amino acids found in proteins. After the binding of a particular amino acid to its tRNA, the tRNA is said to be "charged." In another part of the tRNA molecule, there are three unpaired nucleotides that together are called the anticodon sequence. This sequence plays a crucial role in the formation of the linear array of amino acids that constitute a protein.

Translation

In prokaryotes, which lack a nucleus, the processes of transcription and translation are not spatially separated. When a newly synthesized mRNA molecule begins to emerge from the RNA polymerase complex, a ribosome binds to a specific ribonucleotide sequence near the 5′ end of the mRNA to initiate translation. Thus, transcription and translation occur concurrently in a prokaryotic cell (Fig. 2.16). In contrast, in eukaryotic cells, a mature mRNA molecule leaves the nucleus via special pores in the nuclear membrane and is bound by ribosomes that either remain in the

FIGURE 2.16 Concurrent transcription and translation in prokaryotes. When nascent mRNA emerges from RNA polymerase (yellow ovals), ribosomes (tan, double-lobed shapes) bind to the ribosome-binding site on the mRNA and begin translation. Translation begins before transcription of mRNA is completed. The arrows indicate the direction of transcription.

FIGURE 2.17 Transcription and translation are spatially separated in eukaryotes. Transcription occurs in the nucleus. Primary transcripts produced by RNA polymerase (yellow ovals) are processed to remove introns (grey lines), and the resulting mRNA (green lines) is exported from the nucleus via nuclear pores. Ribosomes (tan, double-lobed shapes) in the cytoplasm or associated with the endoplasmic reticulum translate the mRNA to produce proteins that remain in the cytoplasm or are translocated into the lumen of the endoplasmic reticulum for further processing.

cytoplasm or associate with the endoplasmic reticulum (Fig. 2.17). In addition to removal of introns, before the mRNA leaves the nucleus, it is capped with a modified guanine nucleotide at the 5′ end and a polymer of adenine nucleotides is added to the 3′ end to form a poly(A) tail (Fig. 2.18). The 5′ cap and the 3′ poly(A) tail aid in the binding of ribosomes to the mRNA to begin translation.

Translation requires the interaction of mRNA, charged tRNAs, ribosomes, and a large number of proteins (factors) that facilitate the initiation,

FIGURE 2.18 Modification of the ends of a primary RNA transcript in the nucleus. A modified guanine nucleotide cap is added to the 5′ end of the transcript, and a polyadenylation signal in the RNA sequence specifies the addition of a polymer of 50 to 250 adenine (A) nucleotides to the 3′ end to form a poly(A) tail. The modified ends aid in the transport of the mature mRNA from the nucleus and in the binding of ribosomes to the mRNA and increase the stability of the mRNA.

FIGURE 2.19 Schematic representation of the initiation of translation in prokaryotes. The mRNA binds to the small ribosomal subunit. For some mRNAs, the Shine-Dalgarno sequence near the 5′ end of the mRNA base pairs with a sequence near the 3′ end of the rRNA of the small ribosomal subunit. The anticodon (UAC) of the initiator fMet-tRNA^{fMet} base pairs with the start codon (AUG) of the mRNA. The large ribosomal subunit combines with the initiator tRNA–mRNA–small ribosomal subunit complex to form the initiation complex. The amino acid methionine of the initiator tRNA is formylated (CHO) at the amino group in prokaryotes (not depicted). After translation, the initial formyl-methionine is removed from the protein chain.

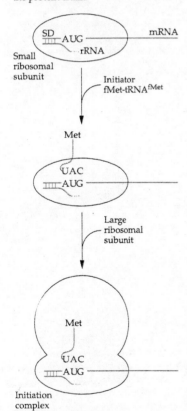

elongation, and termination of the polypeptide chain. In prokaryotes, translation is initiated by the binding of a small ribosomal subunit to an mRNA by base pairing between a sequence of about 8 nucleotides (a Shine-Dalgarno sequence) that is located near the 5′ end of the mRNA and a complementary sequence near the 3′ end of the rRNA of the small ribosomal subunit. The 3′-UAC-5′ anticodon of a specific initiator tRNA, fMet-tRNA^{fMet}, where f represents a formyl moiety that is bound to the methionine residue, binds to a 5′-AUG-3′ codon (start codon) of the mRNA. Proteins (initiation factors) facilitate the binding of the initiator tRNA to the mRNA–small ribosomal subunit complex. A large ribosomal subunit then combines with the fMet-tRNA^{fMet}–mRNA–small subunit complex to form the initiation complex (Fig. 2.19).

In eukaryotes, translation is initiated by the binding of a particular charged initiator tRNA, Met-tRNA^{Met}, along with initiation factors, to a small ribosomal subunit. Next, the 5′ capped end of an mRNA, which is combined with specific proteins, associates with the initiator tRNA–small ribosomal subunit complex, and the complex migrates along the mRNA until an AUG sequence (initiator, or start codon) is encountered. The 3′ poly(A) tail of the mRNA facilitates the interaction between the mRNA and the ribosome. When the UAC anticodon sequence of the initiator Met-tRNA^{Met} base pairs with the AUG sequence of the mRNA, the migration stops, and the large ribosomal subunit joins the complex to form the initiation complex (Fig. 2.20).

The elongation and termination phases of translation are very similar in prokaryotes and eukaryotes. The elongation process entails the formation of a peptide bond between adjacent amino acids, with the order of the amino acids being determined by the order of codons of the mRNA (Fig. 2.21). More specifically, after the initiation complex is formed, the second set of three nucleotides (triplet, or codon) in the mRNA that immediately follows the AUG codon dictates the anticodon sequence and, therefore, the charged tRNA that will bind to the ribosome complex. Uncharged tRNAs do not bind efficiently to ribosomes. For example, if the second nucleotide triplet in the mRNA is CUG, then the charged tRNA with the anticodon sequence 3′-GAC-5′ will bind. This charged tRNA carries the amino acid leucine. Once this charged tRNA is in place, a peptide bond is formed between the carboxyl group of the methionine and the amino group of the leucine. The leucine remains bound to its tRNA. Peptide bond formation is catalyzed by activity exclusively associated with the large rRNA. The formation of the peptide bond "discharges" the initiator tRNA because the bond between the

carboxyl group of methionine and its tRNA is cleaved to make the carboxyl group available for peptide bond formation. The uncharged tRNA is ejected from the ribosomal complex. The methionine–leucine–tRNALeu–mRNA combination shifts (translocates) along the ribosome to the site vacated by the initiator tRNA, and as a consequence, the next codon of the mRNA is available for binding by another charged tRNA with the appropriate anticodon sequence. If the third codon is UUU, then the charged tRNA with an AAA anticodon will bind. In this case, the tRNA with an AAA anticodon carries the amino acid phenylalanine. Once this charged tRNA is in place, the linkage between the carboxyl group of leucine and its tRNA is broken and a peptide bond is formed between the carboxyl group of the leucine and the amino group of the phenylalanine. After ejection of the uncharged tRNALeu, the "peptidyl" tRNAPhe, with the attached methionine–leucine–phenylalanine amino acid polymer and the mRNA, is translocated to the peptidyl site (P site), and the next codon is available for binding by the appropriately charged tRNA in the aminoacyl site (A site).

The succession of operations that includes binding of a charged tRNA by means of anticodon–codon pairing, peptide bond formation, ejection of an uncharged tRNA, and translocation continues until all the amino acids that are encoded by the mRNA are linked together. Translation occurs in a 5′-to-3′ direction along the mRNA at a rate of about 15 amino acids per second. When the 5′ end of the mRNA is free of a ribosome, it can combine with another initiation complex. A single mRNA can be translated simultaneously by a number of ribosomes, with each ribosome producing a polypeptide chain. In rapidly growing *E. coli* cells, the entire population of approximately 20,000 ribosomes per cell is capable of producing about 30,000 polypeptides per minute. Parenthetically, the average bacterial structural gene with about 1,000 base pairs (bp) encodes a protein with 333 amino acids because 3 bases code for each amino acid. With a mean molecular weight of an amino acid being about 105, the molecular weight of an average bacterial protein is about 35,000.

The elongation process continues until a UAA, UAG, or UGA codon (stop codon, or termination codon) is encountered (Fig. 2.22). There are no naturally occurring tRNAs with anticodons that are complementary to these codons. However, a protein(s) (termination factor, or release factor) recognizes a stop codon and binds to the ribosome. After binding of a termination factor, the bond between the last tRNA, which has the complete chain of amino acids linked to it, and its amino acid is broken, resulting in dissociation of the uncharged tRNA, the complete protein, and the mRNA from the ribosome. In addition, a ribosome-releasing factor separates the ribosomal subunits so that they can be recycled for the translation of other mRNAs.

After translation, a protein may be modified in various ways. In both prokaryotes and eukaryotes, the methionine at the N terminus is cleaved from most proteins, leaving the second encoded amino acid as the N-terminal moiety. In eukaryotes, certain proteins are selectively cleaved at defined sites (processed) to make smaller protein chains that have discrete functions. In other instances, especially in eukaryotes, phosphate groups, lipids, carbohydrates, or other low-molecular-weight groups are enzymatically added to certain amino acids of a protein. These chemical additions (posttranslational modifications) create proteins that mediate specific cellular activities.

FIGURE 2.20 Schematic representation of the initiation of translation in eukaryotes. The initiator tRNA (Met-tRNAMet) binds to a small ribosomal subunit, and then the mRNA moves along the complex until the anticodon (UAC) of the initiator tRNA base pairs with the start codon (AUG) of the mRNA. The large ribosomal subunit combines with the mRNA–initiator tRNA–small ribosomal subunit complex to form the initiation complex.

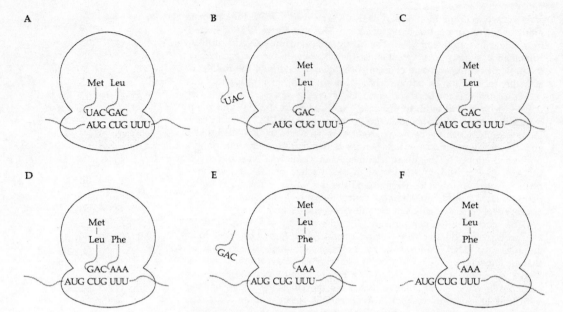

FIGURE 2.21 Schematic representation of the elongation phase of translation. (A) The second codon (CUG) base pairs with the anticodon (GAC) of Leu-tRNA^Leu. (B) The methionine of the initiator tRNA is joined to the leucine of Leu-tRNA^Leu by a peptide bond, and the uncharged initiator tRNA is ejected from the ribosome. (C) Translocation of the peptidyl-tRNA and the mRNA to the peptidyl site from the aminoacyl site opens the aminoacyl site for the next codon (UUU). (D) The third codon (UUU) base pairs with the anticodon (AAA) of Phe-tRNA^Phe. (E) The leucine of the peptidyl-tRNA is joined to the phenylalanine of the Phe-tRNA^Phe by a peptide bond, and the uncharged Leu-tRNA^Leu is ejected from the ribosome. (F) Translocation of the peptidyl-tRNA and mRNA to the peptidyl site from the aminoacyl site opens the aminoacyl site for the next codon and codon–anticodon interaction.

The complete genetic code consists of 64 codons. Three of these codons are reserved for stops, and one (AUG) is used for initiation (Table 2.1). When a methionine residue occurs internally in a protein, the codon AUG is recognized by another Met-tRNA^Met that is neither formylated nor the initiator tRNA. There is one codon (UGG) for the amino acid tryptophan. For the rest of the amino acids that are found in proteins, there are at least two, usually four, and sometimes as many as six codons. For example, there are six codons (UUA, UUG, CUU, CUC, CUA, and CUG) for the amino acid leucine. Different codons are used to different extents in different organisms (Table 2.1). Of the four codons for glycine, GGA is used about 26% of the time by human structural genes and about 9% of the time by protein-coding genes of *E. coli*. The stop codons are also used to different extents in different organisms. In humans, the frequencies of usage of UAA, UAG, and UGA are 0.22, 0.17, and 0.61, respectively, whereas in *E. coli*, they are 0.62, 0.09, and 0.30, respectively. The differences in codon usage notwithstanding, the genetic code, with a few rare exceptions, is the same in all organisms.

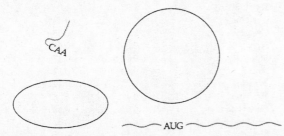

FIGURE 2.22 Schematic representation of the termination of translation. The stop codon (UAG) interacts with a termination factor that leads to the termination of translation. The last tRNA is cleaved from the peptide chain and ejected. The mRNA and the finished peptide are released. The ribosomes are prepared for recycling by a ribosome-releasing factor.

TABLE 2.1 Genetic code and codon usage in *E. coli* and humans

Codon	Amino acid	Frequency of use in:	
		E. coli	Humans
GGG	Glycine	0.13	0.23
GGA	Glycine	0.09	0.26
GGU	Glycine	0.38	0.18
GGC	Glycine	0.40	0.33
GAG	Glutamic acid	0.30	0.59
GAA	Glutamic acid	0.70	0.41
GAU	Aspartic acid	0.59	0.44
GAC	Aspartic acid	0.41	0.56
GUG	Valine	0.34	0.48
GUA	Valine	0.17	0.10
GUU	Valine	0.29	0.17
GUC	Valine	0.20	0.25
GCG	Alanine	0.34	0.10
GCA	Alanine	0.22	0.22
GCU	Alanine	0.19	0.28

(continued)

TABLE 2.1 Genetic code and codon usage in *E. coli* and humans *(continued)*

Codon	Amino acid	Frequency of use in:	
		E. coli	Humans
GCC	Alanine	0.25	0.40
AAG	Lysine	0.24	0.60
AAA	Lysine	0.76	0.40
AAU	Asparagine	0.39	0.44
AAC	Asparagine	0.61	0.56
AUG	Methionine	1.00	1.00
AUA	Isoleucine	0.07	0.14
AUU	Isoleucine	0.47	0.35
AUC	Isoleucine	0.46	0.51
ACG	Threonine	0.23	0.12
ACA	Threonine	0.12	0.27
ACU	Threonine	0.21	0.23
ACC	Threonine	0.43	0.38
UGG	Tryptophan	1.00	1.00
UGU	Cysteine	0.43	0.42
UGC	Cysteine	0.57	0.58
UGA	Stop	0.30	0.61
UAG	Stop	0.09	0.17
UAA	Stop	0.62	0.22
UAU	Tyrosine	0.53	0.42
UAC	Tyrosine	0.47	0.58
UUU	Phenylalanine	0.51	0.43
UUC	Phenylalanine	0.49	0.57
UCG	Serine	0.13	0.06
UCA	Serine	0.12	0.15
UCU	Serine	0.19	0.17
UCC	Serine	0.17	0.23
AGU	Serine	0.13	0.14
AGC	Serine	0.27	0.25
CGG	Arginine	0.08	0.19
CGA	Arginine	0.05	0.10
CGU	Arginine	0.42	0.09
CGC	Arginine	0.37	0.19
AGG	Arginine	0.03	0.22
AGA	Arginine	0.04	0.21
CAG	Glutamine	0.69	0.73
CAA	Glutamine	0.31	0.27
CAU	Histidine	0.52	0.41
CAC	Histidine	0.48	0.59
CUG	Leucine	0.55	0.43
CUA	Leucine	0.03	0.07
CUU	Leucine	0.10	0.12
CUC	Leucine	0.10	0.20
UUG	Leucine	0.11	0.12
UUA	Leucine	0.11	0.06
CCG	Proline	0.55	0.11
CCA	Proline	0.20	0.27
CCU	Proline	0.16	0.29
CCC	Proline	0.10	0.33

Regulation of mRNA Transcription in Bacteria

In bacteria, the production of amino acids, nucleotides, and other essential metabolites; replication; transcription; translation; cell growth; catabolic pathways; energy-generating systems; and responses to environmental changes all depend on proteins. However, the energy resources of a cell are not sufficient to support the transcription and translation (expression) of all of its structural genes at the same time. Consequently, only those genes that encode proteins that maintain basic cellular functions are expressed continuously. The transcription of the remaining structural genes is regulated. If a protein(s) is required by a cell, then a signaling system initiates transcription (the "on" state) of the pertinent structural gene(s). Alternatively, if a protein(s) is not needed, transcription of the protein-coding gene(s) is turned off (the "off" state).

Frequently, bacterial structural genes that encode proteins required for several steps in a single metabolic pathway are contiguous in the chromosome. This arrangement is called an operon. Generally, an operon is under the control of a single promoter, and its transcription gives rise to one large mRNA. The placement of a stop codon for one protein close to the start codon of the next protein within a multigene mRNA generates a set of discrete proteins during translation. Note that a ribosome-binding site (a Shine-Dalgarno sequence) precedes each start codon.

For many of the structural genes of *E. coli*, the promoter region has two DNA-binding sites for RNA polymerase; more specifically, the binding sites are recognized by the component of the RNA polymerase complex known as the sigma factor. Frequently, one of these sites tends to have the sequence $_{\text{ATATTA}}^{\text{TATAAT}}$ (a Pribnow box), and the other is usually $_{\text{AACTGT}}^{\text{TTGACA}}$. The Pribnow box and the TTGACA sequence are located about 10 bp (the −10 region) and 35 bp (the −35 region), respectively, upstream from the site of initiation of transcription (the +1 nucleotide) (Fig. 2.23). A promoter containing a Pribnow box and the TTGACA sequence is recognized by the sigma factor RpoD (also called sigma-70 [σ^{70}] because it has a molecular mass of 70 kilodaltons). Many bacteria are capable of producing several different sigma factors, each of which recognizes a different promoter sequence. For example, *E. coli* can produce seven different sigma factors, each of which initiates the transcription of a specific subset of genes, although there is some overlap among these sigma factors in the promoter sequences that they recognize (Table 2.2). RpoD, together with RNA polymerase, binds to the promoters of genes that encode proteins or RNA molecules that are required for essential or "housekeeping" processes. Other sigma factors direct RNA polymerase to the promoters of genes that encode more specialized functions, such as proteins required for adaptation to environmental stresses (RpoS) or for nitrogen metabolism (RpoN).

Nucleotide sequences in and around the RNA polymerase-binding site often play an essential role in determining whether an operon is transcribed. This regulatory region is usually referred to as the operator region. A plethora of elaborate regulatory systems that control the on and off states of various operons have evolved. For example, when a regulatory protein called a repressor binds to an operator region and prevents RNA polymerase from binding to the promoter or moving along the DNA, transcription is blocked

A

B

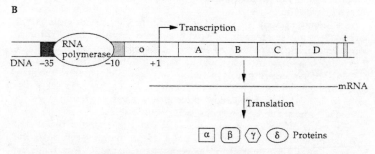

FIGURE 2.23 Schematic representation of a bacterial transcription unit. **(A)** The structural genes (A, B, C, and D) of an operon are under the transcriptional control of an operator (o) and a promoter (p) region. RNA polymerase binds to regions that are 10 (–10) and 35 (–35) bp from the site of initiation of transcription (+1) (right-angled arrow). The t denotes a transcription termination signal sequence. After transcription of the operon, the proteins of the operon (α, β, γ, and δ) are produced during translation. **(B)** Same as panel A, except that binding of RNA polymerase to the promoter region is shown.

(Fig. 2.24). However, in some cases, specific low-molecular-weight compounds (effectors) bind to a particular repressor protein and change its conformation, thus preventing it from binding to its operator region. When an effector-repressor complex fails to bind to an operator region, RNA poly-

TABLE 2.2 Sigma factors produced by *E. coli*

Sigma factor	Synonym(s)	-35 region	-10 region	Function of genes controlled by sigma factor
RpoD	σ^{70}	TTGACA	TATAAT	Most genes required during growth phase
RpoS	σ^{38}	—	CTACACT	Stationary phase and stress response
RpoN	σ^{54}	YTGGCAC (–24 region)	TTGCW (–12 region)	Nitrogen metabolism
RpoH	σ^{32}	TCTCNCCCTTGAA	CCCCATNTA	Heat shock response
RpoF	σ^{28}, FliA	CTAAA	CCGATAT	Flagellum synthesis and chemotaxis
RpoE	σ^{24}	GAANTT	YCTGA	Response to misfolded proteins in the periplasm
RpoFecI	σ^{19}	GAAAAT	—	Iron transport

The DNA-binding sequences shown are the consensus sequences for each sigma factor recognition site. A consensus sequence represents the nucleotides most frequently found at each position as determined by comparing the nucleotide sequences of many different promoters recognized by the sigma factor. Rarely, however, are all of the nucleotides in a given recognition site exactly as represented by the consensus sequence. N = A, T, G, or C; Y = T or C; W = A or T; —, no consensus sequence.

MILESTONE

The Dependence of Cell-Free Protein Synthesis in *E. coli* upon Naturally Occurring or Synthetic Polyribonucleotides

M. W. NIRENBERG and J. H. MATTHAEI
Proc. Natl. Acad. Sci. USA **47**:1588–1602, 1961

An Intermediate in the Biosynthesis of Polyphenylalanine Directed by Synthetic Template RNA

M. W. NIRENBERG, J. H. MATTHAEI, and O. W. JONES
Proc. Natl. Acad. Sci. USA **48**:104–109, 1962

By the early 1960s, due in large part to the efforts of Watson and Crick, it was known that the sequence of bases in DNA contained the genetic code. However, an outstanding question was how nucleotide sequences were decoded to produce proteins with precise sequences of amino acids. Specifically, how could the arrangement of four different nucleotides (i.e., A, T, G, and C) in a sequence determine the combination and linear order of 20 different amino acids that were known to be found in proteins? In a series of papers published in 1961 and 1962, Marshall W. Nirenberg and his colleague J. Heinrich Matthaei at the National Institutes of Health described a cell-free system that allowed them to add various components that might be required to synthesize a protein to a reaction under controlled conditions.

Included in the reaction mixture were ribosomes and soluble RNA (later determined to be the source of aminoacyl-tRNAs) extracted from *E. coli* and radiolabeled amino acids. Only when a simple, synthetic RNA polymer, polyuridylic acid [poly(U)] was added to the reaction, was radiolabeled L-phenylalanine incorporated into a polypeptide identified as poly-L-phenylalanine. "The synthetic polynucleotide appears to contain the code for the synthesis of a protein containing only one amino acid....Polyuridylic acid appears to function as a synthetic template or messenger RNA." Polyphenylalanine could not be produced from any other polynucleotide tested, e.g., poly(A), poly(C), or poly(A·U). Furthermore, phenylalanyl-tRNA was required for the transfer of phenylalanine to the polypeptide chain. Nirenberg, Matthaei, and Jones

suggested that, "since a sequence of one or more uridylic acid residues in poly-U is the code for phenylalanine in this system, it is probable that phenylalanine-sRNA [tRNA] contains a complementary sequence of one or more adenylic acid residues which base-pair with the template." Not only had the first "word" of the genetic code been discovered, but also a mechanism was proposed by which the "letters" in mRNA were interpreted to produce a protein. In a subsequent paper (*Proc. Natl. Acad. Sci. USA* **48**:666–677, 1962), Matthaei et al. showed that an amino acid coding unit contains a minimum of three nucleotides and that the genetic code is at least partially degenerate (two coding units composed of different nucleotides specified the same amino acid) and contains "nonsense words" that do not encode amino acids but likely "serve as periods." Nirenberg, together with H. G. Khorana, who showed that polyribonucleic acids with precise sequences of nucleotides could produce polypeptides with predicted sequences of amino acids, and R. W. Holley, who worked out the structure and function of tRNA, was awarded the Nobel Prize in physiology or medicine in 1968 for the cracking of the genetic code.

merase can bind to the promoter and move along the DNA, and the operon is transcribed. Effector molecules that block repression are generally broken down by cellular activity. When the levels of an effector molecule are reduced, the repressor proteins can bind to the operator region and the off state is reestablished. In many cases an operator region is specific for its particular operon; however, there are many examples of different operons with similar operator sequences that are controlled by the same regulatory protein. The proteins encoded in these operons are usually involved in related cellular processes.

By way of illustration, if a cell has the enzymatic capability of catabolizing a particular sugar, it is a waste of cellular resources to synthesize the enzymes that break down the sugar if the sugar is not present in the medium. On the other hand, if the sugar is available and is the only carbon source, then the enzymes that are responsible for its cellular utilization are essential. In this case, the sugar acts as an effector, preventing the repressor from binding to the operator region and thus enabling the operon to be transcribed. When the amount of sugar is depleted, the

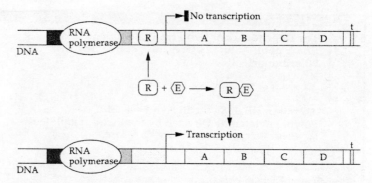

FIGURE 2.24 Induction of the on state for transcription of a bacterial operon. The repressor protein (R) binds to the operator region and blocks transcription. The binding of an effector molecule (E) to the repressor protein changes the conformation of the repressor protein. The repressor protein–effector (RE) complex cannot bind to the operator region; thus, RNA polymerase can transcribe the operon.

repressor protein binds to the operator region and prevents transcription of the operon.

For other operons, transcription may be the normal state because the repressor protein is inactive. In these cases, a specific effector molecule (corepressor) attaches to an inactive repressor and causes a conformational change that enables the repressor–corepressor complex to bind to its corresponding operator region and turn off the transcription of the operon (Fig. 2.25). When the concentration of the corepressor decreases, the on state for the operon resumes because the repressor by itself is unable to bind to the operator.

FIGURE 2.25 Induction of the off state for transcription of a bacterial operon. The binding of a corepressor molecule (C) to an inactive repressor protein (IR) changes the conformation of the repressor protein. The corepressor–repressor protein complex (IR-C) binds to the operator region and blocks transcription of the operon by RNA polymerase.

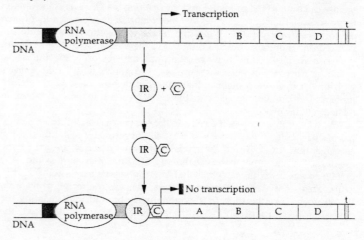

The regulation of transcription by a repressor protein is called a negatively controlled system. In a positively controlled system, a regulatory protein increases the rate of transcription instead of repressing it. Briefly, a protein (activator protein, or activator) binds to the operator region and attracts RNA polymerase to the adjacent promoter region; consequently, transcription of the operon is enhanced (Fig. 2.26). A bound activator protein does not block the movement of RNA polymerase along the DNA. Rather, it can be viewed as "greasing the wheels" for transcription. Activators are specific for particular activator sites. In some instances, an effector molecule converts an active activator to an inactive one and diminishes the rate of transcription of the operon (Fig. 2.26). In other cases, an effector molecule activates an inactive activator by altering the conformation of the activator so that it has an increased binding affinity for the operator sequence. Understanding how the transcription of a bacterial operon is regulated requires detailed molecular studies of mutations that affect a regulatory system and in vitro analyses of the various protein- and DNA-binding sites.

Regulation of mRNA Transcription in Eukaryotes

Most active eukaryotic cells transcribe a common (basal) set of structural genes that maintain routine (housekeeping) cellular functions. In some cells, specific structural genes are transcribed and translated, giving the tissue or organ its unique properties. For example, the genes that encode the α and β subunits of adult hemoglobin are expressed only in the cells that develop into red blood cells. The numbers of cell-specific mRNA transcripts range from a few sequences in some cells to dozens of different sequences in others. The ability of cells to turn on (activate) or turn off (repress) transcription of particular structural genes is essential for maintaining cell specificity, for conserving cellular energy, and for enabling cells to respond to developmental cues or environmental changes.

There are a number of diverse, highly specific processes that activate or repress the transcription of various eukaryotic structural genes. In general,

FIGURE 2.26 Activation and deactivation of a bacterial operon. An activator protein (Act) binds to an activating site and enhances the rate of transcription of the operon. When an effector molecule (E) binds to the activator protein, the Act–E complex does not bind to the activating site. The rate of transcription of the operon is diminished when the activating site is not occupied by the activating protein.

the control of transcription in eukaryotes is mediated by proteins that are collectively classified as transcription factors. Many transcription factors bind directly to DNA sequences that are frequently less than 10 bp in length. The naming of these protein-binding sites is idiosyncratic. However, for the most part, they are called boxes, DNA modules, initiator elements, or response elements. Unlike the situation in prokaryotes, operons are almost never found in the genomes of eukaryotes. Consequently, each eukaryotic structural gene has its own set of response elements. Moreover, in addition to DNA–protein interactions, protein–protein associations are important for regulating eukaryotic transcription.

In addition to specific response elements, a representative eukaryotic structural gene has a promoter sequence that binds to a core set of proteins that are minimally required for transcription initiation. A eukaryotic promoter consists of a TATA sequence (TATA box, or Hogness box), a CCAAT sequence ("cat" box), and a sequence of repeated GC nucleotides (GC box) that lie about –25, –75, and –90 bp, respectively, from the site of initiation of transcription (+1) (Fig. 2.27). The first step in the initiation of transcription of eukaryotic structural genes with a TATA promoter is the binding of transcription factor IID (TFIID, or TATA-binding protein [TBP]), which is a complex of at least 14 proteins, to an available TATA sequence. Subsequently, other transcription factors bind to TFIID and the DNA adjacent to the TATA box. Then, RNA polymerase II, which is oriented toward the structural gene, binds to the transcription complex. With the aid of additional transcription factors, transcription is initiated at the correct starting point (the +1 nucleotide) (Fig. 2.28). Clearly, if a TATA sequence is deleted or grossly altered, then transcription of the structural gene cannot occur. Transcription factors that are specific for the CCAAT and GC response elements have been identified. In addition, enhancer sequences that increase the rate of transcription of structural genes are located hundreds or even thousands of base pairs from the +1 base pair. Folding, looping, or bending of the chromosomal DNA may bring DNA regions, which in the elongated state are far apart, close to one another. Also, transcription factors that bind to certain enhancers or response elements may form a chain of proteins that create bridges from one DNA site to another.

Some repressed (nonexpressed) structural genes are activated by a cascade of events that is triggered by a specific extracellular signal, such as a temperature increase or the presence of a hormone. For example, a hormone that is released into the circulatory system comes into contact with a specific cell type that has a receptor on its outer surface that binds the hormone and facilitates the entry of the hormone into the cell. Once inside the

FIGURE 2.27 Promoter and initiator elements of some eukaryotic structural genes. The negative numbers designate the locations of nucleotide pairs in the DNA that lie upstream from the site of initiation (+1) of transcription. The right-angled arrow indicates the site of initiation and the direction of transcription. The locations of the transcription elements are not drawn to scale.

FIGURE 2.28 Formation of an RNA polymerase II transcription initiation complex at a TATA box. Transcription factor TFIID binds to a TATA box, and in sequence, other transcription factors and RNA polymerase II bind to form a protein aggregate that is responsible for initiating transcription. The right-angled arrow indicates the site of initiation and the direction of transcription.

cell, the hormone interacts with a cytoplasmic protein and changes the conformation of the protein. In this altered state, the protein is now able to enter the nucleus, where it binds to an exclusive response element that initiates transcription of the target gene.

Some proteins bind to response elements and prevent transcription. For example, there is a class of about 18 vertebrate genes that are actively transcribed in nerve cells (neurons) and turned off in nonneuronal cells. Each of these neuron-active genes has a 24-bp response element that lies upstream of its transcription initiation site. This DNA sequence is called a neuron-restrictive silencer element (NRSE). In nonneuronal cells, a protein called neuron-restrictive silencer factor (NRSF) is synthesized, binds to each NRSE, and prevents transcription of each member of this set of genes.

Conversely, NRSF is not produced by neuronal cells, and therefore, each gene with an NRSE is transcribed.

On the whole, the regulation of transcription in eukaryotes is complex. A structural gene may have a number of different response elements that can be activated in different cell types by different signals at different times in the life cycle of an organism. Alternatively, some structural genes are under the preferential control of a unique transcription factor. For the off state, specific proteins can interact with certain response elements and prevent transcription, or in a more general way, some proteins obstruct transcription by binding to the transcription complex either before initiation or during the elongation process.

More generalized control of gene expression that influences larger regions of the chromosomes is mediated by the state of chromosome structure. A very large amount of chromosomal DNA must be packaged into the nucleus of a eukaryotic cell. To facilitate this, the DNA is bound by specific proteins called histones that interact with each other to compact (condense) the chromosomes into a smaller volume. DNA with its associated packaging proteins is known as chromatin. Some regions of the chromosomes are tightly packed (heterochromatin), while other regions are less condensed (euchromatin). Highly condensed DNA is less accessible to regulatory proteins that activate transcription, and therefore, the genes in these regions are usually not expressed or are expressed only at a low level. Chromatin structure, however, is dynamic, and condensed regions can be "relaxed" by the addition of chemical groups, such as an acetyl group to amino acids in the packaging proteins or methyl groups to specific sites in the nucleotide sequences to which the proteins bind. Unpacking of the chromatin generally increases transcription of genes in the region.

Protein Secretion Pathways

Bacteria and eukaryotic cells have specialized systems for exporting certain proteins (secretory proteins) to the external environment. Generally, secretory proteins are required for acquiring nutrients, cell-to-cell communication, protection, and structures that reside on the outer surface of the cell membrane. The primary impediment to the release of a secretory protein is a membrane. The processes that facilitate secretion of proteins through such a formidable barrier are similar among all organisms, although there are significant differences between organisms. For example, gram-negative and gram-positive bacteria do not have the same secretory pathways. A secreted protein in gram-negative bacteria must pass through an inner membrane, a periplasmic space, and an outer membrane to exit the cell, whereas in gram-positive bacteria, secretory proteins are transported only across a single cytoplasmic membrane. In contrast, the secretory system in higher organisms is more complex. Unlike prokaryotic proteins, many eukaryotic proteins require a number of highly specific modifications, such as glycosylation, acetylation, sulfation, and phosphorylation, to produce functional secretory proteins. Some of these protein modifications and various processing steps are carried out in the endoplasmic reticulum, and others take place in the Golgi apparatus, where proteins are also sorted according to their final cellular destinations, including those that exit

through the cell membrane. The property that distinguishes a protein that remains in the cytoplasm from one that is secreted is often an amino acid sequence (a signal peptide, signal sequence, leader sequence, or leader peptide) at its N terminus.

In gram-positive bacteria, the signal peptide of some secretory proteins makes direct contact with a membrane-bound assembly of proteins (a secretion complex, or Sec complex) that facilitates the passage of these proteins through the membrane and their release to the external environment (Fig. 2.29). Alternatively, for other secretory proteins, a group of proteins called a signal recognition complex binds to a signal peptide, and this combination attaches to a membrane-bound signal recognition complex receptor before making contact with the Sec complex (Fig. 2.29). In both cases, the secretory protein is translocated through a channel formed by the Sec complex, and its release depends on removal of the signal peptide by a membrane-bound enzyme called a signal peptidase. Subsequently, proteins that have crossed the cytoplasmic membrane readily pass through the porous cell wall, where they encounter metal ions and other components that promote proper folding and molecular stabilization.

Gram-negative bacteria have multiple pathways for the secretion of various proteins. Some of these systems (Sec-dependent pathways) use the

FIGURE 2.29 Schematic representation of secretion in gram-positive bacteria. A signal recognition particle (SRP) binds to the signal peptide of a secretory protein, and this complex binds to a membrane protein that directs the secretory protein (1) to the Sec complex. There is also an SRP-independent pathway (2), where a signal peptide alone makes contact with the Sec complex. The secretory protein is translocated through a channel within the Sec complex (3), and the signal peptide is removed by a signal peptidase(s). Proper folding of the secretory protein occurs as it passes through the cell wall (4).

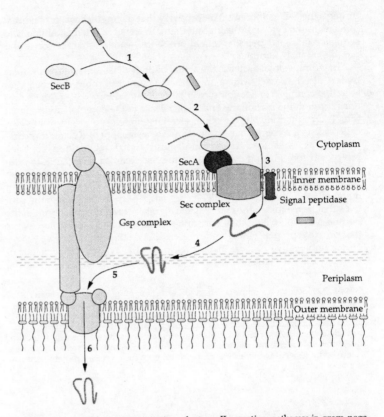

FIGURE 2.30 Schematic representation of a type II secretion pathway in gram-negative bacteria. The SecB protein binds to a secretory protein in the cytoplasm (1), SecB attaches to the SecA protein that is part of the Sec complex of the inner membrane (2), and the secretory protein is translocated through the inner membrane (3). A signal peptidase removes the signal peptide, and the secretory protein is properly folded in the periplasm (4); the secretory protein combines with the Gsp complex (5); and it is translocated to the external environment (6).

same membrane-bound Sec complex for transmitting a secretory protein through the inner membrane into the periplasm. Collectively, the Sec-dependent pathways are designated the general secretion pathway. In these instances, a cytoplasmic protein (SecB) binds an amino acid sequence (domain) of a secretory protein that has a signal peptide. In turn, the SecB protein combines with a protein (SecA) of the membrane-bound Sec complex. The secretory protein is translocated into the periplasm, and the signal peptide is removed. At this point, the secretory protein encounters various periplasmic proteins that ensure proper folding. Thereafter, Sec-dependent secretory proteins exit through the outer membrane by different routes. A region of some proteins is capable of forming a channel in the outer membrane that allows part of the remaining protein to be selectively

Cytoplasm

Inner membrane

Periplasm

Outer membrane

FIGURE 2.31 The type III secretion system is made up of about 20 different proteins that form a continuous channel through the inner and outer membranes of gram-negative bacteria. The type III secretion system is used by bacterial pathogens to secrete toxins and other proteins into plant and animal host cells. A hollow needle-like protein structure extends from the bacterial surface into the host cell.

extruded (autotransporter pathway). In these cases, proteolytic cleavage releases the functional portion of the protein to the external environment. Other proteins are able to pass through an outer membrane channel that is formed by a separate protein (single accessory pathway). Another pathway (chaperone/usher pathway) is used by specific proteins that form fimbriae on the surface of the bacterial cell. A fourth general secretion pathway branch called the type II secretion pathway consists of a protein complex (the Gsp complex) that spans the periplasmic space and forms a channel through the outer membrane. Most secreted proteins pass through the type II pathway. In these cases, secretory proteins earmarked for the type II pathway are first transported to the periplasmic space via the Sec-dependent pathway, where they bind to the Gsp complex and are shunted through the outer membrane (Fig. 2.30). Other Sec-dependent pathways have been found in various gram-negative bacteria. In contrast to the type II pathway, the type I and type III secretion pathways are Sec independent, and each has its own protein complex that extends from the inner to the outer membrane, forming a continuous channel from the bacterial cytoplasm to the external environment. For example, bacterial flagellar proteins reach the outer surface of the cell by means of a type III secretion pathway. Type III secretion pathways are often used by bacterial pathogens to secrete bacterial proteins into the cytoplasm of eukaryotic host cells (Fig. 2.31). Signal peptides are recognized by the Sec-independent systems but are not necessarily cleaved during the secretion process.

FIGURE 2.32 Schematic representation of the secretion pathway in eukaryotes. **(A)** A signal recognition particle (SRP) binds to the signal sequence of a secretory protein. **(B)** The SRP attaches to an SRP receptor on the endoplasmic reticulum (ER) membrane. **(C)** The secretory protein is translocated into the lumen of the ER, and a signal peptidase removes the signal sequence. **(D)** The secretory protein is folded, partially modified, and packaged in a transport vesicle intended for the Golgi network. **(E)** The ER-released vesicle carrying the secretory protein enters the Golgi network at the *cis* face and passes through the Golgi stack, where it is further modified; after it is sorted, a plasma membrane-specific vesicle is formed at the *trans* face of the Golgi network. The secretory transport vesicle fuses with the plasma membrane and releases the secretory protein to the extracellular environment.

Protein secretion is basically the same in all eukaryotic organisms from yeast to plant and animal cells. Briefly, the signal sequence of a secretory protein is bound by a signal recognition particle during protein synthesis; the signal recognition particle attaches to a receptor on the membrane of the endoplasmic reticulum, and the secretory protein passes through a channel in the membrane as translation proceeds; a signal peptidase removes the signal sequence; and the secretory protein is released into the lumen of the endoplasmic reticulum, where it is folded and, if required, glycosylated. A vesicle containing a processed secretory protein buds off from the endoplasmic reticulum and is transported to and fuses with the *cis* face of the Golgi apparatus (Fig. 2.32). Additional processing, glycosylations, and posttranslation modifications take place in the Golgi stack. The secretory protein then emerges from the *trans* face of the Golgi apparatus enclosed in a vesicle that is transported to and fuses with the plasma membrane, where the contents are released to the external environment (Fig. 2.32). In eukaryotic organisms, some proteins are secreted continuously (constitutive secretion). Others remain in vesicles (mature secretory granules) near the plasma membrane and are released only after a hormone or membrane depolarization signal is received.

SUMMARY

A DNA molecule has two polynucleotide strands that form an antiparallel double helix. The monomeric unit of a DNA strand is a nucleotide that consists of an base, a deoxyribose sugar, and a phosphate group. The successive nucleotides of a DNA strand are linked by phosphodiester bonds, and the two strands of DNA are held together by hydrogen bonds between specific complementary pairs of bases. During replication, which is mediated by a number of different proteins, including DNA polymerases, each DNA strand acts as a template for the production of a complementary strand.

Proteins are vital for the maintenance of all biological functions. A protein consists of a specific sequence of amino acids that are linked by peptide bonds. The sequence of amino acids for a protein is encoded in the DNA. The process of decoding genetic information is carried out by RNA molecules, including mRNA, tRNA, and rRNA; various enzymes; and an assortment of protein factors. All RNA is transcribed from DNA. Sequences of DNA in combination with protein factors ensure that transcription is initiated at a precise starting point, that the appropriate strand is used as the template, and that termination occurs at a specified nucleotide site. In eukaryotic organisms, most structural genes consist of coding regions (exons) separated by noncoding segments (introns). Primary transcripts contain both exons and introns. However, a processing system removes the introns and joins the exons, in the proper order, to form a functional mRNA. An mRNA carries the code for the sequence of amino acids of a protein.

Translation of mRNA to produce a protein occurs on ribosomes that are composed of a large and a small subunit, each containing rRNA and a large number of specific proteins. Translation in prokaryotes is initiated by the joining of an mRNA with a small ribosomal subunit. As a result of codon-to-anticodon complementary base pairing, the initiator tRNA, fMet-tRNAfMet, attaches to the mRNA–small ribosomal subunit complex, which then combines with the large ribosomal subunit to form an initiation complex. Translation in eukaryotes is initiated by the combining of a unique initiator tRNA which carries the amino acid methionine, Met-tRNAMet, with a small ribosomal subunit and then by the threading of an mRNA through the initiator tRNA–small ribosomal subunit complex until the first AUG sequence in the mRNA pairs with the anticodon of the initiator tRNA. The large ribosomal subunit joins the initiator tRNA–small ribosomal subunit–mRNA complex to form an initiation complex that is ready for the translation of the mRNA sequence.

After the formation of the initiation complex, the elongation phase of translation is very similar in prokaryotes and eukaryotes. The next three nucleotides in the mRNA pair with the anticodon of a tRNA that carries its specific amino acid. The first amino acid, methionine, is cleaved from the initiator tRNA and joined to the second amino acid by a peptide bond. The "empty" initiator tRNA is ejected from the ribosome, the ribosome complex shifts, and the tRNA to which the growing peptide is attached occupies the site vacated by the ejected initiator tRNA. As a consequence of the shift (translocation), the next codon of the mRNA is available to pair with the appropriate anticodon of a tRNA that carries its specific amino acid that will be joined to the growing peptide. By repeating these steps, a polypeptide with a specific sequence of amino acids is formed. Translation is terminated when one of three stop codons is encountered in the mRNA on a ribosome. A termination factor, rather than a tRNA, recognizes the stop codon, and the bond between the last tRNA and the completed amino acid chain is cleaved, causing the tRNA, mRNA, and completed protein to be released.

Only the RNAs and proteins that are essential for maintaining routine cellular functions are synthesized continuously. To conserve cellular resources, transcription of the remaining genes occurs only when a particular protein is required and is turned off when the protein is no longer needed. In prokaryotes, transcription is initiated by the binding of RNA polymerase to the −10 and −35 elements of the promoter region of an operon. Regulatory proteins that bind to operator sequences in and around the promoter region control the activity of RNA polymerase at the promoter and thereby control transcription initiation. Repressors prevent transcription initiation by blocking RNA polymerase binding to the promoter or movement along the DNA, while activators enhance the binding of RNA polymerase to a promoter sequence. The activities of regulatory proteins are controlled by small effector molecules that increase or decrease their binding to the operator sequence. In eukaryotes, RNA polymerase II, which transcribes structural genes, binds to an array of proteins called transcription factors that attach, in sequence, to a TATA sequence of a promoter region. Other transcription factors that bind to DNA elements of eukaryotic structural genes are responsible for turning on or turning off transcription. The expression of eukaryotic genes is also influenced by the local conformation of chromosomal DNA. Regions that are highly compacted by specific DNA-associated proteins are generally not transcribed, while more loosely packed regions contain genes that are transcriptionally active.

Prokaryotes and eukaryotes have specialized systems for exporting proteins across a cytoplasmic membrane. Secreted prokaryotic proteins have a sequence of amino acids at their N-terminal ends that targets the protein either to the general secretory pathway or to more specialized protein complexes that transport specific proteins. Eukaryotic proteins that are to be secreted are synthesized on ribosomes associated with the endoplasmic reticulum and are first secreted into the lumen of the endoplasmic reticulum via an N-terminal signal sequence, where they are cleaved, folded, and chemically modified. After further processing in the Golgi apparatus, the proteins are transported to the cytoplasmic membrane in membrane vesicles and, following fusion of the vesicle and cytoplasmic membranes, are released into the external environment.

REFERENCES

Browning, D. F., and S. J. Busby. 2004. The regulation of bacterial transcription initiation. *Nat. Rev. Microbiol.* 2:57–65.

Dever, T. E. 2002. Gene-specific regulation by general translation factors. *Cell* 108:545–556.

Ghosh, P. 2004. Process of protein transport by the type III secretion system. *Microbiol. Mol. Biol. Rev.* 68:771–795.

Henkin, T. M. 2000. Transcription termination control in bacteria. *Curr. Opin. Microbiol.* 3:149–153.

Juven-Gershon, T., J.-Y. Hsu, J. W. M. Theisen, and J. T. Kadonaga. 2008. The RNA polymerase II core promoter—the gateway to transcription. *Curr. Opin. Cell Biol.* 20:253–259.

Koenigsberger, C., J. J. Chicca II, M. C. Amoureux, G. M. Edelman, and

F. S. Jones. 2000. Differential regulation by multiple promoters of the gene encoding the neuron-restrictive silencer factor. *Proc. Natl. Acad. Sci. USA* 97:2291–2296.

Kozak, M. 2005. Regulation of translation via mRNA structure in prokaryotes and eukaryotes. *Gene* 361:13–37.

Maniatis, T., and B. Tasic. 2002. Alternative pre-mRNA splicing and proteome expansion in metazoans. *Nature* 418:236–243.

Morse, R. H. 2007. Transcription factor access to promoter elements. *J. Cell. Biochem.* 102:560–570.

Petry, S., A. Weixlbaumer, and V. Ramakrishnan. 2008. The termination of translation. *Curr. Opin. Struct. Biol.* 18:70–77.

Saier, M. H., Jr. 2006. Protein secretion and membrane insertion systems in

gram-negative bacteria. *J. Membr. Biol.* 214:75–90.

Schoenherr, C. J., and D. J. Anderson. 1995. The neuron-restrictive silencer factor (NRSF): a coordinate repressor of multiple neuron-specific genes. *Science* 267:1360–1363.

Watson, J. D., and F. H. C. Crick. 1953. Genetical implications of the structure of deoxyribonucleic acid. *Nature* 171:964–967.

Williams, S. K., and J. K. Tyler. 2007. Transcriptional regulation by chromatin disassembly and reassembly. *Curr. Opin. Genet. Dev.* 17:88–93.

Wilson, D. N., and K. H. Nierhaus. 2006. The E-site story: the importance of maintaining two tRNAs on the ribosome during protein synthesis. *Cell. Mol. Life Sci.* 63:2725–2737.

REVIEW QUESTIONS

1. Discuss the basic features of DNA replication.

2. Compare and contrast DNA and RNA.

3. Describe the differences and similarities between prokaryotic and eukaryotic structural genes.

4. Describe the elongation phase of translation.

5. Deduce the most likely DNA coding sequence for the following human protein: MAGGTWYQLFPRKMWNDSTLHP FILPMNVAG.

6. Determine the amino acid sequence encoded by the following mRNA: GCGAUCGACGAUGUUUCUAAAAGUAUC UCAUCGAAAUGAGGGUUCGUAAUAGCGACC CGGGCGG.

7. What is an operon? What is the biological significance of an operon?

8. How is transcription initiation controlled in bacterial cells?

9. Describe the major DNA elements that are responsible for the transcription of eukaryotic structural genes.

10. How are proteins transported across the cytoplasmic membrane of gram-positive bacterial cells?

11. Describe the type II secretion system of gram-negative bacterial cells.

12. How are secretory proteins processed in eukaryotic cells?

Recombinant DNA Technology

RECOMBINANT DNA TECHNOLOGY, which is also called gene cloning or molecular cloning, is a general term that encompasses a number of experimental protocols leading to the transfer of genetic information (DNA) from one organism to another. There is no single set of methods that can be used to meet this objective; however, a recombinant DNA experiment often has the following format (Fig. 3.1).

- The DNA (cloned DNA, insert DNA, target DNA, or foreign DNA) from a donor organism is extracted, enzymatically cleaved (cut, or digested), and joined (ligated) to another DNA entity (a cloning vector) to form a new, recombined DNA molecule (cloning vector–insert DNA construct, or DNA construct).

- This cloning vector–insert DNA construct is transferred into and maintained within a host cell. The introduction of DNA into a bacterial host cell is called transformation.

- Those host cells that take up the DNA construct (transformed cells) are identified and selected (separated, or isolated) from those that do not.

- If required, a DNA construct can be created so that the protein product encoded by the cloned DNA sequence is produced in the host cell.

Recombinant DNA technology was developed from discoveries in molecular biology, nucleic acid enzymology, and the molecular genetics of both bacterial viruses (bacteriophages) and bacterial extrachromosomal DNA elements (plasmids). However, recombinant DNA technology would not exist without the availability of enzymes that recognize specific double-stranded DNA sequences and cleave the DNA in both strands at these sequences (restriction enzymes, or restriction endonucleases). Nucleases that cut nucleic acid molecules internally are endonucleases, and those that degrade from the ends of nucleic acids are exonucleases.

FIGURE 3.1 Recombinant DNA-cloning procedure. DNA from a source organism is cleaved with a restriction endonuclease and inserted into a cloning vector. The cloning vector–insert (target) DNA construct is introduced into a host cell, and those cells that carry the construct are identified and grown. If required, the cloned gene can be expressed (transcribed and translated) in the host cell, and the protein (recombinant protein) can be harvested.

Restriction Endonucleases

For molecular cloning, both the source DNA that contains the target sequence and the cloning vector must be consistently cut into discrete and reproducible fragments. It was only after bacterial enzymes that cut DNA molecules internally at specific base pair sequences were discovered that molecular cloning became feasible. These enzymes are formally designated type II restriction endonucleases. Despite the fact that there are other kinds of restriction endonucleases (type I, type III, and type IV), the type II restriction endonucleases are commonly called restriction endonucleases or simply restriction enzymes.

One of the first type II restriction endonucleases to be characterized was from the bacterium *Escherichia coli*, and it was originally designated *Eco*RI. More recently, it has been proposed that the use of italics for naming restriction endonucleases be abandoned. Here, we have implemented this recommendation. EcoRI is a homodimeric protein (it is made up of two identical proteins) that binds to a DNA region with a specific palindromic sequence (recognition site, or binding site). In other words, the sequences of nucleotides in the two strands of the binding site are identical when either is read in the same polarity, i.e., 5′ to 3′. The EcoRI recognition sequence consists of 6 base pairs (bp) and is cut between the guanine and adenine residues on each strand (Fig. 3.2). EcoRI specifically cleaves the internucleotide bond between the oxygen of the 3′ carbon of the sugar of one nucleotide and the phosphate group attached to the 5′ carbon of the sugar of the adjacent nucleotide. The symmetrical staggered cleavage of DNA by EcoRI produces two single-stranded, complementary cut ends, each with extensions of 4 nucleotides, known as sticky ends. In this case,

FIGURE 3.2 Symmetrical, staggered cleavage of a short fragment of DNA by the type II restriction endonuclease EcoRI. The large arrows show the sites of cleavage in the DNA backbone. S, deoxyribose sugar; P, phosphate group; OH, hydroxyl group. The EcoRI recognition sequence is highlighted by the dashed line.

each single-stranded extension terminates with a 5′ phosphate group, and the 3′ hydroxyl group of the opposite strand is recessed.

In addition to EcoRI, more than 3,700 type II restriction endonucleases with about 250 different recognition sites have been isolated from various bacteria. The naming protocol for these enzymes is the same as that for EcoRI; the genus is the capitalized letter, and the first two letters of the species name are in lowercase letters. The strain designation is occasionally added to the name, such as R in EcoRI, or the serotype of the source bacterium is sometimes noted, such as d in HindIII. The Roman numerals are used to designate the order of characterization of different restriction endonucleases from the same organism. For example, HpaI and HpaII are the first and second type II restriction endonucleases that were isolated from *Haemophilus parainfluenzae*.

The palindromic sequences where most type II restriction endonucleases bind and cut a DNA molecule are within the recognition sites. Some restriction endonucleases digest (cleave) DNA, leaving 5′ phosphate extensions (protruding ends, or sticky ends) with recessed 3′ hydroxyl ends; some leave 3′ hydroxyl extensions with recessed 5′ phosphate ends; and some cut the backbones of both strands within a recognition site to produce blunt-ended (flush-ended) DNA molecules (Fig. 3.3). The lengths of the recognition sites for different enzymes can be four, five, six, eight, or more nucleotide pairs (Table 3.1). Because of the frequency with which their recognition sites occur in DNA, restriction endonucleases that cleave within sites of four (four-cutters) and six (six-cutters) nucleotide pairs are used for most of the common molecular-cloning protocols. The importance of the type II restriction endonucleases for gene cloning cannot be overstated.

FIGURE 3.3 Blunt-end cleavage of a short fragment of DNA by the type II restriction endonuclease HindII. The large arrows show the sites of cleavage in the DNA backbone. For abbreviations, see the legend to Fig. 3.2. The HindII recognition sequence is highlighted.

TABLE 3.1 Recognition sequences of some restriction endonucleases

Enzyme	Recognition site	Type of cut end
EcoRI	G↓A—A—T—T—C C—T—T—A—A↑G	5′ phosphate extension
BamHI	G↓G—A—T—C—C C—C—T—A—G↑G	5′ phosphate extension
PstI	C—T—G—C—A↓G G↑A—C—G—T—C	3′ hydroxyl extension
Sau3AI	↓G—A—T—C C—T—A—G↑	5′ phosphate extension
PvuII	C—A—G↓C—T—G G—T—C↑G—A—C	Blunt end
HpaI	G—T—T↓A—A—C C—A—A↑T—T—G	Blunt end
HaeIII	G—G↓C—C C—C↑G—G	Blunt end
NotI	G↓C—G—G—C—C—G—C C—G—C—C—G—G—C↑G	5′ phosphate extension

Arrows denote cleavage sites.

When a DNA sample is treated with one of these enzymes, the same set of fragments is always produced, assuming that all of the recognition sites are cleaved. In addition, ready access to a variety of restriction endonucleases adds versatility to gene-cloning strategies.

Type IIS restriction endonucleases form a subgroup of the type II category of restriction enzymes and are occasionally used for cloning and other molecular studies, such as multiplex polony sequencing, that are discussed in chapter 4. These enzymes have the fascinating feature of cutting DNA, usually in both strands, a fixed number of nucleotides away from one end of the recognition site. Moreover, any particular sequence of nucleotides may be present between the binding sequence and the cut sites. The cleavages for most type IIS restriction enzymes are staggered. For example, the FokI restriction endonuclease binds to $\frac{GGATG}{CCTAC}$ and cuts 9 nucleotides downstream on the upper strand and 13 nucleotides downstream on the lower strand, producing a recessed 3′ hydroxyl end and a 4-nucleotide extension at the 5′ phosphate end. One representation of the recognition sequence and cut sites of the FokI restriction endonuclease is $\frac{GGATGNNNNNNNNN}{CCTACNNNNNNNNNNNNN}$NNNN, where N denotes A, C, G, or T. Of course, with this single-letter code, it is understood that the nucleotides (N) opposite each other are base paired. A simpler notation is $\frac{GGATG(N)_9}{CCTAC(N)_{13}}$, and perhaps the simplest is GGATG(9/13). Examples of some type IIS restriction endonucleases are shown in Table 3.2. It should be noted that a few type IIS restriction endonucleases cleave DNA both upstream and downstream from their recognition sites.

Under natural conditions, bacteria use restriction endonucleases to cleave foreign DNA, such as that of infecting bacterial viruses (bacteriophages), and have developed systems that protect their own DNA from being degraded. Most often, methylation of the cytosine residues of a restriction endonuclease site in the host DNA prevents restriction endonucleases from cutting at these sites, but the nonmethylated sites of foreign DNA are vulnerable to attack. With the characterization of large numbers of restriction endonucleases from various bacteria, interesting relationships have been observed. In some instances, different phosphodiester bonds

TABLE 3.2 Some examples of type IIS restriction endonucleases

Restriction endonuclease	Recognition sequence
AcuI	5' CTGAAG (N)$_{16}$
	3' GACTTC (N)$_{14}$
BfuAI	5' ACCTGC (N)$_4$
	3' TGGACG (N)$_8$
BsmBI	5' CGTCTC (N)$_1$
	3' GCAGAG (N)$_5$
EciI	5' GGCGGA (N)$_{11}$
	3' CCGCCT (N)$_9$
FokI	5' GGATG (N)$_9$
	3' CCTAC (N)$_{13}$
HgaI	5' GACGC (N)$_5$
	3' CTGCG (N)$_{10}$
MlyI	5' GAGTC (N)$_5$
	3' CTCAG (N)$_5$
MmeI	5' TCCRAC (N)$_{20}$
	3' AGGYTG (N)$_{18}$

Recognition sequences are shown with locations of downstream cleavage sites. N = A, T, G, or C; R = A or G; Y = T or C. The single-letter codes $\frac{R}{Y}$ represent the base pair $\frac{A}{T}$ or $\frac{G}{C}$, and $\frac{N}{N}$ represents $\frac{A}{T}$, $\frac{T}{A}$, $\frac{G}{C}$, or $\frac{C}{G}$.

within the same recognition site are cleaved by restriction endonucleases from different organisms. For example, the restriction enzymes XmaI and SmaI both recognize the sequence $\frac{CCCGGG}{GGGCCC}$, but XmaI cleaves after the first 5' cytosine in each strand and produces 5' phosphate extensions whereas SmaI generates blunt ends by cleaving between the $\frac{CG}{GC}$ base pair in the middle of the recognition site. The first restriction endonuclease that is discovered to bind to a particular recognition site is designated the prototype. Any additional restriction endonucleases that attack the same sequence as the prototype are called isoschizomers. For example, the restriction endonucleases XhoI and PaeR7I from different organisms both have the same recognition sequences and cleavage locations. Isoschizomers that cleave at different positions within the same recognition site are neoschizomers (Fig. 3.4). On the other hand, restriction endonucleases that produce the same nucleotide extensions but have different recognition sites are designated isocaudomers, e.g., BamHI and Sau3AI (Table 3.1). In some cases, a restriction endonuclease will cleave a sequence only if the cytosines of the recognition site are not methylated whereas another restriction endonuclease will cut the same sequence if these cytosines are methylated. For example, HpaII cleaves only nonmethylated $\frac{CCGG}{GGCC}$ sites, and MspI, an isoschizomer of HpaII, cuts this sequence regardless of cytosine methylation. This pair of restriction endonucleases is often used to determine the methylation status of genomic DNA. If a DNA molecule is not cut by HpaII but is cut by MspI, then the recognition site is methylated. If both restriction endonucleases cleave a DNA molecule, then the site(s) is not methylated.

Physical maps that designate the relative positions of restriction endonuclease sites on a specific piece of DNA can be constructed by treating the DNA molecule singly with different restriction endonucleases and then with combinations of the same restriction endonucleases. The positions of the cleavage sites can be deduced from an analysis of fragment sizes, which are determined by agarose gel electrophoresis (Box 3.1). By way of illustration, the fragment sizes produced by various digestions are shown

FIGURE 3.4 Neoschizomers. Four restriction endonucleases bind to the same recognition site and cleave at different positions. The restriction endonucleases and cleavage sites (arrows) are color coded: KasI, red; NarI, blue; SfoI, black; BbeI, green. A number of other restriction endonucleases, such as NdaI, Mly113I, MchI, BinSII, DinI, EgeI, and EheI, that bind to and cleave this sequence are not shown.

in Fig. 3.5A. It can be deduced that this linear piece of DNA has two BamHI sites and two EcoRI sites in a definite order with a specified number of base pairs separating the sites. More specifically, the sizes of fragments produced in each single digestion can be compared with those from double digestions to determine the positions of the restriction endonuclease sites and to generate a restriction endonuclease site map (restriction endonuclease map). In the example shown in Fig. 3.5, the analysis goes as follows. Because each single digestion produces three fragments from a linear DNA molecule, the original piece of DNA must contain two sites for each of the restriction endonucleases. The 3,000-bp fragment that

BOX 3.1

Gel Electrophoresis

Gel electrophoresis is a commonly used technique for resolving proteins or nucleic acids. In general, a sample of one particular type of macromolecule (protein, DNA, or RNA) is placed in a well at or near the end of a gel matrix (gel). The composition of an electrophoresis gel is a semisolid open meshwork of interlinked linear strands. A gel is cast as a thin slab with a number of sample wells. After the wells of a gel are loaded with sample, an electric field is applied across the gel, and charged macromolecules of the same size are driven together in the direction of the anode through the gel as discrete invisible bands of material. The distance that a band moves into a gel depends on the mass of its macromolecules and the size of the openings (pore size) of the gel. The smaller macromolecules travel further than the larger ones.

The progress of gel electrophoresis is monitored by observing the migration of a visible dye (tracking dye) through the gel. The tracking dye is a charged, low-molecular-weight compound that is loaded into each sample well at the start of a run. When the tracking dye reaches the end of the gel, the run is terminated. The bands, which are aligned in a lane under each well, are visualized by staining the gel with a dye that is specific for protein, DNA, or RNA. Discrete bands are observed when there is enough material present in a band to bind the dye to make the band visible and when the individual macromolecules of a

sample have distinctly different sizes. Otherwise, a band is not detected. If there is little or no difference among the sizes of the macromolecules in a concentrated sample, a smear of stained material is observed. The intensity of a stained band reflects the frequency of occurrence of a macromolecule in a sample.

The molecular mass (molecular weight) of a gel-fractionated macromolecule (band) is determined from a standard curve that is based on a set of macromolecules of known molecular mass (size markers) that covers the separation range of the gel system and is run in one or both of the outside lanes (calibrator lanes) of the same gel as the samples. The logarithm of the molecular mass of a size marker is related to its relative mobility (R_f) through a gel. The value of R_f is defined as the distance traveled by a band divided by the distance traveled by the tracking dye (ion front). The relationship between the logarithm of the molecular mass of each size marker and its R_f value is plotted. Then, with this standard curve, a molecular mass is calculated for each band in a lane. The units of molecular mass for proteins and double-stranded and single-stranded nucleic acids are daltons, base pairs, and bases, respectively. The size markers are included in the same gel as the samples because the extent of mobility of a macromolecule(s) varies from one electrophoretic run to the next.

Polyacrylamide is the preferred gel system for separating proteins.

Copolymerization of monomeric acrylamide and the cross-linker bisacrylamide forms a lattice of cross-linked, linear polyacrylamide strands. The pore size of a polyacrylamide gel is determined by the concentration of acrylamide and the ratio of acrylamide to bisacrylamide. For many applications, a protein sample is treated with the anionic detergent sodium dodecyl sulfate (SDS) before electrophoresis. The SDS binds to proteins and dissociates most multichain proteins. Each SDS-coated protein chain has a similar charge-to-mass ratio. Consequently, during electrophoresis, the separation of the SDS–protein chains is based primarily on size, and the effect of conformation is eliminated. SDS–polyacrylamide gel electrophoresis with a 10% polyacrylamide gel resolves proteins that range from 20 to 200 kilodaltons (kDa).

Agarose, which is a polysaccharide from seaweed, is used routinely as the gel matrix for the electrophoretic separation of medium-size nucleic acid molecules. A 1.0% agarose gel can resolve duplex DNA chains that range from about 600 to 10,000 bp. Specialized agarose gel electrophoresis systems are available for fractionating DNA molecules with millions of base pairs, denatured DNA, and denatured RNA. In addition, for specific purposes, polyacrylamide gels are used for separating DNA molecules. For example, DNA chains that are as small as 6 bases and that differ from each other by 1 nucleotide can be resolved with a 20% polyacrylamide gel.

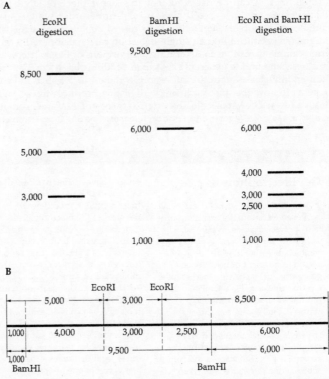

FIGURE 3.5 Mapping of restriction endonuclease sites. **(A)** Restriction endonuclease digestions and electrophoretic separation of fragments. A purified, linear piece of DNA is cut with EcoRI and BamHI separately (single digestions) and then with both enzymes together (double digestion). The horizontal lines under the digestion conditions represent schematically the locations of the DNA fragments (bands) in the lanes of the gel after electrophoresis and staining of the DNA with ethidium bromide. The numbers denote the lengths of the digestion products (fragments) in base pairs. **(B)** Restriction endonuclease map derived from the digestions and electrophoretic separation shown in panel A.

is produced by the single EcoRI digestion remains intact after the double digestion, whereas the 8,500- and 5,000-bp EcoRI fragments are cleaved. Therefore, the two EcoRI sites are 3,000 bp apart with no intervening BamHI site, and there is a single BamHI site within each of the 8,500- and 5,000-bp EcoRI fragments. The 9,500-bp fragment that is produced by the single BamHI digestion is cleaved by EcoRI in the double digestion into three pieces (2,500 + 3,000 + 4,000 = 9,500 bp). Therefore, the two BamHI sites lie 2,500 and 4,000 bp to either side of the EcoRI sites. Digestion with BamHI cleaves the 8,500-bp EcoRI fragment into 2,500- and 6,000-bp fragments, and one of the EcoRI sites is 2,500 bp from a BamHI site, so the 6,000-bp region must include one of the ends of the original molecule. Using the same logic, we also note that digestion with BamHI cuts the 5,000-bp EcoRI fragment into 1,000- and 4,000-bp fragments and that one of the EcoRI sites is 4,000 bp from a BamHI site; therefore, the 1,000-bp

TABLE 3.3 DNA fragment sizes (in kilobase pairs) after single and double restriction endonuclease digestions of a plasmid

EcoRI	BamHI	HindIII	HaeII	EcoRI + HaeII	BamHI + HaeII	HindIII + HaeII	EcoRI + HindIII	EcoRI + BamHI	BamHI + HindIII
12.0	12.0	12.0	6.0	5.0	6.0	6.0	6.5	10.5	8.0
			4.0	4.0	4.0	2.5	5.5	1.5	4.0
			2.0	2.0	1.5	2.0			
				1.0	0.5	1.5			

region must include the other end of the original molecule. In the final map (Fig. 3.5B), the assigned locations of the restriction endonuclease sites are consistent with the fragment lengths that were observed in each of the digestion reactions.

The process of formulating a restriction endonuclease map for circular DNA is, in principle, the same as with linear DNA, except that each cleavage produces a fragment. In other words, three pieces are formed when three sites are cut, and so on. With the data in Table 3.3, the deduction of a restriction endonuclease map of a circular plasmid is as follows. The source DNA is a 12-kilobase-pair (kb) circle with single EcoRI, BamHI, and HindIII sites and three HaeII sites. Digestion with EcoRI, BamHI, or HindIII separately produces a single 12-kb fragment, while digestion with HaeII produces three fragments. The results of the EcoRI and HaeII double digestion indicate that the EcoRI site lies within the 6.0-kb HaeII fragment, because the 2.0-kb and 4.0-kb HaeII fragments remain intact and the sum of the two new pieces (5.0 kb + 1.0 kb) is 6.0 kb. Based on the BamHI and HaeII double digestion, the BamHI site lies within the 2.0-kb HaeII region. The BamHI and EcoRI double digestion places these sites 1.5 kb apart; therefore, the 6.0-kb and 2.0-kb HaeII fragments are adjacent. The data do not support any other positions for the BamHI and EcoRI sites. The order of the HaeII segments around the circular molecule is 6.0 kb-4.0 kb-2.0 kb. The same reasoning localizes the HindIII site to the 4.0-kb HaeII fragment, and the results from the BamHI and HindIII and/or EcoRI and HindIII double digestions complete the restriction endonuclease map (Fig. 3.6).

For some restriction endonuclease mapping experiments, the sum of the fragments of some multiple digestions is less than the total length of the starting DNA because the fortuitous locations of some sites produce fragments of the same size. Under these conditions, two different fragments with the same length that migrate to the same location in a gel after electrophoresis often stain more heavily than a band with only one kind of fragment. This difference in staining intensity gives an indication that coincidental fragments have been produced by restriction endonuclease digestion. Generally, computer programs are used to configure restriction endonuclease maps for large DNA molecules with many single and multiple digestions. Also, for very large DNA molecules, specialized electrophoresis systems are used to separate the large number of restriction endonuclease digestion products.

The resolution of fragments for restriction endonuclease mapping can be enhanced by labeling the pieces of DNA, usually at the 5' ends, with a radioactive compound or fluorescent dye and determining their lengths after electrophoretic separation with autoradiography or fluorography, respectively. A common 5'-end-labeling procedure entails dephosphorylation of the 5' ends of a linear DNA molecule with calf intestine alkaline

FIGURE 3.6 Restriction endonuclease map for the digestion products presented in Table 3.3. The circular DNA has 12,000 bp (12 kb). With one of the HaeII sites arbitrarily placed at position 0/12.0 kb, the locations of the other mapped restriction endonuclease sites are marked. The nucleotide positions of the sites are in parentheses.

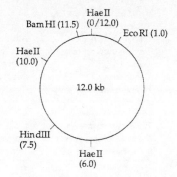

phosphatase and the addition of radiolabeled γ-phosphate from adenosine triphosphate (ATP) to the 5' OH ends by T4 polynucleotide kinase. The labeled DNA fragments are separated from unincorporated label by column chromatography before gel electrophoresis. Parenthetically, recombinant DNA technology requires many different enzymes with various activities. Some of these are listed in Table 3.4.

Restriction endonuclease cleavage is important in molecular cloning for inserting target DNA into a cloning vector. When two different DNA samples are digested with the same restriction endonuclease that produces a staggered cut, i.e., the same 5' or 3' extension or sticky end, and then mixed together, new DNA combinations can be formed as a result of base pairing between the extension (overhang) regions (Fig. 3.7). However, restriction enzymes alone are not sufficient for molecular cloning. First, when the extended ends that are created by restriction enzyme (e.g., BamHI) cleavage are aligned, the hydrogen bonds of the four bases that pair are not strong enough to keep two DNA molecules together. A means of re-forming the internucleotide linkage between the 3' hydroxyl group and the 5' phosphate group in the backbone at the two broken bond sites (nicks) is required. This problem is resolved by using the enzyme DNA ligase, usually from bacteriophage T4. This enzyme catalyzes the formation of phosphodiester bonds at the ends of DNA strands that are already held together by the base pairing of two extensions. DNA ligase also joins blunt ends that come in contact when they both bind to the enzyme (Fig. 3.8). The reaction conditions for DNA ligations depend on whether the DNA molecules have extensions or blunt ends. With protruding ends, the reaction is often carried out at low temperatures for long periods to ensure that the extensions remain base paired. Blunt-end ligations require 10 to 100 times more T4 DNA ligase

TABLE 3.4 Some of the enzymes used for recombinant DNA technology

Enzyme	Activity
Alkaline phosphatase	Removes 5' phosphate groups of DNA molecules; bacterial alkaline phosphatase is more stable but less active than calf intestinal alkaline phosphatase
DNase I	Degrades double-stranded DNA by hydrolyzing internal phosphodiester linkages
E. coli exonuclease III	Sequentially removes nucleotides from 3' OH ends of DNA molecules, except from protruding 3' OH termini
Klenow fragment	Proteolytic product of E. coli DNA polymerase I that has both polymerase and 3' exonuclease activities and no 5' exonuclease activity because fractionation of the digestion products removes the fragment with the 5' exonuclease activity; a Klenow fragment with only DNA polymerase activity due to a mutation in the 3' exonuclease sequence is also available
Mung bean nuclease	Single-stranded DNA and RNA endonuclease
Nuclease BAL 31	Degrades both 3' and 5' ends of DNA without internal cleavages
Poly(A) polymerase	Adds AMP from ATP to the 3' end of mRNA
Reverse transcriptase	Retroviral RNA-directed DNA polymerase
RNase H	Degrades the RNA strand of a DNA–RNA hybrid molecule
S1 nuclease	Degrades single-stranded DNA
T4 polynucleotide kinase	Catalyzes the transfer of the terminal (γ) phosphate from a nucleoside 5' triphosphate to a 5' hydroxyl group of a polynucleotide
T4 DNA polymerase	DNA polymerase and 3' exonuclease activities
T7 DNA polymerase	DNA polymerase and 3' exonuclease activities
Taq DNA polymerase	Heat-stable DNA polymerase from Thermus aquaticus
β-Agarase I	Digests agarose; is used to retrieve separated DNA molecules from agarose gels

FIGURE 3.7 Annealing complementary extensions after staggered cleavage with a type II restriction endonuclease. Two different DNA fragments are cut with the restriction endonuclease BamHI, mixed, and annealed. Not all of the possible combinations of annealed DNAs are shown. The four fragments that are generated by the BamHI digestion can anneal to one another to form any of six different DNA molecules. A break in the phosphodiester bond in one strand of duplex DNA is called a nick. The hydrogen bonds of the four base pairs between nicks on opposite strands are not strong enough to hold DNA molecules together for long periods in solution. A, C, G, and T represent nucleotides.

than do ligations of DNA molecules with extensions and are conducted at room temperature because stable base pairing is not required.

Second, the ability to join different DNA molecules is not by itself useful unless the new DNA combination (i.e., recombinant DNA) can be perpetuated in a host cell. Thus, the ligated construct must contain the biological information for cellular maintenance. This requirement is usually provided on cloning vectors that were developed to overcome this problem.

Third, digestion of the source DNA containing the gene of interest with a restriction endonuclease produces a mixture of DNA molecules, and a number of different DNA constructs are formed after ligation with a cloning vector. Consequently, there has to be a way of identifying the DNA combination in a host cell that contains the target DNA sequence. Screening procedures have been devised to detect host cells carrying a specific cloning vector–DNA insert construct.

Plasmid Cloning Vectors

Plasmids are self-replicating, double-stranded, circular DNA molecules that are maintained in bacteria as independent extrachromosomal entities.

FIGURE 3.8 Mode of action of T4 DNA ligase. The enzyme T4 DNA ligase forms phosphodiester bonds by joining 5' phosphate and 3' hydroxyl groups at nicks in the backbone of double-stranded DNA. **(A)** Ligation of sticky-ended DNA; **(B)** ligation of blunt-ended DNA. A, C, G, and T represent nucleotides.

Virtually all bacterial genera have natural plasmids. Some plasmids carry information for their own transfer from one cell to another (e.g., F plasmids), others encode resistance to antibiotics (R plasmids), others carry specific sets of genes for the utilization of unusual metabolites (degradative plasmids), and some have no apparent functional coding genes (cryptic plasmids). Although they are not typically essential for bacterial cell survival under laboratory conditions, plasmids often carry genes that are advantageous under particular conditions. Plasmids can range in size from less than 1 kb to more than 500 kb. Each plasmid has a sequence that functions as an origin of DNA replication; without this site, it cannot replicate in a host cell.

Some plasmids are represented by 10 to 100 copies per host cell; these are called high-copy-number plasmids. Others maintain one to four copies per cell and are called low-copy-number plasmids. Seldom does the population of plasmids in a bacterium make up more than approximately 0.1 to 5.0% of the total DNA. When two or more different plasmids cannot coexist in the same host cell, they are said to belong to the same incompatibility group, but plasmids from different incompatibility groups can be maintained together in the same cell. This coexistence is independent of the copy numbers of the individual plasmids. Some microorganisms have been found to contain as many as 8 to 10 different plasmids. In these instances, each plasmid can carry out different functions and have its own unique copy number, and each belongs to a different incompatibility group. Some plasmids, because of the specificity of their origin of replication, can replicate in only one species of host cell. Other plasmids have less specific ori-

gins of replication and can replicate in a number of bacterial species. These plasmids are called narrow- and broad-host-range plasmids, respectively.

As autonomous, self-replicating genetic elements, plasmids have the basic attributes to make them potential vectors for carrying cloned DNA. However, naturally occurring (unmodified, or nonengineered) plasmids often lack several important features that are required for a high-quality cloning vector. The more important features are (1) a choice of unique (single) restriction endonuclease recognition sites into which the insert DNA can be cloned and (2) one or more selectable genetic markers for identifying recipient cells that carry the cloning vector–insert DNA construct. In other words, plasmid cloning vectors have to be genetically engineered.

Plasmid Cloning Vector pBR322

In the 1980s, one of the best-studied and most often used "general-purpose" plasmid cloning vectors was pBR322. In general, plasmid cloning vectors are designated by a lowercase p, which stands for plasmid, and some abbreviation that may be descriptive or, as is the case with pBR322, anecdotal. The "BR" of pBR322 recognizes the work of the researchers F. Bolivar and R. Rodriguez, who created the plasmid, and 322 is a numerical designation that has relevance to these workers. Plasmid pBR322 contains 4,361 bp. As shown in Fig. 3.9, pBR322 carries two antibiotic resistance genes. One confers resistance to ampicillin (Ampr), and the other confers resistance to tetracycline (Tetr). This plasmid also has unique BamHI, HindIII, and SalI recognition sites within the Tetr gene; a unique PstI site in the Ampr gene; a unique EcoRI site that is not within any coding DNA; and

MILESTONE

Cleavage of DNA by RI Restriction Endonuclease Generates Cohesive Ends

J. E. MERTZ and R. W. DAVIS
Proc. Natl. Acad. Sci. USA **69**:3370–3374, 1972

Recombinant DNA technology requires a vector to carry cloned DNA, the specific joining of vector and cloned (insert) DNA molecules to form a vector–insert DNA construct, the introduction of the vector–insert DNA construct into a host cell, and the identification of host cells that acquired the cloned DNA. Without type II restriction endonucleases, it would be impossible to do recombinant DNA technology routinely. These enzymes facilitate the development of vectors (see, e.g., Bolivar et al., *Gene* 2:95–113, 1977) and are essential for cloning genes into vectors. In 1968, M. Meselson and R.

Yuan (*Nature* 217:1110–1114) showed that the capability of a strain of *E. coli* to prevent (restrict) the development of a bacterial virus (bacteriophage) was due to a host cell enzyme that cleaved the DNA of the infecting bacteriophage. The study done by Mertz and Davis established that the RI restriction endonuclease from *E. coli*, which is now called EcoRI, cut DNA at a specific site and produced complementary extensions. Briefly, they showed that after circular DNA was linearized by treatment with EcoRI, some of the molecules formed hydrogen-bonded circular DNA molecules, which were converted to cova-

lently closed circular DNA molecules by treating the sample with a DNA ligase. The extensions of all of the cut DNA molecules were the same and were estimated to be 4 to 6 nucleotides long, with the recognition site being six nucleotide pairs. Mertz and Davis concluded that "any two DNA molecules with RI sites can be 'recombined' at their restriction sites by the sequential action of RI endonuclease and DNA ligase to generate hybrid DNA molecules." The discovery that EcoRI created cohesive ends was one of the most important contributions to the development of recombinant DNA technology because it provided, according to Mertz and Davis, a "simple way...to generate specifically oriented recombinant DNA molecules in vitro."

A

B

FIGURE 3.9 Plasmid pBR322. **(A)** Genetic map of the plasmid cloning vector pBR322. Unique HindIII, SalI, BamHI, and PstI recognition sites are present in the Ampr and Tetr genes. The unique EcoRI site is just outside the Tetr gene. The origin of replication functions in the bacterium *E. coli*. The complete DNA sequence of pBR322 consists of 4,361 bp. **(B)** Electron micrograph of plasmid pBR322. Magnification, ×100,000. Source: K. G. Murti. © Visuals Unlimited.

an origin of DNA replication that functions only in *E. coli*, is maintained at a high copy number in *E. coli*, and cannot be readily transferred to other bacteria.

How does pBR322 work as a cloning vector? Purified, closed circular pBR322 molecules are cut with a restriction enzyme that lies within either of the antibiotic resistance genes and cleaves the plasmid DNA only once to create single, linear, sticky-ended DNA molecules. These linear molecules are combined with prepared target DNA from a source organism. This DNA has been cut with the same restriction enzyme, which generates the same sticky ends as those on the plasmid DNA. The DNA mixture is then treated with T4 DNA ligase in the presence of ATP. Under these conditions, a number of different ligated combinations are produced, including the original closed circular plasmid DNA. To reduce the amount of this particular unwanted ligation product, the cleaved plasmid DNA preparation is treated with the enzyme alkaline phosphatase to remove the 5′ phosphate groups from the linearized plasmid DNA. As a consequence, T4 DNA ligase cannot join the ends of the dephosphorylated linear plasmid DNA (Fig. 3.10). However, the two phosphodiester bonds that are formed by T4 DNA ligase after the ligation and circularization of alkaline phosphatase-treated plasmid DNA with restriction endonuclease-digested source DNA, which provides the phosphate groups, are sufficient to hold the two molecules together, despite the presence of two nicks (Fig. 3.10). After transformation, these nicks are sealed by the host cell DNA ligase system. Digested fragments from the source DNA are also joined to each other by T4 DNA ligase. However, these unwanted ligation products do not contain an origin of replication and therefore will not replicate following introduction into a host cell.

Transformation and Selection

The next step in a recombinant DNA experiment requires the uptake of the cloned plasmid DNA by a bacterial cell, usually *E. coli*. The process of introducing purified DNA into a bacterial cell is called transformation, and a cell that is capable of taking up DNA is said to be competent. Competence occurs naturally in many bacteria. In different bacterial species, usually when cell density is high or starvation is impending, a set of proteins is produced that facilitates the uptake of DNA molecules. This phenomenon allows genes to be transferred between different bacteria. A natural transformation process often entails (1) the binding of double-stranded DNA to components of the cell wall; (2) entry of the DNA into an inner compartment (periplasm), where it is protected from enzymes that degrade nucleic acids (nucleases); (3) transmission of one strand into the cytoplasm while the other one is degraded; and (4) if the DNA is a linear molecule, integration into the host chromosome. If the introduced DNA is a plasmid, it is maintained in the cytoplasm after the second strand is synthesized. Competence and transformation are not intrinsic properties of *E. coli*. However, competence can be induced in *E. coli* by various special treatments, such as cold calcium chloride, which in turn enhance the acquisition of DNA by the cell. A brief heat shock facilitates the uptake of exogenous DNA molecules.

Two parameters—transformation frequency and transformation efficiency—are used to assess the success of DNA transformation. The transformation frequency is the ratio of transformed cells to the total number of

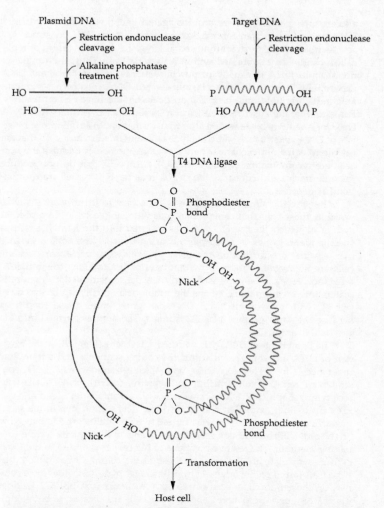

FIGURE 3.10 Cloning foreign DNA into a plasmid vector. After restriction endonuclease cleavage and alkaline phosphatase treatment, the plasmid DNA is ligated to the restriction endonuclease-digested target DNA, and two of the four nicks are sealed. This molecular configuration is stable, and the two DNA molecules are covalently joined. After introduction into a host cell, ensuing replication cycles produce new complete circular DNA molecules with no nicks.

treated cells. The transformation efficiency is the number of transformed cells as a function of the amount of DNA that was originally added to the cells. Generally, transformation is an inefficient process, with typically no more than 1 cell in 1,000 being transformed. After transformation, most of the cells have not acquired a new plasmid. Furthermore, a few cells are transformed by recircularized plasmid DNA that escaped dephosphorylation by

alkaline phosphatase, others acquire ligated and nonligated nonplasmid DNA, and a few are transformed by the plasmid–insert DNA construct.

As noted earlier, extrachromosomal DNA that lacks an origin of replication cannot be maintained within a bacterial cell. Thus, the uptake of nonplasmid DNA is usually of no consequence in a recombinant DNA experiment. To ensure that a plasmid–cloned DNA construct is perpetuated in its original form, the *E. coli* host cells should have certain features. For example, the absence of restriction endonucleases ensures that DNA constructs will not be degraded after transformation. In addition, the integrity of DNA constructs is more likely to be maintained in host cells that are unable to carry out exchanges between DNA molecules because the host cells are recombination negative (RecA⁻). Also, cells that do not produce the endonuclease encoded by the *endA1* gene have increased transformation frequencies.

After the transformation step, it is necessary to identify, as easily as possible, those cells that contain plasmids with cloned DNA. In a pBR322 system in which the target DNA was inserted into the BamHI site, this specific identification is accomplished using the two antibiotic resistance markers that are carried on the plasmid. Following transformation, the cells are incubated in medium without antibiotics to allow the antibiotic resistance genes to be expressed, and then the transformation mixture is plated onto medium that contains the antibiotic ampicillin. Cells that carry pBR322 with or without insert DNA can grow under these conditions because the Ampr gene on pBR322 is intact. The nontransformed cells are sensitive to ampicillin.

The BamHI site of pBR322 is within the Tetr gene (Fig. 3.9), so the insertion of DNA into this gene disrupts the coding sequence and tetracycline resistance is lost. Therefore, cells with these plasmid–cloned DNA constructs are resistant to ampicillin and sensitive to tetracycline. Cells with recircularized pBR322 DNA, however, have an intact Tetr gene and are resistant to both ampicillin and tetracycline. The second step in the selection scheme distinguishes between these two possibilities. Cells that grow on the ampicillin-containing medium are transferred to a tetracycline-containing medium. The relative positions of the cells transferred to the tetracycline–agar plate are the same as those of the colonies from which they were transferred on the original ampicillin–agar plate. Cells that form colonies on the tetracycline–agar plates carry recircularized pBR322 without insert DNA, because as noted above, these cells are resistant to both ampicillin and tetracycline. Those cells that do not grow on the tetracycline–agar plates, however, are sensitive to tetracycline and carry pBR322–cloned DNA constructs (Fig. 3.11).

Individual cultures that are sensitive to tetracycline are established from each of the colonies on the ampicillin–agar plates. Later, additional screening procedures can be conducted to verify that these cells, called transformants, carry the desired pBR322–cloned DNA construct. The HindIII and SalI sites in the tetracycline resistance gene and the PstI site in the ampicillin resistance gene of pBR322 provide alternative potential cloning locations. When the PstI recognition site is used for cloning, the principle of the selection scheme is the same but the antibiotic sensitivities are reversed; thus, the first set of plates contains tetracycline and the second set contains ampicillin.

The pBR322 selection scheme for identifying transformed cells with insert DNA–vector constructs relies on replica plating. This technique,

which can be used in many different ways for various purposes, was originally devised to isolate mutant bacterial colonies that require a supplement for growth, i.e., auxotrophic mutants (Fig. 3.12).

Other Plasmid Cloning Vectors

The plasmid pBR322 was a well-conceived cloning vector. However, it has only a few unique cloning sites, and the selection procedure is time-consuming. Thus, inevitably, other systems were developed. For example, the

FIGURE 3.11 Strategy for selecting host cells that have been transformed with pBR322. (1) The transformation mixture, which contains three cell types, viz., nontransformed cells, cells with the intact original plasmid, and cells with DNA cloned into the BamHI site of pBR322, is plated on complete medium with ampicillin. (2) The mixture is diluted beforehand to ensure separate colonies are formed on the agar. The nontransformed cells (Amps) are killed. The cells with the intact plasmid and cloned DNA–plasmid constructs are Ampr and therefore form colonies. Samples of the surviving colonies on the ampicillin plate are transferred to a plate with complete medium and tetracycline, keeping the same position of each colony on the second plate, i.e., replica plating. Only cells with intact plasmids (Tetr) will form colonies in the presence of tetracycline. (3) The colonies that did not grow on the tetracycline plate (dashed circles) but grew on the ampicillin plate carry pBR322 with DNA that was cloned into the BamHI site. The colonies with cloned DNA inserts are picked from the original plate, pooled, and grown. The red square represents an orientation marker that keeps the master and replica plates aligned.

No plasmid
Amps Tets

Intact plasmid
Ampr Tetr

Cloned plasmid
Ampr Tets

1 | Plate on complete medium with ampicillin

Only Ampr cells survive and grow

2 | Replica plate on complete medium with tetracycline

3 | Pick, pool, and grow cells from Ampr Tets colonies

Only Tetr cells survive and grow

Cells with pBR322-cloned DNA inserts

A

Orientation marker — Handle
— Disk
— Velveteen

B

FIGURE 3.12 Screening bacterial colonies for mutant strains by replica plating. **(A)** Replica-plating (colony transfer) device; **(B)** replica-plating technique. Cells from each separated colony on a master plate (1) adhere to the velveteen of the replica-plating device after it is gently pressed against the agar surface (2). The adhering cells are transferred (3), in succession, to a petri plate with complete medium (4) and to one with selective medium (5). The pattern of the colonies is consistent among the replicated plates because the orientation markers (red squares) are aligned for each transfer. In this example, minimal medium is the selective medium used to identify colonies that require a nutritional supplement for growth, i.e., auxotrophic mutants. The missing colony (dashed circle) on the minimal medium (5) denotes an auxotrophic mutation. The equivalent location on the plate with complete medium (4) has the colony with the auxotrophic mutation that can be picked and grown (6). Further analysis of the isolated strain is necessary to determine the nature of the auxotrophic mutation.

plasmid pUC19 is 2,686 bp long and contains an Amp^r gene; a segment of the β-galactosidase gene *(lacZ')* of the lactose operon of *E. coli* under the control of the regulatable *lac* promoter; a *lacI* gene that produces a repressor protein that regulates the expression of the *lacZ'* gene from the *lac* promoter; a short DNA sequence with many unique cloning sites (e.g., EcoRI, SacI, KpnI, XmaI, SmaI, BamHI, XbaI, SalI, HincII, AccI, BspMI, PstI, SphI, and HindIII), which is called a multiple cloning site (multiple cloning

sequence, multicloning site, or polylinker); and the origin of DNA replication from pBR322 (Fig. 3.13).

The pUC19 selection procedure has the following rationale. When cells carrying unmodified pUC19 are grown in the presence of isopropyl-β-D-thiogalactopyranoside (IPTG), which is an inducer of the *lac* operon, the protein product of the *lacI* gene can no longer bind to the promoter–operator region of the *lacZ'* gene, so the *lacZ'* gene in the plasmid is transcribed and translated. The LacZ' protein combines with a protein (LacZα) that is encoded by chromosomal DNA to form an active hybrid β-galactosidase. In pUC19, the multiple cloning site is incorporated into the *lacZ'* gene in the plasmid without interfering with the production of the functional hybrid β-galactosidase. Finally, if the substrate 5-bromo-4-chloro-3-indolyl-β-D-galactopyranoside (X-Gal) is present in the medium, it is hydrolyzed by this hybrid β-galactosidase to a blue product. Under these conditions, colonies containing unmodified pUC19 appear blue.

For a pUC19 cloning experiment, DNA from a source organism is cut with one of the restriction endonucleases for which there is a recognition site in the multiple cloning site (Fig. 3.14). This source DNA is mixed with pUC19 plasmid DNA that has been treated with the same restriction endonuclease and then with alkaline phosphatase. After ligation with T4 DNA ligase, the reaction mixture is introduced by transformation into a host cell which can synthesize that part of β-galactosidase (LacZα) that combines with the product of the *lacZ'* gene to form a functional enzyme. The treated host cells are plated onto medium that contains ampicillin, IPTG, and X-Gal.

Nontransformed cells cannot grow in the presence of ampicillin. Cells with recircularized plasmids can grow with ampicillin in the medium, and because they can form functional β-galactosidase, they produce blue colonies. In contrast, host cells that carry a plasmid–cloned DNA construct produce white colonies on the same medium. The reason for this is that, usually, DNA inserted into a restriction endonuclease site within the multiple cloning site disrupts the correct sequence of DNA codons (reading frame) of the *lacZ'* gene and prevents the production of a functional LacZ' protein, so no active hybrid β-galactosidase is produced (Fig. 3.14). In the

FIGURE 3.13 Genetic map of the plasmid cloning vector pUC19. The multiple cloning site contains unique sites for the restriction endonucleases that are used for the insertion of cloned DNA. The plasmid contains an Ampr gene, an origin of replication that functions in *E. coli*, and the *lacI* gene, which produces a repressor that blocks the transcription of the *lacZ'* gene in the absence of the inducer IPTG. The complete DNA sequence of pUC19 is 2,686 bp long.

FIGURE 3.14 Plasmid pUC19 multiple cloning site. The multiple cloning site (upper-case nucleotides) is inserted into the *lacZ'* gene (lowercase nucleotides). Some of the unique restriction endonuclease sites of the multiple cloning site are named and demarcated by horizontal lines. The double arrows mark the *lacZ'*–multiple cloning site DNA sequence that encodes the first 26 amino acids of the hybrid LacZ' protein. Insertion of DNA into any of the unique restriction endonuclease sites of the multiple cloning site changes the reading frame of the *lacZ'* gene and prevents the correct translation of the LacZ' protein.

absence of β-galactosidase activity, the X-Gal in the medium is not converted to the blue compound, so these colonies remain white. The white (positive) colonies subsequently must be screened to identify those that carry a specific target DNA sequence.

In addition to ampicillin and tetracycline, other antibiotics are used as selective agents in various cloning vectors (Table 3.5). Moreover, a number of inventive selection systems have been devised to identify cells with insert–vector constructs. For example, a vector that is derived from the pUC series carries a gene that, when expressed, encodes a protein that kills the cell (suicide protein). This cell-killing gene is fused in the correct reading frame to the *lacZ'* gene so that it is transcribed from the regulatable *lacZ'* gene promoter. A cell with an intact plasmid and no IPTG in the medium does not synthesize the suicide protein. Cells with a plasmid and no insert, in the presence of IPTG, synthesize the suicide protein and are killed. With an insert and IPTG, a nonfunctional suicide protein is produced because the insert, in all likelihood, disrupts the reading frame of the suicide gene. Nontransformed cells are sensitive to an antibiotic, whereas transformed cells have as part of the vector a gene that confers resistance to the antibiotic. In other words, in this case, the only surviving cells in the presence of IPTG and antibiotic are those that carry a plasmid with a DNA insert.

Although a number of vectors have ingenious designs, in principle they all retain the two basic requirements of recombinant DNA technology. There is both a choice of cloning sites and an easy way of identifying cells with plasmid–cloned DNA constructs. It should be noted that unique restriction endonuclease sites have a dual function in recombinant DNA research. They are required for inserting DNA into a cloning vector, and they allow an inserted DNA sequence to be recovered from the vector. In other words, after a piece of DNA has been cloned into a plasmid that was cut with the same restriction endonuclease, it can be retrieved by cutting the purified plasmid–cloned DNA construct with that restriction endonuclease because the insertion event recreates the recognition site at each end of the cloned DNA sequence. A recovered DNA fragment can be cloned into specialized cloning vectors for DNA sequencing or vectors that have been specifically

designed to achieve high levels of expression (transcription and translation) of the cloned gene. In fact, thousands of vectors have been developed for a variety of purposes and for many different organisms.

Even though *E. coli,* which is well-known as a laboratory organism, is used for all routine molecular-cloning procedures, other bacteria, such as *Bacillus subtilis* and *Agrobacterium tumefaciens,* often act as the final host cells. For many applications, cloning vectors that function in *E. coli* may be provided with a second origin of replication that enables the plasmid to replicate in the alternative host cell. With these shuttle cloning vectors, the initial cloning steps are conducted with *E. coli* before the fully developed construct is introduced into a different host cell. In addition, a number of plasmid vectors have been constructed with a single broad-host-range origin of DNA replication instead of a narrow-host-range origin of replication. These vectors can be used with a variety of microorganisms.

Shuttle vectors have some drawbacks. The addition of a segment of DNA containing the second origin of replication increases the size of the vector and reduces the amount of DNA that can be inserted, and in some instances, shuttle vectors are not efficiently propagated in the host cell. Also, broad-host-range cloning vectors can be unstable and can be lost from a preferred host cell. To overcome these limitations, a system was devised for cloning a DNA insert into an *E. coli*-based plasmid and then combining the part of the plasmid that carries both the cloned DNA and an antibiotic resistance gene with a part of a host cell-specific plasmid carrying its own origin of replication. The first step in the creation of this shuttle vector requires engineering two different recognition sites for the restriction endonuclease SfiI. The sequence of this site is $\frac{\text{GGCCNNNNNGGCC}}{\text{CCGGNNNNNCCGG}}$, where N represents any base pair (Fig. 3.15A). Two different SfiI sites (SfiI$_x$ and SfiI$_y$) are designed to have different variable sequences so that after digestion with SfiI, the extensions of the SfiI$_x$ site are not complementary to those of the SfiI$_y$ site (Fig. 3.15B). Next, the two SfiI sequences are inserted into both the *E. coli*-based and host cell-specific plasmids so that they flank the region containing the antibiotic resistance gene and the cloning site on the *E. coli*-based plasmid (Fig. 3.16A) and the origin of replication on the host cell-specific plasmid (Fig. 3.16B). After a DNA sequence is cloned into the *E. coli*-based plasmid and the construct is grown in *E. coli,* the *E. coli*-based and host cell-specific plasmids are purified separately, mixed, and digested with SfiI. The SfiI$_x$–SfiI$_x$ and SfiI$_y$–SfiI$_y$ extensions base pair, and after ligation, several different "chimeric" circular DNA molecules are formed. The

TABLE 3.5 Some antibiotics commonly used as selective agents

Antibiotic (abbreviations)	Description
Ampicillin (Ap, Amp)	Inhibits cell wall formation; inactivated by β-lactamase
Hygromycin B (HygB)	Blocks translocation from amino acyl site to peptidyl site; inactivated by a phosphotransferase
Kanamycin (Km, Kan)	Binds to 30S subunit and prevents translocation from aminoacyl-tRNA site to peptidyl site; inactivated by a phosphotransferase
Neomycin (Nm, Neo)	Binds to 30S subunit and inhibits protein synthesis; inactivated by a phosphotransferase
Streptomycin (Sm, Str)	Blocks protein initiation complex formation and causes misreading during translation; inactivated by a phosphotransferase
Tetracycline (Tc, Tet)	Prevents binding of aminoacyl-tRNA to 30S ribosomal subunit; resistance gene encodes an inner cell membrane protein that passes the antibiotic out of the cell and blocks the passage of the antibiotic through the cell wall

A

B

SfiI$_x$

FIGURE 3.15 **(A)** SfiI recognition site. The arrows mark the cleavage sites, and $\frac{N}{N}$ represents any base pair. **(B)** The SfiI$_x$ and SfiI$_y$ recognition sites are designed so that after digestion with the restriction endonuclease SfiI, the SfiI$_x$ extensions will not base pair with the SfiI$_y$ extensions. The nucleotide differences between the SfiI$_x$ (red) and SfiI$_y$ (orange) recognition sites are noted.

mixture is transformed into the host cell and selected on medium containing an antibiotic, i.e., chloramphenicol. Cells without any plasmid and those with plasmids without the chloramphenicol resistance gene cannot grow in the presence of chloramphenicol. Also, plasmids that do not carry an origin of replication or that carry the origin of replication from the *E. coli*-based plasmid are not replicated in the host cell and therefore are not maintained. Only cells transformed with a chimeric plasmid that carries the part of the *E. coli*-based plasmid with the chloramphenicol resistance gene and the cloned gene joined to the fragment of the host cell-specific plasmid that contains the origin of replication that functions in the host cell are resistant to chloramphenicol and, consequently, can grow (Fig. 3.16C). The "SfiI$_x$–SfiI$_y$" procedure, which can be adapted for any host cell that has a plasmid, is called vector backbone exchange.

Creating and Screening a Library

Making a Genomic Library

One of the fundamental objectives of molecular biotechnology is the isolation of genes that encode proteins for industrial, agricultural, and medical applications. In prokaryotic organisms, structural genes form a continuous coding domain in the genomic DNA, whereas in eukaryotes, the coding regions (exons) of structural genes are separated by noncoding regions (introns). Consequently, different cloning strategies have to be used for cloning prokaryotic and eukaryotic genes.

In a prokaryote, the desired sequence (target DNA, or gene of interest) is typically a minuscule portion (about 0.02%) of the total chromosomal DNA. The problem, then, is how to clone and select the targeted DNA sequence. To do this, the complete DNA of an organism, i.e., the genome, is cut with a restriction endonuclease, and each fragment is inserted into a vector. Then, the specific clone that carries the target DNA sequence must be identified, isolated, and characterized. The process of subdividing genomic DNA into clonable elements and inserting them into host cells is called creating a library (clone bank, gene bank, or genomic library). A complete library, by definition, contains all of the genomic DNA of the source organism.

One way to create a genomic library is to first treat the DNA from a source organism with a four-cutter restriction endonuclease, e.g., Sau3AI, which theoretically cleaves the DNA approximately once in every 256 bp. The conditions of the digestion reaction are set to give a partial, not a complete, digestion. In this way, all possible fragment sizes are generated (Fig. 3.17). Partial digestions are carried out with a low concentration of restriction endonuclease or shortened incubation times. The fragments become smaller as the reaction period is extended (Fig. 3.18). To ensure that the entire genome, or most of it, is contained within the clones of a library, the sum of the inserted DNA in the clones of the library should be three or more times the amount of DNA in the genome. For example, if a genome has 4×10^6 bp and the average size of an insert is 1,000 bp, then 12,000 clones are required for threefold coverage, i.e., $3[(4 \times 10^6)/10^3]$. For the human genome (3.3×10^9 bp), about 80,000 bacterial artificial chromosome (BAC) clones that have an average insert size of 150,000 bp compose a library with fourfold coverage, i.e., $4[(3.3 \times 10^9)/(15 \times 10^4)]$. From a statistical perspective, the relationship $N = \ln(1 - P)/\ln(1 - f)$ (where N is the number of clones, P is the probability of finding a specific gene, and f is the ratio of the length of the

FIGURE 3.16 Vector backbone exchange. Shown are an *E. coli*-based plasmid with a cloned DNA sequence, a chloramphenicol resistance gene (Cmr), and an *E. coli*-specific origin of replication (*ori*E) **(A)** and a host cell-specific plasmid with a host-specific origin of replication (*ori*H) and an erythromycin resistance gene (Eryr) **(B)** that have each been engineered with SfiI$_x$ and SfiI$_y$ recognition sites. Treatment of the plasmids shown in panels A and B with SfiI generates two fragments from each plasmid with SfiI$_x$ and SfiI$_y$ extensions. Several different circular chimeric DNA molecules are formed after base pairing between complementary extensions and ligation (not shown). **(C)** After transformation of the mixture of chimeric DNA molecules into the host cell, only cells carrying a chimeric plasmid that has an origin of replication that functions in the host cell, as well as the cloned DNA sequence and the chloramphenicol resistance gene from the *E. coli*-based plasmid, will be selected on medium containing chloramphenicol.

average insert to the size of the entire genome) provides an estimate of the number of clones that is necessary for a comprehensive genomic library. On this basis, about 700,000 clones are required for a 99% chance of discovering a particular sequence in a human genomic library with an average insert size of 20 kb. Finally, because restriction endonuclease sites are not randomly located, some fragments may be too large to be cloned. When this occurs, it may be difficult or even impossible to find a specific target DNA sequence because the library is incomplete. This problem can be overcome by forming libraries with different restriction endonucleases. Clearly, the

FIGURE 3.17 Partial digestion of a fragment of DNA with a type II restriction endo-nuclease. Partial digestions are usually performed by varying either the length of time or the amount of enzyme used for the digestion. In some of the DNA molecules, the restriction endonuclease has cut at all sites (each labeled RE1). In other molecules, fewer cleavages have occurred. The desired outcome is a sample with DNA molecules of all possible lengths.

number of clones in a genomic library depends on the extent of the coverage, the size of the genome of the organism (Table 3.6), and the average size of the insert in the vector.

After a library is created, the clone(s) with the target sequence must be identified. Four popular methods of identification are used: DNA hybridization with a labeled DNA probe followed by radiographic screening for the probe label, immunological screening for the protein product, assaying for protein activity, and functional (genetic) complementation.

Screening by DNA Hybridization

The presence of a target nucleotide sequence in a DNA sample can be determined with a DNA probe. This procedure, called DNA hybridization, depends on the formation of stable base pairs between the probe and the target sequence. DNA hybridization is feasible because naturally occurring double-stranded DNA can be converted into single-stranded DNA by heat or alkali treatment. Heating DNA breaks the hydrogen bonds that hold the

FIGURE 3.18 Effect of increasing the time of restriction endonuclease digestion of a DNA sample. **(A)** The restriction endonuclease sites (arrows) of a DNA molecule are shown. **(B)** As the duration of restriction endonuclease treatment is extended, cleavage occurs at an increased number of sites (lanes 1 to 5). Lane 1 represents the size of the DNA molecule at the time of addition of restriction endonuclease. Lanes 2 to 5 depict the extents of DNA cleavage after increasing exposures to restriction endonuclease.

TABLE 3.6 DNA contents of various organisms

Organism	Genome size (millions of base pairs)
Mycoplasma genitalium	0.58
Methanococcus jannaschii	1.66
Haemophilus influenzae Rd	1.83
Neisseria meningitidis	2.27
Lactococcus lactis	2.36
Mycobacterium leprae	3.26
Vibrio cholerae	4.00
B. subtilis	4.20
E. coli K-12	4.60
E. coli O157:H7	5.50
Pseudomonas aeruginosa	6.30
Mesorhizobium loti	7.59
Saccharomyces cerevisiae	13
Caenorhabditis elegans	97
Arabidopsis thaliana	125
Drosophila melanogaster	165
Fugu rubripes	400
Solanum tuberosum	840
Zea mays	2,700
Mus musculus	3,000
Homo sapiens	3,300
Hordeum vulgare	5,500
Triticum aestivum	17,300

1 Prepare target DNA

ATCGTAGTCGTAGGTCGGTTAGCTTGAACC TTTCCCCAAAAGGGGGCCCCCTTTTAAAA
TAGCATCAGCATCCAGCCAATCGAACTTGG AAAGGGGTTTTCCCCCGGGGGAAAATTTT

 Extract
 ─── Denature ───
 Immobilize

ATCGTAGTCGTAGGTCGGTTAGCTTGAACC TTTCCCCAAAAGGGGGCCCCCTTTTAAAA

 TAGCATCAGCATCCAGCCAATCGAACTTGG AAAGGGGTTTTCCCCCGGGGGAAAATTTT

2 Prepare probe DNA

TAGGTCGG
ATCCAGCC

 Label
 Denature

TAGGTCGG*

 ATCCAGCC*

3 Hybridization

 ATCCAGCC*
 ATCGTAGTCGTAGGTCGGTTAGCTTGAACC TTTCCCCAAAAGGGGGCCCCCTTTTAAAA

 TAGGTCGG*
 TAGCATCAGCATCCAGCCAATCGAACTTGG AAAGGGGTTTTCCCCCGGGGGAAAATTTT

FIGURE 3.19 DNA hybridization. (1) The DNA of samples containing the putative
target DNA is denatured, and the single strands are kept apart, usually by binding
them to a solid support, such as a nitrocellulose or nylon membrane. (2) The probe,
which is often 100 to 1,000 bp in length, is labeled, denatured, and mixed with the
denatured putative target DNA under hybridization conditions. (3) After the
hybridization reaction, the membrane is washed to remove nonhybridized probe
DNA and assayed for the presence of any hybridized labeled tag. If the probe does
not hybridize, no label is detected. The asterisks denote the labeled tags (signal) of
the probe DNA.

bases together (denaturation) but does not affect the phosphodiester bonds
of the DNA backbone. If the heated solution is rapidly cooled, the strands
remain single stranded. However, if the temperature of a heated DNA solu-
tion is lowered slowly, the double-stranded, helical conformation of DNA
can be reestablished because of the base pairing of complementary nucle-
otides (renaturation). The process of heating and slowly cooling double-
stranded DNA is called annealing. When DNA fragments from different
sources with some shared (homologous) sequences are mixed, heated to
100°C, and slowly cooled, there will be some hybrid DNA molecules
among the annealed products, that is, double-stranded DNA in which the
strands come from the different sources.

In general, for a DNA hybridization assay, the target DNA is denatured
and the single strands are irreversibly bound to a matrix, e.g., nitrocellulose
or nylon. Then, the single strands of a DNA probe, which are labeled with
either a radioisotope or another tagging system, are incubated with the

bound DNA sample. If the sequence of nucleotides in the DNA probe is complementary to a nucleotide sequence in the sample, then base pairing, i.e., hybridization, occurs (Fig. 3.19). The hybridization can be detected by autoradiography (Box 3.2) or other visualization procedures depending on the nature of the probe label. If the nucleotide sequence of the probe does not base pair with a DNA sequence in the sample, then no hybridization occurs and the assay gives a negative result. Generally, probes range in length from 100 to more than 1,000 bp, although both larger and smaller probes can be used. Depending on the conditions of the hybridization reaction, stable base pairing requires a match of >80% within a segment of 50 bases.

DNA probes can be labeled in various ways. One strategy, which is called the random-primer method, utilizes a mixture of synthetic random oligonucleotides (oligomers) containing all possible combinations of sequences of 6 nucleotides (hexamers) that act as primers for DNA synthesis. On the basis of the chance occurrence of complementary sequences, some of the oligomers in the sample will hybridize to complementary sequences on the unlabeled probe DNA template (Fig. 3.20). After the oligomer sample is mixed with the denatured probe template DNA, the four deoxyribonucleotides (deoxyribonucleoside triphosphates [dNTPs]) and a portion of *E. coli* DNA polymerase I called the Klenow fragment are added. The dNTPs are deoxyadenosine triphosphate (dATP), deoxyribosylthymine triphosphate (dTTP), deoxyguanosine triphosphate (dGTP), and

BOX 3.2

Autoradiography

Autoradiography is used to detect the location of a radiolabeled entity in a cell or sample of fractionated macromolecules. In principle, autoradiography consists of placing a radioactive source next to a radiosensitive photographic film that contains silver bromide. The energy from the decay of the radioisotope hits the photographic emulsion and produces electrons that are trapped by specks of silver bromide crystals in the emulsion. The negatively charged specks attract silver ions, and metallic silver is formed. The grains of metallic silver are visualized by developing the photographic film. Thus, an exposed dark region on a developed film indicates that the underlying material was radiolabeled. Parenthetically, fluorography is the term used for the exposure of light-sensitive photographic film to molecules that directly or indirectly generate light as the source of energy that reduces silver in the photographic emulsion.

Proteins and nucleic acids that are radiolabeled and separated by gel electrophoresis can be visualized by placing an X-ray film on a dried gel and developing the film after a suitable exposure time. All autoradiographic steps are carried out in the dark to avoid inadvertent exposure of the X-ray film to light. A number of autoradiographic techniques have been devised for the quantitative and qualitative analysis of proteins and nucleic acids.

One of the major applications of autoradiography is the detection of the hybridization of a radiolabeled DNA probe to a DNA molecule that has been electrophoretically fractionated. However, DNA molecules in a gel are not accessible to hybridization with a DNA probe. Consequently, the DNA molecules in the gel are transferred by blotting or electrotransfer to a nitrocellulose or nylon membrane. The transfer process retains the same positions on the membrane as the DNA molecules had in the gel. The DNA molecules that are transferred to

a membrane are denatured, bound to the membrane, and hybridized with a radiolabeled DNA probe. Autoradiography of the membrane reveals whether the probe hybridized to a particular DNA band(s).

The transfer of DNA from a gel to a membrane is called Southern blotting (Southern DNA blotting) after Edwin Southern, who devised the original DNA blotting strategy. Northern blotting and Western blotting are methods for the transfer of RNA and protein, respectively, from a gel to a membrane. The terms "Northern" and "Western" have nothing to do with direction and were coined by molecular biologists both to give Edwin Southern further credit for developing the notion of blotting macromolecules from a gel to a membrane and to distinguish the macromolecules that are transferred. The designations "Northern" and "Western" are also examples of molecular biology humor.

FIGURE 3.20 Production of labeled probe DNA by the random-primer method. The duplex DNA containing the sequence that is to act as the probe is denatured, and an oligonucleotide sample containing all possible sequences of 6 nucleotides is added. It is a statistical certainty that some of the molecules of the oligonucleotide mixture will hybridize to the unlabeled, denatured probe DNA. In the presence of Klenow fragment and the four dNTPs, one of which is labeled with a tag (*), the base-paired oligonucleotides act as primers for DNA synthesis. The synthesized DNA is labeled and used as a probe to detect the presence of a DNA sequence in a DNA sample. In this case, the labeled probe consists of a number of separate DNA molecules that together constitute almost the entire sequence of the original unlabeled template DNA.

deoxycytidine triphosphate (dCTP). The Klenow fragment retains both DNA polymerase and 3' exonuclease activities but lacks the 5' exonuclease activity that is normally associated with *E. coli* DNA polymerase I (Fig. 3.21). The 3' exonuclease is retained because it reduces the misincorporation of erroneous dNTPs during the synthesis of the new DNA strand; however, 5' exonuclease activity is abolished because it would degrade some of the newly synthesized DNA. With the available 3' hydroxyl groups provided by the base-paired random primers and the strands of the probe as templates, new DNA synthesis occurs (Fig. 3.20). If a radioactive label is used, then one of the dNTPs contains the isotope ^{32}P in the α-position phosphate. Autoradiography is used to determine whether the labeled probe sequences hybridize to sequences of a target DNA sample. Often today, the deoxyribonucleotides, including the labeled dNTP, are incorporated into the probe sequence using the polymerase chain reaction (PCR), generating high yields of labeled probe DNA (see chapter 4).

For nonisotopic detection of hybridization, biotin can be attached to one of the four dNTPs that are incorporated during the DNA synthesis step. When a biotin-labeled probe hybridizes to the sample DNA, detection

FIGURE 3.21 Schematic representation of the enzymatic activities of *E. coli* DNA polymerase I. **(A)** The polymerase (red) adds deoxyribonucleotides to the 3' hydroxyl groups of the growing chains. **(B)** The 5' exonuclease (blue) removes successive nucleotides from 5' phosphate ends. **(C)** The 3' exonuclease (yellow) removes successive nucleotides from 3' hydroxyl ends.

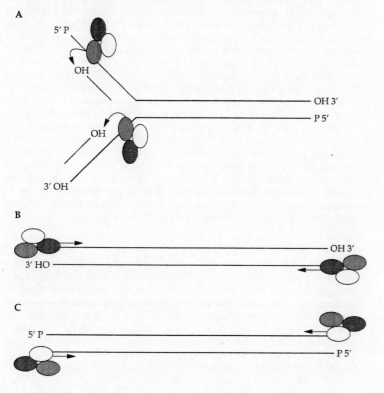

is based on the binding of an intermediary compound (e.g., streptavidin) to biotin (see chapter 9). The intermediary compound carries an appropriate enzyme that, depending on the assay system, may either form a chromogenic (colored) molecule that can be visualized directly or produce a chemiluminescent response that can be detected by autoradiography.

There are at least two possible sources of probes for screening a genomic library. First, cloned DNA from a closely related organism (a heterologous probe) can be used. In this case, the conditions of the hybridization reaction can be adjusted to permit considerable mismatch between the probe and the target DNA to compensate for the natural differences between the two sequences. Second, a probe can be produced by chemical synthesis. The nucleotide sequence of a synthetic probe is based on the probable nucleotide sequence that is deduced from the known amino acid sequence of the protein encoded by the target gene.

Genomic libraries are often screened by plating out the transformed cells on the growth medium of a master plate and then transferring samples of each colony to a solid matrix, such as a nitrocellulose or nylon membrane. The cells on the membrane are broken open (lysed), the protein is removed, and the DNA is bound to the membrane. At this stage, a labeled probe is added, and if hybridization occurs, signals are observed on an autoradiograph. The colonies from the master plate that correspond to samples containing hybridized DNA are then isolated and cultured (Fig. 3.22). Because most libraries are created from partial digestions of genomic DNA, a number of colonies may give a positive response to the probe. The next task is to determine which clone, if any, contains the complete sequence of the target gene. Preliminary analyses that use the results of gel electrophoresis and restriction endonuclease mapping reveal the length of each insert and identify those inserts that are the same and those that share overlapping sequences. If an insert in any one of the clones is large enough to include the full gene, then the complete gene can be recognized after DNA sequencing because it will have start and stop codons and a contiguous set of nucleotides that code for the target protein. Alternatively, a gene can be assembled by using overlapping sequences from different clones.

Unfortunately, there is no guarantee that the complete sequence of a target gene will be present in a particular library. If the search for an intact gene fails, then another library can be created with a different restriction endonuclease and screened with either the original probe or probes derived from the first library. On the other hand, as discussed below, libraries that contain DNA fragments larger than the average prokaryotic gene can be created with specialized vectors to increase the chance that some members of the library will carry a complete version of the target gene.

Screening by Immunological Assay

Alternative methods are used to screen a library when a DNA probe is not available. For example, if a cloned DNA sequence is transcribed and translated, the presence of the protein, or even part of it, can be determined by an immunological assay. Technically, this procedure has much in common with a DNA hybridization assay. All the clones of the library are grown on several master plates. A sample of each colony is transferred to a known position on a matrix, where the cells are lysed and the released proteins are attached to the matrix. The matrix with the bound proteins is treated with an antibody (primary antibody) that specifically binds to the protein

FIGURE 3.22 Screening a library with a labeled DNA probe (colony hybridization). Cells from the transformation reaction are plated onto solid agar medium under conditions that permit transformed, but not nontransformed, cells to grow. (1) From each discrete colony formed on the master plate, a sample is transferred to a solid matrix, such as a nitrocellulose or nylon membrane. The pattern of the colonies on the master plate is retained on the matrix. (2) The cells on the matrix are lysed, and the released DNA is denatured, deproteinized, and irreversibly bound to the matrix. (3) A labeled DNA probe is added to the matrix under hybridization conditions. After the nonhybridized probe molecules are washed away, the matrix is processed by autoradiography to determine which cells have bound labeled DNA. (4) A colony on the master plate that corresponds to the region of positive response on the X-ray film is identified. Cells from the positive colony on the master plate are subcultured because they may carry the desired plasmid–cloned DNA construct.

encoded by the target gene. Following the interaction of the primary antibody with the target protein (antigen), any unbound antibody is washed away, and the matrix is treated with a second antibody (secondary antibody) that is specific for the primary antibody. In many assay systems, the secondary antibody has an enzyme, such as alkaline phosphatase, attached to it. After the matrix is washed, a colorless substrate is added. If the secondary antibody has bound to the primary antibody, the colorless substrate is hydrolyzed by the attached enzyme and produces a colored compound that accumulates at the site of the reaction (Fig. 3.23).

The colonies on the master plate that correspond to positive results (colored spots) on the matrix contain either an intact gene or a portion of the gene that is large enough to produce a protein product that is recog-

nized by the primary antibody. After detection by immunoassay of genomic DNA libraries, the positive clones must be characterized to determine which, if any, carry a complete gene.

Screening by Protein Activity

DNA hybridization and immunological assays work well for many kinds of genes and gene products. If the target gene produces an enzyme that is not normally made by the host cell, a direct (in situ) plate assay can be

FIGURE 3.23 Immunological screening of a gene library (colony immunoassay). Cells from the transformation reaction are plated onto solid agar medium under conditions that permit transformed, but not nontransformed, cells to grow. (1) From the discrete colonies formed on this master plate, a sample from each colony is transferred to a solid matrix, such as a nitrocellulose or nylon membrane. (2) The cells on the matrix are lysed, and their proteins are bound to the matrix. (3) The matrix is treated with a primary antibody that binds only to the target protein. (4) Unbound primary antibody is washed away, and the matrix is treated with a secondary antibody that binds only to the primary antibody. (5) Any unbound secondary antibody is washed away, and a colorimetric reaction is carried out. The reaction can occur only if the secondary antibody, which is attached to an enzyme (E) that performs the reaction, is present. (6) A colony on the master plate that corresponds to a positive response on the matrix is identified. Cells from the positive colony on the master plate are subcultured because they may carry the plasmid–insert DNA construct that encodes the protein that binds the primary antibody.

devised to identify members of a library that carry the particular gene encoding that enzyme. The genes for α-amylase, endoglucanase, β-glucosidase, and many other enzymes from various organisms have been isolated in this way. This approach has proven effective for isolating genes encoding biotechnologically useful enzymes from microorganisms present in environmental samples. Most of the organisms contained in these samples cannot be grown in the laboratory, outside of their natural environment. However, the total genomic DNA from these organisms can be extracted directly from the sample, for example, a soil sample, and used to prepare a metagenomic library that can be expressed in a host bacterium, such as *E. coli*, and screened for target protein activity. This technique has enabled the isolation of many novel proteins with interesting properties without the need to first culture the natural host microorganism.

In some cases, the cells of a genomic library are plated onto medium supplemented with a specific substrate; if the substrate is hydrolyzed, a colorimetric reaction identifies the colony that carries the target gene (Fig. 3.24). For example, to detect a cloned bacterial lipase gene, transformed cells are grown in the presence of trioleoglycerol and the fluorescent dye rhodamine B. As a result of hydrolysis of the substrate, positive colonies have orange fluorescent halos when viewed under ultraviolet light. Other detection systems do not rely on a colorimetric reaction for discovering a particular gene. For example, a transformed cell with a conjugated bile acid hydrolase gene from *Lactobacillus plantarum* was detected by growing the members of the genomic library in the presence of bile salts. In this case, a hydrolase-positive colony was easily identified because it became surrounded with a ring of precipitated, free bile acids.

Functional (genetic) complementation is another useful way of isolating genes that encode enzymes. In this procedure, the host cell does not have the enzyme activity of interest because the gene encoding the enzyme carries a mutation that abolishes the activity of the enzyme. Next, a DNA library is constructed that carries fragments of genomic DNA from an organism that has the desired enzyme activity. Host cells with the genetic deficiency are transformed with plasmids of the DNA library, and transformed cells that have restored normal enzyme function are selected (Fig. 3.25). The genomic DNA that is used to prepare the library can be from a variety of donor organisms, such as the wild-type strain of the host bacterium that carries a functional copy of the gene encoding the enzyme, a different organism that can be either another prokaryote or perhaps a eukaryote, or uncultured organisms that are present in an environmental sample. *E. coli* and yeast cells with mutations that affect various biochemical pathways have frequently been used as host cells for functional complementation gene cloning. In many of these experiments, the protein derived from the cloned gene enables the host cell to grow on minimal medium; whereas growth of the mutant cells requires the addition of a specific compound to the medium. Furthermore, genes that play a role in antibiotic biosynthesis, root nodulation, and other processes have been isolated in this way.

In practice, the availability of genomic sequences from a great number of organisms, in which the protein coding regions have been identified and in many cases assigned a known or predicted function, has rendered library screening unnecessary for some applications. Where the nucleotide sequence of a gene of interest is known, the gene can be cloned by designing short oligonucleotide primers that bind specifically to complementary sequences

Colony expressing functional enzyme from cloned gene produces a colored product

Medium containing substrate for enzyme

FIGURE 3.24 Screening a genomic library for enzyme activity. Cells of a genomic library are plated onto solid medium containing the substrate for the enzyme of interest. If a functional enzyme is produced by a colony that carries a cloned gene encoding the enzyme, the substrate is converted to a colored product that can be easily detected. Note that other, noncolored colonies on the medium also contain fragments of the genomic library, but they do not carry the gene for the enzyme of interest.

FIGURE 3.25 Gene cloning by functional complementation. Host cells that are defective in a certain function, e.g., A−, are transformed with plasmids from a genomic library derived from cells that are normal with respect to function A, i.e., A+. Only transformed cells that carry a cloned gene that confers the A+ function will grow on minimal medium. The cells that show complementation are isolated, and the insert of the vector is studied to characterize the gene that corrects the defect in the mutant host cells.

within the target gene in a sample of genomic DNA and from which DNA synthesis can be initiated in a reaction known as the PCR (see chapter 4).

Cloning DNA Sequences That Encode Eukaryotic Proteins

Special strategies are required for cloning and expressing eukaryotic coding regions in prokaryotic cells. Basically, a eukaryotic structural gene will not function in a prokaryotic organism because there is no mechanism for removing introns from transcribed RNA. Moreover, a eukaryotic DNA sequence needs prokaryotic transcriptional and translational control sequences to be properly expressed. Parenthetically, a cloned prokaryotic

gene also has the same constraint unless the insert carries regulatory sequences that are compatible with the transcription and translation systems of the host cell. For eukaryotic genes, the "intron problem" is overcome by synthesizing double-stranded DNA copies (complementary DNA [cDNA]) of purified messenger RNA (mRNA) molecules that lack introns and cloning the cDNA molecules into a vector to create a cDNA library. Often, a cDNA library represents the mRNA sequences from a single specific tissue.

Functional eukaryotic mRNA does not have introns because they have been removed by the splicing machinery of the eukaryotic cell. The mRNA has a G cap at the 5' end and, usually, a string of up to 200 adenine residues [poly(A) tail] at the 3' end. The poly(A) tail provides the means for separating the mRNA fraction of a tissue from the more abundant ribosomal RNA (rRNA) and transfer RNA (tRNA). Short chains of 15 thymidine residues (oligodeoxythymidylic acid [oligo(dT), or dT_{15}]) are attached to cellulose beads, and the oligo(dT)–cellulose beads are packed into a column. Total RNA extracted from eukaryotic cells or tissues is passed through the oligo(dT)–cellulose column, and the poly(A) tails of the mRNA molecules bind by base pairing to the oligo(dT) chains. The tRNA and rRNA molecules, which lack poly(A) tails, pass through the column. The mRNA is removed (eluted) from the column by treatment with a buffer that breaks the A:T hydrogen bonds, thereby releasing the base-paired mRNAs (Fig. 3.26).

Before the mRNA molecules can be cloned into a vector, they must be converted to double-stranded DNA. This synthesis is accomplished by using, in succession, two different kinds of nucleic acid polymerases. Reverse transcriptase synthesizes the first DNA strand, and *E. coli* DNA polymerase I synthesizes the second (Fig. 3.27). After the mRNA fraction is purified, short unattached sequences of oligo(dT) molecules are added to the sample, along with the enzyme reverse transcriptase and the four dNTPs. An oligo(dT) molecule base pairs with the adenine residues of the poly(A) tail of an mRNA and provides an available 3' hydroxyl group to prime the synthesis of the first cDNA strand.

Reverse transcriptase, which is encoded by certain RNA viruses (retroviruses), uses an RNA strand as a template while directing deoxyribonucleotides into the growing chain. Thus, when an A, G, C, or U nucleotide of the template RNA strand is encountered, the complementary deoxyribonucleotide (i.e., T, C, G, or A) is incorporated into the growing DNA strand. Unfortunately, full-length first cDNA strands are not always produced by reverse transcriptase in vitro. Incomplete first DNA strands are due to the inability of reverse transcriptase to proceed to the ends of long mRNA templates, frequent pausing of the enzyme during synthesis, and intrastrand base-paired configurations (secondary structure) impeding synthesis.

The second, complementary DNA strands are generated by treating the RNA–DNA (heteroduplex) molecules with ribonuclease H (RNase H), which nicks the mRNA strands, thereby providing a free 3' hydroxyl group for initiation of DNA synthesis. As synthesis of the second strand progresses from the nicks, the 5' exonuclease activity of DNA polymerase I removes any nucleotides that are encountered. The eventual length of the second strand depends on the length of the first DNA strand and the location of the nick in the mRNA molecule relative to the 3' end of the first DNA strand. The synthesis of second strands is often initiated several nucleotides from the 5' end of the mRNA. However, obtaining some full-length cDNAs for cloning is usually not a problem because most eukaryotic mRNAs have

FIGURE 3.26 Schematic representation of oligo(dT)–cellulose separation of polyade-nylated mRNA from total cellular RNA.

noncoding leader sequences that range from 40 to 80 nucleotides in length and precede the coding sequence. In other words, a few of the cDNAs will have a complete protein coding sequence and a truncated leader sequence. After the second DNA strand synthesis is terminated, the ends of the cDNA molecules are blunt-ended (end repaired, or polished) with T4 DNA polymerase, which removes 3′ extensions and fills in from 3′ recessed ends. Chemically synthesized adaptors with extensions for a restriction endonuclease recognition sequence are ligated to the ends of the cDNA molecules to facilitate cloning of the cDNAs into a vector (Fig. 3.27).

A cDNA library is screened by DNA hybridization to identify clones that carry a specific plasmid–cDNA construct. Positive clones must be examined further to determine which one(s) carries the complete coding sequence for the target protein. Once a full-length cDNA is discovered, the sequence can be retrieved and cloned into a vector that is designed to support its expression in a prokaryotic cell.

As noted above, the standard cDNA synthesis protocols produce both complete (full-length) and incomplete molecules. Unfortunately, much time and effort can be spent on identifying clones of a cDNA library with full-length sequences. Various strategies have been devised to overcome

A

B

FIGURE 3.27 Synthesis of cDNA. **(A)** Oligo(dT) primer is added to a purified mRNA preparation, and reverse transcriptase with the four dNTPs is used for the production of a complementary (cDNA) strand from the RNA template. Reverse transcriptase does not always produce full-length cDNA copies from every mRNA template due to mRNA secondary structure, i.e., hairpin loops or other factors. For second-strand DNA synthesis, the mRNA is nicked by RNase H, which creates initiation sites for *E. coli* DNA polymerase I. The 5′ exonuclease activity of DNA polymerase I removes both RNA and DNA sequences that are encountered as synthesis from the nick closest to the 5′ end of the mRNA progresses. **(B)** The cDNA molecules are end repaired with T4 DNA polymerase, and adaptors containing restriction enzyme recognition sequences are ligated to the ends to increase the efficiency of cloning.

this inconvenience. A method for generating full-length cDNA molecules that is based on PCR is presented in chapter 4. Here, a multistep procedure for capturing full-length first-strand cDNAs that are used as templates for the synthesis of second strands is described (Fig. 3.28). Briefly, the primer for first-strand DNA synthesis is a polydeoxythymidylic acid [poly(dT)] sequence at the 3' end of a synthetic nucleic acid sequence that also contains a recognition site for a restriction endonuclease. This dual-function oligonucleotide is called a primer–adaptor. The disaccharide trehalose is added to the reverse transcriptase reaction to stabilize the enzyme and allow DNA synthesis to proceed at a high temperature. Secondary structure (due to intrastrand base pairing) in the mRNAs is disrupted by high temperature, and the likelihood that complete molecules will be synthesized is increased. In addition, one of the four dNTPs in the reverse transcriptase reaction mixture is 5-methyl-dCTP, which is incorporated into the growing strand. The presence of methyl groups in one strand (hemimethylation) of double-stranded DNA protects the DNA from being cleaved by certain restriction endonucleases. This DNA modification is important for the final step of the procedure.

After the first strand is synthesized, biotin is chemically attached to the ribose sugars of the cap nucleotide at the 5' end and the nucleotide at the 3' end of the mRNA molecules. Deoxyribose is not biotinylated under these conditions. Next, the hybrid RNA–DNA molecules are treated with RNase I. This enzyme cleaves single-stranded RNA; it does not attack RNA that is base paired with DNA or DNA strands. As a result, both the 5' single-stranded regions of the mRNAs with incomplete cDNAs and the nonpaired segments of the poly(A) tails of the mRNA molecules are degraded. The mRNA strands of completely synthesized cDNA strands are not affected by this enzyme. The sample is then mixed with streptavidin-coated magnetic beads. Biotin has a high affinity for streptavidin. After RNase I treatment, the only biotinylated RNA–DNA hybrid molecules that remain are those with a biotinylated cap. In other words, only full-length cDNAs are captured because the 5' end of the mRNA is base paired with the cDNA and is therefore protected from cleavage by RNase I, leaving the biotin molecule attached. A magnet is used to separate out the beads from solution. Next, the RNA of the streptavidin-bound RNA–DNA hybrids is hydrolyzed with RNase H, which cuts base-paired RNA and releases the full-length cDNA strands into solution.

Since the sequences at the 3' ends of the first-strand cDNAs are not known, a string of guanine nucleotides is added to the 3' hydroxyl ends to provide a complementary sequence for a DNA primer that initiates the synthesis of second cDNA strands. The addition of the guanine nucleotides is performed by the enzyme terminal deoxynucleotidyl transferase, which adds dNTPs sequentially by phosphodiester bond formation to the 3' hydroxyl end of a polynucleotide in the absence of a template strand. If only one type of dNTP is present in the terminal transferase reaction mixture, in this case dGTP, a homopolymeric tail is formed. After polydeoxyguanylic acid [poly(dG)] tailing, a polydeoxycytidylic acid [poly(dC)] primer–adaptor is added that base pairs with the poly(dG) tail and provides an available 3' hydroxyl group for second-strand cDNA synthesis. The adaptor portion of this oligonucleotide contains the sequence for another restriction endonuclease site. Second-strand cDNA synthesis is carried out at high temperatures with thermostabilized DNA polymerase, RNase H, and DNA ligase. As with the synthesis of the first cDNA strand,

FIGURE 3.28 Schematic representation of a method for selecting and cloning full-length cDNA molecules. (1) Purified mRNA (blue) is mixed with an oligonucleotide (primer–adaptor) with an oligo(dT) sequence and restriction endonuclease site (yellow). (2) Reverse transcriptase synthesizes the first cDNA strand (red) with 5-methyl-dCTP (red boxes) as one of the four dNTPs. Both incomplete and complete DNA strands are synthesized. (3) Biotin (light-blue boxes labeled B) is attached to the ends of mRNA molecules. RNase I-susceptible regions are marked by square brackets. (4) Single-stranded segments of RNA are degraded by RNase I. (5) Biotinylated molecules bind to streptavidin-coated magnetic beads (pink). After RNase I treatment, full-length RNA–DNA hybrids are biotinylated, and therefore, they bind to streptavidin. Incomplete cDNAs are not biotinylated and do not bind to streptavidin. (6) RNase H treatment degrades the RNA of streptavidin-bound RNA–DNA hybrids and releases full-length, first-strand cDNA molecules. (7) A poly(dG) tail is added to the 3′ hydroxyl end of the first cDNA strand. (8) An oligonucleotide (primer–adaptor) with an oligodeoxycytidylic acid [oligo(dC)] sequence and a restriction endonuclease site (green) pairs with the oligodeoxyguanylic acid [oligo(dG)] tail and provides a 3′ hydroxyl group for synthesis of the second DNA strand by DNA polymerase. (9) During the synthesis of the second cDNA strand by DNA polymerase, none of the dNTPs are methylated; RNase H removes any remaining base-paired RNA, and DNA ligase joins DNA segments that were synthesized internally from bits of mRNA that escaped degradation. The oligo(dC) primer–adaptor sequence acts as a template for DNA synthesis from the 3′ hydroxyl group at the end of the poly(dG) tail. (10) The final full-length cDNAs are cut with two restriction endonucleases, one for each end, and cloned into a vector that has complementary extensions. Hemimethylation protects the cDNA from cleavage by the restriction endonucleases that are used for cloning because these enzymes cannot cut methylated restriction endonuclease sites.

the high temperature diminishes intrastrand folding and increases the efficiency of synthesis of a full-length strand. The dCTP in the dNTP mixture used for second-strand synthesis is not methylated. RNase H removes any RNA that escaped the previous treatment, and DNA ligase joins segments that were primed by remaining bits of RNA. The final product is a full-length, double-stranded cDNA that is furnished with nonmethylated restriction endonuclease recognition sites at both ends. These sites are cleaved with the appropriate restriction endonucleases and cloned into a vector that has complementary extensions. Hemimethylation, generated by incorporation of methylated nucleotides during the synthesis of the first cDNA strand, protects a cDNA from cleavage if it contains the same restriction endonuclease sites that are used for cloning because the restriction endonucleases do not cut at methylated sites.

Vectors for Cloning Large Pieces of DNA

Bacteriophage λ Vectors

The plasmid-based vectors used for cloning DNA molecules generally carry up to 10 kb of inserted DNA. However, for the formation of a library, it is often helpful to be able to maintain larger pieces of DNA. To this end, various high-capacity cloning systems have been developed (Table 3.7). The *E. coli* virus (bacteriophage, or phage) λ has been engineered to be a vector for inserts in the range of 15 to 20 kb.

After bacteriophage λ infects *E. coli* by injection of its DNA, two possibilities exist. It can enter a lytic cycle that, after 20 minutes, leads to the lysis of the host cell and the release of about 100 phage particles. Alternatively, the injected bacteriophage λ DNA can be integrated into the *E. coli* chromosome as a prophage and can be maintained more or less indefinitely as a benign guest (lysogen) through successive cell divisions (Fig. 3.29). However, under conditions of nutritional or environmental stress, the chromosomally integrated bacteriophage λ DNA is excised and enters a lytic cycle. The bacteriophage λ DNA is about 50 kb in length, of which approximately 20 kb is essential for the integration–excision (I/E) events. For forming genomic libraries, it was reasoned that this 20 kb of DNA could be replaced with 20 kb of cloned DNA and, subsequently, this recombined DNA molecule could be perpetuated as a "recombinant" bacteriophage λ through compulsory lytic cycles.

To appreciate how bacteriophage λ cloning systems function, some understanding of the molecular aspects of the lytic cycle is necessary. An

TABLE 3.7 Insert capacities of some commonly used vector systems

Vector system	Host cell	Insert capacity (kb)
Plasmid	*E. coli*	0.1–10
Bacteriophage λ	λ/*E. coli*	10–20
Cosmid	*E. coli*	35–45
Fosmid	*E. coli*	35–45
Bacteriophage P1	*E. coli*	80–100
BAC	*E. coli*	50–300
P1 bacteriophage-derived artificial chromosome	*E. coli*	100–300
Yeast artificial chromosome	Yeast	100–2,000
Human artificial chromosome	Cultured human cells	>2,000

FIGURE 3.29 Life cycle of bacteriophage λ. Lysogeny occurs when the bacteriophage λ genome (red) becomes integrated into the host chromosome (blue); otherwise, the lytic cycle is initiated, resulting in the production and release by cell lysis of about 100 bacteriophage particles about 20 minutes after infection.

infective bacteriophage λ consists of a tubular protein tail with a protein tail fiber and a protein head packed with 50 kb of DNA. The production and assembly of the heads and tails and the packaging of DNA are a highly coordinated sequence of events. The DNA within the head of a λ particle is a 50-kb linear molecule with a 12-base single-stranded extension at the 5′ end of each strand. These extensions are called cohesive (cos) ends because they contain sequences that are complementary to each other. After the injection of the λ DNA through the tail into *E. coli*, the cos ends base pair to form a circular DNA molecule. During the early phase of the lytic cycle, DNA replication from the circular molecule creates a linear form of λ DNA that is composed of several contiguous lengths of 50-kb units, i.e., concatemers (Fig. 3.30A). Each newly assembled head is filled with one 50-kb unit of DNA, and finally, the tail assembly is added to complete the formation of an infective particle (Fig. 3.30B). The volume of the bacteriophage λ head is sufficient for about 50 kb. If less than 38 kb of DNA is packed into a head,

a noninfective bacteriophage particle is produced. More than 52 kb of DNA cannot fit into a head. The location of the cos sequences, which are 50 kb apart in the multiple-length linear λ DNA, ensures that each head receives the correct amount of DNA. Located at the opening of the head is an enzyme that recognizes the double-stranded cos sequence and cuts the DNA at this site as the DNA is inserted into the head. By mixing purified empty heads, bacteriophage λ DNA (50 kb), and tail assemblies, infective particles are produced in a reaction tube.

One of the many bacteriophage λ cloning vectors that have been devised has two BamHI sites that flank the I/E region. When purified DNA from this bacteriophage is cut with BamHI, three segments are created. The left arm (L region) contains the genetic information for the production of heads and tails, the right arm (R region) carries the genes for DNA replication and cell lysis, and the middle (I/E) fragment has the genes for the integration and excision processes. The objective of this genetic-engineering

FIGURE 3.30 Packaging of bacteriophage λ DNA into heads during the lytic cycle. (A) DNA replication from the circular form of bacteriophage λ creates a linear form that has contiguous, multiple lengths (concatemers) of bacteriophage DNA with units of approximately 50 kb each. (B) Each newly assembled head is filled with a 50-kb unit of λ DNA before the tail assembly is attached.

A

B

protocol is to replace the middle, I/E, segment of the λ DNA with cloned DNA that is approximately 20 kb in length (Fig. 3.31). The BamHI-treated bacteriophage λ DNA sample is enriched for L and R arms by size fractionation and removal of I/E segments. The source DNA is cut with either BamHI or Sau3AI, and DNA pieces that are 15 to 20 kb in length are isolated. The digested source DNA and the L and R regions are combined and incubated with T4 DNA ligase. Then, empty bacteriophage heads and tail assemblies are added. Under these conditions, 50-kb units of DNA, with insert DNA flanked by L and R regions with cos ends, are packaged into the heads, and infective bacteriophage particles are formed. Other products from the ligation reaction cannot be packaged because they are either too large (>52 kb) or too small (<38 kb). Also, any 50-kb DNA molecules without a functional origin of replication and cos ends cannot be perpetuated. Recombinant bacteriophage λ undergoes lytic cycles and is maintained by growth in *E. coli*.

To identify the recombinant bacteriophage that carries the target gene in the bacteriophage λ library, the individual zones of lysis (plaques), each

FIGURE 3.31 A bacteriophage λ cloning system. Bacteriophage λ is engineered to have two BamHI sites that flank the I/E region. For cloning, the source DNA is cut with BamHI and fractionated by size to isolate pieces that are about 15 to 20 kb long. The bacteriophage λ DNA is also cut with BamHI, and size fractionation removes the I/E segment. The L and R arms, plus the 15- to 20-kb source DNA molecules, are mixed with T4 DNA ligase. The ligation reaction produces a number of different DNA molecules, including ligated source DNA only, combined L and R arms only, and molecules that have a source DNA molecule flanked by L and R arms. The last molecules are packaged into bacteriophage heads in vitro, and infective particles are formed after the addition of tail assemblies. The recombined bacteriophage λ is perpetuated by infection of *E. coli*. Some 50-kb source DNA ligation products may be packaged into heads, but since this DNA lacks both a functional origin of replication and cos ends, it cannot be perpetuated. Other ligation products are either too small or too large to be packaged. For some bacteriophage λ cloning systems (not shown here), high packaging efficiency is achieved by setting the conditions of ligation to favor concatemer formation to imitate how the phage heads are normally filled.

of which contains a recombinant bacteriophage, are lifted onto a matrix and screened with either DNA probes or antibodies. For DNA hybridization, the bacteriophage proteins are removed and the DNA is denatured and bound to a matrix. For immunological assays, the proteins encoded by cloned genes that are synthesized during the lytic cycle, along with bacteriophage and bacterial proteins, are transferred with the plaque and subsequently bound to the matrix. On the basis of the sites on the matrix that give positive responses, corresponding plaques on the original plate are subcultured to provide a source of selected recombinant bacteriophage that is individually cultured in *E. coli*.

Cosmids

Cloning vectors called cosmids can carry about 45 kb of cloned DNA and are maintained as plasmids in *E. coli*. Cosmids combine the properties of plasmids and bacteriophage λ vectors. For example, the commonly used cosmid pLFR-5 has two cos sites (cos ends) from bacteriophage λ flanking a ScaI restriction endonuclease site, a multiple cloning site with six unique recognition sites (HindIII, PstI, SalI, BamHI, SmaI, and EcoRI), an origin of DNA replication, and a Tet^r gene (Fig. 3.32). Pieces of DNA that are approximately 45 kb in length are purified by sucrose density gradient centrifugation from a partial BamHI digestion of the source DNA (Fig. 3.32). The pLFR-5 DNA (~6 kb) is cleaved initially with ScaI and then with BamHI. The final two DNA samples are mixed and ligated. Some of the ligated products have an ~45-kb DNA piece inserted between the two fragments that are derived from the digestions of the pLFR-5 DNA. These molecules are about 50 kb long and have cos sequences that are about 50 kb apart. Consequently, these DNA constructs are successfully packaged into bacteriophage λ heads in vitro. Reconstituted pLFR-5 without inserted DNA is not packaged. After the assembly of bacteriophage particles, the DNA is delivered by infection into *E. coli* (Fig. 3.32). Once inside the host cell, the cos ends, which were cleaved during the in vitro packaging, base pair and enable the linear DNA to circularize. This circular form is stable, and the cloned DNA is maintained as a plasmid–insert DNA construct because the vector DNA contains a complete set of plasmid functions. Moreover, the Tet^r gene allows colonies that carry the cosmid to grow in the presence of tetracycline. Nontransformed cells are sensitive to tetracycline and die.

A fosmid is a kind of cosmid vector that carries up to 40 kb of insert DNA and a cos site for in vitro bacteriophage λ packaging. The difference between a cosmid and a fosmid is that the origin of replication of a fosmid is derived from the *E. coli* F factor (sex plasmid), hence the name. The advantage of fosmids is that they are very stable single-copy vectors, whereas cosmids are maintained at higher copy numbers, which often leads to deletions or rearrangements of parts of the insert DNA.

Other *E. coli* bacteriophages have been used for creating vectors. For example, the genome of the P1 bacteriophage is 115 kb long. The P1 vector system can carry 80 to 100 kb of inserted DNA. The advantages of using cosmids and other vectors derived from bacteriophages are twofold. First, because the capacity of these vectors is greater than that of plasmids, gene clusters and large genes can be cloned. Second, a larger insert in the cloning vehicle means that fewer clones of a genomic library have to be screened for a specific gene.

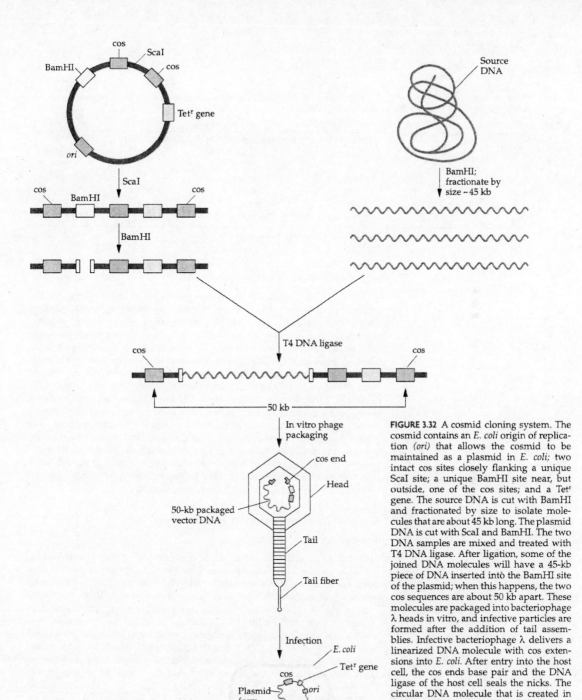

FIGURE 3.32 A cosmid cloning system. The cosmid contains an *E. coli* origin of replication *(ori)* that allows the cosmid to be maintained as a plasmid in *E. coli;* two intact cos sites closely flanking a unique ScaI site; a unique BamHI site near, but outside, one of the cos sites; and a Tet[r] gene. The source DNA is cut with BamHI and fractionated by size to isolate molecules that are about 45 kb long. The plasmid DNA is cut with ScaI and BamHI. The two DNA samples are mixed and treated with T4 DNA ligase. After ligation, some of the joined DNA molecules will have a 45-kb piece of DNA inserted into the BamHI site of the plasmid; when this happens, the two cos sequences are about 50 kb apart. These molecules are packaged into bacteriophage λ heads in vitro, and infective particles are formed after the addition of tail assemblies. Infective bacteriophage λ delivers a linearized DNA molecule with cos extensions into *E. coli.* After entry into the host cell, the cos ends base pair and the DNA ligase of the host cell seals the nicks. The circular DNA molecule that is created in this way persists as a plasmid in the host cell. In this case, transformed cells can be identified because they are resistant to the antibiotic tetracycline.

TABLE 3.8 Estimated numbers of clones required for 99% probability of representation of every DNA region in a genomic library for various organisms and cloning vectors

Organism	Genome size (bp)	No. of clones			
		pBR322 (5 kb)	Bacteriophage λ (17 kb)	Cosmid (35 kb)	BAC (150 kb)
E. coli	4.6×10^6	4,234	1,243	602	138
Yeast	1.23×10^7	11,326	3,329	1,616	375
Fruit fly	1.2×10^8	110,529	32,501	15,787	3,681
Rice	5.7×10^8	525,589	154,521	75,009	17,497
Human	3.3×10^9	3,090,475	898,392	434,053	101,258
Frog	2.3×10^{10}	19,315,480	6,438,493	2,971,610	708,822

For the cloning vectors, the sizes in parentheses are the average sizes of the insert DNA.

High-Capacity Bacterial Vector Systems

A vector system that carries very large inserts (>100 kb) is helpful for the analysis of complex eukaryotic genomes. For example, these types of vector systems are indispensable for creating libraries for genome sequencing and for carrying one or more intact genes on a single insert. In contrast to a small-insert library, a large-insert genomic library is more likely to include all of the genetic material of the organism with fewer clones to maintain (Table 3.8). A low-copy-number E. coli plasmid vector that is based on the P1 bacteriophage cloning system has been devised for cloning DNA molecules that are from 100 to 300 kb in length. The DNA insert–vector constructs of this system are called bacteriophage P1-derived artificial chromosomes. Similarly, the F plasmid (F-factor replicon, sex plasmid, or fertility plasmid) of E. coli, which is present at one or two copies per cell, has been used, along with the lacZ' selection system of the pUC vectors, to construct an extremely stable cloning vector that carries DNA inserts from 50 to 300 kb in length. The F-plasmid-based DNA insert–vector constructs, which are used extensively, are called BACs.

Genetic Transformation of Prokaryotes

Transferring DNA into E. coli

Transformation is the process of introducing free DNA into a bacterial cell. For E. coli, which is the main host cell for recombinant DNA research, the uptake of plasmid DNA is usually achieved by treating mid-log-phase cells with ice-cold calcium chloride ($CaCl_2$) and then exposing them for 2 minutes to a high temperature (42°C). This treatment creates transient openings in the cell wall that enable DNA molecules to enter the cytoplasm. This method has a maximum transformation frequency of about 1 transformed cell per 1,000 cells (i.e., 10^{-3}). The transformation efficiency is approximately 10^7 to 10^8 transformed colonies per microgram of intact plasmid DNA. Although a 100% transformation frequency would be ideal, selection schemes that enable plasmid-transformed cells to be readily identified overcome the drawback of a low transformation frequency. In some other bacteria, competence occurs naturally and, in some cases, can be enhanced by the use of specific growth media or growth conditions. These bacteria are usually easily transformed. Other DNA delivery systems must be used for bacteria that are either refractory to chemically induced competence or are not naturally competent.

Electroporation

The uptake of free DNA can be induced by subjecting bacteria to a high-voltage electric field in the presence of DNA. This procedure is called electroporation, a term that is a contraction of the descriptive phrase "electric-field-mediated membrane permeabilization." The experimental protocols for electroporation are different for various bacterial species. For *E. coli*, the cells (~50 microliters) and DNA are placed in a chamber fitted with electrodes (Fig. 3.33A), and a single pulse of approximately 25 microfarads, 2.5 kilovolts, and 200 ohms is administered for about 4.6 milliseconds. This treatment yields transformation efficiencies of 10^9 transformants per microgram of DNA for small plasmids (~3 kb) and 10^6 for large plasmids (~136 kb). Similar conditions are used to introduce BAC vector DNA into *E. coli*. Thus, electroporation is an effective way to transform *E. coli* with plasmids containing inserts that are longer than 100 kb. Because an appropriate set of electroporation conditions can be found for nearly all bacterial species, this procedure has become standard for transforming many different types of bacteria.

Very little is known about the mechanism of DNA uptake during electroporation (Fig. 3.33B). It has been deduced, along the lines of the explanation of chemically induced transformation, that transient pores are formed in the cell wall as a result of the electroshock and that, after contact with the lipid bilayer of the cell membrane, the DNA is taken into the cell.

FIGURE 3.33 Electroporation. **(A)** Electroporation cuvette with a cell suspension between two electrodes. **(B)** (1) Cells (yellow) and DNA (red) in suspension in an electroporation cuvette prior to the administration of high-voltage electric field (HVEF) pulses. (2) HVEF pulses induce openings in the cells (dashed lines) that allow entry of DNA into the cells. (3) After HVEF pulsing, some cells acquire exogenous DNA, and the HVEF-induced openings are resealed.

Conjugation

For some bacteria, the natural system of transmitting plasmids from one strain to another has been used to transport a plasmid–insert DNA construct from a donor cell to a recipient cell that is not readily transformed. Some plasmids are genetically equipped to form cell-to-cell junctions through which plasmid DNA is transferred from one cell to another. Effective contact between a donor cell and a recipient cell depends on plasmid genes that encode conjugative functions. Moreover, the mechanical transfer of the DNA requires plasmid genes that encode mobilizing functions. Most of the plasmids that are used for recombinant DNA research lack conjugative functions, and therefore, they are not passed to recipient cells by conjugation. However, some nonconjugative plasmid cloning vectors can be mobilized and transferred if the conjugative functions are supplied by a second plasmid in the same cell. In other words, by introducing a plasmid with conjugative functions into a bacterial cell that carries a mobilizable plasmid cloning vector, it is possible to transfer the plasmid cloning vector to a recipient cell that is difficult to transform by other means.

The typical experimental protocol for this procedure entails mixing three strains together. When the cells are close to each other, the conjugative plasmid, which in this case is also mobilizable, can be self-transferred to the cell with the mobilizable plasmid cloning vector. Then, with the help of the conjugative plasmid, the plasmid cloning vector is transferred to a targeted recipient cell. All possible combinations of plasmid transfer occur among the

FIGURE 3.34 Tripartite mating. A helper cell self-transfers a conjugative, mobilizing plasmid with a Tetr gene to a donor cell. The plasmid from the helper cell provides conjugative functions for the nonconjugative, mobilizable plasmid of the donor cell, which carries a kanamycin resistance (Kanr) gene and enables transport of the latter plasmid into the recipient cell. Unlike the recipient cells, neither helper nor donor cells can grow on minimal medium, and they are resistant to kanamycin and sensitive to tetracycline. The selection strategy identifies cells that are able to grow on minimal medium. In this example, the cloning vector is transferred from *E. coli* to *P. putida*. Although it is not shown, each plasmid has an origin of replication. The plasmid from the donor cell replicates in the recipient cell.

E. coli	*E. coli*	*P. putida*
Tetr gene	Tetr gene	
	Kanr gene	Kanr gene
Helper	**Donor**	**Recipient**
Conjugative, mobilizable plasmid	Mobilizable plasmid	Transferred plasmid
No growth on minimal medium	No growth on minimal medium	Grows on minimal medium

cells, but the genetic features of the strains and plasmids are designed to select for the targeted recipient cells that receive the cloning vector. For example, one possible selection procedure uses a helper cell *(E. coli)* that maintains a conjugative, mobilizable plasmid with a Tet^r gene and cannot grow on minimal growth medium; a donor cell *(E. coli)* that also cannot grow on minimal growth medium and carries the nonconjugative, mobilizable plasmid cloning vector that has a kanamycin resistance gene; and a recipient cell *(Pseudomonas putida)* that can grow on minimal growth medium, has no incompatible plasmid, and is sensitive to both tetracycline and kanamycin (Fig. 3.34). After the conjugations are allowed to occur, the cells are grown briefly in complete growth medium in the absence of antibiotics before being transferred to minimal growth medium with kanamycin. Under the latter growth conditions, only the targeted recipient cells that have acquired the plasmid cloning vector can grow. Neither helper nor donor cells can grow on minimal medium, and the recipient cells that did not receive a plasmid from a donor cell cannot grow in the presence of kanamycin. Occasionally, the targeted recipient cell may receive both types of plasmids. However, this rare event can be detected by replica plating onto minimal medium with both tetracycline and kanamycin. Colonies that are formed in the presence of both antibiotics acquire two different plasmids, and those that grow only when kanamycin is present have the cloning vector. Since the transfer of plasmid DNA requires conjugation among three bacterial strains, the process has been designated tripartite mating.

SUMMARY

Recombinant DNA technology comprises a battery of experimental procedures that are used for inserting DNA segments from one organism into a vector, often a bacterial plasmid, and perpetuating the insert DNA–vector DNA combination in a host cell. Large amounts of the insert (cloned) DNA can be retrieved when required. The process would not be possible without type II restriction endonucleases that cleave DNA molecules reproducibly into fragments of discrete sizes. These enzymes bind to specific sequences within a DNA molecule and symmetrically cut phosphodiester bonds of each strand at the recognition site. In addition, many other enzymes, such as T4 DNA ligase and DNA polymerase, are important for cloning genes.

A representative gene-cloning experiment has a number of steps. (1) DNA is isolated from an organism that contains the target gene and is cut with a restriction endonuclease. (2) A DNA cloning vector is cut with the same restriction endonuclease used to digest the source DNA. The cloning vector has only one of these restriction endonuclease sites. (3) The two DNA samples are mixed with T4 DNA ligase, and various combinations of DNA molecules, including vector DNA and DNA from the source organism, are generated by the enzymatic formation of phosphodiester bonds at the ends of DNA strands. (4) Host cells, usually *E. coli*, are transformed with DNA molecules from the ligase reaction, which produces some cells that carry vector–insert DNA constructs. Because the vector has a DNA sequence (origin of replication) that enables it to be replicated in the host cell, the entire construct is perpetuated. Uptake of DNA by *E. coli* is facilitated by

CaCl₂–heat shock treatment, electroporation, or other means. Conjugative and mobilization functions of plasmids are used in some cases to transfer a plasmid–gene construct to a bacterium that is not readily transformed.

Finally, selection schemes are available for identifying cells with vector–insert DNA constructs. Transformed cells are distinguished from nontransformed cells by testing for resistance to specific antibiotics or by observing specifically colored colonies. Cells with a specific cloned target gene are identified by DNA hybridization with a homologous or heterologous probe, by immunological determination of an encoded recombinant protein, by the presence of a specified enzyme activity, or by functional (genetic) complementation. The probability of cloning a complete gene is increased by partially digesting the source DNA with a restriction endonuclease and forming a library of clones consisting of overlapping sequences of an entire genome. Vectors based on bacteriophage λ, bacteriophage P1, P1-derived plasmid (P1 artificial chromosome), and the F plasmid (BAC) have been developed for carrying large pieces of DNA and constructing genomic libraries from both prokaryotic and eukaryotic organisms.

To obtain DNA segments that encode eukaryotic proteins, purified mRNA is used as a template for the enzyme reverse transcriptase to synthesize a cDNA strand; in turn, this strand acts as a template for DNA polymerase to produce a second cDNA strand. After enzymatic treatment, the double-stranded cDNA can be cloned into a vector. Multistep strategies have been devised to increase the likelihood that only full-length cDNA molecules are synthesized and cloned.

REFERENCES

Ammiraju, J. S., M. Luo, J. L. Goicoechea, W. Wang, D. Kudrna, C. Mueller, J. Talag, H. Kim, N. B. Sisneros, B. Blackmon, E. Fang, J. B. Tomkins, D. Brar, D. MacKill, S. McCouch, N. Kurata, G. Lambert, D. W. Galbraith, K. Arumuganathan, K. Rao, J. G. Walling, N. Gill, Y. Yu, P. SanMiguel, C. Soderlund, S. Jackson, and R. A. Wing. 2006. The *Oryza* bacterial artificial chromosome library resource: construction and analysis of 12 deep-coverage large-insert BAC libraries that represent the 10 genome types of the genus *Oryza*. *Genome Res.* 16:140–147.

Bayer, E. A., and M. Wilchek. 1990. Protein biotinylation. *Methods Enzymol.* 184:138–160.

Berger, S. L., and A. R. Kimmel (ed.). 1987. *Methods in Enzymology*, vol. 152. *Guide to Molecular Cloning Techniques*. Academic Press, London, United Kingdom.

Bolivar, F., R. L. Rodriguez, P. J. Greene, M. C. Betlach, H. L. Heyneker, and H. W. Boyer. 1977. Construction and characterization of new cloning vehicles. II. A multipurpose cloning system. *Gene* 2:95–113.

Carninci, P., and Y. Hayashizaki. 1999. High-efficiency full-length cDNA cloning. *Methods Enzymol.* 303:19–44.

Christiaens, H., R. J. Leer, P. H. Pouwels, and W. Verstraete. 1992. Cloning and expression of a conjugated bile acid hydrolase gene from *Lactobacillus plantarum* by using a direct plate assay. *Appl. Environ. Microbiol.* 58:3792–3798.

Frengen, E., D. Weichenhan, B. Zhao, K. Osoegawa, M. van Geel, and P. J. de Jong. 1999. A modular, positive selection bacterial artificial chromosome vector with multiple cloning sites. *Genomics* 58:250–253.

Garfin, D. E. 1995. Electrophoretic methods, p. 53–109. *In* J. A. Glasel and M. P. Deutscher (ed.), *Introduction to Biophysical Methods for Protein and Nucleic Acid Research*. Academic Press, Inc., San Diego, CA.

Geertsma, E. R., and B. Poolman. 2007. High-throughput cloning and expression in recalcitrant bacteria. *Nat. Methods* 4:705–707.

Grinstead, J., and P. M. Bennett (ed.). 1988. *Methods in Microbiology*, vol. 21. *Plasmid Technology*. Academic Press, London, United Kingdom.

Ioannou, A. P., C. T. Amemiya, J. Garnes, P. M. Kroisel, H. Shizuya, C. Chen, M. A. Batzer, and P. J. de Jong. 1994. A new bacteriophage-derived vector for the propagation of large human DNA fragments. *Nat. Genet.* 6:84–89.

Kim, U.-J., B. W. Birren, T. Slepak, V. Mancino, C. Boysen, H.-L. Kang, M. I. Simon, and H. Shizuya. 1996. Construction and characterization of a human bacterial artificial chromosome library. *Genomics* 34:213–218.

Kouker, G., and K. E. Jaeger. 1987. Specific and sensitive plate assay for bacterial lipases. *Appl. Environ. Microbiol.* 53:211–213.

Krzywinski, M., I. Bosdet, D. Smailus, R. Chiu, C. Mathewson, N. Wye, S. Barber, M. Brown-John, S. Chan, S. Chand, A. Cloutier, N. Girn, D. Lee, A. Masson, M. Mayo, T. Olson, P. Pandoh, A. L. Prabhu, E. Schoenmakers, M. Tsai, D. Albertson, W. Lam, C. O. Choy, K. Osoegawa, S. Zhao, P. J. de Jong, J. Schein, S. Jones, and M. A. Marra. 2004. A set of BAC clones spanning the human genome. *Nucleic Acids Res.* 32:3651–3660.

Martin, C., L. Bresnick, R.-R. Juo, J. C. Voyta, and I. Bronstein. 1991. Improved chemiluminescent DNA sequencing. *BioTechniques* 11:110–114.

Meselson, M., and R. Yuan. 1968. DNA restriction enzyme from *E. coli*. *Nature* 217:1110–1114.

Pingoud, A., M. Fuxreiter, V. Pingoud, and W. Wende. 2005. Type II restriction endonucleases: structure and mechanism. *Cell. Mol. Life Sci.* 62:685–707.

Radnedge, L., and H. Richards. 1999. The development of plasmid vectors. *Methods Microbiol.* 29:51–95.

Roberts, R. J. 2005. How restriction enzymes became the workhorses of molecular biology. *Proc. Natl. Acad. Sci. USA* 102:5905–5908.

Roberts, R. J., M. Belfort, T. Bestor, A. S. Bhagwat, T. A. Bickle, J. Bitinaite, R. M. Blumenthal, S. Degtyarev, D. T. Dryden, K. Dybvig, K. Firman, E. S. Gromova, R. I. Gumport, S. E. Halford, S. Hattman, J. Heitman, D. P. Hornby, A. Janulaitis, A. Jeltsch, J. Josephsen, A. Kiss, T. R. Klaenhammer, I. Kobayashi, H. Kong, D. H. Kruger, S. Lacks, M. G. Marinus, M. Miyahara, R. D. Morgan, N. E. Murray, V. Nagaraja, A. Piekarowicz, A. Pingoud, E. Raleigh, D. N. Rao, N. Reich, V. E. Repin, E. U. Selker, P. C. Shaw, D. C. Stein, B. L. Stoddard, W. Szybalski, T. A. Trautner, J. L. Van Etten, J. M. Vitor, G. G. Wilson, and S. Y. Xu. 2003. A nomenclature for restriction enzymes, DNA methyltransferases, homing endonucleases and their genes. *Nucleic Acids Res.* 31:1805–1812.

Roberts, R. J., T. Vincze, J. Posfai, and D. Macelis. 2007. REBASE—enzymes and genes for DNA restriction and modification. *Nucleic Acids Res.* 35:D269–D270.

Sambrook, J., and D. Russell. 2001. *Molecular Cloning: a Laboratory Manual*, 3rd ed. Cold Spring Harbor Laboratory Press, Cold Spring Harbor, NY.

Winnacker, E.-L. 1987. *From Genes to Clones: Introduction to Gene Technology*. VCH, New York, NY.

Zeng, C., N. Kouprina, B. Zhu, A. Cairo, M. Hoek, G. Cross, K. Osoegawa, V. Larionov, and P. de Jong. 2001. Large-insert BAC/YAC libraries for selective re-isolation of genomic regions by homologous recombination in yeast. *Genomics* 77:27–34.

REVIEW QUESTIONS

1. What are type II restriction endonucleases? Why are they important for recombinant DNA technology?

2. When circular double-stranded DNA from the plasmid pCEL1 is digested by various restriction endonucleases and combinations thereof, the following bands (with lengths given in kilobase pairs) are observed: EcoRI, 6.0; BamHI, 6.0; HindIII, 6.0; HaeII, 3.0, 2.0, and 1.0; EcoRI and HaeII, 2.0 and 1.0; EcoRI and HindIII, 3.5 and 2.5; EcoRI and BamHI, 4.5 and 1.5; BamHI and HindIII, 5.0 and 1.0; BamHI and HaeII, 3.0, 1.5, 1.0, and 0.5; and HindIII and HaeII, 3.0, 1.5, 1.0, and 0.5. Construct a restriction endonuclease enzyme site map with this information.

3. Describe how plasmid pBR322 is used as a cloning vector. What are its special features?

4. Describe the principal features of the pUC cloning system.

5. A genomic library of a prokaryotic organism is often constructed by cloning the products of a Sau3AI partial digest of the genomic DNA into a BamHI site of the vector.

 a. Why are two different enzymes used in this experiment?

 b. What is a partial digestion, and how is it performed?

 c. Why is partial digestion often used for constructing genomic libraries?

6. For gene-cloning experiments, why is the cleaved plasmid DNA often treated with alkaline phosphatase prior to the ligation step?

7. Suggest a few different ways that recombinant plasmids can be introduced into a gram-negative bacterium, such as *E. coli*.

8. Outline some of the strategies that are used to detect a cloned target gene within a library in *E. coli*. What conditions must be satisfied for each type of assay?

9. What is a cDNA library?

10. Why would you use a plasmid, bacteriophage λ, cosmid, or BAC as a cloning vector?

11. What is a common mode of action of a type IIS restriction endonuclease?

12. What is replica plating? Outline the basic methodology for replica plating.

13. What is a fosmid?

14. What is a tripartite mating?

15. What is the role of RNase H during cDNA synthesis?

Chemical Synthesis, Amplification, and Sequencing of DNA

TECHNOLOGICAL ADVANCES IN ANY AREA OF SCIENCE have profound effects on research. New protocols spawn novel experiments, and laboratory procedures that were at one time difficult to implement become much easier to perform. The very essence of molecular biotechnology is rooted in a wide range of technical developments, many of which have become commonplace and accessible to both large and small research facilities. For example, it is now standard to chemically synthesize a DNA molecule, amplify DNA using the polymerase chain reaction (PCR), and obtain the nucleotide sequence of DNA. Each of these procedures is derived from basic studies of the structure of DNA and the mechanism of DNA replication. Moreover, these experimental methods are essential for isolating, characterizing, and expressing cloned genes.

Chemical Synthesis of DNA

The ability to chemically synthesize a strand of DNA with a specific sequence of nucleotides easily, inexpensively, and rapidly has contributed significantly to the methodologies of molecular cloning and DNA characterization. Chemically synthesized single-stranded DNA oligonucleotides are used for assembling whole genes, amplifying specific DNA sequences, introducing mutations into cloned genes, screening gene libraries, sequencing DNA, and facilitating gene cloning.

Machines that automate the chemical reactions for DNA synthesis (DNA synthesizers, or "gene machines") have made the production of single-stranded oligonucleotides (\leq50 nucleotides) into a more or less routine procedure. Generally, DNA synthesizers consist of a set of valves and pumps that are programmed to introduce, in the correct order, specified nucleotides and the reagents required for the coupling of each consecutive nucleotide to the growing chain. Chemical DNA synthesis does not follow the biological direction of DNA synthesis; rather, during the chemical process, each incoming nucleotide is coupled to the 5' hydroxyl terminus of the growing chain. All the reactions are carried out in succession in a single

reaction column, and both the duration of each reaction and the washing steps are computer controlled.

The Phosphoramidite Method

Currently, the phosphoramidite method of chemical DNA synthesis is the procedure of choice. Before their introduction into the reaction column, the amino groups of the bases adenine, guanine, and cytosine are derivatized by the addition of benzoyl, isobutyryl, and benzoyl groups, respectively, to prevent undesirable side reactions during chain growth. Thymine is not treated because it lacks an amino group. Solid-phase synthesis, i.e., attachment of the growing DNA strand to a solid support, is used so that all the

FIGURE 4.1 Flowchart for the chemical synthesis of DNA oligonucleotides. After n coupling reactions (cycles), a single-stranded piece of DNA with $n + 1$ nucleotides is produced.

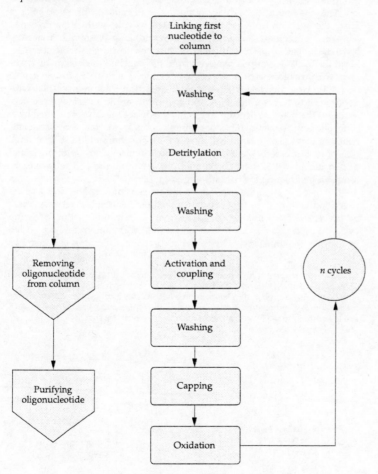

FIGURE 4.2 Starting complex for the chemical synthesis of a DNA strand. The initial nucleoside has a protective DMT group attached to the 5′ hydroxyl group of the deoxyribose moiety and a spacer molecule attached to the hydroxyl group of the 3′ carbon of the deoxyribose. The spacer unit is attached to a solid support, which is usually a CPG bead.

reactions can be conducted in one reaction vessel, the reagents from one reaction step can be readily washed away before the reagents for the next step are added, and the reagents can be used in excess in an attempt to drive the reactions to completion.

The chemical synthesis of DNA is a multistep process (Fig. 4.1). The initial nucleoside (base and sugar only), which will be the 3′-terminal nucleotide of the synthesized strand, is attached to a spacer molecule by its 3′ hydroxyl terminus, and the spacer molecule is covalently attached to an inert support, which is often a controlled-pore glass (CPG) bead (a glass bead with uniformly sized pores) (Fig. 4.2). A dimethoxytrityl (DMT) group is attached to the 5′ terminus of the first nucleoside to prevent the 5′ hydroxyl group from reacting nonspecifically before the addition of the second nucleotide. Each nucleotide that is added to the growing chain has a 5′ DMT protective group and also a diisopropylamine group attached to a 3′ phosphite group that is protected by a β-cyanoethyl (CH_2CH_2CN) group (Fig. 4.3). This molecular assembly is called a phosphoramidite.

After the first nucleoside is bound to the CPG beads, the cycle begins. First, the reaction column is washed extensively with an anhydrous reagent, e.g., acetonitrile, to remove water and any nucleophiles that may be present. The column is flushed with argon to purge the acetonitrile. Next, the 5′ DMT group is removed from the attached nucleoside by treatment with trichloroacetic acid (TCA) to yield a reactive 5′ hydroxyl group (Fig. 4.4). After this detritylation step, the reaction column is washed with acetonitrile to remove the TCA and then with argon to remove the acetonitrile. The machine is programmed to introduce the next prescribed base (phosphoramidite) and tetrazole simultaneously for the activation and coupling steps. The tetrazole activates the phosphoramidite so that its 3′ phosphite forms a covalent bond with the 5′ hydroxyl group of the initial nucleoside (Fig. 4.5). Unincorporated phosphoramidite and tetrazole are removed by flushing the column with argon.

Because not all of the support-bound nucleosides are linked to a phosphoramidite during the first coupling reaction, the unlinked residues must be prevented from linking to the next nucleotide during the following cycle. To do this, acetic anhydride and dimethylaminopyridine are added to acetylate the unreacted 5′ hydroxyl groups (Fig. 4.6). If this capping step

FIGURE 4.3 Structure of a phosphoramidite. Phosphoramidites are available for each of the four bases (A, C, G, and T) that are used for the chemical synthesis of a DNA strand. A diisopropylamine group is attached to the 3′ phosphite group of the nucleoside. A β-cyanoethyl group protects the 3′ phosphite group, and a DMT group is bound to the 5′ hydroxyl group of the deoxyribose sugar.

FIGURE 4.4 Detritylation. The 5′ DMT group is removed by treatment with TCA. In this example, the detritylation of the first nucleoside is depicted.

FIGURE 4.5 Activation and coupling. The activation of a phosphoramidite enables its 3′ phosphite group to attach to the 5′ hydroxyl group of the bound detritylated nucleoside.

FIGURE 4.6 Capping. The available 5' hydroxyl groups of unreacted detritylated nucleosides are acetylated to prevent them from participating in the coupling reaction of the next cycle.

is not carried out, then, after a number of cycles, the growing chains will differ in both length and nucleotide sequence.

At this stage of the process, the linkage between the nucleotides is in the form of a phosphite triester bond, which is unstable and prone to breakage in the presence of either acid or base. Therefore, the phosphite triester is oxidized with an iodine mixture to form the more stable pentavalent phosphate triester (Fig. 4.7). After this oxidation step and a subsequent wash of the reaction column, the cycle of detritylation, phosphoramidite activation, coupling, capping, and oxidation is repeated (Fig. 4.1). This

FIGURE 4.7 Oxidation. The phosphite triester internucleotide linkage is oxidized to the pentavalent phosphate triester. This reaction stabilizes the phosphodiester bond and makes it less susceptible to cleavage under either acidic or basic conditions.

cycling continues with each successive phosphoramidite until the last programmed residue has been added to the growing chain. When the final cycle is completed, the newly synthesized DNA strands are bound to the CPG beads; each phosphate triester contains a β-cyanoethyl group; every guanine, cytosine, and adenine carries its amino-protecting group; and the 5′ terminus of the last nucleotide has a DMT group.

The β-cyanoethyl groups are removed by a chemical treatment in the reaction column. The DNA strands are then cleaved from the spacer molecule, leaving a 3′ hydroxyl terminus. The DNA is eluted from the reaction column, and in succession, the benzoyl and isobutyryl groups are stripped away and the DNA is detritylated. The 5′ terminus of the DNA strand is phosphorylated either by a T4 polynucleotide kinase reaction or by a chemical procedure. Phosphorylation can also be carried out after detritylation while the oligonucleotide is still bound to the support.

To achieve a reasonable overall yield of an oligonucleotide, the coupling efficiency should be greater than 98% at each step. The coupling efficiency of each cycle is determined by spectrophotometrically monitoring released trityl groups. If, for example, the efficiency is 99% at each cycle during the production of a 20-unit oligonucleotide (20-mer), which entails 19 coupling reactions, since the first base is bound to the spacer and is not involved in a coupling step, then 83% (i.e., $0.99^{19} \times 100$) of the product will be 20 nucleotides long. If a 60-mer is synthesized with 99% efficiency at each cycle, then about 55% of the final product will contain all 60 of the nucleotides. With an average coupling efficiency consistently less than 98%, the yield of full-length oligonucleotides diminishes as a function of the required number of cycles (Table 4.1). The coupling efficiency for most commercial DNA synthesizers averages about 99.5% for each step. However, depending on the length and stringency of the end use of an oligonucleotide, it may be necessary to purify the final product using either reverse-phase high-pressure liquid chromatography or gel electrophoresis. These methods separate the longer target oligonucleotides from the shorter "failure" sequences.

Uses of Synthesized Oligonucleotides

Chemically synthesized oligonucleotides (<100-mers) have a myriad of functions. Single-stranded hybridization oligonucleotide probes (20- to 40-mers) can be formulated by deducing the codons from the amino acid sequence of a protein and then used to screen a genomic library for the gene (Fig. 4.8A). Since the actual codons representing a conserved amino acid sequence are unknown because of codon redundancy, especially at the third position, a single arbitrary synthetic probe may not contain sufficient complementary bases (matches) to produce significant hybridization with

TABLE 4.1 Overall yields of chemically synthesized oligonucleotides with different coupling efficiencies

Coupling efficiency (%)	Overall yield of oligonucleotide (%)				
	20-mer	40-mer	60-mer	80-mer	100-mer
90	14	1.6	0.2	0.02	0.003
95	38	14	4.8	1.7	0.6
98	68	46	30	20	14
99	83	68	55	45	37
99.5	91	82	74	67	61

a heterologous sequence. For this reason, a set of mixed probes is often used to screen a genomic library. The formation of a sample of mixed probes is straightforward. Briefly, during chemical DNA synthesis, instead of providing a specific phosphoramidite for a particular nucleotide site, a mixture of different bases is added to the reaction. For example, with the addition of equal concentrations of four different bases for one nucleotide position, four different probes are produced. If two sites are treated this way, 16 (4^2) different probes will be synthesized (Fig. 4.8B); for n sites, there are 4^n different oligonucleotides. Moreover, the frequencies of various probes in the mixture can be skewed by varying the proportions of bases in the reaction mixture for specific sites. As a consequence, in contrast to a single probe, a set of mixed probes is likely to contain sequences that are highly complementary to a heterologous gene. As discussed below, single-stranded oligonucleotides (~17- to 24-mers, or primers) are also required for DNA sequencing and PCR. In some cases, additional sequences are added to the PCR primers as part of the synthesis process to create molecules with restriction endonuclease sites for cloning or sequences that contain regulatory elements for transcription and translation of the amplified DNA after it is inserted into a vector.

Oligonucleotides are extremely useful for both cloning DNA molecules and creating unique cloning sites. For example, linkers are short, double-stranded, blunt-ended DNA molecules with self-complementary (palin-

FIGURE 4.8 (A) All possible DNA sequences deduced from a protein sequence. For simplicity, only 3 amino acids, 2 of which have twofold degeneracy and 1 that has a single codon, are shown. (B) Formation of sets of mixed probes. A question mark denotes a site where equal concentrations of A, C, G, and T are supplied during chemical synthesis. The remaining sites have the same deoxynucleotide (C). Four and 16 different oligonucleotides are produced when there is a 25% probability that any 1 of the 4 nucleotides will be incorporated at one or two sites, respectively.

dromic) strands that contain a restriction endonuclease site (Fig. 4.9A and B). Typically, after complementary single-stranded oligonucleotides are annealed, the resulting double-stranded linker is blunt-end ligated to DNA molecules that are unclonable because they lack a suitable restriction endonuclease site. In practice, during the ligation reaction, the linker molecules are successively added to the ends of the source DNA and to each other. Then, after treatment with the restriction endonuclease corresponding to the linker sequence, the large DNA fragments, i.e., the source DNA with restriction endonuclease extensions, are separated from the remnants of linker DNA and cloned into the comparable site of a cloning vector (Fig. 4.10).

Adaptors are variants of linkers that are often used to create novel cloning sites in vectors. They are short double-stranded DNA molecules that contain one or more restriction endonuclease sites and may have either one blunt end and one extended end or two extended ends. For example, the BamHI–SmaI adaptor (Fig. 4.9C) is inserted into a unique BamHI site of a cloning vector to create a novel SmaI site. The DNA fragment that is to be cloned can be blunt-end ligated into the SmaI site, and after selection, the insert can be retrieved by treating the construct with BamHI (Fig. 4.11). For this procedure to be effective, the cloned DNA fragment must not have the same restriction endonuclease sites as the linker sequence; otherwise, the insert will be cut during restriction endonuclease treatment.

Oligonucleotides are the key components for assembling genes. There are a number of applications for synthetic genes, including large-scale production of proteins, testing protein function after changing specific codons, and creating nucleotide sequences that encode proteins with novel properties. The production of short genes (60 to 80 base pairs [bp]) is technically straightforward and can be accomplished by synthesizing the complementary strands and then annealing them. For the production of longer genes (>300 bp), however, special strategies must be devised because the coupling efficiency of each cycle during chemical DNA synthesis is never 100%. For example, if a gene contains 1,000 bp and the average coupling efficiency is 99.5%, then the proportion of full-length single DNA strands after the last cycle is a minuscule 0.007%. To overcome this problem, synthetic (double-stranded) genes are assembled in modular fashion from oligonucleotides that are about 60 nucleotides in length.

One method for building a synthetic gene requires the initial production of a set of overlapping, complementary oligonucleotides, each of which is usually between 20 and 60 nucleotides long. Each internal section of the gene is made up of a set of oligonucleotides with complementary 3′- and 5′-terminal extensions that are designed to base pair precisely with a different oligonucleotide that has complementary terminal extensions (Fig. 4.12). The oligonucleotides that make up the two ends of a gene are aligned to give blunt ends. Thus, after the gene is assembled, the only remaining requirement to complete the process is sealing the nicks along the backbones of the two strands with T4 DNA ligase. In addition to the protein coding sequence, synthetic genes can be designed with restriction endonuclease sites at their ends to facilitate insertion into a cloning vector and, if necessary, with additional sequences that contain signals for the proper initiation and termination of transcription and translation. To optimize translation, the codons of a gene from one organism can be changed to those that are preferred by the host cell without altering the amino acid sequence.

FIGURE 4.9 Typical linker and adaptor sequences. **(A)** A 6-mer EcoRI linker; **(B)** an 8-mer EcoRI linker; **(C)** a BamHI–SmaI adaptor. Both the BamHI cohesive ends and the SmaI recognition sequence are indicated.

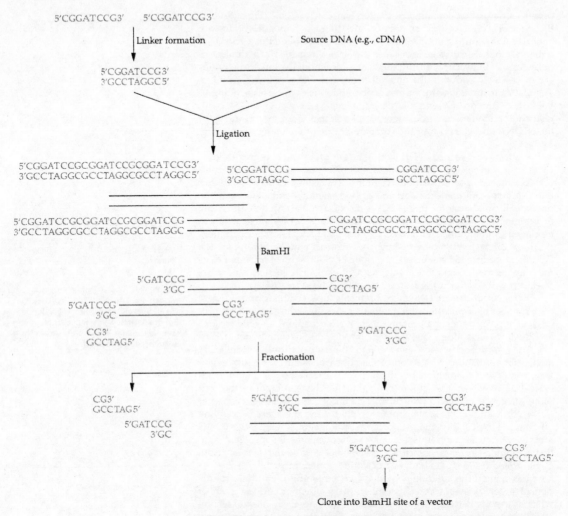

FIGURE 4.10 Cloning with a linker. A palindromic oligonucleotide (red) with a BamHI recognition site base pairs to itself to form a BamHI linker. During the ligation reaction, linkers are successively attached to the source DNA and to each other. The ligation mixture is treated with BamHI. The large DNA molecules are purified and cloned into the BamHI site of a cloning vector. DNA molecules without linkers are not cloned.

Another way to prepare a full-size gene is to synthesize a specified set of overlapping oligonucleotides that are about 60 nucleotides in length with approximately 20-base overlaps (Fig. 4.13). After the 3′ and 5′ extensions are annealed, large gaps still remain, but the base-paired regions are both long enough and stable enough to hold the structure together. After all the oligonucleotides are combined, the gaps are filled by enzymatic DNA synthesis with *Escherichia coli* DNA polymerase I. This enzyme uses

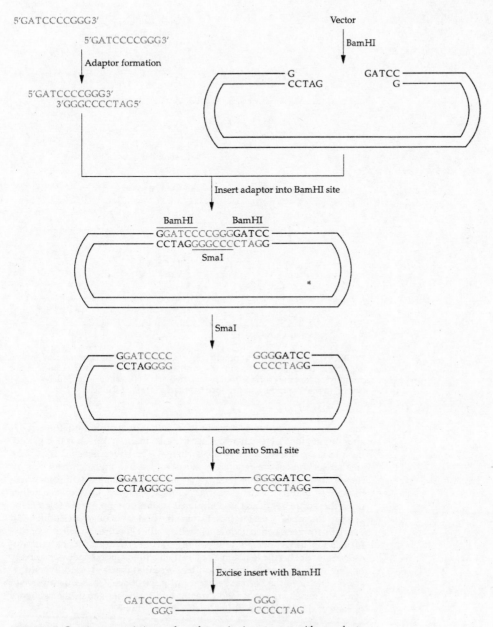

FIGURE 4.11 Creating a restriction endonuclease site in a vector with an adaptor. After self-hybridization, an adaptor molecule (red) with two BamHI 5′ extensions and a SmaI site (BamHI–SmaI adaptor) is formed. The BamHI–SmaI adaptor is inserted into a unique BamHI site of a vector to create a unique SmaI site. DNA (blue) is cloned into the SmaI site by blunt-end ligation. Although the SmaI site is destroyed by the insertion of a DNA molecule, the insert can be retrieved by cutting the vector with BamHI.

FIGURE 4.12 Assembly of a synthetic gene from short oligonucleotides. Individual oligonucleotides (20- to 60-mers) are synthesized chemically. Their sequences are designed so that they form a double-stranded array after annealing. T4 DNA ligase is used to seal the nicks and produce an intact version of the gene.

the 3′ hydroxyl groups as replication initiation points and the single-stranded regions as templates. After the enzymatic synthesis is completed, the nicks are sealed with T4 DNA ligase. For larger genes (≥1,000 bp), smaller sections of the gene are first assembled into units (chunks, or synthons) about 500 bases in length that are then combined with other 500-base units, and in turn, these larger kilobase segments are joined together until the entire sequence is completed. Computer programs (e.g., Gene Design) that make it easier to determine the best set of oligonucleotides and overlaps for gene construction, as well as allow the user to select a particular codon usage, change any codon, and designate restriction endonuclease sites at specific locations, are available both commercially and freely on the Internet. Finally, it is absolutely essential that a chemically synthesized gene have the correct sequence of nucleotides. Consequently, small synthetic genes are sequenced directly, and for larger genes, the sequence of each of the 500-base building blocks is determined.

Polymerase Chain Reaction

PCR is an effective procedure for generating large quantities of a specific DNA sequence in vitro. This amplification, which can be more than a millionfold, is achieved by a three-step cycling process. The essential compo-

FIGURE 4.13 Assembly and in vitro enzymatic DNA synthesis of a gene. Individual oligonucleotides are synthesized chemically. Their sequences are designed to enable them to form a stable molecule, with base-paired regions separated by open regions (gaps). The gaps are filled in by in vitro enzymatic DNA synthesis. The nicks are sealed with T4 DNA ligase.

nents for PCR amplification are (1) two synthetic oligonucleotide primers (~20 nucleotides each) that are complementary to regions on opposite strands that flank the target DNA sequence and that, after annealing to the source DNA, have their 3′ hydroxyl ends oriented toward each other; (2) a template sequence in a DNA sample that lies between the primer-binding sites and that can be from 100 to ~35,000 bp in length; (3) a thermostable DNA polymerase that can withstand being heated to 95°C or higher and that copies the DNA template with high fidelity; and (4) the four deoxyribonucleotides.

A typical PCR process entails a number of cycles for amplifying a specific DNA sequence. Each cycle has three successive steps.

1. Denaturation. The first step in the PCR amplification system is the thermal denaturation of the DNA sample by raising the temperature within a reaction tube to 95°C. In addition to the source template DNA, this reaction tube contains a vast molar excess of the two oligonucleotide primers, a thermostable DNA polymerase (e.g., *Taq* DNA polymerase, isolated from the bacterium *Thermus aquaticus*), and four deoxyribonucleotides. The temperature is maintained for about 1 minute.

2. Renaturation. For the second step, the temperature of the mixture is slowly lowered to ~55°C. During this step, the primers base pair with their complementary sequences in the DNA sample.

3. Synthesis. In the third step, the temperature is raised to ~75°C, which is optimum for the catalytic functioning of *Taq* DNA polymerase. DNA synthesis is initiated at the 3' hydroxyl end of each primer and uses the source DNA as a template (Fig. 4.14).

All steps in a PCR cycle are carried out in an automated block heater that is programmed to change temperatures after a specified period of time. One cycle generally lasts from 3 to 5 minutes.

To understand how the PCR protocol succeeds in amplifying a discrete segment of DNA, it is important to keep in mind the location of each primer-annealing site and its complementary sequence within the strands that are synthesized during each cycle. During the synthesis phase of the first cycle, the newly synthesized DNA from each primer is extended

MILESTONE

DNA Sequencing with Chain-Terminating Inhibitors

F. SANGER, S. NICKLEN, and A. R. COULSON

Proc. Natl. Acad. Sci. USA **74**:5463–5467, 1977

New techniques are the lifeblood of science. They enable researchers to acquire information that was previously inaccessible, and that, in turn, generates insights that stimulate new research and lead to new discoveries. For molecular biotechnology, DNA sequencing and PCR are powerful procedures that have become laboratory mainstays.

DNA sequencing by enzymatic synthesis with chain elongation inhibitors is a relatively simple, accurate, and reliable method. The most definitive form of molecular characterization of a cloned piece of DNA is its sequence. Among other things, the coding content of an insert, potential primer sequences for a PCR, and the presence of a gene mutation can be

determined by DNA sequencing. At the time the Sanger (dideoxy) method was published, most DNA sequencing was carried out by the base-specific chemical-cleavage method devised by A. M. Maxam and W. Gilbert (*Proc. Natl. Acad. Sci. USA* **74**:560–564, 1977). Before the development of these techniques, nucleic acid sequencing was more or less limited to RNA molecules. The sequencing of a DNA molecule required transcribing a DNA fragment into RNA with RNA polymerase and then sequencing the RNA product. In general, RNA sequencing entailed treating a radiolabeled RNA molecule with different ribonucleases, chromatographically separating the digestion products, redigesting the separated products, hydrolyzing the products of the second digestion with

alkali, chromatographically separating the hydrolysis products, determining the sequence of the oligonucleotides, and constructing the sequence based on overlapping stretches of nucleotides. This approach was time-consuming and tedious. With the advent of the dideoxy method, it became obsolete. Now, RNA molecules are usually sequenced by converting them into DNA molecules. The Sanger method superseded the Maxam and Gilbert sequencing procedure when the M13 bacteriophage cloning system, which provided the single-stranded DNA templates required for sequencing, was developed. Sanger and Gilbert received the Nobel Prize in Chemistry in 1980 for this work. The ability to sequence DNA molecules has been, directly and indirectly, responsible for both the dramatic upsurge in studies of the molecular basis of human diseases and the development of diagnostic and therapeutic treatments for these disorders.

FIGURE 4.14 First PCR cycle. The target DNA lies between sequences 1' and 2 on one strand and between sequences 1 and 2' on the complementary strand. Two primers (P1 and P2) are mixed with the sample DNA. The mixture, which also contains *Taq* DNA polymerase and the four deoxyribonucleotides (deoxyribonucleoside triphosphates [dNTPs]), is heated to 95°C to denature the DNA and then slowly cooled to 55°C. The primers, which are present in excess, base pair to the original DNA strands of the sample during the renaturation (annealing) step. The temperature is raised to about 75°C, and DNA synthesis commences from the 3' hydroxyl end of each primer sequence and continues past the region of the template DNA strand that is complementary to the other primer sequence. The products of this reaction are two long strands of DNA (long templates) that serve as additional DNA templates during the second PCR cycle.

beyond the endpoint of the sequence that is complementary to the second primer. These new strands form "long templates" that are used in the second cycle (Fig. 4.14).

During the second cycle, the original DNA strands and the new strands synthesized in the first cycle (long templates) are denatured and then

FIGURE 4.15 Second PCR cycle. The templates for this cycle are the long templates synthesized during the first PCR cycle and the original DNA strands. The primers hybridize to complementary regions in both the original strands and the long templates strands, and DNA synthesis produces more long template strands from the original strands and short template strands from the long template strands. A short template has a primer sequence at one end and the sequence complementary to the other primer at its other end.

hybridized with the primers. The large molar excess of primers in the reaction mixture ensures that they will hybridize to the template DNA before complementary template strands have the chance to reanneal to each other. A second round of synthesis produces long templates from the original strands, as well as some DNA strands that have a primer sequence at one end and terminate with a sequence complementary to the other primer at the other end ("short templates") that were generated from the long templates (Fig. 4.15).

During the third cycle, short templates, long templates, and original strands all hybridize with the primers and are replicated (Fig. 4.16). In subsequent cycles, the short templates preferentially accumulate, and by the 30th cycle, these strands are about a million times more abundant than either the original or long template strands (Fig. 4.17). PCR has become a pervasive technique that is used for innumerable purposes, some of which are described here and many others in the ensuing chapters.

PCR Amplification of Full-Length cDNAs

A PCR-based method that enriches for full-length cDNA molecules entails adding an oligonucleotide that consists of an oligo(dT) sequence followed by a PCR primer sequence at the 5′ end to a purified poly(A) mRNA preparation (Fig. 4.18). The first cDNA strand is synthesized with the enzyme reverse transcriptase, which catalyzes the synthesis of a DNA strand using RNA as a template. When reverse transcriptase reaches the 5′ end of an RNA template, its terminal transferase activity, which does not require a template, adds additional nucleotides that consist predominantly of cytosines. A second oligonucleotide in the reaction mixture that has a poly(dG) sequence at its 3′ end and a PCR primer sequence at the 5′ end base pairs with the poly(dC) tract at the end of each full-length cDNA first strand. Reverse transcriptase uses the sequence of the second oligonucleotide, including the primer sequence, as a template to extend the cDNA first strand at the 3′ end. The reaction conditions prevent tandem repeats from forming at the 5′ ends of the full-length first cDNA strands. Next, reverse and forward PCR primers are added to the reaction mixture, and full-length double-stranded cDNA molecules are generated by PCR. Incomplete cDNA molecules do not have oligo(dC) tracts at their 5′ ends. Consequently, they lack the necessary complementary sequence for the forward primer, and as a result, they are not amplified. Moreover, sequences for restriction endonuclease sites that facilitate cloning into a vector may be included as part of the original oligo(dT)–primer and primer–oligo(dG) oligonucleotide sequences. This PCR amplification strategy has been dubbed SMART (which stands for switching mechanism at 5′ end of RNA transcript) cDNA synthesis by its developers.

Gene Synthesis by PCR

The assembly of a gene by PCR is faster and more economical than filling in overlapping oligonucleotides using DNA polymerase and then sealing the nicks with T4 DNA ligase. One PCR-based protocol for total gene construction starts with two overlapping oligonucleotides (A and B) that represent sequences from the center of the gene (Fig. 4.19). After being annealed, these oligonucleotides have recessed 3′ hydroxyl groups that provide a starting point for DNA synthesis during the elongation phase of a PCR cycle. A double-stranded DNA molecule is formed by a filling-in

FIGURE 4.16 Third PCR cycle. During the renaturation step, the primer sequences hybridize to complementary regions of original, long-template, and short-template strands, and DNA synthesis produces long templates from the original strands and short templates from both the long and short templates.

reaction. This 4-minute cycle is repeated 20 times to maximize the amount of the product that is formed. Next, two additional oligonucleotides (C and D) are added to the mixture. Oligonucleotide C overlaps at its 3′ end with the 5′ end of oligonucleotide A and represents the nucleotide sequence of the gene immediately upstream of the oligonucleotide A sequence. Oligonucleotide D overlaps at its 3′ end with the 5′ end of oligonucleotide B and represents the nucleotide sequence of the gene immediately downstream of the oligonucleotide B sequence. After 20 denaturation, renaturation, and synthesis cycles, a double-stranded DNA with a specific sequence order (CABD) is produced.

Thereafter, pairs of oligonucleotides are added, one of the pair overlapping the upstream sequence of the DNA molecule formed in the previous round and the other overlapping the downstream sequence, and subjected to 20 PCR cycles for each pair added until the entire gene is formed. Generally, the oligonucleotides are about 50 nucleotides long. Thus, the 10

Thirtieth cycle

FIGURE 4.17 Thirtieth PCR cycle. By the 30th cycle, the population of DNA molecules in a reaction tube consists almost entirely of short template strands.

FIGURE 4.18 PCR amplification of full-length cDNAs. An oligonucleotide with oligo(dT) and an added sequence [oligo(dT)–primer] is used by reverse transcriptase to initiate first-strand cDNA synthesis from poly(A) mRNA templates (1). The terminal transferase activity of reverse transcriptase adds mostly deoxycytidines (dCs) to the end of each full-length first-strand cDNA molecule (1). A primer-deoxyguanosine (dG) oligonucleotide that base pairs with the dC tail (2) acts as a template for reverse transcriptase to extend the first-strand cDNA at the 3′ ends (3). Forward and reverse primers that have the same sequences as the primer–dG and oligo(dT)–primer oligonucleotides, respectively, are added to the first-strand cDNA mixture (4), and full-length double-stranded cDNAs are generated by PCR amplification (5).

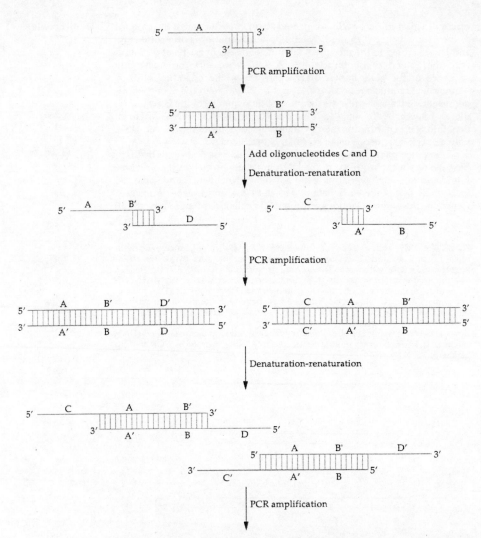

FIGURE 4.19 Gene synthesis by PCR. Overlapping oligonucleotides (A and B) are filled in from the recessed 3′ hydroxyl ends during DNA synthesis. Oligonucleotides (C and D) that are complementary to the ends of the product of the first PCR cycle are added to a sample, overlapping molecules are formed after denaturation and renaturation, and the recessed ends are filled in during DNA synthesis. Next, oligonucleotides (E and F) that overlap the ends of the second-cycle PCR product are added to a sample, and a third PCR cycle is initiated. The final PCR product is a double-stranded DNA molecule with a specified sequence of nucleotides. The pairs of letters with or without a prime (e.g., A′ and A) represent complementary oligonucleotides. Each oligonucleotide corresponds to a sequence from a particular DNA strand.

rounds of 20 4-minute PCR cycles that are required to synthesize a gene with 1,000 bp can be carried out in 1 day. In addition, as with other methods for assembling genes, the last pair of oligonucleotides (i.e., the 5′ and 3′

FIGURE 4.19 *(continued)*

ends of the gene) can be made with supplementary sequences outside the coding region that facilitate the cloning of the gene into a vector and, at the 5′ end, with sequences that enable the gene to be expressed in a host cell.

DNA-Sequencing Techniques

In molecular terms, the definitive understanding of a DNA molecule comes from determining its nucleotide sequence. The function of a gene can often be deduced from its nucleotide sequence. For example, a presumptive amino acid sequence, determined from the nucleotide sequence, can be compared with protein sequences of known genes, and significant sequence

similarity generally indicates a protein with an equivalent function. Also, distinctive coding regions, such as DNA-binding sites, receptor recognition sites, and transmembrane domains, can be ascertained. The nucleotide sequences in noncoding regions (regions that do not encode a protein or RNA molecule) may provide information about the regulation of a gene. In addition, nucleotide sequence information is essential for molecular-cloning studies and for characterizing gene activity.

For more than 3 decades, the dideoxynucleotide procedure developed by Fred Sanger has been used for DNA sequencing. This includes sequencing of DNA fragments containing one to a few genes and also many whole genomes, including the human genome. However, the interest in sequencing large numbers of DNA molecules in less time and at a lower cost has driven the recent development of new sequencing technologies that can process thousands to millions of sequences concurrently (a term often used to describe this is massive parallelization). Many different sequencing technologies are currently being explored; however, those that have reached the commercialization stage are largely based on the principles of sequencing by synthesis, which includes pyrosequencing and sequencing using reversible chain terminators, and on sequencing by ligation. In general, these new, second-generation methods involve repeated cycles of (1) enzymatic addition of nucleotides to a primer based on complementarity to a template DNA fragment and (2) detection and identification of the nucleotide(s) added. The techniques differ in the method by which the nucleotides are extended, employing either DNA polymerase to catalyze the addition of a single nucleotide or ligase to add a short, complementary oligonucleotide, and in the method by which the addition is detected. The development of these promising new technologies notwithstanding, the Sanger dideoxynucleotide procedure is still the most commonly used method today and is well suited for small-scale sequencing projects (in the kilobase-to-megabase range).

Dideoxynucleotide Procedure for Sequencing DNA

A dideoxynucleotide is a human-made molecule that lacks a hydroxyl group at both the 2′ and 3′ carbons of the sugar moiety (Fig. 4.20A). In con-

FIGURE 4.20 (A) A dideoxynucleotide. The 2′ and 3′ carbons of the sugar moiety lack hydroxyl groups. (B) A deoxyribonucleotide.

trast, a natural deoxyribonucleotide has a 3' hydroxyl group on the sugar unit (Fig. 4.20B). Normally, during DNA replication, an incoming natural nucleoside triphosphate is linked by its 5' α-phosphate group to the 3' hydroxyl group of the last nucleotide of the growing chain (Fig. 4.21). However, if a dideoxynucleotide is incorporated at the end of the growing chain, DNA synthesis stops because a phosphodiester bond cannot be formed with the next incoming nucleotide (Fig. 4.22). The termination of DNA synthesis is the quintessential feature of the dideoxynucleotide DNA-sequencing method, although other experimental conditions must be met before a DNA sequence can be determined.

In principle, the first step in the standard laboratory procedure for dideoxynucleotide DNA sequencing entails annealing a synthetic oligo-nucleotide (17- to 24-mer; primer) to a predetermined segment of a strand of the DNA to be sequenced, for example, to a segment of a cloning vector near the insertion site of the cloned DNA. The oligonucleotide acts as a primer by providing a 3' hydroxyl group for the initiation of DNA synthesis. In the original method, the primed DNA sample is partitioned into

FIGURE 4.21 Normal DNA synthesis. An incoming deoxyribonucleotide (deoxyribo-nucleoside triphosphate [dNTP]) base pairs with the complementary nucleotide of the template strand. The internucleotide linkage occurs between the 3' hydroxyl group of the last nucleotide of the growing strand and the α-phosphate group of the incoming nucleotide.

FIGURE 4.22 Blocked DNA synthesis. Chain growth is stopped by the addition of a dideoxynucleotide to the end of the growing strand. The internucleotide linkage between the last nucleotide, which is a dideoxynucleotide, and the next incoming nucleotide cannot be formed because there is no 3′ hydroxyl group on the dideoxynucleotide sugar.

four separate reaction tubes. Each tube contains four deoxyribonucleotides (dATP, dCTP, dGTP, and dTTP), one of which is radiolabeled, and one of the four dideoxynucleotides (dideoxyadenosine triphosphate [ddATP], dideoxycytidine triphosphate [ddCTP], dideoxyguanosine triphosphate [ddGTP], or dideoxythymidine triphosphate [ddTTP]). The concentration of each dideoxynucleotide in each reaction tube is carefully adjusted to ensure that it is incorporated into the mixture of growing chains at every possible site. Recall that chain growth stops as soon as a dideoxynucleotide is incorporated, so each growing chain will eventually contain a dideoxynucleotide at its 3′ terminus. This experimental condition is met in each of the four reaction tubes. Consequently, after enzymatic DNA synthesis with DNA polymerase, each reaction tube will contain a unique set of single-stranded DNA molecules of all possible lengths, each of which includes the primer sequence at its 5′ end (Fig. 4.23).

The synthesis reactions are stopped by the addition of formamide, which prevents DNA strands from base pairing, and the DNA molecules, including the newly synthesized DNA molecules, are separated by polyacrylamide gel electrophoresis. This separation procedure resolves pieces of DNA that differ in size by as little as a single nucleotide. An autoradiograph of the gel shows only the radiolabeled DNA fragments that were produced during the enzymatic DNA synthesis step. Each of the four lanes in the gel and the autoradiograph corresponds to a reaction tube that contained one of the four dideoxynucleotides.

The sequence of a segment of DNA is determined by noting the order of the bands, as accurately as possible, from the bottom to the top of the

autoradiograph. In the example shown in Fig. 4.24, the first 6 bases of the sequenced DNA are AGCTGC. In this case, the fastest-migrating band (the radiolabeled fragment closest to the bottom), which corresponds to the smallest DNA fragment, is in the ddATP lane, the next band is in the ddGTP lane, the next is in the ddCTP lane, the next is in the ddTTP lane, and so on. Up to 500 bands can be resolved reliably on most autoradiographs. Usually, the primer sequence is positioned about 10 to 20 nucleotides away from the target DNA so that the researcher can recognize the known sequence at the start of the autoradiograph and thereby identify precisely the first nucleotide of the target DNA.

Although the procedure described above is still used for some specialized applications, in practice, the entire procedure has been automated and typically uses nucleotides labeled with fluorescent dyes that are detected using a laser, rather than radiolabeled nucleotides which are visualized on an autoradiograph. Automated DNA sequencing minimizes manual manipulations and increases the rate of acquiring sequence data, which is essential for assembling vast amounts of nucleotide sequence data from whole prokaryotic and eukaryotic genomes. Automated sequence analysis can be carried out with four different fluorescent dyes, one for each dideoxynucleotide reaction, or with the same fluorescent dye for each dideoxynucleotide in each reaction mixture. In some cases, the primer, rather than a dideoxynucleotide, is labeled with a fluorescent dye. With a four-fluorescent-dye system, the samples at the completion of each reaction are pooled,

FIGURE 4.23 Primer extension during DNA synthesis in the presence of dideoxynucleotides. Each of the four reaction tubes contains a unique set of nucleotide extensions attached to the primer, because when a dideoxynucleotide is incorporated into the growing strand, it terminates the synthesis. A few full-length DNA molecules will be synthesized in each reaction tube. dNTP, deoxyribonucleoside triphosphate.

Contents of reaction tube	Size of primer and extension	Primer and sequence of extension
ddATP + four dNTPs	Primer + 3	Primer – dGdCddA
	Primer + 7	Primer – dGdCdAdTdCdGddA
	Primer + 8	Primer – dGdCdAdTdCdGdAddA
ddCTP + four dNTPs	Primer + 2	Primer – dGddC
	Primer + 5	Primer – dGdCdAdTddC
ddGTP + four dNTPs	Primer + 1	Primer – ddG
	Primer + 6	Primer – dGdCdAdTdCddG
ddTTP + four dNTPs	Primer + 4	Primer – dGdCdAddT
	Primer + 9	Primer – dGdCdAdTdCdGdAdAddT

FIGURE 4.24 Simulated autoradiograph of a dideoxynucleotide DNA-sequencing gel. Each lane of the gel was loaded with the contents of one of the four reaction tubes, which contained either ddATP, ddCTP, ddGTP, or ddTTP. By convention, the bands of the autoradiograph are read from the bottom to the top. In this example, the results of the sequence determination are shown on the right.

and the fragments are separated in a single lane of a polyacrylamide gel or polymer-filled capillary tube. This type of analysis is called "four-color, one-lane" detection. Alternatively, with one fluorescent dye marker, each sample is run in a separate lane; this is "one-color, four-lane" detection.

Each fluorescent dye emits a narrow spectrum of light with a distinctive peak when it is struck by an argon ion laser beam. The beam scans a fixed location near the bottom of the electrophoretic matrix. As each successive labeled fragment passes through the beam, excitation by the laser causes an emission with specific spectral features that is detected by a photomultiplier tube. The emission data are recorded and stored in a computer. After a run is completed, the succession of fluorescent signals is converted to nucleotide sequence information. For a four-color, one-lane system, each fluorescent dye emits a different wavelength, and the order of spectral responses in a single lane corresponds to the sequence of nucleotides (Fig. 4.25 and 4.26A to C). In other words, each dye represents a particular nucleotide. With a one-color, four-lane system, the fluorescent signals from the dideoxynucleotide-terminated fragments are recorded in succession across the four lanes. In this case, the overall order of the fluorescent signals as a function of each lane corresponds to a nucleotide sequence. Parenthetically, DNA sequencing with radioactive label is equivalent to the one-color, four-lane format (Fig. 4.26D).

FIGURE 4.25 Automated fluorescent-dye terminator Sanger DNA sequencing. Fragments that are synthesized with a primer (highlighted in pale green) from a DNA template (highlighted in pale blue) and terminated with fluorescent dideoxynucleotides are separated by capillary electrophoresis. A detector records each successive laser-induced fluorescent signal (not shown). The successive fluorescent signals are represented as a sequencing chromatogram (colored peaks). In this case, the fluorescence for dideoxyadenosine (ddA), dideoxyribosylthymine (ddT), dideoxyguanosine (ddG), and dideoxycytidine (ddC) are green, purple, orange, and blue, respectively. Commercial automated DNA sequencers run 96 (Applied Biosystems 3730xl) and 384 (GE Healthcare MegaBACE 4550) samples concurrently.

Generally, automated DNA-sequencing systems can read with high accuracy about 500 bases per run; under optimal conditions, one instrument can resolve about 20,000 bases per hour. The electrophoretic matrix for separating dideoxynucleotide-terminated products may be a slab gel or a liquid polymer in a capillary tube. Automated capillary DNA-sequencing machines handle larger numbers of samples with faster separations than do units that analyze slab gels.

To produce large amounts of dideoxynucleotide-terminated fragments from small amounts of template DNA, PCR-based cycle sequencing is commonly used. The setup and components for this method are the same as those for the standard automated dideoxynucleotide sequencing protocol except that a thermostable DNA polymerase is required because the process entails 25 or more cycles of denaturation, annealing, and elongation

FIGURE 4.26 DNA sequence determination by the dideoxynucleotide procedure. **(A and B)** Computer readout (A) of the nucleotide sequence from a four-color, one-lane sequencing gel (B). The numbers denote nucleotide positions. **(C)** Electrophoretic separation of the fluorescently labeled dideoxynucleotide fragments in a single lane that correspond to the nucleotide sequence shown in panel A. **(D)** Autoradiograph of a four-lane, one-label sequencing gel for the nucleotide sequence shown in panel A. Redrawn from a figure supplied by Applied Biosystems.

(Fig. 4.27). Since there is only a single primer in each dideoxynucleotide reaction, the amplification of fragments is linear. The high temperature both reduces intrastrand base pairing (secondary structure), which blocks strand elongation, and minimizes false priming due to incomplete base pairing (mismatching) between the primer and DNA template. After the last cycle, formamide-treated samples are run in either one or four lanes, depending on the format of the experiment, and the sequence is determined. Under optimal conditions, cycle sequencing resolves between 600 and 800 nucleotides at a time.

Primer Walking

The entire sequence of pieces of DNA longer than about 500 bp cannot typically be obtained in a single run in most sequencing systems, and therefore, a number of different strategies are used to obtain the complete sequence of large DNA fragments. In one commonly used strategy, the dideoxynucleotide sequencing reactions are carried out to determine the identity and order of the first 500 or so nucleotides of the DNA. On the basis of this analysis, a second primer that is designed to hybridize to a region about 20 nucleotides upstream from the end of the acquired sequence is chemically synthesized and then used to determine the sequence of the next 500 nucleotides. In a similar manner, a third primer-binding site is selected, another oligonucleotide is synthesized, and the sequence of the next 500 bases is determined (Fig. 4.28). This "primer-walking" strategy proceeds until the entire cloned DNA is sequenced. To ensure that the overall sequence is correct and that there is no ambiguity regarding the identity of any nucleotide, both strands of the DNA must be sequenced. Different initial primers enable sequencing of both strands; one primer binds to the strand at one end of the insert, and the other primer binds to the opposite strand at the other end of the insert. False priming of DNA synthesis can give erroneous and ambig-

Elongation (72°C, 60 s)

Renaturation (~55°C, 30 s)

Denaturation
(95°C, 30 s)

~25 cycles

DNA sequence analysis

FIGURE 4.27 Cycle sequencing. The approximate temperatures and durations of each step are noted. The primer is green, the template DNA is blue, and the dideoxynucleotide-terminated fragments are red.

uous results. This situation may arise if the primer binds to more than one region within the target DNA. To avoid this problem, the primers used for this procedure are generally at least 24 nucleotides long. In addition, stringent annealing conditions do not permit spurious binding of the primer to similar but nonidentical sequences. Primer walking has been used to sequence pieces of DNA that have been cloned into bacteriophage λ (~20 kilobase pairs [kb]) or a cosmid vector (~45 kb).

Pyrosequencing

Pyrosequencing was the first of the second-generation sequencing technologies to be made commercially available and has contributed to the recent rapid output of large amounts of sequence data by the scientific community. The basis of the technique is the detection of pyrophosphate that is released during DNA synthesis. As part of the structure of a deoxynucleoside triphosphate, the phosphate attached to the 5′ carbon of the deoxyribose sugar moiety is designated the α-phosphate, the next phosphate is the β-phosphate, and the third is the γ-phosphate (Fig. 4.29). During replication, the α-phosphate of each incoming complementary nucleotide is joined enzymatically by a phosphodiester linkage to the 3′ OH group of the last

FIGURE 4.28 DNA sequencing by primer walking. **(1)** DNA sequencing is initiated with a primer (P1) that is complementary to a site on a plasmid near the point of insertion of the cloned DNA. **(2)** Based on the segment of the cloned DNA that has just been sequenced, a second primer (P2) that is complementary to a stretch of about 20 nucleotides near the end of that segment is synthesized. **(3)** P2 is used to sequence the next segment of cloned DNA. **(4)** Based on the segment of the cloned DNA that has just been sequenced, a third primer (P3) that is complementary to a stretch of about 20 nucleotides near the end of that segment is synthesized. **(5)** P3 is used to sequence the next segment of cloned DNA. **(6)** Based on the segment of the cloned DNA that has just been sequenced, a fourth primer that is complementary to a stretch of about 20 nucleotides near the end of that segment is synthesized. The process of successively synthesizing and using new primers continues until the entire insert is sequenced.

nucleotide of the growing strand, and the β- and γ-phosphates are cleaved off as a unit that is called pyrophosphate (Fig. 4.29).

The unambiguous detection of pyrophosphate during DNA strand synthesis forms the basis for determining the DNA sequence of a template strand. Specifically, the release of pyrophosphate is correlated with the incorporation of a known nucleotide in the growing DNA strand. A DNA fragment of unknown sequence is engineered at one end with a sequence that is complementary to a primer, and then, after the primer is added, one deoxynucleotide is introduced at a time in the presence of DNA polymerase. Pyrophosphate is formed only when the complementary nucleotide is incorporated at the end of the growing strand. Obviously, nucleotides that are not complementary to the nucleotide in the template strand are not incorporated and no pyrophosphate is formed. Thus, for this system, it was necessary to develop an accurate and rapid method for detecting pyrophosphate.

The strategy for pyrosequencing entails a series of enzymatic reactions (Fig. 4.30). Briefly, the pyrophosphate generated by the incorporation of a nucleotide is combined with adenosine-5′-phosphosulfate by the enzyme

FIGURE 4.29 Phosphodiester bond formation and release of pyrophosphate during the incorporation of a nucleotide at the end of a growing DNA strand. Phosphodiester bond formation occurs between the 3' OH of the deoxyribose sugar of the last incorporated nucleotide and the α-phosphate of the incoming nucleotide (blue arrow). The bond between the α- and β-phosphates is cleaved (green arrow), and pyrophosphate is released (black arrow).

FIGURE 4.30 Pyrosequencing enzyme reactions. Black, nucleotide incorporation and release of pyrophosphate; red, generation of light from pyrophosphate with ATP sulfurylase and luciferase. The DNA sequence is determined by correlating the extent of light emission with a particular nucleotide. Green, breakdown of unincorporated deoxynucleoside triphosphate (dXTP) and any remaining ATP to monophosphates (dXMP) by apyrase. AMP, adenosine monophosphate.

MILESTONE

Specific Enzymatic Amplification of DNA In Vitro: the Polymerase Chain Reaction

K. B. MULLIS, F. A. FALOONA, S. J. SCHARF, R. K. SAIKI, G. T. HORN, and H. A. ERLICH

Cold Spring Harbor Symp. Quant. Biol. **51**:263–273, 1986

PCR, which is the invention of Kary Mullis (U.S. patent 4,683,202), has had a tremendous impact on many research areas, including molecular biotechnology. The capability of generating large amounts of DNA by amplification from segments of cloned or genomic DNA has facilitated the cloning of DNA versions of rare mRNA molecules, screening gene libraries, diagnostic testing for gene mutations, physical mapping of chromosomes, and a myriad of other applications. In fact, the first study using PCR described a diagnostic test for sickle-cell anemia (Saiki et al., *Science* **230**:1350–1354, 1985). PCR was a unique idea that did not replace any existing technology. The power of the method is in its simplicity, sensitivity, and specificity. It utilizes a mechanism similar to that used by our cells to accurately replicate a DNA template, it can detect and produce millions of copies from a single template molecule in a few hours, and under appropriate conditions, it can be used to amplify a specific sequence in a complex mixture of DNA molecules even when other, similar sequences are present. Mullis received the Nobel Prize in Chemistry for his work on PCR in 1993. Since 1986, more than 200,000 published studies have used PCR in one way or another. Moreover, a Google search with the phrase "polymerase chain reaction" yields more than 17,000,000 hits! Its status as an indispensable method is well established, and considering the large number of PCR applications that have already been devised, there seems to be no end to its potential uses.

ATP sulfurylase to form ATP. In turn, ATP drives the conversion of luciferin to oxyluciferin by the enzyme luciferase, which generates light that is recorded by a photon detector. Before the next nucleotide is added to the mixture, ATP and any unincorporated deoxynucleoside triphosphate is degraded to its monophosphate form by the enzyme apyrase, which is an ADP diphosphohydrolase that removes the γ-phosphate from nucleoside triphosphates and the β-phosphate from nucleoside diphosphates (Fig. 4.30). Because the natural nucleotide dATP can participate in the luciferase reaction, deoxyadenosine α-thiotriphosphate (dATPαS), which is used by DNA polymerase but not luciferase, is substituted for dATP in the reaction mixture.

The amount of light generated after the addition of a particular nucleotide tends to be proportional to the number of nucleotides that are incorporated in the growing strand (Fig. 4.31). The incorporation of any single nucleotide produces an amount of light that falls within a limited range that represents the incorporation of one nucleotide, i.e., a 1-mer. A dinucleotide sequence, e.g., AA, TT, CC, or GG, generates a more intense signal that falls within the 2-mer range. This more or less linear relationship holds only for stretches of about eight identical nucleotides in a row (homopolymer tracts). Generally, regardless of the DNA-sequencing chemistry, homopolymer tracts are difficult to sequence accurately.

During each incubation, the amount of the light signal is measured and recorded. At the end of the sequencing run, the light emissions are represented as a bar on a graph (pyrogram) where the y axis reveals whether the incorporation is equivalent to one or more nucleotide units (mers) and the x axis presents the sequence of the strand that is complementary to the template sequence (Fig. 4.31C).

Sequencing Using Reversible Chain Terminators

For pyrosequencing, in which DNA is sequenced by synthesis, that is, by nucleotide extension of a growing DNA strand, each of the 4 nucleotides must be added to the reaction sequentially in separate cycles. This process

would be considerably faster if, for each cycle, all the nucleotides were added together. For this, it is necessary to ensure that the growing DNA strands are extended by only a single nucleotide during each cycle and that the incorporated nucleotides are recognized individually. These objectives can be met with reversible chain terminators and four-color fluorescence, which form the basis of some new sequencing technologies.

One approach entails capping the 3′ carbon of the deoxyribose sugar with a chemical group that blocks subsequent addition of nucleotides and attaching a different fluorophore to each nucleotide at positions that do not interfere with either base pairing or phosphodiester bond formation

FIGURE 4.31 DNA sequence determination by pyrosequencing. **(A)** Template strand (blue background) with primer sequence (blue letters). **(B)** Signal (light) intensities with four pyrosequencing cycles based on the template sequence in panel A. A pyrosequencing cycle consists of four rounds, where one round represents the addition of one of the four deoxynucleotides. Each round is followed by treatment with apyrase. A minus sign denotes no light emission, and the plus signs indicate the relative amount of light released after the introduction of a particular deoxynucleotide. **(C)** Pyrogram based on the data in panel B and the deduced nucleotide sequence of the strand that is complementary to the template sequence in panel A.

A

Template strand

T A T C G T C A G A T T C G G G G G C
A T A G C
Primer

B

Round	Deoxynucleotide*	Signal	Round	Deoxynucleotide*	Signal
1	dTTP	−	9	dTTP	+
2	dATPαS	+	10	dATPαS	++
3	dCTP	−	11	dCTP	−
4	dGTP	+	12	dGTP	+
5	dTTP	+	13	dTTP	−
6	dATPαS	−	14	dATPαS	−
7	dCTP	+	15	dCTP	+++++
8	dGTP	−	16	dGTP	+

*Apyrase is added after each round.

C

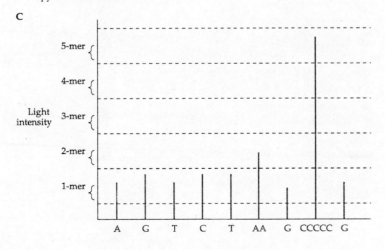

A

Cleavage site

Linker

Primer
sequence

3' blocking group

Cleavage site

Fluorescent dye

B

Primer
sequence

Linker

Cleavage site

3' blocking group

Cleavage site

Fluorescent dye

C

Primer
sequence

Linker

Cleavage site

3' blocking group

Cleavage site

Fluorescent dye

D

Cleavage site

Linker

Primer
sequence

3' blocking group

Cleavage site

Fluorescent dye

(Fig. 4.32). It is essential that both the 3' blocking group and the fluorescent dye be quickly and easily removed. Also, the decapping step must restore a hydroxyl group at the 3' position of the deoxyribose sugars to provide a site for phosphodiester bond formation with the next nucleotide. After fluorescent emissions are recorded, only 30 seconds is required to remove both the 3' blocking group and the fluorescent dye from each incorporated nucleotide and to leave a hydroxyl group at the 3' position of the deoxyribose sugars. Cycles of nucleotide addition to the growing DNA strand by DNA polymerase, acquisition of fluorescence data, and chemical cleavage of the blocking and dye groups are repeated to generate short sequence determinations (reads) of up to 36 nucleotides per run. Currently, read lengths are limited by difficulties in incorporating the fluorescent nucleotides and incomplete cleavage of the dye or blocking groups.

Sequencing by Ligation

In contrast to pyrosequencing and sequencing using reversible terminators, which extend the growing DNA strand by a single base during each cycle, sequencing by ligation extends the DNA strand by ligation of short oligonucleotides in a template-dependent fashion and utilizes the enzyme ligase rather than DNA polymerase. This procedure requires oligonucleotides that are usually 8 (octamers) or 9 (nonamers) nucleotides in length and are partially degenerate. That is, they contain a known (fixed) nucleotide at a specific (query) position and any nucleotide in the other positions. As shown in Fig. 4.33A, one set of nonamers has a fixed nucleotide (A, C, G, or T) in query position 1 and any nucleotide in positions 2 to 9; another set has a fixed nucleotide in query position 2 and any nucleotide in the other eight positions, i.e., 1 and 3 to 9, and so on. Moreover, all the nonamers with the same fixed nucleotide, regardless of position, are tagged at their 3' ends with the same fluorescent dye (Fig. 4.33A). Each of the four different fluorescent dyes emits a distinctive wavelength that can be used to identify the nucleotide in the query position.

A short nucleotide adaptor is joined to the ends of the DNA fragments that are to be sequenced. The adaptor sequences serve as binding sites for anchor primers (Fig. 4.33B). An anchor primer provides a 3' end for ligation

FIGURE 4.32 Addition of reversible terminators to a primer sequence. A blocking group that prevents chain extension is attached to the oxygen of the 3' position of the deoxyribose sugars of each nucleotide. A different fluorescent dye (colored structures) is linked to each nucleotide by means of a blocking group and a linker sequence at position 9 of the purines (guanine [A] and adenine [B]) and position 5 of the pyrimidines (cytosine [C] and uracil [D]). Palladium-catalyzed cleavage (arrows) removes the 3' blocking group and the fluorescent dyes with the restoration of a hydroxyl group at the 3' carbon of each deoxyribose sugar. During the next cycle, the growing strands are extended by one reversible terminator. The template strand is not shown here. Note that the difference between deoxyuridine monophosphate (dUMP) and deoxythymidine monophosphate (dTMP) is the absence of the methyl group at position 5 of the pyrimidine ring of dUMP. The uracil of the modified deoxyuridine triphosphate (dUTP) pairs with adenine of the template strand, and dUMP is joined to the last nucleotide of the growing strand by DNA polymerase. Adapted, with permission, from Fig. 7 of the online Supporting Information supplement at http://www.pnas.org/cgi/content/full/0609513103/DC1 accompanying J. Ju et al., *Proc. Natl. Acad. Sci. USA* **103:**19635–19640, 2006.

A

B

FIGURE 4.33 Sequencing by ligation. **(A)** Sets of nonamers. The fixed position of each nucleotide is denoted by a boldface colored letter. The colored dots represent different fluorescent dyes. The letter N signifies that any nucleotide can occupy that position in the nonamer. There are more than 65,000 different nonamer sequences when one position is fixed and the other eight sites are filled by any of the four nucleotides. **(B)** Representation of the first three cycles of sequencing by ligation of a template sequence. During cycle 1, the anchor primer anneals to the adaptor sequence at the 3′ end of the template sequence. Nonamers with A, T, C, and G in the first query position are added, and the complementary nonamer with A in the first position hybridizes and is ligated to the anchor primer. After the fluorescent signal is recorded, the ligated anchor primer–nonamer strand is released by melting. During the following two cycles, nonamers with T and C in the second and third positions, respectively, are ligated to the anchor primer. In this example, the successive color signals from the fluorescent dyes are red, blue, and orange, which correspond to A, T, and C.

to the 5′ end of an adjacent completely hybridized nonamer. Ligation does not occur if there is a single noncomplementary base pair (mismatch) between a nonamer and template sequence.

A sequencing cycle consists of the following steps. (1) The template DNA is denatured, and the anchor primer binds to its complementary sequence in the adaptor at the 3′ end of the single-stranded template DNA. (2) A pool of nonamers with fixed nucleotides A, G, C, and T at the same query position, say position 1, is added and incubated for a brief period with T4 DNA ligase. (3) The nonligated nonamers and other components are washed away, and the fluorescent signal is recorded. If the nonamer sequence is exactly complementary to the template sequence, then T4 DNA ligase will join the nonamer to the anchor primer (Fig. 4.33B). The identity of the nucleotide in position 1 is determined by the fluorescence produced. (4) The ligated anchor primer–nonamer sequence is removed by increasing

the temperature, and the cycle is repeated using another pool of nonamers with fixed nucleotides A, G, C, and T in query position 2 to identify the nucleotide in the second position on the template. These cycles are repeated to determine the sequences of short regions of DNA.

Large-Scale DNA Sequencing

Generally, DNA-sequencing projects fall into two categories: de novo genome sequencing and resequencing. Sequencing entire genomes that have not been previously sequenced is de novo genome sequencing, whereas resequencing entails comparing a newly determined sequence with a known reference sequence. Some of the applications for both de novo sequencing and resequencing include the identification of pathogenic strains, drug discovery, tests for disease-related mutations, forensic analyses, and development of biological products for commercial and industrial purposes.

Over the past 30 years, the cost of sequencing using the Sanger dideoxynucleotide procedure has been lowered from more than $10 to less than $0.05 per base. In addition, the speed of acquisition of DNA sequences has been increased dramatically by the introduction of automated DNA sequencers that run, depending on the instrument, either 96 or 384 capillary electrophoretic separations concurrently. Generally, these machines generate about 2×10^6 to 3×10^6 bases per day from more than 2,500 different DNA templates. The success of the Sanger dideoxynucleotide method is due to the highly accurate, long sequence reads of about 700 bases per sequencing reaction. These read lengths make it computationally easier to definitively determine overlapping sequences and thereby to assemble the nucleotide sequence of a genome, chromosome, or large gene, and for now, it remains the method of choice for de novo sequencing. However, the method is time-consuming, mainly due to the requirement for electrophoretic separation of the fragments, and expensive due to the relatively large volumes of chemicals that are used. Substantial research funds have been granted by the U.S. National Human Genome Research Institute for developing novel, inexpensive technologies to facilitate large-scale sequencing projects. The nominal objective of these efforts has been christened the "$1,000 genome." In other words, the goal is to reduce the cost of sequencing any human genome to $1,000. The National Human Genome Research Institute has targeted a "$100,000 genome" for 2009 and the "$1,000 genome" for 2014. In 2005, the sequencing of a human genome required about 10 months at a cost of about 15×10^6, which is obviously less than the 15 years and the 2.7×10^9 that were required to assemble the first human genome sequence (completed in 2003). The expectation is that a "$1,000 genome" would allow assessment of the risks of genetic diseases on an individual basis, as well as optimization of drug treatments for each patient, and of course, a "$1,000 genome" would mean that genome sequencing of microorganisms would cost a few dollars and that of single genes would cost pennies.

Shotgun Cloning Strategy for Sequencing Genomes

The shotgun cloning strategy has been used for de novo sequencing of thousands of prokaryotic, eukaryotic, and viral genomes. First, genomic DNA is randomly fragmented by sonication, nebulization, or hydrodynamic shearing. Breaking DNA by a physical method leaves extended (frayed)

A

B

C

FIGURE 4.34 Repair of the ends of frayed DNA (end repair) and phosphorylation of blunt-end DNA. **(A)** DNA polymerase fills in from recessed 3′ ends. **(B)** 3′ exonuclease degrades 3′ extensions. **(C)** T4 polynucleotide kinase phosphorylates the 5′ ends of the blunt-end fragments. Note that fragments with different combinations of extensions and recessed ends are not shown here. In all of these cases, the polymerase and/or 3′-exonuclease activity produces blunt-end DNA molecules.

ends that make cloning extremely inefficient. Consequently, the fragments are enzymatically blunt ended (end repaired, or polished) by filling in 3′ recessed ends with T4 DNA polymerase in the presence of the four deoxyribonucleotides and removing protruding 3′ ends with 3′ exonuclease activity (Fig. 4.34A and B). To facilitate ligation, the 5′ ends of the polished genomic fragments are phosphorylated with T4 polynucleotide kinase (Fig. 4.34C).

Next, the fragments are separated into small (~1-kb), medium (~8-kb), and large (~40-kb) fractions with which three libraries are created by cloning the small- and medium-size pieces into plasmids and the large, 40-kb fragments into a fosmid vector. Alternatively, the different-size DNA fractions may be isolated first and then end repaired separately before being cloned into different vectors. After transformation of *E. coli* with the library, colonies with cloned DNA are picked and grown. Vector DNA is purified from each library and amplified. Depending on the DNA sequencer, either 96 or 384 sequencing templates are analyzed concurrently. To achieve a high degree of accuracy, each nucleotide site in a genome should be sequenced at least 6 to 10 different times from different fragments. The extent of sequencing redundancy is called coverage, or depth of coverage.

A computer program, called a base caller, assesses the fluorescence chromatogram of each read and designates the nucleotides that most likely correspond to unambiguous peaks. After ignoring primer and vector sequences and removing low-quality base calls that commonly occur at the beginnings and ends of the chromatograms, another program, called an assembler, finds extensive overlapping segments. The process of generating successive overlapping sequences produces long, contiguous stretches of nucleotides (contigs).

Although assemblers are extremely effective, repetitive elements that in actuality occupy different genomic locations may be assigned to the same genomic region. This creates false contigs. This problem is overcome by using sequence information from both ends of an insert (paired ends, or mate pairs). Paired ends from the three libraries are situated ~1, ~8, or ~40 kb apart, respectively. The assembler identifies sets of paired ends that, in turn, are used to order and orient contigs. This process is called scaffolding (Fig. 4.35). Linking contigs together may also be confounded by incomplete genomic libraries that are often due to certain sequences not being replicated in *E. coli*. Additional cloning and sequencing may be required to complete the overall sequence. After the assembly process is completed, any small gaps between contigs that remain are resolved (gap closure, or finishing) either by PCR of high-molecular-weight genomic DNA across each gap, followed by sequencing the amplification product, or by primer walking. The sequences adjacent to the gaps provide the information for the primer sequences.

The genomes of more than 800 organisms, mostly bacteria, have been entirely sequenced by the shotgun strategy (Fig. 4.36), and incomplete (draft) versions of the genomes of more than 2,000 organisms are in the process of

FIGURE 4.35 Scaffolding. A scaffold of three contigs (black) is detected by paired end sequences. The paired ends are matched by color. The dashed lines represent the different distances between the paired ends.

Paired ends

Contigs

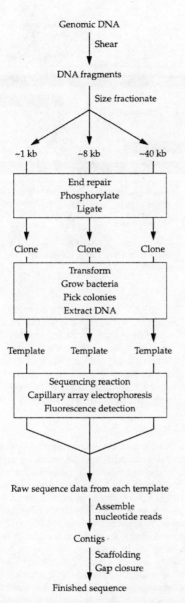

FIGURE 4.36 Flow diagram for whole-genome shotgun DNA sequencing. Samples of genomic DNA may be fragmented under different conditions to enhance the yield of small (~1-kb), medium (~8-kb), and large (~40-kb) pieces. It takes about 4 weeks to go from genomic DNA to purified templates. The time from the acquisition of raw sequence data to a finished (completed) sequence depends on the size of the genome, the extent of coverage, and the number of DNA sequencers that are used for the project. The procedures for cloning, colony selection, and template preparation apply to each library.

Adaptor A

PCR primer site
(20 nucleotides)

Left-specific
sequencing
primer site
(20 nucleotides)

Key sequence
(4 nucleotides)

Adaptor B

Key sequence
(4 nucleotides)

Right-specific
sequencing
primer site
(20 nucleotides)

PCR primer site
(20 nucleotides)

Biotin

FIGURE 4.37 Features of adaptors A and B that are used for template preparation, PCR amplification, and sequencing using a cyclic array-sequencing strategy with the 454 sequencing platform.

being finished. One major DNA-sequencing center (Joint Genome Institute, Walnut Creek, CA [http://www.jgi.doe.gov]) has 70 instruments that each analyze 96 samples at a time and run 24 hours a day, 7 days a week, along with another 40 instruments that each process 384 sequencing samples concurrently and run 24 hours a day, 5 days a week. The monthly output is about 2.8×10^9 bases. Under these conditions, with six-times coverage and 1 month to prepare the sequencing samples, it would take about 8 months to determine the genomic sequence of a single person.

Cyclic Array Sequencing

Cloning of large numbers of DNA fragments into plasmids, transforming the plasmids into bacterial cells, and then picking and extracting the plasmids from thousands to millions of colonies for sequencing using the Sanger dideoxynucleotide method is very time-consuming and expensive, even though many of these steps have been automated. To reduce the time and cost of large-scale sequencing, cyclic array sequencing strategies have been developed that (1) prepare libraries of DNA fragments for sequencing in vitro, (2) immobilize the sequencing templates in a dense array on a surface so that very small volumes of reagents are required for the sequencing reactions, and (3) utilize a sequencing-by-synthesis approach so that hundreds of millions of sequences can be acquired simultaneously (in parallel). In comparison to the 8 months required to sequence a human genome using the shotgun cloning–Sanger sequencing approach, cyclic array sequencing can provide the sequence of a human genome in 2 months.

Cell-free methods have been developed to construct libraries of sequencing templates that circumvent the requirement for preparation of clone libraries in bacterial cells. Instead, PCR is used to produce clonal clusters containing millions of copies of each template DNA molecule that are separated from other sequences. The term "polony," which is a contrac-

tion of *polymerase colony*, has been coined to represent multiple copies of the same nucleotide sequence that are confined to an entity, such as within a bead or on a solid or gel surface. One cyclic array-sequencing strategy entails capturing the PCR-amplified sequencing templates on the surface of a small bead, arraying the beads in wells of a plate, and then using pyrosequencing to determine the sequences of the captured templates. This strategy is often referred to as 454 sequencing after the company (454 Life Sciences) that developed the technology.

The source DNA is fragmented to an average size of about 350 bp. The frayed ends are blunt ended, and the 5′ ends are phosphorylated. Two nonphosphorylated adaptor sequences (A and B) are ligated to the polished, phosphorylated genomic DNA fragments (Fig. 4.37). The adaptors have sequences for PCR amplification of the genomic sequence, for priming the sequencing reaction, and for calibrating the signal output of the sequencing reaction. The elements of the long arm of adaptor A, reading from the 3′ end, consist of a 4-nucleotide calibration (key) sequence, a 20-nucleotide sequencing primer site (left-template-specific primer; left-specific sequencing primer), and a 20-nucleotide PCR primer site (primer A). Adaptor B has a key sequence, a sequencing primer site (right-template-specific primer; right-specific sequencing primer), a PCR primer site (primer B), and a biotin tag on the 5′ end (Fig. 4.37). Because the adaptors are not phosphorylated, during ligation, the 5′ phosphate end of the genomic DNA is joined to the 3′ hydroxyl group of an adaptor with a nick (gap) remaining at the 3′ hydroxyl end of the genomic DNA. Complete double-stranded DNA molecules are formed by filling in from the 3′ ends of the genomic DNA with a DNA polymerase that lacks exonuclease activity. The short adaptor strands are displaced during replication, and the long arms of the adaptors act as the templates (Fig. 4.38A).

After ligation and filling in, a genomic DNA fragment may be flanked on each end by (1) an A and B adaptor, (2) only adaptor A, or (3) only adaptor B (Fig. 4.38B). The next step is designed to recover single-stranded DNA with adaptors A and B on each end of the genomic DNA fragment, i.e., A–genomic DNA–B. Streptavidin beads are added to the DNA sample, and the biotin on adaptor B binds to the streptavidin beads. Thus, both the A–genomic DNA–B and B–genomic DNA–B molecules are immobilized. On the other hand, the A–genomic DNA–A molecules do not bind and are subsequently washed away. Next, after denaturation, only the nonbiotinylated strands of the A–genomic DNA–B molecules are released and collected. The biotinylated strands that remain bound to the streptavidin beads under these conditions are discarded (Fig. 4.38B).

During the next phase of the procedure, each collected genomic sequence is individually amplified. To this end, 20-nucleotide oligomers with a sequence that is complementary to the PCR primer site of adaptor B are bound at their 5′ ends to beads (DNA capture beads). Each DNA capture bead carries more than 10^7 of these oligomers. Then, the isolated A–genomic DNA–B strands are mixed with the DNA capture beads in a ratio that allows only one DNA strand to base pair with one of the oligomers on a bead (Fig. 4.39). Next, the beads and PCR reagents, including PCR primers that anneal to sequences that are part of adaptors A and B, are stirred vigorously with oil to create a water-in-oil emulsion. The conditions are set so that there is a single bead, along with PCR components, in a water droplet within an oil globule (Fig. 4.40A). In other words, each oil globule is a separate reaction chamber. There may be as many as 1,000 of

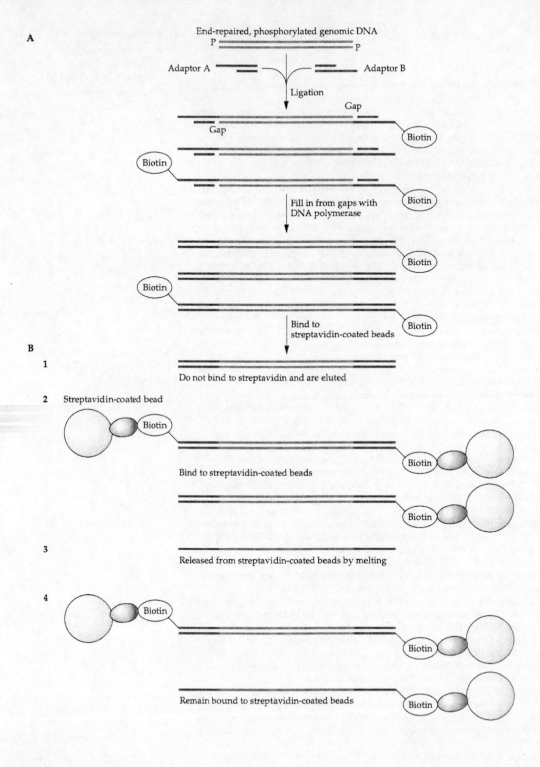

A

End-repaired, phosphorylated genomic DNA

P ══════════════════════ P

Adaptor A ━━━━ ━━━━ Adaptor B

Ligation

Gap

Gap

Biotin

Biotin

Biotin

Fill in from gaps with
DNA polymerase

Biotin

Biotin

Biotin

Bind to
streptavidin-coated beads

B

1

Do not bind to streptavidin and are eluted

2 Streptavidin-coated bead

Biotin

Biotin

Bind to streptavidin-coated beads

Biotin

3

Released from streptavidin-coated beads by melting

4

Biotin

Biotin

Remain bound to streptavidin-coated beads

Biotin

FIGURE 4.38 Preparation of single-stranded genomic DNA fragments for the 454 sequencing platform. (A) The frayed ends of genomic fragments are polished (end repaired), phosphorylated, and ligated with adaptors A and B. (B) The ligation products are mixed with streptavidin-coated beads. (1) The adaptor A–genomic DNA–adaptor A molecules do not bind to the streptavidin-coated beads and are washed out. (2) The DNA molecules with biotin tags bind to the streptavidin-coated beads. (3) The adaptor A–genomic DNA–adaptor B strands without a biotin tag are released by melting, concentrated, and retained for sequencing. (4) DNA molecules with biotin tags remain bound to the streptavidin-coated beads and are discarded.

these PCR "microreactors" per microliter. This form of PCR has been designated emulsion PCR.

During PCR cycling in each microreactor, strands with the same sequence as the isolated A–genomic DNA–B molecule are synthesized and base pair with the immobilized oligomers. This is followed by the synthesis of a complete complementary strand from the 3' ends of the oligomers (Fig. 4.40B to D). After 20 to 30 cycles, each bead has about 10^7 bound DNA molecules that are complementary to the original hybridized A–genomic DNA–B strand. Following PCR, the emulsion is broken, the beads are collected, and all the free DNA molecules are washed away. DNA strands that are base paired with the bound DNA strands are removed by melting them. Since not all of the DNA capture beads become enclosed in a PCR microreactor, it is necessary to concentrate the beads with attached full-length DNA extensions. These beads are enriched by hybridization to oligomers that are bound to magnetic beads and are complementary to the adaptor A sequence at the free 3' end of each full-length immobilized DNA molecule. All the DNA capture beads that do not hybridize are discarded. The DNA capture beads that are held by the oligomer attached to the magnetic beads are released by melting them. Finally, the magnetic beads are removed with a magnet. At this point, in preparation for DNA sequencing, a protein that binds to single-stranded

FIGURE 4.39 DNA capture bead. Oligomers that are complementary to the PCR amplification sequence of adaptor B are attached at their 5' ends to a bead. Each DNA capture bead hybridizes with only one adaptor A–genomic DNA–adaptor B strand. The inset highlights the available 3' end of the immobilized oligomer.

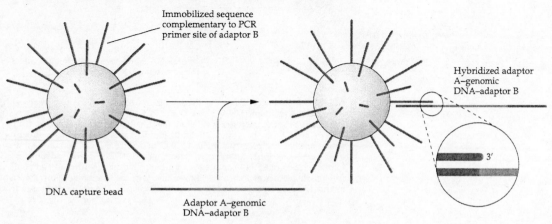

Immobilized sequence complementary to PCR primer site of adaptor B

Hybridized adaptor A–genomic DNA–adaptor B

3'

DNA capture bead

Adaptor A–genomic DNA–adaptor B

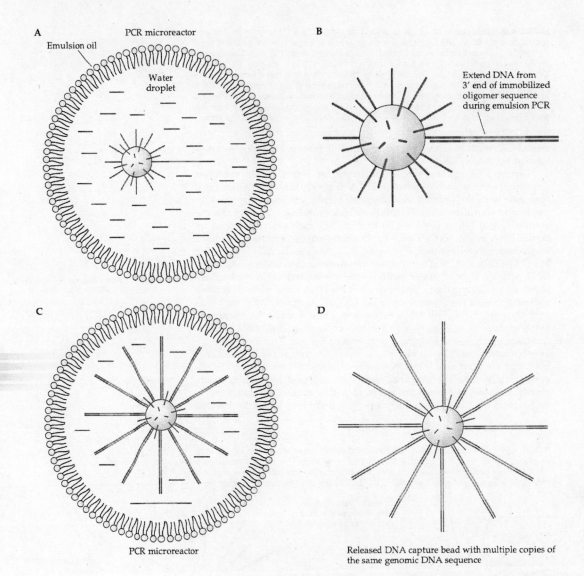

A

Emulsion oil

PCR microreactor

Water droplet

B

Extend DNA from 3′ end of immobilized oligomer sequence during emulsion PCR

C

PCR microreactor

D

Released DNA capture bead with multiple copies of the same genomic DNA sequence

FIGURE 4.40 Emulsion PCR. **(A)** Representation of a DNA capture bead with a hybridized A–genomic DNA–B strand and PCR amplification primers in a water-in-oil droplet (PCR microreactor) before the initiation of the PCR cycles. **(B)** DNA capture bead with the original hybridized adaptor A–genomic DNA–adaptor B strand and the complementary sequence extended from the 3′ end of the immobilized oligomer. Blue, adaptor A; green, genomic DNA; red, adaptor B. **(C)** Representation of a DNA capture bead during PCR cycling with many immobilized full-length sequences that are complementary to the originally hybridized DNA strand. **(D)** A DNA capture bead with many copies of the same genomic sequence.

DNA, a sequencing primer that is complementary to the left-template-specific sequence of adaptor A, and DNA polymerase are added to the DNA capture beads. Although sample preparation may seem excessive, the actual process takes only 2 to 3 days. By contrast, cloning, growing bacteria, and preparing vector DNA for conventional whole-genome shotgun sequencing requires from 20 to 30 days.

Pyrosequencing can be used to determine the nucleotide sequence by cycles of single-nucleotide addition followed by detection of light emission to determine which incorporated nucleotide releases pyrophosphate. The sequencing reactions are carried out in wells that hold picoliter volumes. (One picoliter is one millionth of a millionth of a liter.) Two other types of beads, in addition to the DNA capture beads (~28-μm diameter), are used to enhance the efficiency of the sequencing reaction. First, for pyrosequencing, luciferase and ATP sulfurylase are bound to small beads (2.8-μm diameter). Second, microparticles (0.8-μm diameter), without any immobilized molecules, are used to maintain uniformity within the reaction wells and to support the DNA capture beads. The beads are mixed and applied to a plate that has 2.6×10^6 or 0.8×10^6 wells, depending on the size of the plate. Each hexagonal well is only large enough to accommodate one DNA capture bead (Fig. 4.41). Optic fibers mounted next to the plate transmit the light signal, which corresponds to the incorporation of a particular nucleotide, from each of the wells to a sensor. The succession of signal outputs (flow signals) that corresponds to the sequence of incorporated nucleotides from each well is captured and stored in a computer.

A single sequencing round consists of flooding the wells, in succession, with one of the four deoxyribonucleotides, pyrosequencing reagents, and finally apyrase. This process is repeated for each nucleotide. The duration of a round is about 60 seconds. The "key" sequence on the adaptors is used to locate the wells with DNA capture beads and to calibrate the signal

FIGURE 4.41 Wells of a PicoTiterPlate used for 454 sequencing. Reproduced with the kind permission of Roche Diagnostics North America, Indianapolis, IN.

output. Generally, high-quality sequence information is generated from 200 to 300 bases before the accuracy of the read drops off. At the end of a run, the flow signal data from the wells are combined, and an assembler determines the most likely sets of contiguous nucleotides. This platform generates about 25×10^6 raw base reads in 4.5 hours, which is about 10 times coverage for a genome with 2×10^6 bp. A range of large-scale sequencing projects have demonstrated the utility of this approach, for example, the sequencing of a human genome (the genome of the Nobel laureate James Watson was used as a test case) and the sequencing of DNA in complex environmental samples that contain many microbial genomes with the aim of identifying candidate pathogens responsible for the mysterious collapse of honeybee colonies. Sequencing of the Neanderthal genome showed that PCR amplification of sequencing templates is especially useful when only small amounts of low-quality template are available, as is usually the case for ancient DNA samples.

Other cyclic array-sequencing strategies use emulsion PCR, or another PCR-based method, for clonal amplification of sequencing templates in combination with sequencing by ligation or sequencing by base extension using reversible chain terminators. Methods for sequencing single DNA molecules without amplification are also being explored. One of these approaches envisions translocating a DNA molecule through a very small channel (nanopore) and reading the nucleotide sequence from the successive perturbations of electrical conductance caused by specific base pairs. An advantage of nanopore sequencing is that extensive template preparation is not required. Moreover, hypothetically, sequence information could be generated in microseconds. Finally, notwithstanding the advances in large-scale DNA sequencing, it will be remarkable if any group ever wins the daunting $10 million challenge, called the X Prize, for devising a platform that will sequence 100 human genomes with 99.999% accuracy in 10 days for no more than $10,000 per genome.

SUMMARY

In addition to the various gene-cloning techniques, a number of other procedures, such as the chemical synthesis, amplification, and sequencing of DNA, are fundamental tools of molecular biotechnology. The chemical synthesis of DNA using phosphoramidites is a stepwise method that produces single-stranded DNA molecules (oligonucleotides). A high efficiency of phosphodiester bond formation (coupling) is mandatory. Otherwise, at the end of the process, the sample contains very few full-length molecules. The most commonly used chemically synthesized oligonucleotides range from about 10- to 30-mers. Although the yields are low, for special applications, oligonucleotides with 80 to 100 nucleotides can be produced. To make double-stranded DNA molecules, the complementary strands are synthesized separately and then mixed together. Oligonucleotides are used as probes for screening gene libraries, as linkers and adaptors for cloning genes and adding novel restriction endonuclease sites to vectors, as primers for dideoxynucleotide DNA sequencing and PCR, and for assembling genes.

PCR is an invaluable procedure that has innumerable applications. With this technique, specific segments of DNA are amplified over a millionfold. This amplification is achieved with two primers that hybridize to segments of DNA on opposite strands and have their 3' hydroxyl ends facing each other. The primers flank the target sequence. The process entails 30 or more successive cycles, with each cycle consisting of denaturation, renaturation, and in vitro DNA synthesis. Because it would be tedious and costly to add DNA polymerase at the end of each cycle, a DNA polymerase that is not inactivated at the high denaturation temperature (95°C) is used throughout. During the DNA renaturation step, the primer sequences, which are present in excess, hybridize to the sample DNA in the first cycle and to primer sites in the amplified DNA product molecules in subsequent cycles. In the DNA synthesis step, a new DNA strand that is complementary to its template strand grows from the 3' end of the primer. Among its various applications, PCR can be used to detect a specific nucleotide sequence in a biological sample, to obtain large amounts of a

particular DNA sequence either for cloning or for DNA sequencing, or to assemble a synthetic gene.

Among other uses, knowledge of the complete sequence of a gene enables researchers to both optimize the function of a coding sequence in a particular host cell and maximize the production of an economically important protein. The dideoxynucleotide method that was developed by Sanger and his colleagues is routinely used to sequence DNA. This technique relies on the in vitro incorporation of a dideoxynucleotide into a growing DNA strand. A dideoxynucleotide terminates the synthesis of a strand because it does not have a 3' hydroxyl group. In a sequencing experiment, four DNA synthesis reactions, each with a different dideoxynucleotide, are carried out independently. The DNA fragments of different lengths that are produced during each reaction are separated electrophoretically in an individual lane of a polyacrylamide gel. The pattern of separation of the synthesized radiolabeled fragments is used to determine the nucleotide sequence of the growing strand. Automated DNA sequencers that detect fluorescent dyes are now used routinely for both small- and large-scale sequencing projects. A common format entails using dideoxynucleotides that are each labeled with a different fluorescent dye, i.e., a one-lane, four-color detection system. In this case, the dideoxynucleotide reaction products are generated using a thermostable polymerase and a PCR-based approach, mixed, and then separated in a single lane of a polyacrylamide gel or a polymer-filled capillary tube. The sequence of fluorescent signals is recorded and converted to the corresponding nucleotide sequence.

Pyrosequencing entails correlating the release of pyrophosphate, which is recorded as the extent of an emission of light, with the incorporation of a particular nucleotide into a growing DNA strand. Pyrophosphate is enzymatically combined with adenosine-5'-phosphosulfate to form ATP, which in turn acts as a substrate for luciferase, which causes the emission of light. Sequencing using reversible chain terminators also reveals the sequence of a DNA fragment by detecting single-nucleotide extensions; however, in contrast to pyrosequencing, the 4 nucleotides are added to the reaction together

in each cycle, and after the unincorporated nucleotides are washed away, the nucleotide incorporated by DNA polymerase is distinguished by its fluorescent signal. The fluorescent dye and a blocking group that prevents addition of more than 1 nucleotide during each cycle are chemically cleaved, and the cycle is repeated. In another method, short sequences can be determined by ligating degenerate oligonucleotides that have a known nucleotide at the query position to an anchor primer in a DNA template-dependent fashion. The identity of the nucleotide in the query position is determined by the corresponding fluorescent signal.

Traditionally, large-scale DNA sequencing of genomes has relied on the four-color Sanger dideoxynucleotide method and instruments that run 94 or 364 capillary gels in parallel. The Sanger method generates sequence lengths from 600 to 800 bases, and effective software exists for assembling long contigs from the sequence data. Also, mate pairs and other strategies facilitate the ordering of the contigs. Finally, gaps are closed by various methods, such as primer walking, to produce a finished sequence. Although the whole-genome shotgun strategy has been the method of choice for sequencing genomes, novel, massively parallel DNA-sequencing platforms have been developed to significantly reduce the cost of sequencing and to enhance the speed of sequence data acquisition. The ostensible objective of these "next-generation" technologies is the $1,000 genome, which denotes the anticipated cost of sequencing a human genome. To date, massive parallelization has been achieved with cyclic array-sequencing approaches that array clusters, each containing millions of copies of a single PCR-amplified sequence, on a surface and then acquire hundreds of millions of sequences simultaneously using one of the non-Sanger sequencing methods described above. In addition, assemblers have been developed that efficiently and accurately construct contigs from data based on short nucleotide reads from about 25 to 200 nucleotides in length. Various strategies for sequencing single DNA molecules, such as nanopore DNA sequencing, are in the early stages of development.

REFERENCES

Alphey, L. 1997. *DNA Sequencing: from Experimental Methods to Bioinformatics.* BIOS Scientific Publishers Ltd., New York, NY.

Blazej, R. G., P. Kumaresan, and R. A. Mathies. 2006. Microfabricated bioprocessor for integrated nanoliter-scale Sanger DNA sequencing. *Proc. Natl. Acad. Sci. USA* **103:**7240–7245.

Chan, E. Y. 2005. Advances in sequencing technology. *Mutat. Res.* **573:**13–40.

Chen, E. Y., and P. H. Seeburg. 1985. Supercoil sequencing: a fast and simple method for sequencing plasmid DNA. *DNA* **4:**165–170.

Climie, S., and D. V. Santi. 1990. Chemical synthesis of the thymidylate synthase gene. *Proc. Natl. Acad. Sci. USA* **87:**633–637.

Cox-Foster, D. L., S. Conlan, E. C. Holmes, G. Palacios, J. D. Evans, N. A. Moran, P. L. Quan, T. Briese, M. Hornig, D. M. Geiser, V. Martinson, D. vanEngelsdorp, A. L. Kalkstein, A.

Drysdale, J. Hui, J. Zhai, L. Cui, S. K. Hutchison, J. F. Simons, M. Egholm, J. S. Pettis, and W. I. Lipkin. 2007. A metagenomic survey of microbes in honey bee colony collapse disorder. *Science* **318:**283–287.

Di Donato, A., M. de Nigris, N. Russo, S. Di Biase, and G. D'Alessio. 1993. A method for synthesizing genes and cDNAs by the polymerase chain reaction. *Anal. Biochem.* **212:**291–293.

Dressman, D., H. Yan, G. Traverso, K. W. Kinzler, and B. Vogelstein. 2003.

Transforming single DNA molecules into fluorescent magnetic particles for detection and enumeration of genetic variations. *Proc. Natl. Acad. Sci. USA* **100**:8817–8822.

Erlich, H. A., D. Gelfand, and J. J. Sninsky. 1991. Recent advances in the polymerase chain reaction. *Science* **252**:1643–1651.

Fakhrai-Rad, H., N. Pourmand, and M. Ronaghi. 2002. Pyrosequencing: an accurate detection platform for single nucleotide polymorphisms. *Hum. Mutat.* **19**:479–485.

Fan, J. B., M. S. Chee, and K. L. Gunderson. 2006. Highly parallel genomic assays. *Nat. Rev. Genet.* **7**:632–644.

Feng, L., W. W. Chan, S. L. Roderick, and D. E. Cohen. 2000. High-level expression and mutagenesis of recombinant human phosphatidylcholine transfer protein using a synthetic gene: evidence for a C-terminal membrane binding domain. *Biochemistry* **39**:15399–15409.

Green, R. E., J. Krause, S. E. Ptak, A. W. Briggs, M. T. Ronan, J. F. Simons, L. Du, M. Egholm, J. M. Rothberg, M. Paunovic, and S. Pääbo. 2006. Analysis of one million base pairs of Neanderthal DNA. *Nature* **444**:330–336.

Imanishi, M., Y. Hori, M. Nagaoka, and Y. Sugiura. 2001. Design of novel zinc finger proteins: towards artificial control of specific gene expression. *Eur. J. Pharm. Sci.* **13**:91–97.

Itakura, K., J. J. Rossi, and R. B. Wallace. 1984. Synthesis and use of synthetic oligonucleotides. *Annu. Rev. Biochem.* **53**:323–356.

Jarvie, T. 2005. Next generation sequencing technologies. *Drug Discov. Today: Technol.* **2**:255–260.

Jones, H. M., A. Kubo, and R. S. Stephens. 2000. Design, expression and functional characterization of a synthetic gene encoding the *Chlamydia trachomatis* major outer membrane protein. *Gene* **258**:173–181.

Ju, J., D. H. Kim, L. Bi, Q. Meng, X. Bai, Z. Li, X. Li, M. S. Marma, S. Shi,

J. Wu, J. R. Edwards, A. Romu, and N. J. Turro. 2006. Four-color DNA sequencing by synthesis using cleavable fluorescent nucleotide reversible terminators. *Proc. Natl. Acad. Sci. USA* **103**:19635–19640.

Leamon, J. H., M. S. Braverman, and J. M. Rothberg. 2007. High-throughput, massively parallel DNA sequencing technology for the era of personalized medicine. *Gene Ther. Regul.* **3**:15–31.

Levene, M. J., J. Korlach, S. W. Turner, M. Foquet, H. G. Craighead, and W. W. Webb. 2003. Zero-mode waveguides for single-molecule analysis at high concentrations. *Science* **299**:682–686.

Margulies, M., M. Egholm, W. E. Altman, S. Attiya, J. S. Bader, L. A. Bemben, J. Berka, M. S. Braverman, Y. J. Chen, Z. Chen, S. B. Dewell, L. Du, J. M. Fierro, X. V. Gomes, B. C. Godwin, W. He, S. Helgesen, C. H. Ho, G. P. Irzyk, S. C. Jando, M. L. Alenquer, T. P. Jarvie, K. B. Jirage, J. B. Kim, J. R. Knight, J. R. Lanza, J. H. Leamon, S. M. Lefkowitz, M. Lei, J. Li, K. L. Lohman, H. Lu, V. B. Makhijani, K. E. McDade, M. P. McKenna, E. W. Myers, E. Nickerson, J. R. Nobile, R. Plant, B. P. Puc, M. T. Ronan, G. T. Roth, G. J. Sarkis, J. F. Simons, J. W. Simpson, M. Srinivasan, K. R. Tartaro, A. Tomasz, K. A. Vogt, G. A. Volkmer, S. H. Wang, Y. Wang, M. P. Weiner, P. Yu, R. F. Begley, and J. M. Rothberg. 2005. Genome sequencing in microfabricated high-density picolitre reactors. *Nature* **437**:376–380.

Maxam, A. M., and W. Gilbert. 1977. A new method for sequencing DNA. *Proc. Natl. Acad. Sci. USA* **74**:560–564.

Metzker, M. L. 2005. Emerging technologies in DNA sequencing. *Genome Res.* **15**:1767–1776.

Mullis, K. B., F. Ferré, and R. A. Gibbs (ed.). 1994. *The Polymerase Chain Reaction.* Birkhäuser, Boston, MA.

Rhee, M., and M. A. Burns. 2006. Nanopore sequencing technology: research trends and applications. *Trends Biotechnol.* **24**:580–586.

Richardson, S. M., S. J. Wheelan, R. M. Yarrington, and J. D. Boeke. 2006. GeneDesign: rapid, automated design of multikilobase synthetic genes. *Genome Res.* **16**:550–556.

Rothberg, J. M., and J. H. Leamon. 2008. The development and impact of 454 sequencing. *Nat. Biotechnol.* **26**:1117–1124.

Saiki, R. K., D. H. Gelfand, S. Stoffel, S. Scharf, R. Higuchi, G. T. Horn, K. B. Mullis, and H. A. Erlich. 1988. Primer-directed enzymatic amplification of DNA with a thermostable DNA polymerase. *Science* **239**:487–491.

Saiki, R. K., S. Scharf, F. Faloona, K. B. Mullis, G. T. Horn, H. A. Erlich, and N. Arnheim. 1985. Enzymatic amplification of beta-globin genomic sequences and restriction site analysis for diagnosis of sickle cell anemia. *Science* **230**:1350–1354.

Sanger, F., S. Nicklen, and A. R. Coulson. 1977. DNA sequencing with chain-terminating inhibitors. *Proc. Natl. Acad. Sci. USA* **74**:5463–5467.

Shendure, J., and H. Ji. 2008. Next-generation DNA sequencing. *Nat. Biotechnol.* **26**:1135–1145.

Shendure, J., R. D. Mitra, C. Varma, and G. M. Church. 2004. Advanced sequencing technologies: methods and goals. *Nat. Rev. Genet.* **5**:335–344.

Shendure, J., G. J. Porreca, N. B. Reppas, X. Lin, J. P. McCutcheon, A. M. Rosenbaum, M. D. Wang, K. Zhang, R. D. Mitra, and G. M. Church. 2005. Accurate multiplex polony sequencing of an evolved bacterial genome. *Science* **309**:1728–1732.

Wheeler, D. A., M. Srinivasan, M. Egholm, Y. Shen, L. Chen, A. McGuire, W. He, Y. J. Chen, V. Makhijani, G. T. Roth, X. Gomes, K. Tartaro, F. Niazi, C. L. Turcotte, G. P. Irzyk, J. R. Lupski, C. Chinault, X. Z. Song, Y. Liu, Y. Yuan, L. Nazareth, X. Qin, D. M. Muzny, M. Margulies, G. M. Weinstock, R. A. Gibbs, and J. M. Rothberg. 2008. The complete genome of an individual by massively parallel DNA sequencing. *Nature* **452**:872–877.

REVIEW QUESTIONS

1. If your new DNA synthesizer has an average coupling efficiency of 98.5%, what overall synthesis yield would you expect after the synthesis of a 50-mer DNA hybridization probe?

2. Suggest two different strategies for synthesizing a 0.5-kb gene. Discuss the advantages and disadvantages of both methods.

3. What is a linker? How is it used?

4. What are the essential components of a PCR used to amplify a specific sequence of DNA?

5. Outline the steps in a PCR cycle.

6. Discuss the significance of long templates and short templates and their prevalence as the number of cycles increases during PCR.

7. Discuss how PCR is used to synthesize a gene.

8. What is a primer? What are the key requirements of an effective primer? Describe some of the techniques that require primers.

9. What is a dideoxynucleotide? How is it used to determine the sequence of a DNA molecule?

10. Why is it necessary to make DNA single stranded before determining its sequence?

11. Draw the autoradiograph derived from dideoxynucleotide sequencing of CCTGATCTTAGCCAT.

12. Outline the basic features of pyrosequencing.

13. How are incorporated nucleotides recognized after each cycle of sequencing by synthesis using reversible chain terminators? How does this differ from pyrosequencing?

14. How are short sequences of a DNA fragment determined using oligonucleotides and DNA ligase?

15. Describe the basic features of whole-genome shotgun sequencing.

16. What are the advantages of cycle array sequencing compared to the shotgun cloning method for large-scale sequencing?

17. Describe how a million or more copies of the same DNA molecule are attached to a single bead.

Bioinformatics, Genomics, and Proteomics

Molecular Databases

SCIENTIFIC INFORMATION IS GENERALLY PRESENTED for expert scrutiny in peer-reviewed articles that are published in professional periodicals. However, in the mid- to late 1980s, molecular biology journals were devoting more and more pages to DNA, RNA, and protein sequences derived from individually cloned genes. Moreover, anyone who wanted to conduct comparative analyses of nucleotide or amino acid sequences among related genes or proteins, as well as other kinds of analyses, had the unenviable task of typing out all the sequences from the relevant publications. The GenBank database was established in 1982 in anticipation of the increasing availability of DNA sequences. Its purpose was the collection, management, storage, and distribution of sequence data. At first, submissions to GenBank were sporadic, but almost complete compliance was achieved when many journals made database submission a prerequisite for publication. From that point on, the database became an integral part of sequence-based research. Initially, access to the GenBank database was through servers that were linked to NSFnet (National Science Foundation Network). By current standards, the original GenBank interface was primitive, and the download times were interminable. From 1990 to 1995, large-scale projects, such as genetic and physical mapping of the human genome, partial sequencing of thousands of complementary DNAs (cDNAs) (expressed sequence tags [ESTs]), and sequencing of entire genomes, required additional databases and the expansion of the existing databases for storing and retrieving information. NSFnet was replaced in 1995 by the Internet (World Wide Web). Thereafter, submissions, access, and especially retrieval (data mining) of stored molecular information became rapid and easy. The visual aspects of the online sites improved dramatically, and links among relevant databases were established. Ready access through the Internet led to the creation of specialized databases for gene-specific mutations, regulatory sequences, mitochondrial genes and functions, specific

human genetic diseases, protein–protein interactions, protein structures, gene expression data, and many other types of data (Table 5.1).

Generally, the area of research that generates, analyzes, and manages the mountains of information about genome sequences and all the genes that are transcribed in various cell types and tissues has been designated genomics. Studies of the entire protein populations of various cell types and tissues and the numerous protein–protein interactions has been dubbed proteomics. As new methods were implemented and research targets became more focused, other "omics," such as metagenomics, functional genomics (transcriptomics), and metabolomics, emerged. Generally, the suffix "omics" implies large-scale, whole-genome experimentation, with the analysis of many samples at one time. As a consequence of this high throughput, there is heavy reliance on computers and computer programs for assembling, analyzing, archiving, and distributing genomic data. Diverse computer resources have been developed to handle the various kinds of genomic information.

The amount of information generated from massively parallel experimental systems is huge. For example, since its inception, the sequence information in GenBank has been doubling every 18 months (Fig. 5.1). More specifically, after 25 years, GenBank contained more than 80 billion nucleotide bases from about 80 million sequences derived from more than 100,000 different organisms. Currently, there are more than 900 molecular databases that range from major DNA and protein sequence repositories (e.g., GenBank, Ensembl, UCSC Gene Browser, Genome Database, Universal Protein Resource, and the Ribosomal Database Project) that provide genomic and proteomic data to bibliographic and informational resources (e.g., OMIM, PubMed, RefSeq, and Gene Clinics).

Clearly, the proliferation of molecular databases would not have been possible without either high-speed computers or the programmers who develop the means whereby the information can be used by the scientific community. Because of its distinctive nature, the extensive use of computers for storage and analysis of molecular data has become known as bioinformatics. Broadly speaking, bioinformatics is the development and application of computational tools for the submission, storage, organization, archiving, acquisition, analysis, and visualization of biological and medical data. Database contents are routinely accessed through Internet sites that have tutorials (e.g., http://www.ncbi.nlm.nih.gov/Education/) with instructions for accessing the information and explanations of how to use the software tools for sequence similarity searches, gene prediction, and many other kinds of analyses. Most molecular databases are designed to meet the needs of researchers and are not meant for curious visitors. There are, however, many useful websites that provide overviews of genomics, proteomics, bioinformatics, and other related topics.

In sum, the adage "necessity is the mother of invention," which was coined by Richard Franck (1624–1708), aptly encapsulates how bioinformatics has advanced both genomic and proteomic research. Programs are written to analyze and visualize the experimental data, and accessible databases have been developed that are augmented with additional descriptive features (annotations) and linked to other sources of data to combine as much relevant material as possible. Information is now accessible that

TABLE 5.1 Types of molecular databases

Bibliographic resources
Cellular regulation
Chromosome aberrations
Comparative genomics
Gene expression
Gene identification and structure
Gene mutation
Gene sequences
Genetic and physical maps
Genetic disorders
Genomic variants
Genomic sequences
Intermolecular interactions
Metabolic pathways
Protein motifs
Protein sequences
Protein structure
Proteome resources
RNA sequences
Transgenic organisms

FIGURE 5.1 Growth of the base pair content and sequence records in the GenBank DNA database. Note that the *y* axes are logarithmic scales.

would have been impossible to obtain in the past, and importantly, novel studies can be contemplated that previously were considered impossible.

Metagenomics

For more than 100 years, the identification of microorganisms and the characterization of their biological functions have required cultivating each strain in the laboratory. In the 1990s, with the emergence of techniques to extract DNA directly from environmental samples, such as soil and seawater, researchers began to examine the sequence diversity of microorganisms using the universal 16S ribosomal RNA gene as a taxonomic marker. These studies revealed that less than 1% of all bacterial species could be cultured, and therefore, novel genes that might be of considerable interest for basic and applied research were inaccessible using methods that depended on growth of bacteria in the laboratory. Considering the wealth of biotechnologically important genes and proteins that had been obtained from the relatively few culturable microorganisms, the possibility of harvesting useful genes from the much greater number of unculturable microorganisms was exciting, if not daunting. With the development of high-efficiency cloning, robotic workstations that handle thousands of transformed cells, inexpensive DNA sequencing, microbial DNA sequence databases, and bioinformatics resources for processing, standardizing, and storing information, it has become possible to access the genomes of uncultured organisms from environmental and clinical samples. The study of the collective genomes in these samples is known as metagenomics.

The primary objective of a metagenomic project is to construct a comprehensive DNA library from all the microorganisms of a particular ecosystem or location (Table 5.2). The metagenomic clones can be characterized in various ways (Fig. 5.2). One tactic entails sequencing the entire library using the shotgun sequencing strategy with the aim of assembling contig-

uous sequences of DNA (contigs) from as many different genomes as possible and identifying both novel and homologous gene sequences. For example, a massive study that included 50 ocean samples from locations in the North Atlantic through the Panama Canal to the South Pacific yielded 6.3×10^9 bases of sequence. Analysis of the assembled and nonassembled sequences indicated that there might be as many as 400 new bacterial species among the samples, with about 1×10^6 genes that lack significant sequence similarity with any known gene. The analysis also revealed sequences encoding potentially novel forms of many proteins, including proteins for repair of ultraviolet light-induced DNA damage and RuBisCO (ribulose bisphosphate carboxylase), an enzyme that is important for carbon fixation.

Sequence-based metagenomic projects are especially effective with microbial communities that have relatively few species. For example, some bacteria are able to thrive on pyrite (iron sulfide) ore sediments and are associated with extremely acidic runoff from metal and coal mines (acid mine drainage). Not only is this acidic water (often pH <1.0) harmful to aquatic and terrestrial ecosystems, but it leaches out environmentally hazardous heavy metal contaminants, such as copper, lead, zinc, and cadmium, from the ore sediments and mine tailings. The toxic runoff often continues long after the mining operation has been abandoned. Thus, there is considerable interest in learning more about the metabolic pathways of the microorganisms found in these environments and how they survive under such conditions. This information may contribute to more effective control measures for curtailing the production of acid. In one metagenomic study of an abandoned mine site in California, the nearly complete genomes of the two major bacterial species (*Leptospirillum* group II and *Ferroplasma* type II) and partial genomes of three other microbes were cloned and assembled. Although more research is required to determine the metabolic dynamics of this microbial community, gene assignments for the different genomes indicated that a rare member of the assemblage, *Leptospirillum* group III, plays a critical role. It may be the only organism that fixes atmospheric nitrogen in this environment, and as a result, it acts as the primary source of nitrogenous compounds and ammonia for the other microorganisms.

Metagenomic libraries are frequently screened for enzyme activity to identify novel enzymes with biotechnological potential (Fig. 5.2). Selection for growth of transformed *Escherichia coli* cells on particular substrates, complementation tests, and, most often, simple indicator systems are used

TABLE 5.2 Sources of some metagenomic libraries

Abandoned metal and coal mines
Arctic plankton
Freshwater lakes and rivers
High-temperature springs and mudholes
Intestinal microbial communities from insects, humans, and mice
Marine sponges
Oceans
Sediments of all types
Sewage sludge
Soils of all types

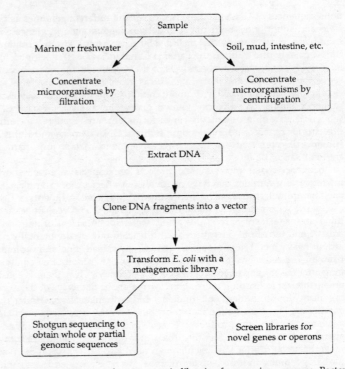

FIGURE 5.2 Construction of metagenomic libraries from various sources. Bacteria from marine or freshwater samples are concentrated by using a 0.1- to 0.8-μm-pore-size filter, and viruses are concentrated by using a <0.1-μm filter before the DNA is extracted and then fragmented. Libraries containing small DNA fragments, inserted into a plasmid, are screened for novel genes, while libraries containing larger DNA fragments, inserted into a fosmid, cosmid, or bacterial artificial chromosome vector, are screened for operons encoding protein complexes or metabolic pathways.

for these studies. In one example, a metagenomic library was screened for cloned lipase genes by growing transformed cells on agar plates that were supplemented with various triglyceride substrates, such as tricaprylin, and isolating colonies that were surrounded by a clear zone, i.e., a halo. The halo indicated that the colony produced and secreted an enzyme that digested tricaprylin. Relatively large DNA fragments (typically between 5 and 40 kilobase pairs [kb]) must be cloned to ensure that all genes encoding proteins in the pathway for catabolism of a substrate, often encoded in a polycistronic operon, are present in a transformed cell. These function-based metagenomic projects have identified a myriad of enzymes (Table 5.3).

The availability of robotic systems for maintaining and transferring transformed cells has been extremely helpful for expression-based studies, because on average, about 10^4 to 10^6 metagenomic clones must be screened to detect one or two positive colonies. However, there is an inherent limita-

tion with the host cell, usually *E. coli,* for selection schemes that depend on transcription and translation of the cloned gene. Computer modeling using codon usage and other transcription and translation features from the genes of many different microorganisms suggests that only 40% of the heterologous genes will be expressed in *E. coli.* Consequently, to increase the likelihood of identifying additional novel genes, broad-host-range vectors and other host cells are being used for constructing and maintaining metagenomic libraries.

Specialized gene expression systems aid in detecting metagenomic clones that carry genes with certain functions. One example of this type of strategy has been called substrate-induced gene expression (SIGEX) screening (Fig. 5.3). As the name suggests, this procedure identifies catabolic genes that are expressed when their promoters are activated in the presence of particular substrates and relies on the cloning of regulatory elements that are often found upstream of the catabolic genes that they control. The system utilizes a vector that contains the green fluorescent protein (*gfp*) gene under the control of the *lac* promoter (*p^{lac}*) in a pUC-based plasmid, designated p18GFP (Fig. 5.3A). The cloning site lies between the *lac* promoter and the *gfp* gene. DNA from a microbial community is fragmented and cloned into p18GFP. The cells are grown in the presence of ampicillin, to prevent the growth of untransformed cells, and IPTG (isopropyl-β-D-thiogalactopyranoside), which induces the expression of green fluorescent protein from the *lac* promoter. Cells that produce green fluorescent protein in the presence of IPTG are those that carry plasmids without inserts (i.e., self-ligated plasmids), plasmids with inserts that do not prevent transcription of *gfp* from the *lac* promoter (for example, the insert does not contain a transcriptional terminator), or plasmids with inserts containing promoters that are constitutively active. Transformed cells of interest in this procedure are those that do not produce green fluorescent protein in the presence of IPTG

TABLE 5.3 Some of the gene–encoded enzymes identified in metagenomic libraries

α-Amylases
Antibiotic resistance enzymes
Antibiotic synthesis enzymes (e.g., polyketide synthases)
Aromatic hydrocarbon catabolic enzymes
Cellulases
Chitinases
Dehydrogenases
1,4-α-Glucan branching enzymes
Lipases, esterases
Nitrilases
Oxidoreductases
Pectin lyases
Proteases
Vitamin biosynthesis enzymes
Xylanases

Relevant feature carried on metagenomic insert sequence	Response to inducer	
	IPTG	Substrate
None	GFP	ND
Constitutive promoter or *p^lac* activity not disrupted	GFP	ND
No promoter	No GFP	No GFP
Substrate-inducible promoter	No GFP	GFP

because they carry plasmids with inserts that do not induce expression of *gfp* under these conditions. To remove cells that produce green fluorescent protein in the presence of IPTG, the transformed cells are subjected to fluorescence-activated cell sorting (FACS). Briefly, FACS consists of streaming cells in single file past a laser beam that detects the excitation of a fluorochrome that is either attached to or, as in this example, inside the cell and sorts fluorescent and nonfluorescent cells into separate collection vessels (Fig. 5.3B). Accordingly, with SIGEX screening, the cells with green fluorescent protein, which fluoresces green when exposed to blue light, are separated from the cells that do not synthesize green fluorescent protein and, therefore, do not fluoresce.

The green fluorescent protein-negative cells are then grown in the presence of a low-molecular-weight substrate, for example, benzoate. The purpose of this step is to identify the metagenomic clones that carry cloned DNA segments that are required for activation of catabolic genes by the interaction of the target substrate, e.g., benzoate. Regulatory elements, including genes encoding regulatory proteins and the DNA elements that they bind to in the presence of the target substrate, are usually close to the promoter of the catabolic operon, and therefore, at least a portion of the catabolic operon is likely to also be present on the cloned segment. If a catabolic operon is activated by the substrate and transcription continues through the *gfp* gene, then green fluorescent protein will be produced. Consequently, a second round of FACS is carried out, and the cells that express green fluorescent protein in the presence of the substrate are retained (Fig. 5.3B). This procedure enables rapid, high-throughput screening of a metagenomic library with various substrates. An initial test of SIGEX with a groundwater metagenomic library yielded seven different operons that were induced by benzoate and two induced by naphthalene.

Bioinformatics systems are being developed to handle the vast amount of data derived from metagenomic projects. For example, an Internet resource that has been called CAMERA, which stands for Community Cyberinfrastructure for Advanced Marine Microbial Ecology and Analysis (http://camera.calit2.net), provides extensive sequence and ecological databases, as well as the computational tools for analyzing marine metagenomic

FIGURE 5.3 SIGEX system for isolating catabolic genes from metagenomic libraries. **(A)** A SIGEX vector, designated p18GFP, contains the *gfp* gene encoding green fluorescent protein (GFP) under the control of the IPTG-inducible promoter p^{lac} (top plasmid). Metagenomic DNA fragments are inserted into the multiple cloning site (MCS) between p^{lac} and *gfp*. If an inserted fragment contains a constitutive promoter that is active in the host cell and drives expression of *gfp* or a sequence that does not disrupt the activity of p^{lac} (e.g., a sequence carrying a transcriptional terminator), then the cells carrying these constructs will emit green fluorescence in the presence of the inducer, IPTG. If the insert carries a promoter and regulatory elements that are activated only in the presence of a substrate of interest, e.g., benzoate, and drive *gfp* expression, then these cells will emit green fluorescence when the substrate is added. ND, not determined because cells that express *gfp* in the presence of IPTG are removed in the first SIGEX screening step. **(B)** Metagenomic libraries are prepared in p18GFP and initially screened using FACS to remove clones that emit green fluorescence in the absence of a catabolic substrate. Nonfluorescent cells are collected, grown in the presence of a substrate of interest, and then screened again by FACS to identify clones that carry substrate-inducible regulatory elements. The inserts from clones that emit green fluorescence only in the presence of the substrate are analyzed to identify full or partial sequences encoding catabolic enzymes. Additional experiments may be required to isolate entire catabolic operons.

MILESTONE

Multiplexed Biochemical Assays with Biological Chips
S. P. FODOR, R. P. RAVA, X. C. HUANG, A. C. PEASE, C. P. HOLMES,
and C. L. ADAMS
Nature **364**:555–556, 1993

**Quantitative Monitoring of Gene Expression Patterns
with a Complementary DNA Microarray**
M. SCHENA, D. SHALON, R. W. DAVIS, and P. O. BROWN
Science **270**:467–470, 1995

Fodor et al. described the basic features of an oligonucleotide microarray fabricated by photolithography. In the words of the authors, "Recently, we have developed new technologies to synthesize and assay biological molecules in a miniaturized format. The method uses light to direct the combinatorial chemical synthesis of biopolymers on a solid support. The identity and location of each biopolymer is known, and its interaction with a molecular binding agent can be measured. These miniature biological arrays, or chips, can then be used for a variety of multiplexed biochemical assays...." In a later article (S. P. A. Fodor, *Science* **277**:393–395, 1997), Fodor noted that "the applications [of oligonucleotide microarrays] appear to be only limited by imagination." Over a short period, DNA microarrays have become a standard component in the tool kits of both molecular biologists and biotechnologists.

Schena et al. showed the utility of a robotic printed (spotted) cDNA microarray for analyzing gene expression on a large scale. By current standards, a 45-cDNA microarray seems modest. However, in 1995, it was a spectacular demonstration of a new technology.

In sum, although not necessarily the first articles using or describing multiple assay formats, the Fodor et al. and Schena et al. publications showed that DNA microarray platforms had come of age.

libraries. Researchers will also be able to correlate species abundance and gene frequencies with environmental and physicochemical information for a better appreciation of the dynamics of marine microbial communities. In a broader context, algorithms have been developed to detect prokaryotic gene sequences, to recognize DNA sequences that are specific for particular microbial species, and to distinguish members of known gene families. In sum, the metagenomics approach has begun to reveal an immense amount of information about the vast microbial world that barely a decade ago was considered beyond reach.

Functional Genomics

Genomics encompasses the study of all features of genomes and individual genes at the DNA level, including mutations, polymorphisms, and phylogenetic relationships that are based on sequence differences. Another aspect of genomics that is often called functional genomics (or transcriptomics) is concerned with the patterns of transcription, either qualitatively to determine which genes are expressed or quantitatively to measure changes in the levels of transcription of genes. Transcription at the whole-genome level is assessed as a function of clinical conditions, as a consequence of mutations, in response to natural or toxic agents, in different cells or tissues, or at different times during biological processes, such as cell division or the development of an organism. One of the aims of gene expression studies is to discover the genes that are up- and downregulated under specific conditions (the transcriptome). In the past, the transcription of only one or a few genes could be followed at a time. Currently, functional genomics methodology can track the simultaneous transcription of thousands of genes (gene expression profiling) of either a cell or a tissue sample. The main experimental approaches for determining gene expres-

sion profiles are DNA microarrays and serial analysis of gene expression (SAGE). Because of the large amount of data that is generated from these experiments, special computational tools are required for obtaining, storing, and analyzing the results.

DNA Microarray Technology

A DNA microarray (DNA chip, or gene chip) experiment consists of hybridizing a nucleic acid sample (target) derived from the messenger RNAs (mRNAs) of a cell or tissue to single-stranded DNA sequences (probes) that are bound in an ordered arrangement to a solid platform. One type of DNA microarray is constructed by spotting polymerase chain reaction (PCR)-amplified cDNA sequences from the mRNAs of a single cell or all or specific sets of the coding sequences of an organism onto a glass slide or nylon membrane. In this case, about 10,000 different probes can be arrayed in a 1-cm^2 area.

An alternative microarray system utilizes sets of oligonucleotides as probes, usually representing thousands of genes. For one commonly used platform, the probes are synthesized directly (in situ) on a solid surface (quartz wafer) by a light-directed process known as photolithography. Thousands of copies of an oligonucleotide with the same specific nucleotide sequence are synthesized in a predefined position (probe cell or feature) on the array surface. For this type of microarray, the probes are typically 10 to 40 nucleotides, and several probes with different sequences for each gene will be synthesized on the microarray. Longer oligonucleotides up to 100 nucleotides can also be used. A complete whole-genome oligonucleotide array may contain more than 500,000 probes representing as many as 30,000 genes.

Generally, the design of the probes (probe set) for a microarray depends on the objective of the experiment and the degree of resolution that is required. Computer programs determine probe sequences that are specific for their target sequences, are least likely to hybridize with nontarget sequences (cross-hybridize), have no secondary structure (foldback) that would prevent hybridization with the target sequence, and have similar melting (annealing) temperatures, so that all target sequences can bind to their complementary probe sequences under the same conditions. Oligonucleotide microarrays may consist of probes that represent an entire genome, a single chromosome, selected genomic regions, or selected coding regions from one or several different organisms. Repetitive sequences are not included in genomic DNA microarrays.

Typically, for most gene expression profiling experiments that utilize microarrays, mRNA is extracted from cells or tissues and purified, and cDNA is synthesized using reverse transcriptase and the extracted mRNA as a template. Usually, mRNA is extracted from two or more sources whose expression profiles are compared; for example, from diseased versus normal tissue or from cells grown under different conditions. The cDNA from each source is labeled with a different fluorophore by incorporating fluorescently labeled nucleotides during cDNA synthesis. For example, a green-emitting fluorescent dye (Cy3) is used for the normal (reference) sample and a red-emitting fluorescent dye (Cy5) for the test sample (Fig. 5.4). After being labeled, the cDNA samples are mixed and hybridized to

FIGURE 5.4 Gene expression profiling with a DNA microarray. mRNA is extracted from two samples (sample 1 and sample 2), and during reverse transcription, the first cDNA strands are labeled with the fluorescent dyes Cy3 and Cy5, respectively. The cDNA samples are mixed and hybridized to an ordered array of either gene sequences or gene-specific oligonucleotides. After the hybridization reaction, each probe cell is scanned for both fluorescent dyes and the separate emissions are recorded. Probe cells that produce only a green or red emission represent genes that are transcribed only in samples 1 and 2, respectively; yellow emissions denote genes that are active in both samples; and no emissions (black) represent genes that are not transcribed in either sample.

FIGURE 5.5 Fluorescence image of a DNA microarray hybridized with Cy3- and Cy5-labeled cDNA. Reproduced from http://biotech.biology.arizona.edu/Resources/DNA_analysis.html. Courtesy of N. Anderson, University of Arizona.

the same microarray. A laser scanner determines the intensities of Cy5 and Cy3 for each probe cell. The probe cells have different colors depending on the amounts of Cy3 and Cy5 that are present, and the ratio of red (Cy5) to green (Cy3) fluorescence intensity of a probe cell indicates the relative expression levels of the represented gene in the two samples (Fig. 5.5). To avoid variation due to inherent and sequence-specific differences in labeling efficiencies between Cy3 and Cy5, reference and test samples are often reverse labeled and hybridized to another microarray. In the above example, reverse labeling (dye swapping) would entail labeling the reference sample with Cy5 and the test sample with Cy3. Alternatively, for some microarray platforms, the target sequences from each source are labeled with the same fluorescent dye, and reference and test samples are hybridized to different microarrays.

In an alternative strategy, mRNA is purified with an oligo(dT) sequence that binds to the poly(A) tail of eukaryotic mRNA and has a short extension (T7 primer) containing the sequence for the bacteriophage T7 RNA polymerase promoter (Fig. 5.6). The oligo(dT)–T7 sequence primes the synthesis of cDNA from mRNA using reverse transcriptase. Synthesis of the second DNA strand using DNA polymerase results in double-stranded cDNA that contains the T7 RNA polymerase promoter. Next, T7 RNA polymerase is used to produce RNA copies (complementary RNA [cRNA] or antisense RNA) from the second cDNA strand as a template in the presence of biotin-labeled ribonucleotides. This reaction results in linear amplification and biotinylation of cRNA, which is then fragmented into pieces from 50 to 100 nucleotides in length that are optimal for hybridization. After hybridization, the microarray is treated with streptavidin that is bound to the fluorescent protein phycoerythrin. Streptavidin binds specifically to the biotin residues of hybridized cRNA, and hybridization can be detected by emissions from phycoerythrin that are elicited during laser scanning.

Because of the vast amount of data generated by microarray experiments, specialized software has been developed to maximize the output of information. Analyses of two-dye and one-dye hybridized microarrays are similar. A common method by which information is extracted from two-dye hybridized microarrays is summarized here. Each probe cell of a two-dye hybridized microarray is scanned using a confocal scanning microscope. Following laser excitation of the dye, fluorescence emitted from each probe cell, detected at both 532 and 635 nm for Cy3 and Cy5, respectively, is collected through the microscope's objective lens and converted to an electrical signal via a photomultiplier tube. The intensities of fluorescence emitted by both dyes for each probe cell, along with background readings for the microarray, are recorded and stored. Background fluorescence is determined by measuring the fluorescence from blank areas where probe cells have not been spotted and is subtracted from the fluorescence intensities measured for each probe cell. Microarrays are designed with internal controls, that is, specific probes that are used to evaluate the reliability of the hybridization procedure and to ensure that the laser scanner performed properly. At this stage, the microarray data (i.e., the collection of fluorescence intensities of each probe cell) is normalized to correct for variations (systematic errors) caused by technical factors that contribute to the fluorescence intensities of a probe cell and enable comparison among the microarrays of an experiment. To minimize errors, multiple probe cells for each gene are included on a single microarray, and replicate samples are independently prepared under the same conditions

Total RNA

Purification of mRNA

AAAAAAAA T7 primer
TTTTTTTT

First-strand cDNA synthesis

AAAAAAAA
TTTTTTTT

Second-strand cDNA synthesis

AAAAAAAA
TTTTTTTT

Synthesis of biotinylated cRNA

AAAAAAAA
UUUUUUUU

Purification of cRNA

UUUUUUUU

Fragmentation of cRNA

UUUUUUUU UUUUUUUU

Hybridization

Streptavidin-phycoerythrin staining
Scanning

Oligonucleotide
microarray

FIGURE 5.6 Gene expression profiling with an oligonucleotide microarray. mRNA is purified with a poly(dT) sequence that has a T7 RNA polymerase primer sequence extension. After two-stranded cDNA synthesis, the second cDNA strand acts as a template for synthesis of cRNA by T7 RNA polymerase in the presence of ATP, cytidine triphosphate (CTP), guanosine triphosphate (GTP), uridine triphosphate (UTP), biotinylated CTP, and biotinylated UTP. The gray circles represent incorporated biotinylated nucleotides. The biotinylated cRNA is purified, fragmented into pieces from 50 to 100 nucleotides in length, and hybridized to an oligonucleotide microarray. The microarray is treated with streptavidin–phycoerythrin, and the probe cells (black squares) are scanned for emission (yellow) from the biotin-bound streptavidin–phycoerythrin.

and hybridized to different microarrays. Misleading interpretations are caused, in part, by variations in sample preparation, such as growth conditions, RNA extraction, cDNA synthesis and labeling efficiencies, differences in efficiencies of hybridization of the target sequences among replicate microarrays or across a single microarray, variations in the concentrations of probes on different microarrays, or unequal amounts of target sequences applied to different microarrays or unequal distribution of targets on a single microarray. Several methods for normalization are used to calibrate the data among replicate microarrays, such as using the fluorescence intensity of a gene that is not differentially expressed under different conditions as a reference point, including spiked control sequences that are sufficiently different from the target sequences and therefore bind only to a corresponding control probe cell, and adjusting the total fluorescence intensity for each microarray to a similar value under the assumption that a relatively small number of genes are expected to change under different conditions.

One of the major purposes of a microarray experiment is to identify genes whose expression changes in response to a particular biological condition. The response to a biological condition is determined by comparing the fluorescence intensity for each gene (each probe cell), averaged among replicates, under two different conditions and calculating the ratio, commonly expressed as an n-fold change. For effective comparisons, the raw data of the dye emissions of each probe cell of a microarray are often converted to \log_2 ratios (Table 5.4). The sign indicates the dye with the higher intensity. Generally, positive log ratios represent more Cy5 than Cy3 and, therefore, greater expression of the gene in the test sample than in the reference sample. Negative values (more Cy3 than Cy5) indicate a lower level of expression in the test sample than in the reference sample. The log ratios for all probe cells are compiled into a table called an expression matrix.

Microarray analysis is also used to identify genes that are coexpressed under different conditions or over a period of time, with the goal of determining which gene products function in a given pathway. A number of computational strategies are available that organize the data into related groups (clusters). For a clear presentation of the clustered data, ranges of log ratio values are assigned arbitrary colors. Usually, black is designated for a log ratio of zero, dark to bright red for increasing positive log ratios, and dark to bright green for decreasing negative log ratios. In other words, red is frequently used to denote gene overexpression and green to denote underexpression. A visualized representation of a clustered microarray is called a gene expression profile, where the rows represent the reordered genes and the columns represent either conditions or samples (Fig. 5.7).

The gene expression profile in Fig. 5.7, determined by microarray analysis, clearly shows that different genes are transcribed in patients with cirrhosis of the liver than in healthy individuals and in patients with ethanol-induced cirrhosis than in those with cirrhosis induced by the hepatitis

TABLE 5.4 Converting Cy3 and Cy5 intensities to \log_2 ratios

Feature (gene)	Cy3 intensity	Cy5 intensity	Cy5/Cy3	\log_2(Cy5/Cy3)
1	180	10,000	56	+5.81
2	5,400	5,400	1	0
3	8,400	400	0.05	−4.39

−0.3 +0.3

log$_2$ ratio

FIGURE 5.7 Gene expression profile of cirrhotic liver tissue. Columns 1 to 7 and 8 to 15 are liver samples from patients with ethanol- and hepatitis C virus-induced cirrhosis of the liver, respectively. Each patient's sample was compared to normal liver tissue. The cluster consists of 2,965 genes. The asterisks denote patients with severe cirrhosis of the liver. Adapted from Lederer et al., *Virol. J.* **3**:98, 2006.

FIGURE 5.8 Gene expression profile of lymphocyte-specific genes from cirrhotic liver tissue. Columns 1 to 7 and 8 to 15 are liver samples from the patients shown in Fig. 5.7 with ethanol- and hepatitis C virus-induced cirrhosis of the liver, respectively. Each patient's sample was compared to normal liver tissue. The cluster consists of about 70 genes. The asterisks denote patients with severe cirrhosis of the liver. Adapted from Lederer et al., *Virol. J.* **3**:98, 2006.

C virus. Moreover, there is a difference between the genes that are turned on during advanced ethanol-induced liver damage and those in patients with less severe ethanol-induced cirrhosis (Fig. 5.7). No such distinction is evident among individuals with different severities of virus-induced cirrhosis (Fig. 5.7). In addition, information about the transcription of genes that contribute to a particular pathway or cellular activity can be extracted from a gene expression profile. For example, genes that are transcribed during lymphocyte proliferation and activation are highly expressed in virus-induced liver cirrhosis and to a much lesser extent in ethanol-associated cirrhotic samples (Fig. 5.8).

The importance and pervasiveness of DNA microarrays cannot be overstated. In 2007, for example, there were more than 13,000 published journal articles that either used this technology or described methods for enhancing data analysis. Clinical applications for DNA microarrays are being developed. The U.S. Food and Drug Administration granted permission in 2007 for the first commercial diagnostic assay based on a DNA microarray. In this case, a 70-gene expression profile (MammaPrint) distinguishes between patients with breast cancer that is likely to migrate to other sites (metastasize) and those whose cancer has a low risk of metastasis. The reliability and reproducibility of microarrays with different formats and from various laboratories have been major concerns. However, standards for both running microarray experiments and analyzing the data have been proposed by a number of international groups, which should alleviate these problems. Finally, it should be noted that in addition to gene expression studies, DNA microarrays are used to determine the binding sites for DNA-binding proteins (e.g., ChIP-on-chip assays, which use chromatin immunoprecipitation [ChIP] to identify proteins bound to a DNA microarray), the sites where the transcription of genes starts and stops, and many other aspects of genome architecture. This research has shown that a much larger proportion of the eukaryotic genome is transcribed than was previously thought; a number of genes have multiple start and termination sites, some of which are hundreds of kilobases from known sites for many genes; both strands of many genomic regions are transcribed; splicing occurs between RNA molecules; and some transcription factors bind to dozens of sites scattered throughout the genome. In short, whole-genome microarray analysis has revealed greater complexity in the processes that control transcription in a eukaryotic organism than could be predicted through smaller-scale transcriptional analyses.

Serial Analysis of Gene Expression

Unlike DNA microarrays that rely on hybridization and signal detection, SAGE uses recombinant DNA techniques to clone randomly linked short sequences of cDNA prepared from extracted cellular mRNA that can be efficiently sequenced to identify expressed genes (Fig. 5.9). Polyadenylated mRNA is captured by an oligo(dT) sequence that is labeled with biotin and attached to a streptavidin-coated magnetic bead. Double-stranded cDNA is synthesized from the purified mRNA using reverse transcriptase to synthesize the first strand of cDNA from the oligo(dT) primer and mRNA template and then DNA polymerase to synthesize the second, complementary, strand. A strong magnet is used to retain the magnetic beads with attached cDNAs during successive treatments and washings. The cDNAs are cut with the restriction endonuclease NlaIII, which recognizes the

sequence $_{GTAC}^{CATG}$ and cuts outside the G:C base pairs, leaving a 3′ GTAC extension. Since NlaIII cuts, on average, 1 in 256 base pairs (bp), there is a high probability that each cDNA will have at least one NlaIII recognition site. Because the cDNAs are bound to beads, each NlaIII cut site that is closest to the 3′ end of a cDNA is retained, and all unbound fragments are washed away. In the nomenclature developed for SAGE, NlaIII is called an anchoring enzyme. Next, the NlaIII-digested cDNA sample is divided in two. One aliquot is ligated with adaptor A and the other with adaptor B. Both adaptors have a CATG extension that is complementary to the extension produced by NlaIII digestion, a 5-bp recognition site for the restriction endonuclease BsmFI, and a sequence for priming a PCR. The adaptors have different primer sequences to prevent intrastrand base pairing (snap back) during subsequent PCR steps. After the adaptors are ligated to NlaIII-digested cDNA, the products are treated with BsmFI. Unlike NlaIII and other type II restriction endonucleases, this type IIs restriction endonuclease cuts 10 nucleotides downstream from its recognition site in one DNA strand and 14 nucleotides in the other strand regardless of the intervening nucleotide sequence. In SAGE, BsmFI is known as a tagging enzyme, and the segment of cDNA produced by the BsmFI treatment is called a tag. BsmFI digestion releases the adaptor–tag molecules from the beads into solution, from which they can be recovered. The 4-nucleotide extension of the BsmFI-cut DNA is filled in to form a blunt-end molecule, the pools of adaptor A– and adaptor B–tags are mixed, and T4 DNA ligase is added to the mixture. Under these conditions, the blunt ends of two tags are joined to form a two-tag molecule (a ditag) that is flanked by primer sequences. Since ditag formation is completely random, tags from different cDNAs are joined during ligation, and the ditags are readily amplified during PCR using primer sequences present in the adaptors. The amplified ditags are treated with NlaIII to release the adaptor sequences and produce ditags with an NlaIII extension at each end. The NlaIII-digested ditags are ligated to form multiple, randomly joined combinations (concatemers) of ditags. Concatemers that are about 500 bp in length are isolated and cloned in an *E. coli* plasmid. The concatemers are sequenced, the sequence of each tag is recorded, and a specialized "tag to gene" database is searched to identify the corresponding gene. The sequenced tag is derived from the 3′ end of the mRNA and therefore corresponds to the 3′ end of the gene. The number of times each tag is sequenced, which represents its abundance in the initial sample, is determined. Up- and downregulated mRNAs can be identified by comparing the frequencies of tags in different samples. Generally, more than 10,000 unique tags are collected from a single experiment. Over 30 million SAGE tags have been assembled from humans and another 35 million from various organisms. In principle, SAGE can detect all the transcripts in a sample, whereas with a DNA microarray, only the sequences that correspond to probes on the array are identified.

Additional SAGE protocols, such as LongSAGE and SuperSAGE, have been developed to produce longer tags (Table 5.5). Also, other anchoring enzymes, e.g., Sau3AI and other restriction endonucleases that recognize and cleave at specific 4-bp sequences (4-base cutters), have been used to identify transcribed genes that do not have a convenient NlaIII site. An online resource called SAGE Genie (http://cgap.nci.nih.gov/SAGE) is available for matching tags to likely genes, determining the frequency of a tag among various SAGE libraries, and providing other pertinent information.

FIGURE 5.9 SAGE. Poly(A)⁺ mRNA transcripts are isolated by poly(dT) hybridization. The poly(dT) sequence is biotinylated (B) and bound to streptavidin (SA)-coated magnetic beads (yellow circles), or the poly(dT) is attached directly to magnetic beads. Double-stranded cDNA is synthesized from the captured mRNAs and then cut with the restriction endonuclease NlaIII. The fragments of cDNA that are not bound to the magnetic beads are eluted. The NlaIII-cut cDNA sample that is attached to the magnetic beads is divided in two, and one sample is ligated with adaptor A and the other with adaptor B. Each adaptor contains a 4-base extension that is complementary to the 4-base extension produced by cleavage with NlaIII, a recognition site for the restriction endonuclease BsmFI, and its specific primer sequence (primer A and primer B). The ligated "adaptor–NlaIII-cut" molecules are treated with BsmFI, which cleaves the DNA 10 and 14 nucleotides downstream from its recognition site (open arrows). The extensions of the BsmFI fragments are filled in by DNA synthesis, and the mixture is blunt-end ligated. Some of the ligated molecules consist of two joined segments from different cDNAs (ditags) that are flanked by sequences for primers A and B. The ditags are amplified by PCR and then treated with NlaIII to remove the primer sequences and generate sticky ends. Ligation of NlaIII-cut ditags forms concatemers of various ditags. Concatemers with about 20 ditags (~500 bp) are purified and cloned into a plasmid vector. The concatemers are sequenced, and the individual tags are identified. The likely corresponding gene is determined by a similarity search, and the frequency of each tag in the sample is recorded.

FIGURE 5.9 *(continued)*

TABLE 5.5 Different SAGE systems

System	Tagging enzyme	Recognition site	Tag (bp)
SAGE	BsmFI	GGGAC (N)$_{10}$	10–14
		CCCTG (N)$_{14}$	
LongSAGE	MmeI	TCCRAC (N)$_{21}$	17–21
		AGGYTG (N)$_{19}$	
SuperSAGE	EcoP15I	CAGCAG (N)$_{25}$	26
		GTCGTC (N)$_{27}$	

Proteomics

Proteomics is the comprehensive study of all the proteins, i.e., the proteome, of a cell, tissue, body fluid, or organism from a variety of perspectives, including structure, function, expression profiling, and protein–protein interactions. There are a number of good reasons to study the protein complement of cells or tissues. First, proteins comprise the active component of cells. They are the molecular machines that catalyze the synthesis of important metabolites and molecules, monitor the internal and external environment of the cell and mediate responses to environmental perturbations, and make up the structural components of cells. Thus, insight into the proteins that are present in a cell or tissue under particular biological conditions can aid in our understanding of the cell's activities. Although protein-coding sequences can often be identified in genomic sequences, some annotated open reading frames (ORFs) are subsequently found not to encode proteins, and others encode proteins whose functions cannot be predicted from the sequence. Furthermore, posttranslational modifications that influence the protein function and cellular localization of proteins often cannot be predicted from the sequence. On the other hand, a protein's function can sometimes be inferred by determining the conditions under which it is expressed and active. Although expression profiles of protein-

BOX 5.1

How Many Genes Do We Have?

The exact number of genes in the human genome has been difficult to pin down. Before the release of the draft sequences of the human genome in February 2001, it was thought that we have between 80,000 and 100,000 genes. Surprisingly, estimates based on analyses of the draft sequences ranged from 23,000 to 49,000, with a consensus value of about 30,000 genes. By comparison, yeast (S. cerevisiae), fruit flies (D. melanogaster), and roundworms (C. elegans) have about 6,000, 13,600, and 20,000 genes, respectively. Considering our apparent biological complexity, it was perplexing that humans have only 50% more genes than a simple invertebrate and about as many as a tomato. To confound the gene number controversy, some researchers estimated that there were as many as 60,000, 89,000, or, quite possibly, 120,000 human genes.

Clearly, a number of questions come to mind. How are gene numbers predicted? Why do gene counts vary?

What is the likely number of human genes? What is the significance of a low gene number?

One of the obstacles to an accurate human gene count is that protein-coding genes make up only 3 to 5% of the total genome. Although it is a belabored cliché, gene counters are looking for a handful of needles hidden in a large haystack. There must be a precise identification process for any realistic tally of the total number of human genes. Unfortunately, eukaryote gene structure confounds gene enumeration. Exons are usually about 140 nucleotides and are separated by introns that may be thousands of nucleotides in length. Also, the sequences at the 5′ and 3′ ends (5′ and 3′ untranslated regions) of mRNAs are not translated and vary from gene to gene. However, there are some consistent features that aid in the identification of protein-coding regions (ORFs) and that can be readily recognized. The translation start codon ATG distinguishes the first exon at the beginning of a protein-coding gene and is preceded by a

transcription start site. At the 3′ end of most genes, there are a translation stop codon, transcription termination site, and sequence that signals poly(A) tailing. Finally, the splice sites that precede and follow the internal exons are regular motifs.

A number of gene prediction computer programs based on the common gene structures have been devised to scan the genome for possible genes. Generally, these programs are designated ab initio, which means "from the beginning" or, in the context of gene finding, an approach "based on first principles." The ab initio programs predict coding nucleotides with high accuracy and recognize exons with good efficiency but are less than 50% effective at finding complete genes. In addition, the numbers of falsely identified genes (false positives) are high.

Alignments between a comprehensive set of cDNAs and the human genome are another way of identifying genes. Full-length cDNAs, which are derived from extracted cellular mRNA, are an excellent resource

(continued)

coding sequences can be determined using transcriptomics, mRNA levels do not always correlate with protein levels, and interactions between proteins cannot be assessed by these methods. From a practical standpoint, proteomics can be used to track clinical disorders and detect targets for therapeutic treatments.

A number of factors complicate the study of proteins. First, in eukaryotes, there are many more proteins than genes due to alternative splicing, posttranslation modifications, and, to a lesser extent, posttranscriptional modifications to RNA (RNA editing). With about 60 to 70% of the estimated 30,000 human genes (Box 5.1) undergoing alternative splicing, the human proteome may consist of 85,000 or more different proteins. Second, it is impossible to account experimentally for every member of a proteome with a single technique because proteins are susceptible to degradation; have different properties, including different solubilities; and range considerably in abundance. In spite of these drawbacks, effective procedures have been devised for examining most of the components of many proteomes.

Separation and Identification of Proteins

Ordinarily, the study of the proteome of an entire multicellular organism is difficult due to the diverse functions of the many cells/tissues that comprise

BOX 5.1 *(continued)*

(continued) for finding genes because they contain all the exons of a gene. However, variation in the splicing of exons makes accurate gene identification somewhat arduous. More importantly, relatively few complete human cDNAs have been synthesized and sequenced, although techniques have been developed for capturing intact capped mRNAs. The major sources of cDNA sequences are EST databases. These cDNAs are incomplete and concentrated at the 3′ ends of the mRNAs. In addition, the databases contain about 10 to 15 ESTs for each gene. In some studies, a single representative sequence for each cDNA was determined to winnow down the overall number of cDNA sequences that would be needed for scanning genome sequences. The cDNA approach effectively locates exons. However, final gene counts are determined by combining the information about cDNA alignments with results from ab initio analyses. A number of genes are overlooked with this approach, because not all genes are represented in the cDNA databases. Also, miscounting

splice variants as a number of individual genes instead of a single gene can inflate a gene count.

Theoretically, the alignment of the complete genomic sequence of an organism, such as the mouse or puffer fish, to the entire human genome should locate highly conserved sequences that would likely be exons and regulatory elements and produce poor similarity scores for introns and the DNA between genes (intergenic DNA). The principle underlying this comparative genome strategy for gene enumeration is that introns and intergenic DNA are not under the same biological constraint as exons and regulatory regions. Thus, nucleotide changes accumulate in introns and intergenic DNA, with the result that over a long period of time, these sequences in different species diverge from one another. By contrast, the sequence similarity of exons and regulatory elements is maintained between relatively closely related organisms because gene mutations lower reproductive fitness, which makes these sequence deviations less likely to be

passed on from one generation to the next. Generally, on the basis of different gene identification strategies, we probably have about 22,000 genes.

The ENCODE (Encyclopedia of DNA Elements) project is a large collaborative effort that is dedicated to elaborating in fine detail the molecular aspects of the human genome. Some important and exciting discoveries have been made by the ENCODE pilot project, which covered about 1% of the human genome. For example, virtually all the DNA segments under study were transcribed, many coding regions have multiple transcription start sites, and, surprisingly, transcription often goes in both directions within the same segment of DNA. More studies are required to get a broader view of how the human genome functions. However, not only does the ENCODE pilot study point to more human genes being discovered, but the apparent complexity that has been observed strongly suggests that it may be necessary to redefine the current concept of the gene at the molecular level.

the organism. For convenience, the complexity is often reduced by examining the protein complement of a cellular component or organelle, such as the nucleolus, nuclear matrix, lysosome, or endoplasmic reticulum. These protein subsets have been dubbed subproteomes. Because of its high resolving power, two-dimensional polyacrylamide gel electrophoresis (2D PAGE) is frequently used to separate a population of proteins in a sample (Fig. 5.10). Briefly, the proteins in a sample are first separated on the basis of their net charge by electrophoresis through an immobilized pH gradient in one dimension (the first dimension). Amino acids in a polypeptide have ionizable groups that contribute to the net charge of a protein; the degree of ionization (protonation) is influenced by the pH of the solution. In a gel to which an electric current is applied, proteins migrate through a pH gradient until they reach a specific pH (the isoelectric point) where the overall charge of the protein is zero and they no longer move (Fig. 5.10A). However, some proteins migrate to the same position in the pH gradient because they have the same net charge, although they have different molecular weights. These are further separated according to their molecular wieghts by electrophoresis at right angles to the first dimension (the second dimension) through a sodium dodecyl sulfate-polyacrylamide gel (Fig. 5.10B). The separated pro-

FIGURE 5.10 2D PAGE for separation of proteins. **(A)** First dimension. Isoelectric focusing is performed to first separate the proteins in a mixture on the basis of their net charge. The protein mixture is applied to a pH gradient gel. When an electric current is applied, proteins will migrate toward either the anode (+) or cathode (−), depending on their net charge. As proteins move through the pH gradient, they will gain or lose protons until they reach a point in the gel where their net charge is zero. The pH in this position of the gel is known as the isoelectric point and is characteristic of a given protein. At that point, a protein no longer moves in the electric current. **(B)** Second dimension. Several proteins in a sample may have the same isoelectric point and therefore migrate to the same position in the gel in the first dimension. Therefore, proteins are further separated on the basis of differences in their molecular weights (MW) by electrophoresis, at a right angle to the first dimension, through a sodium dodecyl sulfate-polyacrylamide gel.

teins form an array of spots in the gel that is visualized by staining the spots with Coomassie blue or silver protein stain. A 2D polyacrylamide gel can resolve up to 2,000 different proteins. The pattern of stained spots is captured by densitometric scanning. Databases have been established with images of 2D polyacrylamide gels from different cell types. Software packages are available for detecting spots, matching patterns between gels, and quantifying the protein content of the spots. Proteins with either low or high molecular weights, those that are found in cellular membranes, and those that are present in small amounts are not readily resolved by 2D PAGE. Also, highly charged proteins, such as ribosomal proteins and histone proteins, are not separated by standard conditions. The next task after separation of most of the proteins of a proteome or subproteome is to excise the individual proteins from the gel, often using robotics to extract large numbers of proteins, and to identify as many of the proteins as possible. Mass spectrometry (MS) is commonly used for this purpose.

In principle, a mass spectrometer detects the mass of the ionized form of a molecule. For protein identification, proteins are fragmented into peptides that are ionized and separated according to their mass-to-charge (m/z) ratios, and then the abundances and m/z ratios of the ions are measured. The results are presented as a spectrum, with the x axis representing m/z ratios and the y axis representing the abundance of each ion relative to the most abundant ion. In practice, mass spectrometers have different configurations according to the nature (wet or dry) of the sample (analyte), the mode of ionization of the analyte, how the electric field(s) is established for accelerating the ions in order to separate and sort them, and the method for detecting the different masses. Mass spectrometric studies of proteins and peptides have been facilitated by effective ionization methods, such as electrospray ionization (ESI) and matrix-assisted laser desorption ionization (MALDI). Peptide masses are usually determined by MALDI–MS and amino acid sequences by ESI–tandem MS (ESI–MS-MS). MS is an important proteomic tool because analyses are rapid and accurate and require small amounts of starting material. Moreover, computational protocols are available for processing large amounts of MS data.

Protein identification is straightforward because particular databases can be easily searched with either peptide mass or amino acid sequence data. For whole-proteome analysis, the cellular proteins must first be separated, typically by excision of individual protein spots from a 2D polyacrylamide gel following electrophoresis. Each excised protein is then treated with the proteolytic enzyme trypsin, which cleaves on the C-terminal side of lysine and arginine residues. Contaminating salts, polyacrylamide, and other compounds are removed before the peptides are concentrated. MALDI–MS is used regularly to determine the mass (m/z value) of each peptide fragment generated from the excised protein. Briefly, peptides are ionized by mixing them with a matrix consisting of an organic acid and then using a laser to promote ionization. The ions are accelerated through a tube using a high-voltage current, and the time required to reach the ion detector is determined by their molecular masses, with lower-mass ions reaching the detector first. The values of the observed peptide masses are matched with the expected masses of tryptic peptides for all known proteins (Fig. 5.11). This type of analysis is called peptide mass fingerprinting. Online sites (e.g., http://www.expasy.ch/tools/aldente/) are available that rapidly find the set of peptide masses of a known protein that most likely corresponds to those of the unknown protein.

FIGURE 5.11 Peptide mass fingerprinting. A spot containing an unknown protein that was separated by 2D PAGE is excised from the gel and treated with trypsin. Purified trypsin peptides are separated by MALDI–time of flight (TOF) MS. The set of peptide masses from the unknown protein are used to search a database that contains the masses of tryptic peptides for every known sequenced protein, and the best match is determined. The trypsin cleavage sites of known proteins are determined from the amino acid sequence, and consequently, the masses of the tryptic peptides are easy to calculate. Only some of the tryptic peptide masses for the unknown protein are listed in this example.

Alternatively, the amino acid sequence of a peptide can be obtained by ESI–MS-MS and used to search a protein database to identify an unknown protein (Fig. 5.12). With this approach, the peptides derived from a protein spot in a 2D polyacrylamide gel are first separated by mass, and then one of the peptides is selected for sequencing. Fragmentation and ionization of a peptide occur by cleavage along the peptide backbone at amide bonds (peptide bonds) between amino acids. When the charge from ionization is retained at the N terminus, it is designated a b ion, and when it is retained at the C terminus, it is a y ion. Each ion type forms a ladder of subsequences that differ in size and consist of one, two (dipeptide), three (tripeptide), and more amino acids up to the full-length peptide. An amino acid sequence is determined from the mass values of ions of the same type (i.e., b ion or y ion) by calculating the difference in mass (Δm) between subsequences. This difference for members of a y-ion ladder represents the successive loss of an amino acid from the N terminus. For the y-ion subsequences VFDEFK, FDEFK, DEFK, EFK, FK, and K, the difference from one subsequence to the next is the removal of one amino acid from the N terminus. In other words, for amino acid sequencing, the y ions form a reverse mass ladder. The converse holds true for a b-ion spectrum. Each difference of mass is equivalent to the mass of a known amino acid, except for leucine and isoleucine, which have the same mass. For example, with part of a y-ion series, the mass/charge ratios (m/z values) for five consecutive peaks from large to small are 1,171.50, 1,056.48, 942.43, 813.39, and 684.35, and the calculated successive differences are 115.02, 114.05, 129.04, and 129.04. Thus, based on known amino acid masses, the sequence is Asp-Asn-Glu-Glu. Automated programs are available that distinguish the ion types of a scan, remove as much background noise as possible, and calculate the most likely amino acid sequence. Protein identification does not require complete sequencing of all of the peptides. Frequently, partial sequences of two or three peptides are sufficient for effective similarity searches of protein databases.

A system called shotgun proteomics that circumvents cumbersome 2D separation of proteins in a gel uses liquid chromatography combined with MS-MS (LC–MS-MS) for analyzing the proteins of a proteome. In this case, the entire mixture of proteins in a sample is initially treated with a protease. Then, the peptides are separated by LC, and the amino acid sequence of each peptide is determined by MS-MS. Finally, the proteins are identified by database searches. Hundreds and, in some cases, thousands of proteins, including those not well resolved by 2D PAGE, have been recorded for proteomes and subproteomes with this approach.

Protein Expression Profiling

Protein expression profiling is important for pinpointing changes during disease processes, cataloging differences between normal cells and cancer cells that can be used for diagnosis, and tracking cellular responses to toxic agents. Both gel and nongel methods have been developed for comparing the proteins of different samples.

2D differential in-gel electrophoresis is very similar to 2D PAGE; however, rather than separating proteins from different samples on individual gels and then comparing the maps of the separated proteins, proteins from two different samples are differentially labeled and then separated on the same 2D polyacrylamide gel. Typically, proteins of one sample are labeled with the fluorescent dye Cy3 and those of a second sample with Cy5 (Fig. 5.13); the labeled samples are mixed and then run together in the same gel,

FIGURE 5.12 Protein identification by amino acid sequencing using ESI–MS-MS. A spot containing an unknown protein from a 2D polyacrylamide gel is excised and treated with trypsin to produce peptides. The tryptic peptides are separated according to their mass/charge (*m/z*) ratios, and the amino acid sequence of a selected peptide is determined with a mass spectrometer (MS). The selected peptide is fragmented and ionized to generate a ladder of smaller peptides that differ by single amino acids (only the y-ion ladder [y1, y2, etc.] is depicted here). The differences in the masses of the fragmented peptides correspond to the characteristic masses of the amino acids. The unknown protein is identified by searching a protein database with the amino acid sequences from two or more peptides.

which overcomes the variability between separate gel runs. The two dyes carry the same mass and charge, and therefore, a protein labeled with Cy3 migrates to the same position as the identical protein labeled with Cy5. The

Cy3 and Cy5 protein patterns are visualized separately by fluorescence excitation. The images are compared, and any differences are recorded. In addition, the ratio of Cy3 to Cy5 fluorescence for each spot is determined to detect proteins that are either up- or downregulated. Unknown proteins are identified by MS.

The isotope-coded affinity tag (ICAT) method combined with LC–MS-MS is another way of comparing proteins from different sources (Fig. 5.14). An ICAT reagent consists of an affinity tag (biotin), a carbon chain (mass-encoded linker) that is labeled with either eight hydrogen (light form; H) or eight deuterium (heavy form; D) atoms, and a chemical

FIGURE 5.13 The 2D differential in-gel electrophoresis method for quantitative analysis of protein expression. The proteins of two proteomes are labeled with the fluorescent dyes Cy3 and Cy5, respectively. The fluorescence-labeled samples are combined and separated by 2D PAGE. The gel is scanned for each fluorescent dye, and the relative levels of the two dyes in each protein spot are recorded. The gel is stained with a protein dye, and each spot with an unknown protein is excised and treated with trypsin. The peptides are separated by ESI–MS-MS, and the amino acid sequences of some selected peptides are determined. The protein is identified by searching a protein database for a likely match with amino acid sequences from two or more peptides.

group that covalently binds to an amino acid, usually cysteine. Deuterium is a stable isotope of hydrogen that is twice its mass, i.e., 2 daltons. Thus, the mass difference between a peptide that is labeled with a light and a heavy ICAT is 8 daltons. This difference is readily detected by MS.

The proteins of one proteome are labeled with a light ICAT and those of another with a heavy ICAT. The samples are mixed, treated with trypsin, fractionated, and passed through an avidin column to capture biotin, which is present only on ICAT-labeled peptides (both the light and heavy versions). The purified ICAT-labeled peptides are separated by LC before their introduction into a mass spectrometer. The key feature of this technique is that the same ICAT-labeled peptides from the two samples produce a pair of signals with a defined difference in mass due to the light and heavy versions of the labels. The relative amounts of each pair of light and heavy peptides reflect the relative abundances of the source proteins in the original samples. Finally, with ESI–MS-MS, the amino acid sequences of the peptides are determined, and the proteins that match the sequences can be identified. Hundreds of proteins from different samples can be compared in this way.

Protein Microarrays

Conceptually, protein microarrays are similar to DNA microarrays; however, rather than arrays of oligonucleotides or genes, protein microarrays consist of large numbers of proteins individually immobilized in known positions on the coated surface of a glass slide or silicon chip. The proteins arrayed on the surface can be antibodies specific for each protein in an organism, purified recombinant proteins, or short synthetic peptides. There are many ways of attaching a protein to a support surface. The major objective of any coupling system is maintenance of protein structure and function. Some systems bind the proteins to a chemical group that coats the surface of the support. With other protocols, recombinant proteins are prepared with a short amino acid sequence (tag) at the N or C terminus that binds to a recognition sequence on the support. In this case, all the protein molecules are uniformly oriented. In addition, instead of spotting proteins on a flat surface, some microarrays are engineered with tiny depressions (nanowells) that keep each protein moist and prevent mixing with adjacent proteins.

The purpose of protein microarray analyses, for the most part, is to detect, on a large scale, the molecules that a protein interacts with. These interacting molecules can be other proteins, nucleic acid sequences, or low-molecular-weight compounds. Protein populations from different samples can be compared, for example, in control versus treated samples or in normal versus diseased tissues. There are a number of methods for visualizing the interactions on protein microarrays. One common approach is to label the test samples directly with a fluorescent dye and then detect the labeled molecules that bind to the proteins of a microarray with a laser scanner (Fig. 5.15A). A two-dye strategy (e.g., Cy3 or Cy5), similar to that employed for DNA microarray analyses, can be used to compare proteins in two different samples on a single array. "Sandwich style" assays are also performed (Fig. 5.15B). Briefly, proteins in a sample are biotinylated and applied to the microarray. After the microarrays are washed to remove unbound proteins, streptavidin with a conjugated fluorescent dye is added, and the sample proteins that bind to the proteins on the microarray are

FIGURE 5.14 ICAT method for quantitative analysis of protein expression. **(A)** Schematic representation of an ICAT reagent. An ICAT reagent has either all hydrogen (H) or deuterium (D) atoms at sites (X) of a linker sequence. **(B)** ICAT protocol. Proteins are extracted from two proteomes, and one proteome is labeled with the light (H) hydrogen-only ICAT reagent and the other with the heavy (D) deuterium-only ICAT reagent. The samples are combined and treated with trypsin. The ICAT-labeled peptides are captured by affinity chromatography using avidin, which binds to biotin, and fractionated by LC. The ratio of light to heavy (H:D) versions of the same peptide is determined by MS, which provides an estimate of the relative amounts of the protein in the two proteomes. The protein represented by a pair of heavy and light peptides is identified by amino acid sequencing with ESI–MS-MS and searching a protein database with this sequence for a likely match.

detected by laser scanning. In principle, the interpretation of the signals from a protein microarray is very similar to analysis of DNA microarrays.

Broadly speaking, there are three types of protein microarrays: analytical (capture), reverse phase, and functional. Analytical microarrays are used for protein profiling, that is, the detection and quantification of proteins present in a sample, and consist of either protein samples applied to immobilized antibodies or antibody samples applied to immobilized proteins. Antibody microarrays are often probed with proteins from biological sources, such as serum or plasma, or proteins that are secreted from cells in culture to determine disease-specific profiles. For example, antibody microarrays that specifically detect cytokines have been formulated. Cytokines, of which there are a large number, are small, secreted proteins (signaling proteins) that mediate and regulate immune and inflammatory responses, cell death (apoptosis), cell growth, blood vessel formation, and differentiation in humans and other animals. Cytokine antibody microarrays are used to examine cytokines in both normal and diseased states and from a variety of sources after various treatments. A sandwich immunoassay is often used to detect cytokines that bind to immobilized antibodies (Fig. 5.16). After the microarray is treated with a sample containing cytokines, biotinylated cytokine antibodies are added. A biotinylated cytokine antibody will bind to a cytokine that is bound to an immobilized antibody. Streptavidin with an attached fluorescent dye is added next. Then, the signals are detected with a laser scanner and the data are analyzed.

In one study, plasma samples from individuals with Alzheimer disease and those from individuals with no dementia were applied to a microarray made up of antibodies against 120 cytokines. Eighteen cytokines were found to be associated with Alzheimer disease. The levels of 7 of these were

FIGURE 5.15 Protein microarray detection methods. **(A)** Direct labeling. The sample molecules are labeled with a detector reagent, e.g., fluorescent dye. **(B)** Sandwich style assay. The sample molecules are biotinylated, and after the initial incubation, a streptavidin–fluorescent-dye conjugate that binds to biotin to facilitate the detection of sample molecules is applied.

FIGURE 5.16 Detection of cytokines with a cytokine antibody microarray. A cytokine antibody microarray **(1)** is incubated with a sample, and cytokines (solid circles) bind to specific antibodies **(2)**. Free biotinylated cytokine antibodies are added and bind to the corresponding captured cytokine **(3)**. For visualization, a streptavidin–fluorescent-dye conjugate attaches to the biotin of the secondary antibody **(4)**.

higher and 11 were lower in individuals with Alzheimer disease than in the subjects without dementia. The Alzheimer disease-associated cytokines adversely affect blood cell formation, immune responses, apoptosis, and nerve cell signaling. The Alzheimer disease cytokine pattern was also present in individuals with mild cognitive impairment. Currently, there is no definitive method for either predicting Alzheimer disease or determining whether a patient has the disease. Possibly, the Alzheimer disease-specific cytokine signature may provide the basis for a diagnostic test for this degenerative disease that afflicts more than 4 million people in the United States.

In another type of analytical microarray, proteins (antigens) are attached to a solid support and then probed with antibodies, mostly in serum samples. The purpose of these studies is to discover whether the production of antibodies against specific proteins correlates with particular diseases or biological processes. By way of illustration, a microarray with about 5,000 different human proteins was created and used to determine if

serum from ovarian cancer patients has a distinctive set of antibodies in comparison to the antibody population of healthy individuals. The initial results revealed 94 proteins that were specifically recognized by antibodies in the sera from the ovarian cancer patients. With further testing, three proteins were consistently found to be specific for ovarian cancer. The earlier ovarian cancer is diagnosed, the better the chance of survival. Unfortunately, ovarian cancer is currently identified in a late stage. The ovarian-cancer-specific proteins may help in the early detection of the disease.

Antibody microarrays have also been used to determine whether particular posttranslational protein modifications, such as phosphorylation of tyrosine or glycosylation, are associated with specific diseases. To screen for proteins that contain phosphotyrosine, proteins are first captured by primary antibodies immobilized on a microarray, and then the microarray is flooded with biotinylated anti-phosphotyrosine antibody. Next, streptavidin conjugated with a fluorescent dye is added, and the protein spot with the fluorescence is detected (Fig. 5.17A). In a similar manner, glycosyl groups (glycans) present on proteins can be visualized by adding a biotinylated lectin to proteins that are bound to immobilized antibodies on an array (Fig. 5.17B). Lectins are plant glycoproteins that bind to specific carbohydrate moieties on the surfaces of proteins or cell membranes, and many different lectins with affinities for different glycans are available. The use of lectins can facilitate the detection of specific protein glycosylation patterns.

The utility of antibody microarrays has been enhanced by the expansion of libraries that produce highly specific antibodies. For example, clones making antibodies against more than 1,800 human proteins have been isolated, characterized, and validated. The long-term objective of this project is to have available one antibody for each protein from every coding sequence in the human genome, that is, a total of about 22,000 antibodies.

With a reverse-phase microarray, a multiprotein sample, for example, from a cell lysate or tissue specimen, is immobilized in a single spot on a support. Several such multiprotein samples are spotted on the microarray, which is then probed with a single target molecule. This format contrasts with analytical and functional microarrays, in which immobilized spots containing single proteins are probed with multiple targets; hence, the term "reverse" is used. The advantage of the reverse-phase microarray is that a large number of samples can be compared at one time. With a reverse-phase microarray, the presence of specific proteins in multiple complex samples can be readily determined (Fig. 5.18).

Functional protein microarrays feature large sets of individual proteins that are used predominately to determine interactions with other proteins or low-molecular-weight compounds, such as lipids, drugs, and metabolites (Fig. 5.19). Enzymes, such as oxidoreductases, kinases, proteases, and glycosidases, with novel activities that are useful for biotechnology and medicine are likely to be discovered using functional microarrays. Ideally, a functional protein microarray should consist of all possible proteins of a proteome under study. To obtain comprehensive representation of a proteome, a library containing all of the protein coding sequences is first constructed. The term ORF, which stands for open reading frame, is used to represent any protein-coding sequence, and a library of cloned protein-encoding ORFs has been dubbed an ORFeome. Large-scale expression of

FIGURE 5.17 Detection of post-translational modifications with antibody microarrays. **(A)** Detection of tyrosine phosphorylation. An antibody microarray (1) is incubated with a protein sample (2). Biotinylated phosphotyrosine antibody is added (3), and for visualization, a streptavidin–fluorescent-dye conjugate attaches to the biotin of the phosphotyrosine antibody (4). **(B)** Detection of glycan groups. An antibody microarray (1) is incubated with a protein sample (2). A biotinylated molecule (e.g., lectin) that binds to a specific glycan is added (3), and for visualization, a streptavidin–fluorescent-dye conjugate attaches to the biotin of the lectin (4).

the library is followed by purification of each of the proteins, which are subsequently arrayed on a solid support.

The starting point for producing an ORFeome is usually PCR amplification of the coding sequences for cloning into a vector. For prokaryotic organisms, the protein-coding sequences can often be readily identified from genomic sequences. On the other hand, full-length cDNA libraries are the primary sources of the coding sequences of a eukaryotic proteome.

FIGURE 5.18 Reverse-phase microarray format. Multiprotein samples, e.g., cell lysates, are spotted on a solid support (1) and incubated with a known biotinylated antibody (2). A streptavidin–fluorescent-dye conjugate is used to identify samples with bound antibody (3).

A rapid and versatile system for efficient cloning of PCR-generated ORFs without costly and time-consuming restriction endonuclease and ligation reactions is known as recombinational cloning (also known as Gateway cloning technology) and exploits the bacteriophage λ system for integration and excision of viral DNA into the host bacterial genome. Briefly, as background for understanding recombinational cloning, the integration of bacteriophage λ in the *E. coli* chromosome requires a specific attachment sequence in the bacteriophage genome (243-bp *at*tachment *p*hage [*attP*] site) and another sequence in the bacterial genome (25-bp *at*tachment *b*acteria [*attB*] site), plus an *E. coli*-encoded protein called integration host factor and the bacteriophage λ recombination protein integrase (Fig. 5.20A). Recombination between the *attP* and *attB* sequences results in insertion of the phage genome into the bacterial genome to create a prophage with the attachment sites *attL* (100 bp) and *attR* (168 bp) at the left and right ends of the integrated bacteriophage λ DNA, respectively. For subsequent excision of the bacteriophage λ DNA from the bacterial chromosome, recombination between the *attL* and *attR* sites is mediated by integration host factor, integrase, and bacteriophage λ excisionase (Fig. 5.20B). The recombination events occur at precise locations without either the loss or gain of nucleotides.

For recombinational cloning, bacterial λ attachment sites are added to each ORF during PCR amplification. The PCR primers carry modified *attB* sequences that recombine only with specific *attP* sequences. For example, *attB1* recombines only with *attP1*, and *attB2* recombines with *attP2*. One of the primers has the *attB1* sequence, and the other primer has *attB2* (Fig. 5.21). If required, translation start and termination codons can be added to

FIGURE 5.19 Functional protein microarray platform. The individual proteins of a functional protein microarray can be examined for interactions with proteins, lipids, and drugs, among other compounds, and tested for substrate binding and enzyme activities. Here, for convenience, direct labeling of the input sample is depicted as the detection method. However, there are a variety of visualization protocols for different types of samples.

an ORF by including the corresponding nucleotides on the PCR primers. A nucleotide sequence that encodes a short amino acid sequence (affinity tag) that is in frame with each ORF is also included on one of the primers. The affinity tag enables a protein to be selectively purified and may be added to the N and/or C terminus of the protein. Another short sequence encoding an in-frame peptide provides a cut site that is used to remove the affinity tag after the protein is purified.

Following amplification of a specific ORF by PCR using the primer pair, the PCR products carrying the ORF with flanking *attB1* and *attB2*

FIGURE 5.20 Integration **(A)** and excision **(B)** of bacteriophage λ into and from the *E. coli* genome via recombination between attachment (*att*) sites in the bacterial and bacteriophage DNAs.

sequences are mixed with a vector (donor vector) that has *attP1* and *attP2* sites flanking a negative selection gene (*ccdB*) (Fig. 5.22A). When present and expressed, the product of the *ccdB* gene interferes with DNA replication and is toxic to bacterial cells. Integration host factor and integrase are added to the mixture of DNA molecules to catalyze in vitro recombination between the *attB1* and *attP1* sites and between the *attB2* and *attP2* sites. As a consequence of the two recombination events, the *ccdB* gene sequence between the *attP1* and *attP2* sites on the donor vector is replaced by the ORF. The recombination events create new attachment sites flanking the ORF sequence (designated *attL1* and *attL2*), and the plasmid with the *attL1*-ORF-*attL2* sequence is referred to as an entry clone. The mixture of original and recombinant DNA molecules is transformed into *E. coli,* and cells that are transformed with donor vectors that have not undergone recombination retain the *ccdB* gene and therefore do not survive. Host cells carrying the entry clone are positively selected by the presence of a selectable marker. This procedure is repeated to clone each of the ORFs in the proteome.

The next step to obtain functional proteins is the expression of each cloned ORF. For expression, the ORF is transferred from the entry vector to a destination vector that carries a promoter and other expression signals. An entry clone is mixed with a destination vector that has *attR1* and *attR2* sites flanking a *ccdB* gene (Fig. 5.22B). In the presence of integration host factor, integrase, and bacteriophage λ excisionase, the *attL1* and *attL2* sites on the entry clone recombine with the *attR1* and *attR2* sites, respectively, on the destination vector. This results in the replacement of the *ccdB* toxin gene on the destination vector with the ORF from the entry clone, and the resultant plasmid is designated an expression clone. The reaction mixture is transformed into *E. coli,* and a selectable marker is used to isolate transformed cells that carry an expression clone. Cells that carry an intact destination vector or the exchanged entry plasmid (known as a by-product plasmid) will not survive because they carry the *ccdB* gene. Destination vectors are available for maintenance and expression of the ORF in various host cells, such as *E. coli* and yeast, insect, and mammalian cells. For construction of a microarray, each protein encoded by an ORF is isolated by affinity purification using the affinity tag that was encoded on the initial

FIGURE 5.21 Primer pair used to amplify ORFs for recombinational cloning to generate an ORFeome.

FIGURE 5.22 Recombinational cloning. **(A)** Recombination (thin vertical lines) between a PCR-amplified ORF with attachment sites *(attB1* and *attB2)* and a donor vector with *attP1* and *attP2* sites on either side of the *ccdB* gene results in an entry clone in which the ORF is flanked by *attL1* and *attL2* sites. The selectable marker (SM1) selects transformed cells with an entry clone. The protein encoded by *ccdB* is toxic to transformed cells with nonrecombined donor vector molecules. The origin of replication of the donor vector is not shown. **(B)** Recombination (thin vertical lines) between the entry clone with *attL1* and *attL2* sites and a destination vector with *attR1* and *attR2* sites results in an expression clone with *attB1* and *attB2* sites flanking the ORF. The selectable marker (SM2) selects transformed cells with an expression clone. The second plasmid, designated a by-product, has the *ccdB* gene flanked by *attP1* and *attP2* sites. Cells with an intact destination vector that did not undergo recombination or that retain the by-product plasmid are killed by the CcdB protein. Transformed cells with an entry clone, which lacks the SM2 selectable marker, are selected against. The origins of replication and the sequences for expression of the ORF are not shown.

PCR primer used to amplify the ORFs (Fig. 5.21). Protocols have been developed to isolate thousands of proteins in parallel to facilitate the creation of proteomic microarrays.

Protein–Protein Interaction Mapping

Proteins seldom act alone. On average, one protein interacts with five others. Some protein–protein interactions are short-lived, others form

FIGURE 5.23 Two-hybrid assay for detecting pairwise protein interactions. **(A)** The DNA-binding domain of a transcription factor binds to a specific sequence in the regulatory region of a gene, which orients and localizes the activation domain that is required for the initiation of transcription of the gene by RNA polymerase. **(B)** The coding sequences for the DNA-binding domain and the activation domain are fused to DNA X and DNA Y, respectively, and both constructs (hybrid genes) are introduced into a cell. After translation, the DNA-binding domain–protein X fusion protein binds to the regulatory sequence of a reporter gene. However, protein Y (prey) does not interact with protein X (bait), and the reporter gene is not transcribed because the activation domain does not, on its own, associate with RNA polymerase. **(C)** The coding sequence for the activation domain is fused to the DNA for protein Z (DNA Z) and transformed into a cell containing the DNA-binding domain–DNA X fusion construct. The proteins encoded by the cDNAs of the hybrid genes interact, and the activation domain is properly oriented to initiate transcription of the reporter gene, demonstrating a specific protein–protein interaction.

stable multicomponent complexes, and at a higher level of cellular organization, complexes interact with one another. Determining the functional interconnections among the members of a proteome is not an easy task. The strategies for examining protein–protein interactions on a large scale require a number of experimental manipulations, with no guarantee that all potential interactions will be recognized. Notwithstanding the limitations of existing protocols, thousands of protein–protein interactions for proteomes of single-celled and multicellular organisms have been catalogued.

The two-hybrid method that was originally devised for studying the yeast proteome has been used extensively to determine pairwise protein–protein interactions in both eukaryotes and prokaryotes. The underlying principle of this assay is that the physical connection between two proteins reconstitutes an active transcription factor that initiates the expression of a reporter gene. Generally, transcription factors have two domains. One region is required for binding to a specific DNA site (DNA-binding domain), and the other region activates transcription (activation domain) (Fig. 5.23A). These two domains need not be part of the same protein to function as an effective transcription factor. However, the activation domain alone will not bind to RNA polymerase to activate transcription. Connection with the DNA-binding domain is necessary to place the activation domain in the correct orientation and location to initiate transcription by RNA polymerase.

For a two-hybrid system, the coding regions of the DNA-binding and activation domains of a specific transcription factor are isolated and cloned into separate vectors. Often, the Gal4 transcriptional factor from *Saccharomyces cerevisiae* or the bacterial LexA transcription factor is used. A cDNA sequence is cloned in frame with the DNA-binding domain sequence to form a fusion gene that produces a hybrid protein. A protein attached to the DNA-binding domain is called the "bait," or target. This is the target protein for which interacting proteins are to be identified. Another cDNA sequence is cloned adjacent to the activation domain coding sequence. A protein attached to the activation domain is called the "prey" and potentially interacts with the target, or bait, protein. Host cells are transformed with both bait and prey DNA constructs. After expression and translation, if the bait and prey do not interact, then there is no transcription of the reporter gene (Fig. 5.23B). However, if the reporter gene is transcribed, then a physical connection occurred between the bait and prey proteins that brought the DNA-binding and activation domains together and enabled the activation domain to make contact with RNA polymerase (Fig. 5.23C). In other words, there was a specific interaction between the bait and prey proteins. The product of an active reporter gene may either allow a host cell to proliferate in a specific medium or produce a colorimetric response.

A variant of the two-hybrid system has been developed for studying protein interactions in mammalian cells. With this scheme, two genetically altered subunits, α and ω, of an indicator enzyme (β-galactosidase) are unable to associate under normal cellular conditions, and as a result, there is no β-galactosidase activity (Fig. 5.24A). cDNAs are cloned in frame with

FIGURE 5.24 Complementation assay for detecting pairwise protein interactions in mammalian cells. **(A)** Proteins α and ω must combine to produce an active enzyme but are not able to interact spontaneously due to mutations. **(B)** DNA fusion constructs of the gene encoding protein α (gene α) with a cDNA (cDNA X) and the gene encoding protein ω (gene ω) with a cDNA (cDNA Y) are introduced into a cell. Since proteins X (bait) and Y (prey) do not interact, proteins α and ω do not associate, and the activity specified by the α:ω combination is not observed. **(C)** DNA fusion constructs of the gene encoding protein α (gene α) with a cDNA (cDNA X) and the gene encoding protein ω (gene ω) with a cDNA (cDNA Z) are introduced into a cell. Proteins X and Z interact, bringing together proteins α and ω, and the activity specified by the α:ω combination is observed.

A

B

C

the genes for proteins α and ω, and the constructs are tested by transforming both into a mammalian cell (Fig. 5.24B and C). If two cDNA-encoded proteins interact, then proteins α and ω are brought into close proximity, and the formation of a functional β-galactosidase is detected with a colorimetric assay (Fig. 5.24C).

As a first step in a large-scale protein–protein interaction study, two libraries are prepared, each containing thousands of cDNAs generated from total cellular mRNA (or genomic DNA fragments in a study of proteins from a prokaryote). In one case, the cDNAs are cloned into the vector adjacent to the DNA sequence for the DNA-binding domain of the transcription factor Gal4 to form a library of hybrid bait genes. In the other case, the cDNAs are cloned into a different vector containing the sequence for the activation domain to form the prey library. The libraries are typically screened for bait–prey protein interactions in one of two ways. In one method, a library of yeast cells containing the prey–activation domain constructs is arrayed on a grid. The library is then screened for the production of proteins that interact with a hybrid bait protein by introducing individual bait–DNA-binding domain constructs to the arrayed clones by mating (Fig. 5.25A). Alternatively, each yeast clone in a bait library is mated en masse with a mixture of strains in the prey library, and then positive interactions are identified by screening for activation of the reporter gene (Fig. 5.25B). Challenges with using the two-hybrid system for large-scale determination of protein–protein interactions include the inability to clone all possible ORFs in the libraries in frame with the activation and DNA-binding domains, which leads to missed interactions (false negatives) and the detection of interactions that do not normally occur in their natural environments within the original cells and therefore are not biologically relevant (false positives). Nonetheless, this approach has been used to successfully identify interacting proteins in several organisms, including bacteria, viruses, yeast, the fruit fly *Drosophila melanogaster*, the roundworm *Caenorhabditis elegans*, and humans.

Many schemes have been devised to streamline the acquisition of results. Regardless of the protocol, vast numbers of interactions are scored. Specialized computer programs are required to categorize and map all the relationships. As part of this analysis, stringent statistical criteria are used to minimize the numbers of possible false-positive interactions in the final data set. With *D. melanogaster*, an overall protein interaction (interactome) map of 3,000 interactions with 3,522 proteins was delineated. In addition, the nuclear, cytoplasmic, and extracellular locations of 2,268 interactions with 2,346 proteins were mapped. Finally, smaller interacting sets of proteins within cellular regions were noted (Fig. 5.26). Another study with *Drosophila* revealed 710 protein–protein interactions with 641 proteins. Surprisingly, there was little congruence between the two studies. Clearly, the technical reasons for this difference need to be determined. A network of 5,500 protein interactions was constructed for *C. elegans*, and a similar number was determined for *S. cerevisiae*. Protein interaction maps place proteins with unknown functions into contexts that provide clues about

FIGURE 5.25 Large-scale screens for protein interactions using the yeast two-hybrid system. Two libraries are prepared, one containing genomic DNA fragments or cDNAs fused to the coding sequence for the DNA-binding domain of a transcription factor (bait library) and another containing genomic DNA fragments or cDNAs fused to the activation domain of the transcription factor (prey library). Two methods are commonly used to screen for pairwise protein interactions. **(A)** Individual yeast strains in the bait library are mated with each yeast strain in an arrayed prey library. The resulting strains in the array that produce bait and prey proteins that interact are detected by assaying for reporter gene activation (activated cells growing in a multiwell plate are indicated in green). **(B)** Yeast strains in the prey library are mated en masse with individual strains in the bait library. The mixture of strains is screened for reporter gene activity, which identifies strains with interacting bait and prey proteins (green).

A

Individual yeast strain
from bait library

Arrayed prey library

Mate with each yeast
strain in arrayed library

Reporter gene
activation indicates
yeast strains with
interacting bait and
prey proteins

B

Individual yeast strain
from bait library

Mixture of yeast strains
containing prey library

Mate with mixture of yeast
strains in prey library

Reporter gene
activation indicates
yeast strains with
interacting bait and
prey proteins

Cell surface transporters

Calmodulin-
binding
proteins

Calmodulin and
related proteins

Calmodulin-dependent phosphatases

FIGURE 5.26 Protein interaction map of calcium signaling protein clusters of *D. melanogaster*. Individual proteins (solid circles) are not named. The thickness of a connecting line denotes the extent of the interaction rating. Adapted from Giot et al., *Science* **302**:1727–1736, 2003.

their roles in cellular processes and identify proteins with multiple functions.

Instead of studying pairwise protein interactions, the tandem affinity purification (TAP) tag procedure is designed to capture multiprotein clusters and then identify the components by MS (Fig. 5.27). In this case, a cDNA sequence that encodes the target (bait) protein is fused to a DNA sequence that encodes two short amino acid sequences (tags). An amino acid sequence tag binds with high affinity to a specific molecule and facilitates purification of the target protein. A "two-tag" system allows two successive rounds of affinity binding to ensure that the target and its associated proteins are free of any nonspecific proteins. Alternatively, a "one-tag" system with a small protein tag that is immunoprecipitated with a specific antibody requires only a single purification step. In a number of trials, the tags did not alter the functions of various test proteins.

A cDNA–two-tag construct is introduced into a host cell, where it is expressed, and a tagged protein is synthesized. The underlying assumption is that the cellular proteins that normally interact with the native protein in vivo will also combine with the tagged protein. After the cells are lysed, the target protein and any interacting proteins are purified using the affinity tags. The proteins of the cluster are separated according to their molecular weights by PAGE. Individual bands are excised and treated with trypsin, and the proteins are identified by MS. Computer programs are available for generating maps of clusters with common proteins, assigning proteins with shared interrelationships to specific cellular activities, and establishing the links between multiprotein complexes.

FIGURE 5.27 TAP tag procedure for detecting protein–protein interactions. Two DNA sequences (tag 1 and tag 2), each encoding a short amino acid sequence with high affinity for a specific molecule, are cloned together and fused in frame to the 3' end of the coding region of a cDNA (cDNA X). The tagged cDNA construct is introduced into a host cell, where it is transcribed and the mRNA is translated. Other cellular proteins bind to the protein encoded by cDNA X (protein X). The cluster consisting of protein X and its associated proteins is separated from cell components (squares) by the binding of tag 1 to its affinity partner, which is usually fixed to a column that retains the cluster while allowing all noninteracting proteins to flow through. The cluster is eluted from the affinity partner, typically by cleaving off tag 1, and a second purification step is carried out with tag 2 and its affinity partner. The proteins of the cluster are separated by one-dimensional PAGE. Single bands are excised from the gel and treated with trypsin. The protein represented by the tryptic peptides is identified by either peptide mass fingerprinting or searching a protein database with peptide amino acid sequences obtained with ESI–MS-MS.

SUMMARY

Bioinformatics grew as a field of study, for the most part, from the efforts to maintain, organize, analyze, and make accessible large amounts of gene and genomic sequence information. GenBank, a gene sequence database, was established in the early 1980s to cope with the influx of DNA sequences in the scientific literature. By the mid-1990s, a myriad of databases had been developed for genomic sequences, genetic and physical maps, ESTs, and many other types of molecular data. The expansion of the Internet and the availability of browsers led to enhanced pictorial presentation of information stored in databases, and the development of computational tools enabled rapid searching of DNA or protein databases with query sequences and other kinds of sequence analyses. Currently, there are hundreds of public online molecular databases.

Metagenomics is the study of the genome sequences of a complex population of microorganisms. DNA consisting of many different microbial genomes can be extracted directly from environmental samples and sequenced, and the sequences of as many complete genomes as possible can be assembled and analyzed. With sequence database comparisons, the organisms are placed among their phylogenetic relatives, if any exist. By determining the genetic capacities of annotated sequences, physiological profiles can be predicted for organisms that cannot currently be grown in the laboratory. Moreover, variations in the nucleotide sequences of various genes are determined to discover proteins with unusual, and potentially useful, characteristics.

The expression of thousands of genes in cells or tissues can be tracked simultaneously by hybridization of target sequences in extracted cellular mRNA to the bound probes of cDNA or oligonucleotide microarrays. DNA microarrays are used to quantify differences in gene expression among samples, such as between diseased and normal tissues or mutant and wild-type cells, and among cells exposed to different internal or external conditions. Diagnostic tests based on DNA microarray patterns are being developed that detect the expression of genes known to be associated with a diseased state (molecular markers). SAGE relies on sequence information from short segments at the ends of cDNAs derived from a population of mRNAs to assess which genes are up- or downregulated under various conditions.

The comprehensive study of all the proteins of a cell, tissue, body fluid, or organism, i.e., a proteome, is called proteomics. High-throughput methods have been developed to identify most members of a proteome, compare the levels of individual proteins among proteomes, and characterize thousands of

protein–protein interactions within a proteome. There are two main ways of obtaining comparative protein expression profiles. With these approaches, proteomes from two different sources are mixed and analyzed together. For 2D differential in-gel electrophoresis, the proteins of two samples are labeled with two different fluorescent dyes and separated by 2D PAGE. Then, the specific fluorescent emissions from the individual proteins are recorded to determine the relative proportions of the proteins in each sample. In another method, peptides from two different samples are labeled with a heavy form (containing eight deuterium atoms) or a light form (with no deuterium atoms) of an ICAT. The same ICAT-labeled peptides in the two samples produce a pair of signals with a defined difference in mass due to the light and heavy versions of the labels. MS is used to measure the relative abundances of the proteins in the original proteomes.

Protein microarrays consist of a large number of proteins immobilized in a small area on a support to facilitate massively parallel analyses of interactions between proteins, between proteins and low-molecular-weight compounds, and between antibodies and antigens. Based on the immobilized proteins, there are three kinds of protein microarrays: analytical, reverse phase, and functional. Analytical microarrays use immobilized antibodies to capture proteins or immobilized proteins to bind antibodies. Multiprotein complexes, such as cell lysates, are bound to the support for reverse-phase microarrays. Functional protein microarrays contain as many members of a proteome or subproteome as possible to study the activities of proteins by their interactions with other proteins or small molecules. Recombinational cloning is often used to generate libraries containing the ORFs for all of the proteins encoded in a genome.

Protein interaction maps can reveal novel functions for proteins, place proteins with unknown functions among those with known cellular roles, and elucidate new biological pathways and cellular machines. The yeast two-hybrid system detects interactions between two proteins (bait and prey) that bring together the activation and DNA-binding domains of a transcription factor required for the initiation of transcription of a reporter gene. Large networks of protein–protein interactions are revealed by many thousands of pairwise assays. The TAP tag procedure is used to isolate clusters of proteins that associate with a test (bait) protein in vivo. In this method, the individual proteins of a purified protein complex are separated by one-dimensional PAGE and identified by either peptide mass fingerprinting or MS amino acid sequencing and a database similarity search.

REFERENCES

Benson, D. A., I. Karsch-Mizrachi, D. J. Lipman, J. Ostell, and D. L. Wheeler. 2007. GenBank. *Nucleic Acids Res.* 35:D21–D25.

Bertone, P., and M. Snyder. 2005. Advances in functional protein microarray technology. *FEBS J.* 272:5400–5411.

Brasch, M. A., J. L. Hartley, and M. Vidal. 2004. ORFeome cloning and systems biology: standardized mass production of the parts from the parts-list. *Genome Res.* 14:2001–2009.

Buyse, M., S. Loi, L. van't Veer, G. Viale, M. Delorenzi, A. M. Glas, M. S. d'Assignies, J. Bergh, R. Lidereau, P. Ellis, A. Harris, J. Bogaerts, P. Therasse, A. Floore, M. Amakrane, F. Piette, E. Rutgers, C. Sotiriou, F. Cardoso, and M. J. Piccart. 2006. Validation and clinical utility of a 70-gene prognostic signature for women with node-negative breast cancer. *J. Natl. Cancer Inst.* 98:1183–1192.

Charboneau, L., H. Tory, T. Chen, M. Winters, E. F. Petricoin III, L. A. Liotta, and C. P. Paweletz. 2002. Utility of reverse phase protein arrays: applications to signalling pathways and human body arrays. *Brief Funct. Genomic Proteomic* 1:305–315.

Chen, C. S., E. Korobkova, H. Chen, J. Zhu, X. Jian, S. C. Tao, C. He, and H. Zhu. 2008. A proteome chip approach reveals new DNA damage recognition activities in *Escherichia coli*. *Nat. Methods* 5:69–74.

Chung, C. H., S. Levy, P. Chaurand, and D. P. Carbone. 2007. Genomics and proteomics: emerging technologies in clinical cancer research. *Crit. Rev. Oncol. Hematol.* 61:1–25.

Cochrane, G., R. Akhtar, P. Aldebert, N. Althorpe, A. Baldwin, K. Bates, S. Bhattacharyya, J. Bonfield, L. Bower, P. Browne, M. Castro, T. Cox, F. Demiralp, R. Eberhardt, N. Faruque, G. Hoad, M. Jang, T. Kulikova, A. Labarga, R. Leinonen, S. Leonard, Q. Lin, R. Lopez, D. Lorenc, H. McWilliam, G. Mukherjee, F. Nardone, S. Plaister, S. Robinson, S. Sobhany, R. Vaughan, D. Wu, W. Zhu, R. Apweiler, T. Hubbard, and E. Birney. 2008. Priorities for nucleotide trace, sequence and annota-tion data capture at the Ensembl Trace Archive and the EMBL Nucleotide Sequence Database. *Nucleic Acids Res.* 36:D5–D12.

Committee on Metagenomics: Challenges and Functional Applications, National Research Council. 2007. *The New Science of Metagenomics: Revealing the Secrets of Our Microbial Planet*. National Academies Press, Washington, DC.

Daniel, R. 2005. The metagenomics of soil. *Nat. Rev. Microbiol.* 3:470–478.

DeLong, E. F. 2005. Microbial commu-nity genomics in the ocean. *Nat. Rev. Microbiol.* 3:459–469.

Droit, A., G. G. Poirier, and J. M. Hunter. 2005. Experimental and bioin-formatic approaches for interrogating protein-protein interactions to deter-mine protein function. *J. Mol. Endocrinol.* 34:263–280.

Emanuelsson, O., U. Nagalakshmi, D. Zheng, J. S. Rozowsky, A. E. Urban, J. Du, Z. Lian, V. Stolc, S. Weissman, M. Snyder, and M. B. Gerstein. 2007. Assessing the performance of different high-density tiling microarray strate-gies for mapping transcribed regions of the human genome. *Genome Res.* 17:886–897.

Ewing, R. M., P. Chu, F. Elisma, H. Li, P. Taylor, S. Climie, L. McBroom-Cerajewski, M. D. Robinson, L. O'Connor, M. Li, R. Taylor, M. Dharsee, Y. Ho, A. Heilbut, L. Moore, S. Zhang, O. Ornatsky, Y. V. Bukhman, M. Ethier, Y. Sheng, J. Vasilescu, M. Abu-Farha, J. P. Lambert, H. S. Duewel, I. I. Stewart, B. Kuehl, K. Hogue, K. Colwill, K. Gladwish, B. Muskat, R. Kinach, S. L. Adams, M. F. Moran, G. B. Morin, T. Topaloglou, and D. Figeys. 2007. Large-scale mapping of human pro-tein-protein interactions by mass spec-trometry. *Mol. Syst. Biol.* 3:89.

Fields, S. 2005. High-throughput two-hybrid analysis. The promise and the peril. *FEBS J.* 272:5391–5399.

Fodor, S. P., R. P. Rava, X. C. Huang, A. C. Pease, C. P. Holmes, and C. L. Adams. 1993. Multiplexed biochemical assays with biological chips. *Nature* 364:555–556.

Fodor, S. P. A. 1997. TECH.SIGHT/ Techwire. *Science* 277:393–395.

Formstecher, E., S. Aresta, V. Collura, A. Hamburger, A. Meil, A. Trehin, C. Reverdy, V. Betin, S. Maire, C. Brun, B. Jacq, M. Arpin, Y. Bellaiche, S. Bellusci, P. Benaroch, M. Bornens, R. Chanet, P. Chavrier, O. Delattre, V. Doye, R. Fehon, G. Faye, T. Galli, J. A. Girault, B. Goud, J. de Gunzburg, L. Johannes, M. P. Junier, V. Mirouse, A. Mukherjee, D. Papadopoulo, F. Perez, A. Plessis, C. Rossé, S. Saule, D. Stoppa-Lyonnet, A. Vincent, M. White, P. Legrain, J. Wojcik, J. Camonis, and L. Daviet. 2005. Protein interaction mapping: a *Drosophila* case study. *Genome Res.* 15:376–384.

Gentleman, R., F. Hahne, and W. Huber. 2006. *Visualizing Genomic Data*. Bioconductor Project Working Papers, working paper 10. http://www. bepress.com/bioconductor/paper10.

Giot, L., J. S. Bader, C. Brouwer, A. Chaudhuri, B. Kuang, Y. Li, Y. L. Hao, C. E. Ooi, B. Godwin, E. Vitols, G. Vijayadamodar, P. Pochart, H. Machineni, M. Welsh, Y. Kong, B. Zerhusen, R. Malcolm, Z. Varrone, A. Collis, M. Minto, S. Burgess, L. McDaniel, E. Stimpson, F. Spriggs, J. Williams, K. Neurath, N. Ioime, M. Agee, E. Voss, K. Furtak, R. Renzulli, N. Aanensen, S. Carrolla, E. Bickelhaupt, Y. Lazovatsky, A. DaSilva, J. Zhong, C. A. Stanyon, R. L. Finley, Jr., K. P. White, M. Braverman, T. Jarvie, S. Gold, M. Leach, J. Knight, R. A. Shimkats, M. P. McKenna, J. Chant, and J. M. Rothberg. 2003. A protein interaction map of *Drosophila melanogaster*. *Science* 302:1727–1736.

Glas, A. M., A. Floore, L. J. Delahaye, A. T. Witteveen, R. C. Pover, N. Bakx, J. S. Lahti-Domenici, T. J. Bruinsma, M. O. Warmoes, R. Bernards, L. F. Wessels, and L. J. Van't Veer. 2006. Converting a breast cancer microarray signature into a high-throughput diag-nostic test. *BMC Genomics* 7:278.

Haab, B. B. 2006. Applications of anti-body array platforms. *Curr. Opin. Biotechnol.* 17:415–421.

Hall, D. A., J. Ptacek, and M. Snyder. 2007. Protein microarray technology. *Mech. Ageing Dev.* 128:161–167.

Handelsman, J. 2004. Metagenomics: application of genomics to uncultured microorganisms. *Microbiol. Mol. Biol. Rev.* **68**:669–685.

Hartley, J. L., G. F. Temple, and M. A. Brasch. 2000. DNA cloning using in vitro site-specific recombination. *Genome Res.* **10**:1788–1795.

Higgs, P. G., and T. K. Attwood. 2005. *Bioinformatics and Molecular Evolution.* Blackwell Publishing, Malden, MA.

Hoheisel, J. D. 2006. Microarray technology: beyond transcript profiling and genotype analysis. *Nat. Rev. Genet.* **7**:200–210.

Huber, W., A. von Heydebreck, and M. Vingron. 2005. *An Introduction to Low-Level Analysis Methods of DNA Microarray Data.* Bioconductor Project Working Papers, Working Paper 9. http://www.bepress.com/bioconductor/paper9.

Hudson, M. E., I. Pozdnyakova, K. Haines, G. Mor, and M. Snyder. 2007. Identification of differentially expressed proteins in ovarian cancer using high-density protein microarrays. *Proc. Natl. Acad. Sci. USA* **104**:17494–17499.

Huson, D. H., A. F. Auch, J. Qi, and S. C. Schuster. 2007. MEGAN analysis of metagenomic data. *Genome Res.* **17**:377–386.

Ito, T., T. Chiba, R. Ozawa, M. Yoshida, M. Hattori, and Y. Sakaki. 2001. A comprehensive two-hybrid analysis to explore the yeast protein interactome. *Proc. Natl. Acad. Sci. USA* **98**:4569–4574.

Kawasaki, E. S. 2006. The end of the microarray Tower of Babel: will universal standards lead the way? *J. Biomol. Tech.* **17**:200–206.

Köcher, T., and G. Superti-Furga. 2007. Mass spectrometry-based functional proteomics: from molecular machines to protein networks. *Nat. Methods* **4**:807–815.

LaBaer, J., and N. Ramachandran. 2005. Protein microarrays as tools for functional proteomics. *Curr. Opin. Chem. Biol.* **9**:14–19.

Lederer, S. L., K. A. Walters, S. Proll, B. Paeper, S. Robinzon, L. Boix, N. Fausto, J. Bruix, and M. G. Katze. 2006. Distinct cellular responses differentiating alcohol- and hepatitis C

virus-induced liver cirrhosis. *Virol. J.* **3**:98.

Luan, C. H., S. Qiu, J. B. Finley, M. Carson, R. J. Gray, W. Huang, D. Johnson, J. Tsao, J. Reboul, P. Vaglio, D. E. Hill, M. Vidal, L. J. Delucas, and M. Luo. 2004. High-throughput expression of C. elegans proteins. *Genome Res.* **14**:2102–2110.

Lutz, M. W., P. V. Warren, R. W. Gill, and D. B. Searls. 2005. Managing genomic and proteomic knowledge. *Drug Discov. Today* **2**:197–204.

Marcotte, E. M. 2007. How do shotgun proteomics algorithms identify proteins? *Nat. Biotechnol.* **25**:755–757.

Matsumura, H., A. Ito, H. Saitoh, P. Winter, G. Kahl, M. Reuter, D. H. Krüger, and R. Terauchi. 2005. SuperSAGE. *Cell Microbiol.* **7**:11–18.

Mockler, T. C., S. Chan, A. Sundaresan, H. Chen, S. E. Jacobsen, and J. R. Ecker. 2005. Applications of DNA tiling arrays for whole-genome analysis. *Genomics* **85**:1–15.

Morris, J. S., B. N. Clark, and H. B. Gutstein. 2008. *Pinnacle:* a fast, automatic and accurate method for detecting and quantifying protein spots in 2-dimensional gel electrophoresis data. *Bioinformatics* **24**:529–536.

Mulder, N., and R. Apweiler. 2007. InterPro and InterProScan: tools for protein sequence classification and comparison. *Methods Mol. Biol.* **396**:59–70.

Mulder, N. J., R. Apweiler, T. K. Attwood, A. Bairoch, A. Bateman, D. Binns, P. Bork, V. Buillard, L. Cerutti, R. Copley, E. Courcelle, U. Das, L. Daugherty, M. Dibley, R. Finn, W. Fleischmann, J. Gough, D. Haft, N. Hulo, S. Hunter, D. Kahn, A. Kanapin, A. Kejariwal, A. Labarga, P. S. Langendijk-Genevaux, D. Lonsdale, R. Lopez, I. Letunic, M. Madera, J. Maslen, C. McAnulla, J. McDowall, J. Mistry, A. Mitchell, A. N. Nikolskaya, S. Orchard, C. Orengo, R. Petryszak, J. D. Selengut, C. J. Sigrist, P. D. Thomas, F. Valentin, D. Wilson, C. H. Wu, and C. Yeats. 2007. New developments in the InterPro database. *Nucleic Acids Res.* **35**:D224–D228.

Nesvizhskii, A. I., O. Vitek, and R. Aebersold. 2007. Analysis and validation of proteomic data generated by

tandem mass spectrometry. *Nat. Methods* **4**:787–797.

Nishizuka, S., L. Charboneau, L. Young, S. Major, W. C. Reinhold, M. Waltham, H. Kouros-Mehr, K. J. Bussey, J. K. Lee, V. Espina, P. J. Munson, E. Petricoin III, L. A. Liotta, and J. N. Weinstein. 2003. Proteomic profiling of the NCI-60 cancer cell lines using new high-density reverse-phase lysate microarrays. *Proc. Natl. Acad. Sci. USA* **100**:14229–14234.

Noguchi, H., J. Park, and T. Takagi. 2006. MetaGene: prokaryotic gene finding from environmental genome shotgun sequences. *Nucleic Acids Res.* **34**:5623–5630.

Nuwaysir, E. F., W. Huang, T. J. Albert, J. Singh, K. Nuwaysir, A. Pitas, T. Richmond, T. Gorski, J. P. Berg, J. Ballin, M. McCormick, J. Norton, T. Pollock, T. Sumwalt, L. Butcher, D. Porter, M. Molla, C. Hall, F. Blattner, M. R. Sussman, R. L. Wallace, F. Cerrina, and R. D. Green. 2002. Gene expression analysis using oligonucleotide arrays produced by maskless photolithography. *Genome Res.* **12**:1749–1755.

Parrish, J. R., K. D. Gulyas, and R. L. Finley, Jr. 2006. Yeast two-hybrid contributions to interactome mapping. *Curr. Opin. Biotechnol.* **17**:387–393.

Patterson, T. A., E. K. Lobenhofer, S. B. Fulmer-Smentek, P. J. Collins, T. M. Chu, W. Bao, H. Fang, E. S. Kawasaki, J. Hager, I. R. Tikhonova, S. J. Walker, L. Zhang, P. Hurban, F. de Longueville, J. C. Fuscoe, W. Tong, L. Shi, and R. D. Wolfinger. 2006. Performance comparison of one-color and two-color platforms within the MicroArray Quality Control (MAQC) project. *Nat. Biotechnol.* **24**:1140–1150.

Quackenbush, J. 2006. Microarray analysis and tumor classification. *N. Engl. J. Med.* **354**:2463–2472.

Rapp, B. A., and D. L. Wheeler. 2005. Bioinformatics resources from the National Center for Biotechnology Information: an integrated foundation for discovery. *J. Am. Soc. Inf. Sci. Technol.* **56**:538–550.

Ray, S., M. Britschgi, C. Herbert, Y. Takeda-Uchimura, A. Boxer, K. Blennow, L. F. Friedman, D. R. Galasko, M. Jutel, A. Karydas, J. A. Kaye, J. Leszek, B. L. Miller, L. Minthon, J. F. Quinn,

G. D. Rabinovici, W. H. Robinson, M. N. Sabbagh, Y. T. So, D. L. Sparks, M. Tabaton, J. Tinklenberg, J. A. Yesavage, R. Tibshirani, and T. Wyss-Coray. 2007. Classification and prediction of clinical Alzheimer's diagnosis based on plasma signaling proteins. *Nat. Med.* 13:1359–1362.

Riesenfeld, C. S., P. D. Schloss, and J. Handelsman. 2004. Metagenomics: genomic analysis of microbial communities. *Annu. Rev. Genet.* 38:525–552.

Rual, J. F., T. Hirozane-Kishikawa, T. Hao, N. Bertin, S. Li, A. Dricot, N. Li, J. Rosenberg, P. Lamesch, P. O. Vidalain, T. R. Clingingsmith, J. L. Hartley, D. Esposito, D. Cheo, T. Moore, B. Simmons, R. Sequerra, S. Bosak, L. Doucette-Stamm, C. Le Peuch, J. Vandenhaute, M. E. Cusick, J. S. Albala, D. E. Hill, and M. Vidal. 2004. Human ORFeome version 1.1: a platform for reverse proteomics. *Genome Res.* 14:2128–2135.

Rusch, D. B., A. L. Halpern, G. Sutton, K. B. Heidelberg, S. Williamson, S. Yooseph, D. Wu, J. A. Eisen, J. M. Hoffman, K. Remington, K. Beeson, B. Tran, H. Smith, H. Baden-Tillson, C. Stewart, J. Thorpe, J. Freeman, C. Andrews-Pfannkoch, J. E. Venter, K. Li, S. Kravitz, J. F. Heidelberg, T. Utterback, Y. H. Rogers, L. I. Falcón, V. Souza, G. Bonilla-Rosso, L. E. Eguiarte, D. M. Karl, S. Sathyendranath, T. Platt, E. Bermingham, V. Gallardo, G. Tamayo-Castillo, M. R. Ferrari, R. L. Strausberg, K. Nealson, R. Friedman, M. Frazier, and J. C. Venter. 2007. The Sorcerer II Global Ocean Sampling Expedition: northwest Atlantic through eastern tropical Pacific. *PLoS Biol.* 5:e77.

Saha, S., A. B. Sparks, C. Rago, V. Akmaev, C. J. Wang, B. Vogelstein, K. W. Kinzler, and V. E. Velculescu. 2002. Using the transcriptome to annotate the genome. *Nat. Biotechnol.* 20:508–512.

Sanchez-Carbayo, M. 2006. Antibody arrays: technical considerations and clinical applications in cancer. *Clin. Chem.* 52:1651–1659.

Schena, M., D. Shalon, R. W. Davis, and P. O. Brown. 1995. Quantitative monitoring of gene expression patterns with a complementary DNA microarray. *Science* 270:467–470.

Schloss, P. D., and J. Handelsman. 2005. Metagenomics for studying unculturable microorganisms: cutting the Gordian knot. *Genome Biol.* 6:229.

Seshadri, R., S. A. Kravitz, L. Smarr, P. Gilna, and M. Frazier. 2007. CAMERA: a community resource for metagenomics. *PLoS Biol.* 5:e75.

Shi, L., L. H. Reid, W. D. Jones, R. Shippy, J. A. Warrington, S. C. Baker, P. J. Collins, F. de Longueville, E. S. Kawasaki, K. Y. Lee, Y. Luo, Y. A. Sun, J. C. Willey, R. A. Setterquist, G. M. Fischer, W. Tong, Y. P. Dragan, D. J. Dix, F. W. Frueh, F. M. Goodsaid, D. Herman, R. V. Jensen, C. D. Johnson, E. K. Lobenhofer, R. K. Puri, U. Schrf, J. Thierry-Mieg, C. Wang, M. Wilson, P. K. Wolber, L. Zhang, S. Amur, W. Bao, C. C. Barbacioru, A. B. Lucas, V. Bertholet, C. Boysen, B. Bromley, D. Brown, A. Brunner, R. Canales, X. M. Cao, T. A. Cebula, J. J. Chen, J. Cheng, T. M. Chu, E. Chudin, J. Corson, J. C. Corton, L. J. Croner, C. Davies, T. S. Davison, G. Delenstarr, X. Deng, D. Dorris, A. C. Eklund, X. H. Fan, H. Fang, S. Fulmer-Smentek, J. C. Fuscoe, K. Gallagher, W. Ge, L. Guo, X. Guo, J. Hager, P. K. Haje, J. Han, T. Han, H. C. Harbottle, S. C. Harris, E. Hatchwell, C. A. Hauser, S. Hester, H. Hong, P. Hurban, S. A. Jackson, H. Ji, C. R. Knight, W. P. Kuo, J. E. LeClerc, S. Levy, Q. Z. Li, C. Liu, Y. Liu, M. J. Lombardi, Y. Ma, S. R. Magnuson, B. Maqsodi, T. McDaniel, N. Mei, O. Myklebost, B. Ning, N. Novoradovskaya, M. S. Orr, T. W. Osborn, A. Papallo, T. A. Patterson, R. G. Perkins, E. H. Peters, R. Peterson, K. L. Philips, P. S. Pine, L. Pusztai, F. Qian, H. Ren, M. Rosen, B. A. Rosenzweig, R. R. Samaha, M. Schena, G. P. Schroth, S. Shchegrova, D. D. Smith, F. Staedtler, Z. Su, H. Sun, Z. Szallasi, Z. Tezak, D. Thierry-Mieg, K. L. Thompson, I. Tikhonova, Y. Turpaz, B. Vallanat, C. Van, S. J. Walker, S. J. Wang, Y. Wang, R. Wolfinger, A. Wong, J. Wu, C. Xiao, Q. Xie, J. Xu, W. Yang, L. Zhang, S. Zhong, Y. Zong, and W. Slikker, Jr. 2006. The MicroArray Quality Control (MAQC) project shows inter- and intraplatform reproducibility of gene expression measurements. *Nat. Biotechnol.* 24:1151–1161.

Singh-Gasson, S., R. D. Green, Y. Yue, C. Nelson, F. Blattner, M. R. Sussman, and F. Cerrina. 1999. Maskless fabrication of light-directed oligonucleotide microarrays using a digital micromirror array. *Nat. Biotechnol.* 17:974–978.

Steele, H. L., and W. R. Streit. 2005. Metagenomics: advances in ecology and biotechnology. *FEMS Microbiol. Lett.* 247:105–111.

Tyson, G. W., J. Chapman, P. Hugenholtz, E. E. Allen, R. J. Ram, P. M. Richardson, V. V. Solovyev, E. M. Rubin, D. S. Rokhsar, and J. F. Banfield. 2004. Community structure and metabolism through reconstruction of microbial genomes from the environment. *Nature* 428:37–43.

Uchiyama, T., T. Abe, T. Ikemura, and K. Watanabe. 2005. Substrate-induced gene-expression screening of environmental metagenome libraries for isolation of catabolic genes. *Nat. Biotechnol.* 23:88–93.

Uetz, P., L. Giot, G. Cagney, T. A. Mansfield, R. S. Judson, J. R. Knight, D. Lockshon, V. Narayan, M. Srinivasan, P. Pochart, A. Qureshi-Emili, Y. Li, B. Godwin, D. Conover, T. Kalbfleisch, G. Vijayadamodar, M. Yang, M. Johnston, S. Fields, and J. M. Rothberg. 2000. A comprehensive analysis of protein-protein interactions in *Saccharomyces cerevisiae*. *Nature* 403:623–627.

University of Arizona. 22 January 2008, accession date. *The University of Arizona BIOTECH Project.* http://biotech.biology.arizona.edu/Resources/DNA_analysis.html.

Vasilescu, J., and D. Figeys. 2006. Mapping protein-protein interactions by mass spectrometry. *Curr. Opin. Biotechnol.* 17:394–399.

Velculescu, V. E., L. Zhang, B. Vogelstein, and K. W. Kinzler. 1995. Serial analysis of gene expression. *Science* 270:484–487.

Walhout, A. J., G. F. Temple, M. A. Brasch, J. L. Hartley, M. A. Lorson, S. van den Heuvel, and M. Vidal. 2000. GATEWAY recombinational cloning: application to the cloning of large numbers of open reading frames or ORFeomes. *Methods Enzymol.* 328:575–592.

Wang, S. M. 2007. Understanding SAGE data. *Trends Genet.* **23**:42–50.

Wheeler, D. L., T. Barrett, D. A. Benson, S. H. Bryant, K. Canese, V. Chetvernin, D. M. Church, M. DiCuccio, R. Edgar, S. Federhen, L. Y. Geer, Y. Kapustin, O. Khovayko, D. Landsman, D. J. Lipman, T. L. Madden, D. R. Maglott, J. Ostell, V. Miller, K. D. Pruitt, G. D. Schuler, E.

Sequeira, S. T. Sherry, K. Sirotkin, A. Souvorov, G. Starchenko, R. L. Tatusov, T. A. Tatusova, L. Wagner, and E. Yaschenko. 2007. Database resources of the National Center for Biotechnology Information. *Nucleic Acids Res.* **35**:D5–D12.

Whitfield, E. J., M. Pruess, and R. Apweiler. 2006. Bioinformatics database infrastructure for biotechnology

research. *J. Biotechnol.* **124**:629–639.

Xia, X. 2007. *Bioinformatics and the Cell: Modern Computational Approaches in Genomics, Proteomics, and Transcriptomics.* Springer, New York, NY.

Zhou, J., D. K. Thompson, Y. Xu, and J. M. Tiedje. 2004. *Microbial Functional Genomics.* Wiley-Liss, Hoboken, NJ.

REVIEW QUESTIONS

1. The Basic Local Alignment Search Tool (BLAST) finds regions of similarity between sequences. For a brief introduction to a BLAST nucleotide search, go to http://www.ncbi.nlm.nih.gov/blast/Blast.cgi and click on the link labeled "nucleotide blast." Type accession number NM_000492.3, which is the unique identifier assigned to a specific DNA sequence, into the "Enter accession number…" box. In the pull-down menu in the "Database" field, select "Nucleotide collection (nr/nt)." Check the "Show results in a new window" box. Click on "Algorithm parameters," and select 10 from the "Max target sequences" menu. Click on BLAST. From the results of the nucleotide sequence, determine the identity of the gene that has been given accession number NM_000492.3.

2. What is the likely protein that contains the amino acid sequence LSPQMSGEEEDSDLAAKLGMCNREIVR RGA? To answer this question, go to http://www.ncbi.nlm.nih.gov/blast/Blast.cgi and click on the link labeled "Protein blast." Enter the amino acid sequence into the "Enter accession number…" field. Name the job "test" or whatever appeals to you. Check "Show results in a new window." Click on "Algorithm parameters," and select 10 from the "Max target sequences" menu. Click on BLAST. The results should reveal the identity of the protein containing the amino acid sequence.

3. What is a DNA microarray?

4. Describe a cDNA microarray gene expression profiling system.

5. How is the target sample prepared for an oligonucleotide microarray experiment?

6. What is an affinity tag?

7. What are the objectives of gene expression profiling experiments?

8. Describe the SAGE procedure.

9. Find the best gene for the following SAGE tags: ATCGCTTTCT, TTTTGTCATT, and GGCCCCAGTT. Go to the SAGE Anatomic Viewer (http://cgap.nci.nih.gov/SAGE/AnatomicViewer), and under the "Find the Best Gene for a

Tag" heading, enter one of the query tag sequences at a time in the "10 bp tag" box, and then click on Go.

10. Why are there so many more proteins than genes in humans?

11. What are the principal features of 2D PAGE?

12. Describe how unknown members of a proteome can be readily identified.

13. What is a peptide mass fingerprint?

14. Are you curious about the unknown protein in Fig. 5.11? If so, type the peptide masses of the unknown protein as a column in a word processor. Omit the dots. Copy the column to the clipboard. Go to http://www.expasy.org/cgi-bin/aldente/form.cgi. Paste the list of peptide masses into the "Peak list" box. Change "Minimum number of Hits" from four to nine. Enter your e-mail address in the appropriate box. Click on "Submit." An e-mail message should arrive within 10 minutes with the results. What is the unknown protein? You may also want to check out the peptide mass fingerprint program at http://www.matrixscience.com. Click on the link labeled "Mascot." Click on "Peptide Mass Fingerprint." Enter your name and e-mail address. Give a name to the project in the "Search title" field. Paste the peptide masses into the "Query" box. Select 5 in the "Report top" field. Click on "Start Search.…" Note the "Top Score" and other information on the Mascot Search Results page in your browser.

15. The following ladder of y-ion masses (*m/z* ratios) was observed with MS after fragmentation and ionization of a peptide: 1,136, 980, 851, 723, 609, 512, 411, 324, 196, and 99. What is the likely amino acid sequence of the peptide? A list of average amino acid masses can be obtained from a number of online sites. Simply do an online search with the phrase "amino acid masses."

16. What is the ICAT method?

17. Describe the major features of the two-hybrid assay.

18. What is the TAP tag system?

19. What is a protein microarray?

20. Compare and contrast analytical and reverse-phase microarrays.

21. Describe how a library of ORFs that represents a proteome is constructed by recombinational cloning.

22. What types of molecules can be captured by a functional protein microarray?

23. What are the objectives of protein–protein interaction studies?

6

Manipulation of Gene Expression in Prokaryotes

THE PRIMARY OBJECTIVE OF GENE CLONING for biotechnological applications is the expression of the cloned gene in a selected host organism. Unfortunately, the insertion of a gene into a cloning vector does not necessarily ensure that it will be successfully expressed. Moreover, for many commercial purposes, a high rate of production of the protein encoded by the cloned gene is required. In response to the need for a high expression rate, many specialized expression vectors have been created that provide genetic elements for controlling transcription, translation, protein stability, and secretion of the product of the cloned gene from the host cell. The molecular biological features that have been manipulated to modulate gene expression include the promoter and transcription terminator sequences, the strength of the ribosome-binding site, the number of copies of the cloned gene and whether the gene is plasmid borne or integrated into the genome of the host cell, the final cellular location of the synthesized foreign protein, the efficiency of translation in the host organism, and the intrinsic stability within the host cell of the protein encoded by the cloned gene. There is no single strategy for obtaining maximal expression of every cloned gene. Consideration of the distinctive features of a cloned sequence is usually required before an optimal level of expression is found.

The level of foreign-gene expression also depends on the host organism. Currently, although a wide range of both prokaryotic and eukaryotic organisms can express foreign genes, many of the commercially important proteins produced by recombinant DNA technology are synthesized in *Escherichia coli*. The extensive use of *E. coli* is understandable in light of the vast amount of research that has been carried out on its genetics, molecular biology, biochemistry, and physiology. Moreover, foreign proteins can usually be produced by this organism rapidly and inexpensively. However, other host systems, such as *Bacillus subtilis*, yeasts, fungi, and animal, plant, and insect cells, are used to express certain cloned genes. Nevertheless, the strategies that have been elaborated for *E. coli*, in principle, are applicable to all systems.

Gene Expression from Strong and Regulatable Promoters

The minimal requirement for an effective gene expression system is the presence of a strong and regulatable promoter sequence upstream from a cloned gene. A strong promoter is one that has high affinity for RNA polymerase, with the consequence that the adjacent downstream region is frequently transcribed. The ability to regulate a promoter enables the cell (and the researcher) to control the extent of transcription in a precise manner. The promoter from the well-studied *lac* (lactose) operon of *E. coli* has been used extensively for expressing cloned genes. However, other promoters have distinctive properties that make them useful for controlling expression. Thus, many different promoters have been isolated from a range of organisms.

It might seem that a good way to optimize the expression of a cloned gene would be to insert it into a plasmid under the control of a continuously activated strong promoter. However, a high level of continuous expression of a cloned gene is often detrimental to the host cell because it creates an energy drain, thereby impairing essential host cell functions. In addition, all or a portion of the plasmid carrying a continuously (constitutively) expressed cloned gene may be lost after several division cycles, since cells without a plasmid grow faster and eventually take over the culture. Such plasmid instability is a major problem that may prevent the efficient production of a plasmid-borne gene product on a large scale. To overcome this drawback, it is desirable to control transcription in such a way that a cloned gene is expressed only at a specific stage in the host cell growth cycle and only for a specified duration. This objective is achieved by using a strong regulatable promoter. The plasmids constructed to accomplish this task are called expression vectors.

Regulatable Promoters

The most widely used strong regulatable promoters are those from the *E. coli lac* and *trp* (tryptophan) operons; the *tac* promoter, which is constructed from the −10 region (i.e., 10 nucleotide pairs upstream from the site of initiation of transcription) of the *lac* promoter and the −35 region of the *trp* promoter; the leftward, or p^L, promoter from bacteriophage λ; and the gene 10 promoter from bacteriophage T7. Each of these promoters interacts with regulatory proteins (e.g., repressors or inducers), which provide a controllable switch for either turning on or turning off specific transcription of adjacent cloned genes. In addition, each of these promoters is recognized by the major form of the *E. coli* RNA polymerase holoenzyme. This holoenzyme is formed when a protein, called sigma factor, combines with the core proteins of RNA polymerase. Sigma factor directs the binding of the holoenzyme to promoter regions on the DNA.

In the absence of lactose in the growth medium, the *E. coli lac* promoter is repressed (turned off) by the *lac* repressor protein, which prevents the *lac* operon from being transcribed (Fig. 6.1). Induction (turning on) of the *lac* promoter is achieved by the addition of either lactose or isopropyl-β-D-thiogalactopyranoside (IPTG), a synthetic inducer, to the medium (Fig. 6.2). Either of these substances prevents the *lac* repressor from binding to the *lac* operator, thereby enabling transcription to occur. In practice, lactose must be converted to allolactose, by low levels of β-galactosidase that are synthesized when the system is repressed, before it can act as an inducer. The enzyme β-galactosidase is encoded by the *lacZ* gene of the *lac* operon, and

Glucose concentration	Lactose concentration	cAMP concentration	lac regulatory region				Level of transcription	
Low	Low	High	cAMP CAP	CAP box	Promoter	lac repressor Operator	Gene	Low
High	Low	Low		CAP box	Promoter	lac repressor Operator	Gene	Low
High	High	Low		CAP box	Promoter	Operator	Gene	Low
Low	High	High	cAMP CAP	RNA polymerase CAP box	Promoter	Operator	Gene	High

FIGURE 6.1 Diagrammatic representation of the effects of the concentrations of glucose, lactose, and cAMP in the growth medium on the level of transcription from the *E. coli lac* promoter. The arrow indicates the direction of transcription. The *lac* repressor is a tetramer. The cAMP–CAP complex binds to a CAP recognition site (CAP box) on the DNA.

it is primarily involved in the cleavage of lactose into glucose and galactose.

Transcription from the *lac* promoter is also regulated by the binding of the catabolite activator protein (CAP) (also sometimes referred to as the cyclic AMP [cAMP] repressor protein, or CRP) to a region of the DNA (the CAP box) just upstream of the promoter region (Fig. 6.1). When CAP binds to the CAP box, it increases the affinity of the promoter for RNA polymerase, thereby increasing transcription of the genes downstream from the promoter. The affinity of CAP for its binding site on the DNA is enhanced by its association with cAMP, whose level is highest when the amount of glucose in the medium is lowest. Thus, when inducer (lactose or IPTG) is present and there is no repressor bound to the operator, a high intracellular concentration of cAMP can lead to a high level of transcription of the genes downstream of the *lac* promoter. In practice, *lacUV5*, a variant of the *lac* promoter that contains an altered nucleotide sequence in the –10 region and is a stronger promoter than the wild-type *lac* promoter, is usually used in plasmid expression vectors.

The *trp* promoter regulates transcription of the genes that are necessary for the biosynthesis of the amino acid tryptophan. This strong promoter is negatively regulated (turned off) by the *trp* repressor protein complexed with tryptophan, which binds to the *trp* operator and prevents transcription of the *trp* operon. Derepression (turning on) of the *trp* promoter is achieved either by removing tryptophan or by adding 3-indoleacrylic acid to the growth medium. Unfortunately, repression of this promoter is not very efficient: it is "leaky," which leads to a continuous low level of transcription, even when the gene should be turned off. Because of this, this promoter–operator cannot be used to express genes that might be toxic or otherwise deleterious to the growth of *E. coli*.

The *tac* and *trc* promoters are commonly used hybrid constructs that are similar to one another, differing by only a single base pair. Both promoters

A

CH₂OH

Lactose

β-Galactosidase

Allolactose

B

IPTG

FIGURE 6.2 Inducers of the *lac* promoter. **(A)** Lactose, which must be converted to allolactose to be effective; **(B)** IPTG.

contain the −35 region from the *trp* promoter and the −10 region from the *lac* promoter separated by either 16 *(tac)* or 17 *(trc)* base pairs (bp). Both of the promoters are repressed by the *lac* repressor and can be induced (in the same way as the *lac* promoter) by the addition of lactose or IPTG to the medium. It has been estimated that the *tac* and *trc* promoters are three times as strong as the *trp* promoter and 10 times more effective than the *lac* promoter.

The p^L promoter is controlled by the *c*I repressor protein of bacteriophage λ (Fig. 6.3). In practice, a temperature-sensitive mutant of the *c*I repressor, *c*I857, is generally used to regulate p^L-directed transcription. Cells carrying the temperature-sensitive *c*I repressor are first grown at 28 to 30°C, a temperature at which the *c*I repressor prevents transcription directed by the p^L promoter. When the cell culture reaches the desired stage of growth, often the mid-log phase, the temperature is shifted to 42°C. At this temperature, the thermosensitive *c*I repressor is inactivated and transcription can proceed.

The bacteriophage T7 gene 10 promoter requires T7 RNA polymerase for transcription (Fig. 6.4). To utilize this promoter, the T7 RNA polymerase gene is inserted in the *E. coli* chromosome on a bacteriophage λ lysogen under the control of the *E. coli lac* promoter. After cells are transformed by a plasmid with a cloned gene under the control of the T7 promoter, IPTG is added to the medium. Under these conditions, the T7 RNA polymerase gene is induced and synthesized, and the T7 RNA polymerase transcribes the cloned gene. There is often a lag of an hour or more from the time that the T7 RNA polymerase gene is induced until the cloned (target) gene is transcribed. A series of plasmids called pET vectors have been developed to exploit the strength of the T7 promoter.

The effectiveness of deactivating a repressor protein and thereby activating transcription depends on the ratio of the number of repressor protein molecules to the number of copies of the promoter sequences. If there are too many repressor protein molecules, then it is difficult to induce tran-

A

Active cI protein

mRNA

30°C

p^{cI} cI gene TT

o^L p^L Target gene TT

B

Active cI protein

Inactive protein

42°C

mRNA

p^{cI} cI gene TT

o^L p^L Target gene TT

FIGURE 6.3 Regulation of gene expression controlled by the p^L promoter. **(A)** At 30°C, the cI repressor, which is synthesized constitutively under the control of its own promoter (p^{cI}), binds to the operator region (o^L) of the p^L promoter, thereby preventing the target gene from being transcribed. **(B)** At 42°C, the temperature-sensitive cI repressor is synthesized and then inactivated so that it no longer interferes with transcription of the target protein. TT, transcription termination sequence.

scription. Conversely, with too few repressor protein molecules, even when there are more repressor molecules than copies of the promoter, transcription occurs in the absence of induction. In these cases, the promoters are said to be leaky. Various means have been devised to keep these regulatable systems under complete control. For example, the repressor protein gene and the promoter that it regulates may be placed on two different plasmids that maintain different numbers of copies per cell; this arrangement maintains the appropriate ratio between the repressor protein and the promoter. Usually, the repressor gene is placed on a low-copy-number plasmid that maintains about 1 to 8 copies per cell, and the cloned gene with its promoter sequence is inserted into a high-copy-number plasmid that maintains about 30 to 100 copies per cell. Alternatively, the repressor protein gene may be carried as a single gene in the chromosomal DNA, an arrangement that keeps repressor protein levels low. In systems that use the *lac* promoter, a mutant form of the *lacI* gene (*lacI*q) that produces much higher levels of the *lac* repressor is often used to decrease transcriptional leakiness under noninduced conditions, i.e., transcription of a cloned gene in the absence of inducer.

T7 RNA polymerase

p^{T7} Target gene TT

IPTG

lac repressor

mRNA

o^{lac} p^{lac} T7 RNA
polymerase gene TT

mRNA

p^{lacI} lacI gene TT

FIGURE 6.4 Regulation of gene expression controlled by the promoter for gene 10 from bacteriophage T7 (p^{T7}). In the absence of the inducer IPTG, the constitutively produced *lac* repressor, the product of the *lacI* gene, which is under the control of the *lacI* promoter, p^{lacI}, represses the synthesis of the T7 RNA polymerase that is transcriptionally controlled by the *lac* operator (o^{lac}) and *lac* promoter (p^{lac}). In the absence of T7 RNA polymerase, the target gene, which is under the transcriptional control of the T7 gene 10 promoter (p^{T7}), is not transcribed. When lactose or IPTG is added to the medium, it binds to the *lac* repressor, thereby preventing it from repressing the transcription of T7 RNA polymerase. In the presence of T7 RNA polymerase, the target gene is transcribed. TT, transcription termination sequence.

It is generally believed that the spacer region between the –35 and the –10 regions of *E. coli* promoters does not have any specific sequence requirements and acts primarily to position the binding sites for optimal interaction between the sigma factor of RNA polymerase and the promoter

FIGURE 6.5 A portion of the DNA sequence of the *E. coli lac* promoter (p^{lac}) and its mutated, more active, form (p^{mut}). The –10 and –35 residues are indicated by asterisks. The –10, –20 to –13, and –35 regions are indicated.

–35 region –20 to –13 –10 region
region

p^{lac} TTTACA CCGGCTCG | TATGTT

p^{mut} TTTACA TTTATGTT | TATGTT

DNA. However, this spacer region can in fact contribute to the strength of the promoter. When a portion of the spacer region from the *E. coli lac* promoter was deliberately mutated and constructs that yielded the most active promoters were selected, one construct displayed a >40-fold increase in *lac* promoter-directed RNA synthesis in the absence of CRP (and an ~8-fold increase in the presence of CRP, where CRP stimulated RNA synthesis 10-fold). In the mutated promoter with increased activity, the -20 to -13 region of the promoter was altered from a GC-rich (7 out of 8 bp) to an AT-rich (7 out of 8 bp) region (Fig. 6.5). Moreover, when the -20 to -13 region was excised from the mutated *lac* promoter and inserted into the p^R promoter from bacteriophage λ, transcription was enhanced twofold. This is important, because while the *lac* promoter is normally relatively weak in the absence of CRP, the p^R promoter is one of the strongest promoters in *E. coli*. Thus, by substituting an AT-rich region for a GC-rich region, and possibly enabling the promoter region to form a stronger complex with RNA polymerase, the intrinsic strengths of various promoters, even very strong ones, may be increased. These altered promoters may then be utilized as parts of an expression vector.

Increasing Protein Production

Plasmid pCP3 (Fig. 6.6) was created in an effort to obtain the highest possible level of foreign-protein production in a recombinant *E. coli* strain. This plasmid contains the strong p^L promoter, the β-lactamase gene (ampicillin resistance gene) as a selectable marker, a multiple cloning sequence immediately downstream from the promoter, and a temperature-sensitive origin of DNA replication that increases the plasmid's copy number 5- to 10-fold when the growth temperature is increased to 42°C (Fig. 6.7).

E. coli cells that carry the plasmid pCP3 are first grown at 28°C and then shifted to 42°C. At the lower temperature, the *cI* repressor, which is integrated into the host *E. coli* chromosomal DNA, is functional, the p^L promoter is turned off, and the plasmid copy number is normal (about 60 copies per cell). At the higher temperature, the temperature-sensitive *cI* repressor is inactivated, the p^L promoter is active, and the plasmid copy number increases to around 600 copies per cell. These properties make pCP3 a particularly effective expression vector. When the gene for the enzyme T4 DNA ligase is inserted into the multiple cloning site of pCP3, about 20% of the cellular protein produced at 42°C is T4 DNA ligase. This level of expression is much higher than that for even the most abundant native *E. coli* proteins, such as the elongation factor EF-Tu, which have an expression level of about 2%.

Large-Scale Systems

In small culture vessels (1 to 5 liters), induction is readily achieved either by shifting the temperature or by adding a chemical inducer. In pilot plant-size

FIGURE 6.6 Linear representation of *E. coli* expression vector pCP3 with a temperature-sensitive origin of DNA replication (*ori*^{ts}) that causes an increase in the plasmid copy number at 42°C and a p^L promoter controlled by a temperature-sensitive repressor protein, a multiple cloning site (MCS), and an ampicillin resistance (Amp^r) gene.

28°C 42°C

FIGURE 6.7 *E. coli* cells that contain a plasmid with a temperature-sensitive origin of DNA replication contain a limited number of plasmid copies at 28°C, which is greatly amplified when the temperature is shifted to 42°C.

(20 to 200 liters) and industrial-size (>200 liters) bioreactors, however, a shift in temperature requires time (30 to 60 minutes) and energy, both of which can be costly. Similarly, the cost of a chemical inducer, such as IPTG, that is required for the expression of a cloned gene in a large-scale bioreactor can make the overall process uneconomical. To overcome some of the problems associated with the use of the p^L promoter for large-scale fermentations, a two-plasmid system has been developed. The *cI* repressor was placed under the control of the *trp* promoter and inserted into a low-copy-number plasmid (Fig. 6.8). The use of a low-copy-number plasmid ensures that excess *cI* repressor molecules are not produced. A second plasmid carries a cloned gene under the control of the p^L promoter. As shown in Fig. 6.8A, the *trp* promoter is turned on in the absence of tryptophan, so the *cI* repressor protein is synthesized and the p^L promoter is turned off. In contrast, as shown in Fig. 6.8B, the *trp* promoter is turned off in the presence of tryptophan, so the *cI* repressor protein is not synthesized and the p^L promoter is fully active.

With this two-plasmid system, cells can be grown on an inexpensive medium consisting of molasses and casein hydrolysate, which contains only very small amounts of free tryptophan, and then induced to express the cloned gene by the addition of tryptone to the medium. Tryptone contains enough free tryptophan for efficient induction of transcription. In trial runs of this system, cloned β-galactosidase and citrate synthase genes, after induction by addition of tryptone to the medium, represented 21 and 24% of the cellular protein, respectively. Thus, this system provides a potentially inexpensive means of producing proteins from recombinant microorganisms on a large scale.

Several considerations may limit the choice of promoters for the large-scale production of foreign proteins. Chemical inducers can be costly, toxic, or difficult to remove; thermal induction of promoters may induce the production of heat shock proteins, including proteases; nutrient promoters limit the types of media that can be used for cell growth and induction; and oxygen-regulated promoters often have significant basal levels of activity as a consequence of the inherent difficulty in precisely controlling dissolved oxygen levels in the growth medium. On the other hand, promoters that are induced when cells enter stationary phase may be useful in the design of expression vectors that are useful for large-scale applications.

In *E. coli*, the housekeeping RNA polymerase sigma factor, σ^D, recognizes and binds to a well-characterized consensus DNA sequence at approximately −10 and −35 bp (upstream) from the site where transcription

A No tryptophan in the medium

B Tryptophan in the medium

FIGURE 6.8 Dual-plasmid system for controlling the λ p^L promoter by regulating the
cI repressor with tryptophan. The tryptophan promoter (p^{trp}) is inserted next to the
cI gene on one plasmid, and the p^L promoter is placed adjacent to the cloned gene
(gene) on a second plasmid. The wavy arrows denote transcription. **(A)** With no
tryptophan in the medium, the cI gene is transcribed and translated, and the cI
repressor protein binds to the p^L promoter, thereby blocking the transcription of the
cloned gene. **(B)** In the presence of tryptophan, the cI gene is repressed, no cI
product is made, and the cloned gene is transcribed and translated.

is initiated (Fig. 6.9). The stationary-phase sigma factor, σ^S, recognizes a
similar, but not identical, sequence of nucleotides in the same region
upstream of the start of transcription. Despite the similarities between
these two types of promoter sequences, the −35 region appears not to be
important for the functioning of the known stationary-phase promoters.
Assuming that the sequences around the −35 region affect promoter
activity, in one study, researchers generated more than 150 different sta-
tionary-phase promoters in which the DNA sequences upstream of the −10
consensus sequence were partially randomized. These workers found that
a number of these synthetic promoters had three to four times the level of
activity of naturally occurring stationary-phase promoters and had no, or
only a very low level of, background gene expression during exponential
growth. Thus, it is possible to use these promoters as parts of an expression
vector. In this case, the cells would be grown to a high density without

FIGURE 6.9 Consensus sequences of σ^D-dependent (top) and σ^S-dependent (bottom) promoters. The –10 region is shown, including the –13 residue, since it is important for σ^S binding/recognition. The AT-rich region downstream of the –10 region and the AWWWWWTTTTT sequence contribute to σ^S selectivity. N indicates any one of A, C, G, or T, whereas W indicates an A or a T at that position. The –10 and –35 residues are indicated by an asterisk. Modified from Miksch et al., *J. Biotechnol.* **120:**25–37, 2005.

expressing a foreign gene of interest, and as the cells entered stationary phase, gene expression would be rapidly and efficiently induced. Despite its success on a laboratory scale, the effectiveness of this system remains to be demonstrated on a large scale.

Expression in Other Microorganisms

E. coli is not necessarily the microorganism of choice for the expression of all foreign proteins. However, our understanding of the genetics and molecular biology of most other microorganisms is not as well developed. Unfortunately, there is no one vector or promoter–repressor system that gives optimal levels of gene expression in all bacteria, or even in all gram-negative bacteria. Fortunately, many of the strategies that have been developed for *E. coli* are also useful with a variety of other microorganisms. With this in mind, the abilities of various promoters to support transcription in other gram-negative bacteria have been tested. In one study, a set of plasmid expression vectors containing either the *lac*, *tac*, Nm (from the neomycin resistance gene), or S1 (from the ribosomal protein S1 gene of *Sinorhizobium meliloti*) promoter was constructed. The expression of β-galactosidase under the control of each of these promoters was examined (Table 6.1). The results indicated that (1) all of the promoters were active to some extent in each of the bacteria tested, (2) the *tac* promoter was the most active promoter in *E. coli* and the least active promoter in the other bacteria, and (3) Nm was the second least active promoter in *E. coli* and the most active promoter in the other bacteria. Clearly, even though gram-negative organisms may utilize similar DNA sequences to promote transcription, the best promoter for use in a particular organism is not necessarily the one that is most efficient in *E. coli*. Nevertheless, depending on the application, known *E. coli* promoters may be satisfactory for regulating the expression of cloned genes in other gram-negative bacteria.

Lactic acid bacteria, e.g., *Lactococcus* spp., are widely used in the production of foods such as cheese and yogurt. Genetic manipulation of these bacteria is desirable to increase yields or add to the quality of the product. However, any changes must not affect the production process, product palatability and appearance, or other features. For these reasons, it is not acceptable to modulate gene expression by adding chemical inducers or significantly modifying process conditions, such as temperature. In addition, the range of attainable foreign-gene expression is intrinsically limited when only the available constitutive promoters are used. To overcome this limitation, a plasmid library of synthetic promoters for *Lactococcus lactis*

TABLE 6.1 β-Galactosidase activity expressed by gram-negative bacteria carrying a plasmid vector with the E. coli lacZ gene and a heterologous promoter

Promoter	β-Galactosidase activity (U)			
	Escherichia coli	Sinorhizobium meliloti	Rhizobium leguminosarum	Pseudomonas putida
None	16	110	130	150
Nm	1,400	21,800	13,900	16,300
lac	2,000	9,050	6,250	9,800
tac	11,300	2,850	1,150	2,950
S1	40	3,300	1,200	3,350

Adapted from Labes et al., *Gene* 89:37–46, 1990.

was constructed in which the −10 and −35 regions of each promoter were the same but the sequences of the intervening spacer nucleotides were randomized (Fig. 6.10). To assay the strengths of the individual constructs, each synthetic promoter was used to control the expression, in the related bacterium *Leuconostoc lactis,* of the *lacL* and *lacM* genes, which together encode β-galactosidase. To quantify the strengths of the various promoters, the β-galactosidase activity from each construct was measured. Of the 36 different constructed promoters that were tested, the most active promoter was approximately 7,000 times stronger than the least active promoter. DNA sequence analysis revealed that the least active promoters all had changes in the −10 or −35 consensus region. Of the promoters in which the −10 or −35 consensus region remained intact, there was a 400-fold variation in promoter strength. These results indicated that the sequence of the spacer region is important for promoter activity. With this panel of promoters, it is possible to fine-tune the expression of different genes that are introduced in *L. lactis* and, by extension of the principle, the expression of genes introduced in other organisms, as well.

Fusion Proteins

Often, foreign proteins, especially small ones, occur in minute quantities when they are produced in heterologous host cells. This apparently low level of expression is, in many instances, actually due to degradation of the foreign protein. One way to solve this problem is to engineer a DNA construct that encodes a target protein that is in frame with a stable host protein. This combined, single protein, which is called a fusion protein, protects the cloned gene product from attack by host cell proteases. In a number of studies, proteins synthesized from cloned genes have been found to be resistant to degradation when they are part of a fusion protein, whereas when they are expressed as separate proteins, they are susceptible to degradation by proteolytic enzymes (proteolysis). In general, fusion

FIGURE 6.10 Consensus oligonucleotide sequence of *L. lactis* constitutive promoters. The −10 and −35 regions are shown in red, and the spacer region is shown in blue. To generate the library of synthetic promoters, the N sites were composed of 25% (each) A, C, G, and T; R was 50% A and 50% G; and W was 50% A and 50% T.

5'-CATNNNNNAGTTTATTCTTGACANNNNNNNNNNNNNNNNNTGRTATAATANNWNAGTACTGTT
　　　　　　　　　　−35　　　　　　　　　　　　　　　　　−10

proteins are stable because the target proteins are fused with proteins that are not especially susceptible to proteolysis.

Fusion proteins are constructed at the DNA level by ligating a portion of the coding regions of two or more genes. In its simplest form, a fusion vector system entails the insertion of a target gene or gene segment into the coding region of a cloned host gene. Knowledge of the nucleotide sequences of the various coding segments that are joined at the DNA level is essential to ensure that the ligation product maintains the correct reading frame. If the combined DNA has an altered reading frame, i.e., a sequence of successive codons that yields either an incomplete or an incorrect translation product, then a functional version of the protein encoded by the cloned target gene will not be produced. Many strategies have been devised to ensure that a proper reading frame is achieved.

Uses of Fusion Proteins

For some applications, a fusion protein can be a satisfactory end product. For example, a specific antigenic site that is required in large amounts and is part of a fusion protein may be used for research or diagnostic purposes

FIGURE 6.11 A fusion protein cloning vector. The plasmid contains an ampicillin resistance (Amp^r) gene as the selectable marker, a DNA sequence encoding the N-terminal segment of the *E. coli* outer membrane protein *(ompF)*, a restriction endonuclease site (AbcI) for cloning, and a truncated β-galactosidase gene *(lacZ)*. The cloned gene (Gene) is inserted into the AbcI site. After transcription and translation, a tribrid protein is produced consisting of OmpF–target protein–LacZ.

as long as the stabilizing protein does not interfere with the correct folding of the antigenic site. In this case, the fusion protein can be used as an antigen, and any antibodies that are directed against the stabilizing protein can be removed by absorption with this protein alone, thus leaving in the antiserum only those antibodies that bind to the targeted protein sequence.

In one instance, a fusion cloning vector that included the 5'-terminal segment of the *E. coli ompF* gene, which directs the synthesis of an outer membrane protein, and a portion of the *E. coli lacZ* (β-galactosidase) gene was constructed and used to generate antibodies against selected target proteins (Fig. 6.11). The *ompF* gene segment contributed the signals for the initiation of both transcription and translation and for secretion of the fusion protein. Even though the truncated *lacZ* gene lacks the codons for the first 8 amino acids, the shortened protein encoded by this gene fragment is still enzymatically active. This form of the enzyme β-galactosidase is able to function with almost any peptide fused to its N terminus. The *lacZ* gene was cloned on the vector at a location that put it in an altered reading frame with respect to the *ompF* leader sequence. Therefore, no functional β-galactosidase was produced. However, any cloned target DNA that had both *ompF* and *lacZ* in frame would produce a three-part hybrid protein that comprised a portion of the OmpF amino acid sequence, the protein encoded by the cloned target gene, and the functional C-terminal portion of β-galactosidase, whose activity is readily visualized on plates. Such a hybrid protein can be used either as an antigen to produce antibodies that will cross-react with the protein encoded by the cloned gene or as a means of producing large amounts of small, important portions of specific proteins.

In addition to reducing the degradation of polypeptides, a number of fusion proteins have been developed to simplify the purification of recombinant proteins (Table 6.2). This approach is useful for purification of proteins expressed in either prokaryotic or eukaryotic host organisms. For

TABLE 6.2 Some protein fusion systems used to facilitate the purification of foreign proteins in *E. coli* and other host organisms

Fusion partner	Size	Ligand	Elution conditions
ZZ	14 kDa	Immunoglobulin G	Low pH
Histidine tail	6–10 amino acids	Ni^{2+}	Imidazole
Strep tag	10 amino acids	Streptavidin	Iminobiotin
Pinpoint	13 kDa	Streptavidin	Biotin
Maltose-binding protein	40 kDa	Amylose	Maltose
GST	26 kDa	Glutathione	Reduced glutathione
Flag	8 amino acids	Specific monoclonal antibody (MAb)	EDTA or low pH
Poly-arginine	5–6 amino acids	SP-Sephadex	High salt at pH >8.0
c-myc	11 amino acids	Specific MAb	Low pH
S tag	15 amino acids	S fragment of RNase A	Low pH
Calmodulin-binding peptide	26 amino acids	Calmodulin	EGTA and high salt
Cellulose-binding domain	4–20 kDa	Cellulose	Urea or guanidine hydrochloride
Chitin-binding domain	51 amino acids	Chitin	SDS or guanidine hydrochloride
SBP tag	38 amino acids	Streptavidin	Biotin

ZZ, a fragment of *Staphylococcus aureus* protein A; Strep tag, a peptide with affinity for streptavidin; Pinpoint, a protein fragment that is biotinylated and binds streptavidin; GST, glutathione S-transferase; Flag, a peptide recognized by enterokinase; c-myc, a peptide from a protein that is overexpressed in many cancers; S tag, a peptide fragment of ribonuclease (RNase) A; SBP (streptavidin-binding protein), a peptide with affinity for streptavidin; SP-Sephadex, a cation-exchange resin composed of sulfopropyl groups covalently attached to Sephadex beads.

example, a vector that contains the human interleukin-2 gene joined to DNA encoding the marker peptide sequence Asp-Tyr-Lys-Asp-Asp-Asp-Asp-Lys has the dual function of reducing the degradation of the expressed interleukin-2 gene product and then enabling the product to be purified. Interleukin-2 is a biological factor that stimulates both T-cell growth and B-cell antibody synthesis. Following expression of this construct (Fig. 6.12), the secreted fusion protein can be purified in a single step by immunoaffinity chromatography, in which monoclonal antibodies against the marker peptide have been immobilized on a polypropylene (or other solid) support and act as ligands to bind the fusion protein (Fig. 6.13). Because the marker peptide is relatively small, it does not significantly decrease the amount of host cell resources that are available for the production of interleukin-2; thus, the yield of interleukin-2 is not affected by the concomitant synthesis of the marker peptide. In addition, while the fusion protein has the same biological activity as native interleukin-2, to satisfy the government agencies that regulate the use of pharmaceuticals, it is still necessary to remove the marker peptide if the product is to be used for human immunotherapy or other medical purposes. In this system, the marker sequence may be specifically removed by treatment of the fusion protein with bovine intestinal enterokinase (which is a highly specific protease, despite its name).

In many instances antigen-antibody complexes that form during the immunoaffinity process are difficult to separate without the use of denaturing chemicals. As an alternative, it has become very popular to generate a fusion protein containing six or eight histidine residues attached to either the N- or C-terminal end of the target protein. The histidine-tagged protein, along with other cellular proteins, is then passed over an affinity column of nickel–nitrilotriacetic acid. The histidine-tagged protein, but not the other cellular proteins, binds tightly to the column. The bound protein is eventually eluted from the column by the addition of imidazole (the side chain of histidine). With this protocol, some cloned and overexpressed proteins have been purified up to 100-fold with greater than 90% recovery in a single step. In addition, this system can be utilized to purify denatured proteins, for example, following solubilization of inclusion bodies and before the solubilized proteins are renatured.

Cleavage of Fusion Proteins

Depending on its end use, it may be undesirable to produce a fusion protein as the final product. For example, the presence of the host protein segment makes most fusion proteins unsuitable for clinical use and may affect the biological functioning of the target protein. In addition, fusion proteins require more extensive testing before being approved by regulatory agen-

FIGURE 6.12 Schematic representation of the genetic construct used to produce a secreted fusion protein consisting of a marker peptide and interleukin-2. The amino acid sequence of the marker peptide is shown.

1 Concentrate secreted protein mixture

Marker
peptide

Other proteins

2 Prepare immunoaffinity column

Polypropylene
support

Anti-marker
peptide antibody

3 Add secreted protein mixture
 to the column

FIGURE 6.13 Immunoaffinity chromatographic purification of a fusion protein. An antibody that binds to the marker peptide of the fusion protein (anti-marker peptide antibody) is attached to a solid polypropylene support. The secreted proteins are passed through the column containing the bound antibody. The marker peptide portion of the fusion protein is bound to the antibody, and the other proteins pass through. The immunopurified fusion protein can then be selectively eluted from the column by the addition of pure marker peptide.

cies, such as the U.S. Food and Drug Administration. Thus, strategies have been developed to remove the unwanted amino acid sequence from the target protein. One way to do this is to join the gene for the target protein to all or a portion of the gene for another protein (the stabilizing fusion partner) with oligonucleotides that encode short stretches of amino acids that are recognized by a specific nonbacterial protease. The oligonucleotide linkers that code for the protease recognition site may be ligated upstream of the cloned gene (so that the linker peptide will be synthesized at the N-terminual end of the target protein) before the construct is inserted into

a fusion expression vector. For example, an oligonucleotide linker encoding the amino acid sequence Ile-Glu-Gly-Arg can be joined to the cloned gene. Following synthesis and purification of the fusion protein, a blood coagulation factor called X_a can be used to release the target protein from the fusion partner, because factor X_a is a specific protease that cleaves peptide bonds uniquely on the C-terminal side of the Ile-Glu-Gly-Arg sequence (Fig. 6.14). Moreover, because this peptide sequence occurs rather infrequently in native proteins, this approach can be used to recover many different cloned gene products.

The proteases most commonly used to cleave a fusion partner/affinity tag from a protein of interest are enterokinase, tobacco etch virus protease, thrombin, and factor X_a. However, following this cleavage, it is necessary to perform additional purification steps in order to separate both the protease and the fusion protein from the protein of interest. In addition, proteases may cleave the protein of interest at unintended sites, and the cleavage reaction may not go to completion, leaving a portion of the protein of interest still attached to its fusion partner. One way around this problem is through the use of self-splicing inteins. An intein may be defined as an internal segment of a protein that, under specific conditions, catalyzes its own cleavage into two separate polypeptides. Of the more than 100 known inteins, the majority contain a cysteine or serine residue at the N-terminal side of an asparagine residue, with cleavage occurring between these two amino acids. When the N-terminal residue at the cleavage site is cysteine, protein chain cleavage may be initiated by the addition of a sulfhydryl reagent, such as dithiothreitol. This approach typically includes a gene fusion with the gene of interest (encoding the target protein), an intein, and a protein tag (Fig. 6.15). One inexpensive way to commercialize this system is to utilize a chitin-binding domain as the protein tag. In practice, a mixture of cellular proteins is passed through a chitin column to which only the fusion protein binds. The rest of the proteins pass through the column. Then, the column is treated with dithiothreitol, the protein of interest is cleaved at the intein junction and eluted, and the inexpensive used column is discarded. This system has been used to purify Cre recombinase (a tool for chromosome engineering), α-1-antitrypsin (a therapeutic protein), and basic human fibroblast growth factor (a potential therapeutic protein).

Surface Display

Specialized fusion protein systems have been devised for screening complementary DNA (cDNA) libraries that contain very large numbers of dif-

FIGURE 6.14 Proteolytic cleavage of a fusion protein by blood coagulation factor X_a. The factor X_a recognition sequence (X_a linker sequence) lies between the amino acid sequences of two different proteins. A functional cloned-gene protein (with Val at its N terminus) is released after cleavage.

... Thr-Ala-Glu-Gly-Gly-Ser-Ile-Glu-Gly-Arg-Val-His-Leu ...

ferent clones (sometimes up to 5×10^{10}) for proteins that are encoded by rarely occurring cDNAs. Generally, for these libraries, cDNA molecules are cloned into a surface protein (filament protein, or pilus protein) gene of either a filamentous bacteriophage, such as M13, or a bacterium. After transcription and translation, the fusion protein is incorporated into a surface structure of the bacteriophage or bacterium, where it can be identified by an immunological assay. More specifically, fusions are often made with the protein pIII gene from bacteriophage M13. Protein pIII is normally found at the tip of this tubular bacteriophage and is responsible for initiating phage infection of *E. coli* by binding to F pili. A plasmid that contains a small piece of M13 DNA that allows the plasmid (phagemid) to be packaged in vitro into M13 phage particles; a protein pIII gene under the control of a regulatable bacterial promoter, such as the *E. coli lac* promoter; and a cloning site near the 5' end of the pIII gene for insertion of a cDNA or other coding sequence is constructed. The expressed target protein is fused to bacteriophage M13 protein pIII near its N terminus (Fig. 6.16). After M13 replication in *E. coli* cells, the plaques are assayed immunologically using antibodies that detect the presence of the target protein. Recombinant phagemids isolated from positive plaques can then be used as a source of the target cDNA. This is an extremely powerful selection system that has the capability of finding cDNAs for very rarely expressed but important proteins. Finally, it is also possible, although less straightforward and therefore less common, to create recombinant phage in which a target peptide is fused to protein pVIII, the bacteriophage coat protein.

An alternative to the phage surface display of proteins described above is the use of libraries with bacterial surface structures composed of fusion proteins that can be screened for clones that carry specific coding sequences. To export proteins to the surface of a gram-negative bacterium, such as *E. coli*, fusions between the genes for the target protein and for an outer surface protein are created. Bacterial fusion partners that have been used in these types of constructs include outer membrane protein A (OmpA) and peptide-glycan-associated lipoprotein (PAL) from *E. coli*, as well as *Pseudomonas aeruginosa* outer membrane protein F (OprF). With most bacterial surface fusion proteins, the target protein is located at either the N or C terminus of the fusion protein. However, in some instances, short stretches of a target protein can be expressed in the middle of the fusion partner (Fig. 6.17).

In addition to facilitating the screening of large cDNA libraries, surface-displayed proteins can provide an effective means of overexpressing

FIGURE 6.15 (A) Purification of a protein of interest (POI) from an intein-containing fusion protein bound to a chitin chromatography column through a chitin-binding domain (CBD). Cleavage, which is indicated by the arrow, occurs upon the addition of dithiothreitol. (B) Products following intein cleavage, including the released protein of interest.

FIGURE 6.16 Recombinant bacteriophage M13 displaying a fusion protein consisting of the target protein and phage protein pIII.

FIGURE 6.17 Fusion protein between bacterial outer surface protein and a foreign target protein joined to either the N or C terminus **(A)** or foreign peptides inserted into the surface-exposed loops **(B)**. In both cases, the foreign peptide or protein is directed to the outer surface of the bacterial cell.

peptides or proteins. For example, in one study, the amino-acid-repeating epitope (antigenic determinant) Asn-Ala-Asn-Pro of a protein from the parasite *Plasmodium falciparum*, the causative agent of malaria, was inserted into the regions that encode surface-exposed loops of the major outer membrane protein from *P. aeruginosa* (OprF). Whole bacterial cells expressing this fusion protein reacted positively when challenged with monoclonal antibodies against *P. falciparum*. It may, therefore, be possible to use some surface-displayed fusion proteins as vaccines (see chapter 11).

Translation Expression Vectors

Putting a cloned gene under the control of a regulatable, strong promoter, although essential, may not be sufficient to maximize the yield of the cloned gene product. Other factors, such as the efficiency of translation and the stability of the newly synthesized cloned-gene protein, may also affect the amount of product.

In prokaryotic cells, various proteins are not necessarily synthesized with the same efficiency. In fact, they may be produced at very different levels (up to several hundredfold) even if they are encoded within the same polycistronic messenger RNA (mRNA). Differences in translational efficiency and in transcriptional regulation enable the cell to have hundreds or even thousands of copies of some proteins and only a few copies of others.

In part, the molecular basis for differential translation is the presence of a translational initiation signal called a ribosome-binding site in the tran-

scribed mRNA. A ribosome-binding site is a sequence of 6 to 8 nucleotides (e.g., UAAGGAGG) in mRNA that can base pair with a complementary sequence (AUUCCUCC for *E. coli*) on the RNA component of the small ribosomal subunit.

Generally, the stronger the binding of the mRNA to the ribosomal RNA, the greater the efficiency of translational initiation. For this reason, many *E. coli* expression vectors have been designed to ensure that the mRNA of a cloned gene contains a strong ribosome-binding site. In effect, this means that heterologous prokaryotic and eukaryotic genes can be translated readily in *E. coli*. However, certain other conditions must be satisfied for this approach to function properly. First, the ribosome-binding sequence must be located a precise distance from the translational start codon of the cloned gene. (At the RNA level, the translational codon is usually AUG. At the DNA level, the strand that has the ATG sequence is called the coding strand, and the complementary strand, which acts as the template for transcription, is the noncoding strand. By convention, a start codon at the DNA level is designated ATG.) Second, the DNA sequence that includes the ribosome-binding site through the first few codons of the gene of interest must not contain nucleotide sequences that have regions of complementarity and therefore after transcription can fold back, i.e., form intrastrand loops (Fig. 6.18), thereby thwarting the interaction of the mRNA with the ribosome. The local secondary structure of the mRNA, which can either shield or expose the ribosome-binding site, determines the extent to

MILESTONE

The *tac* Promoter: a Functional Hybrid Derived from the *trp* and *lac* Promoters

H. A. DE BOER, L. J. COMSTOCK, and M. VASSER
Proc. Natl. Acad. Sci. USA **80**:21–25, 1983

De Boer and his colleagues began their efforts to construct the *tac* promoter with the idea of combining portions of two different strong and regulatable promoters to create an even stronger promoter that would direct very high levels of foreign-gene expression. When they undertook their studies, although the DNA sequences of a number of prokaryotic promoters, mostly from *E. coli*, were known, the precise features that enabled a promoter to be efficient at directing transcription were not well understood. It was known that almost all mutations that affected the strength of a prokaryotic promoter were found in either the –10 region or

the –35 region, which are approximately 10 or 35 bp upstream of the mRNA transcription start site, respectively. Moreover, only mutations that made an existing promoter more like the consensus sequences for each of these regions, i.e., 5′-TATAAT-3′ for the –10 region and 5′-TTGACA-3′ for the –35 region, increased the strength of the promoter. The consensus sequences had been deduced by comparing the DNA sequences of all known promoters and determining which nucleotides occurred most often. de Boer and his colleagues also knew that the *lacUV5* promoter, which is a stronger variant of the *lac* promoter, had a consensus sequence at its

–10 but not its –35 region, while the *trp* promoter, which normally controls the transcription of genes involved in the biosynthesis of tryptophan, has a consensus sequence at its –35 but not its –10 region. They decided to create a fusion promoter which included the –10 region from the *lac* promoter and the –35 region from the *trp* promoter. They tested this new "*tac*" promoter, as they called it, for its ability to direct the synthesis of the enzyme galactose kinase in *E. coli* and compared it in the same assay system with the *trp* and *lac* promoters. In agreement with their initial idea, the *tac* promoter was found to be approximately 5 times stronger than the *trp* promoter and 10 times stronger than the *lac* promoter. In addition, like the *lac* promoter, the *tac* promoter was repressed by the *lac* repressor and derepressed by IPTG. Thus, this new promoter was not only strong, but also regulatable.

```
            A
        C       G
        G — C
        U — A
        A — U
        U — G
        A       A
        A — U
        A — U
        A — U
        G       A
        G — U
        G — U
        G — U
5' GAACCG ⌐      ⌐ GAACAC 3'
```

FIGURE 6.18 Example of secondary structure of the 5' end of an mRNA that would prevent efficient translation. The ribosome-binding site is GGGGG, the initiator codon is AUG (shown in red), and the first few codons are CAG-CAU-GAU-UUA-UUU. The mRNA is oriented with its 5' end to the left and its 3' end to the right. Note that in addition to the traditional A·U and G·C base pairs in mRNA, G can also base pair to some extent with U.

FIGURE 6.19 The expression vector pKK233-2. The plasmid pKK233-2 codes for the ampicillin resistance (Ampr) gene as a selectable marker gene, the *tac* promoter (p^{tac}), the *lacZ* ribosome-binding site (rbs), three restriction endonuclease cloning sites (NcoI, PstI, and HindIII), and two transcription termination sequences (T1 and T2). The arrow indicates the direction of transcription. The plasmid is not drawn to scale.

which the mRNA can bind to the appropriate sequence on the ribosome and initiate translation. Thus, for each cloned gene, it is important to establish that the ribosome-binding site is properly placed and that the secondary structure of the mRNA does not prevent its access to the ribosome.

A number of convenient vector systems that incorporate both transcriptional and translational signals for the expression of cloned eukaryotic genes in *E. coli* have been developed. One such system is called expression vector pKK233-2 and includes a number of elements, including the following (Fig. 6.19): an ampicillin resistance gene as a selectable marker, the *tac* promoter, the *lacZ* ribosome-binding site, an ATG start codon located 8 nucleotides downstream from the ribosome-binding site, and the transcription terminators T1 and T2 from bacteriophage λ. The cloned gene is inserted into an NcoI, PstI, or HindIII site that lies between the ribosome-binding site and the transcription terminators so that it is in the same reading frame as the ATG start codon. After induction and transcription, the mRNA of a cloned gene is efficiently translated. However, since the nucleotide sequences that encode the amino acids in the N-terminal region of the target protein vary from one gene to another, it is not possible to design a vector that will eliminate the possibility of mRNA fold-back in all instances. Therefore, no single optimized translational initiation region can guarantee a high rate of translation initiation for all cloned genes. Consequently, the expression vectors described above are merely starting points for the optimization of translation initiation.

A cellular incompatibility that can interfere with efficient translation occurs when a cloned gene has codons that are rarely used by the host cell. For example, AGG, AGA, AUA, CUA, and CGA are the least-used codons in *E. coli*. In these cases, the host cell may not produce enough of the transfer RNAs (tRNAs) that recognize these rarely used codons, and the yield of the cloned-gene protein is much lower than expected. An insufficient supply of certain tRNAs may lead to either a reduction in the amount of protein synthesized or the incorporation of incorrect amino acids into the protein. Any codon that is used less than 5 to 10% of the time by the host organism may cause problems. Particularly detrimental to high levels of expression are places where two or more rarely used codons are close or adjacent or appear in the N-terminal portion of the protein. There are several experimental approaches that can be used to alleviate this problem. (1) If the target gene is eukaryotic, it may be cloned and expressed in a eukaryotic host cell. (2) A new version of the target gene containing codons that are more commonly used by the host cell may be chemically synthesized (codon optimization). (3) A host cell that has been engineered to overexpress several rare tRNAs may be employed (Fig. 6.20). In fact, an *E. coli* strain that overproduces the tRNAs *argU*, *ileY*, and *leuW*, which are specific for the codons AGG/AGA, AUA, and CUA, respectively, is available commercially. This cell line is sold for the explicit purpose of expressing a high level of foreign proteins that use these rare *E. coli* codons. With this commercially available *E. coli* cell line, it was possible to overexpress the Ara h2 protein, a peanut allergen, approximately 100-fold over the amount that was synthesized in conventional *E. coli* cells. Using the approach described, it should be possible to produce large quantities of a variety of heterologous proteins that are otherwise difficult to express in *E. coli* hosts (Table 6.3).

A E. coli host cell

Plasmid with
foreign gene

Low level of foreign
gene expression

B E. coli host cell

Overproduced tRNA

Plasmid with
foreign gene

High level of foreign
gene expression

FIGURE 6.20 Schematic representation of the expression of foreign proteins in a typical *E. coli* host cell **(A)** and in an *E. coli* host cell that has been engineered to overexpress several rare tRNAs **(B).**

Increasing Protein Stability

In recent years, it has become almost routine to overproduce a wide range of different foreign proteins in *E. coli* or other host organisms. However, to recover large amounts of purified active protein requires that the protein be as stable as possible. In this regard, there are certainly large differences in the intrinsic stabilities of different proteins. In addition, a protein produced in a heterologous host cell may, for various reasons, be less stable than the same protein produced in its normal cellular environment.

Intrinsic Protein Stability

Under normal growing conditions, the half-lives of different proteins range from a few minutes to hours. The basis for this differential stability is both the extent of disulfide bond formation and the presence of certain amino acids at the N terminus. For example, when specific amino acids were attached to the N terminus of β-galactosidase, the in vitro survival time of the protein varied from approximately 2 minutes to more than 20 hours (Table 6.4). Amino acid additions that extend the intrinsic survival of a

TABLE 6.3 Increases in gene expression that result from altering the codon usage of the wild-type gene (or cDNA) to more closely correspond to the host *E. coli* cell

Protein	Improvement (fold)
Human interleukin-2	16
Clostridium tetani tetanus toxin fragment C	4
Human cardiac troponin T	10–40
Mouse c-FOS protein	>200
Spinach plastocyanin	1.2
Human neurofibromin	3
Human glutathione transferase M2-2	140
Human phosphatidylcholine transfer protein	>100
Human interleukin-6	3
Human interleukin-18	5
Plasmodium vaccine candidate antigen	4

In some cases, only a small number of codons were altered, while in others, the entire gene was synthesized with the optimal codon usage for expression in *E. coli*.

protein can be readily incorporated into cloned genes. Often the presence of a single extra amino acid at the N-terminal end is sufficient to stabilize a target protein, probably by making it less susceptible to degradation by certain cellular proteases. Long-lived proteins can accumulate in cells and thereby increase the yield of the product. This phenomenon occurs in both prokaryotes and eukaryotes.

In contrast to the amino acids at the N terminus, which can increase the stability of a protein, there are internal amino acid sequences that make a protein more susceptible to proteolytic degradation. These regions of the protein, which are called PEST sequences, are rich in proline (P), glutamic acid (E), serine (S), and threonine (T). They are often, but not always, flanked by clusters of positively charged amino acids, such as lysine and arginine, and may act to mark proteins for degradation within the cell. In some instances, it is possible to enhance the stability of a protein by altering its PEST regions by genetic manipulation. Such changes, of course, must not alter the function of the target protein.

TABLE 6.4 Stability of β-galactosidease with certain amino acids added to its N terminus

Amino acid added	Half-life
Met, Ser, Ala	>20 h
Thr, Val, Gly	>20 h
Ile, Glu	>30 min
Tyr, Gln	~10 min
Pro	~7 min
Phe, Leu, Asp, Lys	~3 min
Arg	~2 min

Adapted from Bachmair et al., *Science* **234**:179–186, 1986.

FIGURE 6.21 Regulation of the synthesis of a thioredoxin–target protein fusion in the absence **(A)** or presence **(B)** of tryptophan in the growth medium. The arrows labeled p^{trp} and p^L indicate the direction of transcription. o^{trp}, the operator region where the *trp* repressor protein binds; o^L, the operator region where the *cI* repressor binds; p^{trp}, the *trp* promoter; p^L, the leftward promoter from bacteriophage λ; TT, transcription termination region. The box between the thioredoxin and target genes indicates the DNA region that codes for the peptide that acts as the enterokinase cleavage site; the horseshoes indicate the binding of a repressor protein to its operator region.

Facilitating Protein Folding

Many of the proteins that are produced in *E. coli* accumulate in the form of insoluble, intracellular, biologically inactive inclusion bodies. Although a small amount of biologically active protein can often be recovered from inclusion bodies, the extraction procedure requires expensive and time-consuming protein solubilization and refolding procedures. Since the in vivo insolubility of proteins is often a consequence of their incorrect

folding, various strategies have been devised to avoid this problem. For example, fusion proteins that contain thioredoxin, an 11.7-kilodalton (kDa) protein, as the fusion partner remain soluble even when up to 40% of the cellular protein consists of the fusion protein. With this system, the target gene is cloned into a multiple cloning site just downstream from the thioredoxin gene. Both of these genes are under the control of the p^L promoter on an *E. coli* plasmid vector (Fig. 6.21). The *E. coli* host cell for this system has a *c*I repressor protein construct that consists of a copy of the gene for the *c*I repressor protein under the transcriptional control of the *trp* promoter integrated into the chromosomal DNA. In the absence of tryptophan (Fig. 6.21A), a sufficient amount of *c*I repressor protein is synthesized to prevent transcription from the p^L promoter and therefore prevent the production of the fusion protein. When tryptophan is added to the growth medium (Fig. 6.21B), the *trp* promoter is turned off by the *trp* repressor, the *c*I repressor protein is not synthesized, and the DNA construct encoding the fusion protein is transcribed from the p^L promoter on the plasmid and then translated. In this case, the fusion protein, which consists of thioredoxin and the target protein, is synthesized and accumulates preferentially at osmotically sensitive sites called adhesion zones at the inner periphery of the host *E. coli* cytoplasmic membrane. The soluble fusion protein is selectively released by osmotic shock from *E. coli* cells into the growth medium. If required, the native form of the target protein can be released from the fusion protein by treatment with the enzyme enterokinase. Finally, since thioredoxin is stable at temperatures as high as 80°C, in those instances where the target protein is also stable at high temperatures, the fusion protein may be purified by high-temperature incubation, a condition that denatures most of the other cellular proteins.

In *E. coli* and other gram-negative bacteria, disulfide bond formation takes place in the periplasmic space, which is topologically equivalent to the endoplasmic reticulum in eukaryotes but is a much more oxidizing environment. Disulfide bond formation in *E. coli* requires the participation of two soluble periplasmic enzymes (DsbA and DsbC) and two membrane-bound enzymes (DsbB and DsbD). Unfortunately, foreign proteins that contain three or more disulfides generally do not fold correctly in bacteria and often form inclusion bodies. In these instances, the foreign protein is usually produced in animal or plant cells. However, researchers have devised some strategies to overcome this problem for recalcitrant proteins with a large number of disulfide bonds.

Human tissue plasminogen activator is an important therapeutic protein that is used to remove blood clots. The active form of this protein is a 527-amino-acid serine protease that folds into five distinct structural domains with 35 cysteine residues that participate in the formation of 17 disulfide bonds. The cDNA for human tissue plasminogen activator was cloned downstream of a DNA sequence that encodes a leader peptide that was previously used to facilitate the secretion (to the periplasm) of other eukaryotic proteins. However, in this case, only trace amounts of human tissue plasminogen activator were produced. This low level of activity is thought to reflect the fact that this complex protein is unable to fold properly in *E. coli*. In an attempt to increase the yield of human tissue plasminogen activator, the gene was coexpressed with the gene for either rat or

yeast protein disulfide isomerase, both of which had been found to assist protein folding in other cases; however, this strategy did not affect the amount of active human tissue plasminogen activator that could be obtained. On the other hand, the coexpression of high levels of DsbC (Fig. 6.22) resulted in more than a 100-fold increase in the production of functional human tissue plasminogen activator. Alterations in the levels of the other Dsb proteins did not affect the amount of active human tissue plasminogen activator that could be recovered. To realize the maximum benefit from DsbC overproduction, it was necessary to induce the synthesis of this protein approximately 30 minutes prior to the induction of human tissue plasminogen activator.

Similar research in another laboratory found that while DsbC overproduction had the largest impact on promoting the correct folding of horseradish peroxidase in *E. coli* and preventing its aggregation, the simultaneous overproduction of all four Dsb proteins yielded the greatest amount of properly folded and active horseradish peroxidase. Thus, the experience of several researchers clearly demonstrates that the correct folding and disulfide bond formation of eukaryotic proteins produced in *E. coli* require high levels of the Dsb proteins or possibly other protein disulfide isomerases.

Coexpression Strategies

The expression of some thermolabile foreign proteins in *E. coli* host strains, which are typically grown at 37°C, often results in the formation of inclusion bodies of inactive protein. This occurs because the foreign protein misfolds when it cannot attain its native active conformation. A variety of strategies have been developed, albeit with limited success, to circumvent this problem. Cultivation of recombinant strains at low temperatures, which is beneficial to proper protein folding, often significantly increases the amount of recoverable active protein. However, mesophilic bacteria like *E. coli* grow extremely slowly at low temperatures. In one study, the chaperonin 60 gene *(cpn60)* and the cochaperonin 10 gene *(cpn10)* from the psychrophilic bacterium *Oleispira antarctica* were introduced into a host strain of *E. coli* with the result that the *E. coli* strain gained the ability to grow at a high rate at low temperatures (4 to 10°C). This strain was subsequently transformed with a plasmid encoding a temperature-sensitive esterase. The expression of the temperature-sensitive esterase in the *E. coli* strain carrying the two chaperone genes at 4 to 10°C yielded esterase specific activity that was 180-fold higher than the activity from the native *E. coli* strain (without chaperonins) grown at 37°C. Interestingly, and contrary to expectations, the psychrophile chaperonins do not facilitate the proper folding of the esterase and do not affect its catalytic properties. Although very high levels of expression of the cloned esterase were not attained, this work is an important first step in the development of expression systems for proteins that are sensitive to high temperature and might otherwise be difficult to produce. The next logical step in the development of this system would likely be the construction of an *E. coli* host cell that contains stably integrated copies of these chaperonin genes in the chromosome.

FIGURE 6.22 Schematic representation of the effect of overproduction of the *E. coli* disulfide bond-forming protein (DsbC) on the synthesis of active human tissue plasminogen activator (tPA). **(A)** When too few molecules of DsbC are available, the tPA is folded incorrectly and is inactive. **(B)** Overproduction of DsbC results in correctly folded and active human tPA. In both instances, the tPA is secreted into the periplasm.

Overcoming Oxygen Limitation

E. coli and most other microorganisms that are used to express foreign proteins generally require oxygen for optimal growth. Unfortunately, oxygen has only limited solubility in aqueous media. Thus, as the cell density of a growing culture increases, the cells rapidly deplete the growth medium of dissolved oxygen. When cells become oxygen limited, exponential growth slows and the culture rapidly enters a stationary phase, during which cellular metabolism changes. One consequence of the stationary phase is the production by the host cells of proteases that can degrade foreign proteins. Oxygen dissolves into the growth medium very slowly, so this problem is not always alleviated when large amounts of air or oxygen are added to the growth medium, even with high stirring rates. Modification of the fermenter configuration to optimize the aeration and agitation of cells, and addition of chemicals to the growth medium to increase the solubility of oxygen have been tried in an effort to deal with the limited amount of dissolved oxygen. However, these efforts have met with only limited success.

Use of Protease-Deficient Host Strains

One possible way to stabilize foreign proteins produced in *E. coli* is to develop host strains that are deficient in the production of proteolytic enzymes. However, this is not as simple as it might appear. *E. coli* has at least 25 different proteases, and only a few of them have been studied at the genetic level. Moreover, these proteases are important for the degradation of abnormal or defective proteins, which is a housekeeping function that is necessary for the continued viability of the cells. In one study, strains with mutations in one or more protease genes were constructed. Generally, the strains that were most deficient in overall protease activity grew most slowly. Thus, decreasing protease activity caused cells to be debilitated. However, an *E. coli* strain with mutations in both the gene for the RNA polymerase sigma factor that is responsible for heat shock protein synthesis (*rpoH*) and the gene for a protease that is required for cell growth at high temperatures (*degP*) secreted target proteins that had a 36-fold-greater specific activity than when they were produced in wild-type host cells. This increase in activity reflects a decrease in the proteolytic degradation of these secreted proteins.

Bacterial Hemoglobin

Some strains of the *Vitreoscilla* bacterium, a gram-negative obligate aerobe, normally live in oxygen-poor environments, such as stagnant ponds. To obtain a sufficient amount of oxygen for their growth and metabolism, these organisms synthesize a hemoglobin-like molecule that binds oxygen from the environment and increases the level of available oxygen inside cells. When the gene for this protein was cloned and expressed in *E. coli*, the transformants displayed higher levels of synthesis of both cellular and recombinant proteins, higher levels of cellular respiration, a higher ATP production rate, and higher ATP contents, especially at low levels of oxygen in the growth medium, than did nontransformed cells. In these transformants, the *Vitreoscilla* hemoglobin increases the intracellular effective oxygen concentration, which raises the activities of both cytochrome *d* and cytochrome *o*. This causes an increase in proton pumping, with the

subsequent generation of ATP, thereby providing additional energy for cellular metabolic processes (Fig. 6.23). For this strategy to be effective in different host cells, not only must the *Vitreoscilla* sp. hemoglobin gene be efficiently expressed, but the host cells must also be able to synthesize the heme portion of the hemoglobin molecule. Once these conditions have been met, this strategy can be used to improve growth, as well as foreign-gene expression, in a range of different industrially important bacteria, including *E. coli*, *Streptomyces* spp., *Enterobacter aerogenes*, and *Xanthomonas maltophilia* (Table 6.5).

Limiting Biofilm Formation

In many natural environments, bacteria are commonly found to be associated with solid surfaces and only rarely exist as free-swimming entities. The bacterial cells typically attach to a surface, form a monolayer, and later organize into a biofilm, a mixture of bacterial cells and polysaccharides (typically alginate) that may be as much as 100 to 200 μm thick (Fig. 6.24). When they are part of a biofilm, bacterial cells are generally protected against hostile agents in the environment, such as biocides, bacteriophages, and protozoa.

Bacterial cells that form biofilms, or otherwise produce significant amounts of extracellular polysaccharide, are difficult to transform with plasmid DNA and are typically resistant to high levels of antibiotics (which find it difficult to enter the bacterial cells). These cells are limited in the amount of foreign protein that they can produce, probably reflecting the large amount of cellular resources directed toward polysaccharide synthesis and the limited amounts of nutrients that are able to enter cells within the biofilm.

FIGURE 6.23 Schematic representation of the binding of O_2 by *Vitreoscilla* hemoglobin, the utilization of this O_2 in pumping (by proteins such as cytochromes) H^+ from the cytoplasm to the periplasm, and the subsequent coupling of H^+ uptake (by ATPase) to ATP generation. ADP, adenosine diphosphate.

TABLE 6.5 Use of *Vitreoscilla* hemoglobin for improved production of foreign proteins in bacteria

Type of improvement	Specific effect	Bacterium
Increased protein production	Growth and α-amylase production	*E. coli*
	Total protein content	*E. coli*
	Protein secretion and α-amylase production	*B. subtilis*
Increased chemical production	Growth and biosurfactant production	*Gordonia amarae*
	Acetoin and butanol production	*E. aerogenes*
	Growth and poly-β-hydroxybutyrate production	*E. coli*
Increased antibiotic production	Cephalosporin C	*Acremonium chrysogenum*
	Actinorhodin	*Streptomyces coelicolor*
	Erythromycin	*Saccharopolyspora erythraea*
	Growth and monensin production	*Streptomyces cinnamonensis*
	Chlorotetracycline	*Streptomyces aureofaciens*
Enhanced bioremediation	Growth and degradation of 2,4-dinitrotoluene	*P. aeruginosa*
		Burkholderia sp.
	Degradation of benzoic acid	*X. maltophilia*
	Growth and degradation of benzoic acid	*Burkholderia* sp.
	Degradation of 2-chlorobenzoate	*Burkholderia cepacia*
Enhanced physiology	Growth	*Tremella fuciformis*
	Copper uptake	*E. coli*
	Growth	*E. aerogenes*
	Resistance to sodium nitroprusside	*E. coli*

Adapted from Zhang et al., *Biotechnol. Adv.* 25:123–136, 2007.

FIGURE 6.24 *E. coli* cells in their planktonic form in solution and not interacting with any surface (A), as a monolayer attached to a solid surface (B), and as part of a three-dimensional biofilm attached to a solid surface (C).

Workers have previously tried to limit the formation of biofilms either by adding biofilm-inhibiting chemical agents to the bacterial growth medium or by utilizing new materials to which bacteria adhere less efficiently. However, these approaches have met with only limited success. Another way to limit biofilm formation is to genetically engineer bacterial strains that are deficient in forming biofilms. This was done by creating an *E. coli* strain in which the genes that were involved in the biosynthesis of curli, colanic acid, and bacterial pili were deleted. Pili are required for initial attachment of a bacterial cell to a solid surface, curli are needed for cell-cell and cell-surface attachment, and colanic acid contributes to the three-dimensional structure of the biofilm. When genes involved in these three functions were deleted, the resultant strain of *E. coli* was unable to form biofilms, displayed an increased sensitivity to antibiotics, transformed with a much greater efficiency, and was able to produce a higher level of recombinant protein (Table 6.6). This result indicates that is possible to engineer an *E. coli* host cell to be more efficient at producing foreign proteins. In addition to producing higher levels of recombinant proteins, the use of a bacterial host strain that displays substantially increased sensitivity to common antibiotics may obviate the overuse of antibiotics in the production of foreign proteins. This should make it easier to ensure that the final purified protein product is free of any contaminating antibiotics.

DNA Integration into the Host Chromosome

A plasmid imposes a metabolic load on the cell because of the energy that is used for its replication and for the transcription of RNA and translation

TABLE 6.6 Performance and behavior of wild-type compared to biofilm-minus *E. coli*

Strain	% Adherence to a polystyrene surface	Sensitivity to streptomycin	Sensitivity to rifampin	Transformation efficiency (no. of transformants/μg of plasmid DNA)	Intracellular endoxylanase activity (U/mL)	Extracellular lipase activity (U/mL)
Wild type	30	15	20	3.4×10^5	6.4	7.9
Biofilm-minus mutant	3	1	1	7.9×10^6	7.3	10.0

Antibiotic sensitivity is reported as the relative amount of antibiotic needed to obtain the same amount of bacterial killing. Foreign endoxylanase and lipase genes were introduced on plasmids.

of the proteins that it encodes. For the most part, high-copy-number plasmids impose a greater metabolic load than do low-copy-number plasmids. As a consequence, a fraction of the cell population often loses its plasmids during cell growth. Also, cells that lack plasmids generally grow faster than those that retain them, so plasmidless cells eventually dominate the culture. After a number of generations of cell growth, the loss of plasmid-containing cells diminishes the yield of the cloned gene product. Investigators have devised at least two methods of combating this loss. On a laboratory scale, plasmid-containing cells are maintained by growing the cells in the presence of either an antibiotic or an essential metabolite that enables only plasmid-bearing cells to thrive. But the addition of either antibiotics or metabolites to pilot plant- or industrial-scale fermentations can be extremely costly, and it is imperative that anything that is added to the fermentation, such as an antibiotic or a metabolite, be completely removed before the product is certified as fit for human use. Moreover, for genetically engineered microorganisms that are designed to be released into the environment to remain both effective and environmentally safe, it is essential that the cloned DNA be retained and be neither easily lost nor transferred to other microorganisms. For these reasons, the introduction of cloned DNA directly into the chromosomal DNA of the host organism can overcome the problem of plasmid loss. When DNA is part of the host chromosomal DNA, it is relatively stable and consequently can be maintained for many generations in the absence of selective agents.

The chromosomal integration site of a cloned gene must not be within an essential coding gene. Consequently, the input DNA sequence must be targeted to a specific nonessential site within the chromosome. In addition, to ensure efficient production of the target protein, the input gene should be under the control of a regulatable promoter.

For integration of DNA into a chromosomal site, the input DNA must share some sequence similarity, usually at least 50 nucleotides, with the chromosomal DNA, and there must be a physical exchange (recombination) between the two DNA molecules. Briefly, a generalized protocol for DNA integration includes the following steps.

1. Identify the desired chromosomal integration site, i.e., a segment of DNA on the host chromosome that can be disrupted without affecting the normal functions of the cell.
2. Isolate and clone part or all of the chromosomal integration site.
3. Ligate a cloned gene and a regulatable promoter either into (Fig. 6.25A) or adjacent to (Fig. 6.25B) the cloned chromosomal integration site.

4. Transfer the chromosomal integration fragment–cloned-gene construct into the host cell as part of a plasmid that cannot replicate in the host cell.

5. Select and perpetuate host cells that express the cloned gene. Propagation of the cloned gene can occur only if it has been integrated into the chromosomal DNA of the host cell.

When a host cell is transformed with a nonreplicating plasmid that carries the cloned gene in the middle of a portion of the cloned chromosomal integration site, the DNA on the plasmid can base pair with identical sequences on the host chromosome (Fig. 6.25A). The integration occurs as a result of a host enzyme-catalyzed double crossover. Alternatively, a single crossover that incorporates the entire input plasmid into the host chromosome may occur (not shown). Similarly, insertion of the entire input plasmid DNA occurs when the cloned gene is inserted next to the cloned chromosomal integration site (Fig. 6.25B).

The effectiveness of integration of a cloned gene was examined in *B. subtilis*. The investigators constructed an *E. coli* plasmid that contained an α-amylase gene from *Bacillus amyloliquefaciens* that had been inserted into the middle of a chromosomal DNA fragment from *B. subtilis* but could not replicate in *B. subtilis*. This construct, however, could transform *B. subtilis*. Transformants expressing α-amylase, an enzyme involved in the hydrolysis of starch, were recovered, indicating that the α-amylase gene had been integrated into the *B. subtilis* chromosome and was functioning. The selected transformants were resistant to ampicillin and chloramphenicol. Because both of the antibiotic resistance genes were on the input plasmid, this result indicated that a single recombination event must have occurred and caused the integration of the entire plasmid into the *B. subtilis* chromosomal DNA.

To increase the number of copies of the α-amylase gene that were present on the *B. subtilis* chromosome, the original transformants were grown in the presence of high levels of chloramphenicol. Only cells in which spontaneous DNA duplication of the integrated plasmid had occurred could survive under these conditions. The cells selected for a high level of chloramphenicol resistance were then assayed for α-amylase activity (Table 6.7). With this selection procedure, cells with up to nine copies of the α-amylase gene were identified. The level of enzyme activity expressed from the chromosomally integrated genes far exceeded the activity levels that occurred when the α-amylase gene was present on a multicopy (about 20 to 40 copies per cell) *B. subtilis* plasmid, probably reflecting either the instability of the multicopy plasmid or the energy drain on the transformed cells imposed by the synthesis of the chloramphenicol resistance gene and α-amylase.

In one study, several copies of a foreign gene were inserted into different predetermined sites on the *B. subtilis* chromosome. To do this, a two-step procedure was used for each copy of the foreign gene to be inserted (Fig. 6.26). First, a selectable marker gene, such as an antibiotic resistance gene, was inserted into the middle of a defined but nonessential piece of *B. subtilis* chromosomal DNA on a plasmid vector that could not replicate in *B. subtilis* (Fig. 6.26, step 1). Following transformation of *B. subtilis* with this construct, cells expressing the marker gene were selected. These transformants carried the selectable marker gene integrated at the specified site in the *B. subtilis* chromosomal DNA. Second, the target gene

FIGURE 6.25 Integration of a cloned gene into a chromosomal site. **(A)** The cloned gene has been inserted, on a plasmid, in the middle of a cloned segment of DNA (ab) from the host chromosome. Homologous DNA pairing occurs between plasmid-borne DNA regions a and b and host chromosome DNA regions a' and b', respectively. A double-crossover event (×—×) results in the integration of the cloned gene. **(B)** The cloned gene is inserted adjacent to the cloned DNA from the host chromosome (c). Homologous DNA pairing occurs between plasmid DNA region c and host chromosome DNA region c'. A single recombination event (×) within the paired c–c' DNA region results in the integration of the entire plasmid, including the cloned gene.

with its transcriptional and translational control sequences was inserted into the middle of the piece of *B. subtilis* chromosomal DNA that was used with the marker gene and introduced into the cell on a nonreplicatable

TABLE 6.7 α-Amylase gene copy number and acitvity in *B. subtilis*

No. of copies/genome	Activity (U/mL of mid-log-phase cells)
2	500
5	2,300
7	3,100
8	3,400
9	4,400
Multicopy plasmid	700

Adapted from Kallio et al., *Appl. Micrtobiol. Biotechnol.* **27**:64–71, 1987.

plasmid (Fig. 6.26, step 2). Following transformation of *B. subtilis* with the target gene–plasmid construct, cells that no longer expressed the marker gene were selected after replica plating. These transformants carried the target gene and not the marker gene integrated into the *B. subtilis* chromosomal DNA. To integrate additional copies of the target gene into the host

FIGURE 6.26 Insertion of a foreign gene into a unique predetermined site on the *B. subtilis* chromosome. In step 1, a marker gene is integrated into the host cell chromosomal DNA by homologous recombination. In step 2, the selectable marker gene is replaced by the target gene. The process may then be repeated with different nonessential regions of *B. subtilis* chromosomal DNA.

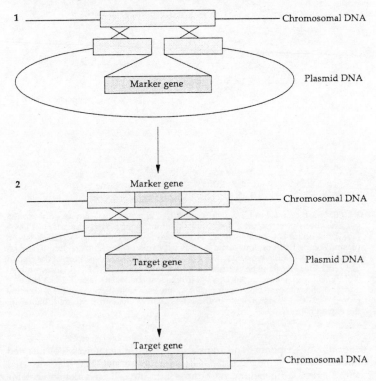

cell chromosomal DNA, the entire procedure was repeated several times with different defined but nonessential regions of *B. subtilis* chromosomal DNA.

Removing Selectable Marker Genes

The integration of a selectable marker gene along with a gene of interest is helpful for identifying transformed cells under laboratory conditions. However, the presence of a selectable marker gene for antibiotic resistance in a genetically modified organism that is released into the environment is not desirable. For organisms that are intended for deliberate release into the environment (e.g., to degrade pollutants), it is desirable to avoid the concomitant proliferation of antibiotic resistance genes in the environment. To ensure that only the cloned gene is integrated into the host chromosome, the cloned gene may be inserted into a DNA fragment (on a plasmid) that is identical to DNA on the host chromosome. Moreover, the input DNA sequence must be targeted to a specific nonessential site within the chromosome or important host functions will be disrupted. However, when no nonessential host genes have been identified, a cloned gene may be introduced into the host chromosome by means of a single crossover that incorporates the entire input plasmid into the host chromosome. This occurs when the cloned gene is inserted (on a plasmid) next to the cloned chromosomal integration site. In this case, any selectable markers on the plasmid (including antibiotic resistance genes) will be inserted into the host chromosomal DNA. To avoid the problems associated with these approaches, several groups of workers have developed "insertion–removal" systems for the selective removal of marker genes from host cell chromosomes. An overview of one of these systems is described below.

When a marker gene is flanked by certain short specific DNA sequences and then inserted into either a plasmid or chromosomal DNA, the gene may be excised by treatment of the construct with an enzyme that recognizes the flanking DNA sequences and removes them (Fig. 6.27). One combination of an enzyme and DNA sequence that is useful for this sort of manipulation is the Cre–*loxP* recombination system, which consists of the Cre recombinase enzyme and two 34-bp *loxP* recombination sites. The marker gene to be removed is flanked by *loxP* sites, and after integration of the plasmid into the chromosomal DNA, the marker gene is removed by the Cre enzyme. A gene encoding the Cre enzyme is located on its own plasmid, which can be introduced into the chromosomally transformed host cells. Marker gene excision is triggered by the addition of IPTG to the growth medium; this derepresses the *lacI* gene (encoding the *lac* repressor), which turns on the *E. coli lac* promoter–operator, which was present upstream of the *Cre* gene, and causes the Cre enzyme to be synthesized. Once there is no longer any need for the Cre enzyme, the plasmid that contains the gene for this enzyme under the control of the *lac* promoter may be removed from the host cells merely by raising the temperature. This plasmid has a temperature-sensitive replicon that allows it to be maintained in the cell at 30°C but not above 37°C.

Although protocols for the excision of marker genes have not as yet been widely implemented, most of the details have been worked out. Given the unease that exists among certain segments of the public in various locales regarding the deliberate release of genetically engineered

FIGURE 6.27 Removal of a selectable marker gene following integration of plasmid DNA into a bacterial chromosome. A single crossover event (×) occurs between chromosomal DNA and a homologous DNA fragment (hatched) on a plasmid, resulting in the integration of the entire plasmid into the chromosomal DNA. The selectable marker gene, which is flanked by *loxP* sites, is excised by the action of the Cre enzyme, leaving one *loxP* site on the integrated plasmid. The Cre enzyme is on a separate plasmid within the same cell under the transcriptional control of the *E. coli lac* promoter so that excision is induced when IPTG is added to the growth medium.

bacteria into the environment, it is essential that the organisms that are released be as benign as possible; removing antibiotic resistance genes is an important step in that direction.

Increasing Secretion

The process of secretion of proteins in *E. coli* entails exit through the inner (cytoplasmic) cell membrane to the periplasm for many proteins and passage through the outer membrane for a few proteins. Directing a foreign protein to the periplasm or the growth medium makes its purification easier and less costly, as many fewer proteins are present there than in the cytoplasm. Moreover, the stability of a cloned protein depends on its cellular location in *E. coli*. For example, recombinant proinsulin is approximately 10 times more stable if it is secreted (exported) into the periplasm than if it is localized in the cytoplasm. In addition, secretion of proteins to the periplasm facilitates the correct formation of disulfide bonds because the periplasm provides an oxidative environment, in contrast to the more reducing environment of the cytoplasm. Table 6.8 indicates the amounts of secreted recombinant pharmaceutical protein attainable in various bacterial systems.

TABLE 6.8 Yields of several secreted recombinant proteins produced in different bacteria

Protein	Yield (per liter)	Host bacterium
Hirudin	>3 g	*E. coli*
Human antibody fragment	1–2 g	*E. coli*
Human insulin-like growth factor	8.5 g	*E. coli*
Monoclonal antibody 5T4	700 mg	*E. coli*
Humanized anti-CD18 F(ab')$_2$	2.5 g	*E. coli*
Human epidermal growth factor	325 mg	*E. coli*
Alkaline phosphatase	5.2 g	*E. coli*
Staphylokinase	340 mg	*B. subtilis*
Human proinsulin	1 g	*B. subtilis*
Human calcitonin precursor	2 g	*Staphylococcus carnosus*
Organophosphohydrolase	1.2 g	*Ralstonia eutropha*
Human CD4 receptor	200 mg	*Streptomyces lividans*
Human insulin	100 mg	*Streptomyces lividans*

Secretion into the Periplasm

Normally, an amino acid sequence called the signal peptide (also called the signal sequence, or leader peptide), located at the N-terminal end of a protein, facilitates its export by enabling the protein to pass through the cell membrane (Fig. 6.28). It is sometimes possible to engineer a protein for secretion to the periplasm by adding the DNA sequence encoding a signal peptide to the cloned gene. When the recombinant protein is secreted into the periplasm, the signal peptide is precisely removed by the cell's secretion apparatus so that the N-terminal end of the target protein is identical to that of the natural protein.

However, the presence of a signal peptide sequence does not necessarily guarantee a high rate of secretion. When the fusion of a target gene to a DNA fragment encoding a signal peptide is ineffective in producing a secreted protein product, alternative strategies need to be employed. One approach that was found to be successful for the secretion of the protein interleukin-2 was the fusion of the interleukin-2 gene downstream from the gene for the entire propeptide maltose-binding protein, rather than just the maltose-binding protein signal sequence, with DNA encoding the factor X$_a$ recognition site as a linker peptide separating the two genes (Fig. 6.29). When this genetic fusion, on a plasmid vector, was used to transform *E. coli* cells, as expected, a large fraction of the fusion protein was found to be localized in the host cell periplasm. Functional interleukin-2 could then be released from the fusion protein by digestion with factor X$_a$.

In many instances, when foreign proteins engineered for secretion are overproduced in *E. coli*, the precursor form is only partially processed, with about half of the secreted proteins retaining the leader peptide and the other half being fully processed to the mature form. This is probably the result of overloading some of the components involved in the secretion process. If this is the case, then it might be possible to increase the ratio of processed to unprocessed proteins by increasing the level of expression of some of the limiting components of the protein secretion pathway. This hypothesis was tested in a series of experiments in which a plasmid containing both the

FIGURE 6.28 Schematic representation of protein secretion. The ribosome is attached to a cellular membrane, and the signal peptide (signal sequence; leader peptide) at the N terminus is transported, by the secretion apparatus, across the cytoplasmic membrane, followed by the rest of the amino acids that constitute the mature protein or peptide. Once the signal peptide has crossed the membrane, it is cleaved by an enzyme, called a signal peptidase, associated with the membrane. Membrane proteins, as well as secreted proteins, generally contain a signal peptide (prior to its removal by processing).

prlA4 and *secE* genes, which encode major components of the molecular apparatus that physically moves proteins across the membrane, was introduced into *E. coli* host cells. Following this augmentation of the host cell secretory machinery, the fraction of the cloned protein (in this case, the cytokine interleukin-6) that was secreted to the periplasm as the processed form with the signal peptide removed increased from about 50% to more than 90%.

In many cases, secretion of heterologous proteins in *E. coli* is dependent on the translational level of the protein. The foreign proteins that were translated most efficiently were not necessarily secreted to the greatest extent. Sometimes too high a level of translation of a foreign protein can overload the cell's secretion machinery and inhibit the secretion of that protein. Thus, one way to ensure that secretion of a target protein occurs most efficiently may be to lower the level of expression of that protein.

Secretion into the Medium

E. coli and other gram-negative microorganisms generally cannot secrete proteins into the surrounding medium because of the presence of an outer membrane that restricts this process. There are at least two solutions to this problem. The first is to use as host organisms gram-positive prokaryotes or eukaryotic cells, both of which lack an outer membrane and therefore can

FIGURE 6.29 Engineering the secretion of interleukin-2. **(A)** Interleukin-2 fused to the *E. coli* maltose-binding protein signal peptide (MBP signal) is not secreted. **(B)** When interleukin-2 is fused to the *E. coli* maltose-binding protein and its signal peptide, with the two proteins joined by a linker peptide, secretion occurs. Subsequently, the maltose-binding protein and the linker peptide are removed by digestion with factor X_a.

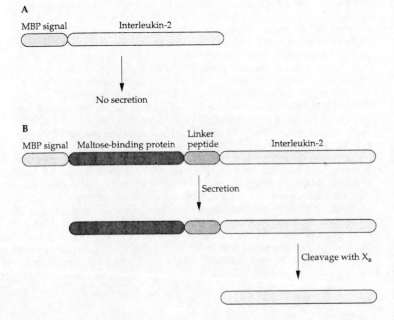

secrete proteins directly into the medium. The second solution entails the use of genetic manipulation to engineer gram-negative bacteria that can secrete proteins directly into the growth medium.

In general, relatively few proteins pass through the outer membrane of *E. coli*. However, some gram-negative bacteria can secrete a bacteriocidal protein called a bacteriocin into the medium. A cascade mechanism is responsible for this specific secretion. A bacteriocin release protein activates phospholipase A, which is present in the bacterial inner membrane, and cleaves membrane phospholipids so that both the inner and outer membranes are permeabilized. Some cytoplasmic and periplasmic proteins are released into the culture medium. Thus, by putting the bacteriocin release protein gene onto a plasmid under the control of a strong regulatable promoter, *E. coli* cells may be permeabilized at will. *E. coli* cells that carry the bacteriocin release protein gene are transformed with another plasmid carrying a cloned gene that has been fused to a secretion signal peptide sequence. The cloned gene is placed under the same transcriptional-regulatory control as the bacteriocin release protein gene so that the two genes can be induced simultaneously, with the target protein being secreted into the medium (Fig. 6.30).

Although secretion of *E. coli* proteins to the growth medium is quite rare, the small protein YebF is naturally secreted to the medium without lysing the cells or permeabilizing the membranes. When various proteins

FIGURE 6.30 *E. coli* cells engineered to secrete a foreign protein to the periplasm by fusing the gene of interest (green) to a secretion signal (**A**) and to the growth medium by permeabilizing cell membranes with a bacteriocin release protein encoded on another plasmid (red) (**B**).

are fused to the C-terminal end of YebF, following the removal of the signal peptide, the entire fusion construct is secreted to the medium. It is believed that the pre-YebF–foreign-protein fusion is first secreted across the *E. coli* cytoplasmic membrane to the periplasm with the concomitant removal of the signal peptide (Fig. 6.31). Next, the leaderless YebF–foreign-protein fusion is secreted from the periplasm to the medium by an unknown process that involves specific amino acids that are part of YebF that interact with an unidentified receptor on the *E. coli* outer membrane. To date, researchers have reported facilitating the secretion to the medium of human interleukin-2 (a 15-kDa hydrophobic protein), bacterial α-amylase (a 48-kDa hydrophilic protein), and alkaline phosphatase (94 kDa), demonstrating that a wide range of proteins may be secreted to the medium using this system. The next step in the development of this system will likely involve engineering a readily cleavable linker region between YebF and the protein of interest so that the protein of interest can be recovered in its native form. In addition, this approach should make it easier to avoid contaminating purified recombinant proteins with *E. coli* lipopolysaccharide, which is a pyrogenic toxin that may be released upon lysis of the bacterial outer membrane and is therefore a serious concern when the proteins are produced for use as therapeutic agents.

YebF is not the only *E. coli* protein that is secreted to the growth medium. The flagellar type III secretion apparatus secretes the protein flagellin to the growth medium. Thus, it is possible to fuse a 173-bp untranslated DNA fragment upstream of the gene encoding flagellin, as well as a transcriptional terminator from the same gene, to a gene encoding a protein of interest, with the result that the protein of interest is efficiently secreted into the medium. However, this system is not applicable to all proteins.

FIGURE 6.31 Secretion, following expression in *E. coli*, of YebF–interleukin-2 fusion protein into the growth medium. The protein synthesized in the cytoplasm includes a signal peptide (yellow) that is excised when the fusion protein is secreted to the periplasm. The YebF–interleukin-2 fusion protein is then secreted from the periplasm, across the outer membrane, to the growth medium. YebF is shown in blue and interleukin-2 in green.

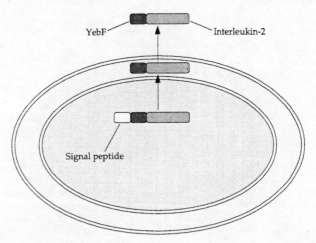

Metabolic Load

The introduction and expression of foreign DNA in a host organism often change the metabolism of the organism in ways that may impair normal cellular functioning (Fig. 6.32). This phenomenon, which is a multifaceted biological response, is due to a metabolic load (metabolic burden; metabolic drain) that is imposed upon the host by the foreign DNA. A metabolic load can occur as the result of a variety of conditions, including the following.

- An increasing plasmid copy number and/or size requires increasing amounts of cellular energy for plasmid replication and maintenance (Table 6.9).
- The limited amount of dissolved oxygen in the growth medium is often insufficient for both host cell metabolism and plasmid maintenance and expression.
- Overproduction of both target and marker proteins may deplete the pools of certain aminoacyl-tRNAs (or even certain amino acids) and/or drain the host cell of its energy (in the form of ATP or GTP).
- When a foreign protein is overexpressed and then exported from the cytoplasm to the cell membrane, the periplasm, or the external medium, it may "jam" export sites and thereby prevent the proper localization of other, essential host cell proteins.
- Host cells with unusual metabolic features, such as a naturally high rate of respiration, e.g., *Azotobacter* spp., are more likely to be affected by these perturbations than are other host cells.
- The foreign protein per se may interfere with the functioning of the host cell, for example, by converting an important and needed metabolic intermediate into a compound that is irrelevant, or even toxic, to the cell.

FIGURE 6.32 Schematic representation of the biological consequences for a host cell of overexpressing a foreign protein and generating a metabolic load. When there is no metabolic load, the cell has access to sufficient energy and resources. The overexpression of a foreign protein—shown here as being analogous to the cell's wearing a heavy backpack—prevents the cell from obtaining sufficient energy and resources for its growth and metabolism so that it is less able to grow rapidly and attain a high density.

One of the most commonly observed consequences of a metabolic load is a decrease in the rate of cell growth after the introduction of foreign DNA (Table 6.9). Sometimes, a metabolic load may result in plasmid-containing cells losing a portion of the plasmid DNA. Even in the presence of selective pressure, all or part of the recombinant gene may be deleted from the plasmid. Since cells growing in the presence of a metabolic load generally have a decreased level of energy for cellular functions, energy-intensive metabolic processes, such as nitrogen fixation and protein synthesis, are invariably adversely affected by a metabolic load. A metabolic load may also lead to changes in the host cell size and shape and to increases in the amount of extracellular polysaccharide produced by the bacterial host cell. This extracellular carbohydrate causes the cells to stick together, making harvesting, e.g., by cross-flow microfiltration procedures, and protein purification more difficult.

Translational errors occur in growing *E. coli* cells at a rate of about 2×10^{-4} to 2×10^{-3} errors per cell per generation. However, when a particular aminoacyl-tRNA becomes limiting, as is often the case when a foreign protein is overexpressed in *E. coli*, there is an increased probability that an incorrect amino acid will be inserted in place of the limiting amino acid. In addition, translational accuracy, which depends upon the availability of GTP as part of a proofreading mechanism, is likely to be further decreased as a consequence of a metabolic load from foreign-protein overexpression. For example, a high level of expression of mouse epidermal growth factor in *E. coli* caused about 10 times the normal amount of incorrect amino acids to be incorporated into the recombinant protein. This frequency of errors diminishes the usefulness of the protein as a therapeutic agent, since (1) the specific activity and stability of the target protein are significantly lowered and (2) the incorrect amino acids may cause the protein to be immunogenic in humans.

A well-designed experiment can minimize the impact of the metabolic load, optimize the yield of the recombinant protein, and enhance the stability of the transformed host cell. For example, the extent of the metabolic load can be reduced by using a low-copy-number rather than a high-copy-number plasmid vector. An even better strategy might be to avoid the use of plasmid vectors altogether and integrate the introduced foreign DNA directly into the chromosomal DNA of the host organism. In this case, plasmid instability will not be a problem. With an integrated cloned gene, without the plasmid vector, the transformed host cell will not waste its resources synthesizing unwanted and unneeded antibiotic resistance

TABLE 6.9 Effect of plasmid copy number on host cell growth rate

E. coli HB101 with plasmid	Plasmid copy no.	Relative specific growth rate
None	0	1.00
A	12	0.92
B	24	0.91
C	60	0.87
D	122	0.82
E	408	0.77

Adapted from Seo and Bailey, *Biotechnol. Bioeng.* 27:1668–1674, 1985.

The different plasmids, designated A, B, C, D, and E, encode only β-lactamase and are all the same size. The growth rates were normalized to the growth rate value for *E. coli* HB101 without a plasmid.

marker gene products. Chromosome integration is particularly important when a genetically engineered organism is destined to be released directly into the environment. The use of strong but regulatable promoters is also an effective means of reducing the metabolic load. In this case, the fermentation process is performed in two stages. During the first, or growth, stage, the promoter controlling the transcription of the target gene is turned off, while during the second, or induction, stage, this promoter is turned on (see chapter 17).

When the codon usage of the foreign gene is different from the codon usage of the host organism, depletion of specific aminoacyl-tRNA pools may be avoided by either completely or partially synthesizing the target gene to better reflect the codon usage of the host organism. However, since this is not a simple procedure, such an approach is likely to be used in only a limited number of instances. Nevertheless, in one study, it was found that levels of the protein streptavidin were 10-fold higher in *E. coli* when expression was directed by a synthetic gene with a G+C content of 54% than when it was directed by the natural gene with a G+C content of 69%.

Although it may at first seem counterintuitive, one way to increase the amount of foreign protein produced during the fermentation process is to accept a modest level of foreign-gene expression—perhaps 5% of the total cell protein—and instead focus on attaining a high host cell density. An organism with a 5% foreign-protein expression level and a low level of metabolic load that can be grown to a density of 40 grams (dry weight) per liter produces more of the target protein than one with a 15% expression level for the same protein and a cell density of only 5 to 10 grams (dry weight) per liter.

SUMMARY

The production of a protein requires that the gene be properly transcribed and then that the mRNA be translated. In prokaryotes, a promoter region is necessary for the initiation of transcription at the correct nucleotide site, and a sequence at the end of the gene (a terminator) is essential for the cessation of transcription. Cloned genes often lack these signals. Consequently, for expression of a cloned gene in a prokaryotic host cell, the appropriate signals recognized by the host must be provided in the correct locations. Moreover, the aim of many biotechnology applications is to produce large amounts of protein, so it is necessary to use a promoter that supports transcription at a high level (strong promoter) and that is compatible with the RNA polymerase of the host cell. However, continuous transcription of a cloned gene drains the energy reserves of the host cell, so it is also necessary to use a promoter system whose activity can be regulated either by the addition of a low-molecular-weight compound or by changing the growth temperature. In addition to utilizing promoters in their native forms, it is possible to alter the DNA to produce promoters with a wide range of activities.

Efficient protein synthesis from a gene depends on specific sequences in its mRNA, and often for cloned genes, other manipulations are required to ensure the stability of the protein and, if necessary, its secretion. As part of the gene-engineering process, a ribosome-binding site is placed in the DNA segment that precedes the translation initiation site (start codon), which also may need to be added. Finally, a termination sequence may be placed at the end of the cloned gene to ensure that translation stops at the correct amino acid. If secretion of the protein is desired, the DNA sequence preceding the cloned gene should include a signal sequence in the same reading frame as the target gene.

Lack of stability of the protein that is encoded by a cloned gene is another complication that is often encountered. For example, the recombinant protein can be degraded by proteolytic enzymes of the host cell. One strategy to overcome this problem is to alter the cloned gene so that it encodes one or more additional amino acids at its N terminus. In this form, the recombinant protein is no longer rapidly degraded. In addition, the amino acids that are added to the recombinant protein can sometimes be used for purifying the fusion protein by, for example, immunoaffinity column chromatography. In these cases, the junction point of a fusion protein is usually designed to be cleaved in vitro either chemically or enzymatically. Fusion proteins may also be used to facilitate the purification of the target protein.

Most microorganisms that are used to express foreign proteins require oxygen for growth. However, oxygen has only limited solubility in water and is rapidly depleted from the growth media of actively growing cultures, especially when

the cultures attain a high cell density. Attempts to deal with the limited amount of dissolved oxygen available for cell growth and maintenance have included (1) utilizing microbial host strains deficient in the production of some proteolytic enzymes that are produced during stationary phase and (2) introducing the gene for the *Vitreoscilla* sp. hemoglobin that binds oxygen from the environment, creating a higher level of intracellular oxygen and thereby causing increases in both host and foreign-protein synthesis.

By increasing the numbers of copies of the cloned gene, the production of the protein is increased, and under these conditions, the stability of the product is often enhanced. However, during scale-up of plasmid-based systems, all or parts of the plasmid can be lost. This plasmid instability is undesirable for commercial systems. To overcome this problem, researchers have developed protocols for integrating a cloned gene into a chromosomal site of the host organism. Under these conditions, the gene is maintained stably as part of the DNA of the host organism.

The introduction and expression of foreign DNA in a host organism often change the metabolism of the organism and thereby impair its normal functioning. This phenomenon is called a metabolic load. A variety of strategies have been developed to minimize the extent of the perturbations caused by a metabolic load and at the same time optimize the yield of the target protein and the stability of the transformed cell.

Proteins produced by gram-negative bacteria may be engineered so that they are secreted to either the periplasm or the external medium by including a sequence encoding a peptide that marks the protein for secretion. This generally facilitates the purification of the protein and ensures that its expression does not interfere with cellular functioning.

Many bacterial cells used to produce recombinant proteins tend to bind to solid surfaces and form biofilms. In this state, bacteria are resistant to high levels of antibiotics and limited in the amount of foreign protein that they can produce. To remedy this, it is possible to genetically engineer bacteria that are unable to form biofilms.

An ideal (plasmid) expression system might include a convenient multiple cloning site in three different reading frames in which to insert the target gene, a strong but regulatable promoter, a selectable marker (to eliminate the large background of nontransformed cells), a replication origin for plasmid maintenance or a site(s) for homologous recombination for integration of the plasmid into the host chromosomal DNA, a secretory signal peptide, and a removable (cleavable) fusion tag that facilitates protein stability and eventual purification. However, both target proteins and expression systems are quite diverse, and investigators tend to develop the set of conditions that optimizes the production of a specific protein in a particular host cell. The differences in detail notwithstanding, the same fundamental strategies may be used to create a variety of different expression systems.

REFERENCES

Amann, E., and J. Brosius. 1985. "ATG vectors" for regulated high-level expression of cloned genes in *Escherichia coli*. *Gene* 40:183–190.

Bachmair, A., D. Finley, and A. Varshavsky. 1986. In vivo half-life of a protein is a function of its amino-terminal residue. *Science* 234:179–186.

Bagdasarian, M. M., E. Amann, R. Lurz, B. Ruckert, and M. Bagdasarian. 1983. Activity of the hybrid *trp-lac* (*tac*) promoter of *Escherichia coli* in *Pseudomonas putida*. Construction of broad-host-range, controlled-expression vectors. *Gene* 26:273–282.

Berlin, Y. A. 1999. DNA splicing by directed ligation (SDL). *Curr. Issues Mol. Biol.* 1:21–30.

Chaitan, K., J. E. Curtis, J. DeModena, U. Rinas, and J. E. Bailey. 1990. Expression of intracellular hemoglobin improves protein synthesis in oxygen-limited *Escherichia coli*. *Bio/Technology* 8:849–853.

Chong, S. R., F. B. Mersha, D. G. Comb, M.E. Scott, D. Landry, L. M. Vence, F. B. Perler, J. Benner, R. B.

Kucera, C. A. Hirvonen, J. J. Pelletier, H. Paulus, and M. Q. Xu. 1997. Single-column purification of free recombinant proteins using a self-cleavable affinity tag derived from a protein splicing element. *Gene* 192:271–281.

Chou, C. H., G. N. Bennett, and K. Y. San. 1994. Effect of modified glucose uptake using genetic engineering techniques on high-level recombinant protein production in *Escherichia coli* dense cultures. *Biotechnol. Bioeng.* 44:952–960.

Cserjan-Puschmann, M., W. Kramer, E. Duerrschmid, G. Striedner, and K. Bayer. 1999. Metabolic approaches for the optimisation of recombinant fermentation processes. *Appl. Microbiol. Biotechnol.* 53:43–50.

de Boer, H. A., L. J. Comstock, and M. Vasser. 1983. The *tac* promoter: a functional hybrid derived from the *trp* and *lac* promoters. *Proc. Natl. Acad. Sci. USA* 80:21–25.

Donovan, R. S., C. W. Robinson, and B. R. Glick. 1996. Optimizing inducer and culture conditions for expression

of foreign proteins under the control of the *lac* promoter. *J. Ind. Microbiol.* 16:145–154.

Ernst, J. F. 1988. Codon usage and gene expression. *Trends Biotechnol.* 6:196–199.

Ferrer, M., T. N. Chernikova, K. N. Timmis, and P. N. Golyshin. 2004. Expression of a temperature-sensitive esterase in a novel chaperone-based *Escherichia coli* strain. *Appl. Environ. Microbiol.* 70:4499–4504.

Geisow, M. J. 1991. Both bane and blessing—inclusion bodies. *Trends Biotechnol.* 9:368–369.

Georgiou, G., and L. Segatori. 2005. Preparative expression of secreted proteins in bacteria: status report and future prospects. *Curr. Opin. Biotechnol.* 16:538–545.

Glick, B. R. 1995. Metabolic load and heterologous gene expression. *Biotechnol. Adv.* 13:247–261.

Goldstein, M. A., and R. H. Doi. 1995. Prokaryotic promoters in biotechnology, p. 105–128. *In* M. R. El-Gewely

(ed.), *Biotechnology Annual Review*, vol. 1. Elsévier Science B.V., Amsterdam, The Netherlands.

Gwynne, D. I., F. P. Buxton, S. A. Williams, S. Garven, and R. W. Davies. 1987. Genetically engineered secretion of active human interferon and a bacterial endoglucanase from *Aspergillus nidulans*. *Bio/Technology* 5:713–719.

Halfmann, G., H. Brailly, A. Bernadac, F. A. Montero-Julian, C. Lazdunski, and D. Baty. 1993. Targeting of interleukin-2 to the periplasm of *Escherichia coli*. *J. Gen. Microbiol.* 139:2465–2473.

Hannig, G., and S. C. Makrides. 1998. Strategies for optimizing heterologous protein expression in *Escherichia coli*. *Trends Biotechnol.* 16:54–60.

Hockney, R. C. 1994. Recent developments in heterologous protein production in *Escherichia coli*. *Trends Biotechnol.* 12:456–463.

Hopp, T. P., K. S. Prickett, V. L. Price, R. T. Libby, C. J. March, D. P. Cerretti, D. L. Urdal, and P. J. Conlon. 1988. A short polypeptide marker sequence useful for recombinant protein identification and purification. *Bio/Technology* 6:1204–1210.

Hsiung, H. M., A. Cantrell, J. Luirink, B. Oudega, A. J. Veros, and G. W. Becker. 1989. Use of bacteriocin release protein in *E. coli* for excretion of human growth hormone into the culture medium. *Bio/Technology* 7:267–271.

Jensen, P. R., and K. Hammer. 1998. The sequence of spacers between the consensus sequences modulates the strength of prokaryotic promoters. *Appl. Environ. Microbiol.* 64:82–87.

Jespers, L. S., J. H. Messens, A. De Keyser, D. Eeckhout, I. Van Den Brande, Y. G. Gansemans, M. J. Lauwereys, G. P. Vlasuk, and P. E. Stanssens. 1995. Surface expression and ligand-based selection of cDNAs fused to filamentous phage gene VI. *Bio/Technology* 13:378–382.

Kallio, P., A. Palva, and I. Palva. 1987. Enhancement of α-amylase production by integrating and amplifying the α-amylase gene of *Bacillus amyloliquefaciens* in the genome of *Bacillus subtilis*. *Appl. Microbiol. Biotechnol.* 27:64–71.

Kurokawa, Y., H. Yanagi, and T. Yura. 2000. Overexpression of protein disulfide isomerase DsbS stabilizes multiple-disulfide-bonded recombinant protein produced and transported to the periplasm in *Escherichia coli*. *Appl. Environ. Microbiol.* 66:3960–3965.

Labes, M., A. Pühler, and R. Simon. 1990. A new family of RSF1010-derived expression and *lac*-fusion broad-host-range vectors for gram-negative bacteria. *Gene* 89:37–46.

Lee, S. Y., J. H. Choi, and Z. Xu. 2003. Microbial cell-surface display. *Trends Biotechnol.* 21:45–52.

Leemans, R., E. Remaut, and W. Fiers. 1987. Broad-host-range expression vector based on the p^L promoter of coliphage 1: regulated synthesis of human interleukin 2 in *Erwinia* and *Serratia* species. *J. Bacteriol.* 169:1899–1904.

Little, M., F. Breitling, B. Micheel, and S. Dübel. 1994. Surface display of antibodies. *Biotechnol. Adv.* 12:539–555.

Liu, M., M. Tolstorukov, V. Zhurkin, S. Garges, and S. Adhaya. 2004. A mutant spacer sequence between −35 and −10 elements makes the P_{lac} promoter hyperactive and cAMP receptor protein-independent. *Proc. Natl. Acad. Sci. USA* 101:6911–6916.

Liu, S. C., D. A. Webster, M. L. Wei, and B. C. Stark. 1996. Genetic engineering to contain the *Vitreoscilla* hemoglobin gene enhances degradation of benzoic acid by *Xanthomonas maltophilia*. *Biotechnol. Bioeng.* 49:101–105.

Looman, A. C., J. Bodlaender, M. de Gruyter, A. Vogelaar, and P. H. van Knippenberg. 1986. Secondary structure as primary determinant of the efficiency of ribosomal binding sites in *Escherichia coli*. *Nucleic Acids Res.* 14:5481–5497.

Majander, K., L. Anton, J. Antikainen, H. Lang, M. Brummer, T. K. Korhonen, and B. Westerlund-Wikström. 2005. Extracellular secretion of polypeptides using a modified *Escherichia coli* flagellar secretion apparatus. *Nat. Biotechnol.* 23:475–481.

Martinez-Morales, F., A. C. Borges, A. Martinez, K. T. Shanmugam, and L. O. Ingram. 1999. Chromosomal integration of heterologous DNA in *Escherichia coli* with precise removal of markers and replicons used during construction. *J. Bacteriol.* 181:7143–7148.

Meerman, H. J., and G. Georgiou. 1994. Construction and characterization of a set of *E. coli* strains deficient in all known loci affecting the proteolytic stability of secreted recombinant proteins. *Bio/Technology* 12:1107–1110.

Mieschendahl, M., and B. Müller-Hill. 1985. F9-coded, temperature-sensitive λ cI857 repressor gene for each construction and regulation of λ promoter-dependent expression systems. *J. Bacteriol.* 164:1366–1369.

Mieschendahl, M., T. Petris, and U. Hanggi. 1986. A novel prophage independent *trp* regulated λ p^L expression system. *Bio/Technology* 4:802–808.

Miksch, G., F. Bettenworth, K. Friehs, E. Flaschel, A. Saalbach, T. Twellmann, and T. W. Nattkemper. 2005. Libraries of synthetic stationary-phase and stress promoters as a tool for fine tuning of expression of recombinant proteins in *Escherichia coli*. *J. Biotechnol.* 120:25–37.

Murby, M., M. Uhlén, and S. Ståhl. 1996. Upstream strategies to minimize proteolytic degradation upon recombinant production in *Escherichia coli*. *Protein Expr. Purif.* 7:129–136.

Nilsson, J., S. Ståhl, J. Lundeberg, M. Uhlén, and P.-Å. Nygren. 1997. Affinity fusion strategies for detection, purification, and immobilization of recombinant proteins. *Protein Expr. Purif.* 11:1–16.

Nygren, P. Å., S. Ståhl, and M. Uhlén. 1994. Engineering proteins to facilitate bioprocessing. *Trends Biotechnol.* 12:184–188.

O'Neil, K. T., and R. H. Hoess. 1995. Phage display: protein engineering by directed evolution. *Curr. Opin. Struct. Biol.* 5:443–449.

Palmeros, B., J. Wild, W. Szybalski, S. LeBorgne, G. Hernández-Chávez, G. Gosset, F. Valle, and F. Bolivar. 2000. A family of removal cassettes designed to obtain antibiotic-resistance-free genomic modifications of *Escherichia coli* and other bacteria. *Gene* 247:255–264.

Pérez-Pérez, J., G. Márquez, J. L. Barbero, and J. Gutiérrez. 1994. Increasing the efficiency of protein export in *Escherichia coli*. *Bio/Technology* 12:178–180.

Qiu, J., J. R. Swartz, and G. Georgiou. 1998. Expression of active human tissue-type plasminogen activator in *Escherichia coli. Appl. Environ. Microbiol.* 64:4891–4896.

Remaut, E., H. Tsao, and W. Fiers. 1983. Improved plasmid vectors with thermoinducible expression and temperature-regulated runaway regulation. *Gene* 22:103–113.

Rogers, S., R. Wells, and M. Rechsteiner. 1986. Amino acid sequences common to rapidly degraded proteins: the PEST hypothesis. *Science* 234:364–368.

Sassenfeld, H. M. 1990. Engineering proteins for purification. *Trends Biotechnol.* 8:88–93.

Schmidt, F. R. 2004. Recombinant expression systems in the pharmaceutical industry. *Appl. Microbiol. Biotechnol.* 65:363–372.

Seo, J. H., and J. E. Bailey. 1985. Effects of recombinant plasmid content on growth properties and cloned gene product formation in *Escherichia coli. Biotechnol. Bioeng.* 27:1668–1674.

Sharma, S. S., S. Chong, and S. W. Harcum. 2006. Intein-mediated protein purification of fusion proteins expressed under high-cell density conditions in *E. coli. J. Biotechnol.* 125:48–56.

Simmons, L. C., and D. G. Yansura. 1996. Translational level is a critical factor for the secretion of heterologous proteins in *Escherichia coli. Nat. Biotechnol.* 14:629–634.

Sung, B. H., C. H. Lee, B. J. Yu, J. H. Lee, J. Y. Lee, M. S. Kim, F. R. Blattner, and S. C. Kim. 2006. Development of a biofilm production-deficient *Escherichia coli* strain as a host for biotechnological applications. *Appl. Environ. Microbiol.* 72:3336–3342.

Talmadge, K., and W. Gilbert. 1982. Cellular location affects protein stability in *Escherichia coli. Proc. Natl. Acad. Sci. USA* 79:1830–1833.

Terpe, K. 2003. Overview of tag protein fusions: from molecular and biochemical fundamentals to commercial systems. *Appl. Microbiol. Biotechnol.* 60:523–533.

Tobias, J. W., T. E. Schrader, G. Rocap, and A. Varshavsky. 1991. The N-end rule in bacteria. *Science* 254:1374–1377.

Weinstock, G. M., C. A. Rhys, M. L. Berman, B. Hampar, D. Jackson, T. J. Silhavy, J. Weisemann, and M. Zweig. 1983. Open reading frame expression vectors: a general method for antigen production in *Escherichia coli* using protein fusion to β-galactosidase. *Proc. Natl. Acad. Sci. USA* 80:4432–4436.

Wilkinson, D. L., and R. G. Harrison. 1991. Predicting the solubility of recombinant proteins in *Escherichia coli. Bio/Technology* 9:443–448.

Wong, R. S. Y., R. A. Wirtz, and R. E. W. Hancock. 1995. *Pseudomonas aeruginosa* outer membrane protein OprF as an expression vector for foreign epitopes: the effects of positioning and length on the antigenicity of the epitope. *Gene* 158:55–60.

Zhang, G., S. Brokx, and J. H. Weiner. 2006. Extracellular accumulation of recombinant proteins fused to the carrier protein YebF in *Escherichia coli. Nat. Biotechnol.* 24:100–104.

Zhang, L., Y. Li, Z. Wang, Y. Xia, W. Chen, and K. Tang. 2007. Recent developments and future prospects of *Vitreoscilla* hemoglobin application in metabolic engineering. *Biotechnol. Adv.* 25:123–136.

REVIEW QUESTIONS

1. Suggest several ways that the expression of a cloned gene can be manipulated for optimal expression.

2. What is *lacI*q, and how is it used?

3. Why is the plasmid that contains the strongest promoter not always the best expression vector?

4. What is the *tac* promoter, and how is it regulated?

5. The *p*L promoter is derived from *E. coli* bacteriophage λ, which cannot infect other bacteria, yet it is sometimes used as part of a broad-host-range expression vector. Explain how the *p*L promoter can be used to promote transcription in organisms other than *E. coli*.

6. Sometimes the strategy for the expression of a target protein in a host organism involves synthesizing the protein as part of a fusion protein. Why is this approach useful? How is a fusion protein created?

7. What are inclusion bodies, and how can their formation be avoided?

8. Why would you want to express a foreign protein on the surface of a bacterium or bacteriophage? How would you do this?

9. How would you manipulate the DNA sequences upstream of a target gene to modulate expression of that gene?

10. How would you avoid some of the problems associated with the limited amount of oxygen that is available to growing *E. coli* cells when a foreign protein is overproduced?

11. A specific target DNA fragment to be integrated into the chromosomal DNA of the host organism can include (1) only the target gene sequence or (2) the entire plasmid, including the target sequence. Explain how each of these results might occur. What are the advantages or disadvantages of the plasmid vector becoming incorporated into the host chromosomal DNA?

12. What factors are responsible for a metabolic load?

13. Suggest a number of different strategies to limit the extent of metabolic load on *E. coli* cells that are designed to overproduce a recombinant protein.

14. During the course of integrating a target gene into the chromosomal DNA of the host bacterium, a marker gene may also be inserted into the chromosomal DNA. What strategy could be used to excise only the marker gene?

15. How do biofilms limit the production of recombinant proteins? How might this limitation be overcome?

16. How can *E. coli* host cells be engineered so that complex proteins with a large number of disulfide bonds are properly folded and therefore produced in an active form rather than as part of an inclusion body?

17. How can *E. coli* host cells be engineered to yield high levels of expression of foreign proteins that contain significant numbers of rare *E. coli* codons?

18. What is the T7 expression system, and how does it work?

19. What features affect the strength of a bacterial promoter?

20. How can a protein of interest be engineered to be secreted to the medium by *E. coli?*

21. What is an intein, and how is it used to purify foreign proteins expressed in *E. coli?*

Heterologous Protein Production in Eukaryotic Cells

ETEROLOGOUS (RECOMBINANT) PROTEINS FROM CLONED DNA origi-
nating from a wide variety of organisms have been successfully
produced using prokaryotic expression systems. Although expres-
sion of any gene from any source organism in a prokaryotic host is theo-
retically possible, in practice, the eukaryotic proteins produced in bacteria
do not always have the desired biological activity or stability. In addition,
despite careful purification procedures, bacterial compounds that are toxic
or that cause a rise in body temperature in humans and animals (pyrogens)
may contaminate the final product. To avoid these problems, investigators
have developed eukaryotic expression systems in fungal, insect, and mam-
malian cells for the production of uncontaminated therapeutic agents for
either humans or animals; large quantities of stable, biologically active
proteins for biochemical, biophysical, and structural studies; and proteins
for industrial processes. Moreover, any human protein intended for med-
ical use must be identical to the natural protein in all its properties. The
inability of prokaryotic organisms to produce authentic versions of eukary-
otic proteins is, for the most part, due to improper posttranslational protein
processing, including improper protein cleavage and folding, and to the
absence of appropriate mechanisms that add chemical groups to specific
amino acid acceptor sites.

Posttranslational Modification of Eukaryotic Proteins

In prokaryotes, the steps in protein synthesis are not compartmentalized,
and therefore, translation of messenger RNA (mRNA) occurs concurrently
with transcription; as soon as the nascent transcript emerges from RNA
polymerase, it is accessible to the ribosome to begin translation. With the
aid of folding proteins, known as chaperones, that bind to polypeptides as
they are being synthesized, proteins are folded into their proper three-
dimensional configuration during synthesis. In contrast, eukaryotes trans-
port mRNA from the nucleus to ribosomes in the cytoplasm or on the
endoplasmic reticulum, where translation occurs. Proteins produced on
ribosomes associated with the endoplasmic reticulum either are inserted in

Preproinsulin polypeptide (inactive)

Proteolytic cleavage

Insulin (active)

FIGURE 7.1 Cleavage of inactive preproinsulin to yield active mature insulin. Proteases remove the leader peptide (L) and an internal peptide (C), yielding a peptide that consists of chains A and B.

the membrane of the endoplasmic reticulum or are secreted into the lumen of the endoplasmic reticulum during synthesis, where they are processed further.

Many proteins, including most of those that are of interest as therapeutic agents for the treatment of human or animal diseases, undergo some type of posttranslational processing that is required for protein activity and stability. Some proteins are produced as inactive precursor polypeptides that must be cleaved by proteases at specific sites to produce the active form of the protein. For example, the small peptide hormone insulin is produced in animal pancreatic cells as a single polypeptide, preproinsulin, that is cleaved to produce two shorter peptides that are joined by disulfide bonds (Fig. 7.1). Production of inactive preproinsulin ensures that the peptide is not active in the pancreatic cells that produce it, but upon secretion, cleaved mature insulin can act on other cells. Similarly, the digestive enzyme trypsinogen, which degrades proteins, is produced as an inactive polypeptide to avoiding digestion of components of the producing cell. Upon secretion into the small intestines, trypsinogen is cleaved by an enteropeptidase to yield the active enzyme trypsin.

Similar to prokaryotes, proper folding of proteins in eukaryotic cells requires the assistance of chaperones. In the endoplasmic reticulum, the chaperones BiP and calnexin bind nascent polypeptides, and protein disulfide isomerases catalyze the formation of disulfide bonds between adjacent cysteine residues. Proper folding is important, not only for the protein to attain a configuration for optimal activity, but also to protect regions of the protein that would otherwise be recognized by proteases that destroy the protein. Quality control systems ensure that only correctly folded proteins are released from the endoplasmic reticulum and transported within vesicles to the Golgi apparatus for further processing. Proteins intended for secretion from the cell are subsequently transported to the cell membrane within specific transport vesicles and released by exocytosis.

The addition of specific sugars (glycosylation) to certain amino acids is a major modification that provides stability and distinctive binding

FIGURE 7.2 Examples of some O-linked oligosaccharides in yeasts (**A**), insects (**B**), and mammals (**C**). O-linked oligosaccharides have a number of arrangements with different combinations of sugars. Some of the more prevalent forms are shown here. S, serine; T, threonine; red circles, mannose; dark-blue squares, *N*-acetylglucosamine; light-blue squares, *N*-acetylgalactosamine; green squares, galactose; orange squares, sialic acid.

properties to a protein. Proper protein glycosylation is important because it contributes to protein conformation by influencing protein folding; can target a protein to a particular location, for example, through interaction with a specific receptor molecule; or can increase protein stability by protecting it from proteases. In the cell, oligosaccharides are attached to newly synthesized proteins in the endoplasmic reticulum and in the Golgi apparatus by specific enzymes known as glycosylases and glycosyltransferases. Different tissues may differentially glycosylate the same protein, thereby increasing protein heterogeneity. Because different sugar modifications can alter the properties of a protein, this presents opportunities for protein engineering to improve the efficacy or to alter the activity of a protein. Therapeutic proteins that require glycosylation for activity include antibodies, blood factors, some interferons, and some hormones.

The most common glycosylations entail the attachment of specific sugars to the hydroxyl group of either serine or threonine (O-linked glycosylation) (Fig. 7.2) and to the amide group of asparagine (N-linked glycosylation) (Fig. 7.3). About 50% of all human proteins are glycosylated. The initial core sugar groups that are added to these amino acid acceptor sites tend to be similar among eukaryotes, although the subsequent elaborations among yeasts, insects, and mammals are quite diverse, especially for N-linked glycosylation. Other amino acid modifications include phosphorylation, acetylation, sulfation, acylation, γ-carboxylation, and the addition of C_{14} and C_{16} fatty acids, i.e., myristoylation (or myristylation) and palmitoylation (or palmitylation), respectively.

Unfortunately, there is no universally effective eukaryotic host cell that performs the correct modifications on every protein. In some cases, a host cell may add unusual sugars to either authentic or spurious amino acid sites and, consequently, create an extremely antigenic protein or possibly one that lacks its proper function. However, even though a recombinant protein may fall short of the stringent properties that are required for a therapeutic agent, it may still be useful for either research or industrial purposes. Different eukaryotic expression systems must be tested to determine which one synthesizes the largest amount of a functional recombinant protein. The choice of an expression system depends primarily on the quality of the recombinant protein that is produced, but the yield of product, ease of use, and cost of production and purification are also important considerations.

General Features of Eukaryotic Expression Systems

The basic requirements for expression of a target protein in a eukaryotic host are similar to those required in prokaryotes. Vectors into which the target gene is cloned for delivery into the host cell can be specialized plasmids designed to be maintained in the eukaryotic host, such as the yeast 2μm plasmid; host-specific viruses, such as the insect baculovirus; or artificial chromosomes, such as the yeast artificial chromosome (YAC). The vector must have a eukaryotic promoter that drives the transcription of the cloned gene of interest, eukaryotic transcriptional and translational stop signals, a sequence that enables polyadenylation of the mRNA, and a selectable eukaryotic marker gene (Fig. 7.4). Because recombinant DNA procedures are technically difficult to carry out with eukaryotic cells, most eukaryotic vectors are shuttle vectors with two origins of replication and selectable marker genes. One set functions in the bacterium *Escherichia coli*,

FIGURE 7.3 Examples of some N-linked oligosaccharides in yeasts **(A)**, insects **(B)**, and mammals **(C)**. All N-linked glycosylations in eukaryotes start with the same initial group, which is subsequently trimmed and then elaborated in diverse ways within and among species. Some yeast sites have 15 or fewer mannose units (core series), and others have more (outer-chain family). In *S. cerevisiae*, the chains frequently have 50 or more mannose units. An asparagine (N) residue next to any amino acid (X) followed by either threonine (T) or serine (S) can be targeted for glycosylation. Red circles, mannose; dark blue squares, *N*-acetylglucosamine; yellow triangles, glucose; green squares, galactose; orange squares, sialic acid; maroon triangle, fucose.

and the other set functions in the eukaryotic host cell. If a eukaryotic expression vector is to be used as a plasmid, i.e., as extrachromosomal replicating DNA, then it must also have a eukaryotic origin of replication. Alternatively, if the vector is designed for stable integration into the host chromosomal DNA, then it must have a sequence that is complementary to

FIGURE 7.4 Generalized eukaryotic expression vector. The major features of a eukaryotic expression vector are a eukaryotic transcription unit with a promoter (*p*), a multiple cloning site (MCS) for a gene of interest, and a DNA segment with termination and polyadenylation signals (*t*); a eukaryotic selectable marker (ESM) gene system; an origin of replication that functions in the eukaryotic cell (*ori*^euk^); an origin of replication that functions in *E. coli* (*ori*^E^); and an *E. coli* selectable marker (Amp^r^) gene.

a segment of host chromosomal DNA to facilitate insertion into a chromosomal site.

The introduction of DNA into bacterial and yeast cells is called transformation. In these systems, the term describes an inherited change due to the acquisition of exogenous (foreign) DNA. However, in animal cells, transformation refers to changes in the growth properties of cells in culture after they become cancerous. To avoid confusion, the word transfection has been chosen to denote inherited changes in animal cells that are due to the addition of exogenous DNA.

Three techniques are commonly used to transform yeasts: electroporation, lithium acetate treatment, and cell wall removal (protoplast formation). Transfection of cultured animal cells is achieved by incubating cells with DNA that has been coprecipitated with either calcium phosphate or diethylaminoethyl (DEAE)–dextran or by electroporation. Electroporation entails subjecting cells to short pulses of electric current, thus creating transient pores through which DNA enters the cell (Fig. 3.33). Viruses, lipid–DNA complexes, and protein–DNA aggregates are also used to transfer exogenous DNA into a recipient animal cell.

Fungus-Based Expression Systems

Fungi share many of the molecular, genetic, and biochemical features of other, "higher" eukaryotes and are therefore a good choice for heterologous protein production. They have growth advantages similar to those of prokaryotes, such as rapid growth in low-cost medium; generally do not require growth factors to be added to the growth medium; can correctly process eukaryotic proteins; and can secrete large amounts of heterologous proteins. Initially, the yeast *Saccharomyces cerevisiae* was used extensively as a host cell for the expression of cloned eukaryotic genes. It has a long history of use in traditional biotechnologies in the brewing and baking industries. Today, a variety of fungal expression systems are available, and they have been optimized for recombinant protein expression. Versatile expression vectors with broad host ranges have been constructed because the optimal host for production of a particular target protein must often be determined experimentally in a number of different systems.

Saccharomyces cerevisiae Expression Systems

High levels of recombinant protein production have been achieved using *S. cerevisiae*. The advantages of using this single-celled yeast are several. First, a great deal is known about the biochemistry, genetics, and cell biology of the fungus. The genome sequence of *S. cerevisiae* was completed in 1996, and it is used extensively in studies as a model organism for cell function. It can be grown rapidly to high cell densities on relatively simple media in both small culture vessels and large-scale bioreactors. Second, several strong promoters have been isolated from the yeast and characterized, and a naturally occurring plasmid, called the 2μm plasmid, can be used as part of an endogenous yeast expression vector system. Third, *S. cerevisiae* is capable of carrying out many posttranslational modifications. Fourth, the yeast normally secretes so few proteins that, when it is engineered for extracellular release of a recombinant protein, the product can be easily purified. Fifth, because of its years of use in the baking and brewing industries, *S. cerevisiae* has been listed by the U.S. Food and Drug

Administration as a "generally recognized as safe" organism. It does not harbor human pathogens or produce fever-stimulating pyrogens. Therefore, the use of the organism for the production of human therapeutic agents (drugs or pharmaceuticals) does not require the same extensive experimentation demanded for unapproved host cells. A number of proteins that have been produced in *S. cerevisiae* are currently being used commercially as vaccines, pharmaceuticals, and diagnostic agents (Table 7.1). For example, at present, more than 50% of the world supply of insulin is produced by *S. cerevisiae*. Engineered *S. cerevisiae* strains are also major producers of a hepatitis B vaccine.

S. cerevisiae vectors. There are three main classes of *S. cerevisiae* expression vectors: episomal, or plasmid, vectors (yeast episomal plasmids [YEps]); integrating vectors (yeast integrating plasmids [YIps]); and YACs. Of these, episomal vectors have been used extensively for the production of either intra- or extracellular heterologous proteins. Typically, the vectors contain features that allow them to function in both bacteria and *S. cerevisiae*. An *E. coli* origin of replication and bacterial antibiotic resistance genes are usually included on the vector, enabling all manipulations to first be performed in *E. coli* before the vector is transferred to *S. cerevisiae* for expression.

The YEp vectors are based on the high-copy-number 2μm plasmid, a small, circular plasmid found in most natural strains of *S. cerevisiae*. The vector replicates independently of the host chromosome via a single origin of replication (autonomous replicating sequence [ARS]/STB loci), and is maintained in more than 30 copies per cell. Many *S. cerevisiae* selection

TABLE 7.1 Recombinant proteins produced by
S. cerevisiae expression systems

Vaccines
 Hepatitis B virus surface antigen
 Malaria circumsporozoite protein
 HIV-1 envelope protein

Diagnostics
 Hepatitis C virus protein
 HIV-1 antigens

Human therapeutic agents
 Epidermal growth factor
 Insulin
 Insulin-like growth factor
 Platelet-derived growth factor
 Proinsulin
 Fibroblast growth factor
 Granulocyte-macrophage colony-stimulating factor
 α_1-Antitrypsin
 Blood coagulation factor XIIIa
 Hirudin
 Human growth factor
 Human serum albumin

HIV-1, human immunodeficiency virus type 1.

TABLE 7.2 Promoters for *S. cerevisiae* expression vectors

Promoter	Expression conditions	Status
Acid phosphatase *(PH05)*	Phosphate-deficient medium	Inducible medium
Alcohol dehydrogenase I *(ADHI)*	2–5% Glucose	Constitutive
Alcohol dehydrogenase II *(ADHII)*	0.1–0.2% Glucose	Inducible
Cytochrome c_1 *(CYC1)*	Glucose	Repressible
Gal-1-P Glc-1-P uridyltransferase	Galactose	Inducible
Galactokinase *(GAL1)*	Galactose	Inducible
Glyceraldehyde-3-phosphate dehydrogenase *(GAPD, GAPDH)*	2–5% Glucose	Constitutive
Metallothionein *(CUP1)*	0.03–0.1 mM Copper	Inducible
Phosphoglycerate kinase *(PGK)*	2–5% Glucose	Constitutive
Triosephosphate isomerase *(TPI)*	2–5% Glucose	Constitutive
UDP-galactose epimerase *(GAL10)*	Galactose	Inducible

schemes rely on mutant host strains that require a particular amino acid (histidine, tryptophan, or leucine) or nucleotide (uracil) for growth. Such strains are said to be auxotrophic because minimal growth medium must be supplemented with a specific nutrient. In practice, the vector is equipped with a functional (wild-type) version of a gene that complements the mutated gene in the host strain. For example, when a YEp with a wild-type *LEU2* gene is transformed into a mutant *leu2* host cell and plated onto medium that lacks leucine, only cells that carry the plasmid will grow.

A number of promoters derived from *S. cerevisiae* genes are available for engineering efficient transcription of heterologous genes in yeast vectors (Table 7.2). Generally, tightly regulatable, inducible promoters are preferred for producing large amounts of recombinant protein at a specific time during large-scale growth. In this context, the galactose-regulated promoters respond rapidly to the addition of galactose with a 1,000-fold increase in transcription. Repressible, constitutive, and hybrid promoters that combine the features of different promoters are also available. Maximal expression depends on efficient termination of transcription. Often, for YEp vectors, the terminator sequence is from the same gene as the promoter.

Many heterologous genes are provided with a DNA coding sequence for an amino acid segment (signal sequence, signal peptide, or leader sequence) that facilitates the passage of the recombinant protein through cell membranes and its release to the external environment. The main reason for this modification is that it is much easier to purify a secreted protein than one from a cell lysate. The most commonly used signal sequence for *S. cerevisiae* is derived from the mating factor α gene. Also, synthetic leader sequences have been created to increase the amount of secreted protein. Other sequences that stabilize the recombinant protein, protect it from proteolytic degradation, and provide a specific amino acid sequence (affinity tag) that is used for selective purification can be fused onto the coding sequence of the heterologous gene. These extra amino acid sequences are equipped with a protease cleavage site so that they can be removed from the recombinant protein after it is purified.

Plasmid-based yeast expression systems are often unstable under large-scale (≥10 liters) growth conditions even in the presence of selection pressure. To remedy this problem, a heterologous gene is integrated into the host genome to provide a more reliable production system. Different approaches have been devised for the integration of a cloned gene together with a

selectable marker gene into an *S. cerevisiae* chromosome. Briefly, a functional selectable marker gene and a heterologous gene equipped with yeast-specific transcription and translation control sequences are inserted between two DNA segments derived from the ends of a nonessential yeast gene. In this instance, the plasmid does not usually carry an origin of replication that functions in yeast cells. The plasmid is cleaved, and the linear fragment is transformed into *S. cerevisiae*. A double recombination event between homologous sequences on the linearized plasmid and a chromosome in the host inserts the piece of DNA with both target and marker genes into a spe-

FIGURE 7.5 Schematic representation of integration of DNA with a YIp vector. A selectable marker gene *(LEU2)* and a gene of interest (GOI) with transcription and translation control elements (not shown) are inserted into a YIp vector between two segments from the ends of a nonessential yeast gene *(A1* and *A2).* The ampicillin resistance (Ampr) gene and the origin of replication *(oriE)* function in *E. coli.* A leucine-requiring *(leu2)* yeast strain is transformed with restriction endonuclease-digested (RE) vector DNA because chromosomal DNA is more likely to recombine with linearized DNA than with circular DNA. The restriction endonuclease sites flank the segments from the nonessential gene. The DNA sequences at the ends of nonessential gene *A* undergo recombination (×) that leads to the incorporation of both the gene of interest and the *LEU2* gene into the corresponding chromosome site. Transformants grow on medium that is not supplemented with leucine. Nonrecombined DNA is degraded.

cific chromosome site (Fig. 7.5). The plasmid DNA is linearized because DNA in this form is more likely than circular DNA to recombine with chromosome DNA. The DNA that is not integrated is lost during successive cell divisions. The major drawback of this strategy is the low yield of recombinant protein from a single gene copy.

To increase the number of copies of an integrated heterologous gene and thereby increase the overall yield of the recombinant protein, the gene can be targeted to yeast repetitive DNA sequences, such as the sequences (ribosomal DNA [rDNA]) encoding ribosomal RNA that are present in approximately 200 copies. Alternatively, the heterologous gene can be integrated into several of the 400 copies of δ sequences in the *S. cerevisiae* genome. The δ sequences are parts of nonessential DNA elements derived from retrotransposons. Briefly, retrotransposons are chromosomal DNA sequences that are transcribed but not translated into protein. The RNA molecules act as templates for the synthesis of DNA by the enzyme reverse transcriptase, and the copied DNA sequences integrate into the chromosome at different sites. In one study, 10 copies of a heterologous gene were inserted into δ sequences and produced a significant amount of the recombinant protein.

A YAC is designed to clone a large segment of DNA (100 kilobase pairs [kb]), which is then maintained as a separate chromosome in the host yeast cell. The YAC system is highly stable and has been used for the physical mapping of human genomic DNA, the analysis of large transcription units, and the formation of genomic libraries containing DNA from individual human chromosomes. A YAC vector mimics a chromosome because it has a sequence that acts as an origin of DNA replication (ARS), a yeast centromere sequence to ensure that after cell division each daughter cell receives a copy of the YAC, and telomere sequences that are present at both ends after linearization of the YAC DNA for stability (Fig. 7.6). In some cases, the input DNA is cloned into a site that disrupts a yeast marker gene. In the absence of the product of the marker gene, a colorimetric response is observed when recipient cells are grown on a specialized medium. Alternatively, some YAC vectors contain a selectable marker gene that is independent of the cloning site. To date, YACs have not been used as expression systems for the commercial production of heterologous proteins, although they have the potential to produce large amounts of either a single protein from multiple copies of the same gene or a heterologous protein with different subunits.

Intracellular production of heterologous proteins in *S. cerevisiae*. Most *S. cerevisiae* intracellular expression systems have the same basic features. Here, the production of the human enzyme superoxide dismutase (SOD) will be used to illustrate the process. Superoxide anion is a by-product of oxygen utilization in aerobic organisms. In humans, this anion helps both to stimulate the inflammatory response of phagocytes and to direct leukocytes to the site of an infection. However, too much of the molecule and its derivatives can cause cellular damage. To minimize these potentially cytotoxic effects, the naturally occurring cytoplasmic enzyme Cu/Zn-SOD scavenges the superoxide radical and combines it with a hydrogen ion to form hydrogen peroxide, which in turn is degraded to water and oxygen by catalase or peroxidase. Superoxide anion is also produced when blood is allowed to reenter an organ (reperfusion) after it has been deprived of blood during a surgical procedure. To prevent this source of superoxide

FIGURE 7.6 YAC cloning system. The YAC plasmid (pYAC) has an *E. coli* selectable marker (Amp^r) gene; an origin of replication that functions in *E. coli* (*ori*^E); and yeast DNA sequences, including *URA3*, *CEN*, *TRP1*, and *ARS*. *CEN* provides centromere function, *ARS* is a yeast autonomous replicating sequence that is equivalent to a yeast origin of replication, *URA3* is a functional gene of the uracil biosynthesis pathway, and *TRP1* is a functional gene of the tryptophan biosynthesis pathway. The T regions are yeast chromosome telomeric sequences. The SmaI site is the cloning insertion site. pYAC is first treated with SmaI, BamHI, and alkaline phosphatase and then ligated with size-fractionated (100-kb) input DNA. The final construct carries cloned DNA and can be stably maintained in double-mutant *ura3* and *trp1* cells.

anion damage, clinicians have speculated that Cu/Zn-SOD could be administered to an organ as it is being reperfused. In addition, Cu/Zn-SOD might act as a therapeutic agent against inflammatory diseases, such as osteoarthritis, rheumatoid arthritis, scleroderma, and ankylosing spondylitis. For both of these uses, an authentic human form of Cu/Zn-SOD is preferred to avoid any adverse immunological responses that might result from using an enzyme from another species.

Initially, a complementary DNA (cDNA) for human Cu/Zn-SOD was cloned into an *E. coli* expression system. As expected, the *E. coli* host cells removed the initiator N-terminal methionine from the Cu/Zn-SOD pro-

tein. However, the next amino acid (alanine) was not acetylated, as it is in human cells. To produce a fully functional protein, the human Cu/Zn-SOD cDNA was cloned into a YEp vector (Fig. 7.7). This YEp vector contained (1) a 2μm plasmid origin of DNA replication, (2) a yeast gene for leucine biosynthesis *(LEU2)* for selection in yeast, (3) an *E. coli* origin of replication, (4) the ampicillin resistance (Ampr) gene for selection in *E. coli,* and (5) the human Cu/Zn-SOD cDNA inserted between the promoter region of the yeast glyceraldehyde phosphate dehydrogenase gene *(GAPDp)* and a sequence containing the signals for transcription termination and polyadenylation of mRNA from the same gene *(GAPDt)*. A leucine-defective *(leu2)* yeast strain was transformed with the vector, and the cells were plated onto medium that lacked leucine. Only cells with the functional *LEU2* gene, which was supplied by the vector, could grow under these conditions. The *GAPD* promoter is transcribed continuously (constitutively) during cell growth. In this experiment, the yeast cells produced high levels of intracellular Cu/Zn-SOD that, like the authentic protein from human cells, had an acetylated N-terminal alanine residue.

Secretion of heterologous proteins by *S. cerevisiae*. All glycosylated proteins of *S. cerevisiae* are secreted, and each must have a leader sequence to pass through the secretory system. Consequently, the coding sequences of recombinant proteins that require either O-linked or N-linked sugars for biological activity must be equipped with a leader sequence. Usually, the leader sequence from the yeast mating type α-factor gene (prepro-α-factor) is inserted immediately in front (upstream) of the cDNA of the gene of interest. Under these conditions, correct disulfide bond formation, proteolytic removal of the leader sequence, and appropriate posttranslational modifications often occur, and an active recombinant protein is secreted. During this process, the leader peptide is removed by an endoprotease that recognizes the dipeptide Lys-Arg. The Lys-Arg codons must be located adjacent to the cDNA sequence so that, following removal of the leader peptide, the recombinant protein will have the correct amino acid residue

FIGURE 7.7 *S. cerevisiae* expression vector. The cDNA for human Cu/Zn-SOD was cloned between the promoter *(GAPDp)* and termination–polyadenylation sequence *(GAPDt)* of the *S. cerevisiae* glyceraldehyde phosphate dehydrogenase gene. The *LEU2* gene that was cloned between segments of the yeast 2μm plasmid DNA encodes a functional enzyme of the leucine biosynthesis pathway. The yeast origin of replication is included in the 2μm plasmid DNA. The ampicillin resistance (Ampr) gene and the *E. coli* origin of replication *(oriE)* are derived from plasmid pBR322.

MILESTONE

Synthesis of Rabbit β-Globin in Cultured Monkey Kidney Cells Following Infection with a SV40 β-Globin Recombinant Genome

R. C. MULLIGAN, B. H. HOWARD, and P. BERG

Nature 277:108–114, 1979

Conceptually, the development of a eukaryotic expression system appears to be a relatively simple matter of assembling the appropriate regulatory sequences, cloning them in the correct order into a vector, and then putting the gene of interest into the precise location that enables it to be expressed. In reality, the development of the first generation of eukaryotic expression vectors was a painstaking process following a trial-and-error approach. Before Mulligan, Howard, and Berg's study, a number of genes had been cloned into the mammalian SV40 vectors, but mature, functional mRNAs were never detected after infection of host cells. This problem was overcome by inserting the rabbit cDNA for β-globin into an SV40 gene that had nearly all of its coding region deleted but retained "all the regions implicated in transcriptional initiation and termina-tion, splicing and polyadenylation...." Both rabbit β-globin mRNA and protein were synthesized in cells that were transfected with this β-globin cDNA–SV40 construct. Mulligan et al. concluded, "The principal conceptual innovation is the decision to leave intact the regions of the vector implicated in...mRNA processing." This study established that an effective eukaryotic expression system could be created by placing the cloned gene under the control of transcription and translation regulatory sequences. It also stimulated additional research that pinpointed in detail the structural prerequisites for the next generation of eukaryotic expression vectors.

at its N terminus. For example, a properly processed and active form of the protein hirudin was synthesized and secreted by an *S. cerevisiae* strain containing a YEp vector that had the prepro-α-factor sequence added to the hirudin coding sequence. The gene for hirudin is from an invertebrate, the leech *Hirudo medicinalis*. This protein is a powerful blood anticoagulant that is not immunogenic in humans.

Over the last 10 years, the amount of heterologous protein that can be produced per liter of yeast culture has increased 100-fold (from about 0.02 to 2 g/liter). This increase is mainly due to improvements in growing cultured cells to high cell densities; the level of protein produced per cell has remained largely unchanged. Although there have been significant advances in techniques to increase the number of copies of a target gene in a host cell and to increase the expression levels of these genes, the overexpressed proteins tend to form intracellular aggregates, often associated with molecular chaperones, rather than to be secreted into the medium, which facilitates purification. Major problems that must be addressed to increase heterologous-protein secretion in yeast cells are the incorrect folding of the polypeptide, the activation of cellular mechanisms to cope with the stress of protein overproduction, and the aberrant processing and release of the protein of interest from the endoplasmic reticulum.

One of the major reasons for producing a recombinant protein for use in human therapeutics in yeast rather than in bacteria is to ensure that the protein is processed correctly following synthesis. Correct protein folding occurs in the endoplasmic reticulum in eukaryotes and is facilitated by a number of different proteins, including molecular chaperones, enzymes for disulfide bond formation, signal transduction proteins that monitor the demand and capacity of the protein-folding machinery, and proteases that clear away improperly folded or aggregated proteins (Fig. 7.8). The eukaryotic enzyme protein disulfide isomerase is instrumental in forming the correct disulfide bonds within a protein. Aberrant disulfide bond formation changes a protein's configuration, which abolishes protein activity and causes instability. Poor yields of overexpressed proteins often occur because

FIGURE 7.8 Summary of protein folding in the endoplasmic reticulum of yeast cells. During synthesis on ribosomes associated with the endoplasmic reticulum (ER), nascent proteins are bound by the chaperones BiP and calnexin, which aid in the correct folding of the protein. Protein disulfide isomerases (PDI) catalyze the formation of disulfide bonds between cysteine amino acids that are nearby in the folded protein. Quality control systems ensure that only correctly folded proteins are released from the ER. Proteins released from the ER are transported to the Golgi apparatus for further processing. Prolonged binding of BiP to misfolded proteins leads to activation of the *S. cerevisiae* transcription factor Hac1, which controls the expression of several proteins that mediate the unfolded-protein response (UPR). Adapted from Gasser et al., *Microb. Cell Fact.* 7:11–29, 2008.

the capacity of the cell to properly fold and secrete proteins has been exceeded. Several strategies have therefore been implemented to increase the host cell's capacity to process higher than normal levels of proteins. For example, the overproduction of molecular chaperones and protein disulfide isomerases might increase the yield of recombinant proteins, especially those with disulfide bonds. To test this hypothesis, the yeast protein disulfide isomerase gene was cloned between the constitutive glyceraldehyde phosphate dehydrogenase promoter and a transcription terminator sequence in a YIp vector, and the entire construct was integrated into a chromosomal site. The modified strain showed a 16-fold increase in protein disulfide isomerase production compared with the wild-type strain. When protein disulfide isomerase-overproducing cells were transformed with a YEp vector carrying the gene for human platelet-derived growth factor B, there was a 10-fold increase in the secretion of recombinant protein over that of transformed cells with normal levels of protein disulfide isomerase. The overproduction of protein disulfide isomerase specifically increases the secretion of proteins with disulfide bonds. Higher levels of secreted products are also obtained for the recombinant proteins human erythropoietin, bovine prochymosin, and leech hirudin in *S. cerevisiae* cells that overexpress the chaperone BiP.

Overexpression of the molecular chaperone BiP or protein disulfide isomerase increased the secretion of some heterologous protein; however, overexpression of a single chaperone may not have the desired outcome

and, in some instances, may increase the degradation of the target protein. This is because proper protein folding requires the coordinated efforts of many interacting factors (Fig. 7.8). Even when levels of one chaperone are adequate, the levels of cochaperones or cofactors may be limiting. The unfolded-protein response of yeast cells coordinates the expression of several chaperones, as well as cochaperones. When the demand for protein folding exceeds the folding capacity of the endoplasmic reticulum, the unfolded-protein response increases the expression of chaperones, protein disulfide isomerase, and other proteins involved in protein secretion. Engineering the proteins of the unfolded-protein response may be a better approach to increase the overall capacity of the cell to fold proteins in a coordinated way by maintaining appropriate ratios of all factors required. Accumulation of unfolded proteins in the endoplasmic reticulum activates the *S. cerevisiae* transcription factor Hac1, which activates the expression of proteins of the unfolded-protein response, and therefore expression of Hac1 was targeted for genetic manipulation. Overexpression of Hac1 in *S. cerevisiae* improved secretion of the important industrial enzyme α-amylase, which is used for starch hydrolysis in a wide range of processes, such as alcohol production, paper recycling, and oil drilling.

Pichia pastoris Expression Systems

Recombinant proteins have been produced successfully in *S. cerevisiae* from cloned genes from many sources. However, in many cases, expression levels are low and protein yields are modest. One of the major drawbacks of using *S. cerevisiae* is the tendency for the yeast to hyperglycosylate heterologous proteins by typically adding 50 to 150 mannose residues in N-linked oligosaccharide side chains that often alter protein function. Although the initial stages of addition of glycan chains to proteins in the lumen of the endoplasmic reticulum are similar in yeast and humans, following transfer of the protein to the Golgi apparatus, further processing differs significantly. The outcome is the production of a sialylated protein in humans and a hypermannosylated protein in yeast, with α-1,3 bonds between the sugar residues that can make the heterologous protein antigenic (Fig. 7.3). Also, proteins that are designed for secretion frequently are retained in the periplasmic space, increasing the time and cost of purification. Finally, *S. cerevisiae* produces ethanol at high cell densities, which is toxic to the cells (the Crabtree effect) and, as a consequence, lowers the quantity of secreted protein. For these reasons, researchers have examined other yeast species and eukaryotic cells that could act as effective host cells for recombinant protein production.

 P. pastoris is a methylotrophic yeast that is able to utilize methanol as a source of energy and carbon. It is an attractive host for recombinant protein production because glycosylation occurs to a lesser extent and the linkages between sugar residues are of the α-1,2 type, which are not allergenic to humans. With these natural characteristics as a starting point, a *P. pastoris* strain was extensively engineered with the aim of developing a "humanized" strain that glycosylates proteins in a manner identical to that of human cells. Both human and yeast cells add the same small (10-residue), branched oligosaccharide to nascent proteins in the endoplasmic reticulum (Fig. 7.9). However, this is the last common precursor between the two cell types, because once the protein is transported to the Golgi apparatus, further processing is different. In the Golgi apparatus, yeast cells add an α-1,6

FIGURE 7.9 Differential processing of glycoproteins in *P. pastoris*, humans, and "humanized" *P. pastoris*. Initial additions of sugar residues to glycoproteins in the endoplasmic reticulum are similar in human and *P. pastoris* cells (**A**). However, further N glycosylation in the Golgi apparatus differs significantly between the two cell types. N-glycans are hypermannosylated in *P. pastoris* (**B**), while in humans, mannose residues are trimmed and specific sugars are added, leading to termination of the oligosaccharide in sialic acid (**C**). *P. pastoris* cells have been engineered to produce enzymes that process glycoproteins in a manner similar to that of human cells. In "humanized" *P. pastoris*, a recombinant glycoprotein produced in the endoplasmic reticulum (**D**) is transported to the Golgi apparatus, where it is further processed to yield a properly sialylated glycoprotein (**E**). Blue squares, N-acetylglucosamine; red circles, mannose; green squares, galactose; orange squares, sialic acid. Adapted from Hamilton and Gerngross, *Curr. Opin. Biotechnol.* **18:**387–392, 2007.

mannose residue to the oligosaccharide, which subsequently leads to hypermannosylation. Mammalian cells, on the other hand, remove some mannose residues from the precursor (trimming) and then sequentially add specific sugars to yield a glycoprotein with an oligosaccharide that terminates in sialic acid. To create a "humanized" strain, the enzyme responsible for addition of the α-1,6 mannose was first eliminated from *P. pastoris* to prevent hypermannosylation. Next, the gene encoding a mannose-trimming enzyme (a mannosidase) from the filamentous fungus *Trichoderma reesei* was inserted into the yeast genome and was found to trim the oligosaccharide to a human-like precursor. Genes encoding enzymes for the sequential addition of sugar residues that terminate the oligosaccharide chains in galactose were also added. It should be noted that the coding sequences for all engineered genes contained a secretion signal for localization of the encoded protein to the Golgi apparatus. Finally, several genes for proteins that catalyze the synthesis, transport to the Golgi apparatus, and addition of sialic acid to the terminal galactose on the protein

precursor were inserted into the *P. pastoris* genome. Properly sialylated recombinant proteins that can be used as human therapeutic agents have been produced by the "humanized" *P. pastoris*, including erythropoietin and antibodies.

During growth on methanol, enzymes required for catabolism of this substrate are expressed at very high levels with alcohol oxidase, the first enzyme in the methanol utilization pathway, encoded by the gene *AOX1*, representing as much as 30% of the cellular protein. Transcription of *AOX1* is tightly regulated; in the absence of methanol, the *AOX1* gene is completely turned off but responds rapidly to the addition of methanol to the medium. Therefore, the *AOX1* promoter is an excellent candidate for producing large amounts of recombinant protein under controlled conditions. Moreover, the induction of the cloned gene can be timed to maximize recombinant protein production during large-scale fermentations. In contrast to *S. cerevisiae*, *P. pastoris* does not synthesize ethanol, which can limit cell yields; therefore, very high cell densities of *P. pastoris* are attained, with the concomitant secretion of large quantities of protein. *P. pastoris* normally secretes very few proteins, thus simplifying the purification of secreted recombinant proteins.

Many *P. pastoris* expression vectors have been devised, each one having more or less the same format. The basic features include a gene of interest under the control of promoter and transcription termination sequences from the *P. pastoris AOX1* gene, an *E. coli* origin of replication and selectable marker gene, and a yeast selectable marker gene (Fig. 7.10). The addition of a signal sequence from either the *P. pastoris* phosphatase *PHO1* gene or another yeast gene facilitates the secretion of a recombinant protein. To avoid the problems of plasmid instability during long-term growth, most *P. pastoris* vectors are designed to be integrated into the host genome, usually within the *AOX1* gene, the *HIS4* gene for histidine biosynthesis, or rDNA. Both the engineered gene of interest and a yeast selectable marker gene are inserted together into a specific chromosome site by either a single (Fig. 7.11A) or a double (Fig. 7.11B) recombination event. The *P. pastoris* expression system has been used to produce more than 100 different biologically active proteins from bacteria, fungi, invertebrates, plants, and mammals, including humans. Many of these proteins, such as the hepatitis B virus surface antigen, human serum albumin, and bovine lysozyme, are identical to the native proteins and thus authentic.

Other Yeast Systems

Authentic heterologous proteins for industrial and pharmaceutical uses have also been generated in other yeasts. For example, the cDNAs for the α- and β-globin chains of human hemoglobin A were each cloned between the methanol oxidase promoter *(MOXp)* and transcription terminator *(MOXt)* sequences of the methylotrophic yeast *Hansenula polymorpha* and placed in tandem in an expression vector. Fortuitous integration into a chromosome yielded an isolate that produced functional hemoglobin A that had the correct tetrameric organization of the two α- and two β-globin chains ($\alpha_2\beta_2$). Also, large amounts of the animal feed enzyme supplement phytase have been produced by transformed *H. polymorpha*.

The thermotolerant dimorphic yeasts *Arxula adeninivorans* and *Yarrowia lipolytica* have demonstrated promising potential as hosts for high levels of heterologous-protein expression. These yeasts can grow at temperatures up

FIGURE 7.10 *P. pastoris* integrating expression vector. The gene of interest (GOI) is cloned between the promoter *(AOX1p)* and termination-polyadenylation sequence *(AOX1t)* of the *P. pastoris* alcohol oxidase 1 gene. The *HIS4* gene encodes a functional histidinol dehydrogenase of the histidine biosynthesis pathway. The ampicillin resistance (Ampr) gene and an origin of replication (*oriE*) function in *E. coli*. The segment marked 3' *AOX1* is a piece of DNA from the 3' end of the alcohol oxidase 1 gene of *P. pastoris*. A double recombination event between the *AOX1p* and 3' *AOX1* regions of the vector and the homologous segments of chromosome DNA results in the insertion of the DNA carrying the gene of interest and the *HIS4* gene.

FIGURE 7.11 Integration of DNA into a specific *P. pastoris* chromosome site by single (**A**) or double (**B**) recombination. (**A**) A single recombination (dashed line) between the *HIS4* gene of an intact circular plasmid and a chromosome *his4* mutant gene results in the integration of the entire vector, including the gene of interest (GOI) with the *AOX1* promoter in the 5′ *AOX1* DNA segment and the transcription–polyadenylation sequence from the *AOX1* gene (TT), into the chromosome. The inserted DNA is flanked by recombined mutant *his4* and functional *HIS4* genes. The dot in the *his4* gene represents the mutation. (**B**) A double recombination (dashed lines) between the cloned 5′ *AOX1* and 3′ *AOX1* DNA segments of a restriction endonuclease (RE) linearized DNA fragment from the vector and the corresponding chromosome regions results in the integration of the gene of interest (GOI) with the *AOX1* promoter in the 5′ *AOX1* segment, the termination–polyadenylation sequence from the *AOX1* gene (TT), and a functional *HIS4* gene. The chromosome *AOX1* coding region is lost as a result of the recombination event.

to 48°C and can survive at higher temperatures (55°C) for several hours. At higher temperatures, the fungi grow in a mycelial form and revert to budding cells below 42°C. Some secreted proteins, such as glucoamylase and invertase, are produced at higher levels in mycelia. Cell morphology also influences posttranslational modification, with O-linked glycosylation predominating in budding cells while N glycosylation occurs in both mycelial and budding cells. An additional advantage of *A. adeninivorans* is the ability to grow on a wide range of inexpensive carbon and nitrogen sources.

Stable chromosomal integration systems have been developed for *A. adeninivorans*, including a promising system based on complementation of

a tryptophan auxotroph. An expression cassette was constructed with the target α-amylase gene *(amyA)* from the bacterium *Bacillus amyloliquefaciens* flanked by the *A. adeninivorans TEF1* promoter, the *S. cerevisiae PHO5* terminator, and the selectable marker *ATRP1* that restores tryptophan biosynthesis in an *A. adeninivorans* tryptophan-auxotrophic strain carrying a deletion in the chromosomal copy of *ATRP1* (Fig. 7.12A). The 25S rDNA sequence was included on the vector with the expression cassette for targeted integration into the yeast chromosome. Following transformation of *A. adeninivorans* with the vector and selection on a medium that did not contain tryptophan, transformants were isolated that synthesized tryptophan, produced high levels of α-amylase, and carried a single copy of the vector with the expression cassette within a chromosomal 25S rDNA site. To increase the number of copies of the expression cassette integrated into the chromosome, a defective promoter was used to drive expression of the *ATRP1* selectable marker (Fig. 7.12B). The integration of multiple copies of the cassette compensated for the low levels of ATRP1 expressed from this

FIGURE 7.12 Constructs for stable integration of target genes into a chromosome of the yeast *A. adeninivorans*. **(A)** The target gene (e.g., the *amyA* gene) is inserted into a vector between the *TEF1* promoter *(p)* and the *PHO5* terminator *(t)*, and the vector is introduced into a strain of *A. adeninivorans* that is unable to synthesize tryptophan. The vector is integrated into a chromosome by homologous recombination between chromosomal and vector 25S rDNA sequences, and expression of the *ATRP1* gene driven by a strong promoter restores tryptophan biosynthesis, enabling survival of the yeast on media lacking tryptophan. **(B)** Expression of low levels of ATRP1 from a defective promoter results in chromosomal integration of multiple copies of the expression cassette. In this construct, the expression cassette, which consists of the target gene and the *ATRP1* gene, is inserted in the middle of the 25S rDNA sequence so that, following a double recombination event, only the expression cassette is integrated into the *A. adeninivorans* genome. Sequences for maintenance *(oriᴱ)* and selection (Ampʳ) in *E. coli* are included on the vector.

FIGURE 7.13 A wide-range yeast vector system for expression of heterologous genes in several different yeast hosts. The basic vector contains a multiple cloning site (MCS) for insertion of selected modules containing appropriate sequences for chromosomal integration (rDNA module), replication (ARS module), selection (Selection module), and expression (Expression module) of a target gene in a variety of yeast host cells (Table 7.3 shows examples of interchangeable modules). Sequences for maintenance (ori^E) and selection (Amp^r) of the vector in *E. coli* are also included.

promoter and resulted in sufficient synthesis of tryptophan to enable growth on medium lacking tryptophan, integration of eight copies of *amyA*, and up to five-fold-higher levels of α-amylase activity. Moreover, by inserting the *ATRP1* and *amyA* genes in the middle of the 25S rDNA sequence on the vector, following a double recombination event, only the expression cassette was integrated into the host chromosome; sequences present on the vector that are required for initial manipulation in *E. coli* were excluded.

It is often necessary to try several host types in order to find the one that produces the highest levels of a biologically active recombinant protein. Differences in the processing and productivity of a particular protein can occur among different yeast strains. For example, both *S. cerevisiae* and *H. polymorpha* produced a truncated version of the heterologous protein interleukin-6 (IL-6), whereas *A. adeninivorans* produced a full-length version of the protein. The construction of a wide-range yeast vector for expression in several fungal species has facilitated this trial-and-error process (Fig. 7.13). The basic vector contains features for propagation and selection in *E. coli* and a multiple cloning site for insertion of interchangeable modules that are chosen for a particular yeast host, including a sequence for vector integration into the fungal genome, a suitable origin of replication, a promoter to drive expression of the heterologous gene, and selectable markers to complement a range of nutritional auxotrophies or to confer resistance to antifungal compounds, such as hygromycin B (Table 7.3). In other words, by selecting from a range of available modules, cus-

tomized vectors can be rapidly and easily constructed for expression of the same gene in several different yeast cells to determine which host is optimal for heterologous-protein production.

Filamentous Fungal Systems

Distinct from unicellular yeasts, filamentous fungi are multicellular, microscopic fungi that produce long, branching strands of cells called hyphae. This group of fungi includes the common mold genera *Penicillium, Rhizopus, Trichoderma,* and *Aspergillus.* Many species of these genera of filamentous fungi are a rich natural resource for commercially important metabolites and enzymes, such as the antibiotic penicillin, the cancer chemotherapeutic agent taxol, and the cellulose-degrading enzyme cellulase, and have also been used as cell factories for the production of recombinant proteins for the food, beverage, pulp and paper, and pharmaceutical industries (Table 7.4). Similar to yeast, filamentous fungi can grow rapidly on inexpensive media, secrete large amounts of proteins, process eukaryotic mRNA, and carry out many posttranslational modifications. However, an additional advantage of using filamentous fungi as hosts for the production of mammalian proteins is their ability to add mammalian-like sugars to proteins, in contrast to yeasts, which typically add sugars with high mannose content.

Several vectors have been constructed with appropriate transcription and translation control elements for the expression of recombinant proteins in filamentous fungi, and some of these are commercially available. To achieve high yields, multiple copies of the target gene are expressed under the control of a strong promoter. Commonly used promoters include the regulatable promoter from the cellobiohydrolase I gene *(cbhI)* from *T. reesei* or the glucoamylase A gene *(glaA)* from *Aspergillus niger,* or the strong constitutive promoter from the glyceraldehyde-3-phosphate dehydrogenase gene *(gpdA)* from *Aspergillus nidulans.* However, yields of recombinant proteins are low, owing in part to degradation by extracellular proteases. The use of protease-deficient strains and gene fusion constructs has improved the output of recombinant proteins to a limited extent. The fusion partner is often a secreted protein that can carry the target protein with it to the secretory apparatus. It may also protect the target protein from degradation. When the human IL-6 gene was initially expressed in *A. nidulans* from the *A. niger glaA* promoter, protein production was very low; however, when it was expressed from the same promoter as a fusion with the secreted glucoamylase A protein, IL-6 yields increased 200-fold, although the yields were still too low for commercial viability, possibly due to degradation by host proteases (Table 7.5). Expression of IL-6 from the strong, constitutive *gpdA* promoter in a protease-deficient host improved the protein yields, but only in a mutant host that was unable to acidify the culture medium. The increased yields of recombinant protein at higher pH were attributed to reduced protease activity and altered fungal morphology. At higher pH, the fungus formed small mycelial pellets that contained more live cells.

This system has been used successfully to produce another human protein, the α_1-proteinase inhibitor, which blocks the activity of neutrophil elastase in the lungs. Individuals deficient in α_1-proteinase inhibitor can develop fatal emphysema because they are unable to prevent elastase

TABLE 7.3 Examples of modules available for wide-range yeast vector systems

Module and gene	Donor
Integration	
25S rDNA	*A. adeninivorans*
18S rDNA	*A. adeninivorans*
18S rDNA	*H. polymorpha*
Replication	
2µm ARS	*S. cerevisiae*
ARS1	*S. cerevisiae*
HARS	*H. polymorpha*
Selection	
URA3	*S. cerevisiae*
LEU2	*S. cerevisiae*
ALEU2m	*A. adeninivorans*
ATRP1m	*A. adeninivorans*
HIS4	*P. pastoris*
Expression	
MOX promoter	*H. polymorpha*
AOX1 promoter	*P. pastoris*
TEF1 promoter	*A. adeninivorans*
GAA promoter	*A. adeninivorans*
RPS7 promoter	*Y. lipolytica*

Adapted from Gellissen et al., *FEMS Yeast Res.,* 5:1079–1096, 2005.

HARS, *Hansenula* ARS.

TABLE 7.4 Some recombinant proteins produced by filamentous fungal expression systems

Recombinant protein	Host cell	Main application
α-Amylase	*A. niger, Aspergillus oryzae*	Starch processing, food industry
Aspartyl protease	*A. nidulans, A. oryzae*	Food industry
Cellulase	*T. reesei*	Textile, pulp and paper industries
Chymosin	*A. niger*	Food industry
Immunoglobulin G	*A. niger*	Pharmaceutical industry
Insulin	*A. niger*	Pharmaceutical industry
Interleukin-6	*A. niger*	Pharmaceutical industry
Laccase	*A. niger, T. reesei*	Textile, pulp and paper industries
Manganese peroxidase	*A. niger*	Chemical industry
Lactoferrin	*A. oryzae*	Pharmaceutical industry
Lipase, thermophilic	*A. oryzae*	Detergent
Lysozyme	*A. niger*	Pharmaceutical industry
Phytase	*T. reesei*	Food industry
Xylanase	*A. niger, T. reesei*	Textile, pulp and paper, food industries

from damaging lung tissue. Purified α_1-proteinase inhibitor is used for replacement therapy; however, it is difficult to obtain sufficient quantities from blood plasma, where it is normally found, and there is a risk of transferring infectious agents with the blood product, making production in fungal hosts an attractive alternative. A 1,230-base-pair cDNA encoding the mature human α_1-proteinase inhibitor gene was cloned into an expression vector under the control of the *gpdA* promoter and fused to the glucoamylase A gene to facilitate the secretion of α_1-proteinase inhibitor (Fig. 7.14). The nucleotide sequence encoding the recognition site for a specific host endoprotease was included between the α_1-proteinase inhibitor gene and the fusion partner for in vivo cleavage of the fusion protein and release of α_1-proteinase inhibitor. Expression of this construct in proteasedeficient, nonacidifying *A. niger* resulted in the secretion of active, stable, glycosylated α_1-proteinase inhibitor to the culture medium, demonstrating the efficacy of using filamentous fungal hosts to produce human proteins of therapeutic value.

Transformation of filamentous fungi may be achieved by a variety of methods, including (1) using protoplasts that have had their cell walls removed to facilitate DNA uptake, (2) *Agrobacterium*-mediated transfer of a vector carrying the target gene in a manner similar to that used to transform plants, (3) electroporation, and (4) biolistic transformation, which "shoots" the target DNA into the cell on a gold or tungsten particle. Not all of these

TABLE 7.5 Production of human interleukin-6 in filamentous fungi

Host cell	Relevant host trait	Promoter (donor)	Fusion partner	Yield (mg/liter)
A. nidulans		*glaA* (*A. niger*)		<0.1
		glaA (*A. niger*)	*glaA*	5
A. niger		*glaA*		<0.1
	Protease deficient	*gpdA*		<0.1
	Protease deficient	*gpdA*	*glaA*	2
	Protease deficient, nonacidifying	*gpdA*	*glaA*	10

Adapted from Punt et al., *Trends Biotechnol.* 20:200–206, 2002.

methods have been successful for all filamentous fungi, and the best strategy to transform a given species must be determined experimentally.

While targeted integration of a foreign gene into the genome of the yeast *S. cerevisiae* via recombination between homologous nucleotide sequences on the vector and in the host genome usually occurs at a high frequency, similar approaches in filamentous fungi have been less successful. An alternative approach exploits another recombination system found in many eukaryotes, including filamentous fungi, known as the nonhomologous-end-joining pathway. In this pathway, the Ku protein binds to the ends of introduced linear DNA and, with the DNA ligase IV-Xrcc4, integrates the fragment carrying the foreign gene at random sites in the fungal host chromosome. This system does not require homology between the introduced DNA and the integration site. Interestingly, when the nonhomologous-end-joining pathway is disrupted through mutations in Ku or the DNA ligase, targeted integration through homologous recombination is improved.

In sum, fungal expression systems play an important role in the production of heterologous proteins for research, industrial, and medical applications. However, experience has shown that no one system is able to produce an authentic version of every heterologous protein. For this and other reasons, gene expression systems that use insect or mammalian cells have been developed.

Baculovirus–Insect Cell Expression Systems

Baculoviruses are a large, diverse group of viruses that specifically infect arthropods, including many insect species, and are not infectious to other animals. During the infection cycle, two forms of baculovirus are produced (Fig. 7.15). The infection is initiated by the occluded form of the virus. In this form, the viral nucleocapsids (virions) are clustered in a matrix that is made up of the protein polyhedrin. The occluded virions packaged in this protein matrix are referred to as a polyhedron and are protected from inactivation by environmental agents. Once the virus is taken up into the midgut of the insect, usually through ingestion of contaminated plant material, the polyhedrin matrix dissolves due to the alkaline gut environment, and the virions enter midgut cells to begin the infection cycle in the nucleus. Within the insect midgut, the infection can spread from cell to cell as viral particles (single nucleocapsids) bud off from an infected cell and infect other midgut cells. This form of the virus, known as the budding form, is not embedded in a polyhedrin matrix and is not infectious to other individual insect hosts, although it can infect cultured insect cells. Plaques produced in insect cell cultures by the budding form of baculovirus have a

FIGURE 7.14 Construct for expression and secretion of the human α_1-proteinase inhibitor in the filamentous fungus *A. niger*. The expression cassette includes the strong constitutive promoter *gpdAp*, the transcriptional terminator from the *TrpC* gene *(TrpCt)*, the cDNA encoding glucoamylase to facilitate secretion, and the coding sequence for the Kex2 recognition site for in vivo removal of the glucoamylase fusion protein by the host Kex2 endoprotease.

| *gdpAp* | Glycoamylase cDNA | KEX2 cleavage | Human α_1-proteinase inhibitor cDNA | *TrpCt* |

different morphology from the occluded form. During the late stages of the infection cycle in the insect host, about 36 to 48 hours after infection, the polyhedrin protein is produced in massive quantities and continues for 4 to 5 days, until the infected cells rupture and the host organism dies. Occluded virions are released and can infect new hosts.

The promoter for the polyhedrin *(polyh)* gene is exceptionally strong, and transcription from this promoter can account for as much as 25% of the mRNA produced in cells infected with the virus. Moreover, the polyhedrin protein is not required for virus production. Consequently, it was reasoned that replacement of the polyhedrin gene with a coding sequence for a heterologous protein, followed by infection of cultured insect cells, would result in the production of large amounts of the heterologous protein. Furthermore, because of the similarity of posttranslational modification systems between insects and mammals, it was thought that the recombinant protein would mimic closely, if not precisely, the authentic form of the original protein. On the basis of these premises, a baculovirus–insect cell expression vector system was devised. Baculoviruses have been highly successful as delivery systems for introducing target genes for production of heterologous proteins in insect cells. More than a thousand different proteins have been produced using this system, including enzymes, transport proteins, receptors, and secreted proteins, for a variety of applications (Table 7.6).

FIGURE 7.15 Budded **(A)** and occluded **(B)** forms of AcMNPV. During budding, a nucleocapsid becomes enveloped by the membrane of an infected cell. A polyhedron consists of clusters of nucleocapsids (occluded virions) embedded in various orientations in a polyhedrin matrix.

The specific baculovirus that has been used extensively as an expression vector is *Autographa californica* multiple nuclear polyhedrosis virus (AcMNPV). *A. californica* (the alfalfa looper) and over 30 other insect species are infected by AcMNPV. This virus also grows well on many insect cell lines. The most commonly used cell line for genetically engineered AcMNPV is derived from the fall armyworm, *Spodoptera frugiperda*. In these cells, the polyhedrin promoter is exceptionally active, and during infections with wild-type baculovirus, high levels of polyhedrin are synthesized. To a lesser extent, the *Bombyx mori* nuclear polyhedrosis virus has been used to express heterologous proteins in silkworm larvae.

Baculovirus Expression Vectors

The first step in the production of a recombinant AcMNPV that will be used to deliver the gene of interest into the insect host cell is to create a transfer vector. The transfer vector is an *E. coli*-based plasmid that carries a segment of DNA from AcMNPV (Fig. 7.16) consisting of the polyhedrin promoter region and an adjacent portion of upstream AcMNPV DNA, a multiple cloning site, the polyhedrin termination and polyadenylation signal regions, and an adjacent portion of downstream AcMNPV DNA. The coding region for the polyhedrin gene has been deleted from this block of DNA. The upstream and downstream AcMNPV DNA segments included on the transfer vector provide regions for homologous recombination with AcMNPV. A gene of interest is inserted into the multiple cloning site between the polyhedrin promoter and termination sequences, and the transfer vector is propagated in *E. coli*.

Next, insect cells in culture are cotransfected with AcMNPV DNA and the transfer vector carrying the cloned gene. Within some of the doubly transfected cells, a double-crossover recombination event occurs at homologous polyhedrin gene sequences on the transfer vector and in the AcMNPV genome, and the cloned gene with polyhedrin promoter and termination regions becomes integrated into the AcMNPV DNA (Fig. 7.17) with the concomitant loss of the polyhedrin gene. Virions lacking the polyhedrin gene produce distinctive zones of cell lysis (occlusion-negative plaques), from which recombinant baculovirus is isolated.

DNA hybridization or a polymerase chain reaction (PCR) assay can be used to confirm the presence of recombinant baculovirus. To facilitate the

TABLE 7.6 Some of the recombinant proteins that have been produced by the baculovirus expression vector system

α-Interferon	G-protein-coupled receptors	Malaria proteins
Adenosine deaminase	HIV-1 envelope protein	Mouse monoclonal antibodies
Anthrax antigen	HSV capsid proteins	Multidrug transporter protein
β-Amyloid precursor protein	Human alkaline phosphatase	Poliovirus proteins
β-Interferon	Human DNA polymerase α	Pseudorabies virus glycoprotein 50
Bovine rhodopsin	Human pancreatic lipase	Rabies virus glycoprotein
Cystic fibrosis transmembrane conductance regulator	Influenza virus hemagglutinin Interleukin-2	Respiratory syncytial virus antigen Simian rotavirus capsid antigen
Dengue virus type 1 antigen	Lassa virus protein	Tissue plasminogen activator
Erythropoietin		

HIV-1, human immunodeficiency virus type 1; HSV, herpes simplex virus.

Vector
DNA

5′ AcMNPV *Pp* MCS *Pt* 3′ AcMNPV DNA
DNA

FIGURE 7.16 Organization of the expression unit of a baculovirus (AcMNPV) transfer vector. The gene of interest is inserted into the multiple cloning site (MCS) that lies between the polyhedrin gene promoter *(Pp)* and polyhedrin gene transcription termination *(Pt)* sequences. The AcMNPV DNA upstream from the polyhedrin promoter (5′ AcMNPV DNA) and downstream from the polyhedrin transcription termination sequence (3′ AcMNPV DNA) provides sequences for integration of the expression unit by homologous recombination into an AcMNPV genome.

detection of recombinant plaques, the *E. coli lacZ* gene, which encodes β-galactosidase, is put under the control of a baculovirus promoter that is turned on during the early to late stages of the infection cycle, and this construct is made part of the DNA unit that is incorporated into the AcMNPV genome. Recombinant plaques turn blue when a chromogenic substrate for β-galactosidase is added to the medium. Additional rounds of infection of insect cells with viruses from occlusion-negative plaques increase the concentration of recombinant viruses. Heterologous protein is harvested 4 to 5 days after host insect cells are infected with a high-titer recombinant baculovirus stock.

Increasing the Yield of Recombinant Baculovirus

The identification of occlusion-negative plaques is subjective, and purification of recombinant baculovirus is tedious due to the low frequency of recombination (~0.1%) between the AcMNPV DNA and the transfer plasmid; therefore, improvements have been made to the original procedure to increase the frequency of recombinant viruses. A very simple yet effective procedure that increases the frequency of recombinant plaques to about 30% involves linearization of the AcMNPV genome before transfection into insect cells. Linearized baculovirus genomes have reduced infectivity, decreasing the number of nonrecombinant plaques, and a double-crossover event between a linearized AcMNPV DNA molecule and a circular transfer vector establishes a closed circular DNA molecule that is infective.

The linearization method was further developed to generate a system that produces an even higher frequency of recombinant baculovirus plaques. The AcMNPV genome was engineered with two Bsu36I sites that were placed on either side of the polyhedrin gene (Fig. 7.18). One is in gene 603 (open reading frame 603 [ORF603]), and the other is in a gene (ORF1629) that is essential for viral replication. When DNA from this modified baculovirus is treated with Bsu36I and transfected into insect cells, no viral replication occurs because a segment of the essential gene (ORF1629) is missing. As part of this system, a transfer vector is constructed with the gene of interest between intact versions of gene 603 and gene 1629. This transfer vector is introduced into insect cells that were previously transfected with linearized, replication-defective AcMNPV DNA that is missing the segment between the two Bsu36I sites. A double-crossover event both reestablishes a functional version of ORF1629 and incorporates the cloned

FIGURE 7.17 Replacement of the AcMNPV polyhedrin gene with an expression unit from a transfer vector. A double crossover event (×) between homologous DNA segments of the transfer vector and the AcMNPV genome results in the integration of the expression unit into the AcMNPV genome. GOI, gene of interest; *Pp*, polyhedrin promoter; *Pt*, polyhedrin polyadenylation and termination sequence.

gene into the AcMNPV genome (Fig. 7.18). With this system, over 90% of the baculovirus plaques are recombinant.

Integration of Target Genes into Baculovirus by Site-Specific Recombination

To eliminate the need to use plaque assays to identify and purify recombinant viruses, several methods have been developed that introduce the target gene into the baculovirus genome at a specific nucleotide sequence by recombination, either in an intermediate bacterial host, such as *E. coli*, or in vitro outside of a host cell. Transfection of insect cells is required only for the production of the heterologous protein. AcMNPV DNA can be maintained in *E. coli* as a plasmid known as a bacmid, which is a baculovirus–plasmid hybrid molecule. In addition to AcMNPV genes, the bacmid contains an origin of replication for propagation in *E. coli*, a kanamycin resistance gene for selection of the bacmid, and an integration site (attachment site) that is inserted into the *lacZ'* gene without impairing its function (Fig. 7.19A). Another component of this system is the transfer vector that carries the gene of interest cloned between the polyhedrin promoter and a terminator sequence. In the transfer vector, the target gene expression unit (expression cassette) and a gentamicin resistance gene are flanked by DNA

FIGURE 7.18 Production of recombinant baculovirus. Single Bsu36I sites are engineered into gene 603 and a gene (1629) that is essential for AcMNPV replication. These genes flank the polyhedrin gene in the AcMNPV genome. After a baculovirus with two engineered Bsu36I sites is treated with Bsu36I, the segment between the Bsu36I sites is deleted. Insect cells are cotransfected with a Bsu36I-treated baculovirus DNA and a transfer vector with a gene of interest under the control of the promoter (*p*) and terminator (*t*) elements of the polyhedrin gene and the complete sequences of both genes 603 and 1629. A double crossover event (dashed lines) generates a recombinant baculovirus with a functional gene 1629. With this system, almost all of the progeny baculoviruses are recombinant.

attachment sequences that can bind to the attachment site in the bacmid (Fig. 7.19B). An ampicillin resistance gene lies outside the expression cassette for selection of the transfer vector.

Bacterial cells carrying a bacmid are cotransformed with the transfer vector and a helper plasmid that encodes the specific proteins (transposi-

tion proteins) that mediate recombination between the attachment sites on the transfer vector and on the bacmid and that carries a tetracycline resistance gene. After recombination, the DNA segment that is bounded by the two attachment sites on the transfer vector (the expression cassette carrying the target gene) is transposed into the attachment site on the bacmid, destroying the reading frame of the *lacZ'* gene (Fig. 7.19C). Consequently, bacteria with recombinant bacmids produce white colonies in the presence of isopropyl-β-D-thiogalactopyranoside (IPTG) and 5-bromo-4-chloro-3-indolyl-β-D-galactopyranoside (X-Gal). Moreover, white colonies that are resistant to kanamycin and gentamicin and sensitive to both ampicillin and tetracycline carry only a recombinant bacmid and no transfer and helper plasmids. After all of these manipulations, the integrity of the cloned gene can be confirmed by PCR. Finally, recombinant bacmid DNA can be transfected into insect cells, where the cloned gene is transcribed and the heterologous protein is produced.

Another method exploits the bacteriophage λ integration system for site-specific recombination of λ DNA into a host bacterial genome. All genetic manipulations to construct the baculovirus expression vector are carried out in vitro before transferring the recombinant virus into the insect host for selection and production of the heterologous protein. First, the AcMNPV genome was engineered to include two different integration sequences (attachment sites attR1 and attR2) derived from bacteriophage λ that flank the *tk* gene encoding the enzyme thymidine kinase from herpes simplex virus (Fig. 7.20A). Thymidine kinase converts the synthetic nucleotide analogue ganciclovir into a product that is toxic to insect cells and was included in the engineered AcMNPV construct for subsequent selection against nonrecombinant viruses. The attR1-*tk*-attR2 DNA segment (cassette) was placed downstream of the polyhedrin gene promoter. Next, the target gene was inserted into a donor plasmid between two attachment sites, attL1 and attL2, that correspond to the attachment sites in the engineered AcMNPV genome (Fig. 7.20B). Integration of the target gene into the AcMNPV genome occurs by recombination between the attachment sites flanking the target gene on the plasmid and flanking the *tk* gene in the AcMNPV genome. Site-specific recombination between the attachment sequences is mediated by the addition of integration enzymes (integrase, excisionase, and integration host factor) derived from bacteriophage λ to the in vitro reaction mixture (Fig. 7.20C). Insect cells are then transfected with the recombinant baculovirus for selection and propagation. Because recombination results in excision of the thymidine kinase gene from the baculovirus genome, only cells transfected with viruses carrying the target gene will survive in the presence of ganciclovir.

Mammalian Glycosylation and Processing of Precursor Proteins in Insect Cells

Although insect cells can process proteins in a manner similar to that of higher eukaryotes, some mammalian proteins produced in *S. frugiperda* cell lines are not authentically glycosylated. For example, insect cells do not normally add galactose and terminal sialic acid residues to N-linked glycoproteins. Where these residues are normally added to mannose residues during the processing of some proteins in mammalian cells, insect cells will

FIGURE 7.19 Construction of a recombinant bacmid. **(A)** An *E. coli* plasmid is incorporated into the AcMNPV genome by a double crossover event (dashed lines) between DNA segments (5′ and 3′) that flank the polyhedrin gene to create a shuttle vector (bacmid) that replicates in both *E. coli* and insect cells. The gene for resistance to kanamycin (Kan^r), an attachment site (att) that is inserted in frame in the *lacZ′* sequence, and an *E. coli* origin of replication (*ori*^E) are introduced as part of the plasmid DNA. **(B)** The transposition proteins encoded by genes of the helper plasmid facilitate the integration (transposition) of the DNA segment of the transfer vector that is bounded by two attachment sequences (attR and attL). The gene for resistance to gentamicin (Gen^r) and a gene of interest (GOI) that is under the control of the promoter (*p*) and transcription terminator (*t*) elements of the polyhedrin gene are inserted into the attachment site (att) of the bacmid. The helper plasmid and transfer vector carry the genes for resistance to tetracycline (Tet^r) and ampicillin (Amp^r), respectively. **(C)** The recombinant bacmid has a disrupted *lacZ′* gene (*). The right-angled arrow denotes the site of initiation of transcription of the cloned gene after transfection of the recombinant bacmid into an insect cell. Cells that are transfected with a recombinant bacmid are not able to produce functional β-galactosidase.

trim the oligosaccharide to produce paucimannose (Fig. 7.21). Consequently, because these residues are usually important for the proper functioning of a protein and improperly glycosylated mammalian proteins may elicit an allergic response when used as human therapeutic agents, the baculovirus system cannot be used for the production of several important mammalian glycoproteins. Host insect cell lines have been constructed with an integrated mammalian β-1,4-galactotransferase gene and a mammalian α-2,6-sialyltransferase gene under the control of a promoter that is active during the early stages of the baculovirus infection cycle. Under test conditions, this system synthesized N-linked glycans with both galactose and sialic acid; however, the position of the sugar residues in the oligosaccharide chain was not identical to that found on the natural human glycoprotein. To ensure the production of "humanized" glycoproteins with accurate glycosylation patterns, an insect cell line was constructed to express five different mammalian glycosyltransferases (Fig. 7.21). Because insect cells do not normally produce cytidine monophosphate (CMP)–sialic acid, the substrate for sialyltransferase and donor molecules for sialic acid residues, cell lines have also been constructed to express sialic acid synthases that produce CMP–sialic acid from N-acetylmannosamine provided in the culture medium. Although cell lines have been improved by the addition of mam-

FIGURE 7.20 Construction of a recombinant baculovirus expression vector in vitro. **(A)** The AcMNPV genome was engineered to carry the thymidine kinase gene *(tk)* between attachment sequences attR1 and attR2 and downstream of the baculovirus polyhedrin gene promoter *(Pp)*. **(B)** The target gene is cloned into a donor plasmid between attachment sequences attL1 and attL2. **(C)** The AcMNPV DNA carrying the *tk* gene and the donor plasmid are combined in a test tube, and integration enzymes are added to catalyze the recombination between corresponding attR and attL sites. Recombination results in the replacement of the *tk* gene with the target gene in the AcMNPV DNA so that, following transfection with the recombinant AcMNPV DNA, the insect cells are resistant to the toxic effects of ganciclovir and express the target gene from the polyhedrin gene promoter.

malian N-glycan-processing capabilities, in some cases it may be preferable to express the protein of interest in a mammalian host.

Further improvements to prevent undesirable processing of heterologous proteins in insect cells using the baculovirus expression system are the removal of the genes encoding chitinase and the protease v-cathepsin from the AcMNPV genome. v-Cathepsin is normally produced late in the infection cycle to facilitate the release of new virions from the insect host. It also reduces the yield of heterologous proteins through proteolytic cleavage. Chitinase is produced in conjunction with v-cathepsin and is thought to function in the proper folding of v-cathepsin and in the degradation of the host exoskeleton. It is secreted at very high levels from baculovirus-infected insect host cells and can compete with secreted target proteins for the secretory apparatus, thereby reducing yields of the target protein. Coexpression of chaperones to ensure proper folding of the target protein has also resulted in increased yields of functional heterologous proteins.

Production of Multiprotein Complexes Using Baculovirus

In many cases, the baculovirus–insect expression system is used to express a single protein of interest. For example, it has been recently tested for the production of hemagglutinin, the dominant antigenic protein on the surface of the influenza virus that has potential to be used as a vaccine against influenza infection (subunit vaccines are discussed in chapter 12). In mice and humans, the purified recombinant hemagglutinin vaccine produced using baculovirus in insect cells was found to be safe and to provide a high level of protection against influenza virus infection. Influenza vaccines in current use are inactivated or attenuated forms of the whole virus; however, protection against influenza virus using these vaccines is short-lived

FIGURE 7.21 N glycosylation of proteins in the Golgi apparatus of insect, human, and "humanized" insect cells. While the sugar residues added to N-glycoproteins in the endoplasmic reticulum are similar in insect and human cells, further processing in the Golgi apparatus yields a trimmed oligosaccharide (paucimannose) in insect cells and an oligosaccharide that terminates in sialic acid in human cells. To produce recombinant proteins for use as human therapeutic agents, "humanized" insect cells have been engineered to express several enzymes that process human glycoproteins accurately. Blue squares, N-acetylglucosamine; red circles, mannose; green squares, galactose; orange squares, sialic acid.

because the antigenic surface proteins, such as hemagglutinin, change rapidly, giving rise to new influenza virus strains against which existing vaccines are not effective. An important advantage of producing a recombinant subunit vaccine using baculovirus is the relative ease with which genes such as the hemagglutinin gene can be cloned and expressed. This allows the rapid and flexible production of vaccines that change on a frequent basis. Currently, whole-virus vaccines must be propagated in chicken eggs and therefore have long production times and are less amenable to change once production has begun. Moreover, because production using eggs is avoided, baculovirus vaccines do not contain egg proteins that can stimulate an allergic response in some individuals.

The simultaneous expression of two or more cloned genes can lead to the formation of functional multimeric protein complexes. This can be accomplished by cotransfecting insect cells with multiple baculoviruses, each engineered to express one target protein, or, using a more manageable approach, by transfection with a single recombinant virus expressing multiple proteins. AcMNPV is particularly amenable to carrying large insertions, up to 38 kb, with several foreign genes due to its flexible envelope. An important example is the production of vaccines known as virus-like particles using AcMNPV. Virus-like particles are comprised of the assembled protein coat of the virus but without the nucleic acid genome (Fig. 7.22A), and while these particles are often infectious (i.e., they can enter cells), they cannot replicate and therefore do not cause disease. One of the shortcomings of using single antigenic proteins as vaccines is that they often have poor immunogenicity, that is, they do not elicit a strong immune response. Researchers have shown that protein vaccines that more closely mimic the overall structure of a virus particle, such as virus-like particles, evoke a stronger response and therefore provide greater protection against subsequent infection. Generally, multiple genes encoding the proteins that make up the virus-like particle are cloned into a transfer vector, and these are then incorporated into the AcMNPV DNA via site-specific recombination either in vitro, as described above, or in *E. coli*. In the latter case, rather than supplying purified enzymes required for recombination in vitro, the recombinase is produced from a gene in the *E. coli* genome. In one study, the genes for three different envelope structural proteins from the human severe acute respiratory syndrome coronavirus (SARS-CoV) were expressed simultaneously at a high level from a single baculovirus vector (Fig. 7.22B). The proteins were found to assemble spontaneously and stably into virus-like particles. Although the envelope proteins were also expressed from three separate baculovirus vectors in a single host cell, stable virus-like particles were not recovered, possibly due to asynchronous expression of sufficient structural components.

Mammalian Cell Expression Systems

Mammalian cell expression systems are important for the production of heterologous proteins with a full complement of posttranslational modifications. Currently, about half of the commercially available therapeutic proteins are produced in mammalian cells. However, there are several major challenges to the production of high levels of heterologous proteins in mammalian cell lines. Generally, these cells are slow growing, have more fastidious growth requirements, and can become contaminated with animal viruses. A number of established mammalian cell lines have been

developed as hosts for heterologous-protein production. Cells derived from African green monkey kidney (COS), baby hamster kidney (BHK), and human embryonic kidney (HEK 293) are used for short-term (transient) gene expression for either rapid production of small amounts of heterologous proteins for evaluating their potential as drug candidates or testing the integrity of constructs during various stages of vector development. Important characteristics of these cells are their receptiveness to transfection, their ability to grow in suspension cultures without addition of serum that contains animal proteins, and their suitability for high-density, large-scale production. The ability to grow in serum-free medium not only reduces costs, but also facilitates purification of the target protein and reduces the risk of contamination with animal-derived material. Chinese hamster ovary (CHO) cells and mouse myeloma cells are most commonly used for long-term (stable) gene expression and when high yields of heterologous proteins are required. About 140 recombinant proteins are currently approved for therapeutic use, most produced in CHO cells that have been adapted for growth in high-density suspension cultures, and many more are in clinical trials. Although mammalian cells have been used for some time to produce therapeutic proteins, especially antibodies, and vectors carrying suitable expression signals have been developed, current efforts are aimed at improving productivity through the development of high-producing cell lines, increasing the stability of production over time, and increasing expression by manipulating the chromosomal environment in which the recombinant genes are integrated.

Vector Design

Most cloning vectors constructed for the expression of heterologous genes in mammalian cells are based on the genomes of viruses that infect mammalian cells. The first vector was based on a simian virus (simian virus 40 [SV40]) that can replicate in several mammalian species. The genome of this virus is a double-stranded DNA molecule of 5.2 kb that carries genes expressed early in the infection cycle that function in the replication of viral DNA (early genes) and genes expressed later in the infection cycle that function in the production of viral capsid proteins (late genes). For use as a

FIGURE 7.22 (A) Virus-like particles are made up of viral coat (capsid) or envelope proteins that assemble to form a structure that resembles the original virus but does not contain the viral genetic material. **(B)** Viral spike (S), membrane (M), and envelope (E) proteins, which comprise the envelope of the human SARS-CoV, can be produced in insect cells using a single recombinant baculovirus vector carrying all three viral genes. Following expression, the S, M, and E proteins self-assemble to form a SARS-CoV virus-like particle that is a candidate vaccine for protection against SARS. *Pp*, polyhedrin promoter; *10p*, baculovirus p10 promoter.

FIGURE 7.23 Generalized mammalian expression vector. The multiple cloning site (MCS) and selectable marker gene (SMG) are under the control of eukaryotic promoter *(p)*, polyadenylation *(pa)*, and termination of transcription (TT) sequences. An intron (I) enhances the production of heterologous protein. Propagation of the vector in *E. coli* and mammalian cells depends on the origins of replication *ori*E and *ori*euk, respectively. The ampicillin resistance (Ampr) gene is used for selecting transformed *E. coli*.

cloning vector, some of the early and late genes are removed and replaced with a target gene under the control of appropriate mammalian expression signals. Although many cloning vectors are based on SV40 DNA, its use is restricted to small inserts because only a limited amount of DNA can be packaged into the viral capsid. Other vectors that can accommodate larger amounts of cloned DNA are derived from adenovirus; bovine papillomavirus, which can be maintained as a multicopy plasmid in some mammalian cells; and adeno-associated virus, which can integrate into specific sites in the host chromosome.

While hundreds of mammalian expression vectors have been developed, they all tend to have the same shared features and are not very different in design from other eukaryotic expression vectors. A representative mammalian expression vector (Fig. 7.23) contains a eukaryotic origin of replication, usually from an animal virus, such as SV40. The promoter sequences that drive expression of the cloned gene(s) and the selectable marker gene(s), and the transcription termination sequences (polyadenylation signals), must be eukaryotic and are frequently taken from either human viruses (cytomegalovirus [CMV], SV40, or herpes simplex virus) or mammalian genes (β-actin, metallothionein, thymidine kinase, or bovine growth hormone). Strong constitutive promoters and efficient polyadenylation signals are preferred. Inducible promoters are often used when continuous synthesis of the heterologous protein is toxic to the host cell. Expression of a gene of interest is often increased by placing the sequence for an intron between the promoter and the multiple cloning site within the transcribed region. The sequences that are required for selection and propagation of a mammalian expression vector in *E. coli* are derived from a standard *E. coli* cloning vector, such as pBR322.

For the best results, a gene of interest must be equipped with translation control sequences (Fig. 7.24). Initiation of translation in higher eukaryotic organisms depends on a specific sequence of nucleotides surrounding the start (AUG) codon in the mRNA called the Kozak sequence, e.g., GCCGCC(A or G)CCAUGG in vertebrates. The corresponding DNA sequence for the Kozak sequence, which is often followed by a signal sequence to facilitate secretion, a protein sequence (tag) to enhance the purification of the heterologous protein, and a proteolytic cleavage sequence that enables the tag to be removed from the heterologous protein,

is placed at the 5' end of the gene of interest. A stop codon is added to ensure that translation ceases at the correct location. Finally, the sequence content of the 5' and 3' untranslated regions (UTRs) is important for efficient translation and mRNA stability. Either synthetic 5' and 3' UTRs or those from the human β-globin gene are used in mammalian expression vectors. The codon content of the gene of interest may also require modification to suit the translational preferences of the host cell.

The majority of mammalian cell expression vectors carry a single gene of interest that encodes a functional polypeptide. However, the active form of some commercially important proteins consists of two different protein chains. For example, human thyroid-stimulating hormone is a two-chain protein (heterodimer), and both hemoglobin and antibodies are tetramers with two copies of each subunit, $\alpha_2\beta_2$ and H_2L_2, respectively. It is possible to clone the gene or cDNA for each subunit of a multimeric protein, synthesize and purify each subunit separately, and then mix the chains together in a test tube. Unfortunately, relatively few multichain proteins are properly assembled in vitro. By contrast, in vivo assembly of dimeric and tetrameric proteins is quite efficient. Consequently, various strategies have been devised for the production of two different recombinant proteins within the same cell.

Two mammalian expression vectors, each with the gene or cDNA for one of the subunits and a different selectable marker gene, can be cotransfected into host cells (Fig. 7.25). The transfected cells are treated with both selecting agents, and the cells that survive carry both vectors. Two-vector systems have been used successfully for the production of authentic dimeric and tetrameric recombinant proteins. However, loss of one of the two vectors in doubly transfected cells is common. Moreover, the two vectors are not always maintained with the same copy number, so one subunit is overproduced relative to the other and yields of the final product are reduced. To overcome these problems, single vectors that carry two cloned genes have been developed. In some instances, the two genes are placed under the control of independent promoters and polyadenylation signals (double-cassette vectors) (Fig. 7.26). Alternatively, to ensure that equal amounts of the recombinant proteins are synthesized, vectors (bicistronic vectors) have been constructed with the two cloned genes separated from each other by a DNA sequence that contains an internal ribosomal entry site (IRES) (Fig. 7.27). Parenthetically, IRESs are found in mammalian virus genomes, and after transcription, they allow simultaneous translation of different proteins from a polycistronic mRNA molecule. Transcription of a "gene α–IRES–gene β" construct is controlled by one promoter and polyadenylation signal. Under these conditions, a single "two-gene" (bicistronic) transcript is synthesized, and translation proceeds from the 5' end of the mRNA to produce one of the chains (chain α)

FIGURE 7.24 Translation control elements. A gene of interest can be fitted with various sequences that enhance translation and facilitate both secretion and purification, such as a Kozak sequence (K), signal sequence (S), protein affinity tag (T), proteolytic cleavage site (P), and stop codon (SC). The 5' and 3' UTRs increase the efficiency of translation and contribute to mRNA stability.

5' UTR K S T P Gene of interest SC 3' UTR

FIGURE 7.25 Two-vector expression system. The cloned genes (gene α and gene β) encode subunits of a protein dimer (αβ). After cotransfection, both subunits (α and β) are synthesized and assembled into a functional protein dimer. Both vectors carry origins of replication for *E. coli* (*ori*E) and mammalian cells (*ori*euk) and a marker (Ampr) gene for selecting transformed *E. coli*. The selectable marker genes (SMG1 and SMG2) and the cloned genes (gene α and gene β) are each under the control of promoter *(p)*, polyadenylation *(pa)*, and termination of transcription (TT) sequences.

and internally from the IRES element to produce the second chain (chain β) (Fig. 7.27). Generally, constructing an effective mammalian expression vector is time-consuming and demands considerable effort to achieve optimum protein production.

Baculovirus Vectors for Protein Production in Mammalian Cells

It is possible to use some of the baculovirus delivery systems that have already been developed to express target proteins in mammalian cells, such as HEK 293, CHO, COS, and human HeLa cells. Although baculoviruses cannot replicate in mammalian cells, they can be transduced into these cells with a transduction efficiency reaching 100% in some cases, where they enter the nucleus and express heterologous genes that were inserted in the viral genome. Both adherent cells growing in a single layer on a solid surface and cells suspended in culture can be transduced. Because baculoviruses cannot replicate in mammalian cells and the polyhedron-deficient strains employed as vectors cannot infect insects, this system presents a safe alternative to some of the other approaches to heterologous-protein expression in mammalian cells.

FIGURE 7.26 Two-gene expression vector. The cloned genes (gene α and gene β) encode subunits of a protein dimer (αβ). The cloned genes are inserted into a vector and are under the control of different eukaryotic promoter *(p)*, polyadenylation *(pa)*, and termination of transcription (TT) sequences. Each subunit is translated from a separate mRNA, and a functional protein dimer (αβ) is assembled. The vector has origins of replication for *E. coli* (*ori*E) and mammalian cells (*ori*euk), a marker gene (Ampr) for selecting transformed *E. coli*, and a selectable marker gene (SMG) that is under the control of eukaryotic promoter *(p)*, polyadenylation *(pa)*, and termination of transcription (TT) sequences.

Appropriate promoter, polyadenylation, and transcription termination sequences that are functional in mammalian cells must be included on the recombinant baculovirus delivery system, as they are for other mammalian expression systems. First, a recombinant AcMNPV vector is constructed to carry the target gene under the control of mammalian cell expression signals, using methods such as site-specific recombination (shown in Fig. 7.20). Next, the titer of the recombinant virus is increased by replication in insect cell lines. Finally, purified recombinant AcMNPV DNA is transduced into mammalian cells. The mechanism of baculovirus uptake by mammalian cells is unclear but seems to involve specific protein interactions. The baculovirus envelope glycoprotein 64 (gp64) may be important, because increasing the levels of this protein, for example, by including additional copies of the gp64 gene in the AcMNPV vector, results in increased transduction. Transduction efficiency and, subsequently, target gene expression, are often variable but can be optimized by incubating the baculovirus and mammalian cells for a longer time and at a lower temperature, by adding the viral inoculum over a period of several days, or by addition of the chemical butyrate or trichostatin A,

FIGURE 7.27 Bicistronic expression vector. The cloned genes (gene α and gene β) encode subunits of a protein dimer (αβ). Each cloned gene is inserted into a vector on either side of a sequence for an IRES. The two genes and the IRES sequence form a transcription unit under the control of a single eukaryotic promoter *(p)*, polyadenylation *(pa)*, and termination of transcription (TT) sequence. Translation of the mRNA occurs from the 5' end and internally (right-angled arrows). Both subunits (α and β) are synthesized and assembled into a functional protein dimer (αβ). The vector carries origins of replication for *E. coli* (*ori*E) and mammalian cells (*ori*euk), a selectable marker (Ampr) for selecting transformed *E. coli*, and a selectable marker gene (SMG) that is under the control of eukaryotic promoter *(p)*, polyadenylation *(pa)*, and termination of transcription (TT) sequences.

which prevents modification of chromatin structure that can inhibit gene expression.

Expression of a heterologous gene from the baculovirus vector in mammalian host cells is typically transient, although it can be sustained for several days to weeks. For stable long-term expression, the target gene is integrated into the host genome. Stable cell lines can be generated by including a selectable marker, such as the gene encoding neomycin phosphotransferase (see below) under the control of an appropriate mammalian promoter, on the AcMNPV vector. Under selective conditions, fragments of baculovirus DNA ranging in size from 5 to 18 kb and containing the target gene were found to be randomly integrated into the mammalian host cell genome, albeit at a relatively low frequency. Integration into host DNA using baculoviruses can be increased significantly by engineering the AcMNPV vector to carry the adeno-associated virus inverted terminal repeat regions (145 base pairs) flanking the target

gene (Fig. 7.28). Similar to the attachment (*att*) sequences used by bacteriophage λ to integrate into specific sites in the bacterial genome (described above), the inverted terminal repeat sequences are used by adeno-associated virus for integration into the host genome. The *rep* gene must also be included, as the encoded protein directs site-specific integration.

Selectable Markers for Mammalian Expression Vectors

For the most part, the systems that are used to select transfected mammalian cells are the same as those for other eukaryotic host cells (Table 7.7). In fact, a number of bacterial marker genes have been adapted for eukaryotic cells. For example, the bacterial *neo* gene, which encodes neomycin phosphotransferase, is often used to select transfected mammalian cells. However, in eukaryotic cells, G-418 (Geneticin), which is phosphorylated by neomycin phosphotransferase, replaces neomycin as the selective agent because neomycin is not an effective inhibitor of eukaryotic protein synthesis.

Some selection schemes are designed not only to identify transfected cells, but to increase heterologous-protein production by amplifying the copy number of the expression vector (Fig. 7.29). The dihydrofolate reductase–methotrexate system falls into this category. Briefly, dihydrofolate reductase catalyzes the reduction of dihydrofolate to tetrahydrofolate, which is required for the production of purines. Methotrexate is a competitive inhibitor of dihydrofolate reductase. Sensitivity to methotrexate can be overcome if the cell produces excess dihydrofolate reductase, and as the methotrexate concentration is increased over a period of time, the dihydrofolate reductase gene in cultured cells is amplified. It is not unusual for methotrexate-resistant cells to have hundreds of dihydrofolate reductase genes. The standard dihydrofolate reductase–methotrexate protocol entails transfecting dihydrofolate reductase-deficient cells with an expression vector carrying a dihydrofolate reductase gene as the selectable marker gene and treating the cells with methotrexate. After the initial selection of transfected cells, the concentration of methotrexate is gradually increased, and eventually cells with very high copy numbers of the expression vector are selected.

FIGURE 7.28 Baculovirus vector for stable expression of target genes in mammalian cells. The target gene with appropriate promoter (*p*) and terminator (*t*) sequences is inserted into an AcMNPV vector between sequences for adeno-associated virus inverted terminal repeats (ITR). Following the transfection of mammalian cells, the protein encoded by the *rep* gene from adeno-associated virus mediates site-directed integration of the target gene into the host genome via the ITR sequences.

rep ITR Target gene ITR

TABLE 7.7 Selective marker gene systems for mammalian cells

Selective agent	Action of selective agent	Marker gene	Action of marker gene protein
Xyl-A	Damages DNA	Adenine deaminase (*ada*)	Deaminates Xyl-A
Blasticidin S	Inhibits protein synthesis	Blasticidin S deaminases (*Bsr, BSD*)	Deaminates blasticidin S
Bleomycin	Breaks DNA strands	Bleomycin-binding protein (*Ble*)	Binds to bleomycin
G-418 (Geneticin)	Inhibits protein synthesis	Neomycin phosphotransferase (*neo*)	Phosphorylates G-418
Histidinol	Produces cytotoxic effects	Histidinol dehydrogenase (*hisD*)	Oxidizes histidinol to histidine
Hygromycin B	Inhibits protein synthesis	Hygromycin B phosphotrans-ferase (*Hph*)	Phosphorylates hygromycin B
MSX	Inhibits glutamine synthesis	Glutamine synthetase (*GS*)	Cells that produce excess glutamine synthetase survive.
MTX	Inhibits DNA synthesis	Dihydrofolate reductase (*dhfr*)	Cells that produce excess dihydro-folate reductase survive.
PALA	Inhibits purine synthesis	Cytosine deaminase (*codA*)	Lowers cytosine levels in the medium by converting cytosine to uracil
Puromycin	Inhibits protein synthesis	Puromycin N-acetyltransferase (*Pac*)	Acetylates puromycin

MSX, methionine sulfoximine; MTX, methotrexate; PALA, N-(phosphoacetyl)-L-aspartate; Xyl-A, 9-β-D-xylofuranosyl adenine.

Engineering Mammalian Cell Hosts for Enhanced Productivity

Several improvements have been made to mammalian cell lines to enhance their productivity by increasing cell growth, vector stability, gene expression, and protein secretion. Conditions in large-scale bioreactors can be stressful for mammalian cells. Depleted nutrients and accumulation of toxic cell waste can limit the viability and density of cells as they respond to stress by inducing cell death, also known as apoptosis. Often chemical inhibitors of cell death pathways are utilized, but recently, genetic means have been explored to construct cell lines in which the apoptotic pathways are inhibited. When cells perceive a variety of stresses, an initial response is the activation of the tumor suppressor protein p53, which is a transcription factor that induces the expression of genes that encode proteins in the apoptotic pathway. One method to improve cell growth and viability under culture conditions in bioreactors is to prevent p53 from activating the cell death response pathway. The mouse double-mutant 2 protein (MDM2) binds to protein p53 and prevents it from acting as a transcription factor (Fig. 7.30). MDM2 also marks p53 for degradation. HEK 293 and CHO cells were transfected with plasmids containing a regulatable *MDM2* gene and cultured under conditions that mimicked the late stages of cell culture and in nutrient-limited medium. Cultures expressing *MDM2* had higher cell densities and delayed cell death compared to nontransfected cells, especially in nutrient-deprived medium.

Many cultured mammalian cells are unable to achieve high cell densities in cultures because toxic metabolic products accumulate in the culture medium and inhibit cell growth. Although efforts are made to optimize the culture conditions, inevitably nutrients essential for optimal cell growth, including oxygen, are reduced. Under low-oxygen conditions, many cells,

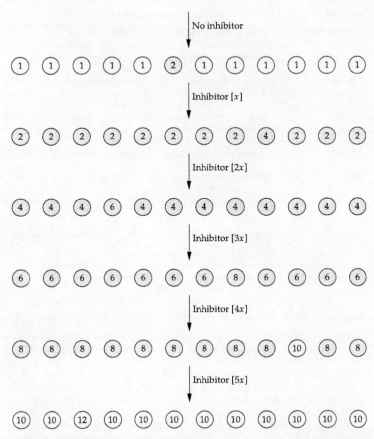

FIGURE 7.29 Schematic representation of the process of selecting for an increased copy number of a gene in cultured cells. As the concentration of an inhibitor of a vital enzyme ($[x]$) is increased, cells with extra copies of the gene that encodes this enzyme survive. The increments of the gene copy number occur by chance among thousands of cells. The circles indicate cells; the numerals indicate numbers of gene copies.

including CHO cells, secrete the acidic waste product lactate as they struggle to obtain energy from glucose. Under these conditions, pyruvate, an intermediate compound produced during the metabolism of glucose, is converted to lactate by lactate dehydrogenase rather than entering into the tricarboxylic acid cycle, where it is further oxidized through the activity of pyruvate carboxylase (Fig. 7.31). Pyruvate carboxylase has a lower level of activity in the absence of oxygen. To counteract the acidification of the medium from lactate secretion, alkaline compounds are typically added; however, they also contribute to reduced cell growth by increasing the osmolality of the medium. A more effective approach may be to either decrease the expression of lactate dehydrogenase or increase the expression

FIGURE 7.30 Strategy to increase yields of recombinant mammalian cells. Cell death (apoptosis), stimulated by the transcription factor p53, can lead to decreased yields of recombinant mammalian cells grown under stressful conditions in large bioreactors. To prevent cell death, the gene encoding MDM2 is introduced into mammalian cells. The MDM2 protein binds to p53 and prevents it from inducing expression of proteins required for apoptosis. Engineered cells not only showed delayed cell death, but also achieved higher cell densities in bioreactors.

and/or the activity of pyruvate carboxylase in host cells. The human pyruvate decarboxylase gene was cloned into an expression vector under the control of the CMV promoter and the SV40 polyadenylation signals and transfected into CHO cells. Under selective conditions, the pyruvate carboxylase gene was stably integrated into the CHO genome and expressed, and the enzyme was detected in the mitochondria, where glucose is degraded. After 7 days in culture, 85% of the CHO cells without the human pyruvate carboxylase gene were viable. In contrast, 96% of the cells that expressed human pyruvate carboxylase were still viable. The rate of lactate production decreased by up to 40% in the engineered cells.

Many of the eukaryotic DNA viruses from which the vectors used in mammalian cells are derived maintain their genomes as multicopy episomal DNA (plasmids) in the host cell nucleus. These viruses produce proteins, such as the large-T antigen in SV40 and the nuclear antigen 1 protein in Epstein-Barr virus, that help to maintain the plasmids in the host nucleus and to ensure that each host cell produced after cell division receives a copy of the plasmid. To increase the copy number of the target gene by increasing the plasmid copy number, HEK 293 cells and other cell lines have been engineered to express the SV40 large-T antigen or Epstein-Barr nuclear antigen 1.

Many heterologous proteins of therapeutic value, such as antibodies and interferon, are secreted. However, the high levels of these proteins that are desirable from a commercial standpoint can quickly overwhelm the capacity of the cell secretory system. Thus, protein processing is a major limiting step in the achievement of high target protein yields. Although high levels of recombinant protein production have been found to increase

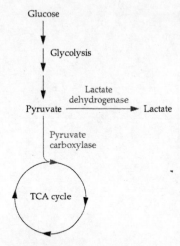

FIGURE 7.31 When oxygen is present, pyruvate, which is formed from glucose during glycolysis, is converted by the enzyme pyruvate carboxylase to an intermediate compound in the tricarboxylic acid (TCA) cycle. This metabolic pathway is important for the generation of cellular energy and for the synthesis of biomolecules required for cell proliferation. However, under low-oxygen conditions, such as those found in large bioreactors, pyruvate carboxylase has a low level of activity. Under these conditions, lactate dehydrogenase converts pyruvate into lactate, which yields a lower level of energy. Cultured cells secrete lactate, thereby acidifying the medium.

the levels of proteins associated with proper protein folding and secretion in the endoplasmic reticulum, the levels are usually not sufficient for optimal protein processing. Researchers have therefore devised methods to increase the capacity for protein secretion by engineering cell lines with enhanced production of components of the secretion apparatus. Although this can be achieved in yeast and insects by transforming host cells with additional copies of the endoplasmic reticulum chaperone proteins BiP and protein disulfide isomerase (described above), they are not very effective in mammalian host cells, possibly because these engineered cell lines overexpress only a single component of the secretion pathway. A more effective strategy may be to simultaneously overexpress several, if not all, of the proteins that make up the secretory mechanism. Simultaneous upregulation of the genes encoding these proteins can be achieved through the enhanced production of the transcription factor X box protein 1 (Xbp-1), a key regulator of the secretory pathway. Normally, full-length, unspliced *xbp-1* mRNA is found in nonstressed cells and is not translated into a stable, functional protein (Fig. 7.32A). However, when unfolded or misfolded proteins accumulate in the endoplasmic reticulum, a ribonuclease is activated that specifically cleaves *xbp-1* mRNA (Fig. 7.32B). This results in the production of a functional transcription factor that activates the expression of a number of proteins of the secretion apparatus. A truncated *xbp-1* gene that encodes an actively translated form of *xbp-1* mRNA (Fig. 7.32C) was overexpressed under the control of the CMV promoter in recombinant CHO cell lines that were previously constructed to express human erythropoietin, human γ-interferon, and human monoclonal antibodies either stably or transiently. Expression of the genes encoding proteins of the secretion apparatus that are controlled by Xbp-1 was found to increase in response to elevated levels of Xbp-1. Although overexpression of Xbp-1 did not increase the production of recombinant proteins in stable cell lines, a significant increase was observed in cell lines engineered to express the target proteins transiently.

Plasmid Integration and Chromosomal Environment

A major consideration for high levels and long-term stability of heterologous-protein production is the site of integration of the gene of interest into the mammalian cell chromosome. Expression of high levels of protein from plasmid vectors is transient and inevitably results in loss of the vector, which cannot be propagated in mammalian cells, or death of the host cell. Stable cell lines in which the target gene is integrated into the chromosome have been generated to overcome this problem. However, the site of integration can have a significant impact on the levels of target protein produced. Genomic DNA is associated with a great number of proteins, including the major histone proteins, around which the DNA is coiled, that compact (condense) the DNA so that it can fit inside the nucleus. The DNA and associated packaging proteins are known as chromatin. While much of the genome is highly condensed (heterochromatin) and contains silent genes or genes with low levels of expression, other regions are less condensed (euchromatin) and contain actively transcribed genes. For enhanced expression and stability, the target gene should be integrated into euchromatin, rather than heterochromatin. Because a larger portion of the genome is in the heterochromatin form, there is a greater chance that the target gene

A Unstressed cells **B** Stressed cells **C** Engineered cells

xbp-1 DNA

xbp-1 RNA

xbp-1 mRNA

Active Xbp-1 transcription
factor not produced

Production of
functional Xbp-1
transcription factor

Overproduction of
functional Xbp-1
transcription factor

Expression of
chaperones and other
proteins of the
secretion apparatus

Overexpression of
chaperones and other
proteins of the
secretion apparatus

FIGURE 7.32 Strategy to increase yields of secreted recombinant proteins from mammalian cells by simultaneously upregulating the expression of several proteins in the secretion apparatus. The expression of chaperones and other proteins of the secretion apparatus is controlled by the transcription factor Xbp-1. **(A)** In unstressed cells, the intron (green box) is not cleaved from the *xbp-1* transcript, and therefore, functional Xbp-1 transcription factor is not produced. **(B)** However, in stressed cells that have accumulated misfolded proteins, an endoribonuclease cleaves the transcript to yield mature *xbp-1* mRNA (the red and blue boxes represent exons) that is translated into a stable, functional transcription factor. **(C)** Recombinant CHO cells were transfected with a truncated gene including only the *xbp-1* exons and overproduced a functional Xbp-1 transcription factor that directed the production of high levels of proteins required for protein secretion.

will be inserted into one of these regions. Therefore, genetic engineering strategies to prevent the surrounding DNA from decreasing transcription of inserted genes are being explored.

These strategies exploit natural cellular processes (known as epigenetic modifications) that contribute to the dynamic state of chromatin. Chromatin structure, that is, the degree of DNA packing, is altered in two general ways. Histone proteins are modified by addition of chemical groups, such as an acetyl group, to specific amino acids, and cytosines at specific sites in the chromosomal DNA can be methylated. Techniques to relax chromatin structure and thereby increase the expression of introduced genes include modifying host strains to express proteins that alter chromatin structure at the site of vector integration or inserting DNA elements that prevent chromosome condensation together with the target gene.

One approach to alter the epigenetic environment surrounding the inserted gene is to increase histone acetylation. The extent of histone acetylation is determined by the relative activities of two host cell enzymes,

histone acetyltransferase, which adds acetyl groups to lysine residues on histone proteins, and histone deacetylase, which removes acetyl groups from the histone. The relative influences of these two enzymes at a given promoter are determined by specific transcription factors that recruit one or the other of the enzymes to the promoter. Increased histone acetylation, which leads to increased gene transcription, can be accomplished either by increasing the expression of histone acetyltransferase or by decreasing the activity of histone deacetylase. Although chemical inhibitors of histone deacetylation, such as butyrate, are often added to the culture medium, they have a broad, genomewide effect on cellular histones and may inhibit cell growth and stimulate apoptosis. A better strategy is to target histone acetyltransferase specifically to the site of target gene insertion to ensure that the target gene is actively and continuously transcribed. One group of researchers created a stable CHO cell line in which histone acetyltransferase was produced as a fusion protein with the LexA protein that binds to specific DNA sequences (Fig. 7.33). To test this fusion protein for the ability to specifically increase expression of integrated target genes, the green fluorescent protein (GFP) reporter gene was employed as a target gene and was integrated into a CHO chromosome under the control of the CMV promoter with the LexA-binding sequence inserted upstream. A gene encoding resistance to the antibiotic Zeocin (a member of the bleomycin/phleomycin family of antibiotics) was coupled to the reporter gene by an IRES element and therefore was also under the control of the CMV promoter. Stable cells with an active CMV promoter were established by addition of Zeocin to the culture medium. Production of GFP, determined by measuring the emission of green fluorescence in a spectrophotometer, was severalfold higher in cells that expressed the LexA–histone acetyltransferase fusion protein than in those that expressed the LexA protein alone (Fig. 7.33A). The LexA protein specifically binds to the LexA recognition site upstream of the gene encoding GFP and brings with it the fused histone acetyltransferase protein that acetylates histones in the promoter region and promotes a higher level of GFP transcription. Moreover, expression remained stable, although at a lower level, for at least 4 months in some of the clones.

To improve expression levels over a longer period, the construct was further modified to include a DNA segment known as a stabilizing and antirepressor (STAR) element on both sides of the expression cassette to block repression (Fig. 7.33B). Repression can occur when heterochromatin forms due to the association of the heterochromatin protein HP1 with methylated histones. This stimulates further histone deacetylation and methylation and, consequently, greater HP1 activity. Insertion of the relatively small (<2-kb) STAR elements was found to counteract the activity of HP1 and other heterochromatin-associated repressor proteins. Flanking the expression cassette with the antirepressor elements resulted in higher levels of GFP expression that were maintained over a longer period of time.

Other DNA elements that improve heterologous-protein expression by modifying heterochromatin structure are the ubiquitous chromatin-opening elements and matrix-associated regions. Ubiquitous chromatin-opening elements are sequences of DNA normally found near the

A

B

FIGURE 7.33 Strategies to increase expression of recombinant proteins in mammalian cells by altering chromatin structure. Local "relaxation" of chromosome condensation, which leads to increased transcription of genes in the region, can be achieved by the addition of an acetyl group to DNA-packing proteins known as histones. Histone acetylation is catalyzed by the enzyme histone acetyltransferase (HAT). **(A)** To increase the expression of a recombinant protein, HAT was directed to the site of target gene (GFP gene) insertion in a mammalian chromosome. HAT was expressed as a fusion protein with the LexA protein that binds to a specific DNA sequence (LexA-BS) inserted upstream of the CMV promoter (P_{CMV}) that directs expression of GFP. Production of the HAT-LexA fusion protein under the control of the SV40 promoter (P_{SV40}) increased expression of GFP sixfold compared to production of the LexA protein alone. **(B)** Insertion of STAR elements on both sides of the expression cassette further increased GFP expression. The gene encoding resistance to the antibiotic Zeocin was included as a selectable marker and was expressed from an IRES. The arrows above the promoter boxes indicate the direction of transcription.

promoters of housekeeping genes that are constitutively expressed at high levels due to enhanced histone acetylation. Inclusion of the ubiquitous chromatin-opening element from the promoter of the highly expressed CHO elongation factor 1 alpha gene in an expression vector increased recombinant protein expression in CHO cells 6- to 35-fold. Matrix-associated regions were also found to enhance the production of heterologous protein in CHO cells. These elements, found in the chromosomes of many eukaryotes, bind to protein complexes in the nucleus that arrange regions of the chromosome into loops. It is thought that these DNA loops contain transcriptionally active genes that are regulated in a coordinated fashion. Although matrix-associated regions from the human β-globin gene and the chicken lysozyme gene were found to increase expression of

a target gene, not all matrix-associated regions have a positive effect on gene expression.

In sum, mammalian cell expression systems are as versatile and effective as other eukaryotic expression systems. However, industrial production of a recombinant protein with engineered mammalian cells is costly. Consequently, less expensive expression systems are favored unless authenticity of an important recombinant protein can be obtained only with mammalian cells.

SUMMARY

A number of heterologous proteins have been successfully synthesized in prokaryotic host cells. However, many proteins require eukaryote-specific posttranslational modifications, such as glycosylation, to be functional. Consequently, expression systems were devised for fungal, insect, and mammalian cells. With respect to the ease and likelihood of obtaining an authentic protein from a cloned gene, each of these systems has distinct merits and shortcomings. In other words, there is no single eukaryotic host cell that is capable of producing an authentic protein from every cloned gene.

All eukaryotic expression vectors have the same basic format. The gene of interest, which may be equipped with sequences that facilitate the secretion and purification of the heterologous protein, is under the control of eukaryotic promoter and polyadenylation and transcription terminator sequences. To simplify both maintenance and recombinant DNA manipulations, eukaryotic expression vectors are routinely maintained in E. coli.

Several different fungus-based expression systems have been developed for the production of heterologous proteins. The yeast S. cerevisiae, which is well characterized genetically and can be grown in large fermenters, has been used extensively for this purpose. Both episomal and integrating expression vectors have been constructed. However, with S. cerevisiae as the host cell, a number of recombinant proteins are hyperglycosylated, and in some cases, protein yields are low because the capacity of the cell to properly fold and secrete proteins has been exceeded. Other yeast and filamentous fungal systems have been developed for the production of heterologous proteins. Of these, the methylotrophic yeast P. pastoris has been used successfully because of the low occurrence of hyperglycosylation, the ease of obtaining high cell densities, and the rapid and strong response of the AOX1 promoter (usually used to drive the gene of interest) to methanol. A "humanized" strain of P. pastoris has been genetically altered to produce glycoproteins with glycosylation patterns that are identical to those found on the same proteins produced in human cells.

A large number of biologically active heterologous proteins have also been produced in insect cells grown in culture using baculoviruses to deliver the gene of interest into the insect host cell. This system is advantageous because posttranslational protein modification is similar in insects and mammals, and the baculoviruses used in these systems do not infect humans or other insect cells. The baculovirus most commonly used as a vector is AcMNPV. A gene of interest is inserted into the AcMNPV genome by homologous or site-specific recombination between sequences on a transfer vector carrying the target gene and the AcMNPV DNA. Recombination occurs either in insect cells doubly transfected with the transfer vector and viral DNA, in E. coli as an intermediate host, or in an in vitro reaction catalyzed by purified integration enzymes. The last two methods eliminate the need to identify and purify recombinant baculoviruses using plaque assays. Once the target gene has been inserted, recombinant AcMNPV DNA is introduced into insect cells for heterologous-protein production. Improved insect host cells have been developed through genetic engineering to increase protein yields and to ensure that target proteins are properly glycosylated. In addition to production of a single protein of interest, the baculovirus–insect expression system is particularly amenable to producing functional multimeric protein complexes, such as virus-like particles, which are effective vaccines.

Many therapeutic proteins that require a full complement of posttranslational modifications are now produced in cultured mammalian cells, such as CHO cells. Most of the vectors that have been developed to introduce foreign genes into mammalian cells are based on mammalian viruses, especially SV40. The viral genome has been altered to remove some viral genes required for replication and viral-protein production and to include suitable mammalian transcription and translation signals to drive expression of the cloned gene. Baculoviruses have also been used to deliver target genes into mammalian cells, although expression of the target gene is usually transient, unless the gene is integrated into the host cell genome to generate a stable cell line. Expression of integrated target genes can be increased by altering the epigenetic state of the insertion site through histone acetylation or insertion of chromatin-relaxing DNA elements. A major challenge for production of high levels of heterologous proteins in mammalian cell lines is preventing cell death, which is often induced by the stressful conditions of large-scale bioreactors. Strategies to improve cell growth and protein yields

include genetically engineering host cells to block the transcription factor that induces apoptosis, to prevent accumulation of toxic metabolites in the culture medium, and to increase expression of proteins required for proper protein folding and secretion.

REFERENCES

Ansari, A., and V. C. Emery. 1998. Baculoviruses, p. 219–233. *In* R. Rabley and J. M. Walker (ed.), *Molecular Biomethods Handbook*. Humana Press Inc., Totowa, NJ.

Barnes, L. M., and A. J. Dickson. 2006. Mammalian cell factories for efficient and stable protein expression. *Curr. Opin. Biotechnol.* 17:381–386.

Berger, I., D. J. Fitzgerald, and T. J. Richmond. 2004. Baculovirus expression system for heterologous multiprotein complexes. *Nat. Biotechnol.* 22:1583–1587.

Bowman, K. K., J. Clark, L. Yu, K. Mortara, K. Radika, J. Wang, and H. Zhan. 2000. Expression, purification, and characterization of deglycosylated human pro-prostate-specific antigen. *Protein Expr. Purif.* 20:405–413.

Cole, E. S., K. Lee, K. Lauziere, C. Kelton, S. Chappel, B. Weintraub, D. Ferrara, P. Peterson, R. Bernasconi, T. Edmunds, S. Richards, L. Dickrell, J. M. Kleeman, J. H. McPherson, and B. M. Pratt. 1993. Recombinant human thyroid stimulating hormone: development of a biotechnology product for detection of metastatic lesions of thyroid carcinoma. *Bio/Technology* 11:1014–1024.

Condreay, J. P., and T. A. Kost. 2007. Baculovirus vectors for insect and mammalian cells. *Curr. Drug Targets* 8:1126–1131.

Cox, M. M. 2008. Progress on baculovirus-derived influenza vaccines. *Curr. Opin. Mol. Ther.* 10:56–61.

Cregg, J. M. 1999. Expression in the methylotrophic yeast *Pichia pastoris*, p. 157–191. *In* J. Fernandez and J. P. Hoeffler (ed.), *Gene Expression Systems: Using Nature for the Art of Expression*. Academic Press, Inc., San Diego, CA.

Figler, R. A., H. Omote, R. K. Nakamoto, and M. K. Al-Shawi. 2000. Use of chemical chaperones in the yeast *Saccharomyces cerevisiae* to enhance heterologous membrane protein expression: high-yield expression and purification of human P-glycoprotein. *Arch. Biochem. Biophys.* 376:34–46.

Gasser, B., M. Saloheimo, U. Rinas, M. Dragosits, E. Rodríguez-Carmona, K. Baumann, M. Giuliani, E. Parrilli, P. Branduardi, C. Lang, D. Porro, P. Ferrer, M. L. Tutino, D. Mattanovich, and A. Villaverde. 2008. Protein folding and conformational stress in microbial cells producing recombinant proteins: a host comparative overview. *Microb. Cell Fact.* 7:11–29.

Gellissen, G., G. Kunze, C. Gaillardin, J. M. Cregg, E. Berardi, M. Veenhuis, and E. van der Klei. 2005. New yeast expression platforms based on methylotrophic *Hansenula polymorpha* and *Pichia pastoris* and on dimorphic *Arxula adeninivorans* and *Yarrowia lipolytica*—a comparison. *FEMS Yeast Res.* 5:1079–1096.

Gurtu, V., G. Yan, and G. Zhang. 1996. IRES bicistronic expression vectors for efficient creation of stable mammalian cell lines. *Biochem. Biophys. Res. Commun.* 229:295–298.

Hallewell, R. A., R. Mills, P. Tekamp-Olson, R. Blacher, S. Rosenberg, F. Otting, F. R. Masiarz, and C. J. Scandella. 1987. Amino terminal acetylation of authentic human Cu,Zn superoxide dismutase produced in yeast. *Bio/Technology* 5:363–366.

Hamilton, S. R., and T. U. Gerngross. 2007. Glycosylation engineering in yeast: the advent of fully humanized yeast. *Curr. Opin. Biotechnol.* 18:387–392.

Jarvis, D. L. 2003. Developing baculovirus-insect cell expression systems for humanized recombinant glycoprotein production. *Virology* 310:1–7.

Karnaukhova, E., Y. Ophir, L. Trinh, N. Dalal, P. J. Punt, B. Golding, and J. Shiloach. 2007. Expression of human α_1-protease inhibitor in *Aspergillus niger. Microb. Cell Fact.* 6:34–44.

Kim, M.-D., S.-K. Rhee, and J.-H. Seo. 2001. Enhanced production of anticoagulant hirudin in recombinant *Saccharomyces cerevisiae* by chromosomal δ-integration. *J. Biotechnol.* 85:41–48.

Kitts, P. A., and R. D. Possee. 1993. A method for producing recombinant baculovirus expression vectors at high frequency. *BioTechniques* 14:810–817.

Kjeldsen, T., M. Hach, P. Balschmidt, S. Havelund, A. F. Pettersson, and J. Markussen. 1998. Prepro-leaders lacking N-linked glycosylation for secretory expression in the yeast *Saccharomyces cerevisiae. Protein Expr. Purif.* 14:309–316.

Kjeldsen, T., A. F. Pettersson, and M. Hach. 1999. Secretory expression and characterization of insulin in *Pichia pastoris. Biotechnol. Appl. Biochem.* 29:79–86.

Kost, T. A., J. P. Condreay, and D. L. Jarvis. 2005. Baculovirus as versatile vectors for protein expression in insect and mammalian cells. *Nat. Biotechnol.* 23:567–575.

Kwaks, T. H. J., and A. P. Otte. 2006. Employing epigenetics to augment the expression of therapeutic proteins in mammalian cells. *Trends Biotechnol.* 24:137–142.

Kwaks, T. H. J., R. G. A. B. Sewalt, R. van Blokland, T. J. Siersma, M. Kasiem, A. Kelder, and A. P. Otte. 2005. Targeting of a histone acetyltransferase domain to a promoter enhances protein expression levels in mammalian cells. *J. Biotechnol.* 115:35–46.

Leahy, D. J., C. E. Dann III, P. Longo, B. Perman, and K. X. Ramyar. 2000. A mammalian expression vector for

expression and purification of secreted proteins for structural studies. *Protein Expr. Purif.* **20**:500–506.

Liang, M., S. Dübel, D. Li, I. Queitsch, W. Li, and E. K. Bautz. 2001. Baculovirus expression cassette vectors for rapid production of complete human IgG from phage display selected antibody fragments. *J. Immunol. Methods* **247**:119–130.

Liu, X., S. N. Constantinescu, Y. Sun, J. S. Bogan, D. Hirsch, R. A. Weinberg, and H. F. Lodish. 2000. Generation of mammalian cells stably expressing multiple genes at predetermined levels. *Anal. Biochem.* **280**:20–28.

Lucas, B. K., L. M. Giere, R. A. DeMarco, A. Shen, V. Chisholm, and C. W. Crowley. 1996. High-level production of recombinant proteins in CHO cells using a dicistronic DHFR intron expression vector. *Nucleic Acids Res.* **24**:1774–1779.

Lucknow, V. A., S. C. Lee, G. F. Barry, and P. O. Olins. 1993. Efficient generation of infectious recombinant baculoviruses by site-specific transposon-mediated insertion of foreign genes into a baculovirus genome propagated in *Escherichia coli. J. Virol.* **67**:4566–4579.

Makrides, S. C. 1999. Components of vectors for gene transfer and expression in mammalian cells. *Protein Expr. Purif.* **17**:183–202.

Malissard, M., S. Zeng, and E. G. Berger. 1999. The yeast expression system for recombinant glycosyltransferases. *Glycoconj. J.* **16**:125–139.

Mayer, A. F., K. Hellmuth, H. Schlieker, R. Lopez-Ulibarri, S. Oertel, U. Dahlems, A. W. Strasser, and A. P. van Loon. 1999. An expression system matures: a highly efficient and cost-effective process for phytase production by recombinant strains of *Hansenula polymorpha. Biotechnol. Bioeng.* **63**:373–381.

Mielke, C., M. Tümmler, D. Schübeler, I. von Hoegen, and H. Hauser. 2000. Stabilized, long-term expression of heterodimeric proteins from tricistronic mRNA. *Gene* **254**:1–8.

Peng, S., M. Sommerfelt, J. Logan, Z. Huang, T. Jilling, K. Kirk, E. Hunter, and E. Sorscher. 1993. One-step affinity isolation of recombinant protein using the baculovirus/insect cell expression system. *Protein Expr. Purif.* **4**:95–100.

PharMingen. 1999. *Baculovirus Expression Vector System Manual,* 6th ed. PharMingen, San Diego, CA.

Punt, P. J., N. van Biezen, A. Conesa, A. Albers, J. Mangnus, and C. van den Hondel. 2002. Filamentous fungi as cell factories for heterologous protein production. *Trends Biotechnol.* **20**:200–206.

Robinson, A. S., V. Hines, and K. D. Wittrup. 1994. Protein disulfide isomerase overexpression increases secretion of foreign proteins in *Saccharomyces cerevisiae. Bio/Technology* **12**:381–384.

Roy, P., M. Mikhailov, and D. H. Bishop. 1997. Baculovirus multigene expression vectors and their use for understanding the assembly process of architecturally complex virus particles. *Gene* **190**:119–129.

Schröder, M. 2008. Engineering eukaryotic protein factories. *Biotechnol. Lett.* **30**:187–196.

Shi, X., and D. L. Jarvis. 2007. Protein N-glycosylation in the baculovirus-insect cell system. *Curr. Drug Targets* **8**:1116–1125.

Steinborn, G., T. Wartmann, G. Gellissen, and G. Kunze. 2007. Construction of an *Arxula adeninivorans* host-vector system based on *trp1* complementation. *J. Biotechnol.* **127**:392–401.

Steinborn, G., G. Gellissen, and G. Kunze. 2007. A novel vector element providing multicopy vector integration in *Arxula adeninivorans. FEMS Yeast Res.* **7**:1197–1205.

Takahashi, K., T. Yuuki, T. Takai, C. Ra, K. Okumura, T. Yokota, and Y. Okumura. 2000. Production of humanized Fab fragment against human high affinity IgE receptor in *Pichia pastoris. Biosci. Biotechnol. Biochem.* **64**:2138–2144.

Whittaker, M. M., and J. W. Whittaker. 2000. Expression of recombinant galactose oxidase by *Pichia pastoris. Protein Expr. Purif.* **20**:105–111.

Wolff, A. M., O. C. Hansen, U. Poulsen, S. Madrid, and P. Stougaard. 2001. Optimization of the production of *Chondrus crispus* hexose oxidase in *Pichia pastoris. Protein Expr. Purif.* **22**:189–199.

REVIEW QUESTIONS

1. What are the major posttranslational modifications of eukaryotic proteins in the endoplasmic reticulum and Golgi apparatus?

2. In general, how do N glycosylation patterns differ among yeast, insects, and mammalian proteins?

3. Describe the features of a eukaryotic expression vector.

4. What are the advantages and disadvantages of the different classes of yeast vectors for producing a biotechnology product?

5. Describe some of the strategies that have been used to increase proper folding and secretion of recombinant proteins from yeast cells.

6. Discuss the salient features of a *P. pastoris* high-expression integrating vector system. How has *P. pastoris* been "humanized"?

7. What are baculoviruses? Describe the strategy of the original baculovirus expression system and how this protocol has been enhanced.

8. Describe two strategies that can be used to insert a target gene into the baculovirus genome that do not require transfection of insect cells.

9. Describe the main features of an extrachromosomal mammalian-cell expression vector.

10. Describe at least two selectable marker systems that are used with mammalian expression vectors.

11. How does a stable mammalian cell line differ from a transient cell line? Describe one way in which a stable cell line can be generated.

12. Why are yields of recombinant proteins produced by mammalian cells in large bioreactors generally low? How can yields be improved?

13. What is chromatin, and how does it affect gene expression? Describe some of the strategies that have been developed to increase expression levels of a target gene that is integrated into a chromosome.

14. What criteria are used to decide if a particular recombinant protein should be produced in a yeast, insect, or mammalian cell system?

Directed Mutagenesis and Protein Engineering

I T IS POSSIBLE WITH RECOMBINANT DNA TECHNOLOGY to isolate the gene (or complementary DNA [cDNA]) for any protein that exists in nature, to express it in a specific host organism, and to produce a purified product that can be used commercially. However, the physical and chemical properties of these "naturally occurring" proteins are often not well suited to an industrial application. In some instances, a protein that is better suited to a particular task may be obtained by using a gene from an organism that grows in an unusual, often extreme, environment. For example, when an enzyme, such as α-amylase, was required to function at a high temperature, the gene for that enzyme was isolated from *Bacillus stearothermophilus*, an organism whose natural niche is a 90°C hot spring. In this case, the cloned gene produced α-amylase that was stable at the high temperatures used in the industrial production of alcohol from starch. In addition to isolating natural genes that encode proteins with useful properties, conventional mutagenesis and selection schemes can be used in an attempt to create and perpetuate a mutant form of a gene that encodes a protein with the desired properties. However, the number of mutant proteins (each with a different amino acid change) that are possible after the alteration of individual nucleotides within a structural gene by conventional mutagenesis is extremely large. In practice, the mutagenesis–selection strategy rarely results in any significant beneficial changes to the targeted protein because most amino acid changes decrease the activity of an enzyme.

By using a set of techniques that change specific amino acids encoded by a cloned gene, proteins with properties that are better suited than those of naturally occurring counterparts can be created for therapeutic and industrial applications. Such "directed evolution" of genes encoding proteins of interest has emerged as a key technology to generate proteins with new and improved properties. For example:

- By altering both the Michaelis constant (K_m), which reflects the "tightness" of substrate binding to the enzyme, and the maximal rate of conversion of the substrate into product under defined conditions (V_{max}) for an enzyme-catalyzed reaction to improve the overall

catalytic efficiency (V_{max}/K_m) of the reaction, where V_{max} equals the total amount of enzyme present (E_0) times the catalytic rate constant (k_{cat})

- By changing the thermal tolerance, pH stability, or both of a protein, enabling the altered protein to be used under conditions that would inactivate the native version
- By modifying the reactivity of an enzyme in nonaqueous solvents so that chemical reactions can be catalyzed under nonphysiological conditions
- By changing an enzyme so that a cofactor is no longer required for certain continuous industrial production processes in which the cofactor must be supplied on a regular basis
- By modifying the substrate-binding site of an enzyme to increase its specificity, thereby decreasing the extent of undesirable side reactions
- By increasing the resistance of a protein to cellular proteases, which simplifies purification and increases the recoverable yield
- By altering the allosteric regulation of an enzyme to diminish the impact of metabolite feedback inhibition and increase the product yield

Directed Mutagenesis Procedures

It is not a simple matter to produce a new protein with specified predetermined properties. However, it is quite feasible to modify the existing properties of known proteins. Theoretically, these changes can be carried out at either the protein or the gene level. However, chemical modifications of proteins generally are harsh, nonspecific, and required repeatedly, for each batch of protein, so it is preferable to manipulate the DNA sequence of a cloned gene to create an altered protein with novel properties. Unfortunately, it is not always possible to know in advance which individual amino acids or short sequences of amino acids contribute to a particular physical, kinetic, or chemical property. For example, a particular property of a protein may be the consequence of two or more amino acid residues that are far apart from each other in the linear sequence but are juxtaposed as a result of the folding of the protein. In this case, two or more amino acid residues may have to be changed to produce a protein with the desired properties. In the not too distant future, computer programs may be able to make accurate predictions of protein function on the basis of deduced amino acid sequences, thereby simplifying the task of producing a protein with specific predetermined properties. At present, although it is relatively straightforward to introduce new coding information into cloned genes, large numbers of novel proteins must often be assayed to determine whether a particular property has been created.

The process for generating amino acid coding changes at the DNA level is called directed mutagenesis. Determining which amino acids of a protein should be changed to attain a specific property is much easier if the three-dimensional structure of the protein, or a similar protein, has been well characterized by X-ray crystallographic analysis and other analytical procedures. However, for many proteins, such detailed information is often lacking, so directed mutagenesis becomes a trial-and-error strategy in which changes are made to those nucleotides that are most likely to yield a

particular change in a protein property. Then, of course, the protein encoded by each mutated gene has to be tested to ascertain whether the mutagenesis process has indeed generated the desired change.

A large number of experimental approaches have been devised for the directed mutagenesis of cloned genes. Some of the methods are designed to mutate, delete, or add specific nucleotides of a cloned gene. Others introduce mutations randomly over a short segment of the cloned gene, thereby creating a panel of mutated proteins among which one or more may have the desired activity.

Oligonucleotide-Directed Mutagenesis with M13 DNA

Oligonucleotide-directed mutagenesis (site-specific mutagenesis) is a straightforward method for producing defined point mutations in a cloned gene (Fig. 8.1). For this procedure, the investigator must know (1) the precise nucleotide sequence in the region of DNA that encodes the messenger RNA (mRNA) codon that is to be changed and (2) the amino acid changes that are being introduced. In an early version of this method, the cloned gene was inserted into the double-stranded form of an M13 bacteriophage vector. The single-stranded form (M13 plus-strand) of the recombinant vector was isolated and mixed with a synthetic oligonucleotide. The oligonucleotide had, except for 1 nucleotide, the sequence exactly complementary to a segment of the cloned gene. The nucleotide difference (i.e., mismatch) coincided precisely with the nucleotide of the mRNA codon that was targeted for change. In Fig. 8.1, the sequence ATT, which encodes the isoleucine codon, AUU, is to be changed to CTT, which encodes the leucine codon, CUU. The oligonucleotide hybridizes to the complementary region of the cloned gene if it is added in an amount much in excess of that of the M13 DNA, if the mismatch is near the middle of the oligonucleotide, and if the mixing is done at a low temperature in the presence of a high concentration of salt. The 3' end of the hybridized oligonucleotide acts as a primer site for the initiation of DNA synthesis that uses the intact M13 strand as the template. The replication, which uses the four deoxyribonucleoside triphosphates, is catalyzed by the Klenow fragment of *Escherichia coli* DNA polymerase I. T4 DNA ligase is added to ensure that the last nucleotide of the synthesized strand is joined to the 5' end of the primer. Since in vitro DNA synthesis is often incomplete, partially double-stranded M13 molecules must be removed from the mixture by sucrose gradient centrifugation.

Each complete double-stranded M13 molecule, now containing the mismatched nucleotide, is introduced into *E. coli* cells by transformation. The infected cells produce M13 virus particles, which eventually lyse the cells and form plaques. Theoretically, because plasmid DNA is replicated semiconservatively, half of the phage that are formed carry the wild-type sequence and the other half contain the mutated sequence that has the specified nucleotide change. Phage produced in the initial transformation step are propagated in *E. coli*, and particles that contain only the mutated gene are identified by DNA hybridization under highly stringent conditions. The original oligonucleotide containing the mismatched nucleotide is the probe in these hybridization experiments and will bind only to the mutated gene under these conditions. After the double-stranded form of M13 is isolated, the mutated gene is excised by digestion with restriction enzymes and then spliced onto an *E. coli* plasmid expression vector. For

FIGURE 8.1 Oligonucleotide-directed mutagenesis. Single-stranded bacteriophage M13 (M13 + strand), carrying a cloned gene, is annealed with a complementary synthetic oligonucleotide containing one mismatched base, i.e., one base that is not complementary to its counterpart in the target DNA. With the oligonucleotide as the primer, DNA synthesis is catalyzed by the Klenow fragment of *E. coli* DNA polymerase I; the cloned gene and the M13 vector are the templates. Synthesis continues until the entire strand is copied. The newly synthesized DNA strand is circularized by T4 DNA ligase. The ligation reaction mixture is used to transform *E. coli*. Both the target DNA with its original sequence and the mutated sequence are present in the progeny M13 phage. dNTPs, deoxynucleoside triphosphates.

further study, the altered protein is expressed in and purified from the *E. coli* cells.

In actuality, when oligonucleotide-directed mutagenesis is used, the expected 50% of the M13 viruses carrying the mutated form of the target gene are not recovered. Rather, for a variety of technical reasons, only around 1% of the plaques actually contain phage carrying the mutated gene. Consequently, the oligonucleotide-directed mutagenesis method has been modified in several ways to enrich for the number of mutant

phage plaques that can be obtained. For example, one approach is to introduce the M13 viral vector carrying the gene that is to be mutagenized into an *E. coli* strain that has two defective enzymes of DNA metabolism (Fig. 8.2). One enzyme is a defective form of dUTPase *(dut)*. Cells without a functional dUTPase have an elevated intracellular level of

FIGURE 8.2 Enrichment of mutated M13 by passage of the parental DNA through a *dut ung* strain of *E. coli*. The target DNA is cloned into the double-stranded replicative form of bacteriophage M13, which is then used to transform a *dut ung* strain of *E. coli*. The *dut* mutation causes the intracellular level of dUTP to be elevated; the high level of nucleotide leads to the incorporation of a few dUTP residues (U). The *ung* mutation prevents the removal of any incorporated uracil residues. Following in vitro oligonucleotide-directed mutagenesis, the double-stranded M13 vector with the mutated DNA is introduced into wild-type *E. coli*. The wild-type *ung* gene product (uracil N-glycosylase) removes any uracil residues from the parental strand, so a significant portion of the parental strand is degraded. The mutated strand remains intact because it does not contain uracil. It serves as a template for DNA replication, thereby enriching the yield of M13 bacteriophage carrying the mutated gene.

dUTP, which in turn causes a few dUTP residues to be incorporated into DNA during replication instead of dTTP. The other enzyme is a defective uracil N-glycosylase *(ung)*. In the absence of functional uracil N-glycosylase, the dUTP residues that were spuriously incorporated into DNA cannot be removed. The single-stranded M13 DNA that is produced by this *E. coli* strain has approximately 1% of its thymidines replaced by uridines. A mismatched oligonucleotide primer is hybridized to this substitution-containing M13 DNA, and the second strand of M13 is prepared by in vitro synthesis and ligation. The double-stranded bacteriophage DNA is next introduced into an *E. coli* strain that contains a functional *ung* gene. The active uracil N-glycosylase in the host cells then removes uridine residues from the transforming M13 DNA (Fig. 8.2). As a result, the original M13 template strand is degraded and only the mutated strand, which contains no dUTP, is replicated. In this way, the yield of M13 bacteriophage carrying a gene with a site-specific mutation is significantly increased.

Oligonucleotide-Directed Mutagenesis with Plasmid DNA

The major drawback to bacteriophage M13 oligonucleotide-directed mutagenesis is the large number of time-consuming steps that need to be performed before the mutated form of the target gene is eventually isolated. As an alternative to the M13 system, a number of protocols that allow oligonucleotide-directed mutagenesis to be performed with plasmid rather than M13 DNA have been developed. With this approach, the need to subclone a target gene from a plasmid into M13 and then, after mutagenesis, clone it back into a plasmid is avoided. In one of the plasmid-based mutagenesis protocols, the target DNA is inserted into a multiple cloning site on a plasmid vector that contains a functional tetracycline resistance gene and a nonfunctional ampicillin resistance (Ampr) gene as the result of a single nucleotide substitution in the middle of the Ampr gene (Fig. 8.3). The vector carrying the target DNA is transformed into *E. coli* host cells to increase the amount of DNA through plasmid replication. Following growth of the transformed cells, the double-stranded plasmid DNA is extracted and then denatured by treatment with an alkaline solution to form single-stranded circular DNA molecules. Three different oligonucleotides that anneal to one of the single-stranded circular DNA molecules are added to the sample of denatured plasmid DNA. One oligonucleotide is designed specifically to alter the target DNA, another is designed to correct the substituted nucleotide in the nonfunctional ampicillin resistance gene, and the third is designed to change a single nucleotide in the tetracycline resistance gene so that the gene will become nonfunctional. The four deoxyribonucleoside triphosphates and T4 DNA polymerase, which has the same activity as the Klenow fragment of *E. coli* DNA polymerase I, are added to the reaction mixture, and the 3′ ends of the annealed oligonucleotides act as primers for DNA synthesis with the intact circular DNA molecule as the template. The nicks in the synthesized strand are sealed by T4 DNA ligase. After synthesis and ligation are complete, the reaction mixture is used to transform *E. coli* cells. Transformants are selected for ampicillin resistance and tetracycline sensitivity. With this procedure, about 90% of the selected transformants have the specified mutation in the target gene. In the remaining transformants, the target gene is unchanged because the oligonucleotide

FIGURE 8.3 Oligonucleotide-directed mutagenesis with plasmid DNA. The target DNA is inserted into the multiple cloning site (MCS) on the vector pALTER. Plasmid DNA isolated from *E. coli* cells is alkaline denatured before the mutagenic oligonucleotide, the ampicillin resistance (Amp^r) oligonucleotide, and the tetracycline sensitivity (Tet^s) oligonucleotide are annealed. The oligonucleotides act as primers for DNA synthesis by T4 DNA polymerase with the original strand as the template. The gaps between the synthesized pieces of DNA are sealed by T4 DNA ligase. The reaction mixture is used to transform *E. coli* host cells, and cells that are Amp^r and Tet^s are selected.

did not anneal to the target gene or it was bypassed during DNA synthesis. The cells with the specified mutation in the target gene are identified by DNA hybridization. All of the plasmids, host bacterial strains, enzymes, oligonucleotides (other than the one needed to alter the target gene), and buffers for this method are sold as a kit, facilitating its widespread use.

PCR-Amplified Oligonucleotide-Directed Mutagenesis

Researchers continually try to develop simpler and faster protocols. For site-specific mutagenesis, the polymerase chain reaction (PCR) can be exploited both to introduce the desired mutation and to enrich for the mutated gene. In fact, kits are often available to simplify the process; a researcher merely adds the target plasmid carrying the gene of interest and forward and reverse PCR primers that are typically 24 to 30 nucleotides in length, and following PCR, a high percentage of the plasmids produced will have the desired mutation. In this case, no special plasmid vectors are required; any plasmid up to approximately 10 kb in length is acceptable. For PCR-based mutagenesis point mutations, nucleotide changes are introduced in the middle of the primer sequence (Fig. 8.4). To create deletion mutations, primers must border the region of target DNA to be deleted on both sides and be perfectly matched to their annealing (or template) sequences. To create mutations with long insertions, a stretch of mismatched nucleotides is added to the 5′ end of one or both primers, while for mutations with short insertions, a stretch of nucleotides is designed in the middle of one of the primers. In all of these procedures, the only absolute requirements are that (1) the nucleotide sequence of the target DNA must be known and (2) the 5′ ends of the primers must be phosphorylated. Following PCR amplification, the linear DNA is circularized by ligation with T4 DNA ligase. The circularized plasmid DNA is then used to transform *E. coli* by any standard procedure. Since this protocol yields a very high frequency of plasmids with the desired mutation, it is not necessary to utilize any enrichment procedures. Rather, screening three or four clones by sequencing the target DNA should be sufficient to find the desired

FIGURE 8.4 Overview of the basic methodology to introduce point mutations, insertions, or deletions into DNA cloned into a plasmid. The forward and reverse primers are shown in red and green, respectively. The solid circles represent template DNA. The dotted lines represent newly synthesized DNA. The X indicates an altered nucleotide(s).

Point mutation Deletion mutation Large insertion mutation Small insertion mutation

mutation. In sum, this procedure introduces a specified mutation (point, insertion, or deletion) into a cloned gene without the need to insert the cloned gene into bacteriophage M13; to use enrichment procedures, such as the *dut ung* system; or to subclone the mutated gene from M13 onto an expression plasmid vector. Given its simplicity and effectiveness, this procedure has come to be widely used.

Error-Prone PCR

Some of the temperature-stable DNA polymerases that are used to amplify target DNA by PCR occasionally insert incorrect nucleotides into the replicating DNA. If one is attempting to amplify a DNA with high fidelity, this is obviously a problem. On the other hand, if the construction of a library of mutants of the target gene is the objective, then this approach is a very powerful method for random mutagenesis. Moreover, with DNA up to 10 kilobase pairs (kb) in size, it is possible to vary the number of alterations per gene from about 1 to about 20 by modifying the DNA template concentration (Fig. 8.5). When error-prone PCR is performed using *Taq* DNA polymerase, which lacks proofreading activity, the error rate may be increased by adding Mn^{2+}, by increasing the concentration of Mg^{2+}, and by adding unequal amounts of the four deoxynucleoside triphosphates to the reaction buffer. Alternatively, high error rates may be achieved with other temperature-stable DNA polymerases in the absence of Mn^{2+} and with balanced amounts of the four deoxynucleoside triphosphates. Following error-prone PCR, the randomly mutagenized DNA is cloned into expression vectors and screened for altered or improved protein activity. The DNA from those clones that encode the desired activity is isolated and sequenced so that the relevant changes to the target DNA may be elaborated. Error-prone PCR has been used to create enzymes with improved solvent and temperature stability and with enhanced specific activity.

Random Mutagenesis with Degenerate Oligonucleotide Primers

Unfortunately, investigators seldom know which specific nucleotide changes need to be introduced into a cloned gene to modify the properties of the target protein. Consequently, they must use methods that generate all the possible amino acid changes at one particular site. For example, oligonucleotide primers can be synthesized with any of the four nucleotides at defined positions. This pattern of sequence degeneracy is generally achieved by programming an automated DNA synthesis reaction to add a low level (usually a few percent) of each of the three alternative nucleotides each time a particular nucleotide is added to the chain (Fig. 8.6). In this way, the oligonucleotide primer preparation contains a heterogeneous set of DNA sequences that will generate a series of mutations that are clustered in a defined portion of the target gene.

This approach has two advantages. (1) Detailed information regarding the roles of particular amino acid residues in the functioning of the protein is not required. (2) Unexpected mutants encoding proteins with a range of interesting and useful properties may be generated because the introduced changes are not limited to one amino acid. Of course, should none of the mutants yield a protein with the properties that are being sought, then it

FIGURE 8.5 Error-prone PCR of a target gene yields a variety of mutated forms of the gene. Mutations are shown in blue. The horizontal arrows represent PCR primers.

FIGURE 8.6 Chemical synthesis of oligonucleotide primers with any of the four nucleotides at defined positions. In this case, the flask with G phosphoramidite consists of a mixture of nucleotides, such as 94% G, 2% A, 2% C, and 2% T, leading to a mixture of oligonucleotides that may have A, C, or T at the sites where G is the specified nucleotide.

may be necessary to repeat the entire procedure with a set of degenerate primers that is complementary to a different region of the gene.

In practice, partially degenerate oligonucleotides may be incorporated into a target gene by a variety of procedures. One strategy entails inserting a target gene into a plasmid between two unique restriction endonuclease sites and using PCR, in separate reactions, to amplify overlapping fragments (Fig. 8.7). The primer pair that is used to amplify the left fragment consists of mismatched oligonucleotides that were synthesized to contain degenerate oligonucleotides and that bind to the lower strand of the target DNA, along with a regular, completely complementary primer that hybridizes to a region of the upper strand that flanks the left unique restriction endonuclease site. For the right fragment, the PCR primers are the mismatched oligonucleotides that were synthesized to contain degenerate oligonucleotides and that bind to the upper strand of the target DNA, along with a primer that is complementary to a region of the lower strand that lies outside the second (right) unique restriction endonuclease site. After PCR amplification, the products are purified and combined. Denaturation and reannealing of the DNA in the mixture produce some DNA molecules that overlap in the target region. DNA polymerase is then used to form complete double-stranded DNA molecules. These molecules are amplified by PCR with a pair of primers that bind to opposite ends of the DNA molecule. The

FIGURE 8.7 Random mutagenesis of a target DNA by using degenerate oligonucle-otides and PCR. The left and right portions of the target DNA are amplified sepa-rately by PCR. The primer pairs are shown by horizontal arrows. A mutation-producing oligonucleotide is shown as a line with three spikes; each spike denotes a position that contains a nucleotide that is not found in the native gene. The amplified frag-ments are purified, denatured to make them single stranded, and then reannealed. Complementary regions of overlap are formed between complementary mutation-producing oligonucleotides. The single-stranded regions are made double stranded with DNA polymerase, and then the entire fragment is amplified by PCR. The resultant product is digested with restriction endonucleases A and B and then cloned into a vector that has been digested with the same enzymes.

amplified DNA is then treated with the two restriction enzymes for which there are unique sites at the ends of the fragment, and the DNA is then cloned into a suitable plasmid vector. This procedure results in the produc-tion of an altered gene that has mutated sites in the region of the overlap of the original oligonucleotides.

MILESTONE

Oligonucleotide-Directed Mutagenesis Using M13-Derived Vectors: an Efficient and General Procedure for the Production of Point Mutations in Any Fragment of DNA
M. J. ZOLLER and M. SMITH
Nucleic Acids Res. **10**:6487–6500, 1982

The technique of oligonucleotide-directed mutagenesis (site-specific mutagenesis) was developed mainly in the laboratory of Michael Smith as incremental changes to the technique of "marker rescue." In the marker rescue procedure, a mutation in a bacteriophage genomic DNA is corrected after the mutant DNA is annealed to a fragment of complementary wild-type DNA. Subsequently, it was demonstrated that a chemically synthesized oligonucleotide annealed to bacteriophage genomic DNA could produce a specific mutation. Unfortunately, these and other early procedures for oligonucleotide-directed mutagenesis required specialized skills and initially could be performed in only a few research laboratories. However, the procedure using bacteriophage M13 described by Zoller and Smith made it a relatively straightforward matter for thousands of laboratories throughout the world to specifically and rapidly alter the DNA sequence of any cloned gene. The key to the success of the protocol developed by Zoller and Smith lay in the use of *E. coli* bacteriophage M13. It was possible to clone foreign DNA into the double-stranded form of the virus, add an oligonucleotide with a specified change to the single-stranded form to produce a mutated DNA copy, and then recover the mutated double-stranded form in a relatively high yield. Since it was originally described, this procedure has been enhanced, simplified, and optimized and has been used by a large number of researchers to specifically modify thousands of different genes.

Random Insertion/Deletion Mutagenesis

The technique of error-prone PCR, which is quite commonly used to introduce random changes into a target gene, is somewhat limited in the types of changes that can be introduced. That is, since errors are typically introduced into DNA at no more than one or two per 1,000 nucleotides, only single nucleotides are replaced within a triplet codon, yielding only a limited number of amino acid changes. As an alternative to error-prone PCR, researchers have developed the technique of random insertion/deletion mutagenesis. With this approach, it is possible to delete a small number of nucleotides at random positions along the gene and, at the same time, insert either specific or random sequences into that position. This method entails the following steps (Fig. 8.8).

1. An isolated gene fragment with different restriction endonuclease sites at each end is ligated at one end to a short nonphosphorylated linker that leaves a small gap in the DNA. The gap is a consequence of the fact that the 5′ nucleotide from the linker is not phosphorylated and therefore cannot be ligated to an adjacent 3′-OH group.
2. After restriction enzyme digestion that creates compatible sticky ends, the gene fragment is cyclized with T4 DNA ligase to create a circular double-stranded gene fragment with a nick in the antisense strand.
3. The nicked strand is degraded by digestion with the enzyme T4 DNA polymerase (which has exonuclease activity).
4. The single-stranded DNA is randomly cleaved at single positions by treating it with a cerium(IV)–ethylenediaminetetraacetic acid (EDTA) complex.
5. The linear single-stranded DNAs are ligated to a linker (containing several additional nucleotides selected for insertion at one end), and the entire mutagenesis library is PCR amplified.

FIGURE 8.8 Schematic representation of random insertion/deletion protocol to introduce random mutations into a gene of interest. The inserted DNA is shown in yellow and the linkers in green. Adapted from Murakami et al., *Nat. Biotechnol.* **20:**76–81, 2002.

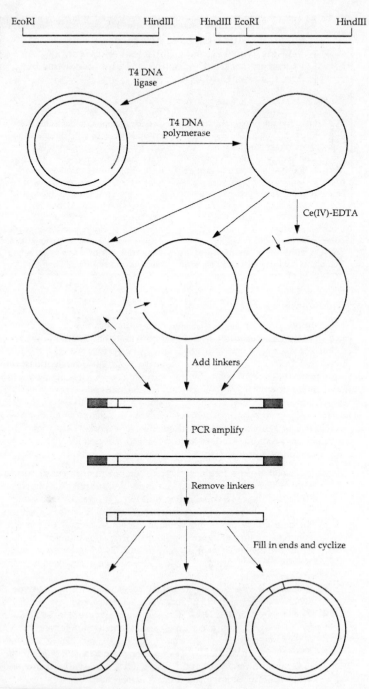

6. The linkers are removed by restriction enzyme digestion.
7. The constructs are made blunt ended by filling in the single-stranded overhangs using the Klenow fragment of *E. coli* DNA polymerase I and then cyclized again by T4 DNA ligase.
8. The amplified products are digested with appropriate restriction enzymes, cloned into a plasmid vector, and then tested for activity.

With this approach, it is possible to insert any small DNA fragment (carried on a linker) into the randomly cleaved single-stranded DNA, with the result that a much greater number of modified genes may be generated than by error-prone PCR. The mutations that are developed by this procedure may be used to select protein variants with a wide range of activities.

DNA Shuffling

Some biologically important proteins, such as α-interferon (IFN-α) (see chapter 10), are encoded by a family of several related genes, with each protein having slightly different biological activity. If all, or at least several, of the genes or cDNAs for a particular protein have been isolated, it is possible to recombine portions of these genes or cDNAs to produce hybrid or chimeric forms (Fig. 8.9). This "DNA shuffling" is done in the hope that some of the hybrid proteins will have unique properties or activities that were not encoded in any of the original sequences. Also, some of the hybrid proteins may combine important attributes of two or more of the original proteins, e.g., high activity and thermostability.

The simplest way to shuffle portions of similar genes is through the use of common restriction enzyme sites (Fig. 8.10). Digestion of two or more of the DNAs that encode the native forms of similar proteins with one or more restriction enzymes that cut the DNAs in the same place, followed by ligation of the mixture of DNA fragments, can potentially generate a large number of hybrids. For example, two DNAs, each of which has three unique restriction enzyme sites, can be recombined (shuffled) to produce 14 different hybrids in addition to the original DNA (Fig. 8.10). Another way to shuffle DNA involves combining several members of a gene family, fragmenting the mixed DNA with deoxyribonuclease I (DNase I), selecting smaller DNA fragments, and PCR amplifying these fragments. During PCR, gene fragments from different members of a gene family cross-prime each other after DNA fragments bind to one another in regions of high homology/complementarity. The final full-length products are obtained by including "terminal primers" in the PCR. After 20 to 30 PCR cycles, a panel of hybrid (full-length) DNAs will be established (Fig. 8.11). The hybrid DNAs are then used to create a library that can be screened for the desired activity (a task that may be the most difficult and labor-intensive part of the entire process). Although DNA shuffling works well with gene families—it is sometimes called molecular breeding—or with genes from different families that nevertheless have a high degree of homology, the technique is not especially useful when proteins have little or no homology. Thus, the DNAs must be very similar to one another or the PCR will not proceed. To remedy this situation and combine the genes of dissimilar proteins, several variations of the DNA-shuffling protocol have been described.

Wild type

Random mutagenesis or error-prone PCR

DNA shuffling

FIGURE 8.9 Schematic representation of the changes introduced into a protein by either random mutagenesis or error-prone PCR, both of which cause single-amino-acid substitutions, and by DNA shuffling, in which genes are formed with large regions from different sources.

FIGURE 8.10 The 14 different hybrid genes that can be generated by combining restriction enzyme fragments from two genes from the same gene family that have three different restriction sites in common. RE, restriction enzyme.

One procedure that was developed to combine the genes of dissimilar proteins and that does not rely on PCR amplification of DNA fragments is called nonhomologous random recombination. In this procedure (Fig. 8.12), DNAs from different sources (either defined or random DNA sequences or a mixture of both) are combined and then partially digested with DNase I. These DNA fragments, which include a wide variety of sizes, are made blunt ended by digestion with the enzyme T4 DNA polymerase. This enzyme both fills in 5' overhanging nucleotides and degrades 3' overhanging nucleotides. The DNA fragments are then mixed with a synthetic DNA fragment that forms a hairpin loop and contains a specific restriction enzyme site before the entire mixture is ligated by the addition of the enzyme T4 DNA ligase to form extended mosaic DNA hairpin molecules of variable lengths. The average length of these hairpin structures is dictated by the ratio between the blunt-ended DNA and the added DNA hairpins, which prevent further concatemerization once they are ligated to the ends. Finally, restriction enzyme digestion removes the hairpin loops so that the resulting sticky-ended DNA fragments can be inserted into plasmid vectors and tested for various activities. Because this process randomly recombines DNA fragments, only a very small fraction of the recombined DNAs are likely to encode the desired activity.

Mutant Proteins with Unusual Amino Acids

Essentially any protein can be altered by substituting one amino acid for another using directed mutagenesis. However, this approach is limited to the 20 amino acids that are normally used in protein synthesis. One way to increase the diversity of the proteins formed after mutagenesis is to introduce synthetic amino acids with unique side chains at specific sites. To do this, *E. coli* was engineered to produce both a novel transfer RNA (tRNA) that is not recognized by any of the existing *E. coli* aminoacyl-tRNA synthetases but nevertheless functions in translation and a new aminoacyl-tRNA synthetase that aminoacylates only that novel tRNA. A novel tRNA and unique aminoacyl-tRNA synthetase pair from the archaebacterium *Methanococcus jannaschii* was used as a starting point for this system. The tyrosine-tRNA synthetase from *M. jannaschii* can add an amino acid to an amber suppressor tRNA that is a mutant of its tyrosine-tRNA. An amber suppressor tRNA is a modified tRNA that can insert an amino acid into a protein in places where the mRNA contains an amber codon, UAG, which normally codes for a stop, i.e., the cessation of protein synthesis. To prevent the translational fusion of proteins whose mRNAs normally code for a stop with a UAG with downstream proteins, suppression is always less than 100% and is often dependent upon the nucleotides surrounding the stop codon. The amino acid specificity of the tyrosine-tRNA synthetase from *M. jannaschii* is altered by random mutagenesis of its gene so that, instead of tyrosine, it places O-methyl-L-tyrosine onto the tRNA. Specifically, a cloned version of the target gene is modified by oligonucleotide-directed mutagenesis so that it contains a 5'-TAG-3' in that portion of the DNA that encodes the amino acid that is targeted for change to O-methyl-L-tyrosine. Once the modified DNA has been selected, it is used to transform an *E. coli* strain that was previously engineered to produce the O-methyl-L-tyrosine-tRNA. The engineered *E. coli* strain inserts O-methyl-L-tyrosine into proteins that contain a UAG stop codon, resulting in a full-length target

protein containing the modified amino acid. Had the mutant gene been expressed in wild-type *E. coli*, a truncated version of the protein would have been produced (Fig. 8.13). This system may be manipulated to insert a variety of different amino acid analogues into specified sites within proteins in the hope of producing functional proteins with altered activities compared with the native form. In a similar approach to this problem, researchers modified a portion of the valine-tRNA synthetase gene so that the altered enzyme was able to insert the nonstandard amino acid aminobutyrate into proteins. While the full potential of these approaches has yet to be realized, it is nevertheless clear that it is now possible to produce proteins containing unusual chemical structures and possibly having unique properties.

Protein Engineering

About 20 of the many thousands of enzymes that have been studied and characterized biochemically account for over 90% of the total amount of enzymes that is currently being used industrially. Table 8.1 lists some of the most important enzymes and their primary uses. A major reason why additional enzymes are not used to any great extent in industrial processes is that an activity that has evolved to perform a particular function for a microorganism, animal, or plant under natural conditions usually is not well suited for a highly specialized industrial application. Most enzymes are easily denatured by exposure to the conditions, such as high temperature and the presence of organic solvents, that are used in many industrial processes. Although thermotolerant enzymes can be isolated from thermophilic microorganisms, these organisms often lack the particular enzyme that is required for use in industrial processes. However, with the availability of directed mutagenesis and gene cloning, these constraints are no longer significant.

Adding Disulfide Bonds

The thermostability of a protein can be increased by creating a molecule that will not readily unfold at elevated temperatures. In addition, these thermostable enzymes are often resistant to denaturation by organic solvents and nonphysiological conditions, such as extremes of pH. The addition of disulfide bonds (through the introduction of specifically placed cysteine residues) can usually significantly increase the stability of a protein (Fig. 8.14). The problem is whether extra disulfide bonds perturb the normal functioning of a protein.

T4 lysozyme. In one study, six variants of the enzyme T4 lysozyme were constructed by oligonucleotide-directed mutagenesis, which introduced new internal disulfide bonds. Specifically, two, four, or six amino acid residues at a time were changed to cysteine, thereby generating one, two, or three disulfide bonds, respectively (Table 8.2). The side chains of the amino acid residues that were targeted to become cysteine residues were known to be spatially close to each other in the active enzyme. This proximity ensured that the overall conformation of the molecule would remain essentially unaffected by the formation of the new disulfide linkages. The targeted amino acids were not involved in the active site of the enzyme, which

Native genes

DNA fragmentation and PCR

Hybrid genes

FIGURE 8.11 Some of the hybrid DNAs that can be generated during PCR amplification of three members of a gene family.

FIGURE 8.12 Schematic representation of nonhomologous random recombination. Different DNAs (shown in different colors) are mixed together, partially digested with DNase I, blunt ended by digestion with T4 DNA polymerase, size fractionated, ligated with synthetic hairpin DNAs to form extended hairpins, restriction enzyme digested to remove the hairpin ends and generate sticky ends, and then ligated into plasmid vectors.

is the portion of the enzyme molecule that is probably most sensitive to small changes in conformation. The newly introduced cysteines created disulfide bonds between positions 3 and 97, 9 and 164, and 21 and 142 of the enzyme, where the numbers denote the amino acid positions in the polypeptide, starting from the N terminus.

After mutagenesis, each mutated gene was identified and expressed in *E. coli*. The engineered enzymes were purified, and the enzymatic activity

FIGURE 8.13 Schematic representation of the production of a protein with a modified (nonstandard amino acid) side chain. The start codon is highlighted in green, and the stop codons are in red. The inserted amino acid analogue is shown in blue.

TABLE 8.1 Some industrial enzymes and their commercial uses

Enzyme	Industrial use(s)
α-Amylase	Beer making, alcohol production
Aminoacylase	Preparation of L-amino acids
Bromelain	Meat tenderizer, juice clarification
Catalase	Antioxidant in prepared foods
Cellulase	Alcohol and glucose production
Ficin	Meat tenderizer, juice clarification
Glucoamylase	Beer making, alcohol production
Glucose isomerase	Manufacture of high-fructose syrups
Glucose oxidase	Antioxidant in prepared foods
Invertase	Sucrose inversion
Lactase	Whey utilization, lactose hydrolysis
Lipase	Cheese making, preparation of flavorings
Papain	Meet tenderizer, juice clarification
Pectinase	Clarifying fruit juices, alcohol production
Protease	Detergent, alcohol production
Rennet	Cheese making

Native protein

Engineered protein

FIGURE 8.14 Schematic representation of the engineering of a protein that contains two engineered disulfide bridges (colored lines in the bottom diagram) that hold together and may stabilize regions of the protein that are often separated in the primary amino acid sequence.

and thermostability of each were determined (Table 8.2). The thermostability of a protein is often defined as the temperature at which the overall structure of the protein is 50% denatured; the state of denaturation can be assessed by monitoring the circular dichroism of the protein in solution. The wild-type (native) form of the enzyme T4 lysozyme has two free cysteine residues that both exist as free sulfhydryl groups, neither of which is involved in a disulfide bond. In the so-called pseudo-wild-type enzyme, these cysteines were changed by oligonucleotide-directed mutagenesis to threonine (Thr) and alanine (Ala) without altering either the activity or the thermostability of the enzyme. Consequently, the pseudo-wild-type sequence provided a standard for comparing variants with potentially thermostabilizing disulfide bonds and also prevented spurious disulfide bonding between the introduced cysteine residues and the naturally occurring ones. The constructed lysozyme derivatives had from one to three disulfide bonds.

The results of this experiment indicate that the thermal stability of the enzyme increases as a result of the presence of disulfide bonds, with the most thermostable variant being the one with the largest number of disulfide bonds, and that some variants (C, E, and F in Table 8.2), which are more thermostable than the wild type or pseudo-wild type, have lost their enzymatic activity. The loss of enzymatic activity in three of the variants probably reflects a distortion of the peptide backbone of the molecule containing a disulfide linkage between residues 21 and 142. Often, the engineering of a protein is a trial-and-error process. Hence, the precise amino acid changes that yield the "best" variant are not always obvious. However, from this experiment, it is clear that increasing disulfide bonds to enhance protein stability is feasible.

Xylanase. In a similar study, the development of a temperature-stable mutant of the enzyme xylanase from *Bacillus circulans* was undertaken. During the making of paper, wood pulp is chemically treated to remove the hemicellulose that would otherwise contribute to the discoloration of the paper product. Unfortunately, this step results in the creation of large amounts of potentially toxic effluent. From an environmental perspective, treatment of wood pulp with xylanase, which degrades hemicellulose, is preferred to pulping. Treatment of wood pulp with this enzyme could lower the amount of bleaching chemical that would otherwise be required as a part of this process. However, the step at which xylanase would be added

TABLE 8.2 Properties of T4 lysozyme and six engineered variants

| Enzyme | Amino acid at position: | | | | | | | No. of -S-S- | % Activity | T_m (°C) |
	3	9	21	54	97	142	164			
wt	Ile	Ile	Thr	Cys	Cys	Thr	Leu	0	100	41.9
pwt	Ile	Ile	Thr	Thr	Ala	Thr	Leu	0	100	41.9
A	Cys	Ile	Thr	Thr	Cys	Thr	Leu	1	96	46.7
B	Ile	Cys	Thr	Thr	Ala	Thr	Cys	1	106	48.3
C	Ile	Ile	Cys	Thr	Aka	Cys	Leu	1	0	52.9
D	Cys	Cys	Thr	Thr	Cys	Thr	Cys	2	95	57.6
E	Ile	Cys	Cys	Thr	Ala	Cys	Cys	2	0	58.9
F	Cys	Cys	Cys	Thr	Cys	Cys	Cys	3	0	65.5

Adapted from Matsumura et al., *Nature* 342:291–293, 1989.

wt, wild-type T4 lysozyme; pwt, pseudo-wild-type enzyme; A through F, six engineered cysteine variants; -S-S-, disulfide bonds; T_m, "melting" temperature (a measure of thermostability).

follows the hot-alkali treatment of the pulp. While it is possible to lower the pH of this material by adding acid, current industry practice is directed toward using less water to cool the pulp, so if xylanase were to be used in this process, it must function efficiently at relatively high temperatures.

Computer modeling of the three-dimensional structure of xylanase was used to predict sites along the polypeptide chain where one, two, or three disulfide bridges could be introduced in order to stabilize the enzyme without disrupting its catalytic activity. All of the eight derivatives of the *B. circulans* xylanase that were generated showed an increase in thermostability compared with the wild type, and three of the eight mutants were as enzymatically active as the wild type at 60°C. Moreover, one mutant, in which a disulfide bridge between the N- and C-terminal ends of the enzyme was introduced, was nearly twice as active as the wild type at 60°C and retained more than 85% of its activity after a 2-hour incubation at 60°C, whereas the wild type lost all of its activity after only 30 minutes at this temperature (Fig. 8.15). These results indicate that the thermostability of other enzymes can be enhanced, provided that sufficiently detailed X-ray crystallographic information is available. The success of the protein engineering and the laboratory testing notwithstanding, it remains to be determined whether a thermostable xylanase can be effectively incorporated into a commercial process for the manufacture of paper.

Human pancreatic RNase. Ribonuclease (RNase) from bull semen can act as an antitumorigenic agent. In both in vitro and in vivo experiments, a dimeric form of this protein is internalized into tumor cells by non-receptor-mediated endocytosis, and when it reaches the cytosol, it selectively degrades ribosomal RNA (rRNA), thereby blocking protein synthesis and causing cell death. The dimeric form of this enzyme consists of two identical subunits covalently joined by two adjacent intersubunit disulfide bridges and stabilized by a small number of noncovalent interactions. The antitumor activity of bull semen RNase is dependent on the dimeric structure of the protein,

FIGURE 8.15 Addition of a disulfide bond between the N and C termini of *B. circulans* xylanase stabilizes the protein. Its activity at room temperature is doubled, and at 60°C it is largely protected against heat inactivation.

A B

FIGURE 8.16 Schematic representation of native monomeric human pancreatic RNase **(A)** and engineered dimeric human pancreatic RNase **(B)**. The native protein was modified by changing glutamine 28 to leucine, arginine 31 to cysteine, arginine 32 to cysteine, and asparagine 34 to lysine. The monomeric enzyme is approximately 13.6 kDa, while the dimeric form is approximately 27.2 kDa.

the only dimeric RNase from the pancreatic-like RNase superfamily of proteins. However, human antibodies against bull semen RNase are often produced following repeated or prolonged use of this therapeutic protein, thereby eventually negating the usefulness and effectiveness of bull semen RNase in treating tumor cells. For this reason, monomeric human pancreatic RNase was engineered to be an antitumorigenic agent.

The amino acid sequence of bull semen RNase is more than 70% identical to the amino acid sequence of human pancreatic RNase and therefore could be used as a model to determine which amino acids might be altered in the human enzyme to participate in dimer formation (Fig. 8.16). When dimeric human pancreatic RNase was formed in *E. coli*, the protein was localized in an insoluble inclusion body (Fig. 8.17). Solubilization of the inclusion body and renaturation of the unfolded protein yielded dimeric human pancreatic RNase that displayed a slightly lower level of antitumorigenic activity than bull semen RNase. Depending on the tumor cell line, up to twice as much of the engineered protein was required. Since the dimeric human pancreatic RNase did not impair the functioning of normal human diploid fibroblast cells, this engineered protein is a good candidate to become an important human therapeutic agent.

Changing Asparagine to Other Amino Acids

When proteins are exposed to high temperatures, asparagine and glutamine residues may undergo deamidation, a reaction that releases ammonia. With the loss of the amide moiety, these amino acids become aspartic acid and glutamic acid, respectively, which have different chemical properties at physiological pH than asparagine and glutamine, resulting in localized changes in the folding of the peptide chain that may lead to a loss of activity.

In one study, the effect of changing some asparagine residues in the *Saccharomyces cerevisiae* enzyme triosephosphate isomerase was examined. This enzyme consists of two identical subunits; each subunit has two asparagine residues that may contribute to the thermosensitivity of the enzyme because they are located at the subunit interface. By oligonucleotide-directed mutagenesis, the asparagine residues at positions 14 and 78 were targeted for change (Table 8.3). Converting either of these asparagine resi-

FIGURE 8.17 Flowchart showing the solubilization and renaturation of the dimeric human pancreatic RNase from *E. coli* inclusion bodies.

dues to threonine or isoleucine enhanced the thermostability of the enzyme, whereas as predicted, changing one of the asparagine residues to aspartic acid reduced thermostability. When both asparagine residues were changed to aspartic acid residues, the resulting enzyme was unstable even at ambient temperature and had low enzymatic activity (data not shown).

The engineered proteins were also tested for their sensitivities to proteolytic digestion. A positive correlation between thermostability and resistance to proteolysis was observed. On the basis of these results, it should be possible to generate thermostable forms of other enzymes by mutating nonessential asparagine codons. In fact, a long-acting human insulin analogue was produced by replacing an aspartic acid residue with glycine. This analogue was recently approved for use as a human therapeutic agent.

Reducing the Number of Free Sulfhydryl Residues

Occasionally, an expressed foreign protein is less active than expected. Protein engineering can be used to increase this activity. For example, when the cDNA for human IFN-β was initially cloned and expressed in *E. coli*, the protein product showed only a disappointing 10% of the antiviral activity of the authentic, glycosylated form. And although reasonable amounts of IFN-β were synthesized, most of the IFN-β was found to exist as dimers and higher oligomers that were inactive.

Analysis of the DNA sequence of the IFN-β gene revealed that the native protein has three cysteine residues, so one or more of these residues could be involved in the intermolecular disulfide bonding that produced the dimers and oligomers in *E. coli* but not in human cells. It was reasoned that conversion of one or more of the cysteine codons into serine codons might result in an IFN-β derivative that would not form oligomers. Serine was chosen to replace cysteine because the structures of the two amino acids are identical, except that serine contains oxygen instead of sulfur and as a result cannot form disulfide bonds.

When this study was undertaken, detailed information about the structure of IFN-β was lacking, so the researchers were forced to rely on data derived from related proteins. In other words, they did not know which of the three cysteine residues contributed to intermolecular disulfide bond formation. However, the locations of the cysteine residues that form the internal disulfide bonds in IFN-α, a structurally similar molecule, were known, so a comparison of the primary amino acid sequence of this mole-

TABLE 8.3 Stability at 100°C of the yeast enzyme triosephosphate isomerase and its engineered derivatives

Enzyme	Amino acid at position:		Half-life (min)
	14	78	
Wild type	Asn	Asn	13
Variant A	Asn	Thr	17
Variant B	Asn	Ile	16
Variant C	Thr	Ile	25
Variant D	Asp	Asn	11

Adapted from Ahern et al., *Proc. Natl. Acad. Sci. USA* 84:657–679, 1987.

Enzyme stability is expressed as the half-life, or rate of enzyme inactivation, at 100°C. A longer half-life indicates a more stable enzyme.

cule with that of IFN-β was made (Fig. 8.18). Alignment of the amino acid sequences of the two protein molecules indicated that Cys-31 and Cys-141 in IFN-β are located in positions similar to those of Cys-29 and Cys-138 in IFN-α. Because Cys-29 and Cys-138 in IFN-α are involved in the formation of an intramolecular disulfide bond, it seemed reasonable to assume that Cys-17 of IFN-β was not involved in intramolecular disulfide bonding and was therefore a good candidate for modification.

This deduction proved to be correct. No multimeric complexes were formed when a Ser-17 variant of IFN-β (Ser-17 IFN-β) was expressed in *E. coli*. Moreover, the Ser-17 IFN-β had a specific activity similar to that of authentic, native IFN-β and was more stable during long-term storage than the native form.

Increasing Enzymatic Activity

In addition to stabilizing an enzyme by directed mutagenesis, it may be feasible to modify its catalytic function. Currently, detailed information about the geometry of the active site of a well-characterized enzyme is required in order to predictably alter enzymatic activity. With such data, researchers are able to deduce which specific changes might be necessary to modulate the substrate-binding specificity of an enzyme (Box 8.1).

Tyrosyl-tRNA synthetase. In an early demonstration of how directed mutagenesis could enhance enzyme activity, the enzyme tyrosyl-tRNA synthetase

FIGURE 8.18 Positions of the cysteine residues and disulfide bonds of IFN-α and IFN-β. The known intramolecular disulfide bond in IFN-α is indicated by a dashed line, and the deduced intramolecular disulfide bond in IFN-β is indicated by a dotted line.

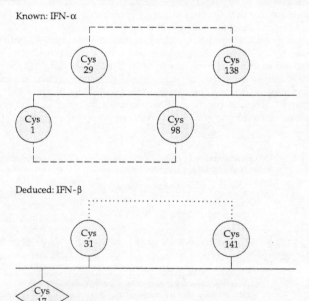

from *B. stearothermophilus* was modified with respect to substrate binding. Tyrosyl-tRNA synthetase catalyzes the aminoacylation of a tRNA that specifically accepts tyrosine (tRNATyr) in a two-step process:

(1) Tyr + ATP → Tyr-A + PP$_i$

(2) Tyr-A + tRNATyr → Tyr-tRNATyr + AMP

In step 1, tyrosine (Tyr) is activated by ATP to yield enzyme-bound tyrosyl adenylate (Tyr-A), with the concomitant formation of pyrophosphate (PP$_i$). In step 2, Tyr-A is hydrolyzed by the free 3′ hydroxyl of the incoming tRNA molecule, so the tyrosine moiety becomes attached to the tRNA, and AMP is released. Both of these reactions take place while the substrates are bound to tyrosyl-tRNA synthetase.

The three-dimensional structure of tyrosyl-tRNA synthetase from *B. stearothermophilus* had already been determined, and the active site had been mapped. With the aid of computer graphics, predictions were made about the effects of changing one or more amino acid residues in the active site on the interaction of the enzyme with the reaction substrates. To test whether these predictions were correct, the gene for tyrosyl-tRNA synthetase was specifically modified by oligonucleotide-directed mutagenesis. A threonine residue at position 51 (Thr-51) was replaced with either an alanine or a proline residue. In the native enzyme, the hydroxyl group of Thr-51 forms a long hydrogen bond with the ring oxygen of the ribose moiety of tyrosine adenylate. It was deduced that the removal of this weak hydrogen bond might improve the affinity of the enzyme for ATP.

BOX 8.1

An Overview of Enzyme Kinetics

In its simplest form, an enzyme-catalyzed reaction may be described by the equation

$$E + S \leftrightarrow ES \rightarrow E + P \qquad (1)$$

where the symbols represent concentrations, E is the enzyme not bound to substrate, S is the unbound substrate, ES is the enzyme–substrate complex, and P is the product of the enzyme-catalyzed reaction. The interaction of E with S to form ES is controlled by the forward rate constant k_1, the dissociation of ES to E and S is controlled by k_{-1}, and the formation of P from ES is controlled by k_2. Thus, the overall rate of an enzyme-catalyzed reaction may be described as follows:

$$dP/dt = v = k_2 ES \qquad (2)$$

Since it is usually quite difficult to directly measure the concentration of

ES, it is necessary to express the rate of the enzyme-catalyzed reaction in terms of parameters that can be readily quantified. The system may also be described, in part, by the following equations:

$$E_0 = E + ES \qquad (3)$$

$$S_0 = S + ES + P \qquad (4)$$

$$v = -dS/dt = k_1 S - k_{-1} ES + k_2 ES \qquad (5)$$

where E_0 and S_0 are the total amount of enzyme and substrate in the system, respectively. From equations 3, 4, and 5, it is possible to derive an expression for the reaction rate in terms of measurable parameters. Thus:

$$v = V_{max} S/(S + K_m) \qquad (6)$$

and

$$V_{max} = E_0 k_{cat} \qquad (7)$$

where V_{max} is the maximum rate that a particular enzyme-catalyzed reaction can attain, K_m is the dissociation con-

stant of the ES complex (generally called the Michaelis constant), and k_{cat} is the catalytic rate constant. Each of these values is dependent upon conditions, including the temperature, pH, and salt concentration. From these equations, it becomes apparent that the greater the value of V_{max} or k_{cat}, the higher the rate of the reaction. Conversely, the greater the value of K_m, the lower the rate of the reaction. Despite differences in mechanisms of action, all enzyme-catalyzed reactions can be characterized by values for V_{max} (or k_{cat}) and K_m under a particular set of conditions. This makes it easy for scientists to rapidly compare the behaviors of different enzymes and substrates. For example, an enzyme with a K_m of 10 mM for a particular substrate has a low affinity for that substrate, whereas an enzyme with a K_m of 1 μM has a high affinity for a particular substrate.

The resultant enzyme variants were characterized by determining their kinetic constants, and some of the observed changes were more dramatic than anticipated (Table 8.4). For the Ala-51 variant, the binding affinity (K_m) of the enzyme for ATP increased approximately twofold, without any significant change in the catalytic rate constant (k_{cat}). By contrast, the enzyme that contained a proline in position 51 bound ATP more than 100-fold more tightly than did the native enzyme. The catalytic efficiency (k_{cat}/K_m) of the aminoacylation reaction was increased with both of the variants. The result obtained with the Pro-51 variant was unexpected, because theoretically, the addition of a proline residue should distort, at least locally, the α-helical polypeptide backbone found in this region. Thus, one might have expected that this conformational change would reduce substrate binding.

This study demonstrates that, even though it may be difficult to predict the precise effect that a particular amino acid change will have on the reaction kinetics, this approach can correctly identify those amino acid side chains that might be altered to improve the kinetic behavior of an enzyme. Moreover, as a consequence of these kinds of experiments, it is clear that the affinity of an enzyme for its substrate, as well as the catalytic efficiency of the enzyme-catalyzed reaction, can be improved by in vitro manipulation of a cloned gene.

Endoprotease. It is often difficult to engineer an enzyme that has a high level of enzymatic activity for one reaction to perform a new and different function that is also at a high level. The enzyme amino acid residues that are optimized for the original activity may interfere with the ability of the enzyme to function optimally for the new activity. To remedy this, one group of researchers argued that, following mutagenesis, it is necessary to simultaneously select for the new/modified activity and against the original enzyme activity. This approach was then used to modify a target gene encoding an endoprotease specific for cleaving between adjacent arginine residues. The gene was first subjected to error-prone PCR, and the modified genes were then cloned so that the encoded modified enzyme was fused to a peptide that displayed the construct on the surfaces of E. coli cells (Fig. 8.19A). Two different substrates were then added. The first substrate was a peptide that contained three arginine residues, each with a positive charge, and two fluorescent dyes, one near each end of the peptide (Fig. 8.19B). The second substrate consisted of a peptide that also contained three arginine residues but only one fluorescent dye near its C terminus. The positive charges guaranteed that the substrate molecules and their cleavage products would become associated with the negatively charged surfaces of the E. coli cells displaying the modified enzymes. The protease

TABLE 8.4 Aminoacylation activity of native (Thr-51) and modified (Ala-51 and pro-51) tyrosyl-tRNA synthetases

Enzyme	k_{cat} (s^{-1})	K_m (mM)	k_{cat}/K_m (s^{-1} M^{-1})
Thr-51	4.7	2.5	1,860
Ala-51	4.0	1.2	3,200
Pro-51	1.8	0.019	95,800

Adapted from Wilkenson et al., *Nature* 307:187–188, 1984.

The units for K_m, the binding constant of the enzyme for ATP, are millimolar units (mM); the units for k_{cat}, the catalytic rate constant, are reciprocal seconds (s^{-1}); and the units for k_{cat}/K_m, the catalytic efficiency, are s^{-1} M^{-1}.

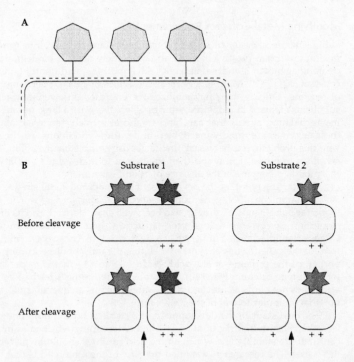

FIGURE 8.19 **(A)** *E. coli* displaying a cloned endoprotease on its surface. The negative charge on the surface of the bacterial cell is shown. **(B)** Positively charged peptide substrates before and after cleavage containing an Ala-Arg bond and two different fluorescent markers (shown in red and green) (substrate 1) and containing an Arg-Arg bond and one fluorescent marker (substrate 2). The arrows indicate the point of cleavage.

activity being selected for cleaves a peptide bond between arginine and alanine, amino acid residues that are located in the middle of substrate 1. The activity being selected against cleaves a peptide bond between arginine and arginine, amino acid residues found in the middle of substrate 2. The cleavage of substrate 1, the new activity being selected for, results in the production of a peptide with three positive charges and carrying a green fluorescent dye (Fig. 8.19B). This peptide binds to the surfaces of cells and is readily detectable using a fluorescent cell sorter. The cleavage of substrate 2, by the original enzyme activity, results in the production of a peptide with two positive charges carrying a red fluorescent dye (Fig. 8.19B) that also binds to cells and is detectable using a fluorescent cell sorter. Following cell sorting, cells that showed both an increase in green fluorescence and a decrease in red fluorescence were isolated and tested further. Cells that displayed this activity encoded the modified enzyme within their plasmid DNA. In this way, one clone was isolated that displayed a >3 million-fold selectivity for cleavage of Ala-Arg bonds compared to Arg-Arg bonds, an enormous change in substrate specificity without any significant decrease in the high catalytic activity used to cleave the original substrate.

Modifying Metal Cofactor Requirements

Subtilisins are a group of serine proteases that are secreted into growth medium by gram-positive bacteria and are widely used as biodegradable cleaning agents in laundry detergents. All subtilisins bind tightly (affinity constant $[K_a]$ = ~10^7 M) to one or more molecules of calcium per molecule of enzyme. Calcium binding stabilizes the enzyme. Unfortunately, since subtilisins are used in industrial settings where there are a large number of metal-chelating agents that can bind to and effectively remove calcium, these enzymes are rapidly inactivated under these conditions. To circumvent this problem, it is necessary first to abolish completely the ability of a subtilisin to bind calcium and then to attempt to increase the stability of this modified enzyme in the absence of bound calcium.

The starting point for the development of a modified subtilisin was the isolated subtilisin BPN' gene from *Bacillus amyloliquefaciens*. Prior to this work, the subtilisin BPN' protein had been well characterized, and its high-resolution X-ray crystallographic structure had been determined. Oligonucleotide-directed mutagenesis was used to construct a mutant form of the gene for this enzyme by deleting the nucleotides encoding the portion of the protein—amino acid residues 75 to 83—that is responsible for binding to calcium (Fig. 8.20). The protein without this stretch of amino acids does not bind calcium and, surprisingly, retains an overall conformation that is similar to that of the native form.

The next steps in the development of a stable subtilisin from one that lacked a calcium-binding domain entailed determining which sites might contribute to stability and which amino acid residues should be placed at these sites. The researchers assumed that any of the amino acids that had previously interacted with the calcium-binding loop in the native form of the enzyme were potential candidates for change. In total, 10 amino acids were considered to be candidates for modification. Moreover, since it was not known a priori which particular amino acid residues might best contribute to stabilizing the enzyme molecule, random mutagenesis was used for each of these sites.

The amino acids selected for mutagenesis came from four separate regions of the protein: the N terminus (residues 2 to 5), the omega loop (residues 36 to 44), an α-helical region (residues 63 to 85), and a β-pleated region (residues 202 to 220). To identify the best amino acid at a particular position, mutant clones were grown in the wells of microtiter plates, heated to 65°C for 1 hour, allowed to cool, and then assayed for subtilisin activity. It was necessary to express the active calcium-free subtilisin in *Bacillus subtilis* because it was lethal when expressed in *E. coli*.

After the initial screening, stabilizing mutations were identified at 7 of the 10 positions that were examined (Table 8.5). When these stabilizing mutations were combined into a single gene, the enzyme that was produced had kinetic properties that were very similar to those of the native form of subtilisin. Moreover, the modified form of subtilisin was nearly 10 times more stable than the native form of the enzyme in the absence of calcium and, surprisingly, about 50% more stable than the native enzyme in the presence of calcium. Although this work was somewhat labor-intensive and painstaking, it demonstrated that complex properties of enzymes that involve a large number of different amino acid residues can be genetically engineered.

High
activity

No
activity

Deleted region

Low
activity

High
activity

FIGURE 8.20 Genetic engineering of calcium-independent subtilisin. The native calcium-containing enzyme is highly active but loses almost all of its activity when the loop that binds the calcium is deleted. After several rounds of random mutagenesis, mutants of the deleted enzyme, each with stabilizing mutations and a low level of activity, are selected. Several of these mutations are combined into a single derivative with the result that a subtilisin that does not require calcium and that has a high level of activity is produced.

Decreasing Protease Sensitivity

Streptokinase, a 47-kilodalton (kDa) protein produced by pathogenic strains of *Streptococcus* bacteria, is a blood clot-dissolving agent. Streptokinase forms a complex with plasminogen that results in the conversion of plasminogen to plasmin, the active protease that degrades fibrin in the blood

TABLE 8.5 Effects of random mutations of selected amino acid residues on the stability of subtilisin BPN lacking a calcium-binding domain

Region of protein	Amino acid residue	Stabilizing mutation	Fold increase in half-life
N terminus	2	Gln→Lys	2.0
	3	Ser→Cys	17.0
	4	None found	None
	5	Pro→Ser	1.2
Omega loop	41	Asp→Ala	1.2
	44	Lys→Asn	1.2
α-Helix	73	Ala→Leu	2.6
	74	None found	None
β-Pleat structure	206	Gln→Cys	17.0
	214	None found	None

Adapted from Strausberg et al., *Bio/Technology* **13**: 669–673, 1995.

The mutations at positions 3 and 206 to Cys occur in the same clone and provide such a high level of stability because of the formation of the disulfide bridge between these residues.

clot. Unfortunately, plasmin also rapidly degrades streptokinase, making it necessary for medical personnel to administer streptokinase as a 30- to 90-minute infusion so that a sufficient level of intact and active streptokinase is maintained. Since it is essential that individuals suffering a heart attack be treated as quickly as possible, a long-lived streptokinase could be administered as a single injection before a person is transported to a hospital. This early treatment might contribute to saving the lives of heart attack victims by quickly restoring blood flow and limiting damage to heart muscles.

Plasmin is a trypsin-like protease that specifically cleaves the peptide bond after a lysine or arginine residue. Plasmin rapidly digests the 414-amino-acid streptokinase protein by cleaving it at lysine 59, near the N terminus, and at lysine 386, near the C terminus. The 328-amino-acid peptide that remains following the digestion by plasmin has approximately 16% of the activity of intact streptokinase in activating plasminogen, and it is slowly degraded by plasmin until no activity remains. To make streptokinase less susceptible to proteolysis by plasmin, the lysine residues at positions 59 and 386 were changed to glutamine by site-specific mutagenesis (Fig. 8.21). Glutamine was chosen to replace lysine because the length of its side chain is similar to that of lysine, so that the three-dimensional structure would not be disturbed, and because glutamine does not have a positive charge. Both single mutants, as well as the double mutant, had the same ability to bind to and activate plasminogen as did the native form of streptokinase. At the same time, in the presence of plasmin, the half-lives of all three mutants were increased compared with native streptokinase, with the double mutant being approximately 21-fold more protease resistant. This work is an important first step in the development of variants of streptokinase with significantly longer half-lives.

Modifying Protein Specificity

FokI endonuclease. Although protein-engineering studies using oligonucleotide-directed mutagenesis have focused on modifying and enhancing existing properties of specialized enzymes, it is conceivable that an enzyme

	Processed size (kDa)	Activity
A	37	Low
B	42	Low
C	40	Low
D	47	High

FIGURE 8.21 Schematic representation of protease (plasmin) sensitivity of streptokinase and some engineered plasmin-resistant derivatives. The green circles indicate positively charged lysine residues where plasmin cuts the peptide chain. The red circles indicate glutamine residues where plasmin does not cut the peptide chain. The horizontal arrows indicate plasmin digestion of streptokinase. The protein size and activity following plasmin digestion are indicated for each derivative. **(A)** Native protein; **(B)** the derivative in which glutamine replaces lysine 386; **(C)** the derivative in which glutamine replaces lysine 59; **(D)** the derivative in which glutamine residues replace lysine 59 and lysine 386.

could be redesigned to produce a unique catalytic entity. For example, new site-specific endonucleases have been created from the relatively nonspecific enzyme FokI endonuclease.

To date, more than 2,500 restriction-modification enzymes from a large number of different organisms have been discovered. Since many of these enzymes recognize the same DNA sequence, there are only about 200 different recognition sites, with the vast majority of the known

enzymes recognizing DNA sequences that are 4 to 6 base pairs (bp) in length. Restriction enzymes that recognize 4 to 6 bp cut DNA relatively frequently and are not as useful for producing large DNA fragments as are restriction endonucleases that recognize DNA sequences that are 8 bp or longer, i.e., rare cutters. Since the discovery of new restriction enzymes is tedious, time-consuming, and unlikely to yield many new enzymes that recognize DNA sequences that are 8 bp or longer, an alternative means of obtaining new rare cutters is to develop them by protein engineering.

The class of proteins that contain unique structural domains that each bind a molecule of Zn^{2+} are called zinc finger proteins. These proteins bind to DNA in a sequence-specific manner by inserting a protein α-helical region into the major groove of the DNA double helix. For example, a mouse protein called Zif268 has three separate zinc finger domains, and each zinc finger interacts with a specific DNA triplet codon. Moreover, since the zinc fingers bind to the DNA independently of one another, they can be linked together in a peptide by genetic engineering so that they will bind to a predetermined site on a DNA fragment. Thus, it is possible to engineer nucleases that can cut DNA at specific sites by fusing several zinc finger-encoding sequences with the portion of the gene for the nonspecific nuclease FokI from the bacterium *Flavobacterium okeanokoites*. To test this idea, a hybrid gene that included six consecutive histidine residues at the N terminus to facilitate purification of the fusion protein, three zinc fingers, a (Gly_4Ser_3) linker peptide to confer flexibility on the fusion protein, and the portion of the FokI gene that encodes the nuclease activity was constructed (Fig. 8.22). After purification of the expressed protein, the N-terminal histidine residues may be removed by treatment with thrombin.

Bacteria that produce restriction enzymes protect their own DNA from being cleaved by these restriction enzymes by synthesizing enzymes that bind to and methylate the restriction enzyme recognition sites on the DNA. However, a host genome would not be protected from digestion by the synthetic FokI hybrid restriction endonuclease. Consequently, during cell growth, the expression of the hybrid enzyme was prevented by placing it under the control of the bacteriophage T7 expression system.

Two FokI hybrid restriction endonucleases, each designed to cleave bacteriophage λ DNA at different single sites, were produced. One cleaved bacteriophage λ DNA at its target site, and the other cleaved λ at the expected site and to a lesser extent at two other sites. The latter result is not entirely surprising, since zinc fingers recognize triplet codons by interacting primarily with two of the three bases. Thus, although these hybrid enzymes are not yet ready for routine laboratory use, the strategy of using zinc finger motifs and a nuclease domain to create unique restriction endonucleases appears promising.

Antibodies. With antibody molecules, large portions of the protein are identical from one antibody to the next. However, a small portion of the amino acids in the peptide chain are hypervariable, giving an antibody

FIGURE 8.22 Gene construct for a zinc finger–FokI hybrid restriction endonuclease.

pT7	His tag	Zinc fingers	Linker	Nuclease domain

molecule a high degree of specificity for the antigenic determinant to which it binds (see chapter 10). By modifying these hypervariable regions of the protein, it should be possible to generate antibodies in vitro that are directed against a wide range of antigenic determinants. The portion of an antibody molecule that contains the ability to bind to an antigenic determinant is sometimes called a Fab fragment; it can bind in the absence of the rest of the antibody molecule and consists of two peptides each with different hypervariable complementarity-determining regions (CDRs) separated by relatively invariant framework regions (Fig. 8.23). Together, the six CDRs (three from the variable part of the light chain and three from the variable part of the heavy chain) determine the specificity of an antibody molecule. Consequently, altering one or more of the amino acid residues in one of the CDRs changes the specificity of the antibody.

Using random mutagenesis with degenerate (mixed) oligonucleotide primers, it was possible to introduce a range of different mutations into the three CDRs of the variable region of an antibody heavy-chain gene (Fig. 8.24). First, one of the CDRs was modified by PCR. Then, in a second PCR, the other two CDRs were modified. Finally, the three altered CDRs were combined in a single DNA fragment. With this approach, the changes could have just as easily been introduced into the gene for the variable portion of an antibody light chain. In one instance, a Fab fragment of a monoclonal antibody that was specific for the compound 11-deoxycortisol was altered as described above to produce a Fab fragment that was specific for cortisol and no longer bound 11-deoxycortisol. Depending on the method used to screen the library of mutagenized Fab genes, this approach can facilitate the creation of Fab fragments directed toward any antigenic determinant.

Increasing Enzyme Stability and Specificity

tPa. The enzyme tissue plasminogen activator (tPA) is a multidomain serine protease that is medically useful for the dissolution of blood clots. However, like streptokinase, tPA is rapidly cleared from the circulation, so that it must be administered by infusion. Therefore, to be effective with this form of delivery, high initial concentrations of tPA must be used. Unfortunately, under these conditions, tPA can cause nonspecific internal bleeding. Thus, a long-lived tPA that has an increased specificity for fibrin in blood clots and is not prone to induce nonspecific bleeding would be desirable. It was found that these three properties could be separately introduced by directed mutagenesis into the gene for the native form of tPA. First, changing Thr-103 to Asn causes the enzyme to persist in rabbit plasma approximately 10 times longer than the native form. Second,

FIGURE 8.23 Structure of a Fab molecule. FR, framework region. C_{H1} and C_L are constant domains from the heavy and light chains of the antibody molecule, respectively. The N-terminal (NH_2) and C-terminal (COOH) ends of each polypeptide, as well as a disulfide bridge (-S-S-), are indicated.

FIGURE 8.24 Schematic representation of the method used to introduce mutations into the three CDR genes of the variable region of a heavy antibody chain. The framework region sequences are in green, and the CDR sequences are in blue. **(A)** The first PCR introduces random mutations into the DNA encoding CDR1. **(B)** The second PCR introduces random mutations into the DNA encoding CDR2 and CDR3. **(C)** The third PCR combines the DNA that was amplified in panels A and B. The circled portion of the DNA indicates the place where random mutations were introduced.

changing amino acids 296 to 299 from Lys-His-Arg-Arg to Ala-Ala-Ala-Ala produces an enzyme that is much more specific for fibrin than is the native form. Third, changing Asn-117 to Gln causes the enzyme to retain the level of fibrinolytic activity found in the native form. Moreover, combining these three mutations in a single construct allows all three activities to be expressed simultaneously (Table 8.6). Additional work is needed to determine whether a modified form of tPA is an acceptable replacement for native tPA.

Fructosyl-amino acid oxidase. Glycation, the nonenzymatic addition of glucosyl residues on the surfaces of blood proteins, such as hemoglobin and albumin, is typically increased in diabetics with high blood glucose levels. Also, since the glycation of blood proteins is not affected by the changes in blood glucose levels that occur following food intake, the levels of glycated proteins serve as good indices for monitoring diabetes patients during therapy. In particular, the hemoglobin A1c (HbA1c) value, an index of the medical condition of diabetes patients, measures the amount of the valine residue at the amino end of the hemoglobin β-subunit that is glycated. One way to measure HbA1c employs the enzyme fructosyl-amino acid oxidase isolated from a strain of *Corynebacterium*. This

TABLE 8.6 Stabilities and activities of various modified versions of tPA

tPA variant	Modification(s)	Stability in plasma	Fibrin binding	Activity in plasma	Activity vs. clots
1	Thr(103)→Asn	10	0.34	0.68	0.56
2	LysHisArgArg(296–299)→AlaAlaAlaAla	0.85	0.93	0.13	1.01
3	Thr(103)→Asn,KysHisargArg(296–299)→AlaAlaAlaAla	5.3	0.33	0.13	0.65
4	Thr(103)→Asn, Ans(117)→Gln	3.4	1.0	1.13	1.17
5	LysHisArgArg(296–299)→AlaAlaAlaAla, Ans(17) Gln	1.2	1.33	0.16	1.38
6	Thr(103)→Asn, LysHisArgArg(296–299)→AlaAlaAlaAla, Asn(117)→Gln	8.3	0.87	0.06	0.85

Adapted from Keyt et al., *Proc. Natl. Acad. Sci. USA* 91:3670–3674, 1994.

All of the values shown are normalized to the wild type. Plasma stability is the reciprocal of the time it takes for plasma clearance, larger numbers indicate a more stable derivative. Fibrin specificity is reflected by a high activity versus clots and a lows activity in plasma.

enzyme is specific for D-fructosyl-L-valine and does not have any activity toward N^ε-fructosyl-L-lysine, the glycated amino acid associated with serum albumin. Thus, the high level of substrate specificity of the *Corynebacterium* enzyme is essential for the accurate enzymatic determination of the amount of HbA1c. The one problem with the *Corynebacterium* enzyme is that it is relatively unstable. To remedy this problem, *E. coli* cells were transformed with a plasmid containing the *Corynebacterium* sp. gene for fructosyl-amino acid oxidase. The transformed E. coli strain was then subjected to repeated rounds of in vivo mutagenesis and screening for stable enzyme activity by measuring the enzyme activity following a 10-minute incubation of the enzyme at a temperature of 47°C. In each round of in vivo mutagenesis, cells were grown in culture and 10,000 cells were plated on medium containing D-fructosyl-L-valine. The fructosyl-amino acid oxidase gene from the most stable clone was isolated and sequenced, and that clone became the starting point for the next round of in vivo mutagenesis. As can be seen in Table 8.7, each successive round produced a more stable enzyme with additional amino acid changes. Importantly, in each round, the enzyme activity remained essentially unchanged; in fact, the mutant selected following four rounds of in vivo mutagenesis had slightly increased activity compared to the starting enzyme. Thus, this simple directed-evolution procedure resulted in an enzyme with significantly increased stability and the possibility of greater practical utility.

Enteropeptidase. The enzyme enteropeptidase (sometimes referred to as enterokinase) is a membrane-bound serine protease from the duodenal mucosa consisting of two polypeptide chains that converts the inactive

TABLE 8.7 Increasing thermostability of fructosyl-amino acid oxidase with increasing rounds of in vivo mutagenesis

Round no.	% Activity remaining after 10 min at 47°C	Changes to wild-type amino acid sequence
0	1	None
1	30	Ala-188→Gly-188, Met-244→Leu-244
2	70	Ala-60→Thr-60, Ala-188→Gly-188, Met-244→Leu-244
3	80	Ala-60→Thr-60, Ala-188→Gly-188, Met-244→Leu-244, Leu-261→Met-261
4	90	Ala-60→Thr-60, Ala-188→Gly-188, Met-244→Leu-244, Asn-27→Ser-257, Leu-261→Met-261

FIGURE 8.25 A target protein with an N-terminal polyhistidine tail, which may be specifically excised by digestion with an enteropeptidase (EP) that recognizes the Asp-Asp-Asp-Asp-Lys sequence.

precursor trypsinogen to active trypsin. The bovine or porcine version of this enzyme is often used to excise polyhistidine tags from recombinant proteins produced in *E. coli*. This is achieved by including a recognition site for enteropeptidase (Asp-Asp-Asp-Asp-Lys) between the polyhistidine tag and the target protein (Fig. 8.25). While this strategy works reasonably well, the enteropeptidases that are currently used to remove polyhistidine tags digest proteins at other amino acid sequences to a significant extent, leading to varying amounts of hydrolysis of the target protein. While this may not be a significant problem when proteins are purified on a laboratory scale, on an industrial scale, anything that lowers the final yield of the target protein is a problem. Therefore, researchers have sought to identify enzymes that recognize the same site as bovine and porcine enteropeptidases but lack their nonspecific peptidase activity. One group of researchers isolated and expressed cDNA encoding enteropeptidase from the medaka *(Oryzias latipes)*, a freshwater teleost fish. The enzyme encoded by this organism has a level of activity comparable to those of the bovine and porcine enzymes toward synthetic substrates containing the Asp-Asp-Asp-Asp-Lys sequence and only about 1/10 the level of activity of the bovine and porcine enzymes against peptide substrates lacking this sequence. To better understand the strict specificity of the medaka enzyme compared to the mammalian enzymes, several mutations were created in the gene for the medaka enzyme by site-specific mutagenesis. Amino acid residues that were conserved in four different mammalian versions of the enzyme but not in the medaka enzyme were identified at five different sites. These sequences were altered in the medaka enzyme to reflect the amino acids used in the mammalian enzymes. When these mutant enzymes were tested, one had about 90% of the activity of the native medaka enzyme against synthetic peptides containing the Asp-Asp-Asp-Asp-Lys sequence and as little as a fifth of the medaka native enzyme's activity against peptides lacking this sequence. In other words, one of the mutant enzymes was significantly better at reducing unwanted nonspecific activities than the native enzyme. This mutant was tested with several different fusion proteins with a histidine tag and an Asp-Asp-Asp-Asp-Lys sequence. In all cases, the enzyme efficiently excised the histidine tag and Asp-Asp-Asp-Asp-Lys sequence without degrading the target protein to any detectable extent. This was in marked contrast to the mammalian enzymes, which in all cases significantly degraded the target proteins. Thus, by changing a single amino acid residue, it was possible to generate an enzyme with an altered specificity that was more beneficial for biotechnological processes.

Altering Multiple Properties

Subtilisin. Generally, directed mutagenesis has been used to alter a single property of a protein. However, changing one property of an enzyme often disrupts other important characteristics. One possible solution to this problem is the "molecular breeding" of new proteins starting from several similar genes. Portions of these genes are recombined by DNA shuffling to produce a large number of new proteins. This approach does not require any prior knowledge of the structure and function of the target protein.

The validity of this concept was tested starting with 26 different subtilisin genes isolated from different *Bacillus* strains. After the DNA was shuffled, a library of chimeras was constructed and transformed into *B. subtilis*. The library of 654 clones that was generated represented only a small portion of the total number of chimeras that could be produced. The enzyme secreted by each clone in the library, as well as each of the 26 parent enzymes, was assayed (in a microtiter plate) for activity at 23°C, thermostability, solvent stability, and pH dependence (Fig. 8.26), traits that are useful in one or more industrial applications. Of the 654 clones tested, 77 produced enzymes that performed as well as or better than the best parent strain at 23°C. For each parameter that was tested, a number of enzymes with improved performance were detected. When these "superior" clones were sequenced, all of the genes were chimeric. In one instance, one of the chimeric genes included eight crossovers that produced a protein with 15 amino acid substitutions compared with the most similar parent. This library, produced by molecular breeding, contains functional genes that are more altered in sequence from the starting sequence than can be achieved by multiple rounds of mutagenesis of a single parent.

Often, the properties that are desirable for use in an industrial process do not exist among naturally occurring enzymes because these properties are not especially useful in nature. For example, an enzyme that is both highly active at 23°C and stable at 70°C is unlikely to have been selected for under natural conditions. However, using molecular breeding should make it easier to develop enzymes with properties that can be used as components of industrial processes.

Peroxidase. The enzyme peroxidase from the ink cap mushroom *Coprinus cinereus* has been used as a dye transfer inhibitor in laundry detergent. This enzyme acts by oxidizing, and therefore decolorizing, free dyes that have leached out of clothing, thereby preventing their uptake by other garments. Unfortunately, under wash conditions using bleach-containing detergents, high pH (10.5), high temperature (50°C), and high peroxide concentration (5 to 10 mM) rapidly inactivate *C. cinereus* peroxidase. To use this enzyme as a dye transfer inhibitor in laundry detergent, it is essential that the enzyme withstand high pH, temperature, and peroxide levels; therefore, a strategy for engineering this enzyme had to be developed.

While it is a relatively straightforward matter to shuffle DNA and isolate hybrid genes with unique properties when two or more similar genes are available, this approach cannot be used when starting with a single gene. Rather, the most effective strategy is probably either random mutagenesis or error-prone PCR. However, one group of researchers utilized an approach that combined either random mutagenesis or error-prone PCR with DNA shuffling (Fig. 8.27). Based on their knowledge of

FIGURE 8.26 Screening and testing a shuffled DNA library of the subtilisin gene family. First, the entire library is plated in a grid formation on agar plates containing 2% skim milk, and the clones that generate a zone of clearance because they have digested the milk proteins are picked, numbered, and cultured. Second, the chosen colonies are grown under different conditions in 96-well microtiter plates before a chromogenic substrate is added. Enzyme activity is quantified by the intensity of the color that is formed.

FIGURE 8.27 Simplified version of a scheme used to generate mutants in which several traits are altered at once. The stars indicate point mutations. The colored regions represent segments generated by site-directed or random mutagenesis after DNA shuffling. Only a small number of protein variants are shown.

the three-dimensional structure of peroxidase from *C. cinereus,* scientists used site-directed mutagenesis to replace solvent-exposed amino acids with those with nonoxidizable side chains and to introduce stabilizing features, such as disulfide bridges, into the protein. To identify other areas of the protein that it might be beneficial to change, the gene was subjected to error-prone PCR, and several beneficial mutants were isolated. When all of the mutations that were successful in improving the properties of the enzyme were combined into a single genetic construct, the resultant enzyme had a 114-fold improvement in thermal stability and a 2.8-fold improvement in oxidative stability. Unfortunately, although these changes were in the right direction, they were insufficient to adequately protect the enzyme against actual wash conditions. Following another round of random mutagenesis, the genes of all of the beneficial mutants were used as a starting point for a round of DNA shuffling. Eventually, an enzyme with a 174-fold increase in thermal stability and a 100-fold increase in oxidative stability compared with the native enzyme was isolated. Not only was the enzyme that was engineered suitable for use as a dye transfer inhibitor in laundry detergent, but this approach may also be used with a variety of enzymes to improve two or more properties at the same time.

SUMMARY

The proper functioning of a protein is due to its conformation, which is a consequence of its amino acid sequence and subunit structure. Certain amino acids in a polypeptide chain play important roles in determining the specificity, thermostability, and other properties of a protein. Changing even a single nucleotide of the gene encoding a target protein can result in the incorporation of an amino acid that can either disrupt the normal activity or enhance a specific property of the protein. With the emergence of recombinant DNA technology, it has become possible to replace nucleotides of a cloned gene and to produce proteins with specific amino acids at defined sites. This procedure is called directed mutagenesis, and it can be performed in various ways. To change a particular amino acid within a protein, the target gene is first subcloned onto bacteriophage M13 DNA. The single-stranded form of this bacteriophage is then copied by using an oligonucleotide primer that is designed to introduce a specified nucleotide into the target gene. *E. coli* cells are transformed with the double-stranded M13, and some of the M13 bacteriophage progeny carry a variant of the cloned gene that contains the mutation. These bacteriophages are identified, the altered gene is subcloned into an expression vector, and the expressed protein is tested for activity. There are also plasmid- and PCR-based strategies for introducing these kinds of changes into cloned genes. In many instances, the amino acid change(s) that might enhance a particular property of a target protein is not known a priori. In these cases, random mutagenesis, error-prone PCR, or DNA shuffling, rather than oligonucleotide-directed mutagenesis, is preferred.

The choice of which amino acid to change is often based on knowledge of the role of a particular amino acid in the functional protein. This knowledge comes from genetic studies or X-ray crystallographic data of the three-dimensional organization of the protein. Specific sites or regions can be altered, or combined, to improve the thermostability, pH tolerance, specificity, allosteric regulation, cofactor requirements, and other properties of enzymes that are used in industrial processes. For example, thermostability has been enhanced by changing amino acids at two sites in the enzyme triosephosphate isomerase, and the protease sensitivity of streptokinase has been decreased by changing two lysine residues to glutamine. Not only are these approaches helpful in engineering new properties for existing proteins, but they can also be used to design unique enzymes.

REFERENCES

Ahern, T. J., J. I. Casal, G. A. Petsko, and A. M. Klibanov. 1987. Control of oligomeric enzyme thermostability by protein engineering. *Proc. Natl. Acad. Sci. USA* 84:675–679.

Andersson, C. I. J., N. Holmberg, J. Farrés, J. E. Bailey, L. Bülow, and P. T. Kallio. 2000. Error-prone PCR of *Vitreoscilla* hemoglobin (VHb) to support the growth of microaerobic *Escherichia coli. Biotechnol. Bioeng.* 70:446–455.

Bittker, J. A., B. V. Le, and D. R. Liu. 2002. Nucleic acid evolution and minimization by nonhomologous random recombination. *Nat. Biotechnol.* 20:1024–1029.

Brange, J., U. Ribel, J. F. Hansen, G. Dodson, M. T. Hansen, S. Havelund, S. G. Melberg, F. Norris, K. Norris, L. Snel, A. R. Sorensen, and H. O. Voigt. 1988. Monomeric insulins obtained by protein engineering and their medical implications. *Nature* 333:679–682.

Chatterjee, R. and L. Yuan. 2006. Directed evolution of metabolic pathways. *Trends Biotechnol.* 24:28–38.

Chen, K., and F. H. Arnold. 1991. Enzyme engineering for nonaqueous solvents: random mutagenesis to enhance activity of subtilisin E in polar organic media. *Bio/Technology* 9:1073–1077.

Cherry, J. R., M. H. Lamsa, P. Schneider, J. Vind, A. Svendsen, A. Jones, and A. H. Pedersen. 1999. Directed evolution of a fungal peroxidase. *Nat. Biotechnol.* 17:379–384.

Döring, V., H. D. Mootz, L. A. Nangle, T. L. Hendrickson, V. de Crécy-Lagard, P. Schimmel, and P. Marlière. 2001. Enlarging the amino acid set of *Escherichia coli* by infiltration of the valine coding pathway. *Science* 292:501–504.

Eijsink, V. G. H., A. Bjørk, S. Gåseidnes, R. Sirevåg, B. Synstad, B. van den Burg, and G. Vriend. 2004. Rational engineering of enzyme stability. *J. Biotechnol.* 113:105–120.

Herlitze, S., and M. Koenen. 1990. A general and rapid mutagenesis method using polymerase chain reaction. *Gene* 91:143–147.

Hermes, J. D., S. M. Parekh, S. C. Blacklow, H. Köster, and J. R. Knowles. 1989. A reliable method for random mutagenesis: the generation of mutant libraries using spiked oligodeoxyribonucleotide primers. *Gene* 84:143–151.

Kaur, J., and R. Sharma. 2006. Directed evolution: an approach to engineer enzymes. *Crit. Rev. Biotechnol.* 26:165–199.

Keyt, B. A., N. F. Paoni, C. J. Refino, L. Berleau, H. Nguyen, A. Chow, J. Lai, L. Peña, C. Pater, J. Ogez, T. Etcheverry, D. Botstein, and W. F. Bennett. 1994. A faster-acting and more potent form of tissue plasminogen activator. *Proc. Natl. Acad. Sci. USA* 91:3670–3674.

Kim, Y.-G., J. Cha, and S. Chandrasegaran. 1996. Hybrid restriction enzymes: zinc finger fusions to FokI cleavage domain. *Proc. Natl. Acad. Sci. USA* 93:1156–1160.

Kirchhoff, F., and R. C. Desrosiers. 1995. Random mutagenesis of short target DNA sequences via PCR with degenerate oligonucleotides. *Methods Mol. Biol.* 57:323–333.

Landt, O., H.-P. Grunert, and U. Hahn. 1990. A general method for rapid site-directed mutagenesis using the polymerase chain reaction. *Gene* 96:125–128.

Mark, D. F., S. D. Lu, A. A. Creasey, R. Yamamoto, and L. S. Lin. 1984. Site-specific mutagenesis of the human fibroblast interferon gene. *Proc. Natl. Acad. Sci. USA* 81:5662–5666.

Matsumura, M., G. Signor, and B. W. Mathews. 1989. Substantial increase of protein stability by multiple disulfide bonds. *Nature* 342:291–293.

Michnick, S. W., and F. H. Arnold. 1999. "Itching" for new strategies in protein engineering. *Nat. Biotechnol.* 17:1159–1160.

Miyazaki, C., Y. Iba, Y. Yamada, H. Takahashi, J. Sawada, and Y. Kurosawa. 1999. Changes in the specificity of antibodies by site-specific mutagenesis followed by random mutagenesis. *Protein Eng.* 12:407–415.

Murakami, H., T. Hohsaka, and M. Sisido. 2002. Random insertion and deletion of arbitrary number of bases for codon-based random mutation of DNAs. *Nat. Biotechnol.* 20:76–81.

Ness, J. E., M. Welch, L. Giver, M. Bueno, J. R. Cherry, T. V. Borchert, W. P. C. Stemmer, and J. Minshull. 1999. DNA shuffling of subgenomic sequences of subtilisin. *Nat. Biotechnol.* 17:893–896.

Nosoh, Y., and T. Sekiguchi. 1990. Protein engineering for thermostability. *Trends Biotechnol.* 8:16–20.

Ogiwara, K., and T. Takahashi. 2007. Specificity of the medaka enteropeptidase serine protease and its usefulness as a biotechnological tool for fusion-protein cleavage. *Proc. Natl. Acad. Sci. USA* 104:7021–7026.

Piccoli, R., S. Di Gaetano, C. De Lorenzo, M. Grauso, C. Monaco, D. Spalletti-Cernia, P. Laccetti, J. Cinátl, J. Matousek, and G. D'Alessio. 1999. A dimeric mutant of human pancreatic ribonuclease with selective cytotoxicity toward malignant cells. *Proc. Natl. Acad. Sci. USA* 96:7768–7773.

Piechocki, M. P., and R. N. Hines. 1994. Oligonucleotide design and optimized protocol for site-directed mutagenesis. *BioTechniques* 16:702–707.

Sakaue, R., and N. Kajiyama. 2003. Thermostabilization of bacterial fructosyl-amino acid oxidase by directed evolution. *Appl. Environ. Microbiol.* 69:139–145.

Smith, M. 1985. In vitro mutagenesis. *Annu. Rev. Genet.* 19:423–462.

Stemmer, W. P. C. 1994. DNA shuffling by random fragmentation and reassembly: in vitro recombination for molecular evolution. *Proc. Natl. Acad. Sci. USA* 91:10747–10751.

Strausberg, S. L., P. A. Alexander, D. T. Gallagher, G. L. Gilliland, B. L. Barnett, and P. N. Bryan. 1995. Directed evolution of a subtilisin with calcium-independent stability. *Bio/Technology* 13:669–673.

Varadarajan, N., J. Gam, M. J. Olsen, G. Georgiou, and B. L. Iverson 2005. Engineering of protease variants exhibiting high catalytic activity and exquisite substrate selectivity. *Proc. Natl. Acad. Sci. USA* 102:6855–6860.

Wakarchuk, W. W., W. L. Sung, R. L. Campbell, A. Cunningham, D. C. Watson, and M. Yaguchi. 1994. Thermostabilization of the *Bacillus circulans* xylanase by the introduction of disulfide bonds. *Protein Eng.* 7:1379–1386.

Wang, L., A. Brock, B. Herberich, and P. G. Schultz. 2001. Expanding the genetic code of *Escherichia coli*. *Science* 292:498–500.

Wetzel, R., L. J. Perry, and C. Veilleux. 1991. Mutations in human interferon gamma affecting inclusion body formation identified by a general immunochemical screen. *Bio/Technology* 9:731–737.

Wilkinson, A. J., A. R. Fersht, D. M. Blow, P. Carter, and G. Winter. 1984. A large increase in enzyme-substrate affinity by protein engineering. *Nature* 307:187–188.

Wu, X.-C., R. Ye, Y. Duan, and S.-L. Wong. 1998. Engineering of plasmin-resistant forms of streptokinase and their production in *Bacillus subtilis*: streptokinase with longer functional half-life. *Appl. Environ. Microbiol.* 64:824–829.

Zoller, M. J., and M. Smith. 1982. Oligonucleotide-directed mutagenesis using M13-derived vectors: an efficient and general procedure for the production of point mutations in any fragment of DNA. *Nucleic Acids Res.* 10:6487–6500.

REVIEW QUESTIONS

1. What physical and chemical properties of enzymes are targets for enhancement by directed mutagenesis?

2. You have cloned a bacterial gene that is expressed in *E. coli*, and now you want to alter its activity. However, because of technical problems with the original M13 protocol, only a very small fraction of the mutagenized clones of this gene actually carry the modified gene; the vast majority of the clones contain the unaltered form of the gene. How would you perform site-specific mutagenesis so that a much larger proportion of the clones have the desired mutation?

3. You have isolated a gene for an enzyme that is expressed in *E. coli*. Describe how you would alter the catalytic activity of the enzyme. Assume that you know the DNA sequence of the gene but do not know anything about which regions of the enzyme are important for catalytic activity.

4. Discuss the advantages and disadvantages of oligonucleotide-directed mutagenesis using either bacteriophage M13 or PCR.

5. Describe a strategy for oligonucleotide-directed mutagenesis that uses plasmid DNA containing the gene of interest.

6. How can degenerate oligonucleotides be used to generate random mutations within a cloned DNA fragment?

7. Describe a strategy for increasing the stability of a protein that has (1) no cysteine residues or (2) an odd number of cysteine residues?

8. How might replacing asparagine with another amino acid residue affect the stability of a protein?

9. How can the cofactor requirements of an enzyme be altered?

10. Describe how you would change the catalytic activity or substrate specificity of an enzyme whose gene you have isolated. Why would you want to do this?

11. What is error-prone PCR, and why is it useful?

12. Outline two ways in which DNA shuffling may be used to generate hybrid genes.

13. How can unusual amino acids be incorporated into proteins, thereby producing an altered form of the target protein?

14. How would you engineer human pancreatic RNase to be an antitumorigenic agent?

15. How would you engineer streptokinase so that it was less sensitive to proteolytic digestion?

16. How can the gene(s) encoding a Fab fragment of a monoclonal antibody be modified so that the specificity of the antibody is altered?

17. What is molecular breeding? How can this approach be used to simultaneously engineer several properties of a protein?

18. Starting from a single enzyme-encoding gene, how can DNA shuffling be used to engineer an enzyme in which several separate and distinct properties have been modified?

19. How would you use PCR-amplified oligonucleotide-directed mutagenesis to create insertion mutants? Deletion mutants?

20. How would you generate random insertion/deletion mutations in a target gene on a plasmid?

21. What is nonhomologous random recombination, and how would you use it to generate modified enzymes?

22. How would you engineer an enzyme with a high level of activity toward one substrate to have a high level of activity for a different substrate and a low level of activity toward the original substrate?

23. How would you ensure that an enteropeptidase cleaved only at the target site within the protein of interest and nowhere else?

This page intentionally left blank

MOLECULAR BIOTECHNOLOGY OF MICROBIAL SYSTEMS

WITH THE ADVENT OF RECOMBINANT DNA TECHNOLOGY, many of the properties of microorganisms that might be useful in a variety of applications can be more readily exploited. In part II, we examine some of the uses for genetically engineered microbial systems.

Currently, bacteria are being genetically manipulated to act as biological factories for the production of pharmaceutical proteins, nucleic acid therapeutic agents, restriction endonucleases, chemical compounds, amino acids, antibiotics, and biopolymers. In some applications, cloned genes have been introduced into bacterial host cells to create novel biosynthetic pathways that produce novel metabolites. Genes and DNA fragments from pathogenic organisms have been isolated and used as probes for the diagnosis of disease in both animals and humans. In other instances, isolated genes and DNA fragments have been used to produce safer and more efficacious vaccines.

Genetic manipulation of microbial systems also entails enhancing the natural ability of certain bacterial strains to carry out specific biological processes. For example, researchers have developed bacterial strains that can degrade environmental pollutants, improve the growth of plant crops, degrade cellulosic biomass into utilizable low-molecular-weight compounds, and prevent the proliferation of specific insect pests.

It is often assumed that the growth of large quantities of microbes is a routine procedure. Successful large-scale production of proteins synthesized

by recombinant microorganisms, however, requires that many different factors be controlled during both the growth phase of the microorganism and the purification process to ensure that high yields of a pure product are obtained.

9

Molecular Diagnostics

THE SUCCESS OF MODERN MEDICINE and agriculture often depends on the ability of workers in these fields to detect the presence of specific viruses, bacteria, fungi, parasites, proteins, and small molecules in humans, animals, plants, water, and soil. For example, the prevention, control, or treatment of infectious disease is generally facilitated by the early and accurate identification of the causative pathogenic organism. Many of these detection procedures require the growth in culture of the potential pathogen and then the analysis of a spectrum of physiological properties that facilitate its identification. Although tests of this type are effective and reasonably specific, they are often slow and costly. These constraints apply to the identification of both bacterial and parasitic (Table 9.1) organisms. In addition, if the pathogenic organism does not grow well or cannot be cultivated, the opportunity to detect the disease-causing organism is severely limited. For example, *Chlamydia trachomatis,* an obligately intracellular bacterium, causes a sexually transmitted disease prevalent in North America and Europe. Clinical diagnosis of chlamydial infection is difficult, because long-term cell culture is required. Frequently, false-negative results (i.e., the diagnosis of the absence of the organism is erroneous) are obtained, and consequently, adequate treatment procedures are not implemented. Certainly, if growth were required for detection, then at best only a few of all known pathogenic organisms could ever be routinely identified. To overcome this major constraint, molecular diagnostic procedures using either immunological or DNA detection methodologies have been devised.

In general, any useful detection strategy must be specific, sensitive, and simple. Specificity means that the assay must yield a positive response for only the target organism or molecule. Sensitivity means that the diagnostic test must identify very small amounts of the target organism or molecule, even in the presence of other potentially interfering organisms or substances. Simplicity is required for the test to be run efficiently, effectively, and inexpensively on a routine basis.

TABLE 9.1 A comparison of some of the methods used to diagnose parasite infection

Method	Advantages	Disadvantages
Microscopic examination	Simple Direct detection of parasite Differentiates morphologically distinct organisms	Slow, laborious, and tedious Low sensitivity Cannot discriminate between similar organisms Requires a high skill level
In vitro culture and mouse inoculation	Detects only viable parasites Measures virulence and infectivity	Slow and expensive Different strains show a range of responses Parasite may lose its viability in the specimen Uses animals
Detection of antibodies in serum	Simple and fast Automatable Can be used to screen a large number of samples	Not always specific Does not distinguish between active and latent infections
DNA hybridization and PCR	Fast, sensitive, and specific Detects parasite directly Can distinguish different species Independent of previous infections Parasites need not be viable Automatable	Expensive and multistep Does not distinguish between live and dead organisms Possible false positives and false negatives

Adapted from Weiss, *Clin. Microbiol Rev.* **8:**113–130, 1995.

It is estimated that worldwide sales of immunodiagnostics accounted for approximately $7.7 billion in 1999, and this figure continues to increase by 5 to 10% per year. The market for DNA-based diagnostic procedures was around $500 million in 1999 and is increasing at around 20 to 30% per year, so that in 2004 it was worth approximately $2 billion. In this chapter, the principles behind some of these molecular diagnostic procedures and the use of these procedures for a variety of applications are discussed.

Immunological Diagnostic Procedures

Many immunological detection methods are sensitive, specific, and simple. They can be used for a wide range of applications, including drug testing, assessment and monitoring of various cancers, detection of specific metabolites, pathogen identification, and monitoring infectious agents. However, there are limitations. For example, if the target is a protein, then the use of antibodies requires that the genes contributing to the presence of the target site be expressed and that the target site not be masked or blocked in any way that would prevent the binding of the antibody.

In principle, traditional diagnostic procedures for infectious agents rely on either a discrete set of traits characteristic of the pathogenic agent or, preferably, one unique, readily distinguishable feature. The clinical microbiologist searches for the smallest number of biological characteristics that

can, with complete certainty, reveal the presence and precise identity of a pathogenic agent. For example, some infectious agents produce distinctive biochemical molecules. The problem is how to determine when the identifying component is present in a biological sample. Often, such a marker molecule can be identified directly in a specialized biochemical assay that is very specific for the marker molecule. The problem with this approach is that it can potentially lead to a proliferation of highly individualized detection systems for different pathogenic organisms. A standardized method of identifying any key marker molecule, regardless of its chemical nature, is preferred. Because antibodies bind with high specificity to discrete target sites (antigens), assays based solely on identifying specific antibody–antigen complexes have abolished the need to devise a unique identification procedure for each particular marker molecule.

ELISA

There are a number of different ways to determine whether an antibody has bound to its target antigen. The enzyme-linked immunosorbent assay (ELISA) is one method, and it is frequently used for diagnostic detection. The ELISA procedure may be either indirect (Fig. 9.1A) or direct (Fig. 9.1B). A generalized indirect ELISA protocol (Fig. 9.1A) has the following steps.

1. Bind the sample being tested for the presence of a specific molecule or organism to a solid support, such as a plastic microtiter plate, which usually contains 96 sample wells. Wash the support to remove unbound molecules.

2. Add a marker-specific antibody (primary antibody directed against the target antigen) to the bound material, and then wash the support to remove unbound primary antibody.

3. Add a second antibody (secondary antibody) that binds specifically to the primary antibody and not to the target molecule. Bound (conjugated) to the secondary antibody is an enzyme, such as alkaline phosphatase, peroxidase, or urease, that can catalyze a reaction that converts a colorless substrate into a colored product. Wash the mixture to remove any unbound secondary antibody–enzyme conjugate.

4. Add the colorless substrate.

5. Observe or measure the amount of colored product.

If the primary antibody does not bind to a target site in the sample, the second washing step removes it. Consequently, the secondary antibody–enzyme conjugate has nothing to bind to and is removed during the third washing step, and the final mixture remains colorless. Conversely, if the target site is present in the sample, then the primary antibody binds to it, the secondary antibody binds to the primary antibody, and the attached enzyme catalyzes the reaction to form an easily detected colored product. Since secondary antibodies that are complexed with an enzyme are available commercially, each new diagnostic test requires only a unique primary antibody. In addition, several secondary antibody molecules, each with several enzyme molecules attached, bind to one primary antibody molecule, thereby amplifying the intensity of the signal.

With a direct ELISA protocol (Fig. 9.1B), a monoclonal antibody specific for the target antigen is first bound to the surface of the microtiter plate. To

FIGURE 9.1 Generalized ELISA protocol for detecting a target antigen. The primary antibody is often obtained from rabbits that have been immunized with the target antigen, while the secondary antibody is from goats immunized with rabbit antibodies. The enzyme (E) is conjugated to the secondary antibody. **(A)** Indirect ELISA; **(B)** direct ELISA.

assess the amount of a particular antigen in a sample, the sample is added to the well of the microtiter plate and allowed to interact with the bound antibody. This is followed by a wash to remove any unbound molecules. Then, the primary antibody and the secondary antibody conjugated to an enzyme are added, as described above, before the presence of bound antigen is visualized.

The principal feature of an ELISA system is the specific binding of the primary antibody to the target site. If the target molecule is, for example, a protein, then a purified preparation of this protein is generally used to generate the antibodies that will be used to detect the target. The resulting antibody mixture, which is found in the serum (antiserum) of an inoculated animal, usually a rabbit, contains a number of different antibodies that would each bind to a different antigenic determinant (epitope) on the target molecule. Such a mixture of antibodies is called a polyclonal preparation. For some diagnostic assays, the use of polyclonal antibodies has two drawbacks: (1) the amounts of the different antibodies within a polyclonal preparation may vary from one batch to the next, and (2) polyclonal antibodies cannot be used to distinguish between two similar targets, e.g., when the difference between the pathogenic form (target) and the nonpathogenic one (nontarget) is a single determinant. However, these problems can be overcome, because it is now possible to generate an antibody preparation that is directed against a single antigenic determinant, namely, a monoclonal antibody. Also, despite these drawbacks, diagnostic assays employing polyclonal antibodies are widely used for a variety of purposes.

Monoclonal Antibodies

In mammals, a complex set of cellular systems has evolved to protect the body from toxic substances and invasion by infectious agents. As part of the defensive response, cells of the lymphatic system can be induced to produce specific proteins (antibodies) that bind to foreign substances (antigens) and—with the help of other immune system proteins, including the complement system—neutralize their biological impact. In response to an immunological challenge, each antibody-producing cell synthesizes and secretes a single antibody that recognizes with high affinity a discrete region (epitope, or antigenic determinant) of the immunizing antigen. Because an antigen generally has several different epitopes, normally several cells of the immune system each produce a different antibody against one of the many epitopes of the antigen. Such a set of antibodies, all of which react with the same antigen, is designated a polyclonal antibody (Fig. 9.2).

Early in the 20th century, although the polyclonal nature of antibodies was not appreciated, it was realized that antibody specificity could be used to prevent infections. Later, antibodies were used as diagnostic agents to determine the presence of toxic substances in clinical samples. Unfortunately, the effectiveness of a polyclonal antibody preparation varies from batch to batch because, in some immunizations, certain antigenic determinants of a particular antigen are strong stimulators of antibody-producing cells, whereas at other times, the immune system responds more actively to different epitopes of the same antigen. Also, individual animals often respond differently to a particular antigen. This variation can affect the abilities of different preparations to neutralize antigens because different epitopes have different potencies (stimulating abilities). Hence, one batch of polyclonal antibody may have a low level of antibody molecules directed against a major epitope and not be as effective as a previous antibody preparation.

Consequently, a fundamental objective for the applied use of antibodies, as diagnostic agents or as components of therapeutic agents, was to discover how to create a cell line that could be grown in culture and that would produce a single type of antibody molecule (monoclonal antibody) with a high affinity for a specific target antigen. Such a cell line would provide a consistent and continuous source of identical antibody molecules. Unfortunately, the B lymphocytes (B cells) that synthesize antibodies do not reproduce in culture. However, it was envisioned that a hybrid cell type could be created to solve this problem. This hybrid would have the B-cell genetic components for producing antibodies and the cell division functions of a compatible cell type to enable the cells to grow in culture. It was known that normal B lymphocytes sometimes become cancer cells (myelomas) that acquire the ability to grow in culture while retaining many of the attributes of B cells. Thus, myeloma cells, especially those that did not produce antibody molecules, became candidates for fusion with antibody-producing B cells. In the mid-1970s, these ideas became reality.

Formation and Selection of Hybrid Cells

The initial step leading to the production of a hybrid cell line that produces a single antibody entails the inoculation of mice with an antigen. After

FIGURE 9.2 Schematic representation of a target antigen. The surface of the antigen depicted has seven (numbered 1 to 7) different antigenic determinants (epitopes). When this antigen is used to immunize an animal, each antigenic determinant elicits the synthesis of a different antibody. Together, the different antibodies that interact with an antigen constitute a polyclonal antibody directed against that antigen.

FIGURE 9.3 The HAT procedure for selecting hybrid spleen–myeloma (hybridoma) cells.

several inoculations over a period of a few weeks, the animals are tested, generally using an ELISA or similar system, to determine whether they have developed an immune response. If they have, they are killed and their spleens are removed, washed, minced, and gently agitated to release individual cells, some of which are antibody-producing B cells. The splenic cell suspension is mixed with a suspension of myeloma cells that are genetically defective for the enzyme hypoxanthine-guanine phosphoribosyltransferase (HGPRT⁻). The combined cell suspensions are mixed with 35% polyethylene glycol for a few minutes and then transferred to a growth medium containing hypoxanthine, aminopterin, and thymidine (HAT medium).

The polyethylene glycol treatment facilitates fusion between cells. Nevertheless, the fusion events are rare and random. There will be myeloma cells, spleen cells, myeloma–spleen fusion cells, myeloma–myeloma fusion cells, and spleen–spleen fusion cells in the mixture. The HAT medium, however, allows only the myeloma–spleen fusion cells to grow, because none of the other cell types can proliferate in this medium. Unfused spleen cells and spleen–spleen fusion cells cannot grow in any culture medium. The HGPRT⁻ myeloma and the myeloma–myeloma fusion cells cannot use hypoxanthine as a precursor for the biosynthesis of the purines guanine and adenine, which are, of course, essential for nucleic acid synthesis. However, they have a second, naturally occurring pathway for purine biosynthesis that utilizes the enzyme dihydrofolate reductase. Therefore, aminopterin is included in the medium because it inhibits dihydrofolate reductase activity. Hence, HGPRT⁻ myeloma and myeloma–myeloma fusion cells are unable to synthesize purines in HAT medium, so they die (Fig. 9.3).

The spleen–myeloma fusion cells survive in HAT medium because the spleen cell contributes a functional HGPRT, which can utilize the exogenous hypoxanthine in the medium even though purine production by means of dihydrofolate reductase is blocked by aminopterin, and because the cell division functions of the myeloma cell are active. Thymidine is provided to overcome the block in pyrimidine production that is caused by the inhibition of dihydrofolate reductase by aminopterin. About 10 to 14 days after the fusion treatment, only spleen–myeloma fusion cells have survived and grown in the HAT medium. These cells are then distributed into the wells of plastic microtiter plates and grown on complete culture medium without HAT.

Identification of Specific Antibody-Producing Hybrid Cell Lines

The next task is to identify those hybrid cells that produce antibody against the immunizing antigen. One common screening procedure uses the culture medium, which contains secreted antibodies. The medium is collected from the wells that have growing cells and is added to a well of another microtiter plate that has been precoated with the target antigen. If the culture medium contains an antibody (primary antibody) that recognizes an epitope of the antigen, it will bind to the antigen and not be washed away during a subsequent washing step. A second antibody (secondary antibody) that is specific for mouse antibodies is added to the wells of the test plate. It will bind to any primary antibody that is bound to the antigen.

Before its use in the immunoassay, the secondary antibody is conjugated to an enzyme that can convert a colorless substrate to a colored compound. The presence of color in one of the test wells indicates that the original culture medium contained an antibody that was specific for the antigen (Fig. 9.4). If the culture medium does not contain an antibody that binds to the antigen, then the first wash will remove the primary antibody. Therefore, when the secondary antibody is added, it has nothing to bind to and is removed by the second washing step. In a well where such a sequence of events occurs, the substrate solution remains colorless.

Those wells of the original microtiter plate whose media give a positive (color) response in the immunoassay may contain a mixture of cell fusions. These cells are therefore diluted with culture medium and seeded into fresh wells to establish cell lines from single cells (clones). After the clones have been cultured, their media are tested again to determine which cell lines (hybrid spleen–myeloma cells, or hybridomas) produce monoclonal antibody molecules that recognize the target antigen. If more than one specific hybridoma is isolated, further tests are conducted to determine whether the different clones produce antibody against the same antigenic determinant. Each monoclonal antibody-producing clone can be maintained, more or less indefinitely, in culture. In addition, samples can be frozen in liquid nitrogen to provide a source of cells for future use.

Because a monoclonal antibody binds to a single discrete site, the specificity of an ELISA protocol can be considerably enhanced by using a monoclonal rather than a polyclonal antibody. Many monoclonal antibodies have been developed for use as immunodiagnostic agents for a variety of compounds and pathogenic organisms (Table 9.2). As an alternative to the

FIGURE 9.4 Screening for the production of a monoclonal antibody. Spleen cells from a mouse that was immunized with a specific antigen are isolated and fused in culture with myeloma cells that do not produce antibodies. Fused cells are selected for the ability to grow on HAT medium, which contains hypoxanthine, aminopterin, and thymidine. Cells that produce a specific antibody to the immunizing antigen (hybridomas) are identified by an immunoassay and individually subcultured. A hybridoma, which grows in culture and secretes a single type of antibody molecules, is the source of a monoclonal antibody.

isolation and synthesis of monoclonal antibodies in hybridoma cells in culture, monoclonal antibodies and parts of antibodies (Fab or Fv fragments) directed against a target antigen may be selected and produced in *Escherichia coli* (see chapter 10).

Biofluorescent and Bioluminescent Systems

Proteins that naturally fluoresce or luminesce, or that can be easily induced to do so, may be used as biological reporters in a variety of ways. For example, genes encoding these bioreporter proteins may be used to engineer cells to produce a measurable signal in response to a particular chemical or physical agent in their environment. In one version of this system, a gene for a fluorescent or luminescent protein is placed under the control of a promoter that responds to certain environmental signals so that when the promoter is activated, a fluorescent or luminescent signal is produced (Fig. 9.5).

Colored Fluorescent Proteins

Green fluorescent protein. The 238-amino-acid-long photoprotein green fluorescent protein, isolated from the jellyfish *Aequorea victoria,* fluoresces green when it is exposed to ultraviolet light. While many fluorescent dyes are phototoxic, the incorporation of green fluorescent protein into cells allows intact living cells to be monitored in real time. The use of this reporter molecule has revolutionized fluorescence microscopy. Among its many uses, researchers have used green fluorescent protein to monitor tumor cells in gene therapy protocols, to assess the responses of specific cell types to various therapeutic drugs and treatments, to monitor protein-protein interactions, and to monitor the fates of individual proteins in different therapies.

Red fluorescent protein. Following the discovery and subsequent successful employment of green fluorescent protein, scientists began to search, both in nature and by directed mutagenesis, for other colored fluorescent proteins. Having multiple colored fluorescent proteins would enable several biological processes to be monitored at the same time. For the practical use of these proteins, it is essential that they be both as stable and as bright as possible. One problem with many of the naturally occurring colored fluorescent proteins is that they often have a tendency to form homodimers or homotetramers. Such multimeric structures can adversely influence the subcellular localization of the proteins, potentially leading to intracellular aggregation and other artifacts. One group of researchers isolated a gene for a red fluorescent protein from *Discosoma* coral and, by means of multiple random mutations, generated a mutant that existed exclusively as a monomer instead of as a tetramer. With each iterative cycle of random mutagenesis, proteins that yielded red fluorescence that was both bright and stable were selected. The production of monomeric red fluorescent protein required 33 mutations. This success notwithstanding, monomeric red fluorescent protein had several drawbacks compared to the native tetrameric form of the protein, including decreased brightness and reduced photostability.

TABLE 9.2 Targets for diagnostic monoclonal antibodies

Polypeptide hormones
Chorionic gonadotropin
Growth hormone
Luteinizing hormone
Follicle-stimulating hormone
Thyroid-stimulating hormone
Prolactin

Tumor markers
Carcinoembryonic antigen
Prostate-specific antigen
Interleukin-2 receptor
Epidermal growth factor receptor

Cytokines
Interleukins 1–8
Colony-stimulating factor

Drug monitoring
Theophylline
Gentamicin
Cyclosporin

Miscellaneous targets
Thyroxine
Vitamin B_{12}
Ferritin
Fibrin degradation products
Tau protein

Infectious disease
Chlamydia
Herpes
Rubella
Hepatitis B
Legionella
Human immunodeficiency virus

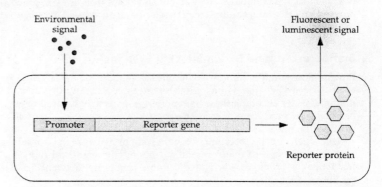

FIGURE 9.5 Schematic representation of a bacterial cell, engineered to respond to a particular environmental compound, producing a detectable fluorescent or bioluminescent signal.

To address some of the above-mentioned problems with monomeric red fluorescent protein, as well as to expand the repertoire of available fluorescent proteins, additional rounds of mutagenesis were performed. First, DNA encoding 7 amino acids from the N terminus of green fluorescent protein was added to the gene for red fluorescent protein (Fig. 9.6). Then, DNA for the 6 amino acids from the green fluorescent protein C terminus was added to the gene for the red fluorescent protein. This construct then became the starting point for several additional rounds of random mutagenesis and directed evolution. Eventually, seven different monomeric colored fluorescent proteins were produced (Fig. 9.7). It is argued that there is no one best colored fluorescent protein. Some are brighter than others, some are more photostable, and some are more sensitive to changes in pH. Thus, various fluorescent proteins may be used for different applications. Moreover, using two or three of these proteins, it is possible to label several different cellular components or cell types at once, thereby increasing the utility of this approach.

Luciferase

The luciferase enzyme, which catalyzes a light-emitting reaction, may be produced by a variety of different organisms, including bacteria, algae, fungi, jellyfish, insects, shrimp, and squid. Luciferase genes from bacteria are termed *lux* genes, while those from other organisms—the most widely studied and utilized being the firefly—are termed *luc* genes. The *lux* system includes five genes, *luxCDABE*, and produces a peak of light at 490 nm. In some applications, all five *lux* genes are utilized as a means of monitoring the presence and concentrations of various compounds in the environment, such as organic compounds, including phenol, salicylate, benzene, trichloroethylene, ammonia, xylene, toluene, and ethylbenezene, or metals, including cobalt, copper, iron, lead, mercury, nickel, and zinc. When all five genes are used, the light-generating system does not require the addition of any other compounds. Therefore, following the addition of a contaminant-containing sample to bacterial cells carrying *luxCDABE,* a quantifiable

amount of bioluminescence is produced within a period of a few minutes to no more than a few hours. In some cases, the reporter system includes only the *luxAB* genes. While *luxA* and *luxB* are together responsible for generating the light signal, this system requires that the substrate decanal be added during the assay procedure.

The firefly luciferase-catalyzed reaction results in the production of light at 550 to 575 nm. Moreover, the system requires the addition of the low-molecular-weight organic compound luciferin as a substrate for the light reaction. Typically, *luc* genes are used in conjunction with eukaryotic cells.

Microbial Biosensors

There is a need for methods that can easily and rapidly detect the large numbers of potentially toxic compounds that contaminate the environment. Once the contaminated sites have been identified and their range has been delineated, there are a number of highly sophisticated analytical techniques available to identify and quantify specific pollutants. Bacteria that are constitutively bioluminescent (i.e., unlike the situation mentioned above, the bioluminescence does not need to be induced) are good candidates for pollutant detectors. In the presence of pollutants, the bioluminescence decreases, providing a clear indication of the presence of the pollutants. Naturally bioluminescent bacteria, such as the marine bacterium *Vibrio fischeri*, require saline conditions and a particular pH range and are therefore not useful for testing terrestrial groundwater. However, structural genes encoding enzymes that lead to bioluminescence *(luxCDABE)* may be inserted into random sites in the chromosomal DNA of a soil bacterium, such as *Pseudomonas fluorescens*. These genes do not contain a transcriptional promoter, so after insertion into the chromosomal DNA of *P. fluorescens,* the only luminescent colonies (visualized in a darkroom) are those in which the *lux* genes are inserted downstream from a constitutive *P. fluorescens* promoter (without disrupting any important bacterial genes). The cells that luminesce to the greatest extent and have a growth rate similar to that of the wild-type strain are selected for testing with various environmental pollutants. To screen water samples for the presence of various pollutants (both metals and organic compounds), a suspension of bioluminescent *P. fluorescens* is mixed with the solution being tested, and after a 15-minute incubation together, the luminescence of the suspension

FIGURE 9.6 Construction of a modified monomeric red fluorescent protein (modified mRFP). The regions of the gene encoding the N and C termini of the green fluorescent protein (GFP) were spliced onto the gene for mRFP following the removal of the portion of the mRFP gene encoding the N terminus and the addition of an oligonucleotide encoding a short linker peptide (L).

Derivative number	1	2	3	4	5	6	7
Emission maximum (nm)	537, 562	553	562	581	585	596	610

FIGURE 9.7 Various colored monomeric fluorescent proteins derived from monomeric red fluorescent protein showing their emission wavelengths and color maxima following excitation. The colors have been called, from derivative 1 through 7, honeydew, banana, orange, tomato, tangerine, strawberry, and cherry, respectively. Adapted from Shaner et al., *Nat. Biotechnol.* **22:**1567–1572, 2004.

is measured in a luminometer (Fig. 9.8). When a test sample contains a low to moderate level of certain pollutants, the cell luminescence is inhibited, presumably because the pollutant directly interferes with bacterial metabolism. Since this procedure is rapid, simple, and inexpensive, it is a good first screen for assessing the presence of pollution at a particular site. After a positive response with a bacterial biosensor, the actual pollutants can be determined by other methods.

In the United States, it has been estimated that there are approximately 87,000 different chemical compounds that need to be tested for estrogenic activity, i.e., steroid-like activity that can disrupt the endocrine system in vertebrates. While a number of different methods exist that could be used to test these compounds, they are too slow for this sort of large-scale screening. Therefore, scientists have developed a simple and sensitive system for the rapid initial screening of these 87,000 compounds. With this system, yeast *(Saccharomyces cerevisiae)* cells have been genetically engineered to produce measurable quantities of light in the presence of extremely low levels of estrogenic compounds (Fig. 9.9). Using this method, in which luminescence is induced, to test for estrogenic compounds, light production could be detected in as little as 1 hour. Moreover, following 6 hours of incubation, the assay attained maximum bioluminescence when the engineered yeast cells were exposed to as little as 5×10^{-11} M 17β-estradiol, a common estrogen. Of course, many estrogenic compounds required higher concentrations in order to be detected. The main drawback of this approach is that the yeast cell wall and transport system facilitate the entry of some compounds into the cell and inhibit the uptake of other compounds. This can skew the results and in some instances may suggest that a compound is not estrogenic when it is unable to efficiently enter yeast cells. Nevertheless, this technique is likely to identify a large number of estrogenic compounds that were deemed nonestrogenic until they were tested with this protocol.

At the same time that some groups of scientists are working to develop and perfect cells as biosensors, others have focused their efforts on automating these systems. Such an automated system might include genetically engineered cells that emit blue-green light (~490 nm) in response to specific

FIGURE 9.8 Assaying for the presence of pollutants with genetically engineered bioluminescent *P. fluorescens*.

compounds, an environment that sustains the cells, a light-tight enclosure, and an integrated circuit for light detection and signal processing. While simple prototypes have been constructed, the difficulties associated with utilizing living cells remain major impediments.

Nucleic Acid Diagnostic Systems

The genetic material of an organism contains the essential information that contributes to its various features and characteristics. For example, bacterial pathogenicity may be due to the presence of a specific gene or set of genes. Similarly, alteration of a gene may cause an inherited genetic disease in humans. In theory, the sequence of nucleotides that contributes to a particular biological characteristic is a distinctive signature that, if detectable, can be used as a definitive diagnostic determinant.

Nucleic acid hybridization is the basis for rapid and reliable assays. The physical basis of these systems is precise nucleotide base pairing and hydrogen bonding between one string of nucleotides and a complementary nucleotide sequence. A general laboratory nucleic acid hybridization scheme is as follows.

1. Bind single-stranded DNA (the target) to a membrane support.
2. Add single-stranded labeled DNA (the probe) under appropriate conditions of temperature and ionic strength to promote base pairing between the probe and the target DNAs.
3. Wash the support to remove excess unbound labeled probe DNA.
4. Detect the hybrid sequences that form between the probe and target DNA.

FIGURE 9.9 Schematic representation of a strain of the yeast *Saccharomyces cerevisiae* that has been engineered to detect low levels of estrogenic substances in the environment. Each yeast cell contains the human estrogen receptor (hER) gene integrated into its chromosomal DNA, one plasmid (pUTK404) that contains constitutively expressed bacterial *luxCDE* genes and the flavin oxidoreductase (*frp*) gene from the bacterium *Vibrio harveyi*, and one plasmid (pUTK407) that contains *luxA* and *luxB* genes under the regulatory control of estrogen response elements (ERE) and constitutive bacterial promoters (not shown). Following the binding of the hER protein to an estrogenic compound, the complex binds to an ERE and activates *luxAB* transcription. Expression of the *luxAB*, *luxCDE*, and *frp* genes leads to the production of a measurable bioluminescent signal. Adapted from Sanseverino et al., *Appl. Environ. Microbiol.* **71**:4455–4460, 2005.

A nucleic acid hybridization diagnostic test has three critical elements: probe DNA, target DNA, and signal detection. This type of detection system can be both extremely specific and highly sensitive.

Hybridization Probes

To be effective, a nucleic acid hybridization probe must have a high degree of specificity. In other words, the probe must hybridize exclusively to the selected target nucleic acid sequence. False positives (i.e., responses in the

absence of the target sequence) and false negatives (i.e., no response when the target is present) severely undermine the utility of a diagnostic procedure. Probes can be specific at different organismic levels. They can distinguish between two or more species, determine particular strains within a given species, or identify differences between genes. Depending on the requirements of the test protocol, probes can be DNA or RNA, long (>100 nucleotides) or short (<50 nucleotides), and chemically synthesized, cloned intact genes, or isolated regions of a gene.

Sequences that might make effective probes can be isolated in a number of ways. For example, the DNA from a pathogenic organism can be cut with a restriction endonuclease and cloned into a plasmid vector. Recombinant plasmids are screened with the genomic DNA from both pathogenic and nonpathogenic strains. Those plasmids that contain sequences that hybridize only to the pathogenic strain form the basis for species-specific, and even strain-specific, probes (Fig. 9.10). Additional hybridization tests with DNA from a wide range of organisms are then conducted to ensure that the candidate probe sequences do not cross-hybridize. Each potential probe is also tested under simulated sample conditions, including the presence of mixed cultures, to determine its level of sensitivity. It is important to note that knowledge of the genomic sequence of a large number of bacterial pathogens (currently several hundred) has facilitated the identification of unique stretches of DNA that could be used as probes.

The ability to perform nucleic acid probe diagnostic assays directly on available samples without either additional culturing or time-consuming extraction procedures is extremely desirable, especially with clinical specimens. Researchers have successfully used probes that hybridize to target DNA from fecal samples, urine, blood, throat washes, and tissue samples without extensive DNA purification. If a target sequence is rare in the working sample, the polymerase chain reaction (PCR) can be used to amplify it.

Diagnosis of Malaria

An example of a diagnostic protocol that utilizes a DNA probe as a means of detection is the procedure developed for the detection of *Plasmodium falciparum*. This parasite causes malaria, a disease that affects about one-third of the world's population. The parasite infects and destroys red blood cells, leading to fever and, in severe cases, damage to the brain, kidneys, and other organs. Sensitive, simple, and inexpensive methods are required to identify the source(s) of the parasite in various localities, to assess the progress of eradication programs, and to facilitate early treatment. Currently, malarial infections are diagnosed by either microscopic examination of blood smears or immunological detection of parasite antigens, effective but labor-intensive and time-consuming processes, especially given the large numbers of samples that need to be examined. Although immunological procedures for *Plasmodium* detection, such as ELISAs, are rapid and amenable to automation, they do not always discriminate between current and past infections, because they are designed simply to detect anti-*Plasmodium* antibodies in the blood of affected individuals.

A DNA diagnostic procedure that selectively measures only current infections, i.e., the presence of DNA-containing organisms, was developed

Pathogenic organism

Chromosomal DNA

Isolate target DNA from the pathogen and clone onto an *E. coli* plasmid

1. Introduce the plasmid into *E. coli*
2. Grow *E. coli* cells
3. Isolate plasmid DNA
4. Isolate target DNA

Generate single-stranded target DNA

Probe

1. Label probe
2. Hybridize

Probe hybridized to target DNA

Bind single-stranded sample DNAs to a solid support

FIGURE 9.10 Overview of the development and use of a DNA hybridization probe.

by using highly repeated DNA (DNA that is present in many copies) from *P. falciparum*. First, a genomic library of the parasite DNA was screened with labeled whole-genome parasite DNA. The most intensely labeled hybridizing colonies were selected because they were expected to contain repetitive DNA. The DNA from each of the selected colonies was then tested for its ability to hybridize with DNA from several other *Plasmodium* species that do not cause malaria. The DNA sequence that was chosen as a specific probe hybridized with *P. falciparum* but not with *Plasmodium vivax*, *Plasmodium cynomolgi*, or human DNA, despite the fact that *P. vivax* causes a less severe form of malaria. This probe can detect as little as 10 picograms of purified *P. falciparum* DNA or 1 nanogram (ng) of *P. falciparum* DNA in blood.

More than 100 different DNA diagnostic probes have been isolated and characterized for the detection of various pathogenic strains of bacteria, viruses, and parasites. For example, probes have been developed for the diagnosis of human bacterial infections caused by *Legionella pneumophila* (respiratory failure), *Salmonella enterica* serovar Typhi (food poisoning), *Campylobacter hyointestinalis* (gastritis), and enterotoxigenic *E. coli* (gastroenteritis). Clearly, this is just the "tip of the iceberg," because in principle, nearly all pathogenic organisms can be detected by this procedure.

Detection of *T. cruzi*

The protozoan parasite *Trypanosoma cruzi* is the causative agent of Chagas disease. In this disease, the parasites invade the liver, spleen, lymph nodes, and central nervous system, where they multiply and destroy the infected cells. *T. cruzi* is quite common in Latin America. It is spread by insects and is responsible for approximately 50,000 deaths per year. Diagnosis of acute Chagas disease is usually made by microscopic examination of a fresh blood sample. Alternatively, a test that takes a longer time but ensures that the parasite has not been overlooked entails feeding a patient's blood to uninfected insects and then examining with a microscope the contents of the insects' intestines for parasites about 30 to 40 days later. Both of these tests are laborious, time-consuming, and costly. Chagas disease can also be diagnosed by immunological tests; however, these tests are notorious for producing false-positive responses. As a possible alternative to these less than satisfactory procedures, several PCR-based assays have been developed. At present, PCR assays for Chagas disease are used as adjuncts to the traditional diagnostic procedures that are currently in widespread use.

In one of the PCR-based assay procedures, a 188-base-pair (bp) DNA fragment that is present in multiple copies in the *T. cruzi* genome but is absent from the genomic DNA of several related parasites is the target sequence. The presence of the amplified 188-bp DNA fragment is readily detected by polyacrylamide gel electrophoresis. In general, with minor variations in the methodology, such as the primer sequences, PCR can facilitate the detection of a wide range of bacteria, viruses, and parasites. Currently, there are several PCR-based diagnostic kits that have been

MILESTONE

Detection of Sickle Cell β^S-Globin Allele by Hybridization with Synthetic Oligonucleotides

B. J. CONNER, A. A. REYES, C. MORIN, K. ITAKURA, R. L. TEPLITZ, and R. B. WALLACE
Proc. Natl. Acad. Sci. USA **80**:278–282, 1983

The development of techniques in the early 1980s for rapid, efficient, and inexpensive chemical synthesis of DNA oligonucleotides opened up the possibility of using radiolabeled oligonucleotides as hybridization probes for the detection of a variety of DNAs, including mutations in human genes. At the time, relatively few human genes or even cDNAs had been isolated. Thus, it was not always easy to find a homologous hybridization probe for a particular human gene. Moreover, even if the relevant cDNAs had been isolated, it was not possible to discriminate by DNA hybridization between wild-type and mutant human genes that had only a single-base-pair difference when the hybridization probe was large (≥100 bp). However, Conner et al. synthesized specific oligonucleotides that could recognize either the wild-type or the mutant DNA. Moreover, oligonucleotides complementary to the sequences of both the wild type and the mutant were synthesized so that it could be determined whether a person was heterozygous, as well as whether a person was homozygous. For sickle-cell anemia, two 19-base-long oligonucleotides were used, one complementary to the normal β-globin gene (β^A) and the other complementary to the sickle-cell gene (β^S). DNA from normal individuals (β^Aβ^A) hybridized only with the β^A probe, DNA from individuals with sickle-cell anemia (β^Sβ^S) hybridized only with the β^S probe, and DNA from heterozygous individuals (β^Aβ^S) hybridized with both probes. This model system was the first demonstration of the feasibility of determining genotypes by DNA hybridization and opened up the possibility of detecting a range of human genetic disorders by hybridization with oligonucleotide probes. This possibility has been realized with the development of a large number of DNA-based gene mutation tests. Although the original strategy has been largely supplanted by newer techniques, such as PCR and OLA, this work was important in establishing that single DNA base pair mutations could be accurately and easily detected.

approved for use by the U.S. Food and Drug Administration for the detection and quantitation of human immunodeficiency virus, *Mycobacterium tuberculosis* (the causative agent of tuberculosis), and *C. trachomatis*.

Nonradioactive Hybridization Procedures

In many research laboratories, nucleic acid hybridization is routinely detected by labeling the probe with a radioactive isotope, commonly phosphorus-32. High specific activity ensures an excellent signal-to-noise ratio. In a standard detection system, a radiolabeled probe is mixed with target DNA that is bound to a membrane support. After the support is washed free of nonhybridized probe DNA, the presence of radioactivity is determined by laying the membrane on X-ray film (autoradiography).

However, phosphorus-32 is short-lived, is potentially dangerous, and requires special laboratory equipment for handling and safe disposal, so nonradioactive systems for indicating hybrid DNA formation have also been developed. The nonradioactive detection systems achieve signal amplification by enzymatic conversion of either chromogenic or chemiluminescent substrates. Chromogenic substrates change color and chemiluminescent substrates give off light when they are converted into a specific product by an appropriate enzyme. The signal is detected, in most of these systems, by incorporating biotin-labeled nucleotides into the DNA probe and following a more or less standard procedure:

1. The biotin-labeled probe is hybridized to the target DNA (Fig. 9.11A).
2. Either avidin, a chicken egg white protein, or streptavidin, a bacterial analogue of avidin, is added (Fig. 9.11B).
3. A biotin-labeled enzyme, such as alkaline phosphatase or peroxidase, is added (Fig. 9.11C).
4. Depending on which biotin-labeled enzyme was used in the previous step, either a chromogenic or a chemiluminescent substrate is added, and either the color change or the light produced as a consequence of the conversion of substrate into product is measured (Fig. 9.11D).

Alternatively, following hybridization with a biotin-labeled probe in step 2 above, a streptavidin–enzyme complex with an available biotin-binding site can be added.

Both avidin and streptavidin bind very tightly (K_d [dissociation constant] = ~10^{-15}) to biotin; in addition, each of these proteins has four separate biotin-binding sites, so a single molecule of avidin or streptavidin can bind both a biotin-labeled enzyme and a biotin-labeled probe. Enzymatic activity is not impaired by biotin labeling or binding to streptavidin. In chromogenic detection systems, the action of the enzyme on the substrate creates a colored insoluble dye that remains at the site of the hybrid DNA. In chemiluminescent systems, enzymatic alteration of the substrate generates a product that emits light at the site of the hybrid DNA.

Nonradioactive systems have other advantages: biotin-labeled DNA is stable for at least 1 year at room temperature, devices that detect chemiluminescence are as sensitive as those that detect radioactive signals, and detection of the emitted light with either X-ray film or a luminometer, or scoring of a color change, can be completed within a few hours. The use of

chemiluminescence, which is more sensitive than chromogenic dyes, is becoming the detection signal system of choice for many nucleic acid probe-based diagnostic assays. For PCR-based assays, the amplification product can be labeled by a fluorescent dye that is bound to the 5′ end of each primer. A fluorescent compound emits light of a longer wavelength after it absorbs light of a shorter wavelength. Fluorescein, which appears green under certain wavelengths of light, and rhodamine, which appears red, are often used for this purpose. After PCR amplification of a target DNA with fluorescence-labeled primers, the primers are separated from the amplification product and the presence of the label is detected (Fig. 9.12). If the target DNA is not present in the sample, then no fluorescent product will be

FIGURE 9.11 Chemiluminescent detection of target DNA. **(A)** A biotin-labeled probe is bound to the target DNA. **(B)** Streptavidin is bound to the biotin molecules. **(C)** Biotin-labeled alkaline phosphatase binds to the streptavidin. **(D)** Alkaline phosphatase converts the substrate into a light-emitting product. B, biotin; AP, alkaline phosphatase.

observed. This system is not only sensitive, it is also quite rapid, since it is not necessary to run a gel to separate the amplified target DNA.

Molecular Beacons

A novel nonradioactive method for detecting specific sequences of nucleic acids involves using "molecular beacon" probes (Fig. 9.13). A typical molecular beacon probe is 25 nucleotides long. The 15 nucleotides in the middle are complementary to the target DNA and are designed so that this single-stranded molecule does not does not form a structure in which these nucleotides base pair with one another. However, the 5 nucleotides at each end are complementary to each other and not to the target DNA. A fluorescent molecule (fluorophore) is attached to the 5′ end, and a nonfluorescent molecule (quencher) that can absorb the energy emitted by the fluorophore before it fluoresces is attached to the 3′ end. In solution at room temperature, the conformation of the molecular beacon ensures that the fluorophore and quencher are close to one another, and the fluorophore is quenched (does not fluoresce). On the other hand, when the 15 middle nucleotides of the molecular beacon probe hybridize to a target DNA or RNA sequence, the fluorophore and quencher are separated from each other and the fluorophore is not quenched, i.e., it fluoresces. With this procedure, care must be taken to maintain the reaction mixture at near-ambient temperatures, since high temperatures can also cause the nucleotides in the intrastrand (hairpin) stem of the molecular beacon to become unpaired, with the result that the molecule fluoresces. For this procedure to be effective, all 15 nucleotides in the molecular beacon probe must be perfectly complementary to the target

FIGURE 9.12 Use of fluorescent dyes that are attached to primers for detecting amplified PCR products. The primers are marked P1 and P2.

DNA or RNA. The sensitivity of this procedure can be improved dramatically if the target DNA is first amplified by PCR.

A number of variations of the basic molecular beacon protocol have been developed. For example, combinations of molecular beacon probes may be used simultaneously provided that each one is complementary to a different target DNA and contains a different-color light-emitting fluorophore (Fig. 9.14). For example, when one wants to determine the genotype of an individual, two different molecular beacon probes are added to a biological sample, such as blood, that contains DNA from that individual. The first molecular beacon probe is labeled with one of the fluorophores (e.g., fluorescein), and all 15 probe nucleotides are exactly complementary to the wild-type sequence (Fig. 9.15). One nucleotide difference is sufficient to prevent hybridization. The second molecular beacon probe is labeled with a different fluorophore (e.g., Texas red), and the 15 probe nucleotides are complementary to the sequence from the mutant form (Fig. 9.15). Following hybridization, the appearance of green fluorescence indicates a homozygous normal genotype, red fluorescence indicates a homozygous mutant genotype, and green and red fluorescence indicates a heterozygous genotype.

DNA Fingerprinting

The DNA from a biological sample left at the scene of a crime can be analyzed and compared with the DNAs of likely suspects. A match between evidence and a particular individual is helpful to the prosecution. In addition, DNA comparisons are used to determine whether individuals have

FIGURE 9.13 Hybridization of a molecular beacon probe to target DNA. If the target sequence is present, the unpaired single-stranded portion of the molecular beacon base pairs with its complementary sequence, thereby separating the fluorophore and quencher moieties. As a result, the fluorescence of the fluorophore is not quenched. Adapted from Tyagi and Kramer, *Nat. Biotechnol.* **14**:303–308, 1996.

Target DNA

Molecular beacon probe

Hybridization

Fluorophore Quencher

Target DNA–probe hybrid

FIGURE 9.14 Molecular-beacon probes with different fluorophores. Beneath each molecular beacon probe is the name of the fluorophore and the wavelength of its maximum emission. Each fluorophore is represented (on the left) by the color of its fluorescence.

FIGURE 9.15 Use of two different molecular beacon probes to distinguish between different genotypes. Once the probe is bound to target DNA, the fluorescence of the fluorophore is no longer quenched.

Homozygous wild type

Homozygous mutant

Heterozygote

been wrongly convicted of a crime. In other instances, DNA analyses help determine paternity and identify victims of disasters. Distinguishing individuals with DNA analysis is called DNA fingerprinting (DNA typing). One approach for determining DNA relationships among humans relies on DNA hybridization to undegraded minisatellite DNA. The probes for this type of analysis consists of human minisatellite DNAs, sequences that occur throughout the human genome and consist of tandemly repeated sequences (Fig. 9.16). The lengths of the repeats range from 9 to 40 bp, and the numbers of repeats in the minisatellites range from about 10 to 30. A minisatellite DNA sequence at a specific chromosome location can have different lengths in different individuals. This variability is due to either a gain or a loss of tandem repeats, probably during DNA replication. These changes do not have any biological effect because minisatellite DNA does not encode any proteins. Unrelated individuals generally have minisatellites that differ in length, but children inherit one set of minisatellite DNA sequences from each parent. For minisatellite DNA typing, the sample DNA is digested with a restriction enzyme, and the fragments are separated on an agarose gel and transferred by blotting them onto a nylon membrane. The membrane is hybridized sequentially with four or five separate labeled minisatellite DNA probes, each of which recognizes a distinct DNA sequence. After each hybridization reaction, the bands in which the probe has bound to the digested DNA sample are visualized by autoradiography, and the banding pattern for each sample is noted (Fig. 9.17). Before the next probe is used, the first probe is completely removed

(stripped) from the membrane. Since each hybridization and autoradiography step can take up to 10 to 14 days, the entire process may take many weeks, and even several months.

A minisatellite DNA pattern (fingerprint) represents the repertoire of the lengths of some of these sequences in an individual. Because of the extensive variability in human minisatellite DNA sequences, the chance of finding two individuals in the population with the same DNA fingerprint is about 1 in 10^5 to 1 in 10^8. Therefore, individuals' DNA banding patterns based on minisatellite DNA sequences are almost as unique as their fingerprints.

RAPD

Not only are DNA banding patterns important for forensic analyses, they are also useful in distinguishing among different plant cultivars. Random amplified polymorphic DNA (RAPD) markers may be used for this purpose. With this procedure, an arbitrary oligonucleotide primer, usually 9 to 10 bp long, that does not contain any palindromic sequences and has a G+C content of 50 to 80% is added to a sample of plant chromosomal DNA; virtually any oligonucleotide sequence will suffice. Because of its short sequence, the added oligonucleotide will pair with the chromosomal DNA at many sites, sometimes including opposite strands on the target DNA. When the 3′ ends of the oligonucleotides on opposite strands of the DNA face each other, the DNA in between can be amplified (Fig. 9.18). Although the sequence of each primer is known, it is not known which oligonucleotide, if any, will be effective in priming the PCR. Whenever a primer can hybridize to both strands of the target DNA in the proper orientation and the two sites are about 100 to 3,000 bp from each other, the intervening DNA region will be amplified via PCR. The DNA fragments of characteristic size that are produced can be visualized following polyacrylamide gel electrophoresis. The number of amplified DNA fragments in a sample is dependent on the primer and the genomic DNA used. Each time that the same primer is used with the same target DNA, the amplified products will be the same. A single nucleotide substitution in a primer will result in a complete change in the RAPD pattern. Thus, the RAPD fingerprints of different plant cultivars can be compared when the same set of oligonucleotide primers is used. To fingerprint the DNAs of two very similar plant strains or cultivars, it is often necessary to perform the RAPD procedure with a number of different arbitrary primers with known

—|ACCGTTCAC|ACCGTTCAC|ACCGTTCAC|ACCGTTCAC|ACCGTTCAC|—

—|ACCGTTCAC|ACCGTTCAC|ACCGTTCAC|ACCGTTCAC|ACCGTTCAC|ACCGTTCAC|—

—|ACCGTTCAC|ACCGTTCAC|ACCGTTCAC|ACCGTTCAC|ACCGTTCAC|ACCGTTCAC|ACCGTTCAC|—

FIGURE 9.16 Schematic representation of human minisatellite DNA. Only one DNA strand is shown. In this example, the repeating unit is 9 bp, and there are 5, 6, and 7 repeating units per cluster (although 10 to 30 repeating units are more common).

sequences until differences are revealed (Fig. 9.19). Like other molecular markers, RAPDs can be used to characterize whole genomes, individual chromosomes, or, less commonly, specific genes. Although the procedure was originally developed for plants, it is also useful in the characterization of microorganisms.

In comparison with other procedures for characterizing complex DNA, the RAPD procedure has a number of advantages. (1) The same (universal) set of oligonucleotide primers can be used for all plant species. (2) No genomic libraries, radioactivity, Southern transfers, or DNA hybridization reactions are required, so a large number of samples may be easily and rapidly characterized. (3) The process can be automated. Moreover, with conventional PCR analysis it is necessary to know the sequence of a specific gene or gene segment that is the target for amplification. On the other hand, amplification in RAPD analysis occurs anywhere in a genome where

FIGURE 9.17 Southern blot of a forensic DNA sample. The DNA samples from the victim, the defendant's shirt, and the defendant were treated with the same restriction enzyme. Here, the banding pattern of the DNA extracted from the blood on the defendant's shirt is identical to the victim's DNA banding pattern and different from the defendant's pattern. The sizes of the DNA molecules in these bands are estimated by comparison with the positions of the sizing standards.

Chromosomal DNA

Region of DNA that is amplified

FIGURE 9.18 Binding of a single random oligonucleotide (arrow) to the chromosomal DNA of an animal, plant, or microbe. When two of the oligonucleotides on opposite strands are oriented facing one another and are 100 to 3,000 bp apart, the intervening DNA is amplified by PCR.

there are two sequences complementary to the primer that are within the length limits of the PCR.

With this technology, scientists were able to distinguish six inbred maize lines from each other, and maize hybrids produced by genetic crossings of these inbred lines were shown to have the PCR products of their parental inbred lines. RAPD markers have also been used to screen different strains of the fungus *Leptosphaeria maculans*, which is the causal agent of blackleg disease in crucifers. Differences between avirulent (non-disease-causing) and virulent (disease-causing) strains could be distinguished on the basis of specific RAPD markers, making it easier for scientists to produce an avirulent strain that could be used as a biological control agent that helps to prevent blackleg disease.

FIGURE 9.19 Ethidium bromide-stained bands following polyacrylamide gel electrophoresis of PCR-amplified plant DNA. Three separate oligonucleotide primers were used to amplify fragments from each of the two cultivars. Cultivars 1 and 2 show identical patterns of bands with oligonucleotides A and C. However, they have different patterns when oligonucleotide B is used; hence, oligonucleotide B can be used to distinguish between cultivars 1 and 2.

Oligonucleotide A		Oligonucleotide B		Oligonucleotide C	
Cultivar 1	Cultivar 2	Cultivar 1	Cultivar 2	Cultivar 1	Cultivar 2

Real-Time PCR

By labeling the DNA that is amplified in a PCR with a fluorescent dye and monitoring the fluorescence that results when the dye bound to double-stranded DNA is irradiated with light of a certain wavelength, it is possible to "watch" the production of PCR products. Moreover, this approach allows one to quantify the amount of a specific DNA fragment in the starting material. Labeling the DNA is achieved using any one of a variety of protocols. In the simplest approach to labeling DNA, researchers add dyes that bind to double-stranded DNA and emit fluorescence, and the fluorescence intensity increases in proportion to the concentration of double-stranded DNA (Fig. 9.20).

Real-time PCR may be described as occurring in four phases (Fig. 9.21). In the first, or linear, phase (Fig. 9.21, phase 1), which generally takes about 10 to 15 cycles, fluorescence emission at each cycle has not yet risen above the background level. In the early exponential phase (Fig. 9.21, phase 2), the amount of fluorescence reaches a threshold at which it is significantly higher than the background. The cycle at which this occurs is known as the threshold cycle (C_T, or CP, depending upon the manufacturer of the PCR equipment). The C_T value is inversely correlated with the amount of target DNA in the original sample. During the exponential phase (Fig. 9.21, phase 3), the amount of product doubles in each cycle under ideal conditions, while in the plateau stage (Fig. 9.21, phase 4), the reaction components become limited and measurements of the fluorescence intensity are no longer useful. To quantitate the amount of target DNA in a sample, a standard curve is first generated by serially diluting a sample with a known number of copies of the target DNA, and assuming all samples are amplified with equal efficiency, the C_T values for each dilution are plotted against the starting amount of sample (Fig. 9.22). The number of copies of a target DNA in a sample can be determined by obtaining the C_T value for the sample and extrapolating the starting amount from the standard curve. In addition, since during the exponential phase the DNA doubles with each cycle, a sample that has four times the number of starting copies of the target sequence compared to another sample would require two fewer cycles of amplification to generate the same number of product strands.

Among its many other uses, real-time PCR has been used to monitor *Cryptosporidium parvum* (a waterborne protozoan parasite that is the causative agent of a range of human diseases, including persistent diarrhea and severe infections, in infected individuals). This approach is likely to replace the more imprecise and time-consuming traditional methods of monitoring *C. parvum* infections, such as histological staining. Similarly, other researchers have reported using real-time PCR to quantitate *S. enterica* contamination in food samples. In this case, food samples (chicken and mung beans were tested) were rinsed with 100 to 250 mL of water or with a physiological saline solution. The liquid was filtered to remove particulate matter and then filtered to capture the *Salmonella* sp. cells. The cells were removed from the filter membrane, lysed, and subjected to real-time PCR. In this case, the entire procedure took only approximately 3 hours and was able to detect and quantitate cell numbers as low as 7×10^2 colony-forming units (i.e., cells) per 100 mL of liquid. Compared to the existing methodology, real-time PCR offers a dramatic improvement in both the sensitivity of detection and the time that it takes to complete the analysis.

FIGURE 9.20 The fluorescent dye SYBR green does not bind to single-stranded DNA (A), binds to double-stranded DNA as it is synthesized (B), and is bound to the double-stranded amplified DNA (C). Only the bound DNA fluoresces.

In addition to its use in the measurement of pathogenic agents in the environment, a variant of real-time PCR may be used to quantitate the levels of a variety of mRNAs in different eukaryotic tissues or prokaryotic cells. In this case, since the initial target is RNA and not DNA, a reverse transcription (RT) step is needed before the real-time PCR. In the first step of real-time RT-PCR, the mRNA sample is reverse transcribed to generate complementary DNA (cDNA). This may be done in the same tube as the subsequent PCR, or the RT reaction and PCR may be carried out in separate tubes. Many of the more traditional methods of monitoring gene expression, including Northern hybridization, ribonuclease (RNase) protection assays, and RNA dot blot hybridizations, are both limited in sensitivity and difficult to quantify. However, with the increasingly popular technique of real-time RT-PCR, it is possible to detect and quantify mRNA levels that are about 10,000- to 100,000-fold lower than those measurable by traditional techniques. With real-time RT-PCR, even a single copy of a transcript may be detected. The very low levels of RNA that are required for this procedure make it the method of choice for monitoring mRNA levels.

Immunoquantitative Real-Time PCR

The detection limits of many commercially available immunological methods for measuring levels of pathogenic microorganisms are often insufficient to

FIGURE 9.21 A plot of Δ*Rn* (normalized fluorescence) versus cycle number in a real-time PCR experiment. Four phases of PCR are shown. (1) A linear phase, where fluorescence emission is not yet above background level. (2) An early exponential phase, where the fluorescence intensity becomes significantly higher than the background. The cycle at which this occurs is generally known as C_T. (3) An exponential phase, where the amount of product doubles in each cycle. (4) A plateau phase, where reaction components are limited and amplification slows down.

FIGURE 9.22 Plot of C_T versus the starting amount of a target nucleotide sequence. Fluorescence detection is linear over several orders of magnitude.

perceive low but still potentially dangerous levels of these organisms. Notwithstanding the high degree of specificity that antibodies provide, it would be advantageous to be able to increase the sensitivity of various immunological assay procedures. One way to do this is to develop a protocol that combines the specificity of antibodies with the sensitivity of PCR. Figure 9.23 compares an ELISA-type protocol with an immunoquantitative real-time PCR procedure. With the ELISA method (Fig. 9.23A), the first antibody is coupled to the surface of a microtiter plate. The added antigen binds to the first antibody. When the second antibody is added, it binds to a different epitope on the antigen. The bound antigen is visualized by the action of alkaline phosphatase, bound to the second antibody, which turns a colorless substrate into a colored product. With the immunoquantitative real-time PCR procedure (Fig. 9.23B), instead of alkaline phosphatase, a streptavidin-biotin complex links the second antibody to a 246-bp DNA fragment with a known sequence. Once the immunological complex has formed, it may be visualized and quantified by performing real-time PCR in the well of the microtiter plate, thereby significantly amplifying the signal from the immunological complex. In fact, it has been estimated that this procedure is approximately 1,000-fold more sensitive than an ELISA.

Ancestry Determination

By examining a number of different single-nucleotide polymorphisms (SNPs) (i.e., minor variations in DNA sequence) in an individual and comparing the pattern of the SNPs to those of other individuals in the population, it is possible to infer information regarding an individual's ancestry. For an analysis of an individual's ancestry, three different types of DNA can be examined: autosomal DNA (which includes all of a person's DNA except for the X and Y chromosomes and mitochondrial DNA), which originates from a combination of a person's parents' DNA; paternal DNA (i.e., the Y chromosome), which is passed on from father to son; and maternal DNA (i.e., mitochondrial DNA and the X chromosome), which is passed on from a mother to all of her children.

To perform an analysis of an individual's ancestry (or for paternity testing or forensic analysis), DNA is typically extracted and purified from buccal swabs (i.e., from cheek cells) or from blood samples. Stretches of DNA are then amplified by PCR using primers that target specific regions of the genome. The DNA samples are then separated by size on a small column by a technique known as capillary electrophoresis (this method has generally replaced gel electrophoresis, which was previously used to separate these small DNA fragments but was slower and less amenable to automation). If the PCR primers are labeled with fluorescent dyes before the PCR amplification reaction, fluorescent samples are eluted from the capillary column in a characteristic pattern of bands (in much the same way that DNA bands form a pattern unique to a particular fragment following gel electrophoresis). The sizes of the amplified DNA bands in specific regions are determined and are referred to as alleles. With autosomal DNA, each person should have two alleles at each site, one from the father and one from the mother. Each known allele has a determined frequency of occurrence in the general population and among various ethnic groups. After testing for approximately 150 to 350 different SNPs, the frequency of certain

FIGURE 9.23 Antigen detection by ELISA with the substrate color change detected spectrophotometrically **(A)** and by immunoquantitative real-time PCR with the amplified DNA detected by measuring the fluorescence of a dye bound to the double-stranded DNA **(B)**.

alleles in an individual is compared to the frequency of those alleles in various ethnic groups. This provides an indication of the ethnic background or ancestry of that individual. For example, this type of testing may indicate that an individual is genetically 70% Northern European, 17% Middle Eastern, and 13% Native American.

Since mitochondrial DNA changes only very little over many generations, characterization of mitochondrial DNA is an ideal means of tracking migrations over many hundreds of generations of human genetic history. Analysis of mitochondrial DNA indicates that the observed genetic variation in human populations may be divided into divisions of ethnically similar individuals called haplotypes. Table 9.3 summarizes the currently accepted mitochondrial DNA haplotypes and the groups associated with these haplotypes. The root of all human lineages is the L groups in Africa. All other groups diverged from these groups after early humans began to migrate out of Africa around 150,000 years ago.

Analysis of parental (Y chromosome) haplotypes has been used to examine the claim that all members of a priestly line of Jewish males called "Kohanim" are descended from the family of the biblical Aaron, the brother of Moses. According to Jewish tradition, membership in this priestly line may be acquired only by males whose biological fathers are Kohanim.

When Y-linked genetic markers were examined among Jews claiming to be Kohanim, as well as men who either were not Jewish or did not claim to be Kohanim, the limited variation in the markers examined was entirely consistent with a 3,300-year-old origin of this priestly line in a single male or a small group of related males. Interestingly, these same Y chromosome genetic markers are found among the Lemba, a South African tribal group claiming paternal kinship with the Jews of Yemen.

By mid-2008, there were nearly 30 companies marketing genetic ancestry kits; each test costs from $100 to $900. Moreover, in the few years that they have been available, more than 500,000 people have purchased these tests, and there is every indication that the demand will continue to grow. Some geneticists, anthropologists, and epidemiologists have publicly expressed concern that naïve laypersons, anxious for definitive information about their personal genetic ancestry, often misinterpret the results of these tests. For example, the fact that a particular allele or haplotype is

TABLE 9.3 Human mitochondrial haplotypes and the groups associated with these haplotypes

Haplotype group	Associated traits
A	Originated in Asia ~60,000 years ago; currently found widely in Asia; a precursor of Native Americans
B	Originated in Asia ~50,000 years ago; subgroup B2 is one precursor of Native Americans
C	Originated in Asia ~60,000 years ago; includes the Siberian region of northern Asia and is a precursor of Native Americans
CZ	Found in modern Eurasian populations in northern and eastern Asia, including Siberia
D	Originated in Asia ~60,000 years ago; along with groups A, B, and C, this group is thought to have produced Native Americans; currently found in northern and eastern Asia
E	Not a well-characterized group; currently found among some people in Argentina
F	Originated in eastern Asia; from haplotype group R1; currently found in China and Japan
G	Currently found in northeastern Siberia; also found among indigenous people of Kamchatka
H	Common in the Middle East and northern Africa; ancestor to about half of all Europeans; a prominent subgroup of HV
HV	Originated ~20,000 years ago; a progenitor of groups H and V; commonly found in modern western Europeans
I	Originated ~30,000 years ago; currently found in both southern Europe and northern Africa
J	Originated in Mesopotamia ~10,000 years ago; currently found in Russia and eastern Europe
JT	Derived from group R and a progenitor of groups J and T
K	Originated ~18,000 years ago in Eurasia; currently found in some parts of western Europe
L1	Originated ~150,000 years ago in Africa; this haplotype group represents the group from which all of humankind is thought to descend; currently found in West and Central Africa
L2	Originated from haplotype group L1 in Africa ~70,000 years ago; currently commonly found in sub-Saharan Africa and among American blacks
L3	Originated from haplotype group L1; gave rise to haplotype groups M and N; currently commonly found in East Africa
M	Originated from haplotype group L3 ~80,000 years ago; this group is thought to have migrated into Eurasia ~60,000 years ago; currently found throughout southern Asia
M1	Believed to be the result of migration from North Africa and parts of Asia to sub-Saharan Africa
N	Originated from haplotype group L3 ~80,000 years ago; this haplotype group is believed to be the progenitor of nearly all European haplotype groups; groups B, U, F, HV, H, and V all descend from haplotype group N
N1a	Currently found in Iran and other parts of western and central Asia
N1b	Common in Near and Middle East regions of Asia, as well as among Ashkenazi Jewish people
Pre-HV	Widely represented in the Middle East and parts of eastern Africa; the ancestor of haplotype groups HV, H, and V
Q	Currently found in the southern Pacific region, especially New Guinea and Melanesia
R	Descended from haplotype group N; currently found throughout Asia and Eastern Europe

A

Cytochrome *b*

B

5' ATGACCAACA TTCGAAAATC CCACCCACTA ATAAAAATTA TAAACAACTC 3'

FIGURE 9.24 **(A)** PCR amplification of a portion of mammalian mitochondrial DNA. **(B)** The consensus sequence of the first 50 nucleotides of the cytochrome *b* gene. Minor variations from the consensus sequence are characteristic of specific genera and species of various mammals. Adapted from Hsieh et al., *Forensic Sci. Int.* **122:**7–18, 2001.

quite common in certain populations does not mean that its presence is a definitive diagnostic of membership in those populations. There is often high genetic diversity within populations, and gene flow can readily occur between populations. Thus, a particular allele could have been inherited from a population in which it is less common rather than from the population in which it appears to be "diagnostic," leading some individuals to mistakenly believe that they are genetically part of a particular ethnic or racial group.

Animal Species Determination

In many parts of the world, numerous large mammalian species have been hunted to the verge of extinction because of the trade in their skin, bones, horns, or other body parts. As part of an effort to stem the illegal traffic in wild-animal remains and enforce international conventions designed to prevent this trade, a number of laboratories have been set up to determine the species of origin from powdered animal remains (so prepared because of their supposed medicinal properties). Currently, the method of choice for animal species determination involves DNA typing. More specifically, using PCR, a portion of the animal's cytochrome *b* gene, which is found in the mitochondrial DNA, is amplified and then sequenced (Fig. 9.24). This locus was chosen because it is both sufficiently conserved so that it is present in all mammals and sufficiently polymorphic that members of different, but closely related, species can be distinguished. The primers used in this method amplify a 486-bp DNA fragment, which is sufficient for DNA sequencing and to identify most mammals despite the fact that the sample DNA is often somewhat degraded. To ensure that high-quality data are obtained, it is necessary to (1) start with 20 to 50 ng of DNA template and (2) use a control DNA sample (usually mouse or cow DNA) that is treated in parallel to the target DNA.

Automated DNA Analysis

More than 1,400 different organisms (bacteria, fungi, viruses, and protozoa) have been identified as being pathogenic to humans. Moreover, new patho-

gens are constantly being identified and characterized. To limit the damage from either a natural epidemic or a bioterrorist attack, it is necessary to rapidly identify the organism(s) that is the source of the infectious outbreak so that appropriate public health measures may be instituted as rapidly as possible. In addition to human diseases, it is also important to rapidly identify the causative agents of outbreaks of animal and plant diseases.

By performing a combination of PCR and electrospray ionization mass spectrometry (Fig. 9.25), it is possible to rapidly and accurately identify a wide range of human pathogens. Small aliquots of the DNA that is isolated from a test sample are placed into a number of different wells of a microtiter plate. Each well contains a pair of PCR primers that have been designed to amplify a gene product from a broad group of organisms within a selected domain of microbial life. For example, workers have reported using 12 primers that are targeted to universally conserved sequences and 6 primers that are targeted to broad divisions of microbial life (such as bacilli). The products of each of the PCRs are electrosprayed into a mass spectrometer, and the DNA base sequences of the various samples are determined. This technique allows scientists to very rapidly hone in on the nature of an infectious agent. Of course, this technique is facilitated by the fact that the genomic DNA sequences of a large number of microbes have already been determined. Moreover, with the very rapid progress that has been made recently in DNA sequence analysis, it is reasonable to expect that all known pathogens will be fully sequenced by 2015.

Molecular Diagnosis of Genetic Disease

The ability to diagnose the occurrence of specific inherited diseases in humans at the genetic level makes it possible for individuals to discover whether they or their offspring are at risk. DNA analysis can be used for the identification of carriers of hereditary disorders, for prenatal diagnosis of serious genetic conditions, and for early diagnosis before the onset of symptoms.

Tests at the DNA level are definitive for determining the existence of specific genetic mutations. Previously, genetic testing relied almost exclusively on biochemical assays that scored either the presence or the absence of a gene product. A DNA-based test does not, however, require expression for detection of the mutant gene, thereby making it theoretically possible to develop screening assays for all single-gene diseases.

FIGURE 9.25 Flowchart of an automated system to identify the pathogenic microbes in an environmental sample.

Screening for Cystic Fibrosis

Often, screening for genetic diseases can be rather complex. This reflects the fact that instead of a disease being the consequence of a single alteration to the wild-type DNA, as is the case with sickle-cell anemia (see below), many diseases are caused by any one of a large number of genetic alterations to the normal DNA for that gene. For example, cystic fibrosis, one of the most common lethal autosomal recessive disorders in Europeans and their descendants, with an incidence of approximately 1 in every 2,500 live births and a carrier frequency of approximately 1 in 29, is caused by mutations to the cystic fibrosis transmembrane conductance regulator (CFTR) gene that result in defects in chloride ion transport. There are currently nearly 1,400 known mutations to the CFTR gene that can result in the development of cystic fibrosis. Screening individuals who may be at risk for cystic fibrosis for 1,400 different mutations is a daunting task. Fortunately, some of the mutations that cause cystic fibrosis are much more common than others (Table 9.4). In fact, over 90% of cystic fibrosis patients carry at least one ΔF508 allele, and nearly 50% of cystic fibrosis cases are individuals who are homozygous for ΔF508. Despite the fact that separate tests are required for each mutation, it is estimated that screening individuals for ΔF508 and for the next 20 most common mutations should identify approximately 98% of cystic fibrosis-affected individuals and carriers.

Current diagnostic tests for cystic fibrosis include several different techniques. One of the most widely used methods is allele-specific oligonucleotide dot blots (also called allele-specific hybridization). With this technique, genomic DNA or cDNA from an individual is amplified by PCR and, following transfer to a membrane, is hybridized (separately) to labeled oligonucleotide probes for the mutant (usually ΔF508) and wild-type genes (Fig. 9.26). In this way, it is possible to distinguish between normal individuals, cystic fibrosis carriers, and cystic fibrosis-affected individuals (Fig. 9.27). With this technique, the probe or the probe–target complex may be labeled in a variety of ways, including the use of radioactivity, enzymes that produce color change when acting on certain substrates (see the discussion of the ELISA procedure above), and fluorescent dyes. This technique may be automated and is currently commercially

TABLE 9.4 The most common mutations of the CFTR protein that lead to cystic fibrosis

Mutation designation	Amino acid change to the CFTR protein
ΔF508	Deletion of phenylalanine at position 508
G542X	Replacement of glycine at position 542 by a stop codon
W1282X	Replacement of tryptophan at position 1282 by a stop codon
N1303K	Replacement of asparagine at position 1303 by lysine
1717-1G>A	Replacement of glycine by alanine at the last nucleotide in the intron proceeding nucleotide 1717 in the cDNA
R553X	Replacement of arginine at position 553 by a stop codon
I148T	Replacement of isoleucine at position 148 by threonine
3120+1G>A	Replacement of glycine by alanine at the first nucleotide in the intron following nucleotide 3120 in the cDNA

Adapted from Eshaque and Dixon, *Biotechnol. Adv.* 24:86–93, 2006.
Amino acids are numbered starting at the N-terminal end of the protein.

A Hybridization

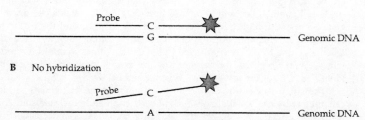

B No hybridization

FIGURE 9.26 Labeled oligonucleotide probe hybridizes to a completely complementary genomic DNA but, under stringent conditions **(A)**, not to a DNA sequence in which one of the bases in the middle has been altered **(B)**. In this case, the probe was designed to hybridize to wild-type DNA. Other probes, designed to hybridize to the genomic DNA of known mutations, would not bind to the wild-type DNA.

available in a kit form that can detect 12 frequent and 17 rare cystic fibrosis mutations.

Another method that has been marketed as a kit is based on the PCR amplification of specific alleles. Using this protocol, several PCRs are performed simultaneously for each DNA sample—the primers anneal to different regions for different mutations. Following amplification, the presence of a DNA band of a particular size indicates that a specific mutation is present. In this case, different-size DNA fragments are typically separated either by gel electrophoresis or by capillary electrophoresis. This test is quite rapid, and it has the ability to detect a variety of different mutations. However, it does not distinguish between homozygotes and heterozygotes, so a positive response must be followed up by additional tests to determine whether a positive test is indicative of a cystic fibrosis gene carrier or affected individual.

The PCR/OLA procedure (described in detail below) is also commonly used to detect cystic fibrosis mutations. This technique is considered to be highly accurate compared to many other protocols and has the highest detection rate of any of the diagnostic tests for this disease. Moreover, it is readily amenable to automation. Notwithstanding the success with all of the procedures mentioned above, researchers continue to refine and develop these and other approaches to the diagnosis of cystic fibrosis.

Sickle-Cell Anemia

Sickle-cell anemia is a genetic disease that is the result of a single-nucleotide change in the codon for the sixth amino acid of the β chain of the hemoglobin molecule. In individuals homozygous for the defect (S/S), the shape of the red blood cells is irregular (sickle shaped) because the conformation of the hemoglobin molecule is distorted by a single amino acid change from glutamic acid to valine. The biological ramifications of this genetic alteration are severe anemia and progressive damage to the heart, lungs, brain, joints, and major organ systems. The anemia is caused by the inability of the mutated hemoglobin to carry sufficient oxygen. The life expectancy for S/S homozygotes is quite short. Heterozygous individuals (A/S) (genetic carriers) have normal-shape red blood cells and no symptoms unless they are subjected to extreme conditions, such as high altitude

or extremes of temperature, that lower the oxygen supply. If both parents are heterozygous, there is a 25% chance that a child of theirs will have sickle-cell anemia, i.e., will be an S/S homozygote. The sickle-cell anemia gene occurs with high frequency among black Africans and their descendants and in Hispanic populations. Carrier screening for the sickle-cell anemia gene is routinely conducted in the United States so that those individuals who are at risk for transmitting the gene to their offspring can be identified. One of the test systems is described below.

The single-nucleotide change in the β-globin gene that causes sickle-cell anemia by chance abolishes a CvnI restriction endonuclease site. This restriction enzyme recognizes the sequence CCTNAGG and cleaves the DNA between the C and the T. (The letter N indicates that any one of the four nucleotides can occupy this position.) In the normal gene, the DNA sequence is CCTGAGG, whereas in the sickle-cell anemia gene, the sequence is CCTGTGG. This difference forms the basis for a DNA diagnostic assay (Fig. 9.28A).

After two oligonucleotide primer sequences that flank the CvnI site are added, a small amount of sample DNA can be amplified by PCR (Fig. 9.28B). The amplified DNA is digested with CvnI (Fig. 9.28C), and the cleavage products are separated by gel electrophoresis and visualized by ethidium bromide staining of the DNA in the gel. If the CvnI site is present, a specific set of DNA fragments is observed (Fig. 9.28D). A different profile of DNA fragments occurs if the CvnI site is absent. By this procedure, the genetic makeup of a tested person can be determined quickly, directly, and easily. Moreover, because of the fortuitous loss of the CvnI site, this assay functions without the need for a target–probe hybridization reaction.

The PCR/OLA Procedure

Obviously, not all genetic changes that produce defective genes affect existing restriction endonuclease sites. Therefore, other strategies for detecting single-nucleotide changes are required. One of these procedures

FIGURE 9.27 Allele-specific oligonucleotide dot blot to diagnose individuals who are either carriers of a mutant CFTR gene (heterozygotes) or affected by the disease (homozygotes). The dark dot blot indicates that the labeled oligonucleotide has bound to the individual's DNA.

combines PCR with an oligonucleotide ligation assay (OLA); not surprisingly, it is called PCR/OLA.

Let us assume that in a normal gene at a specific site (say, nucleotide number 106) the nucleotide pair is A·T; in the mutant form, the nucleotide pair at this site is G·C. Knowledge of the sequence of nucleotides on both sides of position 106 enables the design and use of two short (20-nucleotide) adjacent oligonucleotide sequences that are complementary to one of the two native DNA strands (Fig. 9.29). The essential feature of this pair of oligonucleotides is that one of them (probe X) has as its last base at the 3'

FIGURE 9.28 Detection of the sickle-cell anemia gene at the DNA level. (A) A portion of the sequence of the wild-type (HbA) and sickle-cell (HbS) human β-globin gene. The amino acids (numbered from the N-terminal end of the peptide chain) encoded by this portion of the DNA are shown above the DNA sequence. (B) PCR amplification of the portion of the β-globin gene containing the CvnI recognition site that is altered in the mutant gene. (C) CvnI digestion of the PCR products. The normal (wild-type) gene has three CvnI sites between the PCR primers, and the mutant gene has two. (D) Size distribution of fragments following gel electrophoresis of CvnI-digested PCR-amplified β-globin DNA. AA, homozygous condition for the normal β-globin gene; AS, heterozygous condition; SS, homozygous condition for the sickle-cell anemia β-globin gene.

A

Pro-5 Glu-6 Glu-7
—CCTGAGGAG— HbA

Pro-5 Val-6 Glu-7
—CCTGTGGAG— HbS

B

Primer Normal sequence

Primer

Primer Sickle-cell anemia sequence

Primer

C Amplified normal sequence

CvnI CvnI CvnI

256 bp | 201 bp | 181 bp | 88 bp

Amplified sickle-cell anemia sequence

CvnI CvnI

256 bp | 382 bp | 88 bp

D

Size, bp	Genotype		
	AA	AS	SS
382		▭	▭
256	▭	▭	▭
201	▭	▭	
181	▭	▭	
88	▭	▭	▭

A Synthesize a pair of oligonucleotide probes

B Hybridize probes to PCR-amplified DNA

C Add ligase to hybridized DNA

D Bind probes to streptavidin; wash

E Add antidigoxigenin antibody–alkaline phosphatase conjugate; wash; add substrate

FIGURE 9.29 PCR/OLA procedure. B, biotin; D, digoxigenin; AP, alkaline phosphatase; SA, streptavidin; A, adenine; C, cytosine; G, guanine; T, thymine.

end the nucleotide that is complementary to the nucleotide at position 106 of the normal sequence. The other oligonucleotide (probe Y) starts at its 5' end with a nucleotide that is complementary to the nucleotide immediately adjacent to position 106. When these two probes are hybridized with target DNA containing the normal sequence (which has been amplified by PCR), the nucleotide at the 3' end of probe X base pairs with the target DNA, and probe Y is aligned so that its 5' end lies next to the 3' end of probe X. The addition of DNA ligase to the reaction covalently joins probe X and probe Y. By contrast, when these two probes are hybridized to mutant DNA in which the nucleotide at position 106 is altered, the nucleotide at the 3' end of probe X is mismatched and is not able to pair with nucleotide 106 in the target DNA sequence; probe Y, however, is perfectly aligned. In this case, DNA ligase cannot join probe X and probe Y because of the single-nucleotide misalignment.

Other oligonucleotides (probes) can also be chemically synthesized to give a perfect base pair match when nucleotide 106 is mutated. Obviously, with this second set of probes, ligation occurs when they are hybridized to target DNA that contains the mutant nucleotide, whereas with normal target DNA, the single nucleotide pair mismatch prevents the ligation of the probes. In short, PCR/OLA is designed to distinguish between two possibilities: ligation and no ligation of two input probes.

To determine whether ligation has occurred between two indicator probes, probe X is labeled at its 5' end with biotin and probe Y is labeled at its 3' end with digoxigenin. The low-molecular-weight compound digoxigenin serves as an antibody-binding indicator. After the hybridization and ligation steps are carried out, the DNA is denatured to release the hybridized probes, and the entire mixture is transferred to a small plastic well that has been coated with streptavidin. The well is then washed to remove unbound material, so only the biotin-labeled probe DNA remains bound. Next, antidigoxigenin antibodies, which have been previously coupled to alkaline phosphatase, are added to the well. After an additional washing step to remove unbound conjugated antidigoxigenin antibodies, a colorless chromogenic substrate is added. The appearance of color in the well indicates that antidigoxigenin antibodies have bound to digoxigenin and that the digoxigenin-labeled probe was ligated to the biotinylated probe. If no color appears, then no ligation occurred.

With two pairs of probes, it is possible to ascertain the genetic makeup of any tested individual at a particular site. For example, heterozygous individuals yield positive results with both pairs of probes. The DNA from people with two copies of the normal gene gives a positive response only with the set of probes that contains the nucleotide complementary to the nucleotide at the normal site. Finally, DNA from individuals with two altered gene copies will give a positive response only with the set of probes that is designed to detect the mutant site. To minimize the amount of the original sample DNA that is required for the assay, the segment of the target DNA sequence that contains the nucleotide site to be tested is amplified by PCR before the hybridization reaction.

Overall, the PCR/OLA system is rapid, sensitive, and highly specific. It has even been automated with a robotic workstation to carry out the steps of the assay procedures. Under these conditions, as many as 1,200 ligation reactions can be conducted per day.

The ligase chain reaction assay is a simpler, albeit less sensitive, variant of the PCR/OLA system. Sample DNA is mixed with an excess amount of

a pair of OLA indicator probes (as described above) in the presence of a heat-resistant DNA ligase. After an initial ligation reaction at 65°C, the temperature is raised to 94°C to denature the probe–target DNA hybrid and then lowered to 65°C to allow hybridization of the free, nonligated OLA indicator probes to the target DNA. The cycle is repeated 20 times. If the OLA indicator probes match the target DNA perfectly, then ligation will occur at 65°C during each cycle, and after 20 cycles, enough ligation product (probe X joined to probe Y) will accumulate to be observed by either gel electrophoresis or an ELISA detection system. If no ligation

FIGURE 9.30 Schematic representation of the functioning of a padlock probe. **(A)** When the bases at the 5′ and 3′ ends of the probes are completely paired to the target DNA, ligation can take place. When there is a single-base mismatch at the 3′ end of the probe, ligation cannot occur and the probe assumes a conformation that does not allow hybridization. **(B)** Under stringent conditions, the ligated probe remains bound to the target DNA, which is bound to the surface of a 96-well micro-titer plate. The nonligated probe is removed during washing. The bound probe is detected by interaction with the reporter molecules. If the reporter is biotin, then avidin and a biotinylated enzyme, such as alkaline phosphatase, are added sequentially. A colored well indicates that the probe is present and bound to the target DNA or RNA.

FIGURE 9.31 Detection of a single-base mutation with fluorescence-labeled PCR primers. **(A)** Primers P1 and P2 amplify DNA from the wild-type sequence. The same primers cannot amplify DNA from the mutant sequence because primer P1 is mismatched with this DNA. Primer P1 is labeled at its 5′ end with rhodamine (red). Primer P2 is unlabeled. **(B)** Primers P3 and P2 amplify DNA from the mutant but not the wild-type sequence. Primer P3 is labeled at its 5′ end with fluorescein (green). Primer P2 is unlabeled. The plus and minus signs denote wild-type and mutant sites, respectively. The genotypes 1/1, 1/2, and 2/2 produce PCR products that contain rhodamine only, rhodamine and fluorescein, and fluorescein only and that fluoresce red, yellow, and green, respectively.

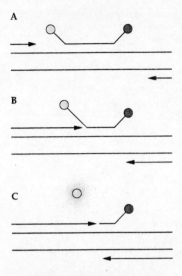

FIGURE 9.32 TaqMan assay. **(A)** A TaqMan probe that is complementary to the wild-type DNA is added prior to PCR amplification of the DNA sequence. The probe contains a fluorescent dye attached to its 5′ end (green) and a quencher attached to its 3′ end (blue). When the probe is intact, the quencher interacts with the fluorophore, quenching its fluorescence. The PCR primers are indicated by arrows. **(B)** In the extension phase of PCR, the TaqMan probe is displaced by the growing DNA strand. **(C)** Subsequently, the 5′ fluorescent dye is cleaved from the probe by the 5′ nuclease activity of the *Taq* polymerase, leading to a dramatic increase in the fluorescence of the reporter dye (shown as a starburst of color from the dye).

occurs because of a mismatch, then no joined probe product will be produced or detected.

Padlock Probes

A padlock probe is an oligonucleotide that is complementary to a target (DNA or RNA) sequence at its 5′ and 3′ ends but not in its middle region (Fig. 9.30). When a padlock probe hybridizes to its target sequence, the 5′ and 3′ ends of the probe come into close proximity with one another and the middle portion loops out. Following hybridization, if the probe is exactly complementary to the target sequence, the 5′ and 3′ ends of the probe can be joined to one another by DNA ligase. The fact that two sequences (actually two ends of the same oligonucleotide) must bind to the target ensures a high "specificity of detection." For DNA ligation to occur, both sequences must hybridize perfectly to the target; this makes it possible to easily detect allelic sequence variants. If there is a mismatch at either end, no ligation occurs. Following the ligation reaction, the probe–target hybrid can be detected because of reporter molecules, such as biotin or digoxigenin, that are attached to the middle (linker) portion of the padlock probe. Padlock probes typically have sequences approximately 15 to 20 nucleotides in length at the 5′ and 3′ ends that are complementary to the target sequence and a middle region of approximately 50 nucleotides. This procedure has become popular with researchers, as it is simpler, with fewer steps than the OLA procedure. In addition, the procedure requires one oligonucleotide compared to two for OLA, and it is amenable to automation.

Genotyping with Fluorescence-Labeled PCR Primers

PCR primers labeled with different fluorescent dyes can be used in the development of nonradioactive color-based detection systems. To distinguish between mutant and wild-type DNAs, PCR is performed with two different primers. One is exactly complementary to the wild-type DNA and is labeled at its 5′ end with rhodamine (red). The other is complementary to the mutant DNA and is labeled at its 5′ end with fluorescein (green) (Fig. 9.31). In both cases, amplification is programmed by a third, unlabeled primer that is complementary to the opposite strand. Since PCR amplification can occur only when the primer is exactly complementary to the target DNA, the presence of these three primers in the same reaction mixture will result in the amplification of either the wild-type or the mutant DNA or both, depending on which target DNAs are initially present to act as PCR templates. If an individual is homozygous for the wild-type DNA, after PCR and removal of unincorporated primer, the reaction mixture will fluoresce red; if he or she is homozygous for the mutant DNA, the reaction mixture will fluoresce green; and if he or she has both mutant and wild-type DNA (i.e., is heterozygous), the reaction mixture will fluoresce yellow. This assay can be automated and adapted for any single-nucleotide target site of any gene that has been sequenced. The problem with this technique is that it is limited to detecting an SNP. Analysis of multiple loci is not possible, since the presence of many different PCR primers in one reaction tube could lead to large numbers of cross-reactions among primer pairs, with a large number of non-specific PCR products being formed.

TaqMan Assay

The TaqMan protocol is used to check individuals for the presence of SNPs that are indicative of any of a variety of genetic diseases (Fig. 9.32). Made popular by one particular company, it is based on the 5′ nuclease activity of *Taq* polymerase, which is commonly used to amplify DNA in PCR applications. To simultaneously monitor wild-type and mutant alleles, two TaqMan probes are utilized. Each probe is exactly complementary to either the wild-type or the mutant DNA sequence, and each probe has a different fluorescent dye attached to its 5′ end. Intact probes, whether bound or unbound to cDNA, do not fluoresce because of the presence of the quencher molecule at the 3′ end of the probe. As PCR proceeds from primers flanking the probe hybridization site, the TaqMan probe is displaced by the growing DNA strand, and the 5′ nuclease activity of the *Taq* polymerase degrades the 5′ end of the TaqMan probe, thereby releasing the fluorescent dye and removing it from the proximity of the quencher molecule. Thus, only TaqMan probes that were previously bound to target DNA will be degraded and subsequently fluoresce. Any mismatched probes, due to mutations in the region where the TaqMan probe binds, will be displaced but not cleaved, so they will not fluoresce. By monitoring the fluorescence at two different wavelengths (one for each TaqMan probe), it is possible to distinguish the wild type, heterozygotes (carrying one mutant and one wild-type gene), and individuals that are homozygous for the target mutation. In fact, this technique may be used to assay for two or three mutations at the same time. The only requirements for the successful employment of the technique are that (1) the precise DNA sequences of the target DNAs must be known and (2) the fluorescent dyes must have well-separated, nonoverlapping fluorescence maxima.

SUMMARY

To be effective, a diagnostic test must be (1) specific for the target molecule, (2) sensitive enough to detect minute levels of the target, and (3) technically simple, with unequivocal results that can be obtained readily. There are two categories of molecular diagnostic techniques. One category relies on the specificity of an antibody for a particular antigen. The other uses nucleic acid hybridization or PCR to detect a specific nucleic acid sequence.

A common assay that uses antibodies is the ELISA. In this procedure, (1) a sample is bound to a solid support, (2) a primary antibody specific for the target antigen is added and binds to the target antigen, (3) a secondary antibody–enzyme conjugate that binds to the primary antibody is added, and (4) a colorless substrate that is transformed into a colored compound by the enzyme in the conjugate is added. The appearance of a color response in an ELISA indicates the presence of the target molecule in the sample.

ELISAs have been used for detecting various proteins, identifying viruses and bacteria, and determining the presence of low-molecular-weight compounds in a wide range of biological samples. To increase the specificity of the primary antibody and to ensure the reliability of the antibody preparation, monoclonal antibodies are often used for diagnostic ELISAs.

Nucleic acid hybridization can be a highly sensitive and specific method for detecting the presence of a nucleic acid sequence in a biological sample. This method has been used to develop diagnostic assays for disease-causing organisms in a clinical setting and other organisms in the environment.

Because a nucleic acid detection assay is directed toward a known DNA sequence, primers for PCR can be synthesized and then used to amplify the target sequence. The detection assay can be run in a nonradioactive system, such as the biotin–streptavidin–chemiluminescence protocol, or the amplified PCR product can be scored by gel electrophoresis. Also, a PCR product can be labeled with a fluorescent dye that is attached to the 5′ end of the primer.

One way to characterize forensic samples is by DNA fingerprinting. In this technique, human minisatellite DNA, which does not encode any proteins and is highly variable in sequence, is usually used as a hybridization probe. The extensive variability of human minisatellite DNA sequences means that each human being produces a unique set of hybridized DNA bands.

To characterize plant DNA, a set of arbitrary oligonucleotide primers can be used to amplify random segments of the plant DNA by PCR and, after electrophoresis, to produce a specific set of DNA bands. This procedure is called the RAPD procedure. Any particular set of primer sequences will produce a unique collection of amplified DNA fragments that is characteristic of the genomic DNA of a particular plant cultivar.

DNA diagnostic assays can also be used to detect the presence of a single-nucleotide change in a particular gene. One of these methods distinguishes between the ligation and the absence of ligation of two oligonucleotides. A single-nucleotide mismatch at the junction of the hybridized oligonucleotides prevents ligation. In general, the use of PCR increases the resolution of nucleic acid diagnostic tests and should also decrease the overall costs of these assays.

The development of molecular diagnostic assays is a growing and dynamic field. Although the technical details of various tests may differ, the general principles have been established. At present, PCR has contributed significantly to overcoming the problem of the limited availability of target DNA. The use of PCR for probe systems has eliminated most concerns about the sensitivity of the detection signal, with the result that nonradioactive chromogenic, chemiluminescent, or fluorescent systems can be used reliably for certain assays. Moreover, in a number of tests, PCR treatment and electrophoretic analysis are sufficient to determine the presence of either a genetic mutation or an infectious agent in the targeted sample. Undoubtedly, many novel DNA-based systems will be created for the diagnosis of most, if not all, of the common genetic, infectious, and malignant diseases.

REFERENCES

Banér, J., M. Nilsson, A. Isaksson, M. Mendel-Hartvig, D.-O. Antson, and U. Landegren. 2001. More keys to padlock probes: mechanisms for high-throughput nucleic acid analysis. *Curr. Opin. Biotechnol.* 12:11–15.

Barker, R. H., L. Suebsaeng, W. Rooney, G. C. Alecrim, H. V. Dourado, and D. F. Wirth. 1986. Specific DNA probe for the diagnosis of *Plasmodium falciparum* malaria. *Science* 231:1434–1436.

Bolnick, D. A., D. Fullwiley, T. Duster, R. S. Cooper, J. H. Fujimura, J. Kahn, J. S. Kaufman, J. Marks, A. Morning, A. Nelson, P. Ossorio, J. Reardon, S. M. Reverby, and K. TallBear. 2007. The science and business of genetic ancestry testing. *Science* 318:399–400.

Boonham, N., J. Tomlinson, and R. Mumford. 2007. Microarrays for rapid identification of plant viruses. *Annu. Rev. Phytopathol.* 45:307–328.

Bugawan, T. L., R. K. Saiki, C. H. Levenson, R. M. Watson, and H. A. Erlich. 1988. The use of non-radioactive oligonucleotide probes to analyze enzymatically amplified DNA for prenatal diagnosis and forensic HLA typing. *Bio/Technology* 6:943–947.

Campbell, R. E., O. Tour, A. E. Palmer, P. A. Steinbach, G. S. Baird, D. A. Zacharias, and R. Y. Tsien. 2002. A monomeric red fluorescent protein. *Proc. Natl. Acad. Sci. USA* 12:7877–7882.

Cao, W. 2004. Recent developments in ligase-mediated amplification and detection. *Trends Biotechnol.* 22:38–44.

Carlson, D. P., C. Superko, J. Mackey, M. E. Gaskill, and P. Hansen. 1990. Chemiluminescent detection of nucleic acid hybridization. *Focus* 12:9–12.

Caskey, C. T. 1987. Disease diagnosis by recombinant DNA methods. *Science* 236:1223–1229.

Chehab, F. F., and Y. W. Kan. 1989. Detection of specific DNA sequences by fluorescence amplification: a color complementation assay. *Proc. Natl. Acad. Sci. USA* 86:9178–9182.

Claustres, M. 2005. Frequency and nature of mutations and methods to detect them, p. 9–31. *In* G. R. Taylor and I. N. M. Day (ed.), *Guide to Mutation Detection.* John Wiley & Sons, Inc., New York, NY.

Debenham, P. G. 1992. Probing identity: the changing face of DNA fingerprinting. *Trends Biotechnol.* 10:96–102.

Erlich, H. A., D. Gelfand, and J. J. Sninsky. 1991. Recent advances in the polymerase chain reaction. *Science* 252:1643–1651.

Eshaque, B., and B. Dixon. 2006. Technology platforms for molecular diagnosis of cystic fibrosis. *Biotechnol. Adv.* 24:86–93.

Gillam, I. C. 1987. Non-radioactive probes for specific DNA sequences. *Trends Biotechnol.* 5:332–334.

Godiwala, N. T., A. Vandewalle, H. D. Ward, and B. A. Leav. 2006. Quantification of in vitro and in vivo *Cryptosporidium parvum* infection by using real-time PCR. *Appl. Environ. Microbiol.* 72:4484–4488.

Hardenbol, P., J. Banér, M. Jain, M. Nilsson, E. A. Namsaraev, G. A. Karlin-Neumann, H. Fakhari-Rad, M. Ronaghi, T. D. Willis, U. Landegren, and R. W. Davis. 2003. Multiplexed genotyping with sequence-tagged molecular inversion probes. *Nat. Biotechnol.* 21:673–678.

Hsieh, H.-M., H.-L. Chiang, L.-C. Tsai, S.-Y. Lai, N.-E. Huang, A. Linacre, and J. C.-I. Lee. 2001. Cytochrome *b* gene for species identification of conservation animals. *Forensic Sci. Int.* 122:7–18.

Jeffreys, A. J., A. MacLeod, K. Tamaki, D. L. Neil, and D. G. Monckton. 1991. Minisatellite repeat coding as a digital approach to DNA typing. *Nature* 354:204–209.

Kingsbury, D. T. 1987. DNA probes in the diagnosis of genetic and infectious diseases. *Trends Biotechnol.* 5:107–111.

Klevan, L., and G. Gebeyehu. 1990. Biotinylated nucleotides for labeling and detecting DNA. *Methods Enzymol.* 184:561–577.

Kohler, G., and C. Milstein. 1975. Continuous cultures of fused cells secreting antibody of predefined specificity. *Nature* 256:495–497.

Kostrikis, L. G., S. Tyagi, M. M. Mhlanga, D. D. Ho, and F. R. Kramer. 1998. Spectral genotyping of human alleles. *Science* 279:1228–1229.

Kuppuswamy, M. N., J. W. Hoffmann, C. K. Kasper, S. G. Spitzer, S. L. Groce, and S. P. Bajaj. 1991. Single nucleotide primer extension to detect genetic diseases: experimental application to hemophilia B (factor IX) and cystic fibrosis genes. *Proc. Natl. Acad. Sci. USA* 88:1143–1147.

Nickerson, D. A., R. Kaiser, S. Lappin, J. Stewart, L. Hood, and U. Landegren. 1990. Automated DNA diagnostic using an ELISA-based oligonucleotide ligation assay. *Proc. Natl. Acad. Sci. USA* 87:8923–8927.

Nivens, D. E., T. E. McKnight, S. A. Moser, S. J. Osbourn, M. L. Simpson, and G. S. Sayler. 2004. Bioluminescent bioreporter integrated circuits: potentially small, rugged and inexpensive whole-cell biosensors for remote environmental monitoring. *J. Appl. Microbiol.* 96:33–46.

Persing, D. H., T. F. Smith, F. C. Tenover, and T. J. White (ed.). 1993. *Diagnostic Molecular Microbiology: Principles and Applications.* American Society for Microbiology, Washington, DC.

Pollard-Knight, D., A. C. Simmonds, A. P. Schaap, H. Akhavan, and M. A. W. Brady. 1990. Nonradioactive DNA detection on Southern blots by enzymatically triggered chemiluminescence. *Anal. Biochem.* 185:353–358.

Rafalski, J. A., and S. V. Tingey. 1993. Genetic diagnostics in plant breeding: RAPDs, microsatellites and machines. *Trends Genet.* 9:275–279.

Rajkovic, A., B. El Moualij, M. Uyttendaele, P. Brolet, W. Zorzi, E. Heinen, E. Foubert, and J. Debevere. 2006. Immunoquantitative real-time PCR for detection and quantification of *Staphylococcus aureus* enterotoxin B in foods. *Appl. Environ. Microbiol.* 72:6593–6599.

Sanseverino, J., R. K. Gupta, A. C. Layton, S. S. Patterson, S. A. Ripp, L. Saidak, M. L. Simpson, T. W. Schultz, and G. S. Sayler. 2005. Use of *Saccharomyces cerevisiae* BLYES expressing bacterial bioluminescence for rapid detection of estrogenic compounds. *Appl. Environ. Microbiol.* 71:4455–4460.

Sayler, G. S., and A. C. Layton. 1990. Environmental application of nucleic acid hybridization. *Annu. Rev. Microbiol.* 44:625–648.

Shaner, N. C., R. E. Campbell, P. A. Steinbach, B. N. G. Giepmans, A. E. Palmer, and R. Y. Tsien. 2004. Improved monomeric red, orange and yellow fluorescent proteins derived from *Discosoma* sp. red fluorescent protein. *Nat. Biotechnol.* 22:1567–1572.

Tyagi, S., and F. R. Kramer. 1996. Molecular beacons: probes that fluoresce upon hybridization. *Nat. Biotechnol.* 14:303–308.

Tyagi, S., D. P. Bratu, and F. R. Kramer. 1998. Multicolor molecular beacons for allele discrimination. *Nat. Biotechnol.* 16:49–53.

Waldmann, T. A. 1991. Monoclonal antibodies in diagnosis and therapy. *Science* 252:1657–1662.

Weiss, J. B. 1995. DNA probes and PCR for diagnosis of parasitic infections. *Clin. Microbiol. Rev.* 8:113–130.

Weitz, H. J., J. M. Ritchie, D. A. Bailey, A. M. Horsburgh, K. Killham, and L. A. Glover. 2001. Construction of a modified mini-Tn5 *lux*CDABE transposon for the development of bacterial biosensors for ecotoxicity testing. *FEMS Microbiol. Lett.* 197:159–165.

White, T. J., R. Madej, and D. H. Persing. 1992. The polymerase chain reaction: clinical applications. *Adv. Clin. Chem.* 29:161–196.

Wolffs, P. F. G., K. Glencross, R. Thibaudeau, and M. W. Griffiths. 2006. Direct quantitation and detection of salmonellae in biological samples without enrichment using two-step filtration and real-time PCR. *Appl. Environ. Microbiol.* 72:3896–3900.

Wong, M. L., and J. F. Medrano. 2005. Real-time PCR for mRNA quantitation. *BioTechniques* 39:75–85.

Yu, K. F., A. Van Deynze, and K. P. Pauls. 1993. Random amplified polymorphic DNA (RAPD) analysis, p. 287–301. *In* B. R. Glick and J. E. Thompson (ed.), *Methods in Plant Molecular Biology and Biotechnology.* CRC Press, Inc., Boca Raton, FL.

REVIEW QUESTIONS

1. Briefly describe how the change in the human β-globin gene that gives rise to sickle-cell anemia can be detected by using PCR.

2. Describe and discuss the PCR/OLA detection protocol.

3. What is an ELISA? How does it work?

4. Describe several types of nonradioactive DNA labels. What are the advantages of nonradioactive detection procedures?

5. You have been given the task of developing a simple, sensitive, and reproducible diagnostic procedure for a double-stranded DNA virus that is devastating a local cattle population. Because effective treatment of this disease depends on early and correct diagnosis, you need to be able to detect the very low levels of this virus that are present in infected animals before the onset of disease symptoms. Briefly explain how you would proceed and why you have chosen a particular course of action.

6. For diagnostic assays, what is meant by sensitivity, specificity, and simplicity?

7. How is Chagas disease currently diagnosed? How might the existing procedures be improved?

8. What is a molecular beacon probe, and how does it work?

9. What is DNA fingerprinting, and how is it used to characterize traces of DNA in forensic samples?

10. What is the RAPD procedure, and how can it be used to characterize plant cultivars?

11. What is a padlock probe, and how is it used?

12. What are monoclonal antibodies? How are they different from polyclonal antibodies?

13. Briefly, explain how the HAT selection for hybridomas works.

14. How can molecular beacon probes be used to (1) detect several genes in the same sample and (2) characterize an individual's genotype for a particular genetic disease, such as sickle-cell anemia?

15. Why is it difficult to screen an individual's chromosomal DNA to assess whether he or she carries a mutation of the CFTR gene that leads to cystic fibrosis?

16. Why is it useful to simultaneously employ several different-color fluorescent proteins?

17. How would you develop microbial biosensors to detect environmental contaminants?

18. What is real-time PCR? What is it used for? How does it work?

19. What is immunoquantitative real-time PCR, and how does it work?

20. What is a padlock probe, and how does it work?

21. What is the TaqMan assay procedure, and how can it be used to assay SNPs?

10

Protein Therapeutics

PRIOR TO THE DEVELOPMENT OF RECOMBINANT DNA TECHNOLOGY, most human protein pharmaceuticals were available in only limited quantities, they were extremely costly to produce, and, in a number of cases, their biological modes of action were not well characterized. When recombinant DNA technology was first developed, it was heralded as a means of producing a whole range of possible human therapeutic agents in sufficient quantities for both efficacy testing and eventual human use. This forecast has turned out to be true. Today, the "genes" (mostly complementary DNAs [cDNAs]) for several thousand different proteins that are potential human therapeutic agents have been cloned. Most of these sequences have been expressed in mammalian as well as bacterial host cells, and currently more than 500 are undergoing clinical testing with human subjects for the treatment of various diseases. More than 250 of these "biotechnology drugs" have been approved for use in the United States or the European Union (Table 10.1). However, it will be several years before many of the other proteins are commercially available, because medical products must first be tested rigorously in animals and then undergo thorough human trials, which can last for several years, before being approved for general use. However, the financial incentive for pharmaceutical companies is considerable. It has been estimated that in 2006 the annual global market for human recombinant protein drugs was about $60 billion. Ten "blockbuster" drugs constitute nearly half of these sales. For example, in 2006, rituximab (Rituxan), a monoclonal antibody used to treat individuals with non-Hodgkin lymphoma, generated nearly $4 billion in sales, while various forms of recombinant human insulin generated around $2.5 billion.

The development of preventive procedures and treatments for human diseases was the outstanding contribution of medicine and science to human well-being in the 20th century. This process, however, is a continuous one. So-called old diseases (e.g., tuberculosis) can reappear if preventive measures are relaxed or if antibiotic-resistant organisms arise. The idea of using antibodies as therapeutic agents has come to fruition in the past several years, and specific antibodies are being tested to attack toxins, bacteria, viruses, and even cancer cells. An antibody may be viewed as a

TABLE 10.1 Examples of recombinant proteins that have been approved for human use in the United States or the European Union

Alglucosidase α	Granulocyte-macrophage colony-stimulating factor	Interferon analogues
Anakinra		Interleukin-2
Antihemophilic factor	Hirudin	Interleukin-2 analogues
Darbepoetin α	Human growth hormone	Interleukin-11
Dibotermin	Human growth hormone analogue	Interleukin-11 analogue
DNase I	Hyaluronidase	Keratinocyte growth factor
Drotrecogin α	Insulin	Laronidase
Erythropoietin	Insulin analogue	Novel erythropoiesis-stimulating protein
Factor VIIa	Insulin-like growth factor 1	
Factor VIII	Interferon-α2a	Osteogenic protein
Factor IX	Interferon-α2b	Platelet-derived growth factor
Follicle-stimulating hormone	Interferon-αN3	Stem cell factor
α-Galactosidase	Interferon-β1a	Tissue plasminogen activator
Galsulfase	Interferon-β1b	Thyrotropin-α
Glucagon	Interferon-γ1b	Truncated tissue plasminogen activator
β-Glucocerebrosidase analogue	Interferon-N	

target-seeking missile or as a magic bullet that either can directly neutralize an offending agent or, if equipped with a warhead or poison arrow, can destroy a specific target cell.

Pharmaceuticals

Isolation of Interferon cDNAs

A number of different strategies have been used to isolate either the genes or cDNAs for human proteins. In some cases, the target protein is isolated and a portion of the amino acid sequence is determined. From this information, a DNA coding sequence is deduced. The appropriate oligonucleotide is synthesized and used as a DNA hybridization probe to isolate the gene or cDNA from either a genomic or a cDNA library. Alternatively, antibodies are raised against the purified protein and used to screen a gene expression library. For human proteins that are synthesized primarily in a single tissue, a cDNA library from the messenger RNA (mRNA) of that tissue is enriched for the target DNA sequence. For example, the major protein synthesized by the islets of Langerhans of the pancreas is insulin; 70% of the mRNA fraction isolated from these cells encodes insulin.

Before the completion of sequencing of the human genome in 2001, it was often necessary to devise innovative approaches to isolate human genes or cDNAs, especially when the proteins encoded were found in very low concentrations or when the site of synthesis was not known. The human interferon (IFN) proteins, which include IFN-α, IFN-β, and IFN-γ, are naturally occurring proteins, each one with somewhat different biological activity. When the IFN cDNAs were initially isolated in the early 1980s, very little was known about the encoded proteins (IFN was originally thought to be a single protein), so a novel scheme had to be devised to overcome the scarcity of both the mRNAs and the proteins. Also, at the time, *Escherichia coli* expression vectors for eukaryotic cDNAs were not readily available, so it was necessary to devise an indirect scheme to iso-

late IFN cDNA. The isolation of IFN cDNAs included the following steps (Fig. 10.1).

1. Size-fractionated mRNA was isolated from human leukocytes, reverse transcribed, and inserted into the PstI site of plasmid pBR322.
2. The approximately 6,000 clones that were produced following transformation of *E. coli* were divided into 12 pools of 512 clones each. Pools of clones, rather than individual clones, were tested to speed up the identification process.
3. The plasmid DNA from each pool was hybridized to a crude IFN mRNA preparation.
4. The input mRNA that hybridized to the plasmid DNA was separated from the cloned DNA–mRNA hybrids and translated in a cell-free protein synthesis system.
5. Each translation mixture was then assayed for IFN antiviral activity. The pools that showed IFN activity contained at least one clone with a cDNA that hybridized to IFN mRNA.
6. Positive pools were divided into eight subgroups of 64 clones each and retested (i.e., steps 3 to 5 were repeated). This subgrouping process was repeated until a clone with the complete cDNA for a human IFN was identified.

Subsequently, whenever large quantities of the IFN were required, the IFN cDNAs could be subcloned into an *E. coli* expression vector and expressed at high levels.

Human Interferons

After the isolation of the first IFN gene, researchers found that there are a number of different IFNs. On the basis of chemical and biological properties, the IFNs can be classified, as noted above, into three different groups: IFN-α, IFN-β, and IFN-γ. The proteins IFN-α and IFN-β are synthesized in cells that have been exposed to viruses or viral RNA; IFN-γ is synthesized in response to cell growth-stimulating agents. IFN-α is encoded by a family

FIGURE 10.1 Overview of the protocol used to isolate IFN cDNA.

of 13 different (but similar) genes, IFN-β is encoded by two genes, and IFN-γ is encoded by a single gene. The IFN-α subtypes have different specificities. For example, the antiviral activities of IFN-α2 and IFN-α1 are approximately the same when assessed with a virus-challenged bovine cell line, but IFN-α2 is seven times more effective than IFN-α1 when human cells are treated with virus. IFN-α2 is 30 times less effective than IFN-α1 when mouse cells are used in this assay.

Interferon gene shuffling. Several research groups have attempted to engineer IFNs with combined properties based on different members of the IFN-α gene family that vary in the extents and specificities of their antiviral activities. Theoretically, this can be achieved by splicing a portion of one IFN-α gene with a DNA sequence from a different IFN-α gene to create, after translation, a hybrid protein that exhibits novel properties, i.e., properties different from either of the contributing genes.

In one study, hybrid genes from IFN-α2 and IFN-α3 were constructed in an effort to create proteins with novel IFN activities. Comparison of the sequences of the two IFN-α cDNAs indicated that they had common restriction sites at positions 60, 92, and 150. Digestion of both cDNAs at these sites and ligation of the DNA fragments yielded a number of hybrid derivatives of the original genes (Fig. 10.2). These hybrids were expressed in *E. coli*, and the resultant proteins were purified and examined for various biological functions. When tested for the extent of protection of mammalian cells in culture against viral infection, some of the hybrid IFNs were found to have greater activity than the parental molecules. In addition, many of the hybrid IFNs induced test cells to synthesize (2′-5′)-oligoisoadenylate synthetase. This enzyme generates (2′-5′)-linked oligonucleotides, which in turn activate a latent cellular endoribonuclease that cleaves viral mRNA. Other hybrid IFNs had an antiproliferative activity against various human cancers that was greater than that of either of the parental molecules. More recently, additional hybrid IFN molecules have been generated by a variation of the above-mentioned procedure. In this case, the entire IFN-α cDNA family was PCR amplified and then digested with DNase into small DNA fragments (~50 to 60 nucleotides long) before the fragments were shuffled and amplified by PCR (Fig. 10.3). This procedure works because the PCR mixture contains many overlapping single-stranded DNAs that can act as PCR primers (see "Chemical Synthesis of DNA" in chapter 4). Following testing of the many shuffled IFN cDNAs, it is possible to select hybrid IFNs with vastly improved antiviral or antiproliferative activities. In fact, some hybrid IFNs have recently undergone successful clinical trials (Box 10.1) and have been approved for use as human therapeutic agents. The strategy for creating hybrid IFNs can also be applied to other gene families whose products have therapeutic potential.

Longer-acting interferons. Hepatitis C virus infection is one of the most common causes of liver disease, which affects nearly 200 million people worldwide. Many of these individuals eventually develop either cirrhosis of the liver or hepatocellular carcinoma. Therapeutic agents that maximize early antiviral response and maintain viral suppression throughout the course of therapy have the best chance of achieving lasting eradication of the virus from an infected individual. One effective treatment for hepatitis C includes the combined use of the antiviral chemical compound ribavirin with IFN-α. Longer-acting IFNs are needed to minimize the side effects

FIGURE 10.2 Structure of the IFN-α2 and IFN-α3 genes and four hybrid genes. Comparison of the sequences of the IFN-α2 and IFN-α3 genes shows shared restriction enzyme sites (RE1, RE2, and RE3). Digestion of the genes at the indicated restriction sites and ligation of the resulting fragments generate a number of different hybrid IFN genes, of which four possibilities are shown.

from IFN treatment, lower the required dosage, and decrease the required frequency of the treatments. One approach to creating long-acting IFNs includes PEGylation. PEGylation entails covalently attaching polyethylene glycol (PEG) to proteins. The binding is typically achieved by incubation of a reactive derivative of PEG with the target protein molecule. PEGylation increases the size of IFN in solution, thereby prolonging its circulatory time by reducing its renal clearance. A simpler means of generating longer-acting IFNs is to fuse an IFN gene with the gene for a stable protein, such as human serum albumin, that, after translation, produces a stable hybrid protein. This combination has been called the albumin–interferon hybrid molecule (Zalbin, formerly Albuferon), and it retains all of the biological activity of the native IFN molecule (Fig. 10.4). Native IFN levels in the blood of a treated patient typically decrease rapidly, so that 2 days after administration, they are undetectable. On the other hand, with the albumin-interferon hybrid molecule, the drug (in this case, the fusion protein) in serum remains at a therapeutically effective level for a much longer time, so that it needs to be administered no more than once every 2 weeks. The initial clinical trials of the albumin-interferon hybrid molecule have all been positive. Phase III clinical trials of the albumin-interferon hybrid molecule began in late 2006. If these trials are successful, then the albumin-interferon hybrid molecule may be available for general use some time in 2010.

Human Growth Hormone

Human growth hormone (somatotropin) is a 191-amino-acid pituitary protein with a molecular mass of 22,125 daltons (Da) that stimulates the

1. PCR amplify IFN cDNAs
2. Partially digest IFN cDNAs with DNase
3. Assemble chimeric cDNAs by PCR synthesis

FIGURE 10.3 Construction of hybrid IFN-α genes. The resultant IFN-α gene-shuffled libraries are tested for antiproliferative and antiviral activities.

production of insulin-like growth factor 1. Insulin-like growth factor 1 is an essential component of the promotion of growth in children, and in adults, it controls metabolism. Human growth hormone was one of the first therapeutic proteins in the world to be approved for human use. The recombinant form of the protein is produced in *E. coli* and is identical to native pituitary-derived human growth hormone. Infants and children who lack sufficient endogenous levels of human growth hormone, patients with chronic renal insufficiency (defective kidneys), and individuals with Turner syndrome respond to treatment with growth hormone, which stimulates tissue and bone growth, increases protein synthesis and mineral retention, and decreases body fat storage.

The first recombinant growth hormone was called somatrem (Protropin); it was produced and marketed by Genentech beginning in 1985. It had an amino acid sequence that was identical to that of human growth hormone, except that there was an extra methionine residue at the N-terminal end of the peptide chain (which was thought to prolong its half-life). It was discontinued in the late 1990s.

Treatment of children with human growth hormone typically entails daily injections during the years when the child is growing. The cost of the treatment varies depending on the country and the size of the child but is generally approximately $10,000 to $30,000 per year. In addition, in 2004, the U.S. Food and Drug Administration (FDA) approved the use of recombinant human growth hormone for individuals whose short stature was

BOX 10.1

Clinical Trials

After the discovery of a new drug or course of treatment, and before it is made available to the public, it is essential that extensive studies and analysis of its safety and efficacy be conducted and then reviewed by an impartial agency. Although a large number of countries have developed their own approaches to test new therapeutics, the "gold standard" for clinical trials is the set of requirements established by the FDA. This process is briefly described here.

The preclinical phase of therapeutic drug development (i.e., the initial stage of the process of bringing a new therapeutic agent to market) entails thorough and extensive laboratory research on the mode of action, structure, and other biochemical and physical properties of a potential new drug. Scientists working at universities, research institutes, and drug and biotechnology companies are continually discovering and testing new molecules, as well as new uses for known compounds. However, it is impossible to know with any certainty which avenues of research will eventually bear fruit. Once a promising result has been obtained in the laboratory, and it has been shown to be reproducible, sufficient quantities of a highly purified version of the potential therapeutic compound must be produced so that it can be tested on small animals, such as mice. If the animal tests are positive and there is no evidence of any serious side effects, the organization seeking to commercialize the research

files an "investigational new drug" application with the FDA. This is an application to begin the process of clinical trials. Based on the preclinical research data that are provided, about 85% of these applications are approved.

Clinical trials are conducted in three distinct phases (described below), generally requiring a total of about 7 to 9 years at a cost of approximately $75 million to $100 million to complete. At each stage, various compounds are dropped from consideration based on the results obtained. Eventually, approximately 20% of the compounds that looked promising based on preclinical results will, after a careful review of all the data, finally be approved. This slow and expensive process is claimed to be "the most effective method ever devised to assess the efficacy of a treatment."

The three phases of the FDA review process are as follows.

Phase I: With between 10 and 100 healthy people, the safety of the drug and, starting with very low doses, the highest dosages that can be administered are assessed. When there is a chance that serious side effects may result, individuals affected with the disorder that the drug is designed to alleviate may be used.

Phase II: With 50 to 500 affected patients, the optimal dosing regimen is determined. A control group is used so that it is possible to clearly distinguish between the effects of the drug and the natural

remission of the disease. The use of a control group also helps to delineate real from apparent side effects of the treatment.

Phase III: Depending upon the disease, approximately 300 to 30,000 patients who have the disease are tested. After it is established that the drug is not harmful and the optimal dosing regimen has been determined, the effectiveness of the treatment needs to be proven.

The requirement for careful and thorough clinical trials ensures both the safety and efficacy of approved drugs. However, since the costs of both the preclinical research and the clinical trials are borne by pharmaceutical companies, this system makes it difficult for small companies that discover a new product to eventually bring that product to market without the involvement of a large corporation with significant financial resources. Furthermore, the high cost of clinical trials and the low probability of a new drug's being approved mean that it is unlikely that therapeutic agents will even be considered for clinical trials unless there is a strong possibility that there will be significant financial gains from the sale of that agent. This financial disincentive may discourage research on therapeutic agents for diseases that either affect only a relatively small number of people or affect only populations in poor, underdeveloped countries.

caused by a variety of medical conditions other than human growth hormone deficiency.

The strategy of designing a protein by either functional domain shuffling or directed mutagenesis can be used to augment or constrain its mode of action. For example, native human growth hormone binds to both growth hormone and prolactin receptors that occur on a number of different cell types. To avoid unwanted side effects during therapy, it is desirable that human growth hormone bind only to growth hormone receptors. Because the segment of the growth hormone molecule that binds to the growth hormone receptor overlaps but is not identical to the portion of the

FIGURE 10.4 Schematic representation of the synthesis of the albumin–interferon fusion protein (Zalbin, formerly Albuferon), which includes human serum albumin (HSA) (red) at the N terminus and human IFN-α2b (blue) at the C terminus. Modified from http://www.hgsi.com/albinterferon-alfa-2b.html with permission.

molecule that binds to the prolactin receptor, it should be possible to selectively decrease the binding to the prolactin receptor.

Site-specific mutagenesis of the cloned human growth hormone cDNA was used to change some of the amino acid side chains that act as ligands for Zn^{2+} (i.e., His-18, His-21, and Glu-174), because the ion is required for the high-affinity binding of human growth hormone to the prolactin receptor (Fig. 10.5). As hoped, these modifications yielded human growth hormone derivatives that bound to the growth hormone receptor but not to the prolactin receptor. These derivatives are being tested for safety and efficacy in humans.

FIGURE 10.5 Schematic representation of native and modified human growth hormone. Oligonucleotide-directed mutagenesis was used to alter human growth hormone so that it no longer bound to the prolactin receptor but retained its specificity for the growth hormone receptor.

As a consequence of its relatively short half-life in plasma, human growth hormone therapy currently requires subcutaneous injection once a day. This treatment is both inconvenient and expensive. Therefore, it would be advantageous to have a long-lasting form of human growth hormone. To this end, the extracellular domain of the human growth hormone receptor was fused to human growth hormone using a 20-amino-acid-long linker peptide consisting of four repeats of the amino acids Gly_4Ser (Fig. 10.6). This construct has a very strong tendency to dimerize as the growth hormone moiety from one molecule binds with the receptor portion of another molecule. When this growth hormone construct was tested in rats, a single injection promoted growth for 10 days (compared to the usual requirement in rats for daily injections). It is thought that the dimerization of the growth hormone construct stabilizes human growth hormone in vivo so that it is cleared from plasma approximately 300 times more slowly than free human growth hormone. Under these conditions, the active monomeric form (Fig.10.6A) is slowly released from the inactive dimeric growth hormone (Fig.10.6B), allowing it to bind to the growth hormone receptor (Fig.10.6C). This experiment is certainly intriguing. It remains to be determined whether humans respond in a similar manner to the dimerized complex.

Another method that has been devised to prolong the active lifetime of human growth hormone includes fusing the coding sequences for the C-terminal end of human growth hormone (~22 kDa) with the N-terminal end of human serum albumin (~67 kDa). This fusion protein is called Albutropin (Fig. 10.7); it has a molecular mass of ~89 kDa and is produced by a strain of yeast that has been genetically modified so that the proteins that it produces have a minimal number of posttranslational modifications. The stabilization of the human growth hormone portion of Albutropin reflects the stability of human serum albumin, which has a half-life in serum of about 19 days. Albutropin has been shown to be effective in both

FIGURE 10.6 Derivatization of growth hormone by coupling it to a portion of the growth hormone receptor using a 20-amino-acid peptide. (A) Monomeric derivative; (B) dimeric derivative; (C) monomeric derivative bound to a growth hormone receptor.

Human
serum
albumin

COOH

Human
growth
hormone

H₂N

FIGURE 10.7 Schematic representation of the fusion protein Albutropin, which includes human serum albumin (red) at the N terminus and human growth hormone (blue) at the C terminus.

rats and monkeys, in which high levels of the protein in serum were observed 5 days after it was administered (Fig. 10.8). Moreover, Albutropin has successfully completed phase I clinical trials.

Tumor Necrosis Factor Alpha

While a number of studies have clearly shown that tumor necrosis factor alpha (TNF-α) is a potent antitumor agent, it has not been widely used in this capacity because of its severe toxicity. If TNF-α could be delivered directly to its site of action, i.e., the tumor, then lower doses could be used and the unwanted side effects would be diminished. To develop a version of TNF-α with tumor specificity, DNA encoding the peptide Cys-Asn-Gly-Arg-Cys-Gly (which targets a tumor cell surface protein) was fused to TNF-α DNA. The fusion protein contained a 6-amino-acid extension at its N-terminal end (Fig. 10.9). In mice, the cytotoxic activities of Cys-Asn-Gly-Arg-Cys-Gly–TNF-α and TNF-α were identical, indicating that the additional amino acids did not prevent protein folding, combining of three subunits to form a trimer, or binding to receptors. However, the modified version of TNF-α was 12 to 15 times more effective at inhibiting tumor growth than the unmodified form. Moreover, a higher percentage of mice with lymphoma survived after treatment with the modified factor (Fig. 10.10). In addition, all the mice that were treated with the modified factor and survived for 30 days survived a second and third challenge with mouse lymphoma cells. These data indicate that there is a significant benefit, at least in mice, to fusing TNF-α with a short targeting peptide. Nevertheless, this work must be regarded as preliminary until its efficacy is demonstrated in humans.

FIGURE 10.8 Intravenous concentration in monkeys of either human growth hormone or Albutropin following subcutaneous injection.

A B

FIGURE 10.9 Schematic representation of TNF-α (blue) without **(A)** and with **(B)** a 6-amino-acid peptide (red) fused to its N terminus. The protein structure shown is hypothetical; only the numbers of amino acid residues (shown as circles) are accurately depicted.

Enzymes

DNase I

Cystic fibrosis is one of the most common fatal hereditary diseases among Europeans and their descendants, with approximately 30,000 diagnosed cases in the United States and another 23,000 cases in Canada and Europe. It is estimated that a mutant cystic fibrosis gene is carried by 1 in 29 Europeans, 1 in 65 African Americans, and 1 in 150 Asians. Individuals with cystic fibrosis are highly susceptible to bacterial infections in their lungs. Antibiotic treatment of patients who have these recurring infections eventually leads to the selection of antibiotic-resistant bacteria. The presence of bacteria, some alive and some lysed, contributes to the accumulation of a thick mucus in the lungs of these patients, making breathing very difficult and acting as a source for further infection. The thick mucus in the

FIGURE 10.10 Survival of lymphoma-bearing mice following treatment with 3 μg of either TNF-α or Cys-Asn-Gly-Arg-Cys-Gly–TNF-α (CNGRCG–TNF) as a function of the number of days after treatment.

lungs is the result of the combination of the alginate that is secreted by the living bacteria, the DNA that is released from lysed bacterial cells, and degenerating leukocytes that accumulate in response to the infection, as well as filamentous actin derived from the cytoskeletons of damaged epithelial cells (Fig. 10.11). To address this problem, scientists at the U.S. biotechnology company Genentech isolated the gene for the human enzyme deoxyribonuclease I (DNase I) and subsequently expressed the gene in Chinese hamster ovary (CHO) cells in culture. DNase I can hydrolyze long polymeric DNA chains into much shorter oligonucleotides. The purified enzyme was delivered in an aerosol mist to the lungs of patients with cystic fibrosis. The DNase I decreased the viscosity and adhesivity of the mucus in the lungs and made it easier for these patients to breathe. While this treatment is not a cure for cystic fibrosis, it nevertheless relieves the most severe symptom of the disease in most patients. The enzyme was approved for use by the FDA in 1994; it had sales of approximately $100 million in 2000.

The monomeric form of actin binds very tightly to DNase I (inhibitor constant $[K_i]$ = ~1 nM) and inhibits its ability to cleave DNA (Fig. 10.12). This interaction limits the effectiveness of DNase I as a therapeutic agent. On the basis of X-ray crystallographic studies, it was possible to predict which amino acid residues of DNase I interacted with actin and were therefore possible targets for change by directed mutagenesis. For example, changing amino acid 144 from alanine to arginine or amino acid 65 from tyrosine to arginine decreased the binding of DNase I to actin up to 10,000-fold. In addition, the actin-resistant mutants had 10- to 50-fold more DNase I activity than the native enzyme. It is not known whether any additional benefit might be realized by combining the amino acid changes from several actin-resistant mutants. The clinical efficacy of a DNase I mutant enzyme that does not bind actin still remains to be demonstrated.

Alginate Lyase

Alginate is a polysaccharide polymer that is produced by a wide range of seaweeds and both soil and marine bacteria. Alginate is composed of chains of the sugars β-D-mannuronate and α-L-guluronate. The properties of a particular alginate depend on the relative amounts and distribution of these two saccharides. For example, stretches of α-L-guluronate residues form both interchain and intrachain cross-links by binding calcium ions, and the β-D-mannuronate residues bind other metal ions. The cross-linked alginate polymer forms an elastic gel. In general, the structure of an alg-

FIGURE 10.11 Schematic representation of a portion of a human lung occluded by a combination of live alginate-secreting bacterial cells, lysed bacterial cells, and leukocytes and their released DNA. This matrix may be digested by alginate lyase or DNase I.

Blocked airway Open airway

Alginase or DNase

inate polymer is related to its viscosity, which is in turn directly proportional to its molecular size.

The excretion of alginate by mucoid strains of *Pseudomonas aeruginosa* that infect the lungs of patients with cystic fibrosis significantly contributes to the viscosity of the mucus in the airways. Once mucoid strains of *P. aeruginosa* have become established in the lungs of cystic fibrosis patients, it is almost impossible to eliminate them by antibiotic treatment. This is because the bacteria form biofilms in which the alginate prevents the antibiotics from coming into contact with the bacterial cells. In one experiment, it was shown that the addition of alginate lyase, which can liquefy bacterial alginate, together with or prior to antibiotic treatment, significantly decreased the number of bacteria found in biofilms (Fig. 10.13). This result suggests that, in addition to the DNase I treatment, depolymerization of the alginate would help clear blocked airways of individuals with cystic fibrosis.

An alginate lyase gene has been isolated from a *Flavobacterium* species, a gram-negative soil bacterium that is a strong producer of this enzyme. A *Flavobacterium* clone bank was constructed in *E. coli* and screened for alginate lyase-producing clones by plating the entire clone bank onto solid medium containing alginate. Following growth, colonies that produced alginate lyase formed a halo around the colony when calcium was added to the plate (Fig. 10.14). In the presence of calcium, all of the alginate in the medium, except in the immediate vicinity of an alginate lyase-positive clone, becomes cross-linked and opaque. Since hydrolyzed alginate chains do not form cross-links, the medium surrounding an alginate lyase-positive clone is transparent. Analysis of a cloned DNA fragment from one of the positive colonies revealed an open reading frame encoding a polypeptide with a molecular mass of approximately 69,000 Da. Detailed biochemical

FIGURE 10.12 Schematic representation of the ternary complex of human DNase I, actin, and DNA.

FIGURE 10.13 Time courses of the killing of bacteria in a biofilm with and without the addition of alginate lyase.

FIGURE 10.14 Schematic representation of the detection of an alginate lyase-producing clone from a clone bank of a *Flavobacterium* sp. in *E. coli*. The alginate that is present in the growth medium is digested by alginase secreted by an *E. coli* clone. The alginate in the vicinity of such a colony is not cross-linked when calcium is added and instead produces a clear zone (halo) surrounding the colony.

and genetic studies indicated that this polypeptide is a precursor of the three different alginate lyases produced by the *Flavobacterium* sp. (Fig. 10.15). After the 69,000-Da precursor is produced, a proteolytic enzyme cleaves off an N-terminal peptide of about 6,000 Da. The 63,000-Da protein can lyse both bacterial and seaweed alginates. Cleavage of the 63,000-Da protein yields a 23,000-Da enzyme that depolymerizes seaweed alginate and a 40,000-Da enzyme that is effective against bacterial alginate. To produce large amounts of the 40,000-Da enzyme, the DNA corresponding to the enzyme was amplified by the polymerase chain reaction (PCR) and then inserted into a *Bacillus subtilis* plasmid vector fused to a *B. subtilis* α-amylase leader peptide to direct the secretion of the protein and placed under the transcriptional control of a penicillinase gene promoter (Fig. 10.16). Transformation of *B. subtilis* cells with this construct yielded colonies with large halos on solid medium containing alginate after calcium was added. When these transformants were grown in liquid medium, the recombinant alginate lyase was secreted into the culture broth. Further tests showed that the enzyme efficiently liquefied alginates that were produced by mucoid strains of *P. aeruginosa* that had been isolated from the lungs of patients with cystic fibrosis. Additional studies are necessary to determine whether recombinant alginate lyase is an effective therapeutic agent.

Phenylalanine Ammonia Lyase

The human genetic disease phenylketonuria results from the impaired functioning of the enzyme phenylalanine hydroxylase. In the United States, approximately 1 of every 12,000 newborns has phenylketonuria. When phenylalanine hydroxylase, which oxidizes phenylalanine to tyrosine, is deficient, the normal cognitive development of an individual is impaired and mental retardation ensues due to a buildup of phenylalanine. Following diagnosis of phenylketonuria, either prenatally or shortly after birth, the

FIGURE 10.15 Processing of the recombinant *Flavobacterium* alginate lyase protein precursor in *E. coli*. A 6-kDa peptide is removed from the N terminus of the 69-kDa precursor to yield a 63-kDa protein that can depolymerize alginate from both seaweed and bacteria. A second cleavage event converts the 63-kDa protein into a 23-kDa protein that is active against seaweed alginate and a 40-kDa protein that hydrolyzes bacterial alginate.

Penicillinase promoter	α-Amylase leader peptide	40,000-Da alginate lyase

FIGURE 10.16 DNA construct encoding the 40,000-Da alginate lyase. The leader peptide from a *B. subtilis* α-amylase gene is fused to the N terminus of the alginate lyase coding sequence. The construct is under the transcriptional control of a *B. subtilis* penicillinase gene expression system.

treatment entails a controlled semisynthetic diet with low levels of phenylalanine through infancy and possibly for life. A possible alternative treatment would be the administration of the enzyme phenylalanine hydroxylase. Unfortunately, phenylalanine hydroxylase is a multienzyme complex that is not very stable and requires a cofactor for activity. On the other hand, phenylalanine ammonia lyase, which converts phenylalanine to ammonia and *trans*-cinnamic acid (Fig. 10.17), is a stable enzyme that does not require a cofactor and could potentially prevent the accumulation of phenylalanine in phenylketonuria patients. To test this concept, the gene for phenylalanine ammonia lyase from the yeast *Rhodosporidium toruloides* was cloned and overexpressed in *E. coli*. Preclinical studies were conducted with mice that were defective in producing phenylalanine ammonia lyase and therefore accumulated phenylalanine. With these mice, plasma phenylalanine levels were lowered when phenylalanine ammonia lyase was injected intravenously or encapsulated enzyme was administered orally. Thus, at least in mice, phenylalanine ammonia lyase is an effective substitute for phenylalanine hydroxylase, and the orally delivered enzyme is sufficiently stable to survive the mouse gastrointestinal tract and still function. Although this report is preliminary, a combination of oral enzyme therapy with phenylalanine ammonia lyase and a less stringent low-phenylalanine diet might serve to improve the quality of life of individuals affected with this disease.

α_1-Antitrypsin

The processing of a number of different pathogenic bacterial or viral precursor proteins by human proteases occurs when the protease recognizes the amino acid sequence –Arg-X-Lys/Arg-Arg↓–, with peptide bond cleavage on the C-terminal side of the C-terminal Arg (as indicated by the arrow), where X is any of the 20 common amino acids. Since this processing step is common to several infectious agents, a therapeutic agent

FIGURE 10.17 Products of the conversion of phenylalanine by phenylalanine hydroxylase and phenylalanine ammonia lyase.

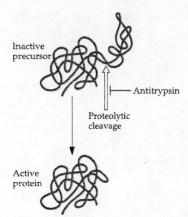

FIGURE 10.18 Schematic representation of α_1-antitrypsin inhibiting the proteolytic cleavage of pathogenic precursor proteins by human proteases.

that targeted the processing enzyme and blocked its activity might act as a broad-spectrum antibacterial and antiviral agent (Fig. 10.18). When a variant of human α_1-antitrypsin was genetically engineered and tested in tissue culture experiments, the protein blocked the processing of human immunodeficiency virus (HIV) type 1 glycoprotein gp160, as well as measles virus protein F_0, and consequently, in both cases, the production of infectious viruses. When the α_1-antitrypsin variant was added to cell cultures, it blocked the production of human cytomegalovirus, a major cause of illness and death in organ transplant recipients and AIDS patients. The α_1-antitrypsin variant is both potent and selective. Against human cytomegalovirus, it is at least 10-fold more effective than any currently used viral inhibitory agent. Its efficacy has been demonstrated in cell culture, but it remains to be determined if the strategy is effective with whole animals.

Glycosidases

The ABO blood group system is based upon the presence or absence of specific carbohydrate residues on the surfaces of erythrocytes, endothelial cells, and some epithelial cells. The monosaccharide that determines blood group A is a terminal α-1,3-linked N-acetylgalactosamine, while the corresponding monosaccharide of blood group B is α-1,3-linked galactose (Fig. 10.19). Group O cells lack both of these monosaccharides at the ends of

FIGURE 10.19 Digestion of the monosaccharides that determine blood groups A and B to obtain the H antigen (i.e., blood group O) with specific glucosidases. AcNH stands for an acetyl moiety covalently bound to a nitrogen atom.

their oligosaccharide chains and instead contain α-1,2-linked fucose, which is designated the H antigen. Plasma from blood group A individuals contains antibodies against the B antigen, blood group B individuals have antibodies against the A antigen, and blood group O individuals have antibodies against both the A and B antigens. In practice, this means that individuals with either anti-A or anti-B antibodies cannot safely receive a blood transfusion containing the incompatible antigen, since this is likely to cause a severe immune response (Table 10.2). As a consequence, blood group AB individuals are said to be universal recipients while those from blood group O are universal donors. Thus, when a blood transfusion is required, it is advantageous to have a large supply of plasma that is from blood group O (e.g., in an emergency situation, there may not be sufficient time to check a patient's blood group). Fortunately, digestion of blood cells from either type A or B with specific glycosidases can cause types A, B, and AB to be converted into type O (Fig. 10.19). These enzymes were found following an extensive screening process of 2,500 fungal and bacterial isolates. Eventually, an active α-N-acetylgalactosamidase, which converts group A to group O, was found in the gram-negative bacterium *Elizabethkingia meningosepticum* and one with α-galactosidase A, which converts group B to group O, was found in *Bacteroides fragilis* (also a gram-negative bacterium). The genes were isolated, characterized, and the proteins were characterized. Both of the enzymes have high specificity for cleaving the appropriate monosaccharide under conditions that maintain the integrity and functioning of the treated red blood cells. Moreover, each enzyme could readily be removed from the treated red blood cells following treatment. While this is a very recent and still preliminary experiment, if this novel approach works effectively in a clinical setting, then it should become a boon for all types of blood transfusions.

Lactic Acid Bacteria

Lactic acid bacteria are widely used in the production and preservation of fermented foods, and many have been given the designation "generally regarded as safe" within the food industry. Many of these organisms are members of the indigenous microflora of the human gut and have been recognized for their health-promoting properties. Some strains of lactic acid bacteria, notably lactobacilli, are used in probiotic products. A probiotic is a live microorganism that is claimed to confer a health benefit by altering the indigenous microflora of the intestinal tract. Lactic acid bacteria have also been used to treat several gastrointestinal disorders, including lactose intolerance, traveler's diarrhea, antibiotic-associated diarrhea, infections caused

TABLE 10.2 Compatible and incompatible blood groups

Donor blood type	Recipient blood type			
	A	B	AB	O
A	Compatible	Incompatible	Compatible	Incompatible
B	Incompatible	Compatible	Compatible	Incompatible
AB	Incompatible	Incompatible	Compatible	Incompatible
O	Compatible	Compatible	Compatible	Compatible

Individuals from one blood group may safely receive a blood transfusion from individuals from a compatible blood group but not from someone from an incompatible blood group.

by various bacterial and viral pathogens, and immunopathological disorders, such as Crohn disease and ulcerative colitis.

In the past few years, lactic acid bacteria have been used as a host system to express various foreign genes with the idea that these bacteria facilitate the delivery of the proteins encoded by the genes to the human gut. In particular, *Lactococcus lactis* has been developed as a host for this purpose. *L. lactis* is a nonpathogenic, noninvasive, noncolonizing gram-positive bacterium that is often used in the production of fermented foods. Moreover, *L. lactis* has been used for many years as a human probiotic.

Interleukin-10

Ulcerative colitis and Crohn disease, both diseases of the intestinal tract, affect approximately 1 in every 500 to 1,000 people in the developed countries of the world. Ulcerative colitis is associated with excess type 2 T helper cell cytokines, including interleukin-4 and interleukin-5, whereas in Crohn disease, type 1 T helper cell cytokines, including TNF-α, IFN-α, and interleukin-2, are overproduced. The treatment for Crohn disease often includes trying to lower the levels of cytokines, especially TNF-α. One approach has been the administration of antibodies against TNF-α. Other workers have targeted interleukin-10 as a means of controlling Crohn disease because it modulates the regulatory T cells that control inflammatory responses to intestinal antigens. However, interleukin-10 is not clinically acceptable because it needs to be administered by either frequent injections or rectal enemas. To overcome this problem, the bacterium *L. lactis* was engineered to synthesize and secrete interleukin-10.

Experiments were performed with mice to test whether interleukin-10-secreting *L. lactis* could be used to treat inflammatory bowel disease (Fig. 10.20). First, interleukin-10-secreting *L. lactis* was fed to mice with ulcerative colitis that had been induced by 5% dextran sulfate in their drinking water. Second, strains of mice that are genetically incapable of synthesizing interleukin-10 and provide an animal model for ulcerative colitis were tested. In both of these cases, the engineered *L. lactis* significantly alleviated

FIGURE 10.20 Schematic representation of the effects of intestinal interleukin-10 (IL-10)-secreting bacteria on inflammatory bowel disease in mice.

the symptoms of the disease, establishing that this approach works in principle. However, these mouse models for inflammatory bowel disease are not identical to the disease in humans, and a large number of questions remain before the treatment is used with humans.

One concern about the use of an interleukin-10-secreting *L. lactis* strain as a therapeutic approach is the possibility that the genetically modified bacterium will be released to the environment. If this were to happen, the plasmid carrying the interleukin-10 gene and any plasmid-borne antibiotic resistance marker genes could be spread to other bacteria in the environment. To prevent this from occurring, a synthetic human interleukin-10 gene that replaced the *L. lactis* thymidylate synthase gene, *thyA*, which is essential for the growth of the bacterium, was inserted into the bacterial chromosome of *L. lactis* by homologous recombination (Fig. 10.21). This strain produced interleukin-10 and grew well in the laboratory when either thymidine or thymine was added to the medium. However, when it was deprived of thymidine and thymine, the viability of the bacterium declined by several orders of magnitude. When this modified bacterium was tested in pigs, whose digestive tract is similar to that of humans, it thrived and actively produced interleukin-10. In addition, laboratory experiments demonstrated that the modified *L. lactis* was extremely unlikely to acquire a thymidylate synthase gene from other bacteria in the environment, confirming both the safety and efficacy of this approach.

Recently, clinical trials with this *L. lactis* strain were initiated. To date, 10 patients with Crohn disease have been treated. So far, a significant decrease in disease activity has been observed, with only minor adverse events. Moreover, bacteria isolated from the patients' feces were not able to grow without the addition of thymidine. In other words, the engineered *L. lactis* did not acquire a thymidylate synthase gene, indicating that the containment strategy was effective. Thus, initial indications are that this strategy appears to be working as well in humans as it did with small animals.

Leptin

It has been estimated that approximately 30% of the North American and 20% of the European populations are overweight. Moreover, North Americans annually spend tens of billions of dollars on various weight reduction schemes, most of which are unsuccessful. However, real weight reduction may be obtained by administration of the protein leptin. Leptin, the product of the *obese (ob)* gene, is a 167-amino-acid protein with a molecular mass of approximately 16 kDa. Leptin is synthesized as a precursor with a 21-amino-acid-long signal peptide that is removed when leptin is secreted. Treatment with recombinant leptin can reduce food intake and

FIGURE 10.21 The genetic construct integrated into the chromosomal DNA of *L. lactis* in place of its thymidylate synthase gene. The promoter (*p^thyA*) is from the thymidylate synthase gene. The interleukin-10 gene was chemically synthesized so that its codon usage was optimized for *L. lactis*, thereby ensuring a high level of protein expression.

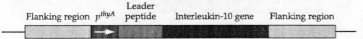

| Flanking region | *p^thyA* | Leader peptide | Interleukin-10 gene | Flanking region |

correct metabolic perturbations in (homozygous) leptin-deficient mice. Leptin also helps to overcome human congenital leptin deficiency. However, when it is introduced subcutaneously, leptin is not particularly effective in obese patients unless their serum leptin concentrations reach levels 20- to 30-fold higher than normal. This response has been attributed to the inefficient transport of leptin across the blood-brain barrier. To overcome this problem, a scheme for the intranasal delivery of leptin has been devised.

When leptin is produced in *E. coli*, it typically forms insoluble inclusion bodies that must be solubilized and renatured before the active protein is generated. This is a time-consuming, inefficient, and expensive process. In one study, the 462-bp cDNA for human leptin without its signal peptide was cloned and expressed under the control of the nisin promoter in *L. lactis* (Fig. 10.22). Nisin is a 34-amino-acid-residue polycyclic peptide that has antibacterial activity and is used as a food preservative. In *L. lactis*, leptin was produced efficiently without the formation of an inclusion body and was secreted from the recombinant bacteria. Intranasal administration of the leptin-producing *L. lactis* strain significantly reduced food intake and body weight in obese mice. This approach opens up the possibility that, if delivered properly, leptin might act as an effective weight loss treatment in humans.

An HIV Inhibitor

Worldwide, the predominant mode of HIV transmission is by heterosexual contact. One possible way to protect women, who currently comprise about half of all new cases of HIV/AIDS, against HIV infection is a topical microbicide, delivered by a live vaginal *Lactobacillus* strain, that prevents HIV infection directly at mucosal surfaces. This strategy seems reasonable because naturally occurring vaginal *Lactobacillus* strains play a protective role in preventing urogenital infections.

The compound cyanovirin N, isolated from the cyanobacterium *Nostoc ellipsosporum*, blocks several steps of HIV infection, preventing virus entry into human cells. Consequently, cyanovirin N is a candidate for a topical microbiocide to prevent HIV infections. To ensure that cyanovirin N would be expressed at a sufficiently high level in a vaginal strain of *Lactobacillus jensenii*, the gene was chemically synthesized to reflect the codon usage found in the bacterium. Typically, the GC content of lactobacilli is about 36%. In addition, during the synthesis of the gene, proline 51 was replaced by a glycine residue to stabilize the cyanovirin N, and four amino acids were added to the N terminus to ensure proper cleavage of the signal sequence (Fig. 10.23). The modified cyanovirin N gene was fused to a strong and constitutive *Lactobacillus* promoter. The final construct was integrated into the chromosomal DNA of a strain of *L. jensenii* and, when it was tested for efficacy, was found to be highly effective at preventing HIV infec-

FIGURE 10.22 Genetic construct used to secrete leptin from *L. lactis.*

FIGURE 10.23 Flowchart of the scheme used to develop a *Lactobacillus* strain that produces and secretes cyanovirin N (CV-N).

tions in mice. Under these conditions, about 4 μg of cyanovirin N per mL was released into the culture medium.

Monoclonal Antibodies

About 100 years ago, horses were inoculated with the bacterium *Corynebacterium diphtheriae,* which causes diphtheria in humans. The resulting crude horse antiserum was used to treat this often fatal childhood disease. In those days, mortality sometimes reached 45%. *C. diphtheriae* infects the throat or tonsils and produces an exotoxin that is lethal to human cells. This exotoxin enters the bloodstream and damages organs that are distant from the primary site of infection. The administration of horse antiserum containing antibodies against the exotoxin provided passive immunity, protecting the patient from a fatal outcome when the antiserum was given within the first few days after the onset of infection.

Unfortunately, this kind of antibody therapy carries considerable risk and is not widely used today. Patients often develop antibodies against the foreign proteins of either whole or partially purified horse antiserum. After a second treatment, the sensitized patient may go into anaphylactic shock and die. As a result, the use of antibodies as therapeutic agents was considered too dangerous for patients and was used only rarely.

However, with the development of hybridoma technology, antibodies are once again seen as potential therapeutic agents. One reason for the renewed interest in therapeutic antibodies is that it is now possible to engi-

TABLE 10.3 Some therapeutic monoclonal antibodies that have been approved for human use in either the United States or the European Union

Approval date	Antibody	Drug name	Antibody type	Therapeutic use
1986	Muromomab	Orthoclone	Murine	Prevention of acute kidney transplant rejection
1994	Abciximab	ReoPro	Chimeric	Prevention of blood clots
1997	Daclizumab	Zenapax	Humanized	Prevention of acute kidney transplant rejection
1998	Rituximab	Rituxan	Chimeric	Treatment of non-Hodgkin lymphoma
1998	Infliximab	Remicade	Chimeric	Treatment of Crohn disease, psoriasis, rheumatoid arthritis
1998	Basiliximab	Simulect	Chimeric	Preventation of transplantation rejection
1998	Palivizumab	Synagis	Humanized	Treatment of viral infections in children
1998	Trastuzumab	Herceptin	Humanized	Treatment of metastatic breast cancer
2000	Gemtuzumab	Mylotarg	Humanized	Treatment of acute myeloid leukemia
2001	Alemtuzumab	Leukosite	Humanized	Treatment of chronic lymphocytic leukemia
2002	Adalimumab	Humira	Human	Treatment of rheumatoid arthritis
2002	Ibritumomab	Zevalin	Chimeric	Treatment of non-Hodgkin lymphoma
2003	Efalzumab	Raptiva	Humanized	Treatment of severe plaque psoriasis
2003	Omalizumab	Xolair	Humanized	Treatment of severe persistent asthma
2003	Tositumomab	Bexxar	Murine + iodine-131	Treatment of non-Hodgkin lymphoma
2004	Cetuximab	Erbitux	Chimeric	Treatment of various cancers
2004	Natalizumab	Tysabri	Humanized	Treatment of multiple sclerosis
2004	Bevacizumab	Avastin	Humanized	Treatment of various cancers
2006	Panitumumab	Vectibix	Human	Treatment of colorectal cancer
2009?	Denosumab		Human	Treatment of osteoporosis

In addition to the monoclonal antibodies listed here, a number of monoclonal antibodies have been approved for diagnostic and imaging purposes. Phase III clinical trials of denosumab were successfully completed in 2008, and in early 2009 the manufacturer applied for FDA approval of denosumab.

neer antibodies with a greatly reduced level of immunogenicity in humans. In addition, this technique can be used to maintain a continuous supply of pure monospecific antibody. However, the problems of cross-reactivity leading to an immune response and anaphylaxis have not been completely overcome. Thus, the recipient might still produce antibodies to a monoclonal antibody that carries mouse (murine) determinants. To avoid this problem, human monoclonal antibodies with both specific immunotherapeutic properties and lowered potential for immunogenicity have been produced. In fact, a number of monoclonal antibodies have been approved for treating human diseases (Table 10.3, Box 10.2, and Box 10.3).

Structure and Function of Antibodies

An antibody molecule (immunoglobulin) consists of two identical light (L) protein chains and two identical heavy (H) protein chains held together by both hydrogen bonding and precisely localized disulfide linkages. The N-terminal regions of the L and H chains together form the antigen recognition site of each antibody. Antibody genes can be readily manipulated because the various functions of an antibody molecule are confined to discrete domains (regions) (Fig. 10.24). The sites that recognize and bind antigens consist of three complementarity-determining regions (CDRs) that lie

BOX 10.2

Trastuzumab: the First Humanized Monoclonal Antibody Approved for the Treatment of Breast Cancer

In 25 to 30% of women with aggressive metastatic breast cancer, there is a genetic alteration in the *HER2* gene that results in the production of an increased amount of human epidermal growth factor receptor 2 (HER2) protein on the surface of the tumor. Overexpression of the HER2 protein can readily be determined by using an immunohistochemistry-based assay. Some years ago, researchers at Genentech isolated a mouse monoclonal antibody with high affinity for the HER2 protein and then (using procedures similar to those described in this chapter) humanized it. The humanized anti-HER2 monoclonal antibody, trastuzumab (Herceptin), contains human FRs and mouse CDRs and is produced commercially using mammalian (CHO) cells grown in sus-

pension culture as the host for the expression of the antibody. Antibodies produced in CHO cells are glycosylated similarly to bona fide human antibodies. After humanization, trastuzumab bound to the HER2 protein with a dissociation constant of approximately 5×10^{-9} M, indicating that the high level of specificity for the substrate had been maintained through the process of humanization.

In the laboratory, and then in initial clinical trials with more than 800 patients, trastuzumab mediated antibody-dependent cellular cytotoxicity (i.e., it told the immune system to target the cancerous cells) and inhibited the proliferation of human tumor cells that overexpressed HER2 (i.e., it stopped the cancerous cells from growing). Trastuzumab was most effective when it was administered together with some of the chemicals that are currently used for the treatment (chemotherapy) of breast cancer, provided that the breast cancer was at a later stage of development. In two

large clinical trials that included over 3,700 women, those who received trastuzumab and chemotherapy had a 52% higher chance that the cancer would not return than those who were treated with chemotherapy alone. Trastuzumab is provided by the manufacturer as a sterile white to pale yellow powder containing 440 mg per vial, and after reconstitution, it is typically administered intravenously over a period of 30 minutes and is taken weekly for 52 weeks. Since a small number of individuals treated with trastuzumab develop heart problems, it is necessary to carefully monitor the cardiac functions of all patients on this therapy, especially older patients and those with a family history of heart problems. In the relatively short time that it has been available, trastuzumab has become a blockbuster drug, with annual sales above $1 billion. In 2006, in the United States, trastuzumab treatment for one individual cost approximately $40,000 for the year.

within the variable (V_H and V_L) regions at the N-terminal ends of the two H and two L chains. The CDRs are the part of an antibody molecule with the greatest variability in amino acid sequence. In addition to the variable regions, each L chain contains one constant region, or domain (C_L), and each H chain has three constant regions, or domains (C_{H1}, C_{H2}, and C_{H3}). When antibodies are digested with the proteolytic enzyme papain, three fragments are released: two identical (Fab) fragments, each of which contains an intact L chain linked by a disulfide bond to the C_{H1} region of the H chain, and one Fc fragment, which consists of two H chain fragments, each containing the C_{H2} and C_{H3} domains and joined by a disulfide bond (Fig. 10.24). The Fab fragment retains the antigen-binding activity. In fact, the N-terminal half of the Fab fragment, which is called the Fv fragment, contains all of the antigen-binding activity of the intact antibody molecule (Fig. 10.24). The amino acid sequence of this portion of the antibody varies considerably from one molecule to another. Each of the constant and variable regions consists of approximately 110 amino acid residues. A complete antibody molecule has a molecular mass of approximately 150 kDa, a Fab fragment is around 50 kDa, and an Fv fragment is about 25 kDa.

In an intact antibody molecule, the Fc portion elicits several immunological responses after antigen–antibody binding occurs.

- The complement cascade is activated. The components of this system break down cell membranes, activate phagocytes, and gen-

erate signals to mobilize other components of the immunological response system.

- Antibody-dependent cell-mediated cytotoxicity (ADCC), which is the result of the binding of the Fc portion of the antibody to an Fc receptor of an ADCC effector cell, is produced. The bound effector cell releases substances that lyse the foreign cell to which the Fab portion of the antibody molecule is bound.
- After the Fab region binds to a soluble antigen, the Fc portion of an antibody can be bound to Fc receptors of phagocytic cells, which engulf and destroy the antibody–antigen complex.

Preventing Rejection of Transplanted Organs

In the 1970s, passive immunization was reconsidered as a way of preventing immunological rejection of a transplanted organ. The rationale was to administer to patients a specific antibody that would bind to certain lymphocytes and diminish the immune response directed against the transplanted organ. The mouse monoclonal antibody OKT3 was approved

BOX 10.3

Rituximab and Ibritumomab: Therapeutic Monoclonal Antibodies That Treat Non-Hodgkin Lymphoma

Non-Hodgkin lymphoma is a malignant growth of B or T cells of the lymph system. It has been estimated by the American Cancer Society that in 2007 alone approximately 63,000 new cases of non-Hodgkin lymphoma were diagnosed, resulting in approximately 19,000 deaths. In fact, about 5 million people worldwide have non-Hodgkin lymphoma, 5 to 10% of these people die every year, and the incidence of the disease is growing. It is the fifth most common cancer (although there are about 29 different lymphomas in this category), with an individual's chance of developing the disease in their lifetime being about 1 in 50.

There are a variety of treatments for patients with non-Hodgkin lymphoma, including radiation therapy, chemotherapy, immunotherapy, bone marrow transplantation, and "watch and wait" for slowly growing cases. In 1997, the FDA approved the use of rituximab (Rituxan) for the treatment

of non-Hodgkin lymphoma. Rituximab is a genetically engineered chimeric (murine/human) monoclonal antibody directed against the CD20 antigen (a protein on the surfaces of B lymphocytes). Following binding of the antibody to CD20, the body's defenses attack and kill the antibody-marked B cells. Stem cells in bone marrow lack CD20, so they are uninhibited by this treatment. Healthy B cells can regenerate from those stem cells, after the completion of the course of rituximab treatment (given once a week for 4 to 8 weeks), and return to normal levels within several months. In 2006, the FDA approved the use of rituximab in combination with CHOP (cyclophosphamide, doxorubicin, vincristine, and prednisone) and other anthracycline-based chemotherapy regimens. In addition, the use of rituximab in combination with the chemical compound methotrexate was approved for the treatment of moderately to severely active rheumatoid arthritis in patients who had been refractory to other treatments.

Notwithstanding some severe side effects in some patients, rituximab has been enormously successful. Hundreds of thousands of people worldwide who did not respond well

to conventional chemotherapy have been successfully treated with rituximab. In fact, while the incidence of non-Hodgkin lymphoma continues to increase, since the introduction of rituximab, mortality from the disease in the United States has declined at a rate of approximately 2.3% a year. In 2002, the FDA approved the use of ibritumomab tiuxetan (Zevalin) together with rituximab. Ibritumomab is also a monoclonal antibody that targets B cells. However, ibritumomab is linked to a chemical chelator molecule (tiuxetan) that binds tightly to radioactive indium-111 or yttrium-90. Thus, a therapeutic regimen with ibritumomab tiuxetan targets tumor cells with a high dose of radiation. In late 2007, treatment with ibritumomab tiuxetan was priced at approximately $24,000 per month, with treatments typically lasting 1 or 2 months. Treatment with ibritumomab tiuxetan is quite toxic, and around half of the treated individuals experience side effects. Therefore, ibritumomab tiuxetan is approved only for patients who have failed to respond to other treatments.

FIGURE 10.24 Structure of an antibody molecule. The H and L chains contain variable regions (V_L and V_H) with their CDRs (CDR1, CDR2, and CDR3) and constant domains (C_L, C_{H1}, C_{H2}, and C_{H3}). The Fv, Fab, and Fc portions of an antibody molecule are delineated. The N-terminal (NH_2) and C-terminal (COOH) ends of each polypeptide chain are indicated.

in 1986 by the FDA for use as an immunosuppressive agent after organ transplantation in humans (Table 10.3). Lymphocytes that differentiate in the thymus are called T cells. Various members of the T-cell population act as immunological helper and effector cells and are responsible for organ rejection. The OKT3 monoclonal antibody binds to a cell surface receptor called CD3, which is present on all T cells. As a result, a full immunological response is blocked, and the transplanted organ is not rejected. Immunosuppression by this means was reasonably effective, although as anticipated, because the antibody was from a mouse, there were some side effects, including fever and rash formation.

Recombinant Antibodies

Hybrid Human–Mouse Monoclonal Antibodies

The modular nature of antibody functions has made it possible to convert a mouse monoclonal antibody into one that has some human segments but still retains its original antigen-binding specificity. This hybrid molecule is called a chimeric antibody (Fig. 10.25), or, with more human sequences, a "humanized" antibody (Fig. 10.26). The difference between a chimeric and a humanized mouse monoclonal antibody depends on which portions of the mouse antibody are removed. The first portion of a mouse monoclonal antibody that was targeted for replacement with a human sequence was

FIGURE 10.25 Genetically engineered chimeric antibody. The V_L and V_H DNA regions from the immunoglobulin L and H genes that encode part of a mouse monoclonal antibody were substituted for the V_L and V_H DNA regions of a human immunoglobulin molecule. The product of the constructed gene is a chimeric (partially humanized) immunoglobulin with the antigen-binding specificity of the mouse monoclonal antibody and both lowered immunogenicity in humans and human Fc effector capabilities.

the mouse Fc fragment. The mouse Fc fragment was chosen because it functions poorly as an effector of immunological responses in humans. It is also the most likely fragment to elicit the production of human antibodies. To diminish immunogenicity and to introduce human Fc effector capabilities, the DNA coding sequences for the Fv regions of both the L and the H chains of a human immunoglobulin were substituted for the Fv DNA sequences for the L and H chains from a specific mouse monoclonal antibody (Fig. 10.25). This replacement of Fv coding regions can be accomplished by using either oligonucleotides with in vitro DNA replication or cloned DNA segments. The DNA constructs for both chimeric chains were cloned into an expression vector and transfected into cultured B lymphocytes, from which the chimeric antibody was collected. Chimeric antibodies are composed of approximately 70% human and 30% mouse DNA sequences.

When a chimeric antibody that contained the binding site from a mouse monoclonal antibody directed against the surfaces of human colon cancer cells was tested in patients with colorectal cancer, it remained in the blood system about six times longer than the complete mouse monoclonal antibody, thereby extending the period of effectiveness. Only 1 patient of the 10 developed a mild immunological reaction to the chimeric antibody. However, in this trial, no antitumor effects were observed, an outcome that

FIGURE 10.26 Genetically engineered humanized antibody. The CDRs (CDR1, CDR2, and CDR3) from the genes for H and L immunoglobulin chains of a mouse monoclonal antibody replace the CDRs of the genes for a human antibody. The product of this constructed gene is an immunoglobulin with the antigen-binding specificity of the mouse monoclonal antibody and all the other properties of a human antibody molecule.

may be due to the low dose levels or to the advanced stage of the cancer in the subjects.

The "humanizing" of mouse and rat monoclonal antibodies has been taken one step further than the formation of chimeric molecules by substituting into human antibodies only the CDRs of the rodent monoclonal antibodies (Fig. 10.26). Humanized antibodies consist of approximately 95% human and 5% mouse DNA sequences. Because these engineered human antibodies have antigen-binding affinities similar to those of the original rodent monoclonal antibodies, they may be more effective therapeutic agents.

The humanizing of rodent monoclonal antibodies may be performed as follows. Starting with a rodent hybridoma cell line, cDNAs for the L and H chains are isolated. The variable regions of these cDNAs are amplified by PCR. The oligonucleotide primers that are used for this amplification are complementary to the sequences at the 5' and 3' ends of the DNA encoding the variable regions. From the nucleotide sequences of the cDNAs for the L and H regions (V_L and V_H), it is possible to delineate the limits of the CDRs. It is usually straightforward to determine where the CDRs begin and end, because these regions are highly variable in sequence while the sequences of the framework regions (FRs) are relatively conserved. On the basis of the sequences of the DNAs encoding the rodent CDRs, six pairs of oligonucleotide PCR primers are synthesized. Each pair of primers is designed to initiate the synthesis of the DNA for one of the six rodent CDRs—three from the L chain and three from the H chain. In addition, each primer includes an extra 12 nucleotides at its 5' end, complementary to the flanking regions within the human framework DNA into which the DNA for the rodent CDRs is targeted (Fig. 10.27). Oligonucleotide-directed mutagenesis is then used to replace, one at a time, the complete DNA sequence for each

FIGURE 10.27 PCR amplification of CDR1 from a rodent monoclonal antibody L chain cDNA. The PCR primers P1 and P2 contain oligonucleotides complementary to the rodent CDR1 DNA. In addition, P1 and P2 each contain 12 nucleotides at their 5′ ends that are complementary to the FRs of human monoclonal L chain cDNAs. Using six separate pairs of oligonucleotide primers—three for the V_L region and three for the V_H region—each of the rodent CDRs is separately amplified by PCR. Then, by PCR, the amplified rodent CDRs are spliced into human antibody genes in place of the resident CDRs. This grafting is made possible by the presence of DNA complementary to the human FRs on the amplified rodent CDR DNAs.

of the human CDRs with the amplified DNA for the rodent CDRs. Thus, it is necessary to carry out six cycles of oligonucleotide-directed mutagenesis, one cycle to replace each CDR. This procedure, in effect, "grafts" the rodent CDRs onto the human antibody framework. The humanized variable-region cDNAs are then cloned into expression vectors, which are then introduced into appropriate host cells, usually either *E. coli* or mammalian cells, for the production of antibodies.

To date, more than 50 different monoclonal antibodies have been humanized. While this technology is clearly effective and widely applicable, it is nevertheless time-consuming and expensive. Probably (as described below) in the future other strategies will be used to produce human antibodies and antibody fragments, such as (1) phage display combinatorial libraries that are constructed from mRNA from human B cells from nonimmunized donors and (2) transgenic mice that express the entire human antibody repertoire.

Human Monoclonal Antibodies

Although most of the immunotherapeutic agents that have been developed have been effective, there are drawbacks to the use of monoclonal antibodies that contain nonhuman sequences. For example, if multiple treatments are required, which is often the case, it is desirable that the antibody contain no or only a very limited amount of nonhuman sequences to prevent immunological cross-reactivity and sensitization of the patient. Unfortunately, it is very difficult to create human monoclonal antibodies for a number of reasons. The human chromosomes of fused human lymphocyte–mouse myeloma cells during hybridoma formation are unstable, and cells that produce a human monoclonal antibody are rarely formed. To date, no human myeloma cell line has been discovered that can replace the mouse myeloma cell line in this procedure. Even if it were possible to form human hybridoma cell lines, it is contrary to accepted norms of medical research to inject humans with a specific antigen for nontherapeutic pur-

Inactivate mouse IgH
and Igκ chain genes

Introduce human IgL loci and
IgH locus into a cell that has
mouse IgH and Igκ genes

XenoMouse

FIGURE 10.28 Generation of a XenoMouse. Mouse antibody genes are inactivated by specific deletions in embryonic stem cells, which are subsequently used to generate transgenic mice unable to make antibodies. The human genes encoding immunoglobulin light and heavy chains are introduced on a YAC into mouse embryonic stem cells. These cells are used to generate transgenic mice able to synthesize both mouse and human antibodies. The mice generated from these two types of manipulation are cross-bred, and mice that can synthesize only human immunoglobulins are selected, immunized, and used to make hybridomas producing human antibodies.

poses and to perform a partial splenectomy to collect antibody-producing cells. Therefore, it has been necessary to devise other approaches for obtaining human monoclonal antibodies.

To address this need, researchers constructed a "XenoMouse" in which (1) the mouse antibody production machinery was inactivated and (2) all of the human immunoglobulin loci (both light and heavy chains) are integrated into a mouse chromosome (Fig. 10.28). The human heavy chain genes and the human κ and λ light chain genes (where κ and λ are different classes of light chain genes) were cloned onto yeast artificial chromosomes (YACs) that can carry very large amounts of foreign DNA. The YACs with the human immunoglobulin genes were then introduced into mouse embryonic stem cells by fusing YAC-containing yeast spheroplasts with the

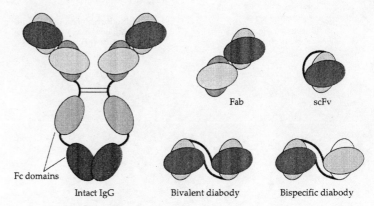

FIGURE 10.29 Schematic representation of active antibodies and antibody fragments.

embryonic stem cells. This procedure yields a large number of embryonic stem cells in which all of the introduced human immunoglobulin genes have become stably integrated into the chromosomal DNA. These transfected cells were used to generate mice containing human immunoglobulin gene loci. Cross-breeding of two mouse lines, one carrying both mouse and human immunoglobulin genes and the other carrying the deleted mouse immunoglobulin genes, produced a mouse strain (called XenoMouse) that expresses only human immunoglobulins. It is now possible, after immunization of a XenoMouse with a particular antigen, to produce a fully human immunoglobulin. The large human antibody repertoire in the XenoMouse has enabled researchers to produce a number of fully human antibodies, many of which are currently at various stages of clinical development. For example, the first fully human monoclonal antibody produced using this technology is panitumumab, which was approved in September 2006 for the treatment of certain forms of colorectal cancer (Table 10.3).

Antibody Fragments

Naturally occurring antibodies are highly specific targeting reagents that provide animals with a powerful means of defending themselves against a wide range of pathogenic organisms and toxins. Immunoglobulin G (IgG) is the main antibody found in mammalian serum, and it is the native form that is almost exclusively used in therapeutic antibodies (Fig. 10.29). The fact that IgG molecules have two identical sites that bind to two identical antigens (i.e., they are bivalent) generally increases their effectiveness in vivo. While the Fc portion of the IgG molecule is important in recruiting cytotoxic effector functions through complement or interaction with specific receptors, Fc-mediated effects are not necessary for all applications and may even sometimes be undesirable. Over the past several years, by manipulating portions of the IgG light and heavy chain cDNAs, researchers have constructed a variety of IgG derivatives or fragments that may be used instead of whole antibody molecules (Fig. 10.29). Some of these molecules, because of their small size, bind more efficiently to targets that are inaccessible to conventional whole antibodies. Others have multiple sites

for binding to the same antigen, while others have binding specificities for two or more target antigens.

Initially, based on Fab and Fv fragments of antibodies, antigen-binding single protein chains (scFv) consisting of only V_L and V_H domains were developed. Single-chain antibodies may be used for a variety of therapeutic and diagnostic applications in which Fc effector functions are not required and when small size is an advantage. Single-chain antibodies have a molecular mass of approximately 27 kDa compared with approximately 150 kDa for IgG molecules. Because of their small size, single-chain antibodies can penetrate and distribute in large tumors more readily than intact antibodies. In addition, a protein-coding sequence can be linked to a single-chain antibody sequence to create a dual-function molecule that can both bind to a specific target and deliver a toxin or some other specific activity to a cell (Fig. 10.30).

Computer simulations of the three-dimensional structure of a potential single-chain antibody showed that the V_L and V_H domains have to be separated by a linker peptide to assume the correct conformation for antigen binding. On the basis of this design constraint, DNA constructs of V_L and V_H sequences from a cDNA of a cloned monoclonal antibody were each ligated to a chemically synthesized DNA linker fragment in the order V_L–linker–V_H. After expression in *E. coli*, the single-chain protein was purified, and both its affinity and specificity were found to be equivalent to those of the original intact monoclonal antibody. Moreover, instead of linking the V_H and V_L chains with a short peptide, amino acids in the FR can be modified to form a disulfide linkage between the two peptides (Fig. 10.30B). The effectiveness of this disulfide-stabilized Fv molecule (V_L-S-S-V_H) coupled to a cancer cell toxin was compared with that of an scFv molecule coupled to the same toxin. The disulfide-stabilized and scFv immunotoxins had the same activity and specificity. However, the former molecule was severalfold more stable than the latter. This suggests that disulfide-stabilized Fv molecules may be more useful than scFv molecules in some therapeutic applications. The two types of molecules have been used in different ways. For example, by altering the number of amino acids in the linker in an scFv molecule (usually to five or fewer amino acids) it is possible to direct the self-assembly of these molecules into either bivalent dimers, called diabodies (Fig. 10.29), trimers (triabodies), or tetramers (tetrabodies). Shortening the linker affects not only the multimerization, but also the stability of the molecule, with molecules with a shorter linker

FIGURE 10.30 Schematic representation of an scFv immunotoxin **(A)** and a disulfide-stabilized Fv immunotoxin **(B)**.

MILESTONE

Synthesis in *E. coli* of a Polypeptide with Human Leukocyte Interferon Activity
S. NAGATA, H. TAIRA, A. HALL, L. JOHNSRUD, M. STREULI, J. ECSÖDI, W. BOLL, K. CANTELL, and C. WEISSMANN
Nature **284**:316–320, 1980

The late 1970s and early 1980s were a time of tremendous excitement in molecular biotechnology. The promise of this new technology was being touted to both the public and large institutional investors. One of the products of the new biotechnology that captured the imagination of a large number of people was IFN, which at the time was seen by many as a possible miracle cure for a wide range of diseases caused by viruses and cancer. Thus, the isolation of a human IFN cDNA and its subsequent expression in *E. coli* were reported in newspapers and magazines around the world.

Several features of IFN made it particularly difficult to synthesize and isolate a cDNA encoding the polypeptide. First, although IFN had been purified more than 80,000-fold, only minuscule amounts were available, so researchers did not even have an accurate estimate of its molecular mass. Second, unlike many other proteins, IFN did not have a chemical or biological activity that was easy to monitor. At the time, its activity was measured by the reduction in the cytopathic effect of an animal virus on cells in culture, which was an extremely complex and time-consuming process. Third, unlike insulin, researchers had no idea if there was one particular human cell that produced high levels of IFN and therefore could serve as a source of mRNA that was enriched for IFN mRNA. These problems notwithstanding, a cDNA encoding IFN was eventually isolated and characterized. Since that time, researchers have discovered that there are several different types of IFNs. Unfortunately, IFN is not the panacea that was dreamed of by both investors and the press. However, the genes for several IFNs have been isolated, and clinical trials have shown that they are effective treatments for a variety of viral diseases.

tending to be more stable. In addition, it is possible to combine two different antigen specificities into a single bispecific diabody (Fig. 10.29).

Most recombinant antibody–toxin combinations (immunotoxins) have been constructed using *Pseudomonas* exotoxin A, which is a 66-kDa protein with three separate domains. Domain I is responsible for cell binding, domain II for translocation of the protein into the cell, and domain III for ADP-ribosylation (Fig. 10.31A). Other protein toxins that have been used include bacterially derived diphtheria toxin and the plant-derived toxin ricin. An immunotoxin is generally synthesized by replacing the N-terminal domain of the toxin, e.g., *Pseudomonas* exotoxin A (domain I), with the single-chain antibody sequence, thereby creating molecules very similar in size to the original toxin with the ability to bind, enter, and kill a specific cell (Fig. 10.31B). A number of immunotoxins that have antitumor activity in vitro and in animal models have been constructed. These include antibodies directed against the p55 subunit of the interleukin-2 receptor, the transferrin receptor, carbohydrate antigens, the epidermal growth factor receptor, and some cancer cell surface proteins. Toxin molecules may also be directed to cancer cells by using a dispecific diabody that is engineered to bind to a surface-specific tumor-associated antigen and then to a toxin molecule, thereby directing the toxin molecule to the tumor (Fig. 10.32). A number of different engineered immunotoxins are currently in clinical trials.

It may be possible to create peptides that are smaller than scFvs and still retain the ability to bind to a specific antigen. The rationale for developing smaller antibody–toxin complexes is that they are more likely to penetrate a tumor and more completely stop tumor growth. Recently, a group of researchers constructed a short peptide (28 amino acids long) that retained the binding specificity of the monoclonal antibody from which it

was derived. It is well established that antibody-binding specificity resides within the six hypervariable loops called CDRs, three from the variable region of the heavy chain and three from the variable region of the light chain (Fig. 10.24 and 10.33). In all antibody molecules, the CDRs are flanked by FRs. Moreover, it was speculated, at least for some antibodies, that the major portion of the antigen-binding site might reside primarily within two CDRs, one from the heavy chain and the other from the light chain. To test this possibility, starting with genes for the variable portion of a monoclonal antibody against a surface protein from Epstein-Barr virus, eight different peptide combinations were synthesized. Each peptide contained at least one CDR3 loop (known to be the major antigen-contacting segment), as well as one other CDR loop and a linker peptide (usually an FR spacer). All eight of these peptides were tested in vitro for the ability to compete with the parental antibody for binding to the Epstein-Barr virus (thought to be the causative agent of Burkitt lymphoma and other cancers) surface protein. One of the peptide combinations, V_HCDR1–V_HFR2–V_LCDR3, appeared to be promising (Fig. 10.33). Next, this peptide was coupled to a toxin molecule, colicin Ia, and the combination was tested both with cells in culture and with mice. In mice, the peptide–colicin adduct efficiently traveled through the circulation and then found and killed the tumor cells expressing the target antigen. Colicin Ia by itself does not affect these tumors to any significant extent. Also, the original monoclonal antibody is unable to penetrate into the tumor. On the other hand, the peptide–colicin adduct accumulated at the cores of the targeted tumors. This very exciting work is at an early stage of development, so a large number of issues remain to be addressed before it can become an effective human therapeutic measure. Nevertheless, the demonstration that a small peptide can mimic the binding specificity of an entire antibody molecule and successfully deliver a cellular toxin to targeted cells may provide the basis for a whole new approach for treating tumors.

Combinatorial Libraries of Antibody Fragments

Hybridoma cells, like most other animal cells in culture, grow relatively slowly, do not attain high cell densities, and require complex and expensive growth media. The cost of monoclonal antibody production is an impediment to their more widespread use as therapeutic agents. To circumvent this problem, attempts have been made to genetically engineer bacteria, plants, and animals to act as "bioreactors" for the production of

FIGURE 10.31 Domain structure of *Pseudomonas* exotoxin A **(A)** and a single-chain antibody–*Pseudomonas* exotoxin A **(B)**. The functions of the various domains are shown.

FIGURE 10.32 Schematic representation of the binding of a diabody to a protein molecule on the surface of a cancerous cell, as well as the binding of a toxin protein molecule to the other portion of the diabody.

monoclonal antibodies. For effective delivery and function of some immunotherapeutic agents, only the antigen-binding region of an antibody (the Fab or Fv fragment) is required. In other words, the Fc portion of an antibody is dispensable for some applications.

An elaborate series of manipulations makes it possible to select, as well as produce, functional antibodies in *E. coli* (Fig. 10.34).

1. cDNA is synthesized from mRNA isolated from mouse antibody-producing cells (B lymphocytes).
2. The H and L chain sequences in the cDNA preparation are amplified separately by PCR.
3. Each amplified cDNA preparation is treated with a specific set of restriction endonucleases and cloned into a bacteriophage λ vector. The cDNA sequences of the H and L chains each have distinctive restriction endonuclease recognition sites, an arrangement that facilitates the directional cloning of each sequence into a separate bacteriophage λ vector. At this stage of the process, many different H and L chain sequences are cloned (Fig. 10.35A and B).
4. The cDNAs of one H and one L chain are cloned into a single "combinatorial" vector, thereby enabling the bacteriophage to coexpress

FIGURE 10.33 Organization of V_H and V_L regions of a monoclonal antibody and the development of a peptide, based on a portion of the CDR and FR of the V_H and V_L regions of the antibody molecule, with a similar binding specificity.

Peptide that binds to target antigen

both chains, thus forming an assembled antibody Fv fragment (Fig. 10.35C).

5. The H and L chains are expressed during the lytic cycle of bacteriophage λ, so that the library of combinatorial bacteriophage clones can be screened for the presence of antigen-binding activity.

The step in which L and H chain cDNAs are combined on one vector creates a vast array of diverse antibody genes, some of which encode unique target-binding sites whose isolation would never have been possible by standard hybridoma procedures. The mammalian antibody repertoire has the potential to produce approximately 10^6 to 10^8 different antibodies. A phage library contains approximately this number of clones, so one combi-

FIGURE 10.34 Procedure to create a combinatorial library of the V_L and V_H regions of antibody chains in *E. coli*. Note that the H and L chains are amplified in separate PCRs.

FIGURE 10.35 DNA constructs of an Fv combinatorial gene library cloned into bacteriophage λ DNA. **(A and B)** Portions of the cDNAs of the L (A) and H (B) chains are separately cloned into bacteriophage λ vectors. **(C)** Each of these libraries is digested with EcoRI, and then the fragments from the H chain library are ligated to the fragments from the L chain library, thereby creating a combinatorial library that contains all possible combinations of L and H chain fragments. p^{lac}, the E. coli lac promoter; RBS, ribosome-binding site.

natorial library can be expected to produce as many different antibodies (in this case, Fv molecules) as any mammal. In addition, once an initial combinatorial library has been constructed, it is possible to shuffle the L and H chains to obtain Fv molecules that recognize unusual epitopes, and even greater variation may be achieved by random mutagenesis of the DNAs in the combinatorial library (see chapter 8). Because millions of bacteriophage plaques can be screened in a relatively short period, the identification of Fv molecules with the desired specificity takes only about 7 to 14 days. By contrast, screening hybridoma cell lines is a slow, time-consuming process.

Because they lyse bacterial host cells, bacteriophage λ vectors are not particularly useful for the production of large quantities of protein. To overcome this drawback, the bacteriophage λ vector was engineered so that the H and L chain DNA sequences were inserted into a site that was flanked by plasmid DNA sequences. This plasmid DNA, containing an H and L chain DNA combination, can be excised from the bacteriophage λ vector and transformed into E. coli (Fig. 10.34). As part of a plasmid, large numbers of Fv fragments can be produced in E. coli cells.

As an alternative to the use of bacteriophage λ, filamentous bacteriophages, such as M13 and fd, have been used for the production of combinatorial libraries (Fig. 10.36). In these cases, the antibody fragment is synthesized as part of a fusion protein that is located on the outer surface of the bacteriophage. A combinatorial library of antibody fragments displayed on the surface of a filamentous bacteriophage can be screened by an enzyme-linked immunosorbent assay-like system. Briefly, samples (aliquots) of the library are added to the wells of a multiwell plate that are coated with the target antigen (Fig. 10.37). The wells are rinsed thoroughly to remove any unbound bacteriophage. Next, an antibody that binds to the

MILESTONE

Construction of a Retrovirus Packaging Mutant and Its Use To Produce Helper-Free Defective Retrovirus

R. MANN, R. C. MULLIGAN, and D. BALTIMORE
Cell 33:153–159, 1983

Human gene therapy has always been a controversial subject. However, most scientists agreed with T. Friedmann and R. Roblin, who in 1972 (*Science* 175:949–955) stated, "In our view, gene therapy may ameliorate some human genetic diseases in the future. For this reason, we believe that research directed at the development of techniques for gene therapy should continue." The essential features of human gene therapy are the delivery of a remedial gene and its expression in a cell type or tissue that cures a disease without risk to either those administering the therapeutic agent or those receiving it. Initially, vectors derived from human viruses seemed likely to be the principal mode for delivering remedial genes because they have specialized mechanisms for entering specific cells. In particular, of the various potential viral vectors, those based on retrovi-

ruses were considered the most promising. However, a native retrovirus is an infectious agent that can cause cell damage and, in some instances, induce cancer. The most significant advance that made human gene therapy possible was the development of a system for packaging a remedial gene into a noninfectious virus particle that retains the capability of attaching to its host cell.

Mann et al. constructed the first retroviral packaging cell line. In essence, they integrated a viral genome from which they had removed a DNA segment that contained the packaging signal into a chromosome of a cell line. Under these conditions, the cell line produced noninfectious virus particles. However, after transfection of these cells with a DNA construct that had a packaging signal and a remedial gene but no retroviral genes, the construct

was packaged into virus particles that in turn could be used to deliver a remedial gene to a particular cell type. This clever strategy was immediately adopted by many other researchers who were working on human gene therapy. Over the years, the original retrovirus cell-packaging line has been enhanced, and the concept has been successfully applied to other viral vectors.

In 1985, as a result of the work of Mann et al. and others, W. F. Anderson, who has been a persistent advocate for human gene therapy, noted, "It now appears that effective delivery-expression systems are becoming available that will allow reasonable attempts at human gene therapy." On 22 May 1989, Anderson and his colleagues initiated the first clinical trial using a gene therapy strategy. To date, gene therapy in general has not been particularly successful; however, as more information accumulates from ongoing studies, it is inevitable that it will become the standard mode of treatment for many diseases.

the drug not being able to reach the targeted site in the whole animal at a concentration sufficient to be effective. Increasing the dose of a drug is not the answer to this problem, because high drug concentrations often have deleterious side effects. A number of different strategies are used to enhance the delivery of a drug to its target site. (1) Drugs may be encapsulated in liposomes, i.e., particles in which the drug is surrounded by a specific lipid surface, that can be targeted to certain organs. (2) Certain toxin genes may be incorporated into tumor-infiltrating lymphocytes. These cells can deliver the incorporated toxin directly to the site of a tumor. (3) A drug can be coupled to a monoclonal antibody that is specific for proteins found only on the surfaces of certain cells, e.g., tumor cells (Fig. 10.40). (4) A prodrug is an inert form of a drug that requires a specific enzyme to be activated. To ensure that the drug is released only in the vicinity of the target cells, the activating enzyme is coupled to a monoclonal antibody directed against specific cell surface antigens (Fig. 10.40).

For this type of therapeutic system to be effective, the monoclonal antibody or single-chain antibody that is complexed with the prodrug-converting enzyme must be available in quantity in a relatively pure form, bind to a protein that is highly specific to the target cell, be stable under physiological conditions but cleared rapidly from circulation, and, when necessary, be able to penetrate into tumor masses so that all of the cells can

A

B

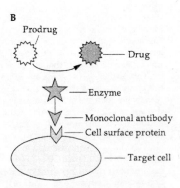

FIGURE 10.40 Schematic representation of a monoclonal antibody-based drug delivery system. **(A)** The drug is coupled to a monoclonal antibody. **(B)** An enzyme that converts an inactive prodrug to an active drug is attached to a monoclonal antibody. The active drug is formed only in the immediate vicinity of the target cells. In both cases, the monoclonal antibody binds to a specific protein on the surface of the target cell.

be exposed to the drug. With this approach, only specifically targeted cells are exposed to the drug, permitting the use of a much lower concentration than if it were administered directly.

Dual-Variable-Domain Antibodies

In some instances, an antibody (particularly one that is conjugated to a toxin or radiochemical) is able to destroy a tumor or pathogen cell. In such cases, it is often advantageous to use antibody fragments, since the Fc portion of the molecule is not only not needed, it may impede or prevent the rest of the molecule from binding to relatively inaccessible antigens. Despite the usefulness of antibody fragments in a variety of applications, a major limitation of using them as therapeutic agents is that, since they lack the Fc portion of the molecule, they are unable to mount a complete immune response. To increase the utility of naturally existing antibodies, as well as to ensure that they are effective initiators of a complete immune response, researchers have created what they have termed "dual-variable-domain immunoglobulins" (Fig. 10.41). These constructs are essentially IgG molecules containing two tandem Fv regions, each with a different specificity. Dual-variable-domain immunoglobulins are bispecific and tetravalent, and they consist entirely of human immunoglobulin sequences. That is, each molecule contains four Fv regions, two identical Fv regions directed against one antigen and two Fv regions directed against another antigen. A dual-variable-domain immunoglobulin specific for both interleukin-12 and interleukin-18 produced in CHO cells showed binding to both of these cytokines, binding each with an affinity similar to that of the original monospecific antibody. In addition, in a biological assay, using a severe combined immunodeficient mouse model engrafted with human peripheral blood mononuclear cells, the interleukin-12/interleukin-18 antibody was as effective at inhibiting induced IFN-γ production as was a combination of the original two monospecific antibodies. Using this strategy, it should be possible to generate full-size bispecific antibodies for a variety of therapeutic purposes.

FIGURE 10.41 Dual-variable-domain immunoglobulin directed against both interleukin-12 (IL-12) and interleukin-18.

FIGURE 10.36 Formation of an Fv antibody combinatorial library in the filamentous bacteriophage M13. Following extraction of mRNA and its conversion to cDNA, the cDNAs for the V_L and V_H regions are amplified (separately) by PCR and then ligated to DNA that encodes a short linker peptide. Each single-chain antibody–DNA construct is cloned into gene 3 of bacteriophage M13. There are three copies of the phage gene 3 protein, which is a phage surface protein, per M13 bacteriophage.

bacteriophage coat protein and is conjugated with an enzyme is added to each well. The wells are rinsed to remove any unbound antibody–enzyme complex. The phage particles bound to the target antigen are recognized by the antibody–enzyme complex. A chromogenic substrate that is cleaved by the bound enzyme is then used to determine which wells contain a phage carrying antibodies to the target antigen. This approach is easier than using plaque assays with bacteriophage λ to select and subsequently purify a bacteriophage producing an antibody fragment that binds to a specific antigen. Once a desired antibody fragment-producing bacteriophage has been isolated, using either bacteriophage λ or M13, the DNA can be isolated and subcloned into an expression vector. These procedures are used to produce mouse, chimeric, or humanized antibodies.

A Combinatorial Library of Full-Length Antibodies

Until recently, all of the combinatorial libraries of antibodies included either single-chain antibodies or Fab fragments and not full-length antibodies.

FIGURE 10.37 Immunological screening of a bacteriophage M13 combinatorial library.

However, for many applications it is advantageous for therapeutic antibodies to be full length. With this in mind, researchers cloned and expressed complete antibody molecules (using either two separate vectors, one encoding a light chain and the other encoding a heavy chain, or a single operon controlling the expression of both the light and heavy chain on a single vector) in *E. coli*.

The process of selecting antibodies with specified affinities would be greatly facilitated if an *E. coli* library could be screened directly for binding to various antigens. To do this, a combinatorial library of full-length antibodies was generated and engineered so that the antibodies were secreted into the periplasm between the inner and outer membranes. In addition, prior to the expression of the antibody molecules, the host *E. coli* was engineered to express a fusion protein that became anchored within the inner membrane (lipoprotein fragment) and also contained a portion of a protein from the *Staphylococcus aureus* protein A that binds specifically to Fc regions (Fig. 10.38). When an IgG molecule is secreted into the periplasm, the fusion protein binds to the Fc region. The tightly bound IgG–fusion protein complex remains intact when the *E. coli* cells are treated with EDTA and lysozyme to remove a portion of the outer membrane. Then, a fluorescently labeled target antigen is added to detect those cells that have expressed an antibody directed against that target antigen. By cell sorting, fluorescently labeled cells are selected. Then, the plasmid DNA that encodes the selected IgG molecules is isolated and expressed in an *E. coli* strain that does not synthesize the membrane-anchored fusion protein. This simple, yet powerful, technique simplifies the selection and production in *E. coli* of full-length monoclonal antibodies.

Shuffling CDR Sequences

Very large libraries of single-chain antibodies can be the sources of a wide range of highly specific human antibodies so that one does not have to resort to using mice for the initial monoclonal antibody. Theoretically, such libraries contain a greater diversity of antibodies than is normally found in the human immune system. To construct a library of this sort, B cells and other antibody-producing cells, from different, nonimmunized individuals

FIGURE 10.38 Schematic representation of the selection of a full-length antibody that binds to a fluorescently labeled target antigen. The Fc portion of the antibody is bound by a fragment of *S. aureus* protein A fused to a portion of an *E. coli* lipoprotein anchored in the inner membrane.

and from different tissues and organs, are collected and pooled before the mRNA is isolated (Fig. 10.39). The isolated mRNA is used to program the synthesis of cDNA, which then becomes a template for the specific PCR amplification of each CDR (separately). The amplified CDRs are mixed with oligonucleotides encoding FRs, a linker, and DNA sequences encoding the variable L and H domains. Overlap extension PCR (see chapter 4) is used to order, join, and amplify H and L antibody chain genes. In addition to being entirely human, the 2×10^9 different single-chain antibodies that have been produced in this way have a very wide range of specificities, reflecting the fact that the CDR sequences have been incorporated in random order and from a variety of sources, i.e., they have been shuffled. There are single-chain antibodies against β-galactosidase, the β subunit of cholera toxin, fluorescein isothiocyanate, human cell surface antigen, human leptin, human prostrate-specific antigen, and streptavidin, among others. Moreover, the dissociation constants (K_ds) for the interaction of the selected antibodies with their target antigens ranged from 0.9×10^{-9} to 420×10^{-9} M^{-1} (where tight binding is represented by a low number). For antibodies, K_ds of around 0.1×10^{-8} to 10×10^{-8} M^{-1} reflect a high degree of specificity for the target antigen. The fact that a very large library of single-chain antibodies, all with high affinity for their target antigens, could easily be generated by this procedure means that the goal of being able to select virtually any antibody from a nonimmunized library has been achieved.

Chemically Linked Monoclonal Antibodies

Drugs that are very effective when tested in cell culture are often much less potent in a whole organism. This difference in potency is typically due to

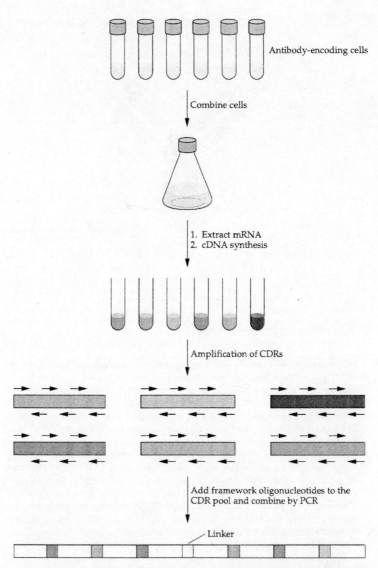

Antibody-encoding cells

Combine cells

1. Extract mRNA
2. cDNA synthesis

Amplification of CDRs

Add framework oligonucleotides to the
CDR pool and combine by PCR

Linker

FIGURE 10.39 Construction of a large library of single-chain antibodies. B cells from several nonimmunized individuals were collected and pooled, the mRNA was isolated and used to program the synthesis of cDNA, oligonucleotide primers containing DNA sequences that included small portions of the FR sequence were added to the cDNA preparation, and all six CDRs were amplified separately by PCR. The amplified CDRs from all six PCRs were mixed together with oligonucleotides encoding the FRs and the linker, and genes encoding the variable L and H domains were synthesized by overlap extension PCR. One of the many possible single-chain antibodies that were synthesized is shown.

mouse monoclonal antibodies by repertoire cloning. *Trends Biotechnol.* 9:169–175.

Chamow, S. M., and A. Ashkenazi. 1996. Immunoadhesins: principles and applications. *Trends Biotechnol.* 14:52–60.

Chester, K. A., and R. E. Hawkins. 1995. Clinical issues in antibody design. *Trends Biotechnol.* 13:294–300.

Collet, T. A., P. Roben, R. O'Kennedy, C. F. Barbas III, D. R. Burton, and R. A. Lerner. 1992. A binary plasmid system for shuffling combinatorial antibody libraries. *Proc. Natl. Acad. Sci. USA* 89:10026–10030.

Cunningham, B. C., and J. A. Wells. 1991. Rational design of receptor-specific variants of human growth hormone. *Proc. Natl. Acad. Sci. USA* 88:3407–3411.

Curnis, F., A. Sacchi, L. Borgna, F. Magni, A. Gasparri, and A. Corti. 2000. Enhancement of tumor necrosis factor α antitumor immunotherapeutic properties by targeted delivery to aminopeptidase N (CD13). *Nat. Biotechnol.* 18:1185–1190.

de Vos, W. M. and J. Hugenholtz. 2004. Engineering metabolic highways in lactococci and other lactic acid bacteria. *Trends Biotechnol.* 22:72–79.

Dübel, S. 2007. Recombinant therapeutic antibodies. *Appl. Microbiol. Biotechnol.* 74:723–729.

Gram, H., L. A. Marconi, C. F. Barbas III, T. A. Collet, R. A. Lerner, and A. S. Kang. 1992. In vitro selection and affinity maturation of antibodies from a naive combinatorial immunoglobulin library. *Proc. Natl. Acad. Sci. USA* 89:3576–3580.

Hanniffy, S., U. Wiedermann, A. Repa, A. Mercenier, C. Daniel, J. Fioamonti, H. Tlaskolova, H. Kozakova, H. Israelsen, S. Madsen, A. Vrang, P. Hols, J. Delcour, P. Bron, M. Kleerebezem, and J. Wells. 2004. Potential and opportunities for use of recombinant lactic acid bacteria in human health. *Adv. Appl. Microbiol.* 56:1–64.

Harris, W. J. 1994. Humanizing monoclonal antibodies for in vivo use. *Anim. Cell Biotechnol.* 6:259–279.

Hodgson, J. 1991. Making monoclonals in microbes. *Bio/Technology* 9:421–425.

Holliger, P. and P. J. Hudson. 2005. Engineered antibody fragments and the rise of single domains. *Nat. Biotechnol.* 23:1126–1136.

Huennekens, F. M. 1994. Tumor targeting: activation of prodrugs by enzyme-monoclonal antibody conjugates. *Trends Biotechnol.* 12:234–239.

Huse, W. D., L. Sastry, S. A. Iverson, A. S. Kang, M. Alting-Mees, D. R. Burton, S. J. Benkovic, and R. A. Lerner. 1989. Generation of a large combinatorial library of the immunoglobulin repertoire in phage lambda. *Science* 246:1275–1281.

Jakobovits, A., R. G. Amado, X. Yang, L. Roskos, and G. Schwab. 2007. From XenoMouse technology to panitumumab, the first fully human antibody product from transgenic mice. *Nat. Biotechnol.* 25:1134–1143.

Jean, F., L. Thomas, S. S. Molloy, G. Liu, M. A. Jarvis, J. A. Nelson, and G. Thomas. 2000. A protein-based therapeutic for human cytomegalovirus infection. *Proc. Natl. Acad. Sci. USA* 97:2864–2869.

Kreitman, R. J. 1999. Immunotoxins in cancer therapy. *Curr. Opin. Immunol.* 11:570–578.

Kufer, P., R. Lutterbrüse, and P. A. Baeuerle. 2004. A revival of bispecific antibodies. *Trends Biotechnol.* 22:238–244.

Little, M., F. Breitling, S. Dübel, P. Fuchs, and M. Braunagel. 1995. Human antibody libraries in *Escherichia coli. J. Biotechnol.* 41:187–195.

Liu, Q. P., G. Sulzenbacher, H. Yuan, E. P. Bennett, G. Pietz, K. Saunders, J. Spence, E. Nudelman, S. B. Levery, T. White, J. M. Neveu, W. S. Lane, Y. Bourne, M. L. Olsson, B. Henrissat, and H. Clausen. 2007. Bacterial glycosidases for the production of universal red blood cells. *Nat. Biotechnol.* 25:454–464.

Liu, X., L. A. Lagenaur, D. A. Simpson, K. P. Essenmacher, C. L. Frazier-Parker, Y. Liu, S. S. Rao, D. H. Hamer, T. P. Parks, P. P. Lee, and Q. Xu. 2006. Engineered vaginal *Lactobacillus* strain for mucosal delivery of the human immunodeficiency virus inhibitor cyanovirin-N. *Antimicrob. Agents Chemother.* 50:3250–3259.

LoBuglio, A. G., R. H. Wheeler, J. Trang, A. Haynes, K. Rogers, E. B. Harvey, L. Sun, J. Ghrayeb, and M. B. Khazaeli. 1989. Mouse/human chimeric monoclonal antibody in man: kinetics and immune response. *Proc. Natl. Acad. Sci. USA* 86:4220–4224.

Lonberg, N. 2005. Human antibodies from transgenic animals. *Nat. Biotechnol.* 23:1117–1125.

Lorenzen, N., P. M. Cupit, K. Einer-Jensen, E. Lorenzen, P. Ahrens, C. J. Secombes, and C. Cunningham. 2000. Immunoprophylaxis in fish by injection of mouse antibody genes. *Nat. Biotechnol.* 18:1177–1180.

Marks, J. D., A. D. Griffiths, M. Malmqvist, T. P. Clackson, J. M. Bye, and G. Winter. 1992. By-passing immunization: building high affinity antibodies by chain shuffling. *Bio/Technology* 10:779–783.

Mazor, Y., T. Van Blarcom, R. Mabry, B. L. Iverson and G. Georgiou. 2007. Isolation of engineered full-length antibodies from libraries expressed in *Escherichia coli. Nat. Biotechnol.* 25:563–565.

Molina, A. 2008. A decade of rituximab: improving survival outcomes in non-Hodgkin's lymphoma. *Annu. Rev. Med.* 59:237–250.

Mullinax, R. L., E. A. Gross, J. R. Amberg, B. N. Hay, H. H. Hogrefe, M. M. Kubitz, A. Greener, M. Alting-Mees, D. Ardourel, J. M. Short, J. A. Sorge, and B. Shopes. 1990. Identification of human antibody fragment clones specific for tetanus toxoid in a bacteriophage λ immunoexpression library. *Proc. Natl. Acad. Sci. USA* 87:8095–8099.

Murata, K., T. Inose, T. Hisano, S. Abe, Y. Yonemoto, T. Yamashita, M. Takagi, K. Sakaguchi, A. Kimura, and T. Imanaka. 1993. Bacterial alginate lyase: enzymology, genetics and application. *J. Ferment. Bioeng.* 76:427–437.

Nagata, S., H. Taira, A. Hall, L. Johnsrud, M. Streuli, J. Ecsödi, W. Boll, K. Cantell, and C. Weissmann. 1980. Synthesis in *E. coli* of a polypeptide with human leukocyte interferon activity. *Nature* 284:316–320.

Osborn, B. L., L. Sekut, M. Corcoran, C. Poortman, B. Sturm, G. Chen, D. Mather, H. L. Lin, and T. J. Parry. 2002. Albutropin: a growth hormone-albumin fusion with improved phar-

macokinetics and pharmacodynamics in rats and monkeys. *Eur. J. Pharmacol.* **456**:149–158.

Plückthun, A. 1991. Antibody engineering: advances from the use of *E. coli* expression systems. *Bio/Technology* **9**:545–551.

Qiu, X.-Q., H. Wang, B. Cai, L.-L. Wang, and S.-T. Yue. 2007. Small antibody mimetics comprising two complementarity-determining regions and a framework region for tumor targeting. *Nat. Biotechnol.* **25**:921–929.

Queen, C., W. P. Schneider, H. E. Selick, P. W. Payne, N. F. Landolf, J. F. Duncan, N. M. Avdalovic, M. Levitt, R. P. Junghans, and T. A. Waldmann. 1989. A humanized antibody that binds to the interleukin 2 receptor. *Proc. Natl. Acad. Sci. USA* **86**:10029–10033.

Reichert, J. M. 2006. Trends in US approvals: new biopharmaceuticals and vaccines. *Trends Biotechnol.* **24**:293–298.

Reichert, J. M., C. J. Rosensweig, L. B. Faden, and M. C. Dewitz. 2005. Monoclonal antibody success in the clinic. *Nat. Biotechnol.* **23**:1073–1078.

Reiter, Y., U. Brinkmann, K. O. Webber, S.-H. Jung, and I. Pastan. 1994. Engineering interchain disulfide bonds into conserved framework regions of Fv fragments: improved biochemical characteristics of recombinant immunotoxins containing disulfide-stabilized Fv. *Protein Eng.* **7**:697–704.

Rubinfeld, B., A. Upadhyay, S. L. Clark, S. E. Fong, V. Smith, H. Koeppen, S. Ross, and P. Polakis. 2006. Identification and immunotherapeutic targeting of antigens induced by chemotherapy. *Nat. Biotechnol.* **24**:205–209.

Sampson, J. H., L. E. Crotty, S. Lee, G. E. Archer, D. M. Ashley, C. J. Wikstrand, L. P. Hale, C. Small, G. Dranoff, A. H. Friedman, H. S. Friedman, and D. D. Bigner. 2000. Unarmed, tumor-specific monoclonal antibody effectively treats brain tumors. *Proc. Natl. Acad. Sci. USA* **97**:7503–7508.

Sarkissian, C. H., Z. Shao, F. Blain, R. Peevers, H. Su, R. Heft, T. M. S. Chang, and C. R. Scriver. 1999. A different approach to treatment of phenylketonuria: phenylalanine degradation with recombinant phenylalanine ammonia lyase. *Proc. Natl. Acad. Sci. USA* **96**:2339–2344.

Söderlind, E., L. Strandberg, P. Jirholt, N. Kobayashi, B. Alexeiva, A.-M. Åberg, A. Nilsson, B. Jansson, M. Ohlin, C. Wingren, L. Danielsson, R. Carlsson, and C. A. K. Borrebaeck. 2000. Recombining germline-derived CDR sequences for creating diverse single-framework antibody libraries. *Nat. Biotechnol.* **18**:852–856.

Steidler, L., W. Hans, L. Schotte, S. Neirynck, F. Obermeier, W. Falk, W. Fiers, and E. Remaut. 2000. Treatment of murine colitis by *Lactococcus lactis* secreting interleukin-10. *Science* **289**:1352–1355.

Steidler, L., S. Neirynck, N. Huyghebaert, V. Snoeck, A. Vermeire, B. Goddeeris, E. Cox, J. P. Remon, and E. Remaut. 2003. Biological containment of genetically modified *Lactococcus lactis* for intestinal delivery of human interleukin 10. *Nat. Biotechnol.* **21**:785–789.

Subramanian, G. M., M. Fiscella, A. Lamousé-Smith, S. Zeuzem, and J. G. McHutchison. 2007. Albuferon α-2b: a generic fusion protein for the treatment of chronic hepatitis C. *Nat. Biotechnol.* **25**:1411–1419.

Taniguchi, T., Y. Fujii-Kuriyama, and M. Muramatsu. 1980. Molecular cloning of human interferon cDNA. *Proc. Natl. Acad. Sci. USA* **77**:4003–4006.

Ulmer, G. S., A. Herzka, K. J. Toy, D. L. Baker, A. H. Dodge, D. Sinicropi, S. Shak, and R. A. Lazarus. 1996. Engineering actin-resistant human DNase I for treatment of cystic fibrosis. *Proc. Natl. Acad. Sci. USA* **93**:8225–8229.

Vaughan, T. J., A. J. Williams, K. Pritchard, J. K. Osbourn, A. R. Pope, J. C. Earnshaw, J. McCafferty, R. A. Hodits, J. Wilton, and K. S. Johnson. 1996. Human antibodies with subnanomolar affinities isolated from a large non-immunized phage display library. *Nat. Biotechnol.* **14**:309–314.

Wilkenson, I. R., E. Ferrandis, P. J. Artymiuk, M. Teillot, C. Soulard, C. Touvay, S. L. Pradananga, S. Justice, Z. Wu, K. C. Leung, C. J. Strasburger, J. R. Sayers, and R. J. Ross. 2007. A ligand-receptor fusion of growth hormone forms a dimer and is a potent long-acting agonist. *Nat. Med.* **13**:1108–1113.

Wu, C., H. Ying, C. Grinnell, S. Bryant, R. Miller, A. Clabbers, S. Bose, D. McCarthy, R.-R. Zhu, L. Santora, R. Davis-Taber, Y. Kunes, E. Fung, A. Schwartz, P. Sakorafas, J. Gu, E. Tarcsa, A. Murtaza, and T. Ghayur. 2007. Simultaneous targeting of multiple disease mediators by a dual-variable-domain immunoglobin. *Nat. Biotechnol.* **25**:1290–1297.

Zahm, J.-M., C. Debordeaux, C. Maurer, D. Hubert, D. Dusser, N. Bonnet, R. A. Lazarus, and E. Puchelle. 2001. Improved activity of an actin-resistant DNase I variant on the cystic fibrosis airway secretions. *Am. J. Respir. Crit. Care Med.* **163**:1153–1157.

REVIEW QUESTIONS

1. Before the sequencing of the human genome, how would you have cloned and expressed a cDNA sequence encoding human IFN? You do not have a DNA hybridization probe for human IFN, although you have isolated a human cell line that can be induced to synthesize IFN approximately 100-fold over background levels. Explain your strategy.

2. What is the Fc portion of an antibody molecule? The Fab portion? The Fv portion? The CDR portion?

3. How are antibody light and heavy chains coordinately synthesized in *E. coli*?

4. How would you modify growth hormone to make it longer-acting?

5. Why would DNase I and alginate lyase be useful for treating cystic fibrosis?

6. How is the production of alginate lyase from a cloned gene detected in *E. coli* transformants?

7. What is a combinatorial cDNA library?

8. How is bacteriophage M13 used to select Fv fragments that bind to specific target antigens?

9. What are disulfide-stabilized and scFv molecules?

10. How are enzymes coupled to monoclonal antibodies or Fv fragments used as therapeutic agents?

11. How are mouse monoclonal antibodies "humanized"? Discuss the reasons for creating humanized monoclonal antibodies.

12. Describe a protocol for producing a therapeutic agent that targets and kills a specific cell type.

13. How would you engineer TNF-α to be a more specific and effective anticancer agent?

14. What would you do to make interleukin-10 more effective for treating inflammatory bowel disease?

15. How can the gene for DNase I be manipulated so that the enzyme becomes more effective for treating cystic fibrosis patients?

16. How would you develop a strategy to protect at-risk women from HIV infection?

17. How might low levels of phenylalanine be attained, other than with a phenylalanine-free diet, in patients with the human genetic disease phenylketonuria?

18. What types of genetic manipulations can be used to generate a very large bacterial library of highly specific single-chain human monoclonal antibodies?

19. How would you engineer a mouse so that it produces only human antibodies?

20. What is a bispecific diabody?

21. How would you design a short peptide so that it retains the antigen-binding specificity of an entire immunoglobulin molecule?

22. How would select antibodies against specific antigens in *E. coli*?

23. What are dual-variable-domain immunoglobulins?

24. How can you use a chemotherapy agent to facilitate the targeting of tumor cells with monoclonal antibodies?

Nucleic Acids as Therapeutic Agents

OFTEN, HUMAN DISORDERS, such as cancer, inflammatory conditions, and both viral and parasitic infections, result from the overproduction of a normal protein. Therapeutic systems using nucleotide sequences are being devised to treat these types of conditions. Theoretically, a small single-stranded nucleotide sequence (oligonucleotide) could hybridize to a specific gene or messenger RNA (mRNA) and diminish transcription or translation, respectively, thereby decreasing the amount of protein that is synthesized. An oligonucleotide that is designed to bind to a gene and block transcription is called an antigene oligonucleotide, and one that base pairs with a specific mRNA is called an antisense oligonucleotide. The binding of an oligonucleotide to a transcription factor that is responsible for the expression of a specific gene could lower both transcription and translation of the target gene. Double-stranded oligonucleotides that attach to DNA-binding proteins could prevent the activation of transcription of specific genes. Also, some synthetic RNA/DNA molecules called aptamers that bind to proteins that are not naturally nucleic acid-binding proteins and prevent them from functioning can be created. Ribozymes, which are natural RNA sequences that bind and cleave specific RNA molecules, could be engineered to target an mRNA and subsequently decrease the amount of a particular protein that is synthesized. In addition, interfering RNAs, small double-stranded RNA molecules that direct the sequence-specific degradation of mRNA, may be used instead of either antisense RNAs (or oligonucleotides) or ribozymes. The potential for nucleic acid therapeutic agents is considerable and is just now beginning to be realized.

Antisense RNA

To be an effective therapeutic agent, an antisense RNA must bind to a specified mRNA and prevent translation of the protein (Fig. 11.1A). The possibility of using an expression vector to produce an antisense RNA that suppresses a pathogenic condition has been examined. For example, episomally based expression vectors that carry the complementary DNA (cDNA)

FIGURE 10.42 Targeting tumor cells for destruction by monoclonal antibody–toxin conjugates. Tumor cells are first treated with the chemotherapeutic agent irinotecan, which induces the synthesis of a unique cell surface protein. Then, a monoclonal antibody directed against the cell surface protein and conjugated to a toxin molecule is added. After binding of the antibody to the cell surface, the toxin is internalized, thereby killing the tumor cell.

Anticancer Antibodies

A number of therapeutic antibodies that are directed against protein antigenic determinants on the surfaces of cancer cells have been selected because the proteins are overexpressed compared to those on noncancerous cells. Unfortunately, (1) antibodies directed against these proteins may also bind to some noncancerous cells expressing the same or a similar antigen and (2) this approach presents researchers with only a limited number of targets for therapeutic antibodies. One way to select for additional cell surface targets would be to identify proteins whose expression is selectively induced in tumor cells exposed to chemotherapeutic drugs. When colorectal cancer cells were treated with the drug irinotecan, which is a topoisomerase inhibitor and is commonly used to treat this type of cancer, several newly synthesized proteins were found on the surfaces of those cells. (Topoisomerases are enzymes that unwind DNA during either DNA replication or mRNA transcription.) The new cell surface proteins were expressed early, prior to any major effects of the chemotherapeutic compound on cell viability. Monoclonal antibodies directed against one newly synthesized cell surface protein (called LY6D/E48) were generated, and then the antibodies were complexed with the cellular toxin auristatin E. The antibody–toxin conjugate was then used to treat tumor cells that were

first treated with irinotecan (Fig. 10.42). Following binding to the cell surface protein, the antibody–toxin conjugate was internalized inside the tumor cell. With this strategy, in six out of eight mice tumors disappeared entirely, while in the other two mice, the tumors were dramatically decreased in size. This exciting approach will have to be tried with larger numbers of animals before it can begin clinical trials. However, provided that it is possible to identify one or more proteins that are specifically induced by chemotherapeutic agents and are not found on the surfaces of nontumor cells, this procedure could become a general strategy that is used to treat a variety of different types of human cancer.

SUMMARY

A large number of proteins that have potential as therapeutic agents have been synthesized from cloned genes in bacteria. Because most of these proteins are from eukaryotic organisms, the strategy for the isolation of a target gene often involves isolating mRNA enriched in the messenger of interest, synthesizing a cDNA library, and subcloning the selected target cDNA into an appropriate expression vector. In some instances, novel and useful variants of these proteins can be constructed either by shuffling functional domains of related genes or by directed replacement of functional domains of the cloned gene. In addition, long-acting and stable variants of some therapeutic proteins have been synthesized.

In some instances, genetically engineered enzymes may be used as therapeutic agents. For example, both recombinant DNase I and alginate lyase have been used in an aerosol form to decrease the viscosity of the mucus found in the lungs of patients with cystic fibrosis. In addition, phenylalanine ammonia lyase may help patients with phenylketonuria as a replacement for phenylalanine hydroxylase, α_1-antitrypsin may be used to limit some infections, and glycosidases may be utilized to convert blood groups A, B, and AB to type O.

The development of recombinant DNA and monoclonal antibody technologies, combined with an understanding of the molecular structure and function of immunoglobulin molecules, has provided specific antibodies as therapeutic agents to treat various diseases. Antibody genes can be readily manipulated because the various functions of an antibody molecule are confined to discrete domains.

Drugs, prodrugs, or enzymes can be coupled to monoclonal antibodies or Fv fragments that are specific for proteins found only on the surfaces of certain cells, e.g., tumor cells. These antibody–drug or antibody–enzyme combinations act as therapeutic agents. However, if the therapy requires multiple treatments, the antibody component should be from a human source to prevent immunological cross-reactivity and sensitization of the patient. To achieve this, rodent monoclonal antibodies are "humanized" by substituting into human antibodies only the CDRs of the rodent monoclonal antibodies. In addition, it has become possible to produce and select human monoclonal antibodies in E. coli and in transgenic mice.

REFERENCES

Adams, G. P. and L. M. Weiner. 2005. Monoclonal antibody therapy of cancer. *Nat. Biotechnol.* **23:**1147–1157.

Alkawash, M. A., J. S. Soothill, and N. L. Schiller. 2006. Alginate lyase enhances antibiotic killing of mucoid *Pseudomonas aeruginosa* in biofilms. *APMIS* **114:**131–138.

Barbas, C. F., III, and D. R. Burton. 1996. Selection and evolution of high-affinity human anti-viral antibodies. *Trends Biotechnol.* **14:**230–234.

Bermúdez-Humarán, L. G., S. Nouaille, V. Zilberfarb, G. Corthier, A. Gruss, P. Langella, and T. Issad. 2007. Effect of intranasal administration of a leptin-secreting *Lactococcus lactis* recombinant on food intake,

body weight, and immune response of mice. *Appl. Environ. Microbiol.* **73:**5300–5307.

Bird, R. E., and B. W. Walker. 1991. Single chain antibody variable regions. *Trends Biotechnol.* **9:**132–137.

Braat, H., P. Rottiers, D. W. Hommes, N. Huyghebaert, E. Remaut, J.-P. Remon, S. J. H. van Deventer, S. Neirynck, M. P. Peppelenbosch, and L. Steidler. 2006. A phase I trial with transgenic bacteria expressing interleukin-10 in Crohn's disease. *Clin. Gastroenterol. Hepatol.* **4:**754–759.

Brideau-Andersen, A. D., X. Huang, S.-C. C. Sun, T. T. Chen, D. Stark, I. J. Sas, L. Zadik, G. N. Dawes, D. R. Guptill, R. McCord, S. Govindarajan,

A. Roy, S. Yang, J. Gao, Y. H. Chen, N. J. Ø. Skartved, A. K. Pedersen, D. Lin, C. P. Locher, I. Rebbarpragada, A. D. Jensen, S. H. Bass, T. L. S. Nissen, S. Viswanathan, G. R. Foster, J. A. Symons, and P. A. Patten. 2007. Directed evolution of gene-shuffled IFN-α molecules with activity profiles tailored for treatment of chronic viral diseases. *Proc. Natl. Acd. Sci. USA* **104:**8269–8274.

Brinkmann, U., L. H. Pai, D. J. FitzGerald, M. Willingham, and I. Pastan. 1991. B3(Fv)-PE38KDEL, a single-chain immunotoxin that causes complete regression of a human carcinoma in mice. *Proc. Natl. Acad. Sci. USA* **88:**8616–8620.

Burton, D. R. 1991. Human and

FIGURE 11.1 Inhibition of translation of specific mRNAs by antisense (AS) nucleic acid molecules. The promoter and polyadenylation regions are marked by *p* and *pa*, respectively; the intron is indicated by the letter A; and the exons are indicated by numbers (1 and 2). **(A)** A cDNA (AS gene) is cloned into an expression vector in reverse orientation, and the construct is transfected into a cell, where the AS RNA is synthesized. The AS RNA hybridizes to the target mRNA, and translation is blocked. **(B)** An AS oligonucleotide is introduced into a cell, and after it hybridizes with the target mRNA, translation is blocked.

FIGURE 11.2 A cDNA for human insulin-like growth factor 1 (ILGF-1) cloned on a vector in the antisense orientation under the transcriptional control of a metallothionein promoter (MT*p*). Following transfection into tumor-causing cells, when low levels of ZnSO₄ are added, the cells have decreased tumorigenicity. The arrows above the gene and promoter indicate the normal direction of transcription. The origin of replication and other plasmid sequences have been omitted for clarity.

sequence for either insulin-like growth factor 1 or insulin-like growth factor 1 receptor were constructed with the cloned sequences oriented so that the transcripts were antisense rather than mRNA (sense) sequences. Insulin-like growth factor 1 is prevalent in malignant glioma, which is the most common form of human brain tumor. Excess production of insulin-like growth factor 1 receptor occurs in prostate carcinoma, which is a significant type of cancer in males. In both vectors, the reverse-oriented cDNAs are under the control of the metallothionein promoter, which is induced by low levels of $ZnSO_4$.

Cultured glioma cells were transfected with the vector that produces the antisense version of the insulin-like growth factor 1 mRNA. In the absence of $ZnSO_4$, the tumorous properties were retained; in contrast, when $ZnSO_4$ was added to the culture medium, these distinctive features were lost (Fig. 11.2). In another experiment, nontransfected glioma cells caused tumors after they were injected into rats, whereas glioma cells that had been transfected with antisense insulin-like growth factor 1 cDNA did not develop tumors.

When mice were injected with rat prostate carcinoma cells that were transfected with the insulin-like growth factor 1 receptor cDNA in the antisense orientation, they developed either small or no tumors, whereas large tumors were formed when mice were treated with either nontransfected or control-transfected rat prostate carcinoma cells. It was assumed that in both cases the antisense RNA hybridized with its complementary mRNA sequence and hindered translation of insulin-like growth factor 1 and insulin-like growth factor 1 receptor, thus preventing the proliferation of the cancer cells.

Antisense Oligonucleotides

The sequence-specific effectiveness of chemically synthesized antisense oligodeoxynucleotides (Fig. 11.1B) relies on hybridization to an accessible nucleotide sequence on the target mRNA, resistance to degradation by cellular nucleases, and ready delivery into cells. Oligonucleotides with about 15 to 24 nucleotides have sufficient specificity to hybridize to a unique mRNA. Potential mRNA target sites are determined by testing a set of antisense oligonucleotides with cells in culture that produce the target mRNA. Those antisense oligonucleotides that diminish the translation of the specified protein are selected. Proteomic analysis of cellular proteins that are labeled with fluorescent dyes during translation can be used to determine if the production of a particular protein is reduced in the presence of an antisense oligonucleotide. There are no general rules for predicting the best target sites in various RNA transcripts. Antisense oligonucleotides that are directed to the 5′ and 3′ ends of mRNAs, intron–exon boundaries, and regions that are naturally double stranded have all been effective.

Since oligodeoxynucleotides are susceptible to degradation by intracellular nucleases, it was important to find ways to synthesize molecules that are resistant to attack by nucleases without affecting the ability of the antisense oligonucleotide to hybridize to a target sequence. To this end, the backbone, pyrimidines, and sugar moiety have been modified (Fig. 11.3). Currently, the most extensively used antisense oligonucleotide has a sulfur group in place of the free oxygen of the phosphodiester bond (Fig. 11.3B). This modification is called a phosphorothioate linkage. Phosphorothioate antisense oligonucleotides are water soluble, polyanionic, and resistant to

endogenous nucleases. In addition, when a phosphorothioate antisense oligonucleotide hybridizes to its target site, the RNA–DNA duplex activates the endogenous enzyme ribonuclease H (RNase H), which cleaves the mRNA component of the hybrid molecule. Clinical trials with several phosphorothioate antisense oligonucleotides, which are considered to be "first-generation" therapeutic agents, have been initiated. Second-generation antisense oligonucleotides typically contain alkyl modifications at the 2′ position of the ribose (Fig. 11.3E) and are generally less toxic and more specific than phosphorothioate-modified molecules. Third-generation antisense oligonucleotides contain a variety of modifications within the ribose ring and/or the phosphate backbone, as well as being less toxic than either first- or second-generation antisense oligonucleotides. One phosphorothioate antisense oligonucleotide has been approved by the U.S. Food and Drug Administration (FDA) to treat cytomegalovirus infections of the retina in patients with acquired immune deficiency syndrome (AIDS). This particular antisense oligonucleotide, called fomivirsen and sold as Vitravene, is administered by injection of 330 µg in a volume of 50 µl directly into an affected eye after the application of a topical or local anesthetic. Fomivirsen treatment is typically once every 2 weeks for 4 weeks, followed by once

MILESTONE

Potent and Specific Genetic Interference by Double-Stranded RNA in *Caenorhabditis elegans*

A. FIRE, S.-Q. XU, M. K. MONTGOMERY, S. A. KOSTAS, S. E. DRIVER, and C. C. MELLO
Nature 391:806-811, 1998

The nematode worm *Caenorhabditis elegans* is studied as a model eukaryotic organism in part because the strains are inexpensive to breed and can be frozen. When the cells are thawed, they remain viable, allowing long-term storage. *C. elegans* has the advantage of being a multicellular eukaryotic organism that is simple enough to be studied in great detail. The developmental fate of every single somatic cell (959 in the adult hermaphrodite; 1,031 in the adult male) has been mapped out, and these patterns of cell lineage are largely invariant between individuals. In addition, *C. elegans* is one of the simplest organisms with a nervous system.

In the late 1990s, Andrew Fire, Craig Mello, and their colleagues were investigating how gene expression is regulated in *C. elegans*. When they injected worms with mRNA molecules encoding a *C. elegans* muscle protein, they did not observe any changes in

the behavior of the worms. Injecting the antisense version of this mRNA also had no effect. However, when they injected sense and antisense RNAs together, they observed that the worms displayed peculiar twitching movements. Similar movements were seen in worms that completely lacked a functioning gene for the muscle protein.

Somehow the added double-stranded RNA molecule was silencing the expression of the gene carrying the same genetic information as that particular RNA. When double-stranded RNA molecules containing portions of the mRNA sequences for several other worm proteins were injected, the expression of these genes was also silenced.

From these experiments, Fire and Mello deduced that double-stranded RNA can silence genes, that this RNAi is specific for the gene whose sequence matches that of the injected RNA molecule, and that RNAi can

spread between cells and even be inherited. In addition, since the injection of even tiny amounts of double-stranded RNA was sufficient to achieve an effect, Fire and Mello proposed that RNAi is a catalytic process.

Fire and Mello's discovery clarified many earlier confusing and apparently contradictory experimental observations and revealed a natural mechanism for controlling the flow of genetic information. Soon after this original report, other workers found interfering RNAs in a number of different systems from worms to mammals to plants. This work opened up a whole new field of research. Workers soon discovered that RNAi can regulate gene expression in hundreds of genes in our genome and that these small RNAs play an important role in animal and plant development and the control of cellular functions. RNAi also appeared to protect the genome against transposons and viruses, and it opened up exciting possibilities for use as a therapeutic agent. In 2006, Fire and Mello received the Nobel Prize in Physiology or Medicine for their pioneering work.

FIGURE 11.3 Modifications to antisense oligonucleotides. **(A)** Phosphodiester linkage; **(B)** phosphorothioate linkage; **(C)** phosphoramidite linkage; **(D)** polyamide linkage (peptide nucleic acid); **(E)** 2'-*O*-methyl ribose; **(F)** C-5 propynylcytosine.

every 4 weeks. Before treatment with fomivirsen is started, it is essential that the presence of cytomegalovirus be absolutely confirmed, since several other infective agents produce similar symptoms.

Antisense oligonucleotides with phosphoramidate and polyamide (peptide) linkages have been synhesized in the expectation that these molecules should be very resistant to nuclease degradation (Fig. 11.3C and D). Furthermore, as mentioned above, chemical groups have been added to the 2' carbon of the sugar moiety and the 5 carbon (C-5) of pyrimidines to both enhance stability and facilitate the binding of the antisense oligonucleotide to its target site (Fig. 11.3E and F).

In one set of experiments, phosphoramidite antisense oligonucleotides were delivered by injecting muscle, followed by a short (less than a second)

electrical pulse. In this case, the antisense oligonucleotide formed highly stable duplexes with the target RNA and did not induce RNase H activity. Since only oligonucleotides targeted to the 5′ untranslated region, and not to the coding portion, of the mRNA were inhibitory, it was surmised that phosphoramidite antisense oligonucleotides prevented translation of the target mRNA.

Several preclinical trials have shown the usefulness of antisense oligonucleotides as therapeutic agents. For example, the narrowing (stenosis) of coronary and carotid arteries that leads to heart attacks and strokes, respectively, is often alleviated by angioplasty, which is a procedure that widens arteries by the insertion of an inflated balloon. However, arterial blockage recurs (restenosis) in about 40% of patients within 6 months because angioplasty induces a healing reaction, which stimulates the proliferation of smooth muscle cells and the secretion of an extracellular matrix in the inner layer of the artery at the site of the treatment. When phosphorothioate antisense oligonucleotides that targeted mRNAs for proteins that are essential for the mammalian cell cycle were applied to rat carotid arteries after angioplasty, restenosis was reduced by about 90%. In addition to postangioplasty restenosis, smooth muscle cell proliferation is implicated in atherosclerosis, hypertension, diabetes mellitus, and the failure of coronary bypass grafts. Presumably, these conditions might be controlled by similar antisense therapeutics.

In another study, a 20-nucleotide phosphorothioate antisense oligonucleotide complementary to the coding region of human apolipoprotein B was used to lower the level of low-density lipoprotein cholesterol in humans. High levels of low-density lipoprotein cholesterol have long been considered a significant risk factor for cardiovascular disease; high levels of apolipoprotein B are also likely associated with cardiovascular risk. Apolipoprotein B, which is produced in the liver, is an essential structural and receptor-binding component of all atherogenic (plaque-causing) lipoproteins. It plays a key role in low-density lipoprotein cholesterol transport and removal. Typically, statins, the most prescribed drug class in the world, are used to lower low-density lipoprotein cholesterol levels. While statins are effective for many individuals, some people continue to have high levels of both low-density lipoprotein cholesterol and apolipoprotein B. Therefore, a 20-nucleotide phosphorothioate antisense oligonucleotide complementary to the coding region of human apolipoprotein B was developed to be an adjunct to statin treatment. While this antisense oligonucleotide has been tested on only 36 individuals (Fig. 11.4), the results to date

FIGURE 11.4 Dosing regimen of an antisense oligonucleotide designed to lower low-density lipoprotein cholesterol. The entire procedure took approximately 10 weeks. The arrows below the horizonal line indicate the times when the antisense oligonucleotide was administered (subcutaneously). Doses of the antisense oligonucleotide ranged from 50 to 400 mg per injection.

Hydrophobic

Hydrophilic

FIGURE 11.5 Schematic representation of a liposome carrying a nucleic acid.

are encouraging, and there is an expectation that this approach may lead to significant reductions in adverse cardiovascular events.

Antisense oligonucleotides have been tested to determine if they can control psoriasis, a disease of uncontrolled epidermal growth that causes red scaly, itchy patches to appear on the skin. Insulin-like growth factor I has been implicated in the pathogenesis of psoriasis because insulin-like growth factor I receptors are present in excess in psoriatic lesions. Thus, antisense oligonucleotide lowering of the mRNA for insulin-like growth factor I receptor might form the basis of a psoriasis therapy. In preliminary experiments, all of the different insulin-like growth factor receptor antisense oligonucleotides tested were 15 nucleotides in length. The potential antisense oligonucleotides were transfected into keratinocytes by using liposomes to facilitate antisense oligonucleotide cellular uptake (Fig. 11.5), and then the level of insulin-like growth factor I receptor mRNA was assessed. The three most active antisense oligonucleotides reduced the insulin-like growth factor I receptor protein concentration by 45 to 65%, while a random oligonucleotide had no effect on the amount of the protein. The selected antisense oligonucleotides were tested with athymic nude mice carrying human psoriatic lesional grafts. When the grafts were injected every 2 days for 20 days with antisense oligonucleotides complementary to the insulin-like growth factor I receptor mRNA, there was a significant reduction (58 to 69%) in both epidermis thickness and the cross-sectional area of the skin lesions. This result is very encouraging and suggests that skin diseases in which a normal protein is overproduced may be appropriate targets for antisense oligonucleotides that can be delivered topically.

Antisense oligonucleotides have also been used to inhibit the synthesis of the transcription factor forkhead box O1 (also called FOXO1) in mice. This protein increases the expression of phosphoenolpyruvate carboxykinase (PEPCK) and glucose-6-phosphatase (G6Pase), both of which are key enzymes in gluconeogenesis. Antisense oligonucleotides cause a reduction in the expression of these genes (approximately 50 to 60%) in both liver and fat tissues, but not in cardiac or skeletal muscle. Thus, the introduction of antisense oligonucleotides complementary to FOXO1 mRNA essentially mimics insulin action and therefore may bypass some of the defects in insulin signaling common among diabetics. To choose the most effective antisense oligonucleotide sequence, 80 different 20-nucleotide-long sequences complementary to various portions of mouse FOXO1 mRNA were tested, using mouse primary hepatocytes in culture, for the ability to inhibit FOXO1 mRNA expression. The positive effects that were reported represent the results of studies with the most effective of the original 80 oligonucleotides. It will now be of interest to determine whether the promising results observed in mice can be extended to humans.

Aberrant splicing of an mRNA occurs when a mutation in an intron is recognized by the RNA-processing system as an authentic splice site, and consequently, a portion of the intron is included as part of the processed mRNA (Fig. 11.6A). The presence of part of an intron disrupts the reading frame, and a truncated protein is produced. As a result, a disease condition may result from a diminished level of normal protein.

It was reasoned that an antisense oligonucleotide that targeted an aberrant splice site could likely prevent splicing at that site and increase the number of joining events between the correct intron–exon splice sequences. This notion was tested with a splice mutation in the second intron of the

A

B

FIGURE 11.6 Correction of a mutant splice site with an antisense oligonucleotide. **(A)** The outcome of a mutation in a splice site is depicted. The numbers denote exons. The first intron is marked with the letter A, and the second intron contains a splice mutation (red dot) that divides the intron into two parts (B1 and B2). The dotted lines span the RNA segments that are removed during RNA processing. There are two possible splicing events: pathway a leads to a functional mRNA, and pathway b leads to an RNA that includes part of the second intron (B2). **(B)** An antisense oligonucleotide (AS) (shown as a red bar) that binds to the mutant splice site prevents RNA processing at the site, and consequently, only functional mRNA is produced.

β-globin gene (Fig. 11.6B). This mutation is responsible for one form of β-thalassemia, which is an inherited blood disorder that leads to loss of red blood cells (anemia). After cells that are homozygous for the intron 2 splice site mutation were transfected with a 2′-*O*-methyl phosphorothioate antisense oligonucleotide that targeted the mutant splice site, the number of normal β-globin chains was increased by about 50%, which theoretically would be beneficial to patients with this genetic defect. Further studies are required to determine if antisense rectification of splice site mutations is an effective therapeutic strategy for thalassemia and other conditions due to similar mutations.

It has recently been shown that it is possible to protect mice against retroviruses by injecting them, intravenously or intraperitoneally, with phosphorothioated antisense oligonucleotides that prevent the conversion of the viral RNA genome into double-stranded DNA. In this system, the added antisense oligonucleotide effectively blocks replication of the retrovirus. When an added antisense oligonucleotide binds to the junction of the polypurine tract (which is present in a broad range of different retroviruses) and the U3 element, a structure is formed which mimics the normal substrate for the virus-encoded enzyme RNase H (Fig. 11.7). This causes

FIGURE 11.7 Schematic representation of the reverse transcription of retroviral RNA (red) to produce double-stranded DNA (the minus strand is light blue, and the plus strand is dark blue). In step 1, a transfer RNA (tRNA) (shown as a blue circle) primes synthesis of the minus strand. The RNA shows U3 and U5 elements and a polypurine tract (PPT). In step 2, a complete RNA–DNA duplex is formed. In step 3, RNase H digests the viral RNA in the RNA–DNA duplex into small pieces (the arrows indicate digestion sites). In step 4, a double-stranded DNA copy of the viral RNA is produced, which can exist as a provirus integrated into a cell's DNA. To block the formation of the minus strand and hence the synthesis of a double-stranded DNA version of the virus, an antisense oligonucleotide that hybridizes to the PPT region is added.

premature cleavage of the viral RNA, resulting in the virus being destroyed before reverse transcription occurs. This strategy has been shown to be effective in protecting mice from retroviruses. In principle, it should also work in humans and on a range of different retroviruses. However, a number of technical obstacles must be overcome before this approach is ready for testing in humans.

Ribozymes

Ribozymes are naturally occurring catalytic RNA molecules (RNA metalloenzymes) that are ~40 to 50 nucleotides in length and have separate catalytic and substrate-binding domains. Compared with protein therapeutics, an important advantage of ribozymes is that they are unlikely to evoke an immune response in a treated animal or human. The substrate-binding sequence combines by nucleotide complementarity and, possibly, non-hydrogen-bond interactions with its target sequence. The catalytic portion cleaves the target RNA at a specific site. By altering the substrate-binding domain, a ribozyme can be engineered to specifically cleave any mRNA sequence (Fig. 11.8). For therapeutic purposes, either hammerhead or hairpin ribozymes—named after the appearance of their secondary structure that results from intrastrand base pairing—may be used. However, some workers have suggested that hammerhead ribozymes are preferable because of their ability to more efficiently recognize, bind to, and cleave a range of different mRNAs.

In practice, an indirect strategy is often used for creating a therapeutic ribozyme, since the large-scale production of synthetic RNA molecules is

FIGURE 11.8 Two-dimensional representation of hammerhead **(A)** and hairpin **(B)** ribozyme–mRNA substrate complexes. The mRNA substrates and ribozymes are shown in red and blue, respectively. A, adenosine; C, cytosine; G, guanosine; U, uridine; Y, a pyrimidine nucleotide (C or U); R, a purine nucleotide (A or G); H, any nucleotide except G; B, any nucleotide except A; V, any nucleotide except U; N and N', any complementary nucleotides. The arrows indicate the points of mRNA cleavage.

difficult and RNA molecules are susceptible to degradation after delivery to a target cell. One approach to overcome these drawbacks entails chemically synthesizing a double-stranded oligodeoxyribonucleotide with a ribozyme catalytic domain (~20 nucleotides) flanked by sequences that hybridize to the target mRNA after it is transcribed. The double-stranded form of the ribozyme oligodeoxyribonucleotide is cloned into a eukaryotic expression vector (usually a retrovirus). Cells are transfected with the construct, and the transcribed ribozyme cleaves the target mRNA, thereby suppressing the translation of the protein that is responsible for a disorder. Since most of the vectors that have been used cannot infect nondividing cells, target cells may be removed from a patient and then grown and transfected in culture before they are returned to the original tissue.

As an alternative to intracellular ribozyme production, ribozymes may be delivered directly to cells by injection or with liposomes, i.e., endogenous delivery. Directly delivered ribozymes may be chemically modified to protect them from rapid breakdown by nucleases. For example, the 2 hydroxyl groups may be modified by alkylation or by substitution with either an amino group or a fluorine atom. These modifications increase the half-life of ribozymes in serum from minutes to days.

Under laboratory conditions, ribozymes can inhibit the expression of a variety of viral genes and significantly inhibit the proliferation of numerous organisms. For example, in cell culture, ribozymes inhibit the expression of (1) human cytomegalovirus transcriptional regulatory proteins, resulting in a 150-fold decrease in viral growth; (2) human herpes simplex virus type 1 transcriptional activator, resulting in a reduction of around 1,000-fold in viral growth; and (3) a reovirus mRNA encoding a protein required for viral proliferation. Moreover, a hammerhead ribozyme was designed to

treat collagen-induced arthritis in mice. A plasmid-encoded ribozyme directed against the mRNA for tumor necrosis factor alpha, which is involved in rheumatoid arthritis, was intravenously injected into affected mice. Following this treatment, there was a significant reduction in the level of the tumor necrosis factor alpha mRNA, as well as a decrease in the collagen-induced arthritis. This type of ribozyme, used so far only with mice, has the potential to become a human therapeutic agent.

The development of resistance in humans to various chemical treatments is a persistent problem for the pharmaceutical industry. Generally, a single mutation that alters the target site is sufficient to void the action of a drug. However, with appropriate ribozyme-based therapeutics, ribozymes for a number of different sites could be used simultaneously, thereby cleaving an mRNA at different sites. The ability to cleave multiple sites on a single viral gene should make it less likely that any single viral mutation will confer resistance.

Deoxyribozymes

To date, no naturally occurring DNA equivalent of ribozymes, i.e., DNA enzymes (deoxyribozymes), has been discovered. However, oligodeoxynucleotides with catalytic activity have been synthesized. The best characterized and most studied of these deoxyribozymes is 10-23 RNase (Fig. 11.9). As a therapeutic agent, a catalytic oligodeoxynucleotide has some advantages over a ribozyme. DNA is approximately 1,000-fold more stable against hydrolytic destruction than protein and is nearly 100,000-fold more stable than RNA. In addition, deoxyribozymes are more efficient at binding and cutting mRNAs than are ribozymes. However, a deoxyribozyme cannot be produced continuously after the vector that encodes it is introduced into a particular tissue, because only ribozymes are produced from the DNA sequence. Therefore, deoxyribozymes must be delivered directly to affected cells. Proof-of-principle experiments have shown that deoxyribonucleotides are effective with cells in culture. For example, deoxyribozymes have been used to cleave mRNA transcribed from the growth-stimulating gene *myc*, which limits the growth of leukemia cells in culture. A deoxyribozyme has also been used to prevent mRNA from a gene called *Egr-1* from being expressed. Production of this mRNA is one reason for the failure of angioplasty—a procedure in which a balloon at the end of a catheter is used to

FIGURE 11.9 Two-dimensional representation of deoxyribozyme 10-23 RNase–mRNA substrate complex. The mRNA substrate and deoxyribozyme are shown in red and blue, respectively. A, adenosine; C, cytosine; G, guanosine; U, uridine; Y, a pyrimidine nucleotide (C or U); R, a purine nucleotide (A or G); N and N', any complementary nucleotides. The arrow indicates the point of mRNA cleavage.

unclog arteries that contain atherosclerotic plaques. When the *Egr-1* mRNA is expressed, the recently unclogged artery is rapidly closed.

Chimeric RNA–DNA Molecules

The ability to convert a mutant base pair of a gene to the wild-type (normal, or correct) version would reverse the consequences of many different genetic conditions. A strategy using a modified RNA–DNA oligonucleotide with 68 nucleotides (chimeric oligonucleotide) has been devised for this purpose. The composition of the chimeric oligonucleotide includes a single mixed oligonucleotide with ribonucleotides and deoxyribonucleotides in a duplex conformation with hairpin caps at the ends of the complementary segments and methylation of the oxygen of the 2′ carbon of the ribose sugars (Fig. 11.10). The rationale for this particular arrangement is based on various experimental observations. First, combined RNA–DNA molecules participate more readily than duplex DNA in homologous nucleic acid pairing reactions. Second, hairpin caps, which do not interfere with the pairing of homologous nucleic acid molecules, protect the molecule from exonucleases. Third, the 2′-O methylation of the ribose units shields the molecule from degradation by RNase H. In addition, the organization of the nucleotides of a chimeric oligonucleotide is important. Ten ribonucleotides flank a central core of five deoxyribonucleotides, and except for the correct base pair, this segment of the chimeric oligonucleotide has the same sequence as the target.

In cell culture, the feasibility of base pair correction with a chimeric oligonucleotide was examined with both a mutated cDNA sequence carried by a plasmid and a mutant site within a chromosomal sequence. In both instances, with high frequencies, the mutant sites were replaced by the correct base pair. However, more studies are required before chimeric oligonucleotides will become effective therapeutic agents.

Aptamers

Aptamers are nucleic acid sequences, RNA or DNA, that bind tightly to proteins, amino acids, drugs, or other molecules. They are typically 15 to 40

FIGURE 11.10 Correction of a single-base-pair mutation by a chimeric oligonucleotide. The double arrow points to the mutant site in the target sequence and the correct base pair in the chimeric oligonucleotide. The mutant and correct nucleotides are underlined. The uppercase letters represent deoxyribonucleotides, and the lowercase letters represent ribonucleotides. The nucleotides of the hairpin caps are shown in red. The vertical line and the 3′ and 5′ designations mark the 3′ and 5′ ends of the chimeric oligonucleotide. Adapted from Yoon et al., *Proc. Natl. Acad. Sci. USA* **93**:2071–2076, 1996.

FIGURE 11.11 Overview of the SELEX procedure for selecting aptamers with high affinity to a target molecule (often a protein). The selected aptamers are typically cycled through this procedure 5 to 15 times.

nucleotides long, have highly organized secondary and tertiary structures, and bind with high affinity ($10^{-12} < K_d < 10^{-9}$, where K_d is the dissociation constant) to their target molecules. Aptamers are attractive as potential therapeutic agents because of their high specificity, relative ease of production, low or no immunogenicity, and long-term stability.

Aptamers that are directed against specific targets are typically selected by a procedure known as SELEX (*s*ystematic *e*volution of *l*igands by *exp*onential enrichment), in which DNA or RNA ligands that bind to the target molecule are selectively enriched (Fig. 11.11). In this procedure, a random DNA sequence is cloned between two particular DNA sequences. The 3' region contains an attachment site for reverse transcriptase primers, and the 5' region contains an attachment site for a polymerase chain reaction (PCR) primer. The double-stranded DNA is converted to RNA using T7 RNA polymerase. The SELEX procedure combines several rounds of binding, partitioning, and amplification of selected nucleotide sequences from an initial pool of up to 10^{16} nucleotide sequence variants. The end

TABLE 11.1 Some proteins against which aptamers have been generated and the affinities of the aptamers for the proteins

Protein	K_d (nM)
Keratinocyte growth factor	0.0003
HIV type 1 reverse transcriptase	0.02
Transforming growth factor β1	0.03
P-Selectin	0.04
VEGF receptor	0.05
Platelet-derived growth factor	0.09
Immunoglobulin E	0.1
Extracellular signal-regulated kinase	0.2
CD4 antigen	0.5
HIV type 1 RNase H	0.5
Factor IXa	0.58
Angiogenin	0.7
Complement factor 5	1.0
Transforming growth factor β2	1.0
Secretory phospholipase A2	2.0
Thrombin	2.0
Angiopoietin 2	2.2
γ-Interferon	2.7
L-Selectin	3.0
Human neutrophil elastase	5.0
Tenascin C	5.0
Integrin	8.0
Hepatitis C virus NS3 protease	10.0
Factor VIIa	11.0
Yersinia pestis tyrosine phosphatase	18.0
Anti-insulin receptor antibody MA20	30.0
Trypanosoma cruzi cell adhesion receptor	172.0

result of this procedure is the selection of aptamers that bind to the target molecule with high affinity. Ultimately, the SELEX procedure yields one (or just a few) unique nucleic acid sequence(s) from the original mixture with high affinity for the target molecule. To make aptamers less sensitive to nuclease digestion, OH residues at the 2′ positions of purines may be replaced with 2′-O-methyl residues. In addition, aptamers may be capped at their 3′ end with a deoxythymidine residue. Table 11.1 lists some of the proteins against which aptamers have been generated, as well as the range of affinities of the aptamer for the target protein.

An aptamer known as pegaptanib received approval from the U.S. FDA in December of 2004 for use as a human therapeutic agent. Pegaptanib is a 30-nucleotide-long aptamer that targets vascular endothelial growth factor (VEGF) and binds to the protein with extremely high affinity ($K_d = 0.05$ nM). This secreted protein promotes the growth of new blood vessels by stimulating the endothelial cells that not only form the walls of the blood vessels, but also transport nutrients and oxygen to the tissues. When retinal pigment epithelial cells begin to senesce from lack of nutrition (ischemia), VEGF acts to stimulate the synthesis of new blood vessels (neovascularization).

Receptor-binding domain

Heparin-binding domain

FIGURE 11.12 Schematic representation of protein VEGF, which contains both a receptor-binding domain and a heparin-binding domain.

However, this process is imperfect, and often the blood vessels do not form properly so that leakage results, causing scarring in the macular region of the retina with the eventual loss of central vision. These physiological changes contribute to age-related macular degeneration, a leading cause of blindness. Pegaptanib was selected to bind to one of the four isoforms of VEGF (VEGF$_{165}$) that is responsible for age-related macular degeneration. The drug is injected directly into the eye every 6 weeks, or about nine times a year. All four forms of VEGF have a receptor-binding domain (Fig. 11.12), while only VEGF$_{165}$ has a heparin-binding domain, which is the specific target for pegaptanib. Pegaptanib is a new type of therapeutic agent with an unusual specificity that can effectively suppress age-related macular degeneration—to date, approximately 95% of the patients receiving pegaptanib were 65 years of age or older.

The safety of aptamers used in clinical trials is a concern, especially when the optimal dose of a particular aptamer is not known. One way to overcome this problem is through the use of aptamer "antidotes." These molecules consist of short oligonucleotides whose sequences are complementary to the aptamers being tested. When antidotes are added to aptamers, they hybridize to the aptamers and inhibit their binding to the clinical target.

Interfering RNAs

Principles

The addition of double-stranded RNA to animal and plant cells reduces the expression of the gene from which the double-stranded RNA sequence is derived. This "gene silencing," which specifically reduces the concentration of a target mRNA by up to 90%, is reversible, since there is no change in the target cells' DNA. This phenomenon has been termed RNA interference (or "RNAi") and occurs naturally in virtually all eukaryotic organisms. RNAi appears to be the same phenomenon as gene silencing in animals or cosuppression in plants. Although all of its biological roles remain to be established, RNAi may protect both animals and plants from viruses and from the accumulation of transposons. A working model for RNAi has been formulated based on experimental analyses (Fig. 11.13). Following the introduction of a double-stranded RNA molecule into a cell, the double-stranded RNA is cleaved by the RNase III-like enzyme Dicer into single-stranded pieces of RNA, approximately 21 to 23 nucleotides in length, that have been called small interfering RNAs (siRNAs). The antisense strand of an siRNA is incorporated into an RNA-induced silencing complex (RISC) that binds to and then cleaves the mRNA. The specific binding of the siRNA to the mRNA that occurs is based on the complementarity of the two RNA sequences. The site of cleavage of the targeted mRNA is between nucleotides 10 and 11 relative to the 5' end of the siRNA (antisense) guide strand. Consistent with this model, the transfection of mammalian cells in culture with duplexes of 21-nucleotide RNA can also mediate RNAi.

Despite the fact that many aspects of RNAi are still not completely understood, it could form the basis for new therapeutic agents. The use of short RNA duplexes may eventually provide an alternative approach to the use of antisense oligonucleotides or ribozymes.

The phenomenon of RNAi is expected to facilitate the development of a wide range of antiviral compounds and therapies utilizing specific siRNAs delivered to the appropriate target cell. Similarly, the expression of endogenous eukaryotic genes may be inhibited by plasmid-driven expression of short hairpin RNAs (shRNAs), which are similar in structure to the microRNAs that often normally regulate gene expression in eukaryotic cells. In fact, there are a number of reports of the use of either siRNA or shRNA to suppress virus replication in tissue culture (Table 11.2). Moreover, it has been successfully demonstrated that RNAi is effective in vivo (with mice), suggesting that, in principle, all viruses may be inactivated by RNAi.

Independently of how an siRNA or shRNA is introduced into a cell, it may have nonspecific effects. For example, introduction of these molecules may inadvertently activate innate cellular immune responses, such as the interferon response. In addition, siRNA or shRNA may also be complementary to nontarget mRNAs. However, several experimental approaches may be utilized to avoid these problems. (1) Off-target effects are most often observed when the siRNA or shRNA concentration is ≥100 nM. By lowering the concentration as much as possible (often to 20 nM or less), off-target

FIGURE 11.13 Overview of the process of RNA interference. Following introduction of double-stranded RNA (dsRNA) into a cell, the Dicer complex binds to the RNA and cleaves it into an siRNA containing approximately 21 bp. The antisense strand (red) becomes part of the RISC, directing the cleavage of the complementary mRNA.

TABLE 11.2 Some examples of suppression of viral replication in tissue culture by RNAi

Severe acute respiratory syndrome-associated coronavirus

Hepatitis C virus

West Nile virus

Coxsackievirus B3

Foot-and-mouth disease virus

Hepatitis A virus

Human rhinovirus 6

Poliovirus

Respiratory syncytial virus

Human parainfluenza virus 3

Vesicular stomatitis virus

Influenza virus

Hepatitis delta virus

Rotavirus

HIV type 1

Hepatitis B virus

Herpes simplex virus type 1

Human cytomegalovirus

Epstein-Barr virus

Human herpesvirus 6B

Murine herpesvirus 68

Human papillomavirus type 18

JC virus

effects are often avoided. (2) Since the interferon response can be induced by double-stranded RNAs with as few as 11 bp that are perfectly complementary, siRNA or shRNA is designed to contain at least a 1-nucleotide bulge (where the bases on opposing strands are noncomplementary) near the center of the molecule (typically around 21 bp). (3) Since siRNA or shRNA can exert a toxic effect when it contains the sequence 5′-UGGC-3′, this sequence should be avoided. (4) Blunt-ended 27-bp RNA duplexes or 29-bp shRNAs with 2 nucleotides overhanging at the 3′ end are much more potent inducers of RNAi than 21-mer siRNAs. The greater level of effectiveness of the slightly longer RNAs may reflect the fact that they are first bound and cleaved by Dicer, which facilitates their entry into the RISC. Using these slightly longer RNAs at low concentrations should avoid side reactions associated with 21-mer siRNAs.

Unlike siRNAs, shRNAs are expressed in vivo as part of a genetic construct that includes a promoter sequence. This means that shRNAs need to be introduced by using strategies different than those used with siRNAs. Thus, shRNAs are typically delivered to their target cells by using viral vectors. Viral vectors that integrate into the chromosomal DNA are generally used when persistent long-term knockdown of gene expression is desired; the most popular choice is lentiviruses. However, with the use of all virus-based vectors, there are serious safety concerns that need to be addressed, and the type of promoter that is used also needs to be optimized.

Applications

Interfering RNAs have already found widespread use as tools in research that is directed toward understanding how gene expression is regulated in natural systems. One company that specializes in producing RNAi directed against human mRNAs advertises, "For each target (human) gene, we provide four plasmids each with a different short hairpin RNAi sequence (shRNA). Our experimentally verified design algorithm minimizes the risk of off target effects and ensures the maximum knock-down. At least one of the four shRNA plasmids will reduce the target mRNA levels in the transfected cells by >70%." With the ready availability of human shRNA libraries, new insights and understanding of many fundamental and disease processes should be rapidly forthcoming. It is hoped that this in turn will lead to a variety of new therapeutic agents and approaches.

In addition to the many reports of successful modification of the gene expression of cells in culture with RNAi, there are an increasing number of reports of the in vivo effectiveness of RNAi. By 2008, siRNAs against a wide range of proteins, viruses, and diseases had been successfully expressed in mice, including siRNAs directed against herpes simplex virus type 2, hepatitis B virus, hepatitis C virus, Huntington disease, metastatic Ewing sarcoma (a form of cancer), respiratory syncytial virus, hepatic cancer, transforming growth factor receptor 2, severe acute respiratory syndrome, heme oxygenase 1, keratinocyte-derived chemokine, tumor necrosis factor alpha, and human epidermal growth factor receptor 2. In addition, in 2008, three different RNAi therapeutics were being tested in clinical trials. All three of these therapeutics target VEGF or its receptor, a cause of age-related macular degeneration (see "Aptamers" above), and at that time, all had successfully completed either phase I or phase II clinical trials.

A

B

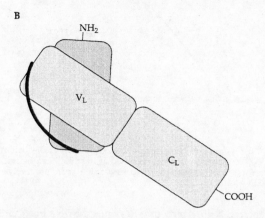

FIGURE 11.14 **(A)** DNA construct of a single-chain antibody against the hemorrhagic septicemia virus G protein. P_{CMV}, cytomegalovirus promoter; TGF, rainbow trout transforming growth factor beta signal peptide; V_H, variable domain from mouse hybridoma heavy chain; spacer, 42 nucleotides encoding a 14-amino-acid spacer connecting V_H and V_L; V_L, variable domain from mouse hybridoma light chain; C_L, constant part of the human light chain gene. **(B)** Schematic representation of the single-chain antibody against the hemorrhagic septicemia virus G protein. The curved black line represents the 14-amino-acid spacer.

Antibody Genes

A major problem with aquaculture is the loss of fish due to bacterial and viral infections. The chemical treatments that protect fish against these disease-causing pathogens are extremely costly and not particularly effective. One way to address this problem is to develop fish that synthesize protective antibodies against particular pathogens. The impetus for this approach came from the observation that rainbow trout could be protected against hemorrhagic septicemia virus by passive immunization through the injection of a monoclonal antibody against the G protein from the virus. Subsequently, a gene encoding a single-chain antibody directed against the hemorrhagic septicemia virus G protein was synthesized. The synthetic gene encoded variable regions from the mouse L and H chains of an anti-G protein monoclonal antibody with a human antibody constant domain fused to the 3′ end of the construct (Fig. 11.14). To mediate secretion in fish cells, the DNA was fused to the gene sequence encoding the signal sequence of rainbow trout transforming growth factor beta. The DNA construct was inserted into a eukaryotic expression vector under the transcriptional control of a constitutive cytomegalovirus promoter. The cloned gene–vector construct was injected into the circulatory system of rainbow trout. When the fish were challenged with the hemorrhagic septicemia virus 11 days after injection of the DNA construct, nearly all of them survived, whereas

FIGURE 11.15 Survival of fish exposed to hemorrhagic septicemia virus 11 days after being injected with DNA encoding an antibody directed against the hemorrhagic septicemia virus G protein (+DNA) compared with control fish that did not receive this DNA construct (–DNA).

the control fish did not (Fig. 11.15). Thirty-nine days after the DNA injection, the plasma concentration of the single-chain antibody remained at a high level. Thus, instead of administering a purified antibody to provide an animal with passive immunity, it is possible to inject an animal with DNA encoding the antibody. Giving an animal the ability to synthesize a specific antibody may be more efficient than depending upon the animal's immune system to produce a similar antibody. However, since it may not be practical to inject large numbers of fish, the next step will be to create transgenic fish with antibody genes that confer passive immunity to various diseases.

Nucleic Acid Delivery

The ultimate effectiveness of any therapeutic agent depends upon the ability to deliver that agent to the tissues where it is required. Systemic introduction of a therapeutic agent often leads to the accumulation of very high levels in tissues where the agent is not required and sometimes results in serious side effects. To this end, viral vectors that deliver small nucleic acids to specific cellular targets have been developed. However, although virus-based gene delivery has been successful, a number of safety concerns have arisen in regard to the use of these vectors. Several approaches have recently been developed as an alternative to virus-based systems, as well as to the systemic introduction of target nucleic acids. There are several methods that have been used to deliver relatively small nucleic acids to animal cells. They include (1) intravenous injection; (2) local injection at the site of the pathology; (3) packaging into cationic liposomes (Fig. 11.5); (4) physical methods, like electroporation, sonoporation, or hydrodynamic pressure; and (5) a number of systems in which the nucleic acid is chemically conjugated to another molecule.

Human Gene Therapy

Most of the experience of managing genetic diseases has been gathered from inherited inborn errors of metabolism and, to a lesser extent, from

disorders with defective structural proteins. The strategies for treating genetic disorders include restrictive or supplemented diets, inhibition of enzyme reactions to prevent the accumulation of toxic molecules, removal of toxic molecules, replacement of defective or absent proteins, restoration of protein activity, selective protein removal, organ and bone marrow transplantation, and nucleic acid-based therapies (Table 11.3).

With the development of recombinant DNA technology, large numbers of enzymes and structural proteins are now available for therapeutic use. Infusions of β-glucosidase, β-galactosidase, α-L-iduronidase, and adenosine deaminase (ADA) in clinical trials have significantly reduced the adverse effects of Gaucher disease, Fabry disease, mucopolysaccharidosis I, and severe combined immunodeficiency disorder (SCID), respectively. This type of treatment, called enzyme replacement therapy, works well when either the enzyme or the structural protein (protein replacement therapy) is delivered to its biological site of action through the bloodstream.

Since the 1940s, when it was discovered that a gene from one strain of bacteria could be transferred to and expressed in another strain, researchers have contemplated the possibility that human genetic diseases might be cured in an analogous manner. Introduction of a normal gene into a cell with a defective gene ought to correct the disorder because the transferred

TABLE 11.3 Strategies for treating genetic disorders

Specially formulated diets
 Restrictive diet to lower the intracellular level of a toxic
 molecule
 Supplemented diet to replace a metabolic deficiency
Inhibition of enzyme reactions
 Enzyme inhibitor to prevent the accumulation of a toxic
 molecule by blocking a step in a metabolic pathway
 that precedes the reaction with a defective enzyme
Removal of toxic molecules
 Dialysis
 Removal of excess cations (chelation)
 Facilitation of excretion by binding a toxic molecule to a
 low-molecular-weight compound
Replacement of defective or missing product
 Enzyme replacement therapy
 Protein replacement therapy
 Cofactor supplementation
Alteration of defective protein by small molecules
 Restoration of partial protein function
 Directed proteolytic degradation of defective protein
Transplantation
 Replacement of a nonfunctional organ transplantation
 Providing a required protein synthesized by blood cells
 (bone marrow transplantation)
Gene therapy
 Rectification of a genetic defect with a functional gene
Nucleic acid therapy
 Blocking translation of mRNA from a mutant gene with
 an oligonucleotide (antisense, ribozyme)
 Correction of a gene mutation with an oligonucleotide

gene provides the required gene product. In theory, gene therapy should provide a persistent in vivo treatment, either in the tissue that is primarily affected by a gene mutation or in deficient cells that acquire a recombinant protein from distant cells that release the therapeutic protein into the circulatory system. Although gene therapy was intended as a cure for genetic disorders, gene products can also be used to treat cancers, infections, and various degenerative disorders.

In 1990, after exhaustive reviews by many different regulating panels in the United States, the first human gene therapy trial was initiated. Two young girls with ADA-deficient SCID received large doses of their own cells that had been engineered to carry a functional *ADA* gene. In both instances, the adverse symptoms were alleviated, indicating that this form of therapy is feasible. One of the patients has been free of SCID for more than 10 years, although she was regularly administered polyethylene glycol–ADA. The second ADA-deficient patient from the original trial and others from additional experiments have not had long-lasting cures. After the initial trials with gene therapy for ADA, a number of gene-based clinical protocols for various conditions were conducted. Unfortunately, these trials failed to establish the effectiveness of any of the treatments. Notwithstanding this lack of success, the trials provided a great deal of information about the methods of gene delivery, the duration of gene expression, and other technical features of gene therapy. Generally, despite the failure to correct a genetic disorder with an exogenous functional gene, this type of clinical research was considered safe. However, in September 1999, the attitude toward gene therapy dramatically changed. Jesse Gelsinger, a healthy 18-year-old with ornithine transcarbamylase deficiency, was given a large dose of a virus carrying the *OTC* gene as part of a clinical trial. Tragically, he died 4 days later of a massive immune response. In another trial, injection of a gene into the heart muscle of a patient with severe coronary artery disease was fatal. As a consequence, although these disastrous outcomes were not predictable, the rigorous requirements for human gene therapy experiments became even more stringent. Researchers, in addition, became disinclined to initiate new trials. However, in 2000, two infants with an X-linked form of SCID (SCID-X1) were successfully treated with the gene encoding the subunit (γc) that is part of various cytokine receptors. These patients were free of symptoms for 10 months and are being monitored to determine if the correction is permanent; of the 11 patients, 4 developed cancer. Also, hemophilic patients expressed an input gene encoding the blood coagulation factor IX for long periods and, importantly, enough of the protein was produced to reduce the extent of the condition from severe to mild.

Although in the broadest sense, the concept of human somatic cell gene therapy is straightforward, there are a number of critical biological considerations. For example, how will the cells that are to be targeted for correction be accessed? How will the therapeutic (remedial) gene be delivered? What proportion of the target cells must acquire the input gene to counteract the disease? Does transcription of the input gene need to be precisely regulated to be effective? Will overexpression of the input gene cause alternative physiological problems? Will the cells with the input gene be maintained indefinitely, or will repeated treatments be required?

Much of the research effort in human gene therapy has been directed to developing efficient and nonimmunogenic systems that deliver a therapeutic gene to a specified cell type. Both viral and nonviral strategies have

been examined in detail. Different types of viruses, including retroviruses, adenovirus, adeno-associated virus, herpes simplex virus, and vaccinia virus, have been engineered as gene transfer vectors. A virus-mediated gene delivery system uses the cell receptor recognition system of the virus for binding to a specific cell type, which is followed by the internalization of the vector DNA and its transport to the cell nucleus. Some viruses have mechanisms for integration of the vector DNA into a chromosome site, and with others, the input DNA is maintained as an extrachromosomal element. Since high efficiency of vector DNA transfer is important, the administered sample of viruses should contain mostly vector viruses with very few, and preferably no, infectious virus particles. To meet this goal, packaging cell lines were constructed for some virus vectors. These cultured cells carry genes that express viral proteins that are necessary for the formation of virus particles but are not capable of producing replication-competent (infectious) viruses. After transfection of a packaging cell line with a vector construct that is equivalent to the length of the wild-type virus genome and that carries the appropriate DNA sequence for packaging into a virus particle, the input DNA is replicated, assembled into viruses, and released into the cell medium. The noninfectious vector viruses are concentrated and prepared for use. Packaging cell lines have been devised for retrovirus vectors (Fig. 11.16) and other viral delivery systems. In some cases, disarmed viral and vector DNAs are cotransfected and only viruses with vector DNA are produced. In other instances, protocols allow the formation of both vector and infectious viruses with the separation of the two types of viruses before use. There are advantages and disadvantages to each of the major viral gene delivery systems. Some vector viruses transduce DNA at high efficiencies but the size of the insert is limited. Retrovirus vectors infect only dividing cells, which, without genetic modification, makes them ineligible for treating disorders of nondividing cells. Some viruses lack cell specificity. However, this particular shortcoming has been countered by designing viruses with cell-specific receptor-binding sites. Many vector viruses are immunogenic, which nullifies repeated treatment with the same viral strain. To overcome this problem, vector viruses with different antigenic determinants may be used for successive treatments. Currently, third- and fourth-generation varieties of vector viruses are being developed with distinctive features for specific illnesses.

Some successful gene therapy experiments using viral vectors have been reported. In phase I clinical trials, a small number of patients have been treated with a recombinant adeno-associated virus vector carrying a human cDNA encoding retinal-pigment epithelium-specific 65-kDa protein (RPE65). The protein encoded by the *RPE65* gene is an important part of the visual cycle, forming part of a pathway that regenerates the visual pigment after exposure to light. Individuals who lack this protein become deficient in 11-*cis* retinal, and their rod photoreceptors are unable to respond to light, eventually leading to blindness. Prior to undertaking these experiments, a strain of Baird dogs with a spontaneous defect in the *RPE65* gene was successfully treated, with a restoration of visual function in the treated dogs. In all instances, the recombinant viral vector carrying the restorative gene was introduced by surgery of the eye into the subretinal space. Although the phase I human experiments were aimed only at determining the safety of this treatment, an improvement in the vision of four of the six patients was observed. This encouraging result notwithstanding, a longer follow-up

FIGURE 11.16 Production of packaged retrovirus vector RNA. The packaging cell line has two separate retroviral gene regions on its chromosomes; one contains the *gag* gene, and the other contains the *pol* and *env* genes. In each of these inserts, transcription is driven by sequences within the 5′ long terminal repeat (5′-LTR) region. Both virus DNA segments lack the encapsidation sequence (ψ⁺) that is required for packaging a retroviral genome into a viral capsid. The packaging cell line synthesizes viral proteins, but because there is no encapsidation sequence within either of the retroviral mRNAs, empty viral capsids are produced. The viral proteins continue to be synthesized after the transfection of a packaging cell line with a full-length retroviral vector carrying a remedial (therapeutic) gene (Gene X) and a selectable marker gene (Neo'). The full-length RNAs from the retrovirus vector sequence are replicated, and because they have an encapsidation region (ψ⁺), they are packaged into viral capsids. The released viral particles are replication defective because they do not have a *pol* gene.

period and clinical trials with many more subjects are required before this procedure can gain FDA approval. However, on the positive side, if the procedure is used to treat younger patients with less severe disease, greater improvements of visual function might be expected.

Notwithstanding the advantages of viral vectors, they are often immunogenic, costly to maintain, and difficult to produce on a large scale without high-level expertise. Consequently, various nonviral gene transfer systems have been devised. The least complicated nonviral gene delivery system is the introduction of pure (naked) DNA constructs directly into the cells of a target tissue. When plasmid DNA was injected into mouse skeletal muscle, some of the cells took up the DNA and a reporter gene was expressed for more than 50 days. However, this approach is limited to accessible tissues and requires large amounts of DNA. Pure DNA constructs that cover the surfaces of 1- to 3-μm-diameter gold particles have been propelled with a gene gun into skin cells (see chapter 18) and into subcutaneous tumor cells. Therapeutic genes delivered in this way were expressed in the targeted tissues. Surrounding a DNA construct with artificial lipid layers that form a lipid sphere with an aqueous core (liposome) facilitates the passage of the DNA through a cell membrane.

To avoid degradation of introduced DNA, DNA–molecular conjugates have been developed. With this approach, poly-L-lysine is chemically linked (conjugated) to a molecule that binds to a specific cell receptor. Next, DNA is added and combines with the poly-L-lysine to form a tightly compacted, twisted, solid ring. With the cell receptor-binding sites arrayed on the outside of the DNA–molecular conjugate, the complexes bound exclusively to the specified cells, but the frequency of transfection was low. To remedy this problem, in addition to a cell receptor-binding amino acid sequence, other short amino acid sequences that facilitate cell membrane fusion and internalization of the DNA–molecular conjugate and both protect the DNA from degradation and direct it to the cell nucleus have been combined into a single polypeptide. The addition of such a multifunctional protein to a DNA–molecular conjugate (Fig. 11.17) could enhance the efficiency of transfection. The current nonviral gene delivery systems have two major limitations: (1) the frequency of transfection is often too low to create a therapeutic effect and (2) the duration of therapeutic gene expression is too brief to provide an effective treatment.

A human artificial chromosome (HAC) would be an exciting therapeutic vector. The DNA-carrying capacity would be very large, which would allow the inclusion of several genes, each with a complete set of regulatory elements. This type of vector should have long-term stability and sustained expression of a therapeutic gene(s) within either a proliferating or a quiescent target cell. HACs (also called human engineered chromosomes) have been created in two ways (Fig. 11.18). First, HACs were assembled by ligation of individual chromosome components, including the chromosome ends (telomeres), centromere, and origins of replication. Telomere and centromere sequences were mixed with high-molecular-weight human DNA that had both origins of replication and a selectable gene marker in the presence of ligase. Cells were transfected with the DNA from the ligation mixture, and those with HACs were selected and maintained. A second method of forming a HAC entails paring down an existing human chromosome by deleting material from within each chromosome arm to form a "minichromosome." HACs have been formed that range in size from 0.7 to 400 megabases. However, before HACs are used for gene

Multifunctional protein Therapeutic gene

DNA–molecular conjugate

FIGURE 11.17 Schematic representation of a DNA–molecular conjugate delivery system. Short peptide sequences (motifs) that facilitate cell-specific binding (red), fusion with the cell membrane and internalization (yellow), protection of the DNA by preventing it from being routed to a lysosome (orange), and entry into the nucleus (dark blue) are attached to poly-L-lysine (light blue). The poly-L-lysine component combines with the DNA containing a therapeutic gene to form a condensed DNA–polylysine ring (medium blue) with the protein motifs facing outward.

therapy, certain issues must be addressed. For example, will HACs be efficiently introduced into the nuclei of target cells? Will effective levels of therapeutic gene expression be maintained for extended periods of time?

Before therapeutic genes are introduced in human beings, the efficacy of using a particular gene along with a specific delivery system is tested on small animals, typically mice. This is intended to ensure not only that the added gene relieves a particular ailment, but also that there are no unexpected side effects that occur as a consequence of the treatment. Recently, researchers reported the administration of a gene to dystrophic and normal mice that helped them to increase both muscle biomass and strength. The growth factor myostatin plays a critical role in regulating skeletal muscle mass. It negatively regulates both the number of myofibers formed in development and the postnatal growth of muscles. It was previously suggested that a number of neuromuscular disorders, including muscular dystrophies and age-related muscle disorders, might be "treated" using gene therapy approaches that prevent or lessen the inhibition of muscle growth by myostatin (Fig. 11.19). This could be achieved by the knockout of myostatin gene expression or by the overexpression of insulin-like growth factor 1, which can increase muscle size and strength. To this end, transgenic mice were created, from both dystrophic and normal mice, by a single postnatal intramuscular injection of adeno-associated virus that resulted in the overexpression of a gene encoding the myostatin inhibitor protein follistatin (Fig. 11.19). This single treatment enhanced muscle mass and strength in normal and dystrophic mice for

FIGURE 11.18 Construction of human artificial chromosomes (HACs). **(A)** Formation of a HAC in vitro by ligation. Chromosome elements (telomere [red] and centromere [blue]) and high-molecular-weight human DNA (green) that has origins of replication and a selectable marker gene (green rectangle) are placed in a ligation reaction mixture. After ligation, the DNA is introduced into cells in culture, and the selectable marker system is used to identify the cells with a functional HAC. The ligation products that do not form a complete chromosome are not maintained through successive cell divisions. **(B)** Formation of a HAC by truncation of a chromosome in situ. The square brackets denote DNA sections that are removed from the chromosome arms to produce a truncated chromosome (minichromosome). Chromosome DNA can be deleted by radiation of human cells and recovered as a minichromosome in a cell hybrid after fusion of rodent and irradiated human cells.

more than 2 years. This therapeutic strategy warrants serious consideration for clinical trials in the treatment of human muscle diseases. One potential concern, other than the safety of the viral vector, is that gene therapy approaches that are intended to treat muscle diseases by increasing muscle mass and strength might also be used for "gene doping" of healthy individuals to enhance athletic performance.

Targeting Systems

Lipids. While the effectiveness of siRNAs for specifically inhibiting gene expression in cultured cells has been demonstrated on numerous occasions, it is difficult to efficiently deliver these RNAs to tissues in vivo. One approach to overcome this difficulty has been to chemically couple an siRNA (at the terminal hydroxyl group of the sense strand RNA) to cholesterol (Fig. 11.20). The siRNA in question is complementary to an mRNA that encodes apolipoprotein B, a molecule involved in the metabolism of

A

B

FIGURE 11.19 Schematic representation of the regulation of muscle growth and development by myostatin in nontransgenic mice (**A**) and in transgenic mice (**B**) that overexpress the protein follistatin.

cholesterol. When the siRNA–cholesterol complex is intravenously injected into mice, it is taken up by the liver, jejunum (part of the small intestine), heart, kidney, lungs, and fat tissue cells. Once this complex is inside the tissue, the sense strand is destroyed and the antisense strand binds to the target mRNA.

With this approach, the level of apolipoprotein B was reduced by more than 50% in the liver and by 70% in the jejunum. This resulted in a significant decrease in the plasma apolipoprotein B level, as well as the total amount of cholesterol. This strategy is an important first step in the development of a method to therapeutically lower cholesterol levels in humans.

A number of other molecules, including some long-chain fatty acids and bile acids, may be used in place of cholesterol to mediate the uptake of siRNAs into cells. A critical factor in mediating the interaction between fatty acid-conjugated siRNAs and lipoprotein particles is the length of the fatty acid alkyl chain. Thus, docosanyl (C_{22}) and stearoyl (C_{18}) conjugates bind more tightly to high-density lipoprotein and subsequently silence gene expression more effectively in vivo than lauroyl (C_{12}) and myristoyl (C_{14}) conjugates. Studies are under way to improve the delivery of lipid-conjugated siRNAs to treat a wide range of diseases.

Bacteria. Bacteria that are normally found in association with various mammalian tissues and cells may be genetically engineered to produce therapeutic shRNAs. The engineered bacteria may then be used as vectors to deliver the therapeutic agent directly to the affected tissues. For example, a nonpathogenic strain of *Escherichia coli* was transformed with the plasmid vector TRIP containing the gene for the protein invasin, which permits

FIGURE 11.20 A conjugate of cholesterol and an siRNA in which the cholesterol is coupled through the 5'-OH of the sense strand of the siRNA. The cholesterol facilitates uptake of the siRNA into specific tissues. The antisense strand becomes part of the RISC and specifies where the mRNA is to be cleaved.

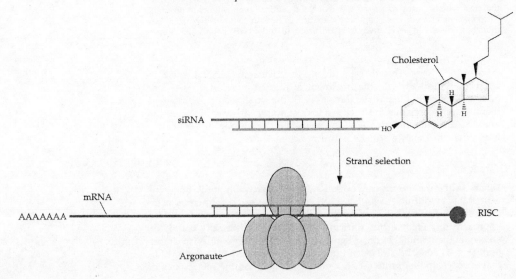

E. coli to enter β1-integrin-positive mammalian cells, and the gene *HlyA*, which encodes listeriolysin O, a protein that enables genetic material to escape from entry vesicles (Fig. 11.21). In addition, the TRIP vector carries an shRNA molecule under the control of a bacterial promoter directed against the mRNA produced by the cancer gene *CTNNB1*. As long as a bacterium is able to enter target mammalian cells and release shRNAs, the shRNA may be directed against any specific mRNAs. The *E. coli* cells act as a vector to transport the shRNAs to where they are required, e.g., cancer cells. This approach has been shown to work both for cancer cells in culture and with mice. With whole animals, the bacteria can be administered orally.

Collagen. The protein polymer collagen, isolated from calf dermis, can be digested, under acidic conditions, by the proteolytic enzyme pepsin to form subunits of approximately 300 kDa each. These rod-like proteins (approximately 300 nm in length by 1.5 nm in diameter) are positively charged and therefore readily interact with and bind to negatively charged siRNAs (Fig. 11.22). These "atelocollagen" particles protect siRNAs from nuclease digestion and also can be injected locally for tissue-targeting delivery of the siRNAs. For example, siRNA–atelocollagen complexes have been efficiently delivered to tumor cells in mice and, after injection, can exist in an intact form for at least 3 days. Furthermore, in mice, siRNA–atelocollagen complexes have been found to inhibit tumor growth in bone cells. This method of packaging siRNA promises to be both reliable and safe, depending on the tissue involved.

FIGURE 11.21 Use of a nonpathogenic strain of *E. coli* to deliver siRNAs to certain tissues. The bacterium was engineered to produce the protein invasin, which permits *E. coli* to enter β1-integrin-positive mammalian cells, as well as the gene *HlyA*, encoding listeriolysin O, which permits the shRNAs synthesized by the bacterium to be released inside the mammalian cell.

FIGURE 11.22 Negatively charged siRNAs bind to positively charged atelocollagen. The complex greatly facilitates the delivery of siRNAs to specific tissues.

Antibodies. It has become relatively straightforward to generate monoclonal antibodies against nearly any target protein; to humanize those antibodies, or their variable regions; and then to produce them in heterologous host cells. Moreover, at the DNA level, it is easy to fuse the antibody gene with the gene for another protein. With this in mind, the gene encoding single-chain Fab fragments that bind specifically to a protein called ErbB2, which is found on the surfaces of breast cancer cells, was fused to the gene for the positively charged nucleic acid-binding protein protamine. The fusion protein binds to the surfaces of cells expressing ErbB2 and at its C terminus carries the 51-amino-acid-long protamine, which readily binds to added siRNAs (Fig. 11.23). In one test of this system,

FIGURE 11.23 A single-chain Fab fragment directed against a mammalian cell surface protein is fused to the positively charged polypeptide protamine, which binds noncovalently to negatively charged siRNAs. The Fab fragment acts to deliver the siRNA to specific cells. Note that a conventional (two-chain) Fab fragment has also been used to deliver siRNAs.

FIGURE 11.24 Schematic representation of the secondary structure of a chimeric RNA molecule consisting of an aptamer and an siRNA. The portion of the aptamer that binds to the target protein and the siRNA portion of the molecule are shaded.

an anti-human immunodeficiency virus (HIV) envelope Fab and an siRNA that is designed to cleave the HIV *gag* mRNA were employed. Using cells in culture, it was possible to reduce the amount of secreted Gag protein (the protein of the nucleocapsid shell around the RNA of a retrovirus) by >70%. This system also works in vivo when the construct is injected either intravenously or directly into tumors. The hope is that by using a combination of specific antibodies (or antibody fragments) that direct siRNAs only to certain cells, and siRNAs that selectively cleave specific target mRNAs, this system can be used to treat a wide range of diseases.

Aptamers. The binding specificity to a target antigen that is a central feature of the functioning of antibodies is also a property of aptamers. Thus, conjugating aptamers, which bind to specific cell surface proteins, to siRNAs that are designed to reduce the expression of certain mRNAs should provide another method of targeting siRNAs to specific tissues or cells. Also, since both aptamers and siRNAs are chemically synthesized RNA oligonucleotides, it should be simple and straightforward to synthesize chimeric RNA molecules that include both the binding specificity of an aptamer and an siRNA that targets a specific mRNA (Fig. 11.24). For example, an aptamer that binds selectively to a prostate-specific membrane antigen (found on prostate cancer cells) was first selected. Then, a 21-bp siRNA directed against mRNAs encoded by either of two genes that are necessary for prostate cells to survive was added to the aptamer sequence. Both activities (i.e., aptamer binding and RNAi) were maintained in the

chimeric molecule. The targeting aptamer did not impair the ability of the siRNA to silence the target gene, and the presence of the siRNA did not affect the ability of the aptamer to bind to its target. This simple but highly effective approach should be amenable to treating a wide range of human diseases provided that (1) silencing specific genes in a population produces therapeutic benefits and (2) there are surface receptors (usually proteins) that distinguish the target cell population and allow the siRNA to be internalized by the cell.

SUMMARY

A number of human disorders that result from the overproduction of a normal protein may be treated by using (1) nucleotide sequences that bind to a specific mRNA and prevent its translation, i.e., an antisense oligonucleotide; (2) RNA sequences that bind and cleave specific RNA molecules, i.e., ribozymes; (3) small RNA molecules, i.e., aptamers, that assume a highly organized secondary and tertiary structure and bind tightly to a wide range of molecules, including proteins, amino acids, and drugs; or (4) small double-stranded RNA molecules that direct the sequence-specific degradation of mRNA, i.e., interfering RNAs. These techniques may also be used to lessen or prevent diseases caused by pathogenic viruses and other disease-causing organisms.

The greatest impediment to the development of nucleic acid-based therapeutic agents is the difficulty in delivering these agents to their target tissue(s). Initially, workers used virus-based delivery systems with some success, although some safety concerns exist in regard to the use of these vectors. Other approaches for the delivery of nucleic acid-based therapeutic agents include intravenous injection; local injection at the site of the pathology; packaging the nucleic acid into cationic liposomes; physical methods, like electroporation, sonoporation, or hydrodynamic pressure; and conjugating the nucleic acid to another molecule, such as a lipid molecule, cholesterol, collagen, an antibody fragment, or an aptamer.

The development of effective treatments for genetic diseases has been elusive because, in many instances, the appropriate gene product cannot be provided to a patient. However, when a normal version of a gene has been identified and cloned, it may be possible that either it or a cDNA derivative can be used to correct the defect in affected individuals. Viral and nonviral systems have been developed for the delivery of therapeutic genes. Viral vectors take advantage of the ability of a virus to penetrate a specific cell, protect the DNA from degradation, and direct it to the cell nucleus. A number of viruses have been engineered for gene therapy applications. Packaging cell lines for some viral systems ensure that virtually no infectious viruses are present in a sample of vector viruses. Nonviral gene delivery systems include injection of pure DNA, bombardment of a target tissue with DNA-coated particles, and cellular uptake of DNA that is enclosed within a lipid envelope. In addition, HACs may find use as vectors for the long-term maintenance and expression of therapeutic genes in human cells. Generally, the major drawbacks of the current generation of gene therapy vector systems are immunogenicity, lack of cell specificity, inefficient gene transfer, and limited therapeutic gene expression.

REFERENCES

Agrawal, S. (ed.). 1996. *Antisense Therapeutics*. Humana Press Inc., Totowa, NJ.

Alton, E., and C. Kitson. 2000. Gene therapy for cystic fibrosis. *Exp. Opin. Investig. Drugs* 9:1523–1535.

Bainbridge, J. W. B., A. J. Smith, S. S. Barker, S. Robbie, R. Henderson, K. Balaggan, A. Viswanathan, G. E. Holder, A. Stockman, N. Tyler, S. Petersen-Jones, S. S. Bhattacharya, A. J. Thrasher, F. W. Fitzke, B. J. Carter, G. S. Rubin, A. T. Moore, and R. R. Ali. 2008. Effect of gene therapy on visual function in Leber's congenital amaurosis. *N. Engl. J. Med.* 358:2231–2239.

Bennett, J., and A. M. Maguire. 2000. Gene therapy for ocular disease. *Mol. Ther.* 1:501–505.

Bramlage, B., E. Luzi, and F. Eckstein. 1998. Designing ribozymes for the inhibition of gene expression. *Trends Biotechnol.* 16:434–438.

Burfeind, P., C. L. Chernicky, F. Rininsland, J. Ilan, and J. Ilan. 1996. Antisense RNA to the type I insulin-like growth factor receptor suppresses tumor growth and prevents invasion by rat prostate cancer cells in vivo. *Proc. Natl. Acad. Sci. USA* 93:7263–7268.

Cairns, M. J., T. M. Hopkins, C. Witherington, L. Wang, and L.-Q. Sun. 1999. Target site selection for an RNA-cleaving catalytic DNA. *Nat. Biotechnol.* 17:480–486.

Cavazzana-Calvo, M., S. Hacein-Bey, G. de Saint Basile, F. Gross, E. Yvon, P. Nusbaum, F. Selz, C. Hue, S. Certain, J. L. Casanova, P. Bousso, F. L. Deist, and A. Fischer. 2000. Gene therapy of human severe combined immunodeficiency (SCID)-X1 disease. *Science* 288:669–672.

Choo, K. H. 2001. Engineering human chromosomes for gene therapy studies. *Trends Mol. Med.* 7:235–237.

Chu, T. C., K. Y. Twu, A. D. Ellington, and M. Levy. 2006. Aptamer mediated siRNA delivery. *Nucleic Acids Res.* 34:e73.

Chuah, M. K., D. Collen, and T. Vanden Driessche. 2001. Gene therapy for hemophilia. *J. Gene Med.* 3:3–20.

Cole-Strauss, A., K. Yoon, Y. Xiang, B. C. Bryne, M. C. Rice, J. Gryn, W. K. Holloman, and E. B. Kmiec. 1996. Correction of the mutation responsible for sickle cell anemia by an RNA-DNA oligonucleotide. *Science* 273:1386–1389.

Cullen, B. R. 2006. Enhancing and confirming the specificity of RNAi experiments. *Nat. Methods* 3:677–681.

Davidson, B. L. 2006. All in the family. *Nat. Biotechnol.* 24:951–952.

De Fougerolles, A., H.-P. Vornlocher, J. Maraganore, and J. Lieberman. 2007. Interfering with disease: a progress report on siRNA-based therapeutics. *Nat. Rev.* 6:443–453.

Dillon, C. P., P. Sandy, A. Nencioni, S. Kissler, D. A. Rubinson, and L. Van Parijs. 2005. RNAi as an experimental and therapeutic tool to study and regulate physiological and disease processes. *Annu. Rev. Physiol.* 67:147–173.

Elbashir, S. M., J. Harborth, W. Lendeckel, A. Yalcin, K. Weber, and T. Tuschi. 2001. Duplexes of 21-nucleotide RNAs mediate RNA interference in cultured mammalian cells. *Nature* 411:494–498.

Elbashir, S. M., W. Lendeckel, and T. Tuschi. 2001. RNA interference is mediated by 21- and 22-nucleotide RNAs. *Genes Dev.* 15:188–200.

Eng, C. M., M. Banikazemi, R. E. Gordon, M. Goldman, R. Phelps, L. Kim, A. Gass, J. Winston, S. Dikman, J. T. Fallon, S. Brodie, C. B. Stacy, D. Mehta, R. Parsons, K. Norton, M. O'Callaghan, and R. J. Desnick. 2001. A phase 1/2 clinical trial of enzyme replacement in Fabry disease: pharmacokinetic, substrate clearance, and safety studies. *Am. J. Hum. Genet.* 68:711–722.

Faria, M., D. G. Spiller, C. Dubertret, J. S. Nelson, M. R. H. White, D. Scherman, C. Hélène, and C. Giovannangeli. 2001. Phosphoramidate oligonucleotides as potent antisense molecules in cells and in vivo. *Nat. Biotechnol.* 19:40–44.

Fichou, Y., and C. Férec. 2006. The potential of oligonucleotides for therapeutic applications. *Trends Biotechnol.* 24:563–570.

Field, A. K. 1998. Viral targets for antisense oligonucleotides: a mini review. *Antivir. Res.* 37:67–81.

Haasnoot, E., M. Westerhout, and B. Berkhout. 2007. RNA interference against viruses: strike and counterstrike. *Nat. Biotechnol.* 25:1435–1443.

Haidet, A. M., L. Rizo, C. Handy, P. Umapathi, A. Eagle, C. Shilling, D. Boue, P. T. Martin, Z. Sahenk, J. R. Mendell, and B. K. Kaspar. 2008. Long-term enhancement of skeletal muscle mass and strength by single gene administration of myostatin inhibitors. *Proc. Natl. Acad. Sci. USA* 105:4318–4322.

Isaacs, F. J., D. J. Dwyer, and J. J. Collins. 2006. RNA synthetic biology. *Nat. Biotechnol.* 24:545–554.

Johnson, W. E. 2007. Assisted suicide for retroviruses. *Nat. Biotechnol.* 25:643–644.

Kay, M. A., C. S. Manno, M. V. Ragni, P. J. Larson, L. B. Couto, A. McClelland, B. Glader, A. J. Chew, S. J. Tai, R. W. Herzog, V. Arruda, F. Johnson, C. Scallan, E. Skarsgard, A. W. Flake, and K. A. High. 2000. Evidence for gene transfer and expression of factor IX in haemophilia B patients treated with an AAV vector. *Nat. Genet.* 24:257–261.

Kim, D.-H., M. A. Behlke, S. D. Rose, M.-S. Chang, S. Choi, and J. J. Rossi. 2005. Synthetic dsRNA Dicer substrates enhance RNAi potency and efficacy. *Nat. Biotechnol.* 23:222–226.

Kono, K., Y. Torikoshi, M. Mitsutomi, T. Itoh, N. Emi, H. Yanagie, and T. Takagishi. 2001. Novel gene delivery systems: complexes of fusigenic polymer-modified liposomes and lipoplexes. *Gene Ther.* 8:5–12.

Lee, J.-H., M. D. Canny, A. De Erkenez, D. Krilleke, Y.-S. Ng, D. T. Shima, A. Pardi, and F. Jucker. 2005. A therapeutic aptamer inhibits angiogenesis by specifically targeting the heparin binding domain of VEGF165. *Proc. Natl. Acad. Sci. USA* 102:18902–18907.

Maguire, A. M., F. Simonelli, E. A. Pierce, E. N. Pugh, F. Mingozzi, J. Bennicelli, S. Banfi, K. A. Marshall, F. Testa, E. M. Surace, S. Rossi, A. Lyubarsky, V. R. Arruda, B. Konkle, E. Stone, J. Sun, J. Jacobs, L. Dell'Osso, R. Hertle, J.-X. Ma, T. M. Redmond, X. Zhu, B. Hauck, O. Zelenaia, K. S. Shindler, M. G. Maguire, J. F. Wright, N. J. Volpe, J. W. McDonnell, A. Auricchio, K. A. High, and J. Bennett. 2008. Safety and efficacy of gene transfer for Leber's congenital amaurosis. *N. Engl. J. Med.* 358:2240–2248.

Matzen, K., L. Elzaouk, A. A. Matskevich, A. Nitzsche, J. Heinrich, and K. Moelling. 2007. RNase H-mediated retrovirus destruction in vivo triggered by oligodeoxynucleotides. *Nat. Biotechnol.* 25:669–674.

McNamara, J. O., II, E. R. Andrechek, Y. Wang, K. D. Viles, R. E. Rempel, E. Gilboa, B. A. Sullenger, and P. H. Giangrande. 2006. Cell type-specific delivery of siRNAs with aptamer-siRNA chimeras. *Nat. Biotechnol.* 24:1005–1015.

Morris, M. C., L. Chaloin, F. Heitz, and G. Divita. 2000. Translocating peptides and proteins and their use for gene delivery. *Curr. Opin. Biotechnol.* 11:461–466.

Nettelbeck, D. M., V. Jérôme, and R. Müller. 2000. Gene therapy: designer promoters for tumour targeting. *Trends Genet.* 16:174–181.

Nimjee, S. M., C. P. Rusconi, and B. A. Sullenger. 2005. Aptamers: an emerging class of therapeutics. *Annu. Rev. Med.* 56:555–583.

Oliveira, S., G. Storm, and R. M. Schiffelers. 2006. Targeted delivery of siRNA. *J. Biomed. Biotechnol.* 2006:1–9.

Pendergast, P. S., H. N. Marsh, D. Grate, J. M. Healy, and M. Stanton. 2005. Nucleic acid aptamers for target validation and therapeutic applications. *J. Biomol. Technol.* 16:224–234.

Putnam, D. A. 1996. Antisense strategies and therapeutic applications. *Am. J. Health Syst. Pharm.* 53:151–160.

Rossi, J. J. 2004. A cholesterol connection in RNAi. *Nature* 432:155–156.

Rossi, J. J. 2005. Receptor-targeted siRNAs. *Nat. Biotechnol.* 23:682–683.

Rubanyi, G. M. 2001. The future of human gene therapy. *Mol. Aspects Med.* 22:113–142.

Sampson, T. 2003. Aptamers and SELEX: the technology. *World Patent Info.* 25:123–129.

Samuel, V. T., C. S. Choi, T. G. Phillips, A. J. Romanelli, J. G. Geisler, S. Bhanot, R. McKay, B. Monia, J. R. Shutter, R. A. Lindberg, G. I. Shulman, and M. M. Veniant. 2006. Targeting Foxo1 in mice using antisense oligonucleotide improves hepatic and peripheral insulin action. *Diabetes* 55:2042–2050.

Scherer, L. J., and J. J. Rossi. 2003. Approaches for the sequence-specific knockdown of mRNA. *Nat. Biotechnol.* 21:1457–1464.

Shahi, S., G. K. Shanmugasundaram, and A. C. Banerjea. 2001. Ribozymes that cleave reovirus genome segment Si also protect cells from pathogenesis caused by reovirus infection. *Proc. Natl. Acad. Sci. USA* 98:4101–4106.

Siolas, D., C. Lerner, J. Burchard, W. Ge, P. S. Linsley, P. J. Paddison, G. J. Hannon, and M. A. Cleary. 2005. Synthetic shRNAs as potent RNAi triggers. *Nat. Biotechnol.* 23:227–231.

Sioud, M., and D. R. Sorensen. 1998. A nuclease-resistant protein kinase Cα ribozyme blocks glioma cell growth. *Nat. Biotechnol.* 16:556–561.

Snøve, O., and J. J. Rossi. 2006. Expressing short hairpin RNAs *in vivo*. *Nat. Methods* 3:689–695.

Song, E., P. Zhu, S.-K. Lee, D. Chowdhury, S. Kussman, D. M. Dykxhoorn, Y. Feng, D. Palliser, D. B. Weiner, P. Shankar, W. A. Marasco,

and J. Lieberman. 2005. Antibody mediated *in vivo* delivery of small interfering RNAs via cell-surface receptors. *Nat. Biotechnol.* 23:709–717.

Soutschek, J., A. Akinc, B. Bramlage, K. Charisse, R. Constien, M. Donoghue, S. Elbashir, A. Geick, P. Hadwiger, J. Harborth, M. John, V. Kesavan, G. Lavine, R. K. Pandey, T. Racie, K. G. Rajeev, I. Röhl, I. Toudjarska, G. Wang, S. Wuschko, D. Bumcrot, V. Koteliansky, S. Limmer, M. Manoharan, and H.-P. Vornlocher. 2004. Therapeutic silencing of an endogenous gene by systematic administration of modified siRNAs. *Nature* 432:173–178.

Takeshita, F., Y. Minakuchi, S. Nagahara, K. Honma, H. Sasaki, K. Hirai, T. Teratani, N. Namatame, Y. Yamamoto, K. Hanai, T. Kato, A. Sano, and T. Ochiya. 2005. Efficient delivery of small interfering RNA to bone-metastatic tumors by using atelocollagen *in vivo*. *Proc. Natl. Acad. Sci. USA* 102:12177–12182.

Trang, P., A. Kilani, J. Kim, and F. Liu. 2000. A ribozyme derived from the catalytic subunit of RNase P from *Escherichia coli* is highly effective in inhibiting replication of herpes simplex virus 1. *J. Mol. Biol.* 301:817–826.

Trang, P., M. Lee, E. Nepomuceno, J. Kim, H. Zhu, and F. Liu. 2000. Effective inhibition of human cytomegalovirus gene expression and replication by a ribozyme derived from the catalytic RNA subunit of RNase P from *Escherichia coli*. *Proc. Natl. Acad.*

Sci. USA 97:5812–5817.

Van Rij, R. P., and R. Andino. 2006. The silent treatment: RNAi as a defense against virus infection in mammals. *Trends Biotechnol.* 24:186–193.

Wolfrum, C., S. Shi, N. K. Jayaprakash, M. Jayaraman, G. Wang, R. J. Pandey, K. G. Rajeev, T. Nakayama, K. Charrise, E. M. Ndungo, T. Zimmermann, V. Koteliansky, M. Manoharan, and M. Stoffel. 2007. Mechanisms and optimization of in vivo delivery of lipophilic siRNAs. *Nat. Biotechnol.* 25:1149–1157.

Wraight, C. J., P. J. White, S. C. McKean, R. D. Fogarty, D. J. Venables, I. J. Liepe, S. R. Edmondson, and G. A. Werther. 2000. Reversal of epidermal hyperproliferation in psoriasis by insulin-like growth factor I receptor antisense oligonucleotides. *Nat. Biotechnol.* 18:521–526.

Xiang, S., J. Fruehauf, and C. J. Li. 2006. Short hairpin RNA-expressing bacteria elicit RNA interference in mammals. *Nat. Biotechnol.* 24:697–702.

Yoon, K., A. Cole-Strauss, and E. B. Kmiec. 1996. Targeted gene correction of episomal DNA in mammalian cells mediated by a chimeric RNA·DNA oligonucleotide. *Proc. Natl. Acad. Sci. USA* 93:2071–2076.

Zamore, P. D., T. Tuschi, P. A. Sharp, and D. P. Bartel. 2001. RNAi: double-stranded RNA directs the ATP-dependent cleavage of mRNA at 21 to 23 nucleotide intervals. *Cell* 101:25–33.

REVIEW QUESTIONS

1. How can antisense oligonucleotides be used to treat psoriasis?

2. What are ribozymes, and how can they be used as human therapeutic agents?

3. What are interfering RNAs, and how might they be used as human therapeutic agents?

4. What is an aptamer, and how is it used as a therapeutic agent?

5. How can antibody genes be used to confer passive immunity?

6. How can interfering RNAs be delivered to specific cells?

7. In developing a new nucleic acid-based therapeutic agent, how would you decide between antisense oligonucleotides, ribozymes, aptamers, and interfering RNA?

8. What are the key attributes of a therapeutic gene delivery system for humans?

9. How can the interferon response, which is usually induced by double-stranded RNA, be avoided when utilizing siRNAs as therapeutic agents?

10. What are some of the advantages and disadvantages of deoxyribozymes compared to ribozymes?

11. How can the progression of age-related macular degeneration be limited using RNA therapeutics?

Vaccines

V ACCINATION PROTECTS A RECIPIENT from pathogenic agents by establishing an immunological resistance to infection. An injected or oral vaccine induces the host to generate antibodies against the disease-causing organism; therefore, during future exposures, the infectious agent is inactivated (neutralized, or killed), its proliferation is prevented, and the disease state is not established.

Over 200 years ago, in 1796, Edward Jenner experimentally tested the folklore-based notion that human infection with a mild cattle disease called cowpox would protect infected individuals against the human disease smallpox. Smallpox is an extremely virulent disease with a high death rate. If one survives, permanent disfigurement, mental derangement, and blindness often follow. Jenner inoculated James Phipps, an 8-year-old boy, with exudate from a cowpox pustule. In two separate trials after the initial vaccination, the boy was fully protected against human smallpox. This country doctor had discovered the principle of vaccination.

Communicable diseases such as tuberculosis, smallpox, cholera, typhus, bubonic plague, and poliomyelitis, have in the past been a scourge for humankind. With the advent of vaccination, antibiotics, and effective public health measures, these epidemic diseases have, for the most part, been brought under control (Table 12.1). Occasionally, however, protective measures become ineffective, and devastating new outbreaks occur. In 1991, a cholera epidemic struck Peru, producing, over the next 3 years, approximately 1 million infections and several thousand deaths. Also, for many current human and animal diseases, there are no vaccines. Today, more than 2 billion humans suffer from diseases that theoretically could be curtailed by vaccination. In addition, new diseases for which vaccines might be useful continue to emerge.

In recent years, in some developed countries, a small but vocal minority of individuals have refused to have their children vaccinated. These individuals argue that many of the previously common illnesses have been vanquished, and they fear the potential side effects of the vaccinations more than the disease itself. In addition, many of these people question modern medicine and instead prefer to rely upon so-called traditional or

TABLE 12.1 Annual cases in Canada from various diseases before and after the introduction of vaccines against the causative agents of the diseases

Disease	Annual no. of cases before vaccine was introduced	No. of cases in 2002
Polio	20,000	0
Diphtheria	9,000	0
Rubella	69,000	16
Mumps	52,000	197
Haemophilus influenzae type b infection	2,000	48
Whooping cough	25,000	2,557
Measles	300,000	7

natural therapies. In fact, the small number of individuals who are not vaccinated benefit from the fact that the vast majority of other people in society have been immunized, thereby making it difficult for many diseases to spread through a community. However, in communities where vaccination levels decrease below a certain level, there is a real danger of some traditional diseases making a comeback.

Modern vaccines typically consist of either a killed (inactivated) or a live, nonvirulent (attenuated) form of an infectious agent. Traditionally, the infectious agent is grown in culture, purified, and either inactivated or attenuated without, of course, losing the ability to evoke an immune response that is effective against the virulent form of the infectious organism. Notwithstanding the considerable success that has been achieved in creating effective vaccines against diseases such as German measles, diphtheria, whooping cough, tetanus, smallpox, and poliomyelitis, there are a number of limitations to the current mode of vaccine production.

- Not all infectious agents can be grown in culture, so no vaccines have been developed for a number of diseases.
- Production of animal and human viruses requires animal cell culture, which is expensive.
- Both the yield and rate of production of animal and human viruses in culture are often quite low, making vaccine production costly.
- Extensive safety precautions are necessary to ensure that laboratory and production personnel are not exposed to a pathogenic agent.
- Batches of vaccine may not be killed or may be insufficiently attenuated during the production process, thereby introducing virulent organisms into the vaccine and inadvertently spreading the disease.
- Attenuated strains may revert, a possibility that requires continual testing to ensure that the reacquisition of virulence has not occurred.
- Not all diseases (e.g., acquired immune deficiency syndrome [AIDS]) are preventable through the use of traditional vaccines.
- Most current vaccines have a limited shelf life and often require refrigeration to maintain potency. This requirement creates storage problems in countries with large, unelectrified rural areas.

Within the last 2 decades, recombinant DNA technology has provided a means of creating a new generation of vaccines that overcome the drawbacks

of traditional vaccines. The availability of gene cloning has enabled research-ers to contemplate various novel strategies for vaccine development.

- Virulence genes could be deleted from an infectious agent that retains the ability to stimulate an immunological response. In this case, the genetically engineered agent could be used as a live vaccine without concern about reversion to virulence, because it is impos-sible for a whole gene to be reacquired spontaneously during growth in pure culture.
- Live nonpathogenic carrier systems that carry discrete antigenic determinants of an unrelated pathogenic agent could be created. In this form, the carrier system facilitates the induction of a strong immunological response directed against the pathogenic agent.
- For infectious agents that cannot be maintained in culture, the genes for the proteins that have critical antigenic determinants can be iso-lated, cloned, and expressed in an alternative host system, such as *Escherichia coli* or a mammalian cell line. These cloned gene proteins can be formulated into a vaccine.
- There are some infectious agents that do not damage host cells directly; instead, the disease condition results when the host immune system attacks its own (infected) cells. For these diseases, it may be possible to create a targeted cell-specific killing system. Although not a true vaccine, this type of system attacks only infected cells, thereby removing the source of the adverse immunological response. In these cases, the gene for a fusion protein is constructed. First, one part of this fusion protein binds to an infected cell. Then, the other part kills the infected cell.

Because of less stringent regulatory requirements, the first vaccines that were produced by recombinant DNA techniques were for animal dis-eases, such as foot-and-mouth disease, rabies, and scours, a diarrheal dis-ease of pigs and cattle. In addition, many more animal vaccines are currently being developed. For human diseases, a large number of recom-binant vaccines are currently in various stages of development, including clinical trials (Table 12.2).

Unfortunately, in comparison to the number of new therapeutic agents, very few recombinant-DNA-based vaccines have been developed. Why, according to the vaccine producers, does it take so long for new vaccines to come to the marketplace? First, while there were 25 major vaccine manufac-turers worldwide in 1970, in 2005 there were only 5. Second, vaccines are currently viewed as "almost a commodity," with little financial incentive to develop new vaccines; in 2005, the worldwide market for preventive vac-cines was approximately $8 billion. Third, the U.S. government is a major purchaser of vaccines, forcing discount prices and thereby decreasing the potential profit. Fourth, in 1980 in the United States, "good manufacturing practices" were introduced into vaccine production, causing manufacturing costs to increase dramatically. Fifth, the transition from conventional to newer processes for vaccine production is expensive and time-consuming (not including clinical trials), so that it is preferable to continue using a more established technology. On the positive side, the focus of the larger vaccine manufacturers on large-scale products has provided smaller biotechnology companies with a number of niche opportunities to develop and market new products. Finally, since most vaccines are intended to protect large

TABLE 12.2 Human disease agents for which recombinant vaccines are currently being developed

Pathogenic agent	Disease
Viruses	
Varicella-zoster viruses	Chicken pox
Cytomegalovirus	Infection in infants and immuno-compromised patients
Dengue virus	Hemorrhagic fever
Hepatitis A virus	High fever, liver damage
Hepatitis B virus	Long-term liver damage
Herpes simplex virus type 2	Genital ulcers
Influenza A and B viruses	Acute respiratory disease
Japanese encephalitis	Encephalitis
Parainfluenza virus	Inflammation of the upper respiratory tract
Rabies virus	Encephalitis
Respiratory syncytial virus	Upper and lower respiratory tract lesions
Rotavirus	Acute infantile gastroenteritis
Yellow fever virus	Lesions of heart, kidney, and liver
Human immunodeficiency virus	AIDS
Bacteria	
Vibrio cholerae	Cholera
E. coli enterotoxin strains	Diarrheal disease
Neisseria gonorrhoeae	Gonorrhea
Haemophilus influenzae	Meningitis, septicemic conditions
Mycobacterium leprae	Leprosy
Neisseria meningitidis	Meningitis
Bordetella pertussis	Whooping cough
Shigella strains	Dysentery
Streptococcus group A	Scarlet fever, rheumatic fever, throat infection
Streptococcus group B	Sepsis, urogenital tract infection
Streptococcus pneumoniae	Pneumonia, meningitis
Clostridium tetani	Tetanus
Mycobacterium tuberculosis	Tuberculosis
Salmonella enterica serovar Typhi	Typhoid fever
Parasites	
Onchocerca volvulus	River blindness
Leishmania spp.	Internal and external lesions
Plasmodium spp.	Malaria
Schistosoma mansoni	Schistosomiasis
Trypanosoma spp.	Sleeping sickness
Wuchereria bancrofti	Filariasis

populations, the very large amounts of money that companies often charge to treat a single individual with some of the newer therapeutic agents (see chapter 10) are unrealistic for pricing of a new vaccine. In fact, it is precisely

in many poorer countries, where most individuals cannot afford to pay very much for treatment or immunization, that vaccines are needed the most.

Subunit Vaccines

Vaccines generally consist of either killed or attenuated forms of the whole pathogenic agent. The antibodies elicited by these vaccines initiate an immune response to inactivate (neutralize) pathogenic organisms by binding to proteins on the outer surface of the agent. So, do vaccines need to contain the whole organism, or will specific portions of pathogenic organisms suffice? For disease-causing viruses, it has been shown that purified outer surface viral proteins, either capsid or envelope proteins (Fig. 12.1), are often sufficient for eliciting neutralizing antibodies in the host organism. Vaccines that use components of a pathogenic organism rather than the whole organism are called "subunit" vaccines; recombinant DNA technology is very well suited for developing new subunit vaccines.

There are advantages and disadvantages to the use of subunit vaccines. On the positive side, using a purified protein(s) as an immunogen ensures that the preparation is stable and safe, is precisely defined chemically, and is free of extraneous proteins and nucleic acids that can initiate undesirable side effects in the host organism. On the negative side, purification of a specific protein can be costly, and in certain instances, an isolated protein may not have the same conformation as it does in situ (within the viral capsid or envelope), with the result that its antigenicity is decreased. Obviously, the decision to produce a subunit vaccine depends on an assessment of several biological and economic factors.

Herpes Simplex Virus

Herpes simplex virus (HSV) has been implicated as a cancer-causing (oncogenic) agent, in addition to its more common roles in causing sexually transmitted disease, severe eye infections, and encephalitis, so prevention of HSV infection by vaccination with either killed or attenuated virus may

FIGURE 12.1 Schematic representation of an animal virus. Viruses generally consist of a relatively small nucleic acid genome (3 to 200 kb of either double- or single-stranded DNA or RNA) within a viral protein capsid that is sometimes, depending on the virus, surrounded by a protein-containing viral envelope (membrane).

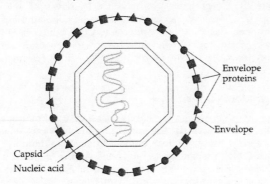

Envelope proteins

Envelope

Capsid

Nucleic acid

FIGURE 12.2 Schematic representation of the development of a subunit vaccine against HSV. The isolated HSV gD protein gene is used to transfect CHO cells. Then, the transfected cells are grown in culture and produce gD protein. Mice inoculated with the purified gD protein are protected against infection by HSV.

put the recipient at risk for cancer. Thus, protection against HSV would be best achieved by a subunit vaccine, which would not be oncogenic.

The primary requirement for creating any subunit vaccine is identification of the component(s) of the infectious agent that elicits antibodies that react against the intact form of the infectious agent. The HSV type 1 (HSV-1) envelope glycoprotein D (gD) is such a component, because after injection into mice, it elicits antibodies that neutralize intact HSV. The HSV-1 gD gene was isolated and then cloned into a mammalian expression vector and expressed in Chinese hamster ovary (CHO) cells (Fig. 12.2), which, unlike the *E. coli* system, properly glycosylate foreign eukaryotic proteins. The complete sequence of the gD gene encodes a protein that becomes bound to the mammalian host cell membrane (Fig. 12.3A). However, a membrane-bound protein is much more difficult to purify than a soluble one. Consequently, the gD gene was modified by removing the nucleotides encoding the C-terminal transmembrane-binding domain (Fig. 12.3B). The modified gene was then transformed into CHO cells, where the product was glycosylated and secreted into the external medium (Fig. 12.2). In laboratory trials, the modified form of gD was effective against both HSV-1 and HSV-2.

Foot-and-Mouth Disease

Foot-and-mouth disease virus (FMDV) has a devastating impact on cattle and swine and is extremely virulent, but for the most part, it has been possible to keep the negative effects of the virus to a minimum by using formalin-killed FMDV preparations as a vaccine. Approximately 1 billion doses of this killed-virus vaccine are used worldwide each year. The availability of the vaccine notwithstanding, in 2001, there was a major outbreak of foot-and-mouth disease in Europe in which tens of thousands of cattle were

A

B

FIGURE 12.3 **(A)** Location in the envelope of HSV-1 gD with the transmembrane domain. **(B)** Extracellular location of a soluble gD without the transmembrane domain.

slaughtered and their carcasses were incinerated in an effort to prevent the virus from spreading.

Research on FMDV found that the major antigenic determinant that induces neutralizing antibodies is capsid viral protein 1 (VP1). Although purified VP1 is a much less potent antigen than intact viral particles, it can still elicit neutralizing antibodies by itself and therefore can protect animals from infection by FMDV. Thus, the gene for VP1 became a target for cloning.

The genome of FMDV is composed of single-stranded RNA (approximately 8,000 nucleotides long). Therefore, for recombinant DNA manipulations, it was necessary first to synthesize a double-stranded complementary DNA (cDNA) of the entire genome (Fig. 12.4). This cDNA was then digested with restriction enzymes, and the fragments were cloned in an *E. coli* expression vector. The product of the VP1 coding sequence was identified immunologically as part of a fusion protein under the control of the p^L promoter–*cI* repressor system. The fusion protein was 396 amino acids long and consisted of a portion of a stabilizing carrier protein, i.e., the bacteriophage MS2 replicase protein, as well as the entire coding sequence of the FMDV VP1 protein (Fig. 12.4). The fusion protein containing the VP1 protein fragment was able to generate neutralizing antibodies to FMDV.

A fusion protein, however, faces more government regulatory hurdles than intact VP1 would because of the potential immunogenic effects of the

FIGURE 12.4 Schematic representation of the development of a subunit vaccine against foot-and-mouth disease. The entire viral RNA is made into cDNA, which is then digested with restriction enzymes. The DNA fragments are cloned into an expression vector in frame with the gene for the *E. coli* bacteriophage MS2 replicative protein. The plasmid constructs are used to transform *E. coli*, and then the stable fusion protein is isolated and used to inoculate animals.

non-VP1 component. Therefore, the VP1 sequence alone will have to be subcloned onto a different expression vector. Nevertheless, a subunit vaccine for foot-and-mouth disease could soon be ready for preclinical trials.

Cholera

The bacterium *Vibrio cholerae,* the causative agent of cholera, colonizes the small intestine and secretes large amounts of a hexameric enterotoxin, which is the actual pathogenic agent. This protein consists of one subunit, the A subunit, that has ADP ribosylation activity and stimulates adenylate cyclase, and five identical B subunits that bind specifically to an intestinal mucosal cell receptor (Fig. 12.5). The A subunit has two functional domains: the A_1 peptide, which contains the toxic activity, and the A_2 peptide, which joins the A subunit to the B subunits. Until a few years ago, a traditional cholera vaccine consisting of phenol-killed *V. cholerae* was in common use. This vaccine generated only moderate protection, typically lasting from about 3 to 6 months. More recently, a vaccine (Dukoral) consisting of heat-inactivated *V. cholerae* Inaba classic strain, heat-inactivated Ogawa classic strain, formalin-inactivated Inaba El Tor strain, formalin-inactivated Ogawa classic strain, and a recombinant cholera toxin B subunit, has come into use. The vaccine is taken orally (two doses 1 week apart), and it is claimed that an additional booster immunization is not required for about 2 years.

SARS

In 2003, there were more or less simultaneous outbreaks in several major cities, including Hong Kong, Singapore, and Toronto, of a new, unknown disease. The first case of this disease, severe acute respiratory syndrome, or SARS, was reported in Guangdong Province, southern People's Republic of China, in November 2002. Given the enormous frequency of air travel, the disease rapidly spread to 29 countries on five continents. With the assistance of the World Health Organization, authorities in affected regions immediately implemented strict infection control procedures, so that by mid-July 2003, the outbreak was effectively contained. However, this was not before a total of 8,096 SARS cases and 774 associated deaths were reported. Within a very short time, scientists had identified a novel coronavirus as the causative agent of the disease. The SARS virus contains a single-stranded plus-sense RNA genome of approximately 30 kb. In nature, the viral spike protein, which is inserted into the viral membrane, binds to

FIGURE 12.5 Schematic representation of hexameric cholera toxin. The A peptide is shown in blue, and the B peptide is shown in green.

B subunit A2 peptide A1 peptide

FIGURE 12.6 Schematic representation of the binding of the SARS virus glycosylated spike protein to a cellular outer surface protein receptor.

a receptor protein that is present on the surfaces of mammalian host cells (Fig. 12.6). Following the binding of the virus to the receptor, the viral and cell membranes can fuse, thereby facilitating the entry of the virus into the cell. The spike protein (or the external portion of the molecule) is an attractive candidate for the development of a subunit vaccine. In practice, it was found that the external portion of the spike protein (i.e., amino acids 318 to 510) could bind efficiently to the host cell receptor protein. Following the determination of the complete nucleotide sequence of the SARS virus in 2003, it was relatively straightforward to express a codon-optimized version of this 192-amino-acid peptide in CHO cells. In addition to encoding the 192-amino-acid spike peptide, the DNA construct introduced into the CHO cells also included a mammalian secretion signal, an N-terminal (*Staphylococcus aureus*) protein A purification tag, and a tobacco etch virus protease cleavage site (Fig. 12.7). The recombinant protein synthesized in CHO cells was secreted into the growth medium, purified by affinity chromatography on a column containing immobilized immunoglobulin G, and then digested with tobacco etch virus protease to remove the protein A purification tag. Using this construct, the spike protein fragment was readily synthesized and purified. To date, the fully glycosylated form of this subunit vaccine candidate has been shown to elicit a strong immune response in mice. It still remains to be seen whether it can protect immunized animals against infection with the SARS virus.

Staphylococcus aureus

The gram-positive bacterium *S. aureus* is a major cause of hospital-acquired infection. This bacterium produces a pore-forming toxin; is a leading cause of infections of the bloodstream, lower respiratory tract, and skin; and, because of the emergence of antibiotic-resistant strains, is a serious public health threat. To address the challenge of treating *S. aureus* infections,

FIGURE 12.7 The main features of a portion of the recombinant plasmid construct used to transfect CHO cells and to produce the fragment of the SARS spike protein that interacts with the host cell receptor.

Signal peptide	Protein A fragment	Protease cleavage site	Spike protein fragment

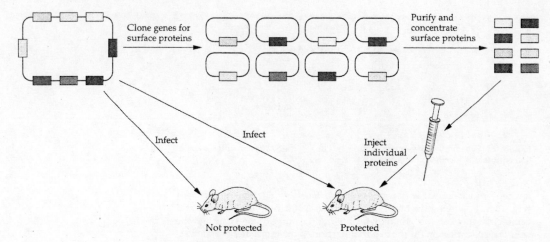

FIGURE 12.8 Development of a vaccine against *S. aureus.*

whole-cell attenuated or killed vaccines have been developed. However, these vaccines have not been particularly effective. Similarly, subunit vaccines composed of individual bacterial surface proteins generate immune responses that afford only partial protection when tested in experimental animals. However, a more effective subunit vaccine has recently been developed to protect individuals against *S. aureus* by combining several of the bacterium's antigens (Fig. 12.8). Starting with one disease-causing strain of *S. aureus*, 23 bacterial outer surface proteins were identified from genomic DNA sequence data. Then, the coding regions of these proteins, minus the signal sequences, were polymerase chain reaction (PCR) amplified and cloned into plasmid vectors that enabled the proteins to be expressed in *E. coli* with a poly-His tag at the N terminus of the protein (to facilitate the purification of the overexpressed protein). The proteins were expressed and purified, and mice were separately immunized with each of the 23 purified proteins. The immunized mice were subsequently challenged by injections of live disease-causing *S. aureus*. Many of the recombinant surface proteins generated an immune response that afforded partial protection against staphylococcal disease, with some proteins affording more protection than others. However, over the long term, immunization with individual surface proteins afforded only modest protection. A mixture of the four proteins that individually generated the most effective antibodies was used to immunize mice and was found to completely protect against the pathogen. The experimental design ensured that only common, and not strain-specific, *S. aureus* surface proteins were used to immunize mice. Thus, it is not surprising that the tetravalent subunit vaccine that was developed was effective against five different clinical isolates (strains) of *S. aureus*. This work represents an important first step in the development of an *S. aureus* vaccine.

Human Papillomavirus

Human papillomavirus is the causative agent of many common sexually transmitted diseases. While most of these infections are benign and often

Type 6 Type 11 Type 16 Type 18

FIGURE 12.9 Schematic representation of the virus-like particles assembled from cloned and overproduced L1 proteins from the capsids of four different strains of human papillomavirus. These virus-like particles are the constituents of a commercial subunit vaccine against the virus.

asymptomatic, persistent infection with some strains of human papillomavirus is associated with the development of cervical and related cancers, as well as genital warts. Since human papillomavirus type 16 is associated with approximately 50% of cervical cancers, a vaccine that prevents human papillomavirus type 16 infection could significantly reduce the incidence of cervical cancer. Moreover, a vaccine that is directed against several different types of human papillomaviruses could effectively prevent nearly all human papillomavirus-induced cervical cancers. To put this into perspective, cervical cancer is the second most commonly diagnosed cancer among women worldwide, accounting for more than 250,000 deaths per year.

In June 2006, the U.S. Food and Drug Administration approved a vaccine that protects women against infection by human papillomavirus types 6, 11, 16, and 18, the types most frequently associated with cervical cancer and genital warts. By the end of 2006, this vaccine had been approved for use in more than 50 countries worldwide. The vaccine, called Gardasil, is quadrivalent, i.e., it contains virus-like particles assembled from the major capsid (L1) proteins of the above-mentioned four types of human papillomavirus (Fig. 12.9 and Box 12.1). It was previously shown that the L1 protein can self-assemble into virus-like particles that resemble papillomavirus virions, and these particles are highly immunogenic, inducing neutralizing antibodies directed against the whole live virus. The gene for the L1 protein from each of the four virus types was cloned and expressed in a recombinant *Saccharomyces cerevisiae* (yeast) strain. Following separate fermentations of the four yeast strains, the viral capsid proteins assembled into virus-like particles (i.e., the viral capsid without any other viral proteins or the viral nucleic acid). These virus-like particles were then purified and combined to form the quadrivalent vaccine.

Peptide Vaccines

The question arises as to whether a small discrete portion (domain) of a protein can act as an effective subunit vaccine and induce the production of neutralizing antibodies. Intuitively, one would expect that only the portions, or domains, of a protein that are accessible to antibody binding, that is, those on the exterior surface of the virus, would be immunologically important and that those located in inaccessible regions inside the virus particle could be ignored if they do not contribute to the conformation of

A Vaccine To Prevent Cervical Cancer

On 15 September 2007, the headline on the front page of *The Globe and Mail*, a Toronto, Canada, newspaper, read, "Should your daughter get the needle?" The article that followed related how the Canadian federal government, in conjunction with the Ontario provincial government, was funding a program that would offer free vaccinations against human papillomavirus to girls in grade 8 (typically 12- and 13-year-olds). The vaccine, which had received approval in the United States a year earlier, provides inoculated women with immunity against the viruses that are responsible for approximately 70% of all cervical cancers and 90% of genital warts. Grade 8 was chosen because, according to officials, it is before most girls become sexually active. The vaccine, sold under the brand name Gardasil, is given by needle in three doses over 6 months and is approved for females between the ages of 9 and

26. The rationale for giving the vaccine at such a young age is related to the fact that once a woman has been exposed to the four strains of the virus for which the vaccine provides protection, the vaccine will no longer be effective. The three doses of vaccine cost about $300 to $400, although those inoculated through this program received the vaccine free of charge. Boys can also get human papillomavirus infections, but testing is still under way to determine whether the vaccine works as well for them.

According to *The Globe and Mail*, "For many parents it's a no-brainer: anything that will protect their daughters from cancer ... is worth the risks." However, at the same time, a small but vocal minority has expressed serious reservations about this program. On one hand, there are individuals who do not trust the medical establishment, the pharmaceutical companies, and/or the government. Others have expressed concerns that some girls will naively believe that this vaccine will protect them against

any and all sexually transmitted diseases and use this as a rationale or excuse for becoming sexually active at an early age. Still others have questioned the potential side effects from the vaccine, despite the fact that extensive clinical trials have shown that they are quite rare. Notwithstanding the concerns of some individuals, the vaccine was initially offered through school inoculation programs to young females in the Canadian provinces of Newfoundland and Labrador, Prince Edward Island, Nova Scotia, and Ontario. However, by September 2008, all of the other provinces in Canada had decided to implement this program. The real benefits of the program (hopefully an enormous reduction in cervical cancer) may not be known for several decades; in the meantime, the debate will continue. Also, since the vaccine does not protect against all strains of human papillomavirus, it is essential that women continue to get an annual Pap test.

the immunogenic domain (Fig. 12.10). If this argument has validity, it is possible that short peptides that mimic epitopes (antigenic determinants) will be immunogenic and could be used as vaccines (peptide vaccines).

However, there are certain limitations to using short peptides as vaccines:

- To be effective, an epitope must consist of a short stretch of contiguous amino acids, which does not always occur naturally.
- The peptide must be able to assume the same conformation as the epitope in the intact viral particle.
- A single epitope may not be sufficiently immunogenic.

Foot-and-Mouth Disease

Potential epitopes of the soluble antigenic FMDV VP1 were identified from the X-ray crystallographic structure, and chemically synthesized domains of the protein were tested as candidate peptide vaccines. Peptides corresponding to amino acids 141 to 160, 151 to 160, and 200 to 213, which are located near the C-terminal end of VP1, and amino acids 9 to 24, 17 to 32, and 25 to 41, which are located near the N-terminal end of VP1, were each bound to a separate inert carrier protein (keyhole limpet hemocyanin) and injected into guinea pigs (Fig. 12.11). Very small peptides are usually rap-

FIGURE 12.10 Generalized envelope-bound protein with external epitopes (1 to 5) that might elicit an immune response.

Exterior

Membrane

Interior

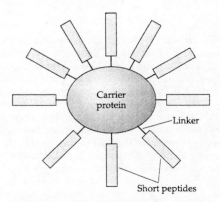

FIGURE 12.11 Structure of a peptide vaccine composed of identical short peptides bound to a carrier protein.

idly degraded unless they are bound to the surface of a larger carrier molecule. A single inoculation with peptide 141 to 160 elicited sufficient antibody to protect animals against subsequent challenges with FMDV. By contrast, inoculation with complete VP1 or peptide 9 to 24, 17 to 32, or 25 to 41 yielded lower levels of neutralizing antibodies.

In an additional experiment, a longer peptide consisting of amino acids 141 to 158 joined to amino acids 200 to 213 by two proline residues elicited high levels of neutralizing antibodies in guinea pigs, even when it was injected without any carrier protein. This "two-peptide" molecule was more effective than either of the single peptides alone and prevented FMDV proliferation in cattle, as well as in guinea pigs.

Although these results were promising, the amount (dose) of peptide material that had to be used to elicit an immunological response was approximately 1,000 times the amount of inactivated FMDV needed to elicit the same response. To overcome this problem, DNA encoding FMDV VP1 peptide 142 to 160 was linked to the gene encoding a highly immunogenic carrier molecule, hepatitis B virus core antigen (HBcAg). When the gene for this fusion protein was expressed in either *E. coli* or animal cells in culture, the protein molecules self-assembled into stable "27-nm particles," with the FMDV VP1 peptide located on the outer surface of the particle. These particles are highly immunogenic in laboratory animals. Therefore, HBcAg may be an effective carrier molecule for such short synthetic peptides. A comparison of the immunogenicities in guinea pigs of a variety of FMDV peptide vaccines, all of which contained the VP1 peptide 142 to 160 sequence, revealed that a fusion protein containing HBcAg and FMDV VP1 amino acids 142 to 160 was approximately 1/10 as immunogenic as inactivated FMDV particles, 35 times more immunogenic than a fusion protein containing *E. coli* β-galactosidase and FMDV VP1 amino acids 137 to 162, and 500 times more immunogenic than the free synthetic peptide composed of amino acids 142 to 160. Because synthetic peptides fused to HBcAg do not interfere with the assembly of the 27-nm hepatitis B virus-like particles, and because these particles are nearly as immunogenic as the intact virus from which the synthetic peptide was derived, this approach may become a general method for the delivery of peptide vaccines.

Malaria

The genus *Plasmodium* consists of approximately 125 known species of parasitic protozoa, 5 of which are known to infect humans and cause malaria. The *Plasmodium* life cycle is very complex. Sporozoites from the saliva of a biting female mosquito are transmitted to either the blood or the lymphatic system and then migrate to the liver and invade liver cells (hepatocytes) (Fig. 12.12). The parasite buds off the hepatocytes in merosomes containing hundreds or thousands of merozoites. These merosomes lodge in pulmonary capillaries and slowly disintegrate there, generally over 2 or 3 days, releasing merozoites. The merozoites invade the red blood cells, where the parasite divides several times to produce new merozoites, which then leave the red blood cells and travel within the bloodstream to invade new red blood cells. The parasite eventually forms gametocytes, which may be ingested by feeding mosquitoes. Fusion of the gametes that develop from gametocytes leads to the formation of new sporozoites in the mosquito that can infect new individuals, spreading the disease.

In the life cycle of the malaria parasite, it is the asexual blood-stage multiplication that is responsible for most of the acute symptoms of the disease. In areas where malaria is endemic, some individuals show considerable resistance to the disease despite the fact that when their blood is examined they are found to carry the parasite. This resistance to the worst symptoms of malaria was shown to be a result of an "antibody-dependent cellular-inhibition" mechanism that inhibits parasite development. In other words, some individuals who were infected with the malaria parasite made antibodies against a parasite protein that prevented the growth of the parasite. Following a detailed study, it was determined that the protective antibodies targeted merozoite surface protein 3. When this protein was examined in different strains of *Plasmodium*, it was observed that while the N-terminal part of the protein varied considerably from one strain to another, the C-terminal end of the protein was highly conserved among the various isolates of the parasite. It was therefore decided to chemically synthesize peptides that corresponded to small portions of the C terminus of merozoite surface protein 3. Human antibodies from individuals who were resistant to the parasite were affinity purified based upon their interaction with one or more of these peptides. The antibodies that bound to the peptides were then tested in an antibody-dependent cellular-inhibition assay. Antibodies directed against peptides B, C, and D (Fig. 12.13) had a major inhibitory effect on parasite growth. Based on the ability of peptides B, C, and D to bind to and select protective antibodies, a peptide representing amino acid residues 181 to 276 of merozoite surface protein 3 was chemically synthesized. This peptide is currently being tested in clinical trials as a novel malaria vaccine. While more research needs to be done, in the future, synthetic peptide vaccines could become highly specific, relatively inexpensive, safe, and effective alternatives to traditional vaccines.

Genetic Immunization: DNA Vaccines

Delivery

A novel strategy that elicits an antibody response without the introduction of an antigen has been developed. In this case, the gene encoding an antigenic protein is introduced into cells of a target animal, where the antigen is synthesized (Table 12.3). In the initial experiments, gold microprojectiles

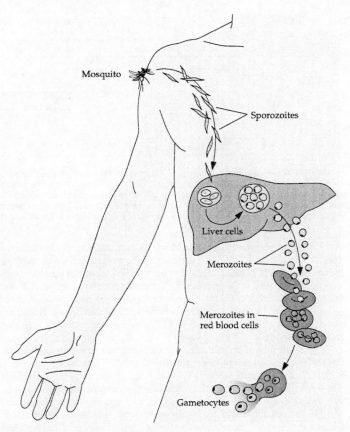

Mosquito

Sporozoites

Liver cells

Merozoites

Merozoites in
red blood cells

Gametocytes

FIGURE 12.12 Infection of an individual with *Plasmodium falciparum* (a malaria-causing parasite) introduced by a mosquito.

were coated with *E. coli* plasmid DNA carrying an antigen gene under the transcriptional control of an animal virus promoter. A biolistic system was used to deliver the microprojectiles into cells in the ears of mice (see chapter 18 for a more detailed description of the biolistic system). Other workers introduced cloned cDNAs into mouse cells by injecting large amounts of the plasmid carrying the target DNA directly into the muscles of test animals. However, effective "genetic immunization" by direct injection into muscles (100 μg per mouse) requires 3 to 4 orders of magnitude more DNA than the biolistic delivery system (10 to 100 ng per mouse). One distinctive feature of genetic immunization is that the costly and time-consuming procedure of either purifying an antigen or creating a recombinant vaccine delivery vehicle is bypassed. Moreover, proteins produced by this procedure are more likely to be correctly posttranslationally modified than are proteins that are produced by different host organisms.

An advantage of genetic immunization, besides bypassing the need for purified protein antigens, is that it can trigger a response against only the

FIGURE 12.13 Schematic representation of *Plasmodium falciparum* merozoite surface protein 3 and peptides corresponding to portions of the C terminus. The peptides, labeled A to F, are drawn to scale, with the numbers above the whole protein indicating the amino acid number (counting from the N terminus). The "final peptide" is currently being tested in clinical trials for efficacy as a malaria vaccine.

protein encoded on the plasmid and not against the plasmid itself. In addition, when plasmid DNA is introduced into a mammalian system, only those genes (or cDNAs) under the control of eukaryotic regulatory signals will be transcribed and translated. Antibiotic resistance genes for maintaining the plasmid in *E. coli* will not be transcribed or translated, and the same vector can be used to deliver different proteins to an individual at the same time, or the administration of the same gene can be repeated a number of times.

The feasibility of genetic immunization has been examined in detail. In one series of experiments, mice were injected in the quadriceps of both legs with an *E. coli* plasmid carrying the cDNA for influenza A virus nucleoprotein under the transcriptional control of either a Rous sarcoma virus or a cytomegalovirus promoter. Although the expression of the nucleoprotein was too low to detect, nucleoprotein-specific antibodies were observed in the blood of the test mice 2 weeks after the initial injection. In comparison to control mice, the nucleoprotein-injected mice were significantly protected against the lethal effects of influenza virus infection (Fig. 12.14). Moreover, the nucleoprotein-injected mice were also protected against a different strain of influenza virus. This cross-protection is in sharp contrast to traditional influenza virus vaccines, which are directed against surface antigens of the virus, so that each vaccine is specific to a single strain of

TABLE 12.3 Advantages of genetic immunization over conventional vaccines

Cultivation of dangerous agents is not required.

Since genetic immunization does not utilize any viral or bacterial strains, there is no chance that an attenuated strain will revert to virulence.

Since no organisms are used, attenuated organisms that many cause disease in young or immunocompromised animals are not a problem.

Approach is independent of whether the microorganism is difficult to grow or attenuate.

Production is inexpensive because protein does not need to be produced or purified.

Storage is inexpensive because of the stability of DNA.

One plasmid could encode several antigens/vaccines, or several plasmids could be mixed together and administered at the same time.

FIGURE 12.14 Survival of DNA-immunized mice. Injected mice were immunized with DNA that contained the influenza A virus nucleoprotein gene under the control of the Rous sarcoma virus promoter on an *E. coli* plasmid. The control mice were injected with plasmid DNA only. The x axis represents the number of days after the animals were challenged with the live influenza virus.

influenza virus. In addition, traditional vaccines work only as long as the antigens on the surface of the virus do not change. Unfortunately, the genes for the surface antigens mutate at a high rate, which creates significant differences among strains. Although core components of the virus, such as the nucleoprotein, are relatively invariant, they can activate the immune system by a mechanism that is different from that of surface antigens.

The fate of the introduced DNA is not known, and it could have the undesirable effect of integrating into the genome of the host cell, possibly disrupting an important gene. However, this risk is currently considered to be extremely low. It is more likely that the DNA will exist for a short period as a nonreplicating extrachromosomal element before it is degraded. To date, genetic immunization has been used primarily to induce immune responses in animals, and to a more limited extent in humans, against a number of pathogenic organisms, including influenza A virus, human immunodeficiency virus (HIV) type 1, bovine herpesvirus 1, rabies virus, *Plasmodium* species (which cause malaria), hepatitis B virus, hepatitis C virus, bovine rotavirus, bovine respiratory syncytial virus, pseudorabies virus, FMDV, Newcastle disease virus, *Clostridium tetani* (which causes tetanus), and *Mycobacterium tuberculosis* (which causes tuberculosis). Several human clinical trials using DNA vaccines are currently ongoing.

One of the problems with the use of DNA vaccines in large animals and humans compared to mice is that the transfection efficiency of introduced plasmid DNA is often insufficient to generate a protective immune response. One approach to deliver foreign DNA to animal cells utilizes biodegradable microscopic (0.3- to 1.5-µm) polymeric particles with a cationic surface that binds the plasmid DNA (Fig. 12.15). Plasmid DNA is bound to the surfaces of these "microparticles" and is slowly released over a period of 2 to 3 weeks after inoculation of an animal. Using microparticles, it was possible to achieve the same biological effect as with naked DNA with about 250-fold less DNA, demonstrating the potential of this approach. In addition, the level of antibodies induced by the expression of

FIGURE 12.15 Schematic representation of the binding of plasmid DNA to the cationic surface of a polymeric microparticle.

plasmid-encoded genes bound to microparticles was significantly enhanced by (i) addition of the vaccine adjuvant aluminum phosphate and (ii) the use of nanoparticles 0.05 μm in diameter that were coated with poly-L-lysine. In contrast to naked DNA, DNA bound to microparticles induced potent cytotoxic T-lymphocyte responses at a low dose.

To date, most DNA vaccines have been delivered either by intramuscular or intradermal injection. Although these vaccines can induce a potent immune response, they do not induce mucosal immunity. Mucosal immunity can prevent pathogens from entering the body, while systemic immunity deals with pathogens only once they are inside the body. This is an important consideration because mucosal surfaces, including the respiratory, intestinal, and urogenital tracts, are the major sites of transmission of many infectious diseases. However, because of the protective barriers of the mucosal surfaces, traditional antigen-based vaccines are largely ineffective unless they are administered with specific agents that penetrate or bind to the mucosa, i.e., mucosal adjuvants.

Mucosal immunity induces a separate and distinct response from systemic immunity. The antibodies produced as part of the mucosal immune response restrict not only mucosal pathogens, but also microorganisms that initially colonize mucosal surfaces and then cause systemic disease. Many mucosal vaccines are live attenuated organisms that infect mucosal surfaces and are effective at inducing mucosal responses. Of these, oral polio vaccines and both attenuated *Salmonella enterica* serovar Typhi Ty21a and *Vibrio cholerae* vaccines are licensed for use in humans.

DNA vaccines that are designed for delivery to mucosal surfaces are similar in principle to those used for intramuscular or intradermal delivery. To increase plasmid uptake and decrease its subsequent degradation, various methods of formulating DNA have been tried. For example, cationic (positively charged) liposomes have been used to deliver DNA (which has a negatively charged phosphate backbone) to the respiratory tract, and DNA entrapment in biodegradable microparticles has been used for the oral delivery of foreign DNA. Moreover, to improve the potency of DNA vaccines for humans, a number of strategies have been devised, including using plasmids that, in addition to encoding a target gene, also express a cytokine(s), such as interleukin-2 (IL-2), IL-10, or IL-12 (which can act as an intercellular mediator in the generation of an immune response).

A range of systems, including liposomes, live vectors (bacteria and viruses), and a wide range of adjuvants that increase the immune response (bacterial toxins, carboxymethylcellulose, lipid derivatives, aluminum salts, and saponins), have been tried for delivery of DNA to different cell types. Of necessity, various optimization strategies are tested in mice before they are tried on larger animals and then on humans, with no guarantee that an approach that works well in mice will also be a successful strategy in humans. Nevertheless, given the many perceived advantages of genetic immunization over the use of conventional vaccines (Table 12.3), this has become a very active area of research. For example, electroporation has been used to increase the transfection of DNA encoding target antigens. With this approach, DNA is injected intramuscularly, and the skeletal muscle is immediately electrically stimulated with a pulse generator. Despite the fact that this procedure, which causes some patient discomfort, results in local tissue injury and inflammation, it is tolerated by patients without the need for any anesthesia, and there do not appear to be any long-term negative side effects to delivering DNA in this way. Most likely,

the electrical pulse increases the transfection efficiency of the added DNA, and it is becoming a method of choice for clinically administering DNA vaccines.

A modified strain of the invasive bacterium *Shigella flexneri* has been developed to facilitate the delivery of DNA into animal cells for genetic immunization (Fig. 12.16). *Shigella* can enter animal epithelial cells, escaping the phagocytic vacuole, and the bacterium can direct plasmid DNA to the nucleus of the host cell, where, if the introduced gene(s) contains a eukaryotic promoter, it is transcribed. *Shigella* is normally a pathogenic organism and would not be an acceptable DNA delivery system. Therefore, to use *Shigella,* it was first necessary to construct a nonpathogenic version of the wild-type organism by (1) engineering the bacterium to be toxin deficient and (2) making a deletion mutation in the *Shigella asd* gene, which encodes the enzyme aspartate β-semialdehyde dehydrogenase. This enzyme is normally involved in the synthesis of the bacterial cell wall constituent diaminopimelic acid; therefore, the mutant cannot grow unless diaminopimelic acid is added to the growth medium. *Shigella* strains with the *asd* mutation can invade animal epithelial cells and deliver their plasmid DNA; however, once present, the *Shigella* cells are unable to proliferate.

Determination of the safety of using *Shigella* as a vector for the delivery of DNA to animal cells must await the results of human trials; however, the results of experiments with guinea pigs are promising. The greatest potential advantage of this approach is that with the *Shigella* system, DNA for

MILESTONE

Protection against Foot-and-Mouth Disease by Immunization with a Chemically Synthesized Peptide Predicted from the Viral Nucleotide Sequence

J. L. BITTLE, R. A. HOUGHTEN, H. ALEXANDER, T. M. SHINNICK, J. G. SUTCLIFFE, R. A. LERNER, D. J. ROWLANDS, and F. BROWN
Nature 298:30–33, 1982

Since Jenner developed the first vaccine over 200 years ago, most human vaccines against viral diseases have included partially killed or attenuated preparations of the disease-causing, or a similar nonpathogenic, version of the virus. While this approach has been undeniably effective and prevents the spread of a number of viral diseases, it is clearly limited. For example, not all viruses can be grown in culture, which precludes the development of vaccines against these viruses; production of traditional vaccines is expensive and potentially dangerous; and not all viral diseases are preventable through the use of these traditional vaccines. With the advent of molecular biotechnology, alternative strategies were examined for developing safer, less expensive, and more effective vaccines that would not have the limitations of using whole viruses, killed or attenuated, as vaccines. Since vaccines immunize individuals by priming their immune systems, it was thought that for some viruses short synthetic peptides might elicit the same antibody response as the antigenic determinants normally found on the external surface of the virus. These peptides were designed with the identical linear sequence of amino acids that made up the viral antigenic determinant in the first place. Of course, this approach could be expected to work only when the amino acids of an antigenic region (epitope) were contiguous.

Bittle et al. isolated and characterized the viral RNA for FMDV and then determined the sequence of VP1, the major antigenic protein of the virus. Based on other experiments, they reasoned that the major antigenic determinants on VP1 would probably be found at either the N- or C-terminal end of the protein. They then chemically synthesized a series of peptides based on the amino acid sequences of the N and C termini, chemically linked these peptides to carrier proteins, and then used them to inoculate rabbits and guinea pigs. With peptides from the C-terminal end of VP1 as antigens, the treated animals synthesized antibodies that protected them against disease from whole foot-and-mouth disease virus. This work established the principle that a protein domain(s) is sufficient to induce antibodies that can neutralize intact virus particles, and hence a new type of vaccine, which after the initial stages of development does not utilize or depend upon the disease-causing virus, is possible.

FIGURE 12.16 Use of nonpathogenic *S. flexneri* to deliver foreign DNA to mammalian epithelial cells. A strain of *Shigella* with a deletion mutation in the *asd* gene, which encodes the enzyme β-semialdehyde dehydrogenase, is unable to proliferate and can be used as a live vector.

vaccination may be delivered orally, greatly simplifying the delivery of a variety of vaccines.

Some limitations of plasmid-based vaccines are (1) the necessity for strong promoters that function in vivo to selectively transcribe the introduced DNA, (2) low levels of foreign-gene expression resulting from differences in codon usage between the introduced gene (often of viral, bacterial, or parasitic origin) and the animal being inoculated, and (3) the presence of antibiotic resistance genetic marker genes on the plasmid vector. To avoid the use of antibiotic resistance marker genes, researchers have developed a series of *m*inimalistic *i*mmunogenically *d*efined *g*ene *e*xpression (MIDGE) vectors (Fig. 12.17). Following insertion of the gene of interest into a MIDGE

FIGURE 12.17 Use of a MIDGE vector to produce a capped linear DNA sequence containing the gene of interest, a promoter, an intron (which facilitates expression of the gene of interest), and a polyadenylation signal.

vector, the antibiotic resistance gene is excised from the vector, and an oligonucleotide cap is added specifically to both ends of the linearized DNA that contains only a promoter/intron, the gene of interest, and a polyadenylation signal. The remaining portion of the plasmid is degraded by exonucleases. The capped ends are resistant to exonuclease digestion. The purified, capped linear MIDGE vector is then used directly for transfection. These vectors have been used successfully as a substitute for plasmid vectors.

Vaccination of rhesus macaques (monkeys) with DNA encoding simian immunodeficiency virus proteins, followed by a booster with a modified vaccinia virus that encoded many of the same proteins, protected the monkeys against infection by simian immunodeficiency virus (Fig. 12.18). The DNA that was injected at 0 and 8 weeks expressed the simian immunodeficiency virus proteins Gag, Pol, Vif, Vpx, and Vpr, as well as the HIV type 1 proteins Env, Tat, and Rev. The recombinant vaccinia virus expressed the simian immunodeficiency virus proteins Gag and Pol and the HIV protein Env, all under the control of vaccinia virus promoters, and was administered at 24 weeks. The protection against simian immunodeficiency virus at 7 months after the booster with the recombinant modified vaccinia virus was much greater than protection with either treatment by itself. This procedure also confers immunity against a mucosal viral challenge. This feature is important because the site of entry of the virus into the simian host is effectively blocked. It is also noteworthy that the immunity was maintained for a long time.

Dental Caries

The gram-positive, facultatively anaerobic bacteria *Streptococcus mutans* and *Streptococcus sobrinus* are considered to be the primary causative agents of dental caries (tooth decay). These organisms colonize tooth surfaces and metabolize sucrose to produce lactic acid, which causes the tooth enamel to become vulnerable to decay. Sucrose is also used to produce a sticky, extracellular, dextran-based polysaccharide (glucan) that facilitates *Streptococcus* cells' adhering to one another and to tooth surfaces, forming plaque. It is the combination of plaque and acid that leads to tooth decay.

Two regions of one of the adhesion proteins found on the surfaces of *S. mutans* and *S. sobrinus* cells are important in the initial adherence of these bacteria to tooth surfaces: one sequence is rich in alanine residues, while the other is rich in proline residues. Another important component of the mechanism of tooth decay is the enzyme glucosyltransferase, which is responsible for the synthesis of glucan, an insoluble extracellular polymer

FIGURE 12.18 Vaccination regimen of rhesus monkeys with DNA containing simian immunodeficiency virus (SIV) genes and vaccinia virus carrying the same genes.

of glucose moieties. A DNA vaccine designed to prevent dental caries included the coding sequences for an alanine- and proline-rich peptide, as well as the C-terminal domain of a *Streptococcus* glucosyltransferase. This C-terminal domain is necessary for the binding of the glucosyltransferase to the bacterial cell surface. This DNA vaccine therefore encoded two separate peptides, both of which facilitate the binding of *Streptococcus* cells to the tooth surface. In an attempt to overcome the tendency of many DNA vaccines to induce only a weak immune response, the DNA vaccine construct contained two additional elements. First, the extracellular domain of cytotoxic T-lymphocyte antigen 4 (CTLA4), which binds to the B7 protein that is expressed on the surfaces of antigen-presenting cells, was included in the construct (Fig. 12.19). Second, the Fc region of an immunoglobulin G molecule, which can bind to the Fc receptor on the antigen-presenting cell, was included in this construct. The use of both of these peptides was designed to specifically target the multidomain fusion protein (Fig. 12.19) to immune system cells and thereby amplify the immune response and enhance the efficacy of the vaccine. In fact, rabbits immunized with this vaccine, either intranasally or intramuscularly, displayed a significantly enhanced, specific systemic and mucosal immune response compared to immunization with only the alanine- and proline-rich peptide fused to the C-terminal domain of glucosyltransferase. Moreover, it was subsequently shown that this DNA vaccine could provide significant protection against dental caries in rats that were challenged with *S. mutans* and *S. sobrinus*. Although the problem of delivering the DNA vaccine to humans still needs to be addressed so that its clinical efficacy can be tested, this is a very promising strategy that could be enormously beneficial to human populations.

FIGURE 12.19 Schematic representation of a multidomain protein encoded by a DNA vaccine. Two domains, the CTLA4 extracellular domain and the immunoglobulin G (IgG) Fc region, are designed to target the other two portions of the molecule, i.e., the glucosyltransferase C-terminal domain and the alanine-proline-rich peptide, to antigen-presenting cells.

Attenuated Vaccines

In some instances, genetic manipulation may be used to construct modified organisms (bacteria or viruses) that are used as live recombinant vaccines. These vaccines are either nonpathogenic organisms that have been engineered to carry and express antigenic determinants from a target pathogenic agent or engineered strains of pathogenic organisms in which the virulence genes have been modified or deleted. In these instances, as part of a bacterium or a virus, the important antigenic determinants are presented to the immune system with a conformation that is very similar to the form of the antigen in the disease-causing organism. Although successful in some cases, purified antigen alone often lacks the native conformation and elicits a weak immunological response.

Cholera

It is usually advantageous to develop a live vaccine, because they are generally much more effective than killed or subunit vaccines. The major requirement for a live vaccine is that no virulent forms be present in the inoculation material. With this objective in mind, a live cholera vaccine has been developed. Cholera, caused by the bacterium *V. cholerae*, is a fast-acting intestinal disease characterized by fever, dehydration, abdominal pain, and diarrhea. It is transmitted by drinking water contaminated with fecal matter. In developing countries, the threat of cholera is a real and significant health concern whenever water purification and sewage disposal systems are inadequate.

Since *V. cholerae* colonizes the surface of the intestinal mucosa, it was reasoned that an effective cholera vaccine should be administered orally and directed to this structure. With this in mind, a strain of *V. cholerae* was created with part of the coding sequence for the A_1 peptide deleted. This strain cannot produce active enterotoxin; therefore, it is nonpathogenic and is a good candidate for a live vaccine.

Specifically, in this experiment, a tetracycline resistance gene was incorporated into the A_1 peptide DNA sequence on the *V. cholerae* chromosome. This insertion inactivated the A_1 peptide activity and also made the strain resistant to tetracycline. Although the A_1 peptide sequence has been disrupted, the strain is not acceptable as a vaccine because the inserted tetracycline resistance gene can excise spontaneously, thereby restoring enterotoxin activity. Consequently, it was necessary to engineer a strain carrying a defective A_1 peptide sequence that could not revert (Fig. 12.20).

1. A plasmid containing the cloned DNA segment for the A_1 peptide was digested with the restriction enzymes ClaI and XbaI, each of which cut only within the A_1 peptide-coding sequence of the insert.
2. To recircularize the plasmid, an XbaI linker was added to the ClaI site and then cut with XbaI.
3. T4 DNA ligase was used to join the plasmid at the XbaI sites, thereby deleting a 550-base-pair segment from the middle of the A_1 peptide-coding region. This deletion removed 183 of the 194 amino acids of the A_1 peptide.
4. Then, by conjugation, the plasmid containing the deleted A_1 peptide-coding sequence was transferred into the *V. cholerae* strain carrying the tetracycline resistance gene within its A_1 peptide DNA sequence.

5. Recombination (a double crossover) between the remaining A_1 coding sequence on the plasmid and the tetracycline resistance gene-disrupted A_1 peptide gene on the chromosome replaced the chromosomal A_1 peptide-coding sequence with the homologous segment on the plasmid carrying the deletion.

6. After growth for a number of generations, the extrachromosomal plasmid, which is unstable in *V. cholerae,* was spontaneously lost.

7. Cells with an integrated defective A_1 peptide were selected on the basis of their tetracycline sensitivity. The desired cells no longer had the tetracycline resistance gene but carried the A_1 peptide sequence with the deletion.

A stable strain with an A_1 peptide sequence containing a deletion was selected in this way. This strain did not produce active enterotoxin but nevertheless retained all the other biochemical features of the pathogenic form of *V. cholerae;* that is, *V. cholerae* with an A_1 peptide containing a deletion is a good vaccine candidate because the bacterium that synthesizes only the A_2 and B peptides is as immunogenic as the native bacterium. When this strain was evaluated in clinical trials to test its effectiveness as a cholera vaccine, the results were equivocal. While the vaccine conferred nearly 90% protection against diarrheal disease in volunteers, it induced side effects in some of those who were tested. This strain may require modification at another chromosomal locus before it can be used as a vaccine.

Salmonella Species

Other attempts to engineer nonpathogenic strains of pathogenic bacteria that could be used as live vaccines have involved deletions in chromosomal regions that code for independent and essential functions. At least two deletions are preferred, because the probability that both sets of functions can be simultaneously reacquired is very small. It is assumed that a "doubly deleted" strain would have a limited ability to proliferate when it is used as a vaccine, thereby curtailing its pathogenicity while allowing it to stimulate an immunological response.

Strains of the genus *Salmonella* cause enteric fever, infant death, typhoid fever, and food poisoning. Therefore, an effective vaccine against these organisms is needed. Deletions in a number of different genes have been used to attenuate various *Salmonella* strains (Table 12.4). These mutations can be grouped into three basic categories: mutations in (1) biosynthetic genes, (2) regulatory genes, and (3) genes involved in virulence. In addition, strains with more than one deletion have been constructed. For example, one double-deletion strain has deletions in the *aro* genes, which encode enzymes involved in the biosynthesis of aromatic compounds, and in the *pur* genes, which encode enzymes involved in purine metabolism. These double-deletion strains, which can be grown on a complete and enriched medium that supplies the missing nutrients, generally establish only low-level infections, since their host cells contain only a very low level of the metabolites that they require for growth. Typically, their virulence is reduced by 100-fold or more. These attenuated *Salmonella* strains are effective oral vaccines for mice, sheep, cattle, chickens, and humans.

Deletion of the *dam* gene, which encodes DNA methylase, may be a highly effective approach to produce avirulent *Salmonella* strains. The *dam* gene is a master switch that regulates the expression of 20 to 40 different *Salmonella* regulatory proteins. Thus, when mice were immunized with

FIGURE 12.20 Strategy for deleting part of the cholera toxin A_1 peptide DNA sequence from a strain of *V. cholerae*. Note that the tetracycline resistance gene is introduced into the gene for the A1 peptide as part of a transposon. This construct no longer makes A1 peptide but cannot be used as a vaccine because it is possible for the transposon to be excised, with the result that A1 synthesis and pathogenicity are restored.

Dam-negative strains of *Salmonella*, they tolerated up to 10,000 times the normally lethal dose. Generally, pathogenic bacteria turn on many of their genes as briefly as possible to avoid detection and attack by the host's immune system. However, with Dam-negative strains, these genes are expressed for much longer periods, making it easier for the host immune system to detect and destroy the invading bacteria. Because many other

TABLE 12.4 Deleted genes and their functions in the development of attenuated strains of *Salmonella* spp.

Deleted gene	Gene function
galE	Synthesis of lipopolysaccharide; decrease toxicity from galactose
aroA, *aroC*, or *aroD*	Synthesis of chorismate, an aromatic amino acid precursor and a PABA precursor; PABA is involved in the synthesis of iron chelators
purA or *purE*	Synthesis of purines
asd	Peptidoglycan and lysine biosynthesis
phoP and *phoQ*	Regulation of acid phosphatases and genes necessary for survival in the microphage
cya	Encodes adenylate cyclase, which is involved in camp synthesis
crp	Enclosed camp receptor; regulates expression of proteins involved in transport and breakdown of carbohydrates and amino acids
cdt	Involved in tissue colonization by the bacterium
dam	Encodes DNA methylase; appears to be a master switch for 20–40 different virulence genes
htrA	Enclosed a stress-induced polypeptide; result in significantly reduced persistence in human tissues

cAMP, cyclic AMP; PABA, *p*-aminobenzoic acid.

gut-colonizing bacteria have *dam* genes, if this approach with *Salmonella* turns out to be as effective as is expected, it may be possible to utilize a similar protocol with a range of pathogenic bacteria.

Leishmania Species

Although the human immune system can respond to infections by protozoan parasites of the genus *Leishmania*, it has been difficult to develop an effective vaccine against these organisms. Attenuated strains of *Leishmania* are sometimes effective as vaccines; however, they often revert to virulence. Also, the attenuated parasite can persist for long periods in an infected but apparently asymptomatic individual. Such individuals can act as reservoirs for the parasite, which can be transferred to other people by an intermediate host. To overcome these problems, an attenuated strain of *Leishmania* that is unable to revert to virulence was created by targeted deletion of an essential metabolic gene, such as the one encoding dihydrofolate reductase–thymidylate synthase. In one of these attenuated strains, *Leishmania major* E10-5A3, the two dihydrofolate reductase–thymidylate synthase genes that are present in wild-type strains were replaced with the genes encoding resistance to the antibiotics G-418 and hygromycin. For growth in culture, it is necessary to add thymidine to the medium that is used to propagate the attenuated (but not the wild-type) strain. In addition, unlike the wild type, the attenuated strain is unable to replicate in macrophages in tissue culture unless thymidine is added to the growth medium (Fig. 12.21). Importantly, the attenuated strain survives for only a few days when inoculated into mice; in that time, it does not cause any disease. Moreover, this period is sufficient to induce substantial immunity against *Leishmania* in BALB/c mice after administration of the wild-type parasite (Fig. 12.22). Since the attenuated parasite did not establish a persistent infection or

FIGURE 12.21 Proliferation of wild-type and attenuated *L. major* in mouse macrophages. At time zero, macrophages were infected with the same amount of stationary-phase *L. major*. The wild-type parasite and the attenuated parasite in the presence of thymidine were able to proliferate, while the attenuated strain did not proliferate in the absence of thymidine in the medium. Adapted from Titus et al., *Proc. Natl. Acad. Sci. USA* **92**:10267–10271, 1995.

cause disease, even in the most susceptible strains of mice tested, it is considered to be a strong candidate vaccine. Following additional experiments with animals, it should be possible to test whether this attenuated parasite is effective as a vaccine in humans.

Herpes Simplex Virus

As with other pathogenic organisms that have been developed as live vaccines, portions of the HSV genome have been deleted. Initially, it was

FIGURE 12.22 Immunity to virulent *L. major* induced in BALB/c mice inoculated with attenuated *L. major*. At time zero, mice that were previously inoculated with attenuated *L. major* were challenged with virulent *L. major*, and the sizes of the parasite-induced lesions were measured at various times. Control mice were not vaccinated with attenuated *L. major*. Adapted from Titus et al., *Proc. Natl. Acad. Sci. USA* **92**:10267–10271, 1995.

thought that a strong immune response could be obtained only if the virus was able to replicate. However, several vaccines based on nonreplicating viruses induce an immune response. Developing an avirulent HSV is important, because subunit vaccines so far have been unsuccessful in inducing immunity against the virus. To prepare a safe and efficacious live HSV vaccine, two deletions at different locations in the viral genome were generated independently and then combined to form a double-deletion virus. This strain is unable to proliferate in host cells, and the probability that both sets of functions can be simultaneously reacquired is very small. This replication-defective strain induces protective immunity that can reduce acute viral shedding and latent infection.

Vector Vaccines

Vaccines Directed against Viruses

Vaccinia virus, in the form of a live vaccine, has led to the eradication of smallpox globally. Vaccinia virus is a member of the poxvirus family. This completely sequenced virus has a double-stranded DNA genome that contains 187 kilobase pairs (kb) and encodes approximately 200 different proteins. Vaccinia virus DNA replicates within the cytoplasm of infected cells. Cytoplasmic, rather than nuclear, replication and transcription are possible because vaccinia virus DNA contains genes for DNA polymerase, RNA polymerase, and the enzymes to cap, methylate, and polyadenylate messenger RNA (mRNA). Thus, if a foreign gene is inserted into the vaccinia virus genome under the control of a vaccinia virus promoter, it will be expressed independently of host regulatory and enzymatic functions. The virus can infect humans and many other vertebrates, as well as invertebrates.

In addition to having a broad host range, vaccinia virus is well characterized at the molecular level, is stable for years after lyophilization (freeze-drying), and is usually a benign virus. For these reasons, it is a strong candidate as a vector vaccine. The function of a vector vaccine is to deliver and express cloned genes encoding antigens that elicit neutralizing antibodies against pathogenic agents. Unfortunately, the vaccinia virus genome is very large and lacks unique restriction sites. Therefore, it is not possible to insert additional DNA directly into the viral genome. Of necessity, the genes for specific antigens must be introduced into the viral genome by in vivo homologous recombination.

1. The DNA sequence coding for a specific antigen, such as HBcAg, is inserted into a plasmid vector immediately downstream of a cloned vaccinia virus promoter and in the middle of a nonessential vaccinia virus gene, such as the gene for the enzyme thymidine kinase (Fig. 12.23A).
2. This plasmid is used to transfect thymidine kinase-negative animal cells in culture, usually chicken embryo fibroblasts, that have previously been infected with wild-type vaccinia virus, which produces a functional thymidine kinase.
3. Recombination between DNA sequences that flank the promoter and the neutralizing antigen gene on the plasmid and the homologous sequences on the viral genome results in the incorporation of the cloned gene into the viral DNA (Fig. 12.23B). Although the recombination event is rare, the absence of thymidine kinase

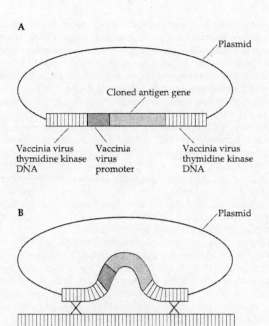

A

Plasmid

Cloned antigen gene

Vaccinia virus
thymidine kinase
DNA

Vaccinia
virus
promoter

Vaccinia virus
thymidine kinase
DNA

B

Plasmid

Vaccinia
virus DNA

Cloned
antigen gene

Vaccinia virus
promoter

Vaccinia virus
DNA

FIGURE 12.23 Method for the integration into vaccinia virus of a gene whose protein product, generally a viral antigen, elicits an immunological response. **(A)** Plasmid carrying a cloned expressible antigen gene. **(B)** A double-crossover event results in the integration of the antigen gene into vaccinia virus DNA.

activity in the host cells and the disruption of the thymidine kinase gene in the recombined virus render the host cells resistant to the otherwise toxic effects of bromodeoxyuridine. This selection scheme enriches for cell lines that carry a recombinant vaccinia virus.

4. The definitive selection of cells with a recombinant vaccinia virus is made by DNA hybridization with a probe for the antigen gene.

Since thymidine kinase-negative mutants of vaccinia virus arise spontaneously at a relatively high frequency of about 1 virus particle in 10^5 to 10^4, a selectable marker is often cotransferred with the target gene. This makes it much easier to distinguish a spontaneous thymidine kinase mutant from a mutant deliberately generated by homologous recombination. In other words, a virus with a spontaneous mutation would not carry the selectable marker, whereas a virus that underwent homologous recombination would.

The *neo* gene, which encodes the enzyme neomycin phosphotransferase II and confers resistance to the kanamycin analogue G-418, is often used as the selectable marker. This gene, unlike some other selectable markers, is quite stable once it is inserted into the vaccinia virus genome.

To avoid disrupting any vaccinia virus genes or the necessity of screening for selectable markers, a novel system has been devised in which every recombinant virus that can form a plaque will contain and express the target gene. Wild-type vaccinia virus contains a gene, *vp37*, that is responsible for the formation of plaques when the virus is grown on an animal cell monolayer (Fig. 12.24A). Deleting the *vp37* gene and replacing it with an *E. coli* marker gene (Fig. 12.24B) creates a vaccinia virus mutant that does not form plaques after 2 to 3 days of growth in cell culture. Target genes are introduced into the mutant vaccinia virus by homologous recombination with a transfer vector that carries the *vp37* gene, as well as the target gene (Fig. 12.24C). If homologous recombination between the non-plaque-forming mutant and the transfer vector occurs, the viruses that can form plaques have acquired the *vp37* gene. Also, the target gene is inserted into the vaccinia virus genome, and the selectable marker gene is lost. Since the *vp37* gene has been deleted in the mutant vaccinia virus, it is impossible for this mutation to revert to the wild type. Therefore, every virus that forms a plaque carries the desired construct. This procedure is simple and straightforward, is applicable to the cloning and expression of any target gene, does not require any extra marker genes, and does not disrupt any vaccinia virus genes.

A number of antigen genes have been successfully inserted into the vaccinia virus genome and subsequently expressed in animal cells in culture. These antigens include rabies virus G protein, hepatitis B surface antigen, Sindbis virus surface proteins, influenza virus NP and HA proteins, vesicular stomatitis virus N and G proteins, and HSV glycoproteins. Several recombinant vaccinia virus vehicles have been shown to be effective vaccines. For example, a recombinant vaccinia virus that expresses the HSV-1 gD (glycoprotein D) gene prevents herpes infections in mice. Another recombinant vaccinia virus that expresses the rabies virus surface antigen gene was able to elicit neutralizing antibodies in foxes, which are major carriers of rabies in Europe, and has been used in the field for some time, including in an area of approximately 10,000 km^2 in Belgium. The vaccinia–rabies virus glycoprotein recombinant virus vaccine that is presently on the market (Raboral) is a live viral vaccine containing 10^8 plaque-forming units (PFU), or live viral particles, per dose. It is constructed by insertion of the DNA copy coding for glycoprotein G of a rabies virus strain into the thymidine kinase gene of a strain of vaccinia virus. Once the vaccine is ingested by a fox, the vaccinia virus begins to replicate and express rabies glycoprotein G, which stimulates the development of immune responses to the rabies glycoprotein. This results in the production of neutralizing antibodies against the rabies virus in the immunized foxes. This immunity typically lasts about 12 months in cubs and 18 months in adult animals.

The use of vector vaccines constructed from vaccinia virus also offers the possibility of vaccinating individuals against several different diseases with one treatment. This may be achieved by using a recombinant vaccinia virus carrying cloned genes encoding a number of different antigens.

The timing of the production of a foreign protein whose gene is carried in a vaccinia virus depends on whether a vaccinia virus promoter functions

A Wild-type vaccinia virus genome

Left flank *vp37* gene Right flank

B Mutant vaccinia virus genome

Left flank *p7.5* Marker gene Right flank

C Vaccinia virus transfer vector

Left flank *vp37* gene *p7.5* MCS Target gene Right flank

FIGURE 12.24 (A) Portion of a wild-type vaccinia virus genome that contains the *vp37* gene that is responsible for plaque formation in host cells. **(B)** Portion of a mutant vaccinia virus genome in which the *vp37* gene has been replaced by a marker gene. **(C)** Portion of a vaccinia virus transfer vector. "Left flank" and "right flank" refer to the DNA sequences that immediately precede and follow the *vp37* gene in the wild-type vaccinia virus genome. The native *vp37* promoter is part of the *vp37* gene sequence (not shown). MCS is a multiple cloning site with seven unique restriction enzyme sites. *p7.5* is a strong early/late vaccinia virus promoter. The target gene is inserted into the multiple cloning site. Subsequently, homologous recombination between the transfer vector (C) and the genomic DNA of the mutant virus (B) results in the replacement of the *E. coli* marker gene with the *vp37* gene, together with a target gene.

during the early or late phase of the infection cycle, and the strength of the promoter determines the amount of an antigen that is produced. For the most part, late promoters for an 11-kilodalton (kDa) protein (p11) and the cowpox virus A-type inclusion protein (pCAE) have been used to achieve high levels of foreign-gene expression. When genes encoding several different foreign proteins are inserted into one vaccinia virus, each is placed under the control of a different vaccinia virus promoter to avoid the possibility of homologous recombination between different portions of the virus genome that might cause the cloned genes to be lost.

A live recombinant viral vaccine has several advantages over killed virus or subunit vaccines. First, the virus can express the authentic antigen(s) in a manner that closely resembles a natural infection. Second, the virus can replicate within the host, thereby amplifying the amount of antigen that activates the release of antibodies from B cells (humoral response) and stimulates the production of T cells (cell-mediated immune response).

A disadvantage of using a live recombinant viral vaccine is that vaccination of an immunosuppressed host, such as an individual with AIDS, can lead to a serious viral infection. One way to avoid this problem may be to

insert the gene encoding human IL-2 into the viral vector. IL-2 enhances the response of the T cells of the immune system, enabling the recipient to limit the proliferation of the viral vector, and thereby decreases the possibility of an unwanted infection.

If the proliferation of vaccinia virus has deleterious effects in certain patients, it would be helpful to kill or inhibit it after vaccination. One approach is to create an interferon-sensitive vaccinia virus—wild-type vaccinia virus is relatively resistant to interferon—whose proliferation is curtailed. Such a virus vector would be susceptible to drug intervention if complications from vaccination with vaccinia virus vectors arose.

The basis of the resistance of vaccinia virus to interferon was not known until a vaccinia virus open reading frame (K3L) was found to encode a 10.5-kDa protein that has an amino acid sequence that is very similar to that of a portion of the 36.1-kDa host cell eukaryotic initiation factor 2a (eIF-2a). The N-terminal regions of both of these proteins contain 87 amino acids that are nearly identical. Moreover, this shared sequence contains a serine residue, amino acid 51, which in eIF-2a is normally phosphorylated by interferon-activated P1 kinase. When this serine residue in eIF-2a is phosphorylated in interferon-treated cells, protein synthesis, and therefore viral replication, is inhibited. Thus, vaccinia virus may avoid inhibition by interferon because the K3L protein acts as a competitive inhibitor of eIF-2a phosphorylation (Fig. 12.25). Therefore, deletion of all or a portion of the K3L gene from vaccinia virus should make the virus sensitive to interferon. A K3L-negative mutant of vaccinia virus was constructed by PCR mutagenesis of the K3L gene carried on a plasmid, followed by homologous recombination to replace the wild-type K3L sequence with the modified version. When the wild-type and mutant versions of vaccinia virus were tested for sensitivity to interferon, the mutant was 10 to 15 times more sensitive to interferon than was the wild-type version (Fig. 12.26). Reinsertion of the wild-type K3L sequence into the mutant virus restored the level of interferon sensitivity found in the wild type. This indicates that K3L is indeed involved in the interferon resistance phenotype of vaccinia virus. This work is an important step in the development of safer vaccinia virus vectors. Moreover, other interferon-resistant viruses may contain sequences comparable to K3L and therefore may be amenable to the construction of interferon-sensitive deletion mutants. Other, comparable approaches to the creation of attenuated strains of vaccinia virus have been developed. For example, a strain of vaccinia virus, constructed to have a mutation in the B8R gene, which encodes an interferon viroreceptor, is less pathogenic for mice than the parental viral strain.

Currently, several veterinary vaccinia virus-based vaccines have been licensed, and clinical studies to test their efficacies in preventing a number of human infectious diseases are under way. This technology is based in part on the development of an attenuated version of the vaccinia virus strain that had previously been used in the eradication of smallpox. To avoid any risk of the vector itself becoming a source of disease, some genetic information was removed from the virus genome so that the viral vector was highly attenuated. This attenuated virus has been used to express a number of viral antigens with the expectation that the recombinant virus would be an effective live vaccine. Protection has been achieved by cloning glycoproteins from porcine pseudorabies virus, hemagglutinin glycoproteins from equine influenza virus, a spike protein from the SARS virus, and a polyprotein of Japanese swine encephalitis virus and then vac-

FIGURE 12.25 Competitive inhibition of the interferon-stimulated phosphorylation (inhibition) of eIF-2a by protein K3L, which is encoded by vaccinia virus and is nearly identical to a portion of eIF-2a. **(A)** In the presence of interferon, a kinase is activated that phosphorylates eIF-2a molecules and thereby prevents them from functioning. **(B)** When vaccinia virus protein K3L is also present, it is phosphorylated instead of the eIF-2a, so the eIF-2a remains active. The thickness of the arrows represents the relative flux through each pathway.

cinating humans to prevent transmission of these viruses. Based on the success of these attenuated vaccinia virus vaccines, it has been proposed that this virus be considered a general delivery system for a wide range of proteins.

For mass vaccination campaigns in developing countries, it would be advantageous to be able to deliver live vaccines in a simple, expeditious, and cost-effective manner. In addition, with mucosally transmitted pathogens, such as HIV, traditional vaccination routes may not induce mucosal immune responses sufficient to provide protective immunity. One possible alternative to traditional vaccination is aerosol immunization, which is potentially safer, easier, and less expensive to administer. To this end, researchers tested the abilities of two attenuated vaccinia virus-based vectors to be delivered effectively by aerosol immunization. In fact, it was found that aerosol delivery was both safe and effective, yielding long-lasting systemic and mucosal immune responses when delivered to rhesus macaques (monkeys). This approach still needs to be tested with humans; however, it could offer an effective means of inoculating large numbers of individuals in the future.

Although much of the work on the development of live viral vaccines has been done with vaccinia virus, other viruses, such as adenovirus, poliovirus, and varicella-zoster virus, are also being tested as potential vaccine vectors. Live attenuated poliovirus can be delivered orally, and such a mucosal vaccine, which is directed to receptors in the lungs or gastrointestinal tract, might also be useful against a range of diseases, including cholera, typhoid fever, influenza, pneumonia, mononucleosis, and rabies. However, the safety and efficacy of any apparently benign virus as a gene delivery and expression system must be firmly established before clinical trials are undertaken.

FIGURE 12.26 Sensitivity of wild-type (K3L⁺) and mutant (K3L⁻) vaccinia virus to interferon. Mouse L929 cells were pretreated with a mixture of mouse alpha and beta interferon for 24 hours before the virus was added. Plates without interferon had approximately 3×10^7 viral plaques per plate. Adapted from Paoletti and Tartaglia, U.S. patent 5,378,457, 1995.

Vaccines Directed against Bacteria

Since the discovery and subsequent widespread dissemination of antibiotics, only a modest amount of research has been directed toward the development of vaccines for bacterial diseases. However, there are good reasons for developing bacterial vaccines:

- Not all bacterial diseases are readily treated with antibiotics.
- The use of antibiotics over the last 40 years has resulted in the proliferation of bacterial strains that are resistant to several antibiotics.
- Reliable refrigeration facilities for the storage of antibiotics are not commonly available in many tropical countries.
- It is often difficult to ensure that individuals receiving antibiotic therapy undergo the full course of treatment.

Given the need to produce vaccines that will be effective against bacterial diseases, the question is, Which strategies are likely to be most effective? In instances where the disease-causing bacterium does not grow well in culture, the development of an attenuated strain is not feasible. For these bacteria, alternative approaches must be used. For example, *Rickettsia rickettsii*, a gram-negative obligately intracellular bacterium that causes Rocky Mountain spotted fever, does not grow in culture. In this case, a cloned 155-kDa protein that is a major surface antigen of *R. rickettsii* was used as a subunit vaccine and was found to protect immunized mice against infection by this disease-causing bacterium.

Tuberculosis. Tuberculosis, one of the most important infectious diseases worldwide, is caused by the bacterium *M. tuberculosis*. The bacterium can form lesions in any tissue or organ, which leads to cell death. The lungs are most commonly affected. Patients suffer fever and loss of body weight, and without treatment, tuberculosis is often fatal. It is estimated that approximately 2 billion people are currently infected with the organism and that approximately 2 million to 3 million deaths a year result from these infec-

tions. Over the past 50 years, antibiotics have been used to treat patients infected with *M. tuberculosis*. However, numerous multidrug-resistant strains of *M. tuberculosis* are now prevalent. In the United States, among HIV patients infected with an antibiotic-resistant strain of *M. tuberculosis*, there is a 50% mortality rate within 60 days. Consequently, a bacterial disease that was thought to be under control has become a serious public health problem in many parts of the world.

Currently, in some countries, bacillus Calmette-Guérin (BCG), an attenuated strain of *Mycobacterium bovis* that was developed between 1906 and 1919, is used as a vaccine against tuberculosis. However, the use of this vaccine has some drawbacks. First, live BCG cells can cause tuberculosis in immunocompromised individuals, such as AIDS patients. Second, individuals treated with BCG respond positively to a common tuberculosis diagnostic test, which makes it impossible to distinguish between individuals infected with *M. tuberculosis* and those inoculated with BCG cells. For these reasons, the BCG strain is not approved for use in a number of countries, including the United States.

In an attempt to determine whether a safer and more effective vaccine against tuberculosis might be developed, the extent of the immunoprotection elicited by purified *M. tuberculosis* extracellular proteins was examined. Following growth of the bacterium in liquid culture, 6 of the most abundant of the approximately 100 secreted proteins (Fig. 12.27) were purified. Each of these proteins was used separately and then in combination to immunize guinea pigs. The immunized animals were then challenged with an aerosol containing approximately 200 cells of live *M. tuberculosis*—a large dose for these animals. The animals were observed for 9 to 10 weeks before their lungs and spleens were examined for the presence of disease-causing organisms. In these experiments, some of the purified protein combinations provided a slightly lower level of protection against weight loss, death, and infection of lungs and spleen than did the live BCG vaccine. Prominent among the proteins that provided protection was the *M. tuberculosis* major secretory protein, a 30-kDa mycolytransferase also known as α-antigen, or antigen 85B. However, a DNA vaccine encoding

FIGURE 12.27 Schematic representation of the development of a multiprotein subunit vaccine for tuberculosis. The six most abundant secreted proteins from *M. tuberculosis* are purified from the growth medium and then tested for the ability to induce antibodies in guinea pigs. The immunized animals are subsequently challenged with *M. tuberculosis*.

FIGURE 12.28 The plasmid construct used to transform BCG to make it a more effective vaccine. The plasmid is isolated from *E. coli* cells and then introduced into BCG by electroporation. *ori* E, *E. coli* origin of replication; *ori* M, *Mycobacterium* origin of replication; Hygr gene, hygromycin resistance gene (and its promoter); P and α-antigen, the promoter and the coding region of the 30-kDa secreted protein.

this protein was even less effective than the purified secreted protein. While this and possibly other *M. tuberculosis*-secreted proteins might eventually be part of a safe and efficacious vaccine for the prevention of tuberculosis in humans, it is necessary to develop a suitable delivery system for them. In theory, the optimal delivery system for an antigen that provides protection against tuberculosis should be (1) able to multiply in the mammalian host, (2) nonpathogenic, and (3) able to express and secrete the protective antigen. All of these requirements are satisfied by the available BCG strain. Therefore, an *E. coli*–mycobacterium shuttle vector that contained the gene for the 30-kDa protein (α-antigen) under the control of its own promoter was introduced into two different BCG strains (Fig. 12.28). Transformed cells produced 2.0- to 5.4-fold more 30-kDa protein than did nontransformed cells. In addition, despite the fact that the introduced genes were plasmid encoded and therefore potentially unstable, transformed cells continued to express a high level of 30-kDa protein after the vaccination of a test animal. In agreement with the hypothesis that the extracellular proteins of intracellular organisms are key immunoprotective molecules, guinea pigs immunized with transformed BCG strains had significantly fewer bacilli in their lungs and spleens. In addition, there were smaller and fewer lesions in their lungs, spleens, and livers, and the survival of the animals was significantly increased, compared with animals vaccinated with a nontransformed BCG strain (Fig. 12.29). This is the first report of a vaccine against tuberculosis that is more potent than the currently available commercial vaccine. This vaccine is currently in clinical trials; if it is successful, it could save tens of thousands of lives. Moreover, it is possible to prepare dried preparations of BCG in which individual bacteria form rod-like structures, 1 to 4 μm long and 0.2 to 0.4 μm in diameter, that may serve as the basis for a live bacterial vaccine that is delivered as an aerosol, thereby facilitating the inoculation of newborn infants.

Bacteria as Antigen Delivery Systems

Antigens that are located on the outer surface of a bacterial cell are more likely to be immunogenic than are those in the cytoplasm. Thus, one strategy

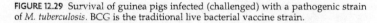

FIGURE 12.29 Survival of guinea pigs infected (challenged) with a pathogenic strain of *M. tuberculosis*. BCG is the traditional live bacterial vaccine strain.

is to place a neutralizing antigen from a pathogenic bacterium on the surface of a live nonpathogenic bacterium. Flagella are made up of filaments of a single protein called flagellin. Under a microscope, they appear as conspicuous threadlike structures on the outer surfaces of some bacteria. If the flagella of a nonpathogenic organism could be made to carry a specific epitope from a pathogenic bacterium, protective immunogenicity might be easily achieved.

This strategy was used to engineer a cholera vaccine (Fig. 12.30). A synthetic oligonucleotide specifying an epitope of the cholera toxin B subunit was inserted into a portion of the *Salmonella* flagellin gene that varies considerably from one strain to another (hypervariable segment). The construct was then introduced into a flagellin-negative strain of *Salmonella*. The epitope, which consisted of amino acid residues 50 to 64 of the cholera toxin B subunit, was shown previously to elicit antibodies directed against intact cholera toxin. The chimeric flagellin functioned normally. Furthermore, the epitope was present at the flagellum surface. Immunization of mice by intraperitoneal injections of approximately 5×10^6 live or formalin-killed "flagellum-engineered" bacteria elicited high levels of antibodies directed against both the peptide, i.e., amino acids 50 to 64, and the intact cholera toxin molecule. Two or three different epitopes can be inserted into a single *Salmonella* flagellin gene, thereby creating a multivalent bacterial vaccine.

Attenuated *Salmonella* strains can be administered orally, which would enable them to deliver a range of bacterial, viral, and parasite antigens to the mucosal immune system. For this purpose, the choice of the promoter that drives the transcription of the foreign antigen is important. If too strong a promoter is used, the metabolic load might constrain bacterial proliferation. Moreover, unlike a closed system, such as a fermentation vessel, shifting the temperature or adding specific metabolites to induce foreign-gene expression is not possible when the bacterial vector is added to a host animal. On the other hand, promoters that respond to environmental signals may provide effective means of controlling the expression of the foreign antigen gene. For example, the *E. coli nirB* promoter, which is

FIGURE 12.30 Using *Salmonella* as an antigen delivery system and a flagellin–antigen fusion protein for presenting the antigen to the host immune system. A flagellin-negative strain of *Salmonella* was transformed with a plasmid containing a synthetic oligonucleotide specifying an epitope of the cholera toxin B subunit inserted into a hypervariable region of a *Salmonella* flagellin gene.

regulated by both nitrite and the oxygen tension of the environment, becomes active under anaerobic conditions. In one series of experiments, the *nirB* promoter was used to direct the expression of the nontoxic immunogenic fragment C of *C. tetani* toxin (tetanus toxin) in an attenuated strain of *Salmonella*. It is estimated that more than 1 million deaths per year in the developing world are the result of *C. tetani* infections. When the engineered *Salmonella* strain was grown aerobically in culture, tetanus toxin fragment C was not synthesized; however, following oral administration of the bacterium to test mice, fragment C was produced, and the animals generated antibodies against the peptide. Thus, the engineered *Salmonella* strain has potential as a live oral tetanus vaccine.

The spiral-shaped, gastrointestinal, and microaerophilic gram-negative bacterium *Helicobacter pylori* is widely distributed among human populations. It is believed to be the causative agent for a number of gastrointestinal diseases, including chronic gastritis, peptic ulcers, gastric lymphoma, and gastric cancer. Among infected individuals, which includes more than half of the world's population, about 10% are at risk of developing peptic ulcers. In recent years, the medical treatment for peptic ulcers has changed from antacids to antibiotics and proton pump inhibitors. The antibiotics eradicate the *H. pylori* infection, while the proton-pump inhibitors block the enzyme hydrogen–potassium ATPase, preventing the production of acid from the parietal cells at the gastric mucosa, which facilitates the healing of the mucosa.

Unfortunately, *H. pylori* is resistant to a number of commonly used antibiotics, including metronidazole, amoxicillin, erythromycin, and clarithromycin. Treatment of *H. pylori* requires multidrug regimens because the organism resides in a layer of mucus that acts as a barrier to antibiotic penetration. In addition, the necessary course of antibiotic treatment is too expensive for populations of less developed countries.

Colonization of the gastrointestinal tract by *H. pylori* is facilitated by the action of an *H. pylori*-encoded urease. This enzyme hydrolyzes urea to carbon dioxide and ammonia, thereby neutralizing stomach acid, making it possible for the bacterium to survive, bind, and function in the host. Urease is a cytosolic and surface-exposed nickel metalloenzyme and is one of the most abundantly expressed proteins in *H. pylori*. The enzyme comprises two subunits, A and B, that assemble into a complex $[(\alpha\beta)3]4$ supramolecular structure. Subunit B is more antigenic, making it a possible

FIGURE 12.31 Schematic representation of an attenuated strain of *S. enterica* serovar Typhi transformed with a plasmid encoding *H. pylori* urease subunits A and B under the transcriptional control of a *Salmonella* promoter (*P*). The arrow indicates the direction of transcription.

vaccine candidate. To develop a vaccine that protects individuals against *H. pylori* infections, the genes encoding *H. pylori* urease subunits A and B were constitutively expressed under the control of a *Salmonella* promoter in a genetically deleted (attenuated) strain of *S. enterica* serovar Typhi (Fig. 12.31). Neither immunization with urease-expressing *S. enterica* serovar Typhi alone nor immunization with the purified urease enzyme plus an adjuvant conferred protection against challenge with a mouse-adapted strain of *H. pylori*. On the other hand, a vaccination protocol that combined both urease-expressing *S. enterica* serovar Typhi and urease plus an adjuvant was protective. While the success of this approach remains to be established in humans, these initial results are nevertheless encouraging and give hope that a human vaccine against *H. pylori* will be developed in the near future.

SUMMARY

Traditionally, vaccines have been either inactivated or attenuated infectious agents (bacteria or viruses) that are injected into an antibody-producing organism to produce immunity. There are a number of drawbacks to these vaccines. For example, not all pathogenic organisms can be grown to the large volumes needed to make a vaccine, there are safety concerns when large volumes of pathogenic organisms are being handled, attenuated strains may revert to the infectious state, inactivation may be incomplete, and shelf life is often dependent on refrigeration.

Recombinant DNA technology has been used in various ways to create reliable vaccines. Immunologically active, noninfectious agents are produced by deleting the genes that cause virulence; with this deletion, a live vaccine would never be able to revert to the infectious form. A gene(s) that encodes the major antigenic determinant(s) from a pathogenic organism can be cloned into the genome of a benign carrier organism (usually a virus or bacterium), which can be used as a vaccine without concern that any pathogenic organisms are present. The genes or segments of genes that encode the major antigenic determinants of pathogenic organisms can be cloned into expression vectors, and large amounts of the product can be harvested, purified, and used as a vaccine. With the last strategy, complete genes produce subunit vaccines, and cloned domains of the major antigenic determinants produce peptide vaccines. Peptide vaccines may also be produced by chemical peptide synthesis. As an alternative to using cloned antigenic proteins or peptides for inoculation, DNA constructs encoding the antigenic protein or peptide may be utilized. These DNA constructs may be delivered directly to animals or humans.

REFERENCES

Agarwal, K., and S. Agarwal. 2008. *Helicobacter pylori* vaccine: from past to future. *Mayo Clin. Proc.* 83:169–175.

Amara, R. R., F. Villinger, J. D. Altman, S. L. Lydy, S. P. O'Neil, S. I. Staprans, D. C. Montefiore, Y. Xu, J. G. Herndon, L. S. Wyatt, M. A. Candido, N. L. Kozyr, P. L. Earl, J. M. Smith, H.-L. Ma, B. D. Grimm, M. L. Hulsey, J. Miller, H. M. McClure, J. M. McNicholl, B. Moss, and H. L. Robinson. 2001. Control of a mucosal challenge and prevention of AIDS by a multiprotein DNA/MVA vaccine. *Science* 292:69–74.

Audran, R., M. Cachat, F. Lurati, S. Soe, O. Leray, G. Corradin, P. Druilhe, and F. Spertini. 2005. Phase I malaria vaccine trial with a long syn- thetic peptide derived from the mero- zoite surface protein 3 antigen. *Infect. Immun.* 73:8017–8026.

Bittle, J. L., R. A. Houghten, H. Alexander, T. M. Shinnick, J. G. Sutcliffe, R. A. Lerner, D. J. Rowlands, and F. Brown. 1982. Protection against foot-and-mouth dis- ease by immunization with a chemi- cally synthesized peptide predicted from the viral nucleotide sequence. *Nature* 298:30–33.

Blancou, J., M. P. Kieny, R. Lathe, J. P. Lecoq, P. P. Pastoret, J. P. Soulebot, and P. Desmettre. 1986. Oral vaccina- tion of the fox against rabies using a live recombinant vaccinia vaccine. *Nature* 322:373–375.

Blasco, R., and B. Moss. 1995. Selection of recombinant vaccinia viruses on the basis of plaque forma- tion. *Gene* 149:157–162.

Boothroyd, J. C., P. E. Highfield, G. A. M. Cross, D. J. Rowlands, P. A. Lowe, F. Brown, and T. J. R. Harris. 1981. Molecular cloning of foot and mouth disease virus genome and nucleotide sequences in the structural protein genes. *Nature* 290:800–802.

Charles, I., and G. Dougan. 1990. Gene expression and the development of live enteric vaccines. *Trends Biotechnol.* 8:117–121.

Chatfield, S. N., I. G. Charles, A. J. Makoff, M. D. Oxer, G. Dougan, D. Pickard, D. Slater, and N. F.

Fairweather. 1992. Use of the *nirB* promoter to direct the stable expression of heterologous antigens in *Salmonella* oral vaccine strains: development of a single-dose oral tetanus vaccine. *Bio/Technology* 10:888–892.

Chow, M., R. Yabrov, J. Bittle, J. Hogle, and D. Baltimore. 1985. Synthetic peptides from four separate regions of the poliovirus type 1 capsid protein VP1 induce neutralizing antibodies. *Proc. Natl. Acad. Sci. USA* 82:910–914.

Cichutek, K. 2000. DNA vaccines: development, standardization and regulation. *Intervirology* 43:331–338.

Clarke, B. E., S. E. Newton, A. R. Carroll, M. J. Francis, G. Appleyard, A. D. Syred, P. E. Highfield, D. J. Rowlands, and F. Brown. 1987. Improved immunogenicity of a peptide epitope after fusion to hepatitis B core protein. *Nature* 330:381–384.

Corbett, M., W. M. Bogers, J. L. Heeney, S. Gerber, C. Genin, A. Didierlaurent, H. Oostermeijer, R. Dubbes, G. Braskamp, S. Lerondel, C. E. Gomez, M. Esteban, R. Wagner, I. Kondova, P. Mooij, S. Ball-Jhagjhoorsingh, N. Beenhakker, G. Koopman, S. van der Burg, J.-P. Kraehenbuhl, and A. Le Pape. 2008. Aerosol immunization with NYVAC and MVA vectored vaccines is safe, simple, and immunogenic. *Proc. Natl. Acad. Sci. USA* 105:2046-2051.

Cremer, K. J., M. Mackett, C. Wohlenberg, A. L. Notkins, and B. Moss. 1985. Vaccinia virus recombinant expressing herpes simplex virus type 1 glycoprotein D prevents latent herpes in mice. *Science* 228:737–740.

Da Costa, X. J., C. A. Jones, and D. M. Knipe. 1999. Immunization against genital herpes with a vaccine virus that has defects in productive and latent infection. *Proc. Natl. Acad. Sci. USA* 96:6994–6998.

DiMarchi, R., G. Brooke, C. Gale, V. Cracknell, T. Doel, and N. Mowat. 1986. Protection of cattle against foot-and-mouth disease by a synthetic peptide. *Science* 232:639–641.

Ferguson, M. 1991. Progress towards rabies control. *Trends Biotechnol.* 9:7–11.

Finkelstein, A., and R. F. Silva. 1989. Live recombinant vaccines for poultry. *Trends Biotechnol.* 7:273–277.

Flexner, C., A. Hugin, and B. Moss. 1987. Prevention of vaccinia virus infection in immunodeficient mice by vector-directed IL-2 expression. *Nature* 330:259–262.

Gómez-Duarte, O. G., D. Bumann, and T. F. Meyer. 1999. The attenuated *Salmonella* vaccine approach for the control of *Helicobacter pylori*-related diseases. *Vaccine* 17:1667–1673.

Heithoff, D. M., R. L. Sinsheimer, D. A. Low, and M. J. Mahan. 1999. An essential role for DNA adenine methylation in bacterial virulence. *Science* 284:967–970.

Horwitz, M. A., B.-W. E. Lee, B. J. Dillon, and G. Harth. 1995. Protective immunity against tuberculosis induced by vaccination with major extracellular proteins of *Mycobacterium tuberculosis*. *Proc. Natl. Acad. Sci. USA* 92:1530–1534.

Horwitz, M. A., G. Harth, B. J. Dillon, and S. Maslesa-Galic. 2000. Recombinant bacillus Calmette-Guérin (BCG) vaccines expressing the *Mycobacterium tuberculosis* 30-kDa major secretory protein induce greater protective immunity against tuberculosis than conventional BCG vaccines in a highly susceptible animal model. *Proc. Natl. Acad. Sci. USA* 97:13853–13858.

Horwitz, M. A., and G. Harth. 2003. A new vaccine against tuberculosis affords greater survival after challenge than current vaccine in the guinea pig model of pulmonary tuberculosis. *Infect. Immun.* 71:1672-1679.

Jia, R., J. H. Guo, M. W. Fan, Z. Bian, Z. Chen, B. Fan, F. Yu, and Q. A. Xu. 2006. Immunogenicity of CTLA4 fusion anti-caries DNA vaccine in rabbits and monkeys. *Vaccine* 24:5192-5200.

Kaper, J. B., H. Lockman, M. M. Baldini, and M. M. Levine. 1984. A recombinant live oral cholera vaccine. *Bio/Technology* 2:345–349.

Kaper, J. B., H. Lockman, M. M. Baldini, and M. M. Levine. 1984. Recombinant nontoxinogenic *Vibrio cholerae* strains as attenuated cholera vaccine candidates. *Nature* 308:655–658.

Kaper, J. B., J. G. Morris, Jr., and M. M. Levine. 1995. Cholera. *Clin. Microbiol. Rev.* 8:48–86.

Kaslow, D. C., S. N. Isaacs, I. A. Quakyi, R. W. Gwadz, B. Moss, and D. B. Keister. 1991. Induction of *Plasmodium falciparum* transmission-blocking antibodies by recombinant vaccinia virus. *Science* 252:1310–1313.

Kirnbauer, R., F. Booy, N. Cheng, D. R. Lowy, and J. T. Schiller. 1992. Papillomavirus L1 major capsid protein self-assembles into virus-like particles that are highly immunogenic. *Proc. Natl. Acad. Sci. USA* 89:12180-12184.

Koutsky, L. A., K. A. Ault, C. M. Wheeler, D. R. Brown, E. Barr, F. B. Alvarez, L. M. Chiacchierini, and K. U. Jansen. 2002. A controlled trial of a human papillomavirus type 16 vaccine. *N. Engl. J. Med.* 347:1645–1650.

Kupper, H., W. Keller, C. Kurz, S. Forss, H. Schaller, R. Franze, K. Strohmaier, O. Marquardt, V. G. Zaslavsky, and P. H. Hofschneider. 1981. Cloning of cDNA of major antigen of foot and mouth disease virus and expression in E. coli. *Nature* 289:555–559.

Lasky, L. A., D. Dowbenko, C. C. Simonsen, and P. W. Berman. 1984. Protection of mice from lethal herpes simplex virus infection by vaccination with a secreted form of cloned glycoprotein D. *Bio/Technology* 2:527–532.

Leitner, W. W., H. Ying, and N. P. Restifo. 2000. DNA and RNA-based vaccines: principles, progress and prospects. *Vaccine* 18:765–777.

Lewis, P. J., and L. A. Babiuk. 1999. DNA vaccines: a review. *Adv. Virus Res.* 54:129–188.

Londoño-Arcila, P., D. Freeman, H. Kleanthous, A. M. O'Dowd, S. Lewis, A. K. Turner, E. L. Rees, T. J. Tibbitts, J. Greenwood, T. P. Monath, and M. J. Darsley. 2002. Attenuated *Salmonella enterica* serovar Typhi expressing urease effectively immunizes mice against *Helicobacter pylori* challenge as part of a heterologousmucosal priming-parenteral boosting vaccination regimen. *Infect. Immun.* 70:5096–5106.

Lowe, R. S., P. M. Keller, B. J. Keech, A. J. Davison, Y. Whang, A. J. Morgan, E. Kieff, and R. W. Ellis. 1987. Varicella-zoster virus as a live vector for the expression of foreign genes. *Proc. Natl. Acad. Sci. USA* 84:3896–3900.

Manoj, S., L. A. Babiuk, and S. van Drunen Littel-van den Hurk. 2004. Approaches to enhance the efficacy of DNA vaccines. *Crit. Rev. Clin. Lab. Sci.* 41:1–39.

McCluskie, M. J., and H. L. Davis. 1999. Mucosal immunization with DNA vaccines. *Microbes Infect.* 1:685–698.

Mekalanos, J. J., and J. C. Sadoff. 1994. Cholera vaccines: fighting an ancient scourge. *Science* 265:1387–1389.

Michel, M.-L., H. L. Davis, M. Schleef, M. Mancini, P. Tiollais, and R. G. Whalen. 1995. DNA-mediated immunization to the hepatitis B surface antigen in mice: aspects of the humoral response mimic hepatitis B viral infection in humans. *Proc. Natl. Acad. Sci. USA* 92:5307–5311.

Miner, J. N., and D. E. Hruby. 1990. Vaccinia virus: a versatile tool for molecular biologists. *Trends Biotechnol.* 8:20–25.

Moss, B. 1991. Vaccinia virus: a tool for research and vaccine development. *Science* 252:1662–1667.

Nabel, G. J., and P. L. Felgner. 1993. Direct gene transfer for immunotherapy and immunization. *Trends Biotechnol.* 11:211–215.

Newton, S. M. C., C. O. Jacob, and B. A. D. Stocker. 1989. Immunoresponse to cholera toxin epitope inserted in *Salmonella* flagellin. *Science* 244:70–72.

Nussenzweig, R. S., and C. A. Long. 1994. Malaria vaccines: multiple targets. *Science* 265:1381–1383.

Oehen, S., H. Hengartner, and R. M. Zinkernagel. 1991. Vaccination for disease. *Science* 251:195–197.

Paoletti, E. 1996. Applications of pox virus vectors to vaccination: an update. *Proc. Natl. Acad. Sci. USA* 93:11349–11353.

Paoletti, E., and J. Tartaglia. January 1995. Interferon sensitive recombinant poxvirus vaccine. U.S. patent 5,378,457.

Rice, J., C. H. Ottensmeier, and F. K. Stevenson. 2008. DNA vaccines: precision tools for activating effective immunity against cancer. *Nat. Rev. Cancer* 8:108–120.

Sheridan, C. 2005. The business of making vaccines. *Nat. Biotechnol.* 23:1359–1366.

Singh, M., M. Briones, G. Ott, and D. O'Hagan. 2000. Cationic microparticles: a potent delivery system for DNA vaccines. *Proc. Natl. Acad. Sci. USA* 97:811–816.

Singh, S., S. Soe, J.-P. Mejia, C. Roussilhon, M. Theisen, G. Corradin, and P. Druilhe. 2004. Identification of a conserved region of *Plasmodium falciparum* MSP3 targeted by biologically active antibodies to improve vaccine design. *J. Infect. Dis.* 190:1010–1018.

Sizemore, D. R., A. A. Branstrom, and J. C. Sadoff. 1995. Attenuated *Shigella* as a DNA delivery vehicle for DNA-mediated immunization. *Science* 270:299–302.

Stover, C. K., V. F. de la Cruz, T. R. Fuerst, J. E. Burlein, L. A. Benson, L. T. Bennett, G. P. Bansal, J. F. Young, M. H. Lee, G. F. Hatfull, S. B. Snapper, R. G. Barletta, W. R. Jacobs, Jr., and B. R. Bloom. 1991. New use of BCG for recombinant vaccines. *Nature* 351:456–460.

Stranger-Jones, Y. K., T. Bae, and O. Schneewind. 2006. Vaccine assembly from surface proteins of *Staphylococcus aureus*. *Proc. Natl. Acad. Sci. USA* 103:16942–16947.

Tang, D.-C., M. DeVit, and S. A. Johnston. 1992. Genetic immunization is a simple method for eliciting an immune response. *Nature* 356:152–154.

Tartaglia, J., and E. Paoletti. 1988. Recombinant vaccinia virus vaccines. *Trends Biotechnol.* 6:43–46.

Titus, R. G., J. G. Gueiros-Filho, L. A. R. De Freitas, and S. M. Beverley. 1995. Development of a safe live *Leishmania* vaccine line by gene replacement. *Proc. Natl. Acad. Sci. USA* 92:10267–10271.

Ulmer, J. B., J. J. Donnelly, S. E., Parker, G. H. Rhodes, P. L. Felgner, V. J. Dwarki, S. H. Gromkowski, R. R. Deck, C. M. DeWitt, A. Friedman, L. A. Hawe, K. R. Leander, D. Martinez, H. C. Perry, J. W. Shiver, D. L. Montgomery, and M. A. Liu. 1993. Heterologous protection against influenza by injection of DNA encoding a viral protein. *Science* 259:1745–1749.

Weeratna, R. D., M. J. McCluskie, L. Comanita, T. Wu, and H. L. Davis. 2001. Optimization strategies for DNA vaccines. *Intervirology* 43:218–226.

Xu, Q. A., F. Yu, M. W. Fan, Z. Bian, Z. Chen, B. Peng, R. Jia, and J. H. Guo. 2007. Protective efficacy of a targeted anti-caries DNA plasmid against cariogenic bacteria infections. *Vaccine* 25:1191–1195.

Zakhartchouk, A. N., C. Sharon, M. Satkunarajah, T. Auperin, S. Viswanathan, G. Mutwiri, M. Petric, R. H.See, R. C. Brunham, B. B. Finlay, C. Cameron, D. J. Kelvin, A. Cochrane, J. M. Rini, and L. A. Babiuk. 2007. Immunogenicity of a receptor-binding domain of SARS coronavirus spike protein in mice: implications for a subunit vaccine. *Vaccine* 25:136–143.

Zimet, G. D., M. L. Shew, and J. A. Kahn. 2008. Appropriate uses of cervical cancer vaccine. *Annu. Rev. Med.* 59:223–236.

REVIEW QUESTIONS

1. Briefly describe a protocol for developing a vaccine against a toxin-producing bacterium.

2. What factors limit the usefulness of conventional vaccines?

3. As part of your work with an international animal health organization, you are given the task of developing a vaccine against a bovine virus that is the cause of tens of thousands of cattle deaths around the world annually. The viral genome consists of a 10-kb linear piece of single-stranded RNA with a poly(A) tail that encodes eight different proteins. The virus does not have a viral envelope, and the major antigenic determinant is the capsid protein viral protein 2. Outline an experimental strategy to develop a vaccine against this virus.

4. Discuss the development of peptide vaccines that are directed against viruses.

5. What is vaccinia virus, and how can it be used to produce unique live recombinant vaccines?

6. As an employee of the World Health Organization, you have to decide on the best strategy for eradicating rabies in wild animal populations. Assuming that you must choose between a peptide and a vaccinia virus-based vaccine, select one type of vaccine and justify your choice.

7. Discuss the advantages of a live recombinant viral vaccine over killed and subunit vaccines.

8. Discuss some of the different strategies that have been used to produce vaccines against cholera.

9. How would you develop a subunit vaccine against HSV?

10. How can bacteria be used as part of a DNA vaccine delivery system?

11. How can vaccinia virus be made more sensitive to interferon? Explain.

12. How would you develop a vaccine against *S. aureus?*

13. Suggest several methods that you could use to deliver DNA for genetic immunization to animal cells.

14. What are MIDGE vectors, and how can they be used to facilitate genetic immunization?

15. How would you develop a vaccine against human papillomavirus?

16. How would you develop an effective DNA vaccine against dental caries?

17. How would you improve the traditional vaccine against tuberculosis?

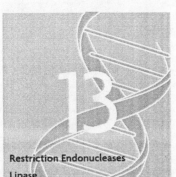

Synthesis of Commercial Products by Recombinant Microorganisms

T O DATE, MOLECULAR BIOTECHNOLOGY RESEARCH has focused largely on the production of a range of different proteins, including enzymes that are used commercially. However, recombinant DNA techniques can also be used to enhance the production of low-molecular-weight compounds, such as vitamins, amino acids, dyes, precursors of biopolymers, and antibiotics. In these cases, the host microorganism is engineered to become a factory for the production of useful metabolites.

Restriction Endonucleases

Recombinant DNA technology would not be possible without a ready supply of different restriction endonucleases. Currently, more than 300 different restriction endonucleases are commercially available, with worldwide sales in 2007 in the range of $350 million. These enzymes occur naturally in many different microorganisms, including species that are aerobic, anaerobic, photosynthetic, diazotrophic, mesophilic, thermophilic, psychrophilic, and either slow or fast growing. For each of these organisms, a detailed fermentation protocol—specifying the temperature, pH, medium composition, and oxygen tension—has to be developed and optimized to achieve the maximum yield of the target restriction enzyme. To avoid having to maintain a large number of different microorganisms, stock a very wide range of microbial growth medium components, design several different types of fermenters, and spend an inordinate amount of time developing optimal growth conditions for a large number of different organisms (one major supplier of restriction enzymes lists 265 different enzymes in its catalog), investigators often clone restriction endonuclease genes into *Escherichia coli*. Exclusive use of *E. coli* allows bioengineers to standardize the production conditions for all restriction endonucleases. In addition, *E. coli* cells grow rapidly to high cell densities and can be engineered to significantly overexpress each target restriction enzyme.

Although the technology for isolating and expressing foreign genes in *E. coli* and some other host organisms is well established, it should be remembered that the host organism is a living entity that can be dramatically

affected by the production or presence of a heterologous protein. For example, overexpression of a heterologous protein may drain the host organism of important metabolic resources and, as a result, adversely affect its growth. In addition, the presence of a heterologous protein may be lethal to the host. For example, restriction endonucleases digest DNA at sites that are present on all DNA molecules. As a result, an organism that expresses a cloned restriction endonuclease gene is likely to have its own DNA degraded unless a protection mechanism is present.

Microorganisms that make restriction endonucleases have evolved a self-protection system. Methylation of one or more of the bases of the DNA within the recognition sequence prevents the homologous restriction endonuclease from cutting the DNA at this site (Fig. 13.1A). Gram-negative microorganisms have an added mode of protection that entails localizing the restriction endonuclease within the periplasmic space and the methylation (modification) enzyme in the cell cytoplasm (Fig. 13.1B). This compartmentalization physically separates the restriction endonuclease from the DNA while ensuring that the modification enzyme has ready access to the chromosomal DNA. In addition to protecting the cell from the toxic effects of the restriction enzyme, this segregation provides a cellular defense against attack by any foreign DNA, such as DNA from a bacterial virus, that might enter the periplasm.

One way to circumvent the problem of host DNA degradation by heterologous restriction endonucleases is to clone and express the genes for both the restriction enzyme and its specific (cognate) modification enzyme in the host organism. Cloning both of these genes into the same organism is technically complex unless both the restriction endonuclease and methylation genes are close to each other on the chromosome. In addition, to prevent the digestion of the host DNA by the restriction endonuclease, it is imperative that, after transformation, the methylation activity be expressed prior to the production of the restriction endonuclease.

One of the first restriction enzyme genes to be cloned (into *E. coli*) encoded the enzyme PstI from *Providencia stuartii*, a gram-negative bacterium (Fig. 13.2). It is important to note that, for a particular genus and species, only some strains encode restriction enzymes. Therefore, in this strategy, in order to easily transform the host *E. coli* strain without degrading the input plasmid DNA, it was necessary to utilize an *E. coli* strain that was unable to synthesize the enzyme EcoRI.

FIGURE 13.1 (A) Protection of DNA from digestion by a restriction endonuclease by prior treatment with methylase, a methylating (modification) enzyme. The asterisks indicate the presence of a methylated base. **(B)** Cytoplasmic localization of modification enzyme (M) and periplasmic localization of restriction endonuclease (R) in gram-negative bacteria.

pBR322

P. stuartii DNA

HindIII

HindIII

T4 DNA ligase

Cloned
DNA

Transform into *E. coli*
Grow in liquid culture
Infect with bacteriophage λ

Only lysis-resistant colonies will grow

FIGURE 13.2 Method for cloning and selecting the gene for the restriction enzyme PstI. The *P. stuartii* chromosomal DNA is digested with HindIII and ligated into the HindIII site of plasmid pBR322. Transformants are grown in liquid medium before being infected with bacteriophage λ. The resistance of some transformants to lysis by λ is due to the presence and expression of a cloned PstI gene and its cognate methylation enzyme.

1. The chromosomal DNA from *P. stuartii* was digested with HindIII and ligated into the HindIII site on plasmid pBR322.
2. Following the introduction of the *P. stuartii* clone bank (library) into *E. coli* HB101 cells, transformants were grown in liquid medium before being infected with bacteriophage λ to test for the production of the restriction enzyme. When a restriction enzyme gene is expressed, the host cells become resistant to the lytic action of DNA bacteriophages such as λ because the restriction endonuclease extensively degrades the infecting bacteriophage DNA.

3. Transformants that were resistant to lysis by λ were grown, and samples were osmotically shocked to release the periplasmic proteins, which were assayed for PstI restriction enzyme activity.

4. Positive clones were assayed for PstI methylase activity.

One positive clone from this experiment contained, within a 4.0-kilobase-pair (kb) DNA fragment, an intact PstI restriction endonuclease and methylation operon, including the *P. stuartii* promoter. In this construct, the natural temporal order of synthesis—the methylation enzyme preceding the restriction endonuclease—was maintained. The level of the PstI restriction enzyme expressed in *E. coli* was approximately 10-fold higher than that in *P. stuartii*. As expected, PstI was localized in the periplasm, and the methylation enzyme was localized in the cytoplasm. Production of PstI using this *E. coli* clone is simpler and more efficient than production with *P. stuartii*.

Another strategy also has been used to isolate the genes for restriction and modification (methylation) enzyme systems. It was developed by a company that eventually became one of the world's leading suppliers of restriction enzymes and consists of the following steps.

1. A clone bank was made from the DNA of a donor organism that had a previously identified restriction endonuclease. The plasmid vector had at least one recognition site for the target restriction endonuclease.

2. The clone bank was introduced into *E. coli* by transformation. This step increased the amount of recombinant plasmid DNA and also allowed the expression of the modification enzyme.

3. Plasmid DNA was isolated from transformed cells that had been grown in liquid media under conditions that selected for the presence of the plasmid.

4. The plasmid DNA preparation was treated with the target restriction endonuclease.

5. *E. coli* cells were transformed with the restriction endonuclease-treated plasmid DNA preparation.

The rationale for this procedure is that the clones that carry and express the target modification enzyme will produce plasmid DNA that is resistant to digestion by the target restriction endonuclease because their DNA will be methylated at the recognition sites. For example, following transformation of *E. coli* by a pBR322–HindIII clone bank of *Desulfovibrio desulfuricans* DNA, plasmid DNA was isolated and digested with the restriction enzyme DdeI (Fig. 13.3). Plasmids that encode and express the DdeI modification enzyme are not digested by DdeI because the eight DdeI recognition sites of pBR322 are methylated. After the DdeI treatment, the remaining plasmid mixture is used to transform *E. coli*. Only intact circular plasmids yield transformants, and these carry the gene for a functional DdeI modification enzyme. All other plasmids are degraded by the restriction endonuclease. The resulting transformants must then be assayed for the DdeI restriction enzyme activity to determine which clones have the genes for both the modification enzyme and the restriction endonuclease. This strategy is effective for any restriction enzyme gene that is physically close to its modification enzyme gene—most restriction enzymes are encoded on the same operon as their cognate modification enzyme—and is cloned into a plasmid vector that has at least one recognition site for the target enzyme.

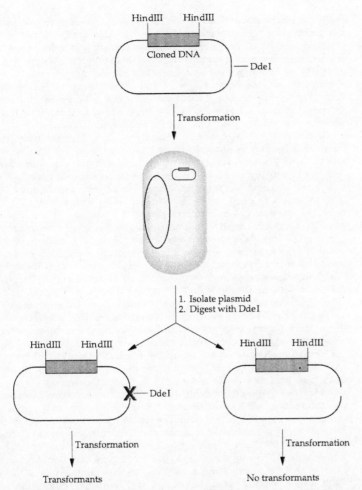

FIGURE 13.3 Scheme for cloning the DdeI modification enzyme. Plasmids with cloned *D. desulfuricans* DNA are used to transform *E. coli* cells. After the cells are grown in liquid culture, the plasmid DNA is isolated and digested with the restriction enzyme DdeI. Plasmids encoding the DdeI modification enzyme will be methylated at the DdeI restriction enzyme recognition site and will not be cut. The intact plasmid DNA is used to transform *E. coli* cells. The final transformants are assayed for the DdeI restriction enzyme and the corresponding methylase.

Lipase

Fatty stains are a persistent problem for the laundry industry. A combination of high temperature and high alkalinity can effectively emulsify and remove many fatty stains. However, these conditions often damage fabrics and also require large amounts of energy. On the other hand, the addition of lipases that are compatible with the wash conditions, such as the enzyme

produced by *Pseudomonas alcaligenes,* may provide an effective solution to this problem. Unfortunately, this enzyme is produced at such low levels that it is prohibitively expensive to use in the cleaning of laundry. Moreover, researchers have found it extremely difficult to overproduce the enzyme in a variety of heterologous hosts, including *Bacillus licheniformis, E. coli, Streptomyces lividans, Aspergillus niger,* and *Kluyveromyces lactis.* The difficulty in overexpressing the *P. alcaligenes* lipase may reflect the requirement for the simultaneous expression of another gene product that is involved in either the secretion or the stabilization of the bacterial lipase.

To isolate the lipase gene from *P. alcaligenes,* as well as any other gene whose expression was linked to lipase gene expression, the enzyme was first purified. The amino acid sequence of the N terminus was determined, and an oligonucleotide probe that corresponded to 11 amino acids from this region of the protein was synthesized. The oligonucleotide probe was used to screen a clone bank of *P. alcaligenes* DNA, with the result that a clone that contained all of the lipase gene and a portion of the additional gene was obtained. The DNA fragment encoding the lipase gene and a portion of the additional gene was used as a hybridization probe to screen another clone bank, with the result that the rest of the second gene was isolated. The two fragments were spliced together (Fig. 13.4), cloned into a broad-host-range expression vector, and used to transform *P. alcaligenes.* The lipase structural gene is called *lipA,* and the second (helper) gene is called *lipB.* When the vector was derived from a low-copy-number plasmid, the lipase activities of the transformants were four- to fivefold greater than that of the wild type, regardless of the presence or absence of the second gene *(lipB).* However, with a high-copy-number plasmid, the lipase activities of the transformants were about 20-fold greater than that of the wild type in the absence of the *lipB* gene and approximately 35-fold greater than that of the wild type in the presence of the *lipB* gene. Since the lipase is secreted into the growth medium, very little purification should be necessary before using it in laundry detergent. Rather, the cells must be removed, and then the growth medium should be concentrated. However, when the production of the growth of this recombinant organism was scaled up from 10 liters to 10,000 liters, considerably less lipase activity was found than was expected. This was attributed to the production, and lack of removal, of large amounts of carbon dioxide in the growth medium. Modification of some of the operating parameters of this large fermenter resulted in a significant decrease in the level of dissolved carbon dioxide and decreased inhibition of lipase accumulation. This work went a long way toward providing lipase of sufficient quality and in sufficient quantity for use in laundry detergent.

Small Biological Molecules

With recombinant DNA technology, it is possible to modify metabolic pathways of organisms either by introducing new genes or by altering existing ones. The goal is to create an organism with a novel enzymatic activity that can convert an existing substrate into a commercial compound that with current technology can be produced only by a combination of chemical treatments and fermentation steps. Early metabolic-engineering experiments typically modified one or two genes in a biosynthetic pathway. However, with the knowledge of the complete DNA sequences of many bacterial genomes and the global information on the expression of bacterial

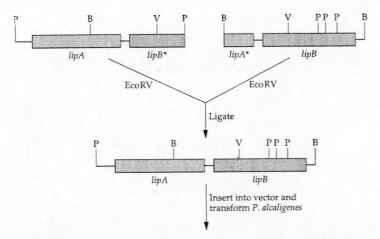

FIGURE 13.4 Splicing together portions of the lipase operon. P, PvuII; B, BclI; V, EcoRV. Partial genes are indicated by asterisks.

genes derived from studies that employ microarrays, proteomics, and metabolomics, it is possible to develop strategies to improve the yield of microbially produced molecules that involve the introduction or modification of an entire panel of related genes.

Synthesis of L-Ascorbic Acid

L-Ascorbic acid (vitamin C) is currently synthesized commercially by an expensive process starting with D-glucose that includes one microbial fermentation step and a number of chemical steps (Fig. 13.5). The last step in this process is the acid-catalyzed conversion of 2-keto-L-gulonic acid (2-KLG) to L-ascorbic acid. Biochemical studies of the metabolic pathways of a number of different microorganisms have shown that it may be possible to synthesize 2-KLG by a different pathway. For example, some bacteria (*Acetobacter, Gluconobacter,* and *Erwinia*) can convert glucose to 2,5-diketo-D-gluconic acid (2,5-DKG), and others (*Corynebacterium, Brevibacterium,* and *Arthrobacter*) have the enzyme 2,5-DKG reductase, which converts 2,5-DKG to 2-KLG.

The current procedure for synthesizing ascorbic acid could be improved by producing 2-KLG from glucose by cofermentation with suitable organisms. Unfortunately, cocultivation has problems of its own. For example, the two fermenting organisms might have different temperature and pH optima. The medium requirements and growth rates also might differ in such a way that the fermentation conditions are optimal for one organism and suboptimal for the other. This situation leads to the eventual "washout" (depletion or loss) of one of the organisms. Some of these incompatibilities may be overcome by utilizing a tandem fermentation process in which the two organisms are cultivated in succession (Fig. 13.6). Of course, this approach requires two separate fermentations rather than one, and if the organisms have different growth requirements, it is difficult to run the process on a continuous basis. Therefore, the best way to convert glucose into

FIGURE 13.5 Commercial synthesis of L-ascorbic acid. Except for the microbial conversion of D-sorbitol to L-sorbose, all the steps are chemical reactions. The microbial conversion is carried out by *Acetobacter suboxydans*, which produces the enzyme sorbitol dehydrogenase.

2-KLG would be to engineer a single microorganism that carried all of the required enzymes. The conversion of D-glucose to 2,5-DKG by *Erwinia herbicola* includes several enzymatic steps, whereas the transformation of 2,5-DKG to 2-KLG by a *Corynebacterium* sp. requires only one. Consequently, the simplest strategy for constructing a single organism that is able to convert D-glucose to 2-KLG is to isolate the 2,5-DKG reductase gene from the *Corynebacterium* sp. and express it in *E. herbicola*.

The first step in cloning the 2,5-DKG reductase gene from the *Corynebacterium* sp. involved purifying the enzyme and determining the sequence of the first 40 amino acids from the N-terminal end of the molecule. On the basis of the known amino acid sequence, two 43-nucleotide DNA hybridization probes, each corresponding to a different portion of the protein molecule, were synthesized. Because 71% of the nucleotides in the *Corynebacterium* sp. are either G or C, the probes were designed to include, where possible, a G or C in the third position of all codons, thereby minimizing the extent of the mismatch between the probe and the target DNA. This approach was taken because at the time that this work was done, mixed probes were not readily available.

A *Corynebacterium* DNA clone bank was screened with these two probes. Any clones that hybridized with only one of the probes were discarded. It was assumed that any DNA that interacted with only one probe was probably not the target DNA. A clone that hybridized with both probes was isolated and then sequenced; it contained the 2,5-DKG reductase gene. The DNA sequences that were upstream of the ATG start signal were

FIGURE 13.6 Biological production of 2-KLG. *Erwinia* has a set of three enzymes that synthesize 2,5-DKG from D-glucose. *Corynebacterium* has an enzyme that converts 2,5-DKG to 2-KLG. Thus, 2-KLG, which is the immediate precursor of L-ascorbic acid, can be produced from D-glucose either by cocultivating these two microorganisms or by genetically engineering *Erwinia* to express the enzyme from *Corynebacterium,* which converts 2,5-DKG to 2-KLG.

deleted and replaced with transcriptional and translational signals that function in *E. coli,* because the regulatory sequences from gram-positive microorganisms, such as *Corynebacterium* spp., are not efficiently utilized by *E. coli.* This construct expressed 2,5-DKG reductase activity in *E. coli* and subsequently was subcloned onto a broad-host-range vector, which was used to transform *E. herbicola,* which is able to use *E. coli* transcriptional and translational signals.

The transformed *Erwinia* cells were able to convert D-glucose directly to 2-KLG. The endogenous *Erwinia* enzymes, localized in the inner membrane of the bacterium, converted glucose to 2,5-DKG, and the cloned 2,5-DKG reductase, localized in the cytoplasm, catalyzed the conversion of 2,5-DKG to 2-KLG (Fig. 13.7). Thus, by genetic manipulation, the metabolic capabilities of two very dissimilar microorganisms were combined into one organism, which was able to produce the end product of the engineered metabolic pathway. This recombinant organism should be useful as a source of 2-KLG for the production of L-ascorbic acid, thereby replacing the first three steps of the currently used process (Fig. 13.5).

The commercial utility of the cloned 2,5-DKG reductase gene product might be improved by replacing certain amino acids of the enzyme to create mutants with increased catalytic activity and enhanced thermal stability. When the 2,5-DKG reductase gene was first isolated, the amino acid residues that contributed to the active site of this enzyme were not known.

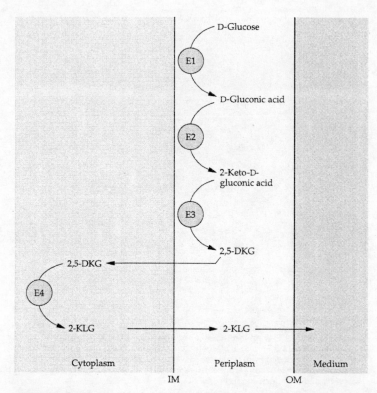

FIGURE 13.7 Conversion of D-glucose to 2-KLG by recombinant *E. herbicola*. The cellular locations of all of the component enzymes are indicated. The enzymes are denoted with the letter E and are numbered consecutively. Enzyme E4 is the introduced 2,5-DKG reductase. The major intermediates in the pathway are named. IM and OM denote the inner and outer membranes, respectively.

However, from the primary amino acid sequence, computer modeling predicted an enzyme structure with an eight-stranded α/β barrel (Fig. 13.8). This structure consisted of eight twisted parallel β-strands arranged close together, surrounded by eight α-helices that were joined to the β-strands through loops of various lengths. This folding pattern had previously been observed for 17 other enzymes whose crystal structures were known. By comparison with the structures of these other proteins, three of the loops that might be involved in substrate binding were identified (Fig. 13.8). Using oligonucleotide-directed mutagenesis, 12 different mutants, each with a single amino acid change in one of these loops, were constructed. Of the 12 mutants, 11 produced enzymes with a lower 2,5-DKG reductase specific activity than that of the native form of the enzyme. The 12th mutant, in which amino acid residue 192 was changed from glutamine to arginine, had approximately twice the activity of the native enzyme. Kinetic studies revealed that this increase in activity resulted from a 1.8-fold increase in the maximal rate of the enzyme-catalyzed reaction (V_{max}) and a 25% decrease in the Michaelis constant (K_m) of the enzyme-catalyzed reaction.

Substrate-binding loops

N terminus

FIGURE 13.8 Predicted structure of 2,5-DKG reductase. The solid arrows indicate β-stranded regions, the solid bars are α-helical regions, and the circles are amino acid residues either at the N or C terminus or involved in loops connecting the β-strands to the α-helices. The three loops that may be involved in substrate binding are indicated. Amino acid residue 192 is shown in yellow.

The reaction catalyzed by 2,5-DKG reductase utilizes reduced nicotin-amide adenine dinucleotide phosphate (NADPH) as a cofactor. However, the cellular concentration of reduced nicotinamide adenine dinucleotide (NADH) is usually about 10-fold greater than that of NADPH, while the financial cost of NADPH is about 10 times higher than that of NADH. To lower the cost of the bacterial production of ascorbic acid, it would be ben-eficial to engineer a version of 2,5-DKG reductase that used NADH instead of NADPH. The only structural difference between NADH and NADPH is the presence or absence of a phosphate group attached to the 2′ site of the adenine moiety. From the three-dimensional structure of 2,5-DKG reductase complexed with NADPH, it appears that 5 amino acid residues interact directly with the 2′ phosphate residue of NADPH. Using cassette mutagen-esis (Fig. 13.9), a total of 40 different mutants of this enzyme were con-structed; in each constructed mutant, 1 of the 5 amino acid residues that computer models suggested interacted with the 2′ phosphate residue was changed to a different amino acid. Following the expression, purification, and kinetic characterization of the 40 mutants in *E. coli*, it was observed that changing three of the five selected amino acids resulted in increases in 2,5-DKG reductase activity with NADH as the cofactor. In the best case, when the arginine residue at position 238 was changed to histidine, there was a sevenfold improvement over the wild type with NADH as a cofactor. Moreover, after two amino acid alterations were combined in one protein, an enzyme that showed even more activity with NADH included a change of the lysine residue at position 232 to glycine, as well as the change of arginine at position 238 to histidine. Also, when the best NADH-active mutant was combined with a double mutant which increased the binding of the substrate, even further improvements in activity with NADH were observed. The activity of the enzyme isolated from the final construct was 72 times higher than the activity of the wild-type enzyme. It now remains

2,5-DKG reductase gene

FIGURE 13.9 Mutagenesis of the *Corynebacterium* sp. 2,5-DKG reductase gene. The isolated gene, on a plasmid, was digested to remove a 57-bp DNA fragment. Then, chemically synthesized 57-bp DNA fragments that contained an alteration in the DNA sequence that coded for one of the amino acids to be changed was spliced into the gene in place of the original fragment. In addition, each 57-bp fragment (or mutagenesis cassette) contained a silent mutation that abolished a PstI site but did not alter the amino acid sequence. The silent mutation facilitated screening against the wild type.

to be seen whether this engineered enzyme can be used as the basis for the economically efficient biological synthesis of ascorbic acid.

Microbial Synthesis of Indigo

A number of bacteria, most notably *Pseudomonas* spp., have the ability to use a variety of organic compounds, such as naphthalene, toluene, xylene, and phenol, as their sole carbon source. In many instances, the genes encoding the enzymes for the degradation of these organic compounds are located on large, naturally occurring plasmids (typically 50 to 200 kb in size). Research on these bacteria often requires detailed genetic and biochemical studies, so that the genes encoding enzymes catalyzing important steps in the pathway can be targeted for modification. Occasionally, despite the original purpose of a study, an unexpected but useful discovery is made. For example, plasmid NAH7 has two separate and distinct operons that allow pseudomonads that contain this plasmid to grow on naphthalene as the sole carbon source. As a first step toward characterizing these genes, NAH7 plasmid DNA was digested with HindIII and the fragments were ligated with linear HindIII-digested plasmid pBR322. This clone bank was introduced into *E. coli* cells, and transformants were selected on the basis of their resistance to ampicillin and sensitivity to tetracycline. All

transformants were then tested for the production of nonvolatile metabolites that might result from the hydrolysis of radiolabeled naphthalene.

During the characterization of one of the transformants that had a 10.5-kb insert and could convert naphthalene to salicylic acid, it was observed that when the minimal growth medium contained tryptophan, it turned blue. A thorough analysis of the blue color revealed that the transformed *E. coli* cells were synthesizing the dye indigo. This synthesis was achieved in four steps (Fig. 13.10):

1. Conversion of tryptophan in the growth medium to indole by the enzyme tryptophanase, which is produced by the *E. coli* host cell
2. Oxidation of indole to *cis*-indole-2,3-dihydrodiol by naphthalene dioxygenase, which is encoded by the DNA that was cloned from the NAH7 plasmid
3. Spontaneous elimination of water
4. Air oxidation to form indigo

Thus, the combination of enzymes from two different pathways and two different organisms resulted in the synthesis of an unexpected compound, the dye indigo. In addition, introduction of the gene for the enzyme xylene oxidase, which is encoded in the TOL plasmid, can convert tryptophan to indoxyl, which then spontaneously oxidizes to indigo (Fig. 13.10).

FIGURE 13.10 Indigo biosynthesis from tryptophan in genetically engineered *E. coli*. Tryptophanase is an *E. coli* enzyme. In pathway A, the naphthalene dioxygenase is derived from the NAH plasmid; in pathway B, the xylene oxidase is from the TOL plasmid. *E. coli* transformants that synthesize indigo contain either pathway A or B, but not both pathways.

Indigo, a commercially important blue pigment that is used to dye both cotton and wool, was originally isolated from plants but is currently synthesized chemically. At present, approximately 13×10^6 kg of indigo, worth more than $250 million, is produced every year. Indigo, the coloring agent in blue jeans, is the largest-selling dye in the world. The ability to produce indigo from bacteria opens the possibility of developing an efficient and economical commercial microbial process for its production. This process would avoid the use of hazardous compounds, such as aniline, formaldehyde, and cyanide, which are needed in the chemical synthesis of indigo.

Despite the environmentally friendly nature of engineering bacteria to make indigo, at the present time, the chemical synthesis of the dye is less expensive, thwarting commercial schemes to produce indigo biologically. One approach to improving indigo production in *E. coli* involves engineering the host strain to overproduce tryptophan, the raw material for the process. However, despite improved efficiency when a tryptophan-overproducing *E. coli* strain is used, the overall process requires additional improvement before it is economically competitive with chemical synthesis.

Synthesis of Amino Acids

Amino acids are used extensively in the food industry as flavor enhancers, antioxidants, and nutritional supplements; in agriculture as feed additives; in medicine in infusion solutions for postoperative treatment; and in the chemical industry as starting materials for the manufacture of polymers and cosmetics (Table 13.1). It is estimated that more than 2.5 million tons of amino acids, worth more than $9 billion, were produced worldwide in 2008. L-Glutamic acid, which is used in the manufacture of the flavor enhancer monosodium glutamate, makes up around half of the total volume.

TABLE 13.1 Commercial applications of amino acids

Amino acid	Application(s)
Alanine	Flavor enhancer
Arginine	Therapy for liver diseases
Aspartic acid	Flavor enhancer; sweetener synthesis
Asparagine	Diuretic
Cysteine	Bread production; therapy for bronchitis; antioxidant
Glutamic acid	Flavor enhancer
Glutamine	Therapy for ulcers
Glycine	Sweetener synthesis
Histidine	Therapy for ulcers; antioxidant
Isoleucine	Intravenous solutions
Leucine	Intravenous solutions
Lysine	Feed additive; food additive
Methionine	Feed additive
Phenylalanine	Infusions; sweetener synthesis
Proline	Intravenous solutions
Serine	Cosmetics
Threonine	Feed additive
Tryptophan	Intravenous solutions; antioxidant
Tyrosine	Intravenous solutions; precursor for L-DOPA
Valine	Intravenous solutions

For the most part, amino acids are commercially produced either by extraction from protein hydrolysates or as fermentation products of either *Corynebacterium* or *Brevibacterium* spp., which are both nonsporulating gram-positive soil bacteria that secrete large amounts of amino acids into the growth medium. Traditionally, the productivity of these organisms has been improved by mutagenesis and subsequent screening for strains that overproduce certain amino acids. However, this way of developing new strains is slow and inefficient. By using detailed biochemical information about the enzymes that are involved in the biosynthesis of various commercially important amino acids, it is more expeditious to isolate and manipulate the specific genes encoding the key components of a particular pathway. However, this type of genetic engineering is not a simple matter. For example, the pathway(s) leading to the biosynthesis of certain amino acids contains a number of different enzymes, each of which may be either activated or inhibited by a number of metabolites present in the cell. This makes it difficult to know which enzyme(s) to manipulate in order to enhance the yield of the end product.

Because most broad-host-range plasmid vectors replicate only in gram-negative organisms, it is necessary to construct expression vectors that are specifically suited for *Corynebacterium* and *Brevibacterium* spp. Such cloning vehicles might take the form of *E. coli–Corynebacterium* shuttle vectors. The *E. coli* portion of the plasmid could encode resistance to the antibiotic tetracycline, chloramphenicol, or kanamycin. Because both *E. coli* and *Corynebacterium* spp. are susceptible to these antibiotics, they could be used as selectable markers in both organisms.

An efficient transformation protocol for *Corynebacterium glutamicum*, the species of *Corynebacterium* often used in these experiments, is still needed. Also, many *C. glutamicum* genes are not efficiently expressed in *E. coli*. Therefore, for selection schemes that depend on gene expression (e.g., complementation), the entire clone bank should be transformed into *C. glutamicum*. Unfortunately, the transformation frequency is very low when DNA is introduced into *C. glutamicum* by either direct transformation or electroporation. However, effective transformation of *C. glutamicum* is achieved when foreign DNA is introduced by conjugation or after the formation of protoplasts, i.e., after removal of the cell wall with lysozyme. The transformation of protoplasts is made possible by adding polyethylene glycol to facilitate the uptake of exogenous plasmid DNA.

Some progress has been made in increasing the amino acid output of *C. glutamicum*. For example, the synthesis of the essential amino acid tryptophan was enhanced by introducing into wild-type *C. glutamicum* cells a second copy of the gene encoding anthranilate synthetase, which is the rate-limiting enzyme in the normal tryptophan biosynthetic pathway (Fig. 13.11). The following protocol describes one way to isolate the anthranilate synthetase gene.

1. A library of *Brevibacterium flavum* chromosomal DNA was cloned into a *C. glutamicum–E. coli* shuttle vector and introduced into a mutant strain of *C. glutamicum* that produced no active anthranilic acid synthetase.
2. The mutant strain was unable to grow on minimal medium unless anthranilic acid was added; therefore, transformants were selected by their ability to grow in the absence of anthranilic acid.
3. The vector carrying the anthranilic acid synthetase gene was then transferred to a wild-type strain of *C. glutamicum*.

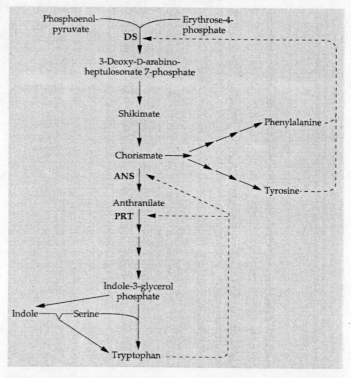

FIGURE 13.11 Simplified pathway and regulation of tryptophan biosynthesis in *C. glutamicum*. The abbreviations DS, ANS, and PRT represent the enzymes 3-deoxy-D-arabino-heptulosonate 7-phosphate synthase, anthranilate synthase, and anthranilate phosphoribosyltransferase, respectively. The solid lines represent the synthetic pathways. The dashed lines denote feedback inhibition. Indole is produced in a side reaction and is converted into tryptophan by the action of tryptophan synthase β.

The amounts of tryptophan produced in the mutant and wild-type *C. glutamicum* strains—one without and one with the vector carrying the cloned anthranilic acid synthetase gene—were measured (Table 13.2). The cloned gene did indeed restore most of the capacity of the mutant to synthesize tryptophan. Moreover, the effect of adding this gene to wild-type *C. glutamicum* was much more dramatic, with the synthesis of tryptophan being increased by approximately 130%. This level of overproduction reflects more efficient utilization of available precursor material. Thus, by cloning an additional gene of an amino acid biosynthesis pathway into an organism, it was possible to generate much more of the end product. An even higher level of tryptophan production was achieved when modified genes for the three key enzymes, 3-deoxy-D-arabino-heptulosonate 7-phosphate synthase, anthranilate synthase, and anthranilate phosphoribosyltransferase, were introduced into *C. glutamicum* cells (Fig. 13.11). The genes encoding these enzymes were mutagenized to render them insensitive to inhibition by the end product (feedback inhibition).

TABLE 13.2 Production of tryptophan under standard growth conditions by certain strains of *C. glutamicum*

Strain	Tryptophan concentration (mg/mL)
Mutant	0.00
Mutant with vector	0.34
Wild type	0.48
Wild type with vector	1.12

Adapted from Ozaki et al., U.S. patent 4,874,698, 1989.

An alternative to producing amino acids in *Corynebacterium* and *Brevibacterium* spp. is to produce them in *E. coli*, where both metabolic pathways and procedures for genetic manipulation are much better characterized. Its relative ease of manipulation makes *E. coli* an attractive host organism for this sort of metabolic engineering.

L-Cysteine, which is one of the most important amino acids in the pharmaceutical, food, and cosmetics industries, has traditionally been obtained by extracting it from acid hydrolysates of human hair and animal feathers. While a number of microorganisms are able to synthesize L-cysteine, high levels cannot be synthesized from glucose because L-cysteine feedback inhibits the enzyme serine (Ser) acetyltransferase, which catalyzes one of the steps in the biosynthesis of L-cysteine (Fig. 13.12). To try to remedy this situation, the methionine residue at position 256 in the *E. coli* serine acetyltransferase amino acid sequence was systematically changed to each of the other 19 amino acids. When *E. coli* was transformed with plasmids carrying *cysE* genes encoding altered serine acetyltransferase, several transformants with altered forms of serine acetyltransferase produced higher levels of L-cysteine than did the wild-type enzyme. Next, plasmids encoding the most effective serine acetyltransferase derivatives were used to transform a strain of *E. coli* that did not degrade L-cysteine. To improve on this modest success, complementary DNAs (cDNAs) encoding feedback inhibition-insensitive serine acetyltransferases from the plant *Arabidopsis thaliana* were expressed in a serine acetyltransferase-deficient and non-L-cysteine-utilizing *E. coli* strain. The transformants included several different strategies and produced a much higher level of L-cysteine than had previously been possible by merely manipulating the *E. coli* serine acetyltransferase gene. Whether the expression of this protein can be further improved and how this affects the synthesis of L-cysteine remain to be determined.

To rationally engineer a bacterium to modify its metabolism so that it overproduces a particular amino acid, it is essential to understand how many of the metabolic pathways of the bacterium are interrelated and regulated. Subsequent systematic reengineering of the metabolism of the organism can then be performed to achieve a much higher yield than would ever be possible by merely modifying one or two genes in the immediate biosynthetic pathway of a particular amino acid. At each stage in the development of the reengineered bacterium, it is possible to monitor the levels of a wide range of transcripts (using microarrays) and metabolites (metabolomics). Moreover, the mRNA and metabolite expression data allow the construction of a detailed computer model that can be used to predict the effects of other possible genetic manipulations on the production of the target amino acid. While this approach is relatively new, such

FIGURE 13.12 Biosynthesis of L-cysteine from L-serine and acetyl-CoA. The dashed arrow indicates feedback inhibition.

rational genetic engineering may be used to engineer bacterial strains for a variety of purposes, in addition to the production of specific amino acids.

To rationally engineer *E. coli* to overproduce L-valine, it was necessary to introduce a large number of mutations into the *E. coli* genome (Fig. 13.13). The flux from glucose to L-valine was first improved by abolishing feedback inhibition by L-valine of the enzyme that converts pyruvate to 2-acetolactate. Then, the subunits of this enzyme were overexpressed by replacing the endogenous promoter with a strong constitutive promoter. Next, the carbon flux toward L-valine was increased. The gene for the enzyme that converts L-threonine to 2-ketobutyrate was knocked out, as were the genes encoding enzymes that convert 2-ketoisovalerate to either pantothenate or L-leucine. In addition, some of the genes that encode enzymes that convert pyruvate to 2-acetolactate were amplified. Subsequently, the expression levels of the genes encoding enzymes that convert 2-acetolactate to L-valine via 2,3-dihydroxyisovalerate and 2-keto-isovalerate were all increased by modifying the regulatory regions of these genes. In addition, the *lrp* gene, encoding the leucine-responsive regulatory protein, was amplified, since some of genes in the L-valine pathway were under the positive transcriptional control of this protein. Finally, the expression of the two genes that encode proteins responsible for the export of L-valine from the bacterial cell was amplified, since it was thought that a low level of these proteins was limiting to L-valine production. Following the extensive metabolic engineering of *E. coli*, the final strain was able to

FIGURE 13.13 Simplified overview of the production of L-valine in rationally engineered *E. coli*. The red X's indicate pathways that were knocked out, the green arrows indicate pathways that were upregulated, and the dashed blue line indicates feedback inhibition. Some arrows represent a single enzymatic step, while other arrows represent several enzymatic steps. The interaction of glucose with other pathways, the export of L-valine from the cell, and several more complex regulatory steps are not shown.

produce 0.378 g of L-valine per g of glucose, which is higher than industrial strains of *C. glutamicum* that have been developed by repeated rounds of random mutagenesis and selection. Moreover, researchers believe that the rationally engineered strain can be further modified with resulting increases in L-valine productivity. Finally, it is important to note that the approach used here should in principle be useful for the overproduction of a wide range of metabolites from bacteria.

Microbial Synthesis of Lycopene

Lycopene ($C_{40}H_{56}$) is a bright red carotenoid pigment (Fig. 13.14) that is commonly found in tomatoes and other fruits, including watermelons, pink grapefruit, pink guavas, papayas, and rose hips. It is a powerful anti-oxidant that has been suggested to decrease low-density lipoprotein oxidation in humans and thereby to lower the risk of atherosclerosis and coronary heart disease. In addition, lycopene, and several carotenoids derived from lycopene, have been proposed as treatments for some types of cancer. It would be useful if lycopene (and carotenoids produced from lycopene) could be produced in microorganisms so that the large-scale-processing problems that exist when lycopene is isolated from tomatoes might be avoided. For the production of lycopene in *E. coli*, the 2-*C*-methyl-D-erythritol 4-phosphate pathway provides the precursors isopentenyl diphosphate and dimethylallyl diphosphate (Fig. 13.15). However, by introducing *Saccharomyces cerevisiae* genes encoding the mevalonate pathway under the control of *E. coli* transcriptional promoters, the levels of these precursor molecules are increased dramatically. By subsequently introducing *Pantoea agglomerans* (a gram-negative bacterium) genes encoding the biosynthesis of lycopene from the above-mentioned precursor metabolites, a relatively high level of lycopene can be produced (Fig. 13.15). With this engineered *E. coli* strain, which contains two additional biosynthetic pathways, it was possible to obtain approximately 60 mg of lycopene per liter of bacterial culture. While additional optimization of this system is still necessary before it can be the basis of a commercial system for lycopene production, this work is an important step in the development of such a system.

Increasing Succinic Acid Production

Succinic acid (succinate) is a dicarboxylic acid that is a component of the citric acid cycle; it is formed from fumarate and reacts to form succinyl-coenzyme A (CoA) (Fig. 13.16). At room temperature, pure succinic acid is a colorless and odorless solid that is moderately soluble in water. Succinic acid is used as a flavoring for foods and beverages and in the production of dyes, perfumes, lacquers, resins, and a variety of medicines. It is currently synthesized by the catalytic hydrogenation of malic acid or its anhydride; however, there is increasing interest in the production of succinic acid from renewable sources by microbial fermentation.

FIGURE 13.14 The chemical structure of lycopene.

FIGURE 13.15 Overview of the production of lycopene in an engineered strain of *E. coli*. The yellow metabolites are normally produced in *E. coli*. The portion of the pathway highlighted in blue represents the enzymes encoded by *S. cerevisiae* genes, as well as some of the metabolites that they produce. The pathway highlighted in green represents enzymes encoded by *P. agglomerans* and the metabolites that they produce. Introduced enzymes are depicted, adjacent to the arrows, by asterisks.

Although a very large number of bacteria synthesize succinic acid, only a few of these organisms, including *Anaerobiospirillum succiniprod-ucens*, *Actinobacillus succinogenes*, and *Mannheimia succiniproducens*, produce the metabolite at high levels. Unfortunately, at the same time that these anaerobic bacteria produce succinic acid, they also produce, and excrete, significant amounts of acetic, formic, and lactic acids. This not only reduces the yield of succinic acid, it also makes the purification process more difficult and costly. To increase the amount of succinic acid produced by *M. succiniproducens*, genes that were known to be involved in the synthesis of acetic, formic, and lactic acids from pyruvic acid were sequentially disrupted (Fig. 13.16), and each mutant was tested for the ability to synthesize succinic (and acetic, formic, and lactic) acid. Using this strategy, it was possible to engineer a strain, under the anaerobic conditions that are normal for the bacterium, to produce 13.5 g of succinic acid per liter of culture compared to 10.5 g per liter for the wild-type bacterium. At the same time, the production of formic and lactic acids was completely

FIGURE 13.16 Overview of the metabolic pathways that lead to the formation of succinic, formic, lactic, and acetic acids under anaerobic conditions in *M. succiniproducens*. The metabolites indicated in green highlight the production of succinic acid from glucose. The metabolites shown in yellow depict the synthesis of unwanted side products. The four genes in red (i.e., *ldhA, pflB, pta,* and *ackA*) were mutated to decrease the flux through this portion of the pathway. The gene in green *(maeB)* may be overproduced in an effort to decrease pyruvic acid and increase succinic acid. *ldh,* lactate dehydrogenase; *pfl,* pyruvate formate lyase; *pta,* phosphotransacetylase; *ack,* acetate kinase; *mae,* malic enzyme.

abolished and the amount of acetic acid was significantly reduced (Fig. 13.17). In addition, when the cells that contained four separate mutations were grown in a fed-batch mode (see chapter 17), the yield of succinic acid increased to 52.4 g per liter while the amount of pyruvate was only 0.8 g per liter. Although this modified strain secreted pyruvic acid into the medium, it is technically simpler to remove pyruvic acid than acetic, formic, or lactic acid. Nevertheless, it is hoped that additional metabolic engineering (e.g., by overproducing MaeB) will both increase the amount of succinic acid and decrease the level of pyruvic acid that this strain produces so that the modified bacterium can be used as a biological "factory" for succinic acid synthesis.

Antibiotics

Since the discovery of penicillin in the late 1920s, more than 12,000 antibiotics with different specificities and a variety of modes of action have been isolated from various microorganisms. The universal use of antibiotics to treat bacterial diseases has resulted in an enormous improvement in human

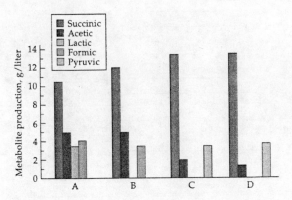

FIGURE 13.17 Formation of succinic, formic, lactic, acetic, and pyruvic acids by wild-type and mutant strains of *M. succiniproducens*. Bars: A, wild type; B, *ldhA* mutant; C, *ldhA* and *pflB* mutant; D, *ldhA, pflB, pta,* and *ackA* mutant.

health and has undoubtedly saved millions of lives. The majority of the most important antibiotics have been isolated from the gram-positive soil bacterium *Streptomyces,* although fungi and other gram-positive and gram-negative bacteria are also sources of antibiotics (Table 13.3). Worldwide, over 100,000 tons of antibiotics is produced per year, with annual gross sales of about $35 billion, including antibiotics used in animal feed and as animal growth promoters. The antibiotic market is driven by the sales of four leading drug classes: the cephalosporins (27%), macrolides (20%), quinolones (17%), and penicillins (17%). Together, these four drug classes account for more than 80% of global antibacterial sales.

An estimated 200 to 300 new antibiotics are discovered each year, primarily through labor-intensive research programs in which many thousands of different microorganisms are screened to find those that produce unique antibiotics. However, with the high costs of development and clinical testing, only the compounds that show significant therapeutic and economic promise are marketed. Therefore, only about 1 to 2% of newly discovered antibiotics are added annually to the disease-fighting arsenal. In fact, the pharmaceutical industry has been reluctant to invest in research and development in this area, and many companies have either abandoned or scaled down their efforts since 1999. In addition, to date, nearly all of the genetic improvements to industrially important antibiotic-producing strains have been achieved by the use of classical mutagenesis and selection. While the yields of antibiotics from many strains have been signifi-

TABLE 13.3 Some of the most common microbially synthesized antibiotics

Amikacin sulfate	Cefotaxime	Chlortetracycline	Kanamycin sulfate	Streptomycin sulfate
Amoxicillin	Cefoxitin	Clarithromycin	Lincomycin HCl	Teicoplanin
Ampicillin	Cefpodoxime proxetil	Clindamycin	Methicillin	Tetracycline HCl
Azithromycin	Ceftazidime	Erythromycin A	Oxytetracycline	Vancomycin HCl
Benzylpenicillin	Ceftriaxone	Flomoxef	Phenoxymethylpenicillin	
Cefaclor	Cefuroxime	Gentamicin sulfate	Rifampin	
Cefixime	Cephalexin	Imipenem	Spiramycin	

cantly improved—the original penicillin-producing fungus isolated by Alexander Fleming yielded 2 units per milliliter of culture, while the strains used today synthesize approximately 70,000 units per milliliter of culture—this yield improvement took many years and required the use of considerable manpower and financial resources. Recombinant DNA technology can have a positive impact on this endeavor in two ways. First, the technology can be used to develop new, structurally unique antibiotics with increased activities against selected targets and decreased side effects. Second, genetic manipulation can be used to relatively rapidly and inexpensively enhance yields and hence lower the cost of production of existing antibiotics.

For the genetic manipulation of *Streptomyces,* it is essential that it can be transformed and that the transformed cells can be readily selected. However, unlike *E. coli, Streptomyces* strains do not exist as individual cells but as extended aggregates called mycelial filaments. The cell wall must be removed to release individual cells (protoplasts) before DNA transformation (Fig. 13.18). Without this step, it would not be possible to distinguish transformed from nontransformed cells, because visible colonies on a solid medium would each have started from a cell aggregate rather than from an individual cell. Thus, colonies that grew in the presence of a selective antibiotic would contain a mixture of transformed and nontransformed cells. However, as a consequence of protoplast formation prior to transformation, all colonies that grow in the presence of a selective antibiotic contain only transformed cells. The uptake of plasmid DNA into *Streptomyces* protoplasts is enhanced by polyethylene glycol. Following transformation, the protoplasts are first plated onto a solid medium to enable the cell walls to regenerate and are then overlaid with a selective medium that often contains either neomycin or thiostrepton, both of which act as selection agents for transformed cells.

Cloning Antibiotic Biosynthesis Genes

The biosynthesis of an antibiotic may include 10 to 30 separate enzyme-catalyzed steps, so cloning all the genes for the synthesis of a particular antibiotic is not an easy task. One strategy for isolating the complete set of antibiotic biosynthesis genes consists of transforming one or more mutant strains that are unable to synthesize the antibiotic with DNA from a clone bank constructed from wild-type chromosomal DNA. Following the introduction of the clone bank DNA into mutant cells, transformants are screened for the ability to produce the antibiotic. Then, the plasmid DNA from the clone that supplies a functional gene and gene product, i.e., complements a mutant strain, is used as a DNA hybridization probe to screen another clone bank of wild-type chromosomal DNA (i.e., one in which the average-size fragment is around 10 kb) to isolate clones with regions that overlap the probe sequence. In this way, DNA segments that are adjacent to and usually bigger than the initial complementing DNA can be identified and cloned. A complete gene cluster can be reconstructed from the overlapping clones. If the antibiotic biosynthesis genes are clustered at a single site on the chromosomal DNA, the genes that are adjacent to the complementing gene are also likely to be involved in the biosynthesis of the target antibiotic. However, if the antibiotic biosynthesis genes are scattered in small clusters at different chromosomal locations, it is necessary to have at least one mutant per gene cluster to obtain a DNA clone that can be used to identify the rest of the genes in the cluster.

Mycelial filaments

Enzymatically
remove cell wall

Protoplasts

Add DNA
and PEG

Transformed cell

Nontransformed cell

Plate cells onto
regeneration medium

Individual
cells

Petri dish

Overlay cells with
selective medium

Colony grown from
an individual cell

FIGURE 13.18 Schematic representation of DNA transformation and selection of transformants of *Streptomyces* strains. The pink circles represent transformed cells, and the green circles represent nontransformed cells. PEG, polyethylene glycol.

The complementation approach has been used to isolate some of the genes for the biosynthesis of the antibiotic undecylprodigiosin from *Streptomyces coelicolor* A3 (Fig. 13.19). In this case, the complementation assay is simple and entails scoring the color of the colonies. Colonies of wild-type organisms are red because of the presence of the antibiotic, and mutant colonies are cream colored. Complementation produces a red colony (Fig. 13.20).

FIGURE 13.19 Chemical structure of the red antibiotic undecylprodigiosin.

In addition to cloning antibiotic biosynthesis genes by complementation, more direct strategies can be employed. One or more of the key enzymes in a biosynthetic pathway can be identified through either genetic or biochemical studies and then purified. The N-terminal amino acid sequence of the enzyme can then be determined, and with this information, oligodeoxyribonucleotide probes for the gene can be prepared. This approach has been used to isolate the gene for isopenicillin N synthetase from *Penicillium chrysogenum*. This enzyme catalyzes the oxidative

FIGURE 13.20 Method for cloning genes involved in the biosynthesis of the antibiotic undecylprodigiosin. Chromosomal DNA from wild-type antibiotic-producing cells is spliced into a *Streptomyces* cloning vector. The clone bank is used to transform a noncolored (i.e., non-antibiotic-producing) mutant of the wild type. Red transformants (in which the mutant has been complemented) are selected, and the plasmid DNA insert is characterized.

condensation of the compound δ-(L-α-aminodipyl)-L-cysteinyl-D-valine to isopenicillin N, a key intermediate in the biosynthesis of penicillins, cephalosporins, and cephamycins (Fig. 13.21).

Despite the difficulty, there are a number of examples of the cloning and transfer of large fragments of DNA encoding entire antibiotic biosynthetic pathways. In these cases, it is usually necessary to use a vector that can accept and maintain pieces of DNA as large as 100 kb. For this purpose, researchers have employed bacterial artificial chromosomes that have been engineered to replicate autonomously in *E. coli* and, when they are introduced into *Streptomyces*, to integrate into the chromosome.

Modulating Gene Expression in Streptomycetes

To improve the productivity of antibiotics produced by *Streptomyces* spp., it is desirable to utilize a regulatory expression system that can suppress the expression of the target gene(s) until the culture reaches a high cell density. It would also be beneficial if the system could be induced simply and inexpensively and if it could function in a range of different *Streptomyces* spp. One regulatable, high-expression *Streptomyces* system that was recently

FIGURE 13.21 Biosynthetic pathway for penicillins and cephalosporins in *P. chrysogenum*. Isopenicillin N synthetase catalyzes the synthesis of isopenicillin N from D-(L-α-aminoadipyl)-L-cysteinyl-D-valine. Isopenicillin N is a precursor in the synthesis of penicillin G, penicillin N, and cephalosporin C.

developed utilizes the nitrilase operon from the actinomycete *Rhodococcus rhodochrous*. In this bacterium, the expression of the enzyme nitrilase (encoded by the *nitA* gene under the control of the *nitA* promoter) is positively regulated by the protein NitR (encoded by *nitR*, which is present in the same operon as *nitA*). NitR forms a complex with the inducer, ε-caprolactam, before the complex binds to the *nitA* promoter, activating the synthesis of both proteins, NitA and NitR. However, to use this system as part of a high-expression vector, a transcription terminator was placed upstream of the *nitA* promoter (to prevent transcriptional read-through from other genes (Fig. 13.22); a multiple cloning site for inserting target DNA was placed downstream of the *nitA* promoter; downstream of the multiple cloning site (and the target gene), the synthetic operon ends with another transcription terminator; and finally, the vector contains the *nitR* gene under the control of the *nitA* promoter in a separate operon. When this expression vector is used, upon the addition of the inducer ε-caprolactam, the inducer–NitR protein complex activates the transcription of both the target gene(s) and *nitR*. The increased level of NitR results in a very high level of production of the target protein(s). While this system is still at a relatively early stage of development, with some target proteins, it has been possible to achieve expression levels as high as approximately 40% of all soluble protein. Moreover, the system functioned well when it was introduced into *S. coelicolor*, *Streptomyces avermitilis*, and *Streptomyces griseus*, bacterial strains that have all previously been used for antibiotic production. However, it still remains to be demonstrated that this expression system can be used as an effective method for increasing the yield of a commercially important antibiotic that is produced in a *Streptomyces* strain.

Synthesis of Novel Antibiotics

New antibiotics with unique properties and specificities may be produced by genetic manipulation of the genes involved in the biosynthesis of existing antibiotics. In one of the first experiments in which a novel antibiotic was produced, researchers began by examining the consequences of placing two slightly different antibiotic production pathways into one organism.

A *Streptomyces* plasmid (pIJ2303) carrying a 32.5-kb fragment of *S. coelicolor* chromosomal DNA contains all of the genes encoding the enzymes

FIGURE 13.22 Overview of a regulatable expression system for use with *Streptomyces* spp. TT, transcription terminator; MCS, multiple cloning site; p^{nitA}, the *nitA* gene promoter. The *nitA* gene encodes nitrilase; *nitR* encodes a positive transcriptional regulatory protein; the inducer is ε-caprolactam.

responsible for the biosynthesis of the antibiotic actinorhodine, starting from acetate. This antibiotic is a member of the family of antibiotics called isochromanequinones (Fig. 13.23). The intact plasmid and various subclones carrying portions of the 32.5-kb DNA fragment (e.g., pIJ2315) were introduced into either *Streptomyces* sp. strain AM-7161, which produces the related antibiotic medermycin, or *Streptomyces violaceoruber* B1140 or Tü22, both of which produce the related antibiotics granaticin and dihydrogranaticin.

Each of the antibiotics actinorhodine, medermycin, granaticin, and dihydrogranaticin (Fig. 13.23) functions as an acid–base indicator, conferring on a growing culture a characteristic color that depends on the pH of the medium (Table 13.4). The pH (and color), in turn, depends on the

FIGURE 13.23 Structures of various isochromanequinone antibiotics produced by *Streptomyces* spp. Wild-type *S. coelicolor* and plasmid pIJ2303 encode actinorhodine, a *Streptomyces* sp. produces medermycin, and *S. violaceoruber* produces both granaticin and dihydrogranaticin. The hybrid antibiotics produced are mederrhodine A and dihydrogranatirhodine.

TABLE 13.4 Antibiotics produced by various *Streptomyces* strains and those transformed with plasmids pIJ2303 and pIJ2315

| Strain/plasmid | Color of culture | | Antibiotic(s) |
	Acidic	Alkaline	
S. coelicolor	Red	Blue	Actinorhodine
Streptomyces sp.	Yellow	Brown	Medermycin
Streptomyces sp./pIJ2303	Red	Blue	Medermycin, actinorhodine
Streptomyces sp./pIJ2315	Red	Purple	Mederrhodine A, medermycin
S. violaceoruber B1140	Red	Blue-purple	Granaticin, dihydrogranaticin
S. violaceoruber B1140/pIJ2303	Red	Blue-purple	Granaticin, dihydrogranaticin, actinorhodine
S. violaceoruber B1140 Tü22	Red	Blue-purple	Granaticin, dihydrogranaticin
S. violaceoruber B1140 Tü22/pIJ2303	Red	Blue-purple	Dihydrogranatirhodine, actinorhodine

Adapted from Hopwood et al., *Nature* 314:642–644, 1985.

compound(s) being synthesized. Mutants of the *S. coelicolor* parental strain that are unable to produce actinorhodine are colorless. The appearance of new colors (in some cases) following the transformation of *Streptomyces* sp. strain AM-7161, or *S. violaceoruber* B1140, or *S. violaceoruber* Tü22 with a plasmid carrying either all or some of the genes encoding the enzymes that synthesize actinorhodine suggests that a novel antibiotic has been produced (Fig. 13.23 and Table 13.4). *Streptomyces* sp. strain AM-7161 and *S. violaceoruber* B1140 transformants containing pIJ2303 produce the antibiotics encoded by both the chromosomal and plasmid DNAs. However, when *S. violaceoruber* Tü22 is transformed with pIJ2303, a new antibiotic—dihydrogranatirhodine—is synthesized, along with actinorhodine. When *Streptomyces* sp. strain AM-7161 is transformed with pIJ2315, a second new antibiotic—mederrhodine A—is produced.

These new antibiotics represent minor structural variants of the preexisting antibiotics actinorhodine, medermycin, granaticin, and hydrogranaticin and probably arise when an intermediate compound from one biosynthetic pathway acts as a substrate for an enzyme from the other pathway. As the biochemistry of various antibiotic biosynthetic pathways has been better understood, it has become possible to design unique antibiotics by genetic manipulation of the genes encoding the relevant enzymes.

Engineering Polyketide Antibiotics

The term "polyketide" defines a class of antibiotics that are synthesized through the successive enzymatic condensation of small carboxylic acids, such as acetate, propionate, and butyrate. Polyketide drugs include the antibiotic erythromycin, the immunosuppressive drug FK506, and the cholesterol-lowering drug lovastatin. While various polyketides are produced by plants and fungi, the majority are produced by actinomycetes as secondary metabolites. To create new polyketide antibiotics, the functioning of the enzymes that synthesize these antibiotics must be understood before the genes encoding the enzymes can be manipulated.

Polyketide antibiotics are synthesized by a complex enzymatic mechanism analogous to that used for the synthesis of long-chain fatty acids. Each condensation cycle results in the formation, on a growing carbon chain, of a β-keto group. Polyketide synthesis consists of a number of steps that are each repeated several times, including ketoreduction, dehydration,

FIGURE 13.24 Schematic representation of polyketide synthase for aromatic polyketides. **(A)** The active site may be on a single polypeptide. **(B)** Alternatively, the enzyme can consist of assemblies of polypeptides with separate and distinct active sites. Both types of enzymes have different domains (regions A through E), and each domain has a separate enzymatic activity.

and enoylreduction of the β-group of the growing polyketide chain. There are two classes of polyketide synthases that are responsible for the synthesis of polyketide antibiotics (Fig. 13.24). The synthases that catalyze the biosynthesis of aromatic polyketides make up one class and generally consist of one polypeptide with an active site for each successive reaction (Fig. 13.24A). The second class includes synthases that are assemblies of several polypeptides that have separate and distinct active sites for every catalyzed step in polyketide biosynthesis (Fig. 13.24B). These enzymes have a number of different domains (regions A through E) (Fig. 13.24), and each domain has a separate enzymatic activity and active site catalyzing a particular step in the process. The complete synthesis of a polyketide antibiotic generally requires the participation of several of these multifunctional enzymes; together, they make up the subunits of the polyketide synthase.

If each of the enzymatic activities that is catalyzed by a domain on a multifunctional polyketide synthase subunit catalyzes only a single biochemical step in the pathway, the loss of any one activity should affect only a single step in the overall synthesis. Moreover, alteration of a catalytic domain whose function has been established should allow researchers to make predictable changes to the structure of the synthesized antibiotic. For example, a detailed knowledge of the genetics and biochemistry of the components involved in the synthesis of the antibiotic erythromycin allowed researchers to alter the biosynthetic genes in a predetermined manner and to produce predictably altered derivatives of erythromycin. Erythromycin is synthesized by *Saccharopolyspora erythraea,* and the entire 56-kb DNA segment that contains the *ery* gene cluster has been sequenced. The erythromycin polyketide synthase was altered in two different ways: either (1) a DNA region that encoded β-ketoreductase activity was deleted or (2) a DNA region encoding enoylreductase was mutated. With the β-ketoreductase deletion, the erythromycin intermediates that accumulated had a carbonyl moiety rather than a hydroxyl group at the C-5 carbon of the ring (Fig. 13.25). Similarly, with the enoylreductase mutation, a carbon–carbon double bond was introduced at positions C-6 and C-7 of the ring (Fig. 13.25). These experiments indicate that once the cluster of genes encoding the biosynthesis of a particular polyketide antibiotic has been isolated and characterized, it is possible, by altering specific DNA frag-

FIGURE 13.25 Altered erythromycin derivatives produced through genetic manipulation. **(A)** A mutation in an enoylreductase gene caused a carbon–carbon double bond to be introduced at positions C-6 and C-7 of the ring (highlighted). **(B)** A deletion in a β-ketoreductase gene caused the erythromycin to have a carbonyl moiety rather than a hydroxyl group at the C-5 carbon of the ring (highlighted). Adapted from Katz and Donadio, *Annu. Rev. Microbiol.* **47:**875–912, 1993.

ments, to modify an antibiotic biosynthesis pathway and thereby to alter the structure of the antibiotic in a predictable manner. Moreover, it is possible to cut and splice DNA fragments and thereby shift polyketide synthase domains around to create novel polyketide antibiotics.

The gene clusters for aromatic polyketides all contain a set of three genes encoding a so-called minimal polyketide synthase. Each minimal polyketide synthase contains the activities for one cycle of polyketide chain elongation. The minimal module has a ketosynthase (with an acyltransferase domain), a chain length factor, and an acyl carrier protein. The minimal polyketide synthase is responsible for the synthesis of the aromatic polyketide backbone. Modifications to the basic structure are catalyzed by other enzymes acting in concert with the minimal polyketide synthase. The order of the modules in a polyketide synthase specifies the sequence of the distinct two-carbon units, and the number of modules determines the size of the polyketide chain. The genes encoding a complete set of these proteins are generally organized into a single cluster (Fig. 13.26). Each minimal polyketide synthase gene cluster encodes the synthesis of a particular antibiotic. By interchanging genes between clusters, new aromatic polyketide antibiotics have been created (Fig. 13.27). This experiment demonstrates the potential of using genetic manipulation to design and produce novel aromatic polyketide antibiotics. This approach promises to dramatically accelerate the process of discovery of new antibiotics.

Improving Antibiotic Production

In addition to being a means of developing new antibiotics, genetic engineering can be used to enhance the yields and rates of production of known antibiotics. The large-scale production of antibiotics by *Streptomyces* spp. is often limited by the amount of oxygen available to the cells. The low solubility of oxygen in aqueous media, combined with the highly dense nature

FIGURE 13.26 Gene clusters for the biosynthesis of the aromatic polyketide antibiotics actinorhodine *(act)*, tetracenomycin *(tcm)*, frenolicin *(fren)*, and griseusin *(gris)*. Each cluster contains genes encoding a minimal polyketide synthase (PKS), which is responsible for the synthesis of the polyketide backbone. The enzymes encoded by the other genes act to modify the growing polyketide chain. Each gene is shown pointed in the direction in which it is transcribed.

FIGURE 13.27 Theoretical biosynthetic pathway for the production of the rationally designed polyketides SEK43 and SEK26 by interchanging gene clusters. *act*, actinorhodine; *tcm*, tetracenomycin; *fren*, frenolicin; *gris*, griseusin; min PKS, minimal polyketide synthase; KR, β-ketoreductase; ARO, aromatase; CYC, cyclase.

of filamentous *Streptomyces* cultures, often results in an oxygen-depleted culture medium, a condition that causes poor cell growth and reduced antibiotic yield. To overcome this problem, it may be possible to improve the design of the bioreactors that are used to grow antibiotic-producing *Streptomyces* cultures and to develop, by genetic manipulation, *Streptomyces* strains that are better able to utilize the available oxygen. These two approaches are not mutually exclusive.

One strategy used by some aerobic microorganisms to cope with oxygen-poor environments is to synthesize a hemoglobin-like molecule that can sequester oxygen from the medium and then deliver it to the cells. For example, the aerobic bacterium *Vitreoscilla* produces a homodimeric heme protein that is functionally similar to eukaryotic hemoglobin. The gene for the *Vitreoscilla* hemoglobin was isolated and subcloned onto a *Streptomyces* plasmid vector. Following expression of the *Vitreoscilla* hemoglobin gene in *S. coelicolor*, the *Vitreoscilla* hemoglobin represented approximately 0.1% of the total cellular protein, even though the expression was controlled by the native *Vitreoscilla* hemoglobin gene promoter rather than by a *Streptomyces* promoter. When both transformed and nontransformed *S. coelicolor* cultures were grown in the presence of a low level of dissolved oxygen (i.e., approximately 5% saturation), the transformed cells with a functional *Vitreoscilla* hemoglobin produced 10 times more actinorhodine per gram (dry weight) of cells and had greater cell densities than did the nontransformed cells. The expression of the *Vitreoscilla* hemoglobin gene in oxygen-starved microbial cells may provide them with a general mechanism for obtaining sufficient oxygen to allow proliferation under otherwise limiting conditions.

The compound 7-aminocephalosporanic acid (7ACA) is synthesized chemically from the antibiotic cephalosporin C (Fig. 13.28) and is used as the starting material for the chemical synthesis of a number of cephem-type antibiotics (cephalosporins). Cephalosporins have few toxic effects on humans and protect against many different bacteria. Unfortunately, there is no known organism that can synthesize 7ACA. However, a novel 7ACA biosynthetic pathway has been constructed in the fungus *Acremonium chrysogenum*, which normally synthesizes only cephalosporin C. The genes involved in this novel engineered pathway consist of a cDNA that encodes D-amino acid oxidase and that comes from the fungus *Fusarium solani* and genomic DNA that encodes cephalosporin acylase and comes from the bacterium *Pseudomonas diminuta*. Both of these genes were subcloned separately onto an *A. chrysogenum* plasmid expression vector under the control of an *A. chrysogenum* promoter. In the first step of this new pathway, cephalosporin C is converted into the compound 7-β-(5-carboxy-5-oxopentanamido)cephalosporanic acid (keto-AD-7ACA) by D-amino acid oxidase (Fig. 13.28). Some of this product reacts with the hydrogen peroxide that is a by-product of the reaction to form 7-β-(4-carboxybutanamido)cephalosporanic acid (GL-7ACA) (Fig. 13.28). Cephalosporin C, keto-AD-7ACA, and GL-7ACA are each hydrolyzed by cephalosporin acylase to form 7ACA. However, in the absence of the D-amino acid oxidase step, only 5% of the cephalosporin C is converted to 7ACA; therefore, both enzymes are essential for high yields of 7ACA. Although the level of 7ACA that could be produced using this system was not sufficient to make this work the basis of a commercially viable process, it nevertheless demonstrates the feasibility of producing 7ACA biologically.

Medically important cephalosporins may be synthesized from either 7ACA or the related compound 7-aminodeacetoxycephalosporanic acid

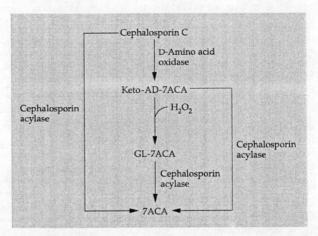

FIGURE 13.28 Genetically engineered biosynthetic pathway for the synthesis of 7ACA from cephalosporin C. The D-amino acid oxidase gene is from the fungus *F. solani*, and the cephalosporin acylase gene is from the bacterium *P. diminuta*.

(7ADCA). Disrupting the functioning of the *A. chrysogenum cefEF* gene results in the accumulation of large amounts of penicillin N (Fig. 13.29). Moreover, when this mutant strain is transformed with a *cefE* gene from *Streptomyces clavuligerus*, penicillin N is converted to deacetoxycephalosporin C (DAOC), which can then be converted to 7ADCA. At this stage of the development of this process, not all of the penicillin N is converted to DAOC; however, it may be possible to further increase the expression of the *cefE* gene. Thus, it is reasonable to expect that transgenic *A. chrysogenum* can eventually be engineered to produce large amounts of 7ADCA.

Many antibiotic-producing organisms are slow growing, require special growth conditions, or yield only small numbers of cells. To overcome these problems, *E. coli* was engineered to produce polyketide antibiotics at rates that are potentially useful for drug production. To do this, three genes (each 10 to 12 kb in length) encoding the components of the polyketide synthase from the bacterium *S. erythraea* were expressed in *E. coli*. Then, a *Bacillus subtilis* gene that produces an enzyme that attaches the cofactor phosophopantetheine to the polyketide synthase was cloned into the engineered *E. coli*. In addition, to supply the polyketide synthase with sufficient building blocks—propionyl-CoA and methylmalonyl-CoA—for polyketide synthesis, the *E. coli* gene encoding an enzyme that breaks down propionyl-CoA was inactivated and an *S. coelicolor* gene for propionyl-CoA carboxylase was introduced. Given the relative ease with which *E. coli* can be genetically manipulated and then grown in large-scale culture, this work may be a significant breakthrough for the development and production of new antibiotics.

Designer Antibiotics

In recent years, there has been an enormous proliferation in the prevalence of antibiotic-resistant bacterial infections. At present in the United States, more deaths are attributable to infections by methicillin-resistant strains of

Staphylococcus aureus than to human immunodeficiency virus/AIDS. An important component of *S. aureus* virulence is the carotenoid pigment staphyloxanthin that is synthesized by the bacterium. As a consequence of the large number of conjugated double bonds that this compound possesses, it can detoxify the reactive oxygen species that are produced by the host immune system in response to the bacterial infection. On the other hand, strains of *S. aureus* that do not contain staphyloxanthin are rapidly inactivated by the reactive oxygen species produced by host neutrophils. This observation suggests that the disruption of *S. aureus* staphyloxanthin synthesis might be a suitable target to prevent the proliferation and toxicity of the bacterium.

In the first committed step in the biosynthesis of *S. aureus* staphyloxanthin, the enzyme dehydrosqualene synthase condenses two molecules of farnesyl diphosphate to produce presqualene diphosphate (Fig. 13.30). In *S. aureus*, this compound is modified to yield dehydrosqualene, which is converted into 4,4'-diaponeurosporene and eventually into staphyloxanthin. Interestingly, the synthesis of cholesterol in humans also proceeds through presqualene diphosphate. In order to determine whether the *S. aureus* enzyme that catalyzed the first committed step could be a target for a designer antibiotic, the bacterial gene was cloned and overexpressed, the enzyme was purified to homogeneity, and its X-ray crystallographic structure was determined to 1.58-Å resolution. Based on the three-dimensional structure of the enzyme, as well as the presence of inhibitors of the human enzyme (from the cholesterol synthesis pathway) that performed the same function, a series of eight chemical inhibitors was designed, synthesized chemically, and tested. Three of the inhibitors, when tested at levels below 1 µM, dramatically blocked the conversion of farnesyl diphosphate to presqualene diphosphate (which is highly pigmented and therefore easy to visualize). In fact, one of the best inhibitors turned out to be a drug candidate that had already undergone preliminary testing in humans for its ability to lower cholesterol levels. Despite the fact that these results are preliminary, the compound that was selected using this strategy caused a 98% decrease in surviving *S. aureus* in infected mice. Thus, while much remains to be done, this work demonstrates that by choosing a nonconventional target it is possible to develop designer antibiotics that render pathogenic bacteria susceptible to human and animal immune systems.

FIGURE 13.29 Synthesis of the compound 7ADCA in a genetically engineered strain of *A. chrysogenum*. The functioning of the endogenous *A. chrysogenum cefEF* gene is disrupted so that penicillin N accumulates. This strain is transformed with a *cefE* gene from *S. clavuligerus*, and the penicillin N is transformed into DAOC, which is subsequently converted to 7ADCA.

Biopolymers

Biopolymers are large, multiunit macromolecules synthesized by microorganisms, plants, and animals. Some of these polymers have physical and chemical properties that are useful to the food-processing, manufacturing, and pharmaceutical industries. The ability to genetically engineer organisms has stimulated researchers to design new biopolymers, replace synthetic polymers with biological equivalents, modify existing biopolymers to enhance their physical and structural characteristics, and find ways to increase the yields and decrease the costs of biopolymers produced by industrial processes.

Xanthan Gum

Xanthomonas campestris is a gram-negative obligatory aerobic soil bacterium that produces the commercially important biopolymer xanthan gum,

FIGURE 13.30 Simplified overview of the biosynthesis of staphyloxanthin in *S. aureus* and cholesterol in humans. The first step (the committed step) is the same in both pathways.

a high-molecular-weight exopolysaccharide, as a by-product of its metabolism. This polymer has a cellulosic backbone made up of a straight-chain polymer of glucose units. Each of its trisaccharide side chains includes one glucuronic acid and two mannose residues, which are attached to every second glucose residue of the backbone (Fig. 13.31). Xanthan gum has high viscosity, is stable in extreme physical and chemical environments, and exhibits physical and chemical properties similar to those of a plastic. In particular, its physical properties make it useful as a stabilizing, emulsifying, thickening, or suspending agent. For successful commercial production of xanthan gum, *X. campestris* should be grown on an inexpensive and

FIGURE 13.31 Structure of xanthan gum. The repeating unit, designated n, forms a chain of glucose units. The trisaccharide is attached to alternate glucose residues of the repeating chain.

plentiful carbon source. Wild-type *X. campestris* can efficiently utilize glucose, sucrose, and starch, but not lactose, as a carbon source.

Whey is a waste by-product of the cheese-making process that consists of water (94 to 95%), lactose (3.5 to 4%), and small amounts of protein, minerals, and low-molecular-weight organic compounds. Enormous quantities of whey are generated by the dairy industry, and its disposal is a major problem. In North America, whey has been used extensively as a "filler" in the preparation of prepared foods; however, with the increasing awareness that large numbers of individuals are lactose intolerant, it is imperative that alternative uses be found for this material. Moreover, disposing of whey by releasing it into rivers and lakes can deplete the amount of available oxygen, thereby killing many of the aquatic organisms. Transporting whey to landfill sites is exceptionally expensive, and potential groundwater contamination by the discarded whey is a major concern. Finally, the costs of removing the solid component of whey are prohibitive. Consequently, many schemes have been devised to use whey in creative ways.

Theoretically, whey could be used as a carbon source for growing industrially important microorganisms. With this in mind, *X. campestris* was genetically engineered to grow on whey. The *E. coli lacZY* genes, which encode the enzymes β-galactosidase and lactose permease, were cloned onto a broad-host-range plasmid under the transcriptional control of an *X. campestris* bacteriophage promoter (Fig. 13.32). This construct was introduced into *E. coli* and then transferred from *E. coli* to *X. campestris* by tripar-

FIGURE 13.32 Engineering *E. coli lacZ* (encoding β-galactosidase) and *lacY* (encoding lactose permease) genes for constitutive expression in *X. campestris (Xc)*.

tite mating. Transformants maintained the plasmid, expressed the enzymes β-galactosidase and lactose permease at high levels, utilized lactose as the sole carbon source, and produced large amounts of xanthan gum with glucose, lactose, or whey as the carbon source (Table 13.5). By contrast, wild-type *X. campestris* produces large amounts of xanthan gum only when grown on glucose (Table 13.5). This system may well be able to convert a nuisance waste product into a substrate for the production of an economically valuable biopolymer.

Melanin

Melanins are a large, diverse family of light-absorbing biopolymers that are synthesized by animals, plants, bacteria, and fungi. It has been suggested that these pigments might be useful as topical sunscreens, sunlight-protective coatings for plastics, or additives for cosmetic products. Currently, melanins are obtained in small quantities either by extraction from natural sources or by chemical synthesis. However, recombinant DNA technology has made it possible to produce a range of melanins with different physical properties inexpensively and on a large scale.

Biochemically, melanins are irregular, somewhat random polymers that are composed of indoles, benzthiazoles, and amino acids. The first step in their synthesis, which is catalyzed by the copper-containing monooxygenase tyrosinase, is the oxidation of tyrosine to dihydroxyphenylalanine quinone. The final stages of the polymerization of melanin are nonenzymatic, and depending on the chemical nature of the nonquinone components that are incorporated into the polymeric structure (typically hydroxylated organic compounds), the end product can be black, brown, yellow, red, or violet.

The genes involved in melanin biosynthesis in the bacterium *Streptomyces antibioticus* have been isolated and analyzed. These genes were

TABLE 13.5 Production of xanthan gum by wild-type and transformed *X. campestris*

X. campestris	Amount of xanthan gum produced (μg/mL) with:		
	0.4% Glucose	0.4% Lactose	10% Whey
Wild type	3,530	245	224
Transformant	3,711	3,608	4,241

Adapted from Fu and Tseng, *Appl. Environ. Microbiol.* **56**:919–923, 1990.

The amount of the product is expressed as micrograms per milliliter of culture grown on a minimal medium either 0.4% glucose or 0.4% lactose added or on diluted whey (10%), which contains approximately 0.44% lactose. The transformant carries the *E. coli lacZY* genes on a plasmid.

selected from a clone bank of *S. antibioticus* DNA on the basis of the ability to change color in the presence of specific compounds that were added to the medium. They consist of two open reading frames (ORFs), one encoding tyrosinase (molecular weight, 30,600) and one (ORF438) encoding a protein of unknown function with a molecular weight of approximately 14,800. To test whether both of these genes are required for melanin production, they were subcloned into an *E. coli* expression vector, where one construct contained only the tyrosinase gene and another carried both the tyrosinase and the ORF438 genes (Fig. 13.33). The vector with the tyrosinase gene directed the synthesis of a larger amount of tyrosinase than did the vector containing both the tyrosinase and the ORF438 genes. However, the amount of tyrosinase was irrelevant, because it turned out that melanin biosynthesis required the products of both genes. The protein encoded by ORF438 may act as a copper donor to apotyrosinase, the inactive precursor form of tyrosinase. Apotyrosinases are activated by acquiring copper ions. Under natural conditions, after dihydroxyphenylalanine quinone is produced by tyrosinase, a variety of low-molecular-weight compounds (nonquinones) can be incorporated into the final polymer. The chemical and physical nature, including the color, of the melanin that is formed after cloning of the key genes into *E. coli* may be manipulated to some extent, to form melanins with different properties, by the addition of different amounts of specific low-molecular-weight compounds to the medium.

Adhesive Protein

Researchers are trying to inexpensively produce an adhesive protein biopolymer, originally isolated from the blue mussel *Mytilus edulis,* in microbial cells. This biopolymer is an exceptionally strong, waterproof adhesive protein, called byssal adhesive, that enables the mussel to attach very tightly to a variety of surfaces. Following its secretion, the byssal adhesive becomes highly cross-linked (randomly), and consequently, the protein cannot be sequenced. Without this information, it is impossible to deduce nucleic acid sequences that might be used for the synthesis of DNA hybridization probes. However, it was possible to isolate an intracellular precursor form of the adhesive protein, called the 130-kilodalton (kDa) precursor protein,

FIGURE 13.33 *E. coli* expression plasmids carrying melanin biosynthesis genes. Plasmid pBGC619 contains the tyrosinase gene. Plasmid pBGC620.3 contains an ORF (ORF438) for melanin synthesis and the tyrosinase gene. Transcription of the cloned genes is under the control of the *E. coli* bacteriophage T7 promoter (p^{T7}). RBS1 and RBS2 denote two different ribosome-binding sites. The plasmids both carry genes that confer resistance to ampicillin (Ampr).

MILESTONE

Production of 2-Keto-L-Gulonate, an Intermediate in L-Ascorbate Synthesis, by a Genetically Modified *Erwinia herbicola*

S. ANDERSON, C. B. MARKS, R. LAZARUS, J. MILLER, K. STAFFORD, J. SEYMOUR, D. LIGHT, W. RASTETTER, and D. ESTELL
Science 230:144–149, 1985

Theoretically, prokaryotes that produce specific metabolites can be genetically manipulated in two different ways. First, the activity or amount of one or more of the enzymes in a pathway encoding the synthesis of a particular metabolite can be modified so that the amount of metabolite that the bacterium produces is increased. Second, foreign genes that produce enzymes that can use an endogenous metabolite as a substrate for the production of another metabolite not normally produced by the host bacterium can be introduced. While these sorts of manipulations are easy in theory, it is not necessarily easy to isolate and manipulate the required genes or to establish the appropriate conditions that enable complex biosynthetic pathways to function properly.

To create a bacterium that synthesized 2-keto-L-gulonic acid, which is the immediate precursor of commercially synthesized vitamin C, Anderson et al. isolated the *Corynebacterium* gene encoding the enzyme that converts 2,5-diketo-D-gluconic acid to 2-keto-L-gulonic acid and transferred it to an *Erwinia* sp., a bacterium that synthesizes 2,5-diketo-D-gluconic acid from D-glucose. The isolation of this gene was difficult because the enzyme had not been previously studied to any great extent. Therefore, before the gene could be isolated, the protein had to be purified and partially sequenced so that DNA hybridization probes based on the amino acid sequence of the protein could be designed. This work is an early example of what some workers have come to call metabolic engineering, which entails taking the genetic information for part of a metabolic pathway from one organism and transferring it into another organism to create a novel metabolic pathway.

that can be analyzed biochemically. It was found that the 130-kDa precursor protein is rich in serine, threonine, lysine, proline (Pro), and tyrosine; 60 to 70% of the amino acids contain a hydroxyl group. Most of the proline residues are hydroxylated to either 3- or 4-hydroxyproline (Hyp), and the majority of the tyrosines are hydroxylated to 3,4-dihydroxyphenylalanine (DOPA). Amino acid sequence analysis of the precursor protein further revealed that it is composed largely of repeating units that consist of a decapeptide with the sequence Ala-Lys-(Pro or Hyp)-Ser-(Tyr or DOPA)-Hyp-Hyp-Thr-DOPA-Lys; 7 of these 10 amino acids are hydroxylated.

The cDNA for the 130-kDa precursor adhesive protein was isolated from a cDNA library that was constructed with messenger RNA (mRNA) isolated from the gland that actively secretes the byssal adhesive. Both the adhesive protein and the cDNA have unusual features that might make cloning, expression, and production of a functional adhesive protein difficult in a heterologous host. First, the highly repetitive nature of the adhesive protein cDNA could make it unstable as a result of homologous recombination and subsequent loss of portions of the cloned sequence. Second, proline, lysine, and tyrosine represent about 70% of the amino acids of the protein; therefore, very high levels of synthesis may not be achievable because the corresponding intracellular aminoacyl-transfer RNA (tRNA) pools might be limiting.

When either complete or partial cDNAs for the adhesive protein were cloned onto yeast expression vectors and introduced into yeast cells, active novel forms of the adhesive protein, ranging from 20 to 100 kDa, were synthesized and represented a significant fraction (2 to 5%) of the total cell protein. Thus, there were no problems concerning either the stability of the cloned cDNA or the production of moderate amounts of the adhesive protein. Considerably higher expression levels were attained when a chemically synthesized adhesive protein gene sequence was expressed in *E. coli* (Fig. 13.34). In this case, repeating DNA units that encode the consensus

decapeptide repeat of the adhesive protein were used to construct a 600-base pair (bp) synthetic gene that encoded a protein with a molecular mass of approximately 25 kDa. The 30-bp repeat, the fundamental building block of the synthetic gene, consisted of codons optimized for *E. coli* expression. The synthetic gene was expressed at very high levels by using the T7 promoter. Notwithstanding the level of expression of the adhesive protein, most microorganisms are limited in their abilities to hydroxylate amino acids posttranslationally, so the final protein might be underhydroxylated. In fact, a number of tyrosine residues of the protein were not converted to DOPA, an outcome that limits the ability of the protein to form cross-links. This deficiency was overcome by creating an in vitro hydroxylation system that used a bacterial tyrosinase in the presence of ascorbic acid to hydroxylate the tyrosine residues to DOPA (Fig. 13.35). Ascorbic acid was included in the reaction mixture to prevent the premature oxidation of the DOPA residues to *o*-quinone. Oxidation must be controlled because it leads to cross-linking of the adhesive protein subunits. Like many other adhesives or glues, the protein adhesive must not be activated (cross-linked) before its actual use.

When the precursor form of the adhesive protein is oxidized, the cross-linked protein can bind to a variety of surfaces, including polystyrene, glass, hydrogel, and collagen. Moreover, the "strength" and specificity of the final adhesive can be manipulated by adding other proteins to the adhesive protein mixture before oxidation and cross-linking. By varying the kinds and amounts of the accessory proteins, adhesives with unique properties can be created. It is anticipated that biopolymeric adhesives will be used extensively in both medicine and dentistry.

More recently, researchers have isolated and expressed in *E. coli* the cDNA for the type 5 foot protein (adhesive protein) from the mussel *Mytilus galloprovincialis*. In this case, the protein that is produced in recombinant *E. coli* cells contains a tag of six histidine residues (to facilitate protein purification), as well as a slightly larger amount of DOPA than is found in the *M. edulis* protein. A higher number of DOPA residues is believed to result in a protein with greater adhesive properties. Unfortunately, the adhesive properties of this protein make it extremely difficult to purify (i.e., it sticks to everything), thereby limiting its commercial possibilities.

Rubber

Natural rubber, *cis*-1,4-polyisoprene, is an extensively used biopolymer that is obtained from a large number of different plants. The biosynthesis

FIGURE 13.34 Synthetic oligonucleotide used in the assembly of a gene for the bioadhesive protein produced by the mussel *M. edulis*. Two oligonucleotides are designed to base pair and form a DNA module with complementary extensions, which base pair to form a linear DNA molecule with a repeating sequence. The repeating units are joined by the enzyme T4 DNA ligase. The amino acid sequence encoded by the DNA repeat is shown. The decapeptide repeating unit contains three hydroxylated amino acids (Tyr, Ser, and Thr) plus three Pro residues which are subsequently hydroxylated.

```
5' CCA ACC TAC AAA GCT AAG CCG TCT TAT CCG 3'
         3' TTT CGA TTC GGC AGA ATA GGC GGT TGG ATG 5'
    Pro–Thr–Tyr–Lys–Ala–Lys–Pro–Ser–Tyr–Pro–Pro–Thr–Tyr
```

FIGURE 13.35 Pathway for in vitro posttranslational hydroxylation of some of the tyrosine residues in the *M. edulis* adhesive protein. Tyrosine is converted to DOPA by the action of the enzyme tyrosinase and then can be oxidized to *o*-quinone by either catechol oxidase or tyrosinase. The oxidation of DOPA to *o*-quinone can be prevented by the addition of ascorbic acid.

of rubber starts from simple sugars and requires approximately 17 enzyme-catalyzed steps, with the final step being the polymerization of isopentenyl pyrophosphate onto an allylic pyrophosphate. The last step is catalyzed by the enzyme rubber polymerase.

Studies have been undertaken to determine whether rubber can be synthesized by genetically engineered microorganisms. As an initial step in this direction, a cDNA library was constructed by using mRNA from the rubber-producing plant *Hevea brasiliensis*. This library was then screened with a short synthetic DNA hybridization probe whose sequence was based on the amino acid sequence of a portion of the rubber polymerase enzyme. Antibodies directed against the purified enzyme were used to prove unequivocally that the cloned cDNA expressed rubber polymerase. This cDNA clone can now be used, possibly in concert with other genes in the rubber synthesis pathway, in an attempt to produce natural rubber in a microbial system. Alternatively, it can be used as a source of rubber polymerase to develop an in vitro catalytic system. In either case, research that might lead to a new synthetic route for the production of rubber is under way.

Polyhydroxyalkanoates

Polyhydroxyalkanoates are a class of biodegradable polymers that are produced by a number of different microorganisms, most notably *Alcaligenes eutrophus*, and used as an intracellular carbon and energy storage material. These compounds have thermoplastic or elastic properties, depending on the polymer composition, and are being considered for use in the synthesis of a range of biodegradable plastics. It has been estimated that by 2012 the U.S. market for biodegradable plastics will be around $1 billion per year.

Poly(3-hydroxybutyric acid) is the most thoroughly studied and characterized polyhydroxyalkanoate. Both the polymer and the *A. eutrophus* genes that encode its synthesis have been characterized. Poly(3-hydroxybutyric acid), its copolymer [poly(3-hydroxybutyrate-co-3-hydroxyvalerate)], and another polyhydroxyalkanoate [poly(3-hydroxyvaleric acid)] are produced commercially in the United Kingdom by the fermentation of *A. eutrophus*.

Although it is possible to produce poly(3-hydroxybutyric acid) as a by-product of the growth of *A. eutrophus,* the organism grows relatively slowly, requires a relatively low growth temperature (so that the fermentation vessel must be cooled), is difficult to lyse [making the purification of poly(3-hydroxybutyric acid) granules difficult], and utilizes only a limited number of carbon sources for growth (making production costs relatively high). On the other hand, when the genes for the biosynthesis of this polymer were transferred to *E. coli,* the resultant transformant grew rapidly to a high cell density and accumulated very large amounts (up to 95% of the dry cell weight) of poly(3-hydroxybutyric acid). Poly(3-hydroxybutyric acid) is synthesized from acetyl-CoA in three steps catalyzed by three enzymes (Fig. 13.36). The operon containing these genes was cloned into a plasmid as part of a 5.2-kb insert. Unfortunately, plasmids expressing the poly(3-hydroxybutyric acid) operon in *E. coli* were unstable. In the absence of selective pressure, such as the addition of antibiotics to the growth medium, about half of the *E. coli* cells lost the plasmid after approximately 50 generations. Plasmid loss of this magnitude, while not a major concern in small-scale batch cultures, becomes more of a problem with large-scale or continuous cultures (see chapter 17). This problem was overcome by inserting the *parB* genetic locus from another plasmid onto plasmids carrying the poly(3-hydroxybutyric acid) operon. This gene mediates plasmid stabilization by postsegregational killing of plasmid-free cells. The modified plasmids were quite stable even though the poly(3-hydroxybutyric acid) was produced constitutively, which places a metabolic load on the cells. An added benefit of producing poly(3-hydroxybutyric acid) in *E. coli* instead of *A. eutrophus* is that when the poly(3-hydroxybutyric acid) is recovered by extraction with an alkaline hypochlorite solution, the polymer is degraded to a much lesser extent than when it is produced in *A. eutrophus.* This is probably because most of the poly(3-hydroxybutyric acid) in *E. coli* is produced in a crystalline state, while in *A. eutrophus* it is amorphous. Nevertheless, the polymers extracted from the two organisms had identical polymer properties. In addition, *E. coli* transformants synthesizing poly(3-hydroxybutyric acid) produced very little acetate, which can be

FIGURE 13.36 Synthesis of poly(3-hydroxybutyric acid) from acetyl-CoA. The enzyme that catalyzes each of the reactions is shown to the right of the arrow.

FIGURE 13.37 Model of the genetically engineered microbial synthesis of the copolymer poly(3-hydroxybutyrate-co-3-hydroxyvalerate).

deleterious for cell growth, presumably because all of the excess acetyl-CoA of the cell was converted to poly(3-hydroxybutyric acid) rather than acetate.

The copolymer poly(3-hydroxybutyrate-co-3-hydroxyvalerate) has properties that are similar to those of polypropylene. Consequently, there is considerable commercial interest in the biological production of poly-(3-hydroxybutyrate-co-3-hydroxyvalerate). However, *E. coli* strains that expressed the three polymer biosynthetic genes synthesized only poly-(3-hydroxybutyric acid) and not the copolymer. This limitation was overcome with *E. coli* cells that were mutated at both the *fadR* and *atoC* loci. The FadR protein is a negative regulator of fatty acid biosynthesis, and the *fadR* mutant activates the glyoxylate shunt, enhancing the capacity for energy metabolism and biosynthesis, which leads to a reduction of acetate excretion and improvement of the biomass yield. The *atoC* gene product is a positive regulator of fatty acid uptake, and the gene product from the *atoC* mutation turns on the synthesis of the proteins encoded by *atoA* and *atoD*, whose gene products facilitate the uptake of propionate from the growth medium into the cell. The propionate is converted to propionyl-CoA and then condensed with acetyl-CoA to form 3-ketovaleryl-CoA, which can be converted into 3-hydroxyvaleryl-CoA before its incorporation into the copolymer (Fig. 13.37). The amount of 3-hydroxyvalerate in the copolymer is dependent on the percentage of propionate used during the fermentation, but it never exceeds 40%.

In addition to engineering the composition of polyhydroxyalkanoate, to produce polymers with specific desired properties, it is also essential that the chain lengths of these polymers be regulated. Some polymerizing enzymes from bacteria such as *Ralstonia eutropha* yield primarily short-chain

polymers with approximately 4 or 5 of the 3-hydroxyalkanoate monomeric units, while other enzymes from different bacteria, including *Pseudomonas oleovorans*, produce medium-chain polymers that include 6 to 14 monomeric units. In addition, mutants of the various steps of fatty acid oxidation can be generated and used to produce monomeric units with a modified composition compared with the wild-type strain. These modified monomers may then be incorporated into the polyhydroxyalkanoate. As a consequence of these manipulations, a wide range of polyhydroxyalkanoates with different physical and chemical properties have been synthesized.

It would be economically advantageous if bacteria could be engineered to efficiently produce polyhydroxyalkanoates using industrial waste products as a carbon source. To achieve this goal, polyhydroxybutyrate biosynthesis genes from a strain of an *Azotobacter* sp. were spliced onto a plasmid under the transcriptional control of the *lac* promoter (Fig. 13.38). The constructed plasmid was introduced into an *E. coli* strain that contained genes for the uptake and assimilation of lactose but that did not encode the *lac* repressor (see chapter 6). Thus, both lactose uptake and assimilation genes, as well as polyhydroxybutyrate biosynthesis genes, were expressed constitutively. The *E. coli* strain that carried the constructed plasmid was able to grow on either 25% lactose (a by-product of cheese making) or corn steep liquor (a by-product of corn [maize] processing) and to produce a significant level of polyhydroxybutyrate. By growing the transformed *E. coli* strain aerobically in a fed-batch culture (see chapter 17), after 24 hours, the cells accumulated polyhydroxybutyrate to 73% of their cell dry weight. Moreover, the physical properties of the polyhydroxybutyrate that was produced were similar to the properties of the polymer isolated from the *Azotobacter* sp. This engineered *E. coli* strain may be a suitable vehicle for producing a variety of polyhydroxyalkanoates from industrial waste products.

Hyaluronic Acid

Hyaluronic acid is a glycosaminoglycan, a polymer consisting of a repeating disaccharide unit of D-glucuronic acid and D-*N*-acetylglucosamine linked by β-1,4 and β-1,3 glycosidic bonds (Fig. 13.39), that in vivo can range in size from 5 to 20 kDa. This polymer is a component of the articular cartilage, where it is present as a coat around the cells; it is important in tissue hydrodynamics, movement, and cell proliferation; and it is used to treat osteoarthritis and to facilitate wound healing. Hyaluronic acid is also used as a component of some cosmetics and skin moisturizers. In 2005, the worldwide market for hyaluronic acid was a little over $1 billion, with most being supplied from rooster combs or the outer capsule of strains of group C *Streptococcus*. Both sources of hyaluronic acid can be problematic.

FIGURE 13.38 *Azotobacter* sp. genes encoding enzymes responsible for the biosynthesis of polyhydroxybutyrate under the transcriptional control of the *E. coli lac* promoter. The arrow indicates the direction of transcription. When a plasmid containing this construct is introduced into an *E. coli* strain that does not encode the *lac* repressor, the *pha* genes are expressed constitutively. *phaA*, 3-ketothiolase; *phaB*, acetoacetyl-CoA reductase; *phaC*, polyhydroxyalkanoate synthase.

FIGURE 13.39 Structure of the repeating disaccharide unit of hyaluronic acid.

The rooster comb-based product can cause severe inflammation in individuals allergic to avian antigens, while the *Streptococcus*-based product is both difficult and expensive to produce. It would therefore be advantageous to have an alternative source of hyaluronic acid.

B. *subtilis* is a well-established industrial bacterium that can secrete large amounts of synthesized products while at the same time being very economical to grow on inexpensive medium on a large scale. In addition, B. *subtilis* does not produce any exo- or endotoxins or the enzyme

FIGURE 13.40 Flowchart of the engineering of B. *subtilis* to produce hyaluronic acid.

Isolate the gene for type A hyaluronic acid synthase from *Streptoccocus pyogenes* by immunologically screening a clone bank

↓

Use PCR to amplify the gene for type C hyaluronic acid synthase (*hasA*) from *S. equisimilis* based on the *S. pyogenes* gene sequence

↓

Create a synthetic operon containing the *hasA* gene and B. *subtilis* analogs of the *hasB* and *hasC* genes under the control of the B. *amyloliquefaciens amyQ* promoter

↓

Introduce the synthetic operon, on a plasmid, into B. *subtilis*

↓

Integrate the synthetic operon into the B. *subtilis* genome

hyaluronidase (which degrades hyaluronic acid). The *Streptococcus equi-similis* gene encoding the last (and key) step in the synthesis of hyaluronic acid was isolated and then overexpressed in *B. subtilis* (Fig. 13.40), along with two *B. subtilis* genes that encode enzymes that provide the metabolites needed for the synthesis of hyaluronic acid. Following the large-scale growth in a bioreactor of this engineered *B. subtilis* strain, the amount of hyaluronic acid that was produced was comparable to the level produced by streptococcal strains (which grow more slowly), and the hyaluronic acid was secreted into the medium and not cell associated (as is the case with streptococcal strains), making it easier to isolate and purify. While this system may require some additional manipulation of the *B. subtilis* host strain to increase the yield of hyaluronic acid, this work is an important step toward the development of a commercial system for the bacterial production of hyaluronic acid.

SUMMARY

In addition to using bacteria as factories for the production of proteins, such as restriction enzymes, it is possible to modify the metabolic pathways of organisms, either by introducing new genes or by altering existing ones. In this way, various organisms can be genetically engineered for the production of a range of low-molecular-weight compounds, such as L-ascorbic acid, indigo, amino acids, antibiotics, lycopene, succinic acid, and the monomeric subunits of various biopolymers, such as xanthan gum, melanin, adhesive protein, rubber, polyhydroxyalkanoates, and hyaluronic acid. Here, the strategy is to insert the genes for one or more specific enzymes into the host organism by transformation with a vector-cloned gene construct. When they are expressed, the inserted genes encode a new pathway or augment a preexisting pathway for the synthesis of a specific compound. In addition, the biosynthesis of a desired compound may often be significantly increased by modulating the metabolic flux of the organism by turning on some pathways and blocking others. Several studies have shown that the creation of such unusual enzymatic pathways is technically feasible. Moreover, recombinant DNA technology has led to the development of new and more efficient synthetic routes for a variety of important compounds.

REFERENCES

Anderson, S., C. B. Marks, R. Lazarus, J. Miller, K. Stafford, J. Seymour, D. Light, W. Rastetter, and D. Estell. 1985. Production of 2-keto-L-gulonate, an intermediate in L-ascorbate synthesis, by a genetically modified *Erwinia herbicola*. *Science* 230:144–149.

Bailey, J. E. 1991. Toward a science of metabolic engineering. *Science* 252:1668–1675.

Banta, S., B. A. Swanson, S. Wu, A. Jarnagin, and S. Anderson. 2002. Alteration of the specificity of the cofactor-binding pocket of *Corynebacterium* 2,5-diketo-D-gluconic acid reductase A. *Protein Eng.* 15:131–140.

Banta, S., B. A. Swanson, S. Wu, A. Jarnagin, and S. Anderson. 2002. Optimizing an artificial metabolic pathway: engineering the cofactor specificity of *Corynebacterium*

2,5-diketo-D-gluconic acid reductase for use in vitamin biosynthesis. *Biochemistry* 41:6226–6236.

Berry, A. 1996. Improving production of aromatic compounds in *Escherichia coli* by metabolic engineering. *Trends Biotechnol.* 14:250–256.

Breukink, E., I. Wiedemann, C. van Kraaij, O. P. Kuipers, H.-G. Sahl, and B. de Kruijff. 1999. Use of the cell wall precursor Lipid II by a pore-forming peptide antibiotic. *Science* 286:2361–2364.

Brooks, J. E., P. D. Nathan, D. Landry, L. A. Sznyter, P. Waite-Rees, C. L. Ives, L. S. Moran, B. E. Slatko, and J. E. Benner. 1991. Characterization of the cloned *Bam*HI restriction modification system: its nucleotide sequence, properties of the methylase, and expression in heterologous hosts. *Nucleic Acids Res.* 19:841–850.

Cohen, G., D. Shiffman, M. Mevarech, and Y. Aharonowitz. 1990. Microbial isopenicillin N synthase genes: structure, function, diversity and evolution. *Trends Biotechnol.* 8:105–111.

della-Cioppa, G., S. J. Garger, G. G. Sverlow, T. H. Turpen, and L. K. Grill. 1990. Melanin production in *Escherichia coli* from a cloned tyrosinase gene. *Bio/Technology* 8:634–638.

Ensley, B. D., B. J. Ratzkin, T. D. Osslund, M. J. Simon, L. P. Wackett, and D. T. Gibson. 1983. Expression of naphthalene oxidation genes in *Escherichia coli* results in the biosynthesis of indigo. *Science* 222:167–169.

Flores, N., J. Xiao, A. Berry, F. Bolivar, and F. Valle. 1996. Pathway engineering for the production of aromatic compounds in *Escherichia coli*. *Nat. Biotechnol.* 14:620–623.

Floss, H. G. 1987. Hybrid antibiotics—the contribution of the new gene combinations. *Trends Biotechnol.* **5**:111–115.

Fu, J.-F., and Y.-H. Tseng. 1990. Construction of lactose-utilizing *Xanthomonas campestris* and production of xanthan gum from whey. *Appl. Environ. Microbiol.* **56**:919–923.

Gerritse, G., R. W. J. Hommes, and W. J. Quax. 1998. Development of a lipase fermentation process that uses a recombinant *Pseudomonas alcaligenes* strain. *Appl. Environ. Microbiol.* **64**:2644–2651.

Hahn, S. K., Y. K. Chang, and S. Y. Lee. 1995. Recovery and characterization of poly(3-hydroxybutyric acid) synthesized in *Alcaligenes eutrophus* and recombinant *Escherichia coli*. *Appl. Environ. Microbiol.* **61**:34–39.

Hazer, B., and A. Steinbüchel. 2007. Increased diversification of polyhydroxyalkanoates by modification reactions for industrial and medical applications. *Appl. Microbiol. Biotechnol.* **74**:1–12.

Herai, S., Y. Hashimoto, H. Higashibata, H. Maseda, H. Ikeda, S. Omura, and M. Kobayashi. 2004. Hyper-inducible expression system for streptomycetes. *Proc. Natl. Acad. Sci. USA* **101**:14031–14035.

Hillemann, D., A. Puhler, and W. Wolleben. 1991. Gene disruption and gene replacement in *Streptomyces* via single stranded DNA transformation of integration vectors. *Nucleic Acids Res.* **19**:727–731.

Hopwood, D. A., M. J. Bibb, C. J. Bruton, K. F. Chater, J. S. Feitelson, and J. A. Gil. 1983. Cloning *Streptomyces* genes for antibiotic production. *Trends Biotechnol.* **1**:42–48.

Hopwood, D. A., F. Malpartida, H. M. Kieser, H. Ikeda, J. Duncan, I. Fujii, B. A. M. Rudd, H. G. Floss, and S. Omura. 1985. Production of hybrid antibiotics by genetic engineering. *Nature* **314**:642–644.

Howard, K. A., C. Card, J. S. Benner, H. L. Callahan, R. Maunus, K. Silber, G. Wilson, and J. E. Brooks. 1986. Cloning the *Dde*I restriction-modification system using a two-step method. *Nucleic Acids Res.* **14**:7939–7951.

Hutchinson, C. R., H. Decker, K. Madduri, S. L. Otten, and L. Tang.

1993. Genetic control of polyketide biosynthesis in the genus *Streptomyces*. *Antonie Leeuwenhoek* **64**:165–176.

Hutchinson, C. R. 1994. Drug synthesis by genetically engineered microorganisms. *Bio/Technology* **12**:375–380.

Hutchinson, C. R., and I. Fujii. 1995. Polyketide synthase gene manipulation: a structure-function approach in engineering novel antibiotics. *Annu. Rev. Microbiol.* **49**:201–238.

Hwang, D. S., H. J. Yoo, J. H. Jun, W. K. Moon, and H. J. Cha. 2004. Expression of functional recombinant mussel adhesive protein Mgfp-5 in *Escherichia coli. Appl. Environ. Microbiol.* **70**:3352–3359.

Ikeda, M., K. Nakanishi, K. Kino, and R. Katsumata. 1994. Fermentative production of tryptophan by a stable recombinant strain of *Corynebacterium glutamicum* with a modified serine-biosynthetic pathway. *Biosci. Biotechnol. Biochem.* **58**:674–678.

Ishida, M., K. Miwa, S. Nakamori, and K. Sano. December 1989. Process for producing L-tryptophan. U.S. patent 4,885,245.

Isogai, T., M. Fukagawa, I. Aramori, M. Iwami, H. Kojo, T. Ono, Y. Ueda, M. Kohsaka, and H. Imanaka. 1991. Construction of a 7-aminocephalosporanic acid (7ACA) biosynthetic operon and direct production of 7ACA in *Acremonium chrysogenum. Bio/Technology* **9**:188–191.

Katz, L., and S. Donadio. 1993. Polyketide synthesis: prospects for hybrid antibiotics. *Annu. Rev. Microbiol.* **47**:875–912.

Kleinkauf, H., and H. von Dohren. 1990. Antibiotics—cloning of biosynthetic pathways. *FEBS Lett.* **268**:405–407.

Krämer, R. 1996. Genetic and physiological approaches for the production of amino acids. *J. Biotechnol.* **45**:1–21.

Lazarus, R. A., M. Hurle, S. Anderson, and D. B. Powers. December 1994. Enzymes for the production of 2-keto-L-gulonic acid. U.S. patent 5,367,544.

Lee, S. J., H. Song, and S. Y. Lee. 2006. Genome-based metabolic engineering of *Mannheimia succiniproducens* for succinic acid production. *Appl. Environ. Microbiol.* **72**:1939–1948.

Lee, S. Y., H. N. Chang, and Y. K. Chang. 1994. Production of poly(β-hydroxybutyric acid) by recombinant *Escherichia coli. Ann. N. Y. Acad. Sci.* **721**:43–53.

Lee, S. Y., K. S. Yim, H. N. Chang, and Y. K. Chang. 1994. Construction of plasmids, estimation of plasmid stability, and use of stable plasmids for the production of poly(β-hydroxybutyric acid) by recombinant *Escherichia coli. J. Biotechnol.* **32**:203–211.

Lee, S. Y., and H. N. Chang. 1995. Production of poly(3-hydroxybutyric acid) by recombinant *Escherichia coli* strains: genetic and fermentation studies. *Can. J. Microbiol.* **41**:207–219.

Liu, C.-I., G. Y. Liu, Y. Song, F. Yin, M. E. Hensler, W.-Y. Jeng, V. Nizet, A. H.-J. Wang, and E. Oldfield. 2008. A cholesterol biosynthesis inhibitor blocks *Staphylococcus aureus* virulence. *Science* **319**:1391–1394.

Magnolo, S. K., D. L. Leenutaphong, J. A. DeModena, J. E. Curtis, J. E. Bailey, J. L. Galazzo, and D. E. Hughes. 1991. Actinorhodin production by *Streptomyces coelicolor* and growth of *Streptomyces lividans* are improved by the expression of a bacterial hemoglobin. *Bio/Technology* **9**:473–476.

Martin, J. F. 1987. Cloning of genes involved in penicillin and cephalosporin biosynthesis. *Trends Biotechnol.* **5**:306–308.

McDaniel, R., S. Ebert-Khosla, D. A. Hopwood, and C. Khosla. 1995. Rational design of aromatic polyketide natural products by recombinant assembly of enzymatic subunits. *Nature* **375**:549–554.

Mermod, N., S. Harayama, and K. N. Timmis. 1986. New route to bacterial production of indigo. *Bio/Technology* **4**:321–324.

Nakamori, S., S.-I. Kobayashi, C. Kobayashi, and H. Takagi. 1998. Overproduction of L-cysteine and L-cystine by *Escherichia coli* strains with a genetically altered serine acetyltransferase. *Appl. Environ. Microbiol.* **64**:1607–1611.

Nikel, P. I., A. de Almeida, E. C. Melillo, M. A. Galvagno, and M. J. Pettinari. 2006. New recombinant *Escherichia coli* strain tailored for the

production of poly(3-hydroxybutyrate) from agroindustrial by-products. *Appl. Environ. Microbiol.* **72**:3949–3954.

Ozaki, A., R. Katsumata, and T. Oka. October 1989. Process for producing tryptophan. U.S. patent 4,874,698.

Park, J. H., K. H. Lee, T. Y. Kim, and S. Y. Lee. 2007. Metabolic engineering of *Escherichia coli* for the production of L-valine based on transcriptome analysis and *in silico* gene knockout simulation. *Proc. Natl. Acad. Sci. USA* **104**:7797–7802.

Pfeifer, B. A., S. J. Admiraal, H. Gramajo, D. E. Cane, and C. Khosla. 2001. Biosynthesis of complex polyketides in a metabolically engineered strain of *E. coli. Science* **291**:1790–1792.

Piekarowicz, A., R. Yuan, and D. C. Stein. 1991. A new method for the rapid identification of genes encoding restriction and modification enzymes. *Nucleic Acids Res.* **19**:1831–1835.

Prieto, M. A., M. B. Kellerhals, G. B. Bozzato, D. Ragnovic, B. Witholt, and B. Kessler. 1999. Engineering of stable recombinant bacteria for production of chiral medium-chain-length poly-3-hydroxyalkanoates. *Appl. Environ. Microbiol.* **65**:3265–3271.

Ren, Q., N. Sierro, M. Kellerhals, B. Kessler, and B. Witholt. 2000. Properties of engineered poly-3-hydroxyalkanoates produced in recombinant *Escherichia coli* strains. *Appl. Environ. Microbiol.* **66**:1311–1320.

Rhie, H. G., and D. Dennis. 1995. Role of *fadR* and *atoC*(Con) mutations in poly(3-hydroxybutyrate-co-3-hydroxyvalerate) synthesis in recombinant *pha*⁺ *Escherichia coli. Appl. Environ.*

Microbiol. **61**:2487–2492.

Salerno, A. J., and I. Goldberg. 1993. Cloning, expression, and characterization of a synthetic analog to the bioadhesive precursor protein of the sea mussel *Mytilus edulis. Appl. Microbiol. Biotechnol.* **39**:221–226.

Schwarzer, A., and A. Puhler. 1991. Manipulation of *Corynebacterium glutamicum* by gene disruption and replacement. *Bio/Technology* **9**:84–87.

Sikora, L. A. January 1991. DNA fragment encoding a rubber polymerase and its use. U.S. patent 4,983,729.

Sosio, M., F. Giusino, C. Cappellano, E. Bossi, A. M. Puglia, and S. Donadio. 2000. Artificial chromosomes for antibiotic-producing actinomycetes. *Nat. Biotechnol.* **18**:343–345.

Stachelhaus, T., A. Schneider, and M. A. Marahiel. 1995. Rational design of peptide antibiotics by targeted replacement of bacterial and fungal domains. *Science* **269**:69–72.

Strausberg, R. L., and R. P. Link. 1990. Protein-based medical adhesives. *Trends Biotechnol.* **8**:53–57.

Takagi, H., N. Awano, S.-I. Kobayashi, M. Noji, K. Saito, and S. Nakamori. 1999. Overproduction of L-cysteine and L-cystine by expression of genes for feedback inhibition-sensitive serine acetyltransferase from *Arabidopsis thaliana* in *Escherichia coli. FEMS Microbiol. Lett.* **179**:453–459.

Terasawa, M., M. Fukushima, Y. Kurusu, and H. Yukawa. 1990. L-Tryptophan production by the application of high expressed tryptophanase in *Escherichia coli. Proc. Biochem. Int.* **25**:172–175.

Velasco, J., J. L. Adrio, M. A. Moreno, B. Díez, G. Soler, and J. L. Barredo. 2000. Environmentally safe production of 7-aminodeactoxycephalosporanic acid (7-ADCA) using recombinant strains of *Acremonium chrysogenum. Nat. Biotechnol.* **18**:857–861.

Walder, R. Y., J. L. Hartley, J. E. Donelson, and J. A. Walder. 1981. Cloning and expression of the *Pst*I restriction-modification system in *Escherichia coli. Proc. Natl. Acad. Sci. USA* **78**:1503–1507.

Weber, J. M., J. O. Leung, S. J. Swanson, K. B. Idler, and J. B. McAlpine. 1991. An erythromycin derivative produced by targeted gene disruption in *Saccharopolyspora erythracea. Science* **252**:114–117.

Widner, B., R. Behr, S. Von Dollen, M. Tang, T. Heu, A. Sloma, D. Sternberg, P. L. DeAngelis, P. H. Weigel, and S. Brown. 2005. Hyaluronic acid production in *Bacillus subtilis. Appl. Environ. Microbiol.* **71**:3747–3752.

Yim, K. S., S. Y. Lee, and H. N. Chang. 1996. Synthesis of poly(3-hydroxybutyate-co-3-hydroxyvalerate) by recombinant *Escherichia coli. Biotechnol. Bioeng.* **49**:495–503.

Yoon, S.-H., J.-E. Kim, S.-H. Lee, H.-M. Park, M.-S. Choi, J.-Y. Kim, S.-H. Lee, Y.-C. Shin, J.-D. Keasling, and S.-W. Kim. 2007. Engineering the lycopene synthetic pathway in *E. coli* by comparison of the carotenoid genes of *Pantoea agglomerans* and *Pantoea ananatis. Appl. Microbiol. Biotechnol.* **74**:131–139.

REVIEW QUESTIONS

1. Describe a strategy for isolating the gene for the restriction endonuclease EcoRI.

2. Outline a strategy for cloning the gene for 2,5-diketo-D-gluconic acid reductase from *Corynebacterium* into *Erwinia*. Why is this useful?

3. Suggest a strategy for improving the commercial utility of a cloned 2,5-diketo-D-gluconic acid reductase gene.

4. How can indigo be produced in *E. coli*?

5. Outline a strategy for increasing the production of the amino acid tryptophan by *C. glutamicum*.

6. Suggest a strategy for isolating some of the genes that are involved in the biosynthesis of the antibiotic undecylprodigiosin, which is normally synthesized by *S. coelicolor*.

7. Why is it difficult to genetically transform various *Streptomyces* spp.? How can this difficulty be overcome?

8. Suggest a simple strategy for increasing the yield of an antibiotic by the genetic manipulation of the *Streptomyces* strain that produces the antibiotic.

9. Suggest an approach for producing modified versions of polyketide antibiotics, such as erythromycin.

10. How can an adhesive protein biopolymer that is normally produced by the blue mussel *M. edulis* be synthesized in *E. coli*?

11. Suggest a scheme for producing poly(3-hydroxybutyric acid) in *E. coli*.

12. What is whey? How can it be used to produce industrially important compounds?

13. How can *E. coli* be engineered to overproduce cysteine?

14. Suggest a scheme for the isolation of a lipase gene from the bacterium *P. alcaligenes*. How might this gene be used in a practical way?

15. How can the very large DNA fragments encoding antibiotic biosynthesis genes be introduced into host bacteria?

16. What strategies can be employed to produce large amounts of either 7ACA or 7ADCA in bacteria?

17. How can *E. coli* be engineered to produce lycopene?

18. How can the level of succinic acid produced by the bacterium *M. succiniproducens* be increased?

19. What is hyaluronic acid? How can it be produced in *B. subtilis*?

20. How can *E. coli* be genetically engineered to overproduce valine?

21. How can foreign proteins be expressed at high levels in *Streptomyces* spp.?

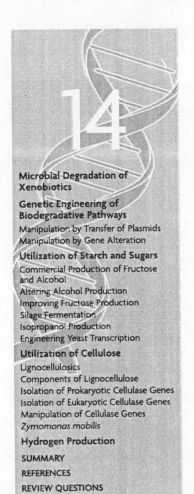

Bioremediation and Biomass Utilization

FOR CENTURIES, HUMANS BELIEVED that atmospheric, terrestrial, and aquatic systems were sufficient to absorb and break down wastes from population centers, industry, and farming. We now know that this is not true. Today, there are two fundamental problems. First, how do we dispose of the large quantities of wastes that are continually being produced? Second, how do we remove the toxic compounds that have been accumulating at dump sites, in the soil, and in water systems over the last few decades? Governments have tried to meet the challenge of environmental contamination by instituting antipollution regulations, but these rules often remain unenforced. Governments have also encouraged the three R's: reduce, reuse, and recycle.

Researchers are currently testing a number of technological strategies, including biotechnological schemes, to deal with large-scale wastes, such as lignocellulosics and toxic substances that persist in ecosystems.

The term "bioremediation" has been introduced to describe the process of using biological agents to remove toxic wastes from the environment. "Biomass" is the term used to describe the materials that are produced by the food and agricultural industries (e.g., starch and lignocellulosics) that were discarded as waste in the past. Biomass is now being considered as a source material for the production of a variety of economically important products.

Microbial Degradation of Xenobiotics

The problem of toxic waste disposal is enormous. Worldwide production in 1985 of just one chemical that is released into the environment—pentachlorophenol—was more than 50,000 tons. Incineration and chemical treatment have been used to break down many toxic chemicals, but these methods are costly and often create new environmental difficulties. With the discovery in the mid-1960s of a number of soil microorganisms that are capable of degrading xenobiotic ("unnatural," or synthetic; from the Greek *xenos*, meaning "foreign") chemicals, such as herbicides, pesticides, refrigerants, solvents, and other organic compounds, the notion that microbial

TABLE 14.1 Some *Pseudomonas* plasmids, their degradative pathways, and sizes

Name of plasmid	Compound(s) degraded	Plasmid size (kilobases)
SAL	Salicylate	60
SAL	Salicylate	68
SAL	Salicylate	72
SAL	Salicylate	83
TOL	Xylene and toluene	113
CAM	Camphor	225
XYL	Xylene	15
NAH	Naphthalene	69
OCT	Octane, D-camphor	~500
NAH7	Naphthalene, salicylate	83
PJP1	2,4-Dichlorophenoxyacetic acid	87
PJP2	2,4-Dichlorophenoxyacetic acid	54
PJB3	2,4-Dichlorophenoxyacetic acid	78
pP51	1,2-Di, 1,4-di-, and 1,2,4-trichlorobenzene	110
pAC31	3,5-Dichlorobenzoate	108
pAC25	3-Chlorobenzoate	102
pWW0	Xylene and toluene	117
pWW100	Biphenyl	200
pWWO	Xylene and toluene	176
pXYL-K	Xylene and toluene	135
pVI150	Phenol	>200
pNL1	Xylene, naphthalene, biphenyl	184
pAC27	3-Chlorobenzoate	110
pHMT112	Benzene	112
pTDN1	Aniline, *m*- and *p*-toluidine	79

Plasmids with the same name encode similar degradative pathways, even though they have different sizes and were described in different laboratories.

degradation might provide an economical and effective means of disposing of toxic chemical wastes gained credence.

Members of the genus *Pseudomonas* are the most predominant group of soil microorganisms that degrade xenobiotic compounds. Biochemical assays have shown that various *Pseudomonas* strains can break down and, as a consequence, detoxify hundreds of different organic compounds. In many cases, one strain can use any of several different related compounds as its sole carbon source.

The biodegradation of complex organic molecules generally requires the concerted efforts of several different enzymes. The genes that code for the enzymes of these biodegradative pathways are sometimes located in the chromosomal DNA, although they are more often found on large (approximately 50- to 200-kilobase) plasmids (Table 14.1). In some organisms, the genes that contribute to the degradative pathway are found in both chromosomal and plasmid DNA.

Degradative bacteria, in most cases, enzymatically convert xenobiotic, nonhalogenated aromatic compounds to either catechol (Fig. 14.1) or protocatechuate (Fig. 14.2). Then, through a series of oxidative cleavage reactions, catechol and protocatechuate are processed to yield either acetyl coenzyme A (acetyl-CoA) and succinate (Fig. 14.3) or pyruvate and acetaldehyde (Fig. 14.4), compounds that are readily metabolized by almost all

FIGURE 14.1 Pathways for the enzymatic conversion of aromatic compounds to catechol by degradative bacteria.

FIGURE 14.2 Pathways for the enzymatic conversion of aromatic compounds to protocatechuate by degradative bacteria.

organisms. Halogenated aromatic compounds, which are the main components of most pesticides and herbicides, are converted to catechol, protocatechuate, hydroquinones, or the corresponding halogenated derivatives

FIGURE 14.3 The *ortho*-cleavage pathway for enzymatic conversion of catechol and protocatechuate to acetyl-CoA and succinate.

by the same enzymes that degrade the nonhalogenated compounds. However, for the halogenated compounds, the rate of degradation is inversely related to the number of halogen atoms that are initially present on the target compound. Dehalogenation, the removal of a halogen substituent from an organic compound, is the critical requirement for detoxification and often occurs by a nonselective dioxygenase reaction that replaces the halogen on a benzene ring with a hydroxyl group. This step may occur either during or after the biodegradation of the original halogenated compound.

FIGURE 14.4 The *meta*-cleavage pathway for the enzymatic conversion of catechol and protocatechuate to pyruvate and acetaldehyde.

Genetic Engineering of Biodegradative Pathways

Despite the ability of many naturally occurring microorganisms to degrade a number of different xenobiotic chemicals, there are limitations to the biological treatment of these waste materials. For example, (1) no single microorganism can degrade all organic wastes; (2) high concentrations of some organic compounds can inhibit the activity or growth of degradative microorganisms; (3) most contaminated sites contain mixtures of chemicals, and an organism that can degrade one or more of the components of the mixture may be inhibited by other components; (4) many nonpolar

compounds adsorb onto particulate matter in soils or sediments and become less available to degradative microorganisms; and (5) microbial biodegradation of organic compounds is often quite slow. One way to address some of these problems is to transfer by conjugation into a recipient strain plasmids that carry genes for different degradative pathways (Fig. 14.5). If two resident plasmids contain homologous regions of DNA, recombination can occur and a single, larger "fusion" plasmid with combined functions can be created. Alternatively, if two plasmids do not contain homologous regions and, in addition, belong to different incompatibility groups, they can coexist within a single bacterium.

Manipulation by Transfer of Plasmids

Bacterial strains with expanded degradative capabilities were first created in the 1970s by Chakrabarty and coworkers. They used different plasmids to construct a bacterial strain that degraded a number of the hydrocarbon components found in petroleum (Fig. 14.5). This strain has been called a "superbug" because of its increased metabolic capabilities. The CAM

FIGURE 14.5 Schematic representation of the development of a bacterial strain that can degrade camphor, octane, xylene, and naphthalene. Strain A, which contains a CAM (camphor-degrading) plasmid, is mated with strain B, which carries an OCT (octane-degrading) plasmid. Following plasmid transfer and homologous recombination between the two plasmids, strain E carries a CAM and OCT biodegradative fusion plasmid. Strain C, which contains an XYL (xylene-degrading) plasmid, is mated with strain D, which contains an NAH (naphthalene-degrading) plasmid, to form strain F, which carries both of these plasmids. Finally, strains E and F are mated to yield strain G, which carries the CAM/OCT fusion plasmid, the XYL plasmid, and the NAH plasmid.

(camphor-degrading) plasmid was transferred by conjugation into a strain carrying the OCT (octane-degrading) plasmid. These two plasmids were incompatible and could not be maintained in the same cell as separate plasmids. However, when recombination occurred between the two plasmids, the resulting single plasmid was perpetuated and carried both camphor- and octane-degradative activities. The NAH (naphthalene-degrading) plasmid was transferred by conjugation into a strain carrying the XYL (xylene-degrading) plasmid. The NAH and XYL plasmids were compatible and could therefore coexist within the same host cell. Finally, the CAM/OCT fusion plasmid was transferred by conjugation into the strain carrying the NAH and XYL plasmids. The final result of these manipulations was the generation of a strain that grew better on crude oil than did any of the single-plasmid strains either alone or in combination.

Although this particular multiple-degradative strain has not been used to clean up oil spills, it has played a critical role in the development of the biotechnology industry. The inventor of this "superbug" was granted a U.S. patent describing its construction and use. This was the first patent ever granted for a genetically engineered microorganism and represented a watershed court decision, because it implied that biotechnology companies could protect their inventions in the same way as the chemical and pharmaceutical industries had in the past.

Most of the degradative bacteria that have been genetically manipulated by plasmid transfer are mesophiles, organisms that grow well only at temperatures between 20 and 40°C. However, rivers, lakes, and oceans that are polluted generally have temperatures that range from 0 to 20°C. To test whether bacteria with enhanced degradative abilities could be created for cold environments, a TOL (toluene-degrading) plasmid from a mesophilic *Pseudomonas putida* strain was transferred by conjugation into a facultative psychrophile, an organism with a low temperature optimum. The host psychrophile was able to degrade salicylate, but not toluene, and to use it as a sole carbon source at temperatures as low as 0°C. The transformed strain carried the introduced TOL plasmid and its own SAL (salicylate-degrading) plasmid and was able to use either salicylate or toluene as its sole carbon source at 0°C (Table 14.2). The wild-type (nontransformed)

TABLE 14.2 Generation times of wild-type (nontransformed) and transformed psychrophilic strains of *P. putida* on salicylate or toluate as the sole carbon source at various temperatures

Temperature (°C)	Generation time (h) for:		
	Wild-type + salicylate	Transformant + salicylate	Transformant + toluate
37	No growth	No growth	No growth
30	2.2	2.5	2.0
25	2.1	3.2	1.3
20	2.6	3.8	1.9
15	3.2	4.2	2.9
10	6.3	5.6	3.3
5	13.9	12.9	12.2
0	28.6	18.1	24.4

Adapted from Kolenc et al., *Appl. Environ. Microbiol.* 54:638–641, 1988.

The wild-type strain is unable to utilize toluate for growth at any temperature because it lacks the enzymes to metabolize the compound.

FIGURE 14.6 The *meta*-cleavage pathway and the *xyl* operon of the toluene- and xylene-degrading plasmid pWWO. Transcription of the *xyl* operon is controlled by the p^m promoter, which is regulated by the XylS gene product, which in turn must be activated by one of the initial pathway substrates. The genes from *xylX* to *xylH* (*X* to *H*) are under the control of the p^m promoter. The *xylS* gene, which is not part of this operon, is constitutively expressed. Some of the primary substrates are benzoate, where R and R' = H; 3-methylbenzoate, where R = H and R' = CH₃; 3-ethylbenzoate, where R = H and R' = CH₂CH₃; and 4-methylbenzoate, where R = CH₃ and R' = H. The *xylXYZ* genes encode toluene dioxygenase, *xylL* encodes dihydroxycyclohexadiene carboxylate dehydrogenase, *xylE* encodes catechol 2,3-dioxygenase, *xylF* encodes hydroxymuconic semialdehyde hydrolase, *xylG* encodes hydroxymuconic semialdehyde dehydrogenase, *xylH* encodes 4-oxalocrotonate tautomerase, *xylI* encodes 4-oxalocrotonate decarboxylase, *xylJ* encodes 2-oxopent-4-enoatehydratase, and *xylK* encodes 2-oxo-4-hydroxypentonate aldolase.

psychrophilic strain was unable to grow at any temperature when toluene (or toluate) was the only carbon source (not shown). This simple experiment indicates the feasibility of engineering psychrophilic degradative bacteria for use in the environment.

Manipulation by Gene Alteration

4-Ethylbenzoate. Bringing together different intact plasmid-based degradative pathways by conjugation is only one way to create bacteria with novel properties. It may also be possible to extend the degradative capability of a strain by altering the genes of an existing degradative pathway. The feasibility of this approach was examined for the toluene- and xylene-degrading pathway of plasmid pWWO. This plasmid encodes a "*meta*-cleavage" pathway involving 12 different genes and enables pseudomonads carrying the plasmid to utilize various alkylbenzoates as carbon sources (Fig. 14.6). The genes in the toluene–xylene pathway of pWWO are part of a single operon, called the *xyl* operon, under the control of the p^m promoter. Transcription from the p^m promoter, by RNA polymerase, is positively regulated by the *xylS* gene product, which is activated by most of the initial

FIGURE 14.7 (A) Protocol used to create a XylS protein that is activated by 4-ethylbenzoate. The p^m promoter is cloned onto plasmid pBR322 and replaces the tetracycline resistance (Tetr) gene promoter to form plasmid pJLR200; the xylS gene and its promoter are spliced onto a broad-host-range plasmid containing a kanamycin resistance (Kanr) gene. E. coli is transformed with both of these plasmids. Transformants are selected by their resistance to both ampicillin (Ampr) and kanamycin and then chemically mutagenized with ethyl methanesulfonate. Only cells with a mutation (S*) in the xylS gene that enables the XylS protein to be activated by 4-ethylbenzoate (EB) can grow on medium that contains both 4-ethylbenzoate and tetracycline, because only these cells are resistant to tetracycline.

substrates, such as benzoate and 3-methylbenzoate, of the pathway (Fig. 14.6). Detailed biochemical and genetic analyses showed that bacteria carrying pWWO could degrade 4-ethylbenzoate, albeit slowly, to 4-ethylcatechol, which accumulated in the medium, but no further. 4-Ethylcatechol

B

FIGURE 14.7 *(continued)* **(B)** Protocol used to create a modified catechol 2,3-dioxygenase that is not inhibited by 4-ethylcatechol. A *P. putida* strain carrying pWWO is transformed with a broad-host-range plasmid carrying the mutated *xylS** gene, whose product can activate the *p^m* promoter. Transformants are chemically mutagenized and then grown on minimal medium that contains 4-ethylbenzoate as the sole carbon source and kanamycin. Any cell that can grow on this medium carries a mutated catechol 2,3-dioxygenase gene. This mutation is indicated by a dot in the middle of the *xyl* gene cluster.

prevented its own degradation by inactivating one of the most important enzymes in the biodegradative pathway, catechol 2,3-dioxygenase, the product of the *xylE* gene. In addition, 4-ethylbenzoate, unlike most other alkylbenzoates, does not activate the XylS protein; consequently, transcription of the operon from the *p^m* promoter did not occur to any significant extent when 4-ethylbenzoate was the only substrate. Thus, there are two major problems with the naturally occurring *meta*-cleavage pathway system: (1) how to overcome the inactivation of an important enzyme in the degradative process by 4-ethylbenzoate and (2) how to induce transcription of the genes of this pathway with 4-ethylbenzoate as the inducer.

To find a mutant that could solve the second problem, a tetracycline resistance gene was placed under the control of the *p^m* promoter on one

plasmid, which also carried an ampicillin resistance gene. The *xylS* gene was cloned onto another plasmid carrying a kanamycin resistance gene. Transformants carrying both of these plasmids were selected on the basis of resistance to both ampicillin and kanamycin (Fig. 14.7A). The *Escherichia coli* cells carrying both of these plasmids were treated with the mutagen ethyl methanesulfonate and plated onto a medium containing both tetracycline and 4-ethylbenzoate. The only cells that could grow on this medium carried an altered XylS protein (S* in Fig. 14.7A) that could interact with 4-ethylbenzoate and cause the tetracycline resistance gene to be transcribed. Thus, the degradative pathway that includes this mutated *xylS* gene can be induced by 4-ethylbenzoate. To address the catechol 2,3-dioxygenase inactivation problem, the mutated *xylS* gene was subcloned onto a broad-host-range plasmid carrying a kanamycin resistance gene and introduced into *P. putida* cells carrying pWWO (Fig. 14.7B). The transformed cells were plated, at a high cell density, onto a minimal medium containing 4-ethylbenzoate as the sole carbon source, kanamycin to select for the presence of the plasmid, and ethyl methanesulfonate. Cells that were able to grow on this medium produced an altered form of the enzyme catechol 2,3-dioxygenase that was not inhibited by 4-ethylcatechol. Additional analysis confirmed that the catechol 2,3-dioxygenase gene on pWWO had been mutated and that mutant versions of both the *xylS* gene and the catechol 2,3-dioxygenase gene were required for the degradation of 4-ethylbenzoate.

An important aspect of this work is the fact that the two genes that were altered, i.e., those encoding XylS and catechol 2,3-dioxygenase, are the major determinants of the range of compounds that can be degraded by this pathway. The work with 4-ethylbenzoate demonstrates that by combining recombinant DNA technology, conventional mutagenesis, and the appropriate selection protocols, novel properties can be added to a degradative pathway.

Trichloroethylene. The compound trichloroethylene is widely used as a solvent and a degreasing agent, and as a result, it is one of the most common contaminants of soil and groundwater. Trichloroethylene persists in the environment for years, is a likely carcinogen, and is regulated in the United States under the Safe Water Drinking Act to a maximum contaminant level of 5 parts per billion. Unfortunately, anaerobic soil bacteria can reductively dehalogenate it to produce vinyl chloride, which is an even more toxic compound.

Studies showed that some of the strains of *P. putida* that could degrade aromatic compounds such as toluene could also degrade trichloroethylene. Genetic studies established that the complete *meta*-cleavage degradative pathway was not necessary to completely detoxify trichloroethylene. In fact, only the enzyme toluene dioxygenase, which normally catalyzes the oxidation of toluene to *cis*-toluene dihydrodiol, was required.

Four genes (Fig. 14.8A) are involved in the production of a functional toluene dioxygenase. These genes were isolated and expressed in *E. coli* under the control of the strong and inducible *tac* promoter. When *E. coli* cells carrying these genes were induced by the addition of isopropyl-β-D-thiogalactopyranoside (IPTG), an inducer of the *tac* promoter, trichloroethylene was efficiently broken down to harmless compounds by the concerted enzymatic activities of the Tod proteins encoded by these four genes (Fig. 14.8B). Although the initial rates of trichloroethylene degradation were

lower with *E. coli* than with the original *P. putida* strain, the *E. coli* cells maintained these rates for longer periods than *P. putida*. It has been speculated that the basis for this difference may be that *E. coli* membranes are not as susceptible to damage from trichloroethylene as *P. putida* membranes are.

In a variation of this experiment, a hybrid *Pseudomonas* strain with elements of two separate degradative pathways was constructed. Bacterial strains that can degrade the compound biphenyl use the enzyme biphenyl dioxygenase. Biphenyl dioxygenase is a multicomponent enzyme encoded by four genes, *bphA1A2A3A4*, where *bphA1* encodes a large subunit of terminal dioxygenase (an iron-sulfur protein), *bphA2* encodes a small subunit of terminal dioxygenase, *bphA3* encodes ferredoxin, and *bphA4* encodes ferredoxin reductase (Fig. 14.9). BphA1 and BphA2 are associated as a heterotetramer and catalyze the introduction of two oxygen atoms into the biphenyl ring. Ferredoxin and ferredoxin reductase act as an electron transfer system from reduced nicotinamide adenine dinucleotide (NADH) to reduce the terminal dioxygenase. Biphenyl dioxygenase is quite similar in both structure and function to the enzyme toluene dioxygenase. Despite the similarities of their enzymes, biphenyl-utilizing pseudomonads cannot grow on toluene, and toluene-utilizing strains cannot grow on biphenyl. However, when the *bphA1* gene (coding for the large subunit of biphenyl dioxygenase) from *P. putida* KF715 was replaced by homologous recombination with the *todC1* gene (coding for the large subunit of the toluene dioxygenase) from *P. putida* F1, the resultant strain (Fig. 14.9) was able to degrade trichloroethylene (Table 14.3). In fact, the engineered strain grew well on a range of aromatic compounds and also was very efficient at

FIGURE 14.8 A cloned toluene dioxygenase operon under the control of the *tac* promoter in *E. coli*. **(A)** Toluene dioxygenase activity is due to the products of four genes (*todA, todB, todC1,* and *todC2*). *todA* encodes a flavoprotein that accepts electrons from NADH and transfers them to a ferredoxin encoded by *todB*, which reduces the terminal dioxygenase that is encoded by *todC1* and *todC2*. These genes are equivalent to the genes *xylXYZ* shown in Fig. 14.7. **(B)** Toluene is converted to *cis*-toluene dihydrodiol by the concerted enzymatic activities of the Tod proteins.

FIGURE 14.9 Creation of a hybrid *Pseudomonas* strain with elements of two separate degradative pathways by replacement, through homologous recombination, of the biphenyl dioxygenase *bphA1* gene with a toluene dioxygenase *todC1* gene.

degrading trichloroethylene, demonstrating that it is possible to rationally engineer bacterial strains that can degrade a number of different compounds. The creation of degradative bacteria with novel biological activities was achieved by slightly different means by the creation of chimeric versions of the *bphA1* gene (Fig. 14.10). In this case, one *bphA1* gene was from a strain of *Pseudomonas pseudoalcaligenes* with the ability to degrade only a narrow range of polychlorinated biphenyls (PCBs), while the other was from *Burkholderia cepacia*, which can degrade a very wide range of PCBs. Some of the hybrid genes encoded an enzyme with a wider degradative ability than either of the original enzymes. The native *bphA1* gene in *P. pseudoalcaligenes* was replaced with hybrid genes by homologous recombination. It now remains to be seen whether these engineered bacterial strains degrade a range of PCBs on a large scale.

Cell surface-expressed enzymes. Currently, detoxification of organophosphate pesticides in the environment is performed by chemical treatment, incineration, or burial in landfill sites. Each of these approaches has serious environmental drawbacks. It would therefore be advantageous if bacteria that are able to degrade these compounds could be utilized in place of the methods that are currently used. Several soil bacteria, including *Pseudomonas diminuta* MG and *Flavobacterium* spp., possess an enzyme, organophosphorus hydrolase, that catalyzes the hydrolysis of many of these pesticides, including methyl and ethyl parathion, paraoxon, chlorpyrifos (Dursban), coumaphos, cyanophos, and diazinon, to environmentally innocuous compounds. Unfortunately, these bacteria, as well as *E. coli* engineered to express organophosphorus hydrolase, degrade these pesticides relatively slowly because of the low rate of uptake into the bacterial cells. Thus, a novel approach was developed to solve this problem. *E. coli* cells were engineered to express organophosphorus hydrolase as part of a fusion pro-

TABLE 14.3 Growth of parental and engineered *Pseudomonas* strains on various aromatic compounds

Strain	Growth on:				
	Biphenyl	Diphenylmethane	Toluene	Benzene	Trichloroethylene
P. putida KF715	+++	+++	−	−	−
P. putida F1	−	−	+++	+++	+
P. putida KF715-D5	++	+	+++	+++	+++

Adapted from Suyama et al., *J. Bacteriol.* **178:**4039–4046, 1996.

In *P. putida* KF715-D5, the *bphA1* gene from *P. putida* KF715 is replaced with the *todC1* gene from *P. putida* F1. +++, good growth; ++ moderate growth; +, poor growth; −, very poor or no growth.

Native genes

FIGURE 14.10 Chimeric (hybrid) *bphA1* genes constructed from *P. pseudoalcaligenes* and *B. cepacia bphA1* genes. The chimeras were constructed by digesting both of the isolated genes with the restriction enzymes shown and then recombining the resultant fragments as indicated. The various transformants carrying these constructs were subsequently assayed for enzymatic (degradative) activity.

tein that contained the *E. coli* lipoprotein signal peptide and the N-terminal portion of the lipoprotein and outer membrane protein A (Fig. 14.11). When this fusion protein was synthesized, it was localized on the outer surface of the bacterium (Fig. 14.12). This eliminated the problem of a low rate of pesticide uptake into the engineered bacterium. Cells with organophosphorus hydrolase on their outer surfaces had approximately seven times higher activity than cells that expressed a similar amount of the enzyme intracellularly. Moreover, the enzyme activity of cells with organophosphorus hydrolase on their surfaces was extremely stable. Nearly 100% of the activity was retained after 1 month at 37°C. This concept is quite promising; however, to date, it has been tested only on a laboratory scale.

Radioactive environments. The 26 countries worldwide that generate electricity from nuclear power plants, as well as those countries that have nuclear weapon programs, have generated thousands of radioactive waste sites. In the United States alone, there are more than 3,000 of these sites, and it has been estimated that, using currently available technology, the cleanup will require around $200 billion and take approximately 70 years. In addition to radioactivity, these sites also often have both organic and metal pollutants. While biodegradation of the organic pollutants is a logical first

FIGURE 14.11 The DNA construct used to produce the fusion protein Lpp–OmpA–OPH. This construct includes the *E. coli lac* promoter, DNA encoding the *E. coli lpp* signal sequence and the first 9 amino acids of the mature *E. coli* lipoprotein, the portion of the *E. coli ompA* gene encoding the transmembrane domain, and the gene *(opd)* for the *Flavobacterium* sp. organophosphorus hydrolase (OPH) and its signal peptide.

step in their remediation, most microorganisms are highly sensitive to the damaging effects of the radiation (Fig. 14.13). Fortunately, the nonpathogenic soil bacterium *Deinococcus radiodurans* is naturally resistant to quite high levels of ionizing radiation. This resistance has been attributed to DNA repair processes that are exceptionally effective at repairing DNA damage. Moreover, any DNA that is introduced into *D. radiodurans*, either as part of a plasmid or inserted into the chromosome, is also protected against high levels of potentially damaging radiation. Since this bacterium can express foreign genes while growing in the presence of continuous radiation, it would appear to be an ideal candidate for the expression of bioremediating proteins in toxic environments that contain radioactive contaminants.

As a first step toward developing a system to remediate organic pollutants that are present in radioactive environments, the four genes that together code for toluene dioxygenase (Fig. 14.8) were placed on a plasmid under the control of a constitutive *D. radiodurans* promoter. The entire plasmid was then inserted into the chromosome of *D. radiodurans* by homologous recombination, a single crossover, between the chromosomal DNA and a chromosomal DNA fragment on the plasmid adjacent to the toluene dioxygenase genes. The integrated toluene dioxygenase was active

FIGURE 14.12 Schematic representation of the fusion protein Lpp–OmpA–OPH anchored in the *E. coli* outer membrane with organophosphorus hydrolase on the outside of the cell and therefore exposed to the external medium. Lpp (shown in red) includes the first 9 amino acids from the *E. coli* lipoprotein. OmpA (shown in black) includes the transmembrane domain (amino acids 46 to 159) of *E. coli* outer membrane protein A. OPH (shown in blue) includes *Flavobacterium* sp. organophosphorus hydrolase and its signal peptide.

FIGURE 14.13 Effect of γ-irradiation on the growth of *E. coli* and *D. radiodurans*.

and conferred upon *D. radiodurans* the ability to degrade toluene, chlorobenzene, and 3,4-dichloro-1-butene irrespective of the presence or absence of high levels of ionizing radiation. The successful expression of toluene dioxygenase, an enzyme with several protein components and including metal and organic cofactors, suggests that many less complex biodegradative enzyme systems could also be expressed in *D. radiodurans*. Since *D. radiodurans* is tolerant of high levels of toluene, and a number of other organic compounds, once this bacterium has been genetically engineered to express the appropriate biodegradation pathway, it should be able to degrade a variety of organic pollutants in a radioactive environment. However, it remains to be seen how these engineered organisms behave under field conditions.

Nitroaromatics. For many years, a large number of different nitroaromatic compounds have been used industrially as dyes, plasticizers, explosives, solvents, and pesticides. Many of these compounds are recalcitrant to breakdown, persist in the environment, and are now considered to be toxic and sometimes carcinogenic pollutants. For example, the compound 4-nitrophenol (Fig. 14.14) is formed by the hydrolysis of the insecticide parathion and is considered to be a priority environmental pollutant, in part because it leads to numerous human health problems. Similarly, the compound 3-methyl-4-nitrophenol (Fig. 14.14) is a toxic breakdown product of the agricultural insecticide fenitrothion.

The bacterium *Burkholderia* sp. strain DNT facilitates the breakdown and detoxification of 2,4-dinitrotoluene. First, the enzyme 2,4-dinitrotoluene dioxygenase removes one nitro group to form 4-methyl-5-nitrocatechol (Fig. 14.14), which is then converted to 2-hydroxy-5-methylquinone by the enzyme 4-methyl-5-nitrocatechol monooxygenase. Unfortunately, the 4-methyl-5-nitrocatechol monooxygenase has a very narrow substrate range, which includes 4-nitrocatechol (Fig. 14.14), as well as 4-methyl-5-nitrocatechol. However, this enzyme cannot efficiently use either of the seemingly similar substrates 4-nitrophenol or 3-methyl-4-nitrophenol. In an effort to expand the substrate range of the enzyme, the *Burkholderia* sp.

	Native enzyme	Modified enzyme
4-Methyl-5-nitrocatechol	+	++
4-Nitrocatechol	+	++
4-Nitrophenol	–	+
3-Methyl-4-nitrophenol	–	+

FIGURE 14.14 Breakdown of nitroaromatic compounds by a strain of *Burkholderia* sp. that produces either the native form or a modified form of the enzyme 4-methyl-5-nitrocatechol monooxygenase.

strain DNT 4-methyl-5-nitrocatechol monooxygenase gene was isolated and subjected to error-prone PCR, and the randomly mutated genes were cloned into a plasmid vector. The library of mutated 4-methyl-5-nitrocatechol monooxygenase genes was transferred into *E. coli* cells by electroporation, and the transformants were screened for activity on agar plates containing 4-nitrophenol. Cells that contained the wild-type gene turned the colonies light brown, while one transformant (of 3,000 tested) turned the colony dark brown, indicating that the 4-nitrophenol was being broken down. When the DNA sequence of the 4-methyl-5-nitrocatechol monooxygenase gene from the transformant that turned the medium dark brown was determined, two amino acids within the encoded protein had been altered. Amino acid 22 was changed from methionine to leucine, and amino acid 380 was changed from leucine to isoleucine. These two amino acid alterations resulted in the altered enzyme having 10 times greater activity toward 4-nitrophenol and 4 times greater activity toward 3-methyl-4-nitrophenol than the native form of the enzyme. In addition, the modified enzyme had about 50% more activity than the native enzyme toward

4-nitrocatechol and 4-methyl-5-nitrocatechol. The changes in activity that were found following the mutagenesis of the 4-methyl-5-nitrocatechol monooxygenase gene are an important first step in developing a bacterium that can effectively degrade 4-nitrophenol and 3-methyl-4-nitrophenol.

Utilization of Starch and Sugars

Starch, the major food reserve polysaccharide in plants, consists of a mixture of linear homopolymers (amylose) and branched homopolymers (amylopectin) of D-glucose. Amylose is made up of linear chains of 1×10^2 to 4×10^5 D-glucose residues linked by α-1,4 bonds (Fig. 14.15A). Amylopectin consists of short linear chains of approximately 17 to 23 glucose units that are linked by α-1,4 bonds and joined by 1,6 linkages and some 1,3 linkages to form a highly branched structure that contains 1×10^4 to 4×10^7 glucose residues (Fig. 14.15B). The degree of branching and the ratio of amylose to amylopectin vary with the source and age of the starch.

FIGURE 14.15 (A) Pathway for the enzymatic hydrolysis of amylose; **(B)** pathway for the enzymatic hydrolysis of amylopectin. The blue circles represent D-glucose residues.

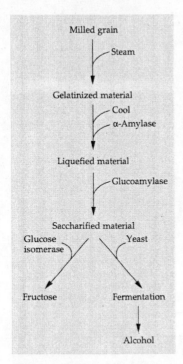

Milled grain

— Steam

Gelatinized material

— Cool
— α-Amylase

Liquefied material

— Glucoamylase

Saccharified material

Glucose Yeast
isomerase

Fructose Fermentation

Alcohol

FIGURE 14.16 Industrial production of fructose and alcohol from starch.

Commercial Production of Fructose and Alcohol

The major use of starch is in the food and brewing industries, where it is usually hydrolyzed to low-molecular-weight components before being converted into other compounds, especially fructose and alcohol. The most important enzymes for breaking down and transforming starch are α-amylase, glucoamylase, and glucose isomerase. Together, these three enzymes account for approximately 30% of the cost of all enzymes currently used for industrial processes.

Fructose and alcohol are produced commercially from starch by multistep processes that include both enzymatic and nonenzymatic reactions, as follows (Fig. 14.16).

1. The procedure begins with the gelatinization of milled grain (often corn [maize], which is approximately 40% starch). This treatment—steam cooking under pressure—exposes the surface area of the starch, thereby making it more readily available for subsequent enzymatic hydrolysis. The product of this process has a gel-like consistency.
2. The gelatinized starch is cooled to 50 to 60°C, and α-amylase is added. In this liquefaction step, the gel-like starch is enzymatically digested by the hydrolysis of the available α-1,4-linkages to form low-molecular-weight polysaccharides. A high temperature is used because enzyme hydrolysis is more rapid at high temperatures and the enzyme does not efficiently penetrate the gelatinized starch at lower temperatures.
3. The final step for the release of glucose includes the addition of glucoamylase and results in the saccharification—complete hydrolysis—of the remaining polysaccharides, including both linear and cross-linked molecules.

The end product of these treatments is glucose, which may be either converted into alcohol as a result of fermentation by yeast cells or transformed into fructose by the enzyme glucose isomerase. The success of the latter enzymatic conversion has led to the replacement of sucrose by fructose, which is much cheaper than sucrose, as a sweetener for prepared foods and beverages in North America. The source of starch for commercial fructose production is generally corn, and the final product is called high-fructose corn syrup or high-fructose syrup, although it contains a mixture of fructose and glucose. High-fructose corn syrup is typically either 90% fructose (for baked goods), 55% fructose (in soft drinks), or 42% fructose (in sports drinks), with the remainder being glucose.

The enzyme α-amylase randomly hydrolyzes α-1,4-linkages in both amylose and amylopectin chains, yielding a mixture of glucose, maltose (two glucose molecules joined by an α-1,4 linkage), maltotriose (three glucose molecules joined by α-1,4 linkages), and a series of α-limit dextrins, which are the portions of the amylopectin chains that contain cross-links (Fig. 14.15). Although α-amylase can be isolated from a variety of microorganisms, it is commonly obtained from *Bacillus amyloliquefaciens* for industrial purposes.

For some applications, the enzyme β-amylase is used in addition to or in place of α-amylase to digest starch. By hydrolyzing alternate α-1,4 linkages from the ends of amylose and amylopectin chains, β-amylase cleavage yields primarily maltose residues and various β-limit dextrins.

MILESTONE

Microorganisms Having Multiple Compatible Degradative Energy-Generating Plasmids and Preparation Thereof
A. M. CHAKRABARTY
U.S. patent 4,259,444, 1981

Before the advent of recombinant DNA technology, one of the ways that DNA could be moved from one microorganism to another was by conjugation, in which entire plasmids were transferred between organisms. Chakrabarty transferred degradative plasmids—plasmids encoding all of the enzymes involved in the biodegradation of a particular compound—from one bacterium to another until he had constructed bacterial strains that contained several degradative plasmids. Each degradative pathway, encoded by the genes on a plasmid, degraded a different organic molecule. Starting with four separate bacteria, Chakrabarty and his coworkers constructed a single bacterium that contained the pathways to degrade camphor, octane, salicylate, and naphthalene. While this work was scientifically interesting and innovative in and of itself (especially since it was conducted in the early 1970s, before the development of most of the techniques of recombinant DNA that are now taken for granted), the key issue for the biotechnology industry was that this invention was awarded a U.S. patent in March 1981, nearly 9 years after the application was first filed. Following the landmark decision by the U.S. Supreme Court in Chakrabarty's favor, it was ruled that genetically engineered microorganisms were inventions that could be patented in the same way as any other invention. As much as any landmark scientific experiment, this court decision and the subsequent award of the patent has become a cornerstone of the development of the biotechnology industry.

The enzyme glucoamylase hydrolyzes α-1,3, α-1,4, and α-1,6 linkages; however, because it is less efficient than α-amylase in cleaving α-1,4 linkages, it is usually used in conjunction with α-amylase. The major role of glucoamylase is digestion of the cross-links of amylopectin, which results in its complete breakdown to glucose. Glucoamylase and other enzymes are used to reduce the carbohydrate (limit dextrin) content of normal beers to produce the so-called light and dry varieties. Although glucoamylase digestion is usually performed prior to the onset of the fermentation, the two steps may be combined. A number of organisms produce glucoamylase, but for industrial purposes, it is usually obtained from the fungus *Aspergillus niger*.

Altering Alcohol Production

The enzymes that are used in the production of alcohol or fructose from milled grain are major components of the overall cost of the process. These enzymes are often used only once and then discarded. Thus, innovative approaches to the inexpensive large-scale production of the enzymes could lower the cost of alcohol or fructose production. There are several ways to achieve this end.

- Each of the enzymes could be overproduced in a fast-growing recombinant microorganism that utilizes an inexpensive substrate, thereby lowering the cost compared with production from native organisms.

- Variants of α-amylase, either naturally occurring or genetically manipulated, that function efficiently at 80 to 90°C could be used to allow the liquefaction step to be performed at this temperature. Heat-resistant α-amylase would speed the hydrolysis of gelatinized starch while decreasing the amount of energy that is required to cool the gelatinized starch to a temperature suitable for starch hydrolysis.

FIGURE 14.17 Detection of a *B. subtilis* clone expressing an α-amylase gene. The halo results from the degradation of the starch in the medium in the vicinity of the clone by secreted α-amylase.

- The α-amylase and glucoamylase genes could be altered so that each enzyme would have the same temperature and pH optimum, thereby enabling the liquefaction and saccharification steps to be performed under the same conditions.
- An enzyme that could efficiently degrade raw starch could be found or engineered, obviating the need for the gelatinization step and thereby saving a large amount of energy.
- A fermentation organism that can synthesize and secrete glucoamylase could be developed, eliminating the need to purify and add this enzyme during fermentation.

A considerable amount of research has been initiated to determine whether these possibilities are feasible.

Genes that code for α-amylase have been isolated from a number of organisms, including *B. amyloliquefaciens* and the high-temperature-tolerant bacterium *Bacillus stearothermophilus*. Briefly, chromosomal DNA was isolated, partially digested with the restriction enzyme Sau3AI, and then ligated to BamHI-digested pUB110 DNA. This plasmid has a unique BamHI site and carries a kanamycin resistance gene. The clone bank was transformed into *Bacillus subtilis*, which does not have α-amylase activity, and transformants were selected for resistance to kanamycin. All transformants were tested for the production and secretion of α-amylase as follows. After the transformants had formed colonies at 65°C on solid medium containing starch, the plates were exposed to iodine vapor. The colonies producing α-amylase were surrounded by a distinctive halo, or clear zone, indicating that the starch in the immediate vicinity of these cells had been hydrolyzed (Fig. 14.17). A positive starch–iodine test signifies that the transformed cell contains an α-amylase gene that is transcribed from its own promoter, because the vector does not carry a promoter. Also, a secretion signal is present, because the substrate is too large to enter the cell, and therefore the halo must be due to the activity of a secreted α-amylase. The availability of α-amylase genes from varied sources will enable researchers to carry out specific genetic modifications that suit the needs of specific industrial processes.

With the aim of bypassing the saccharification step during the production of alcohol from starch, researchers isolated a full-length glucoamylase complementary DNA (cDNA) from the fungus *Aspergillus awamori* and cloned it into a *Saccharomyces cerevisiae* plasmid under the control of the promoter and transcription terminator regulatory signals from the yeast enolase *(ENO1)* gene. A laboratory strain of *S. cerevisiae* that was transformed with the plasmid carrying the glucoamylase cDNA was able to express this activity and to ferment soluble starch to alcohol, thus demonstrating that the approach is feasible.

Unfortunately, this laboratory strain of *S. cerevisiae* has a number of properties that make it ill suited for use in a commercial process, including an inability to tolerate high levels of alcohol, inefficient expression of the glucoamylase cDNA, and loss of plasmids unless special conditions (selective pressure) are used for their maintenance. These problems, however, are not insurmountable. First, the level of glucoamylase expression was increased approximately fivefold by deleting a 175-base-pair (bp) negative regulatory region from the *ENO1* promoter on the plasmid. Second, the plasmid was modified by deleting its yeast origin of replication and adding a segment of DNA that is homologous to a yeast chromosomal site, thereby

converting it to an integrating vector. With this form of the plasmid, the complete glucoamylase construct was incorporated into a chromosomal site and stably maintained. Third, another *S. cerevisiae* strain (brewer's yeast) that tolerates high levels of alcohol was used as the host cell. The integrating vector was used to transform this yeast strain.

As a result of these modifications, investigators created two novel yeast strains that performed better than a naturally occurring amylolytic (starch-hydrolyzing) yeast, *Saccharomyces diastaticus*, which is closely related to *S. cerevisiae* and can hydrolyze and ferment soluble starch (Table 14.4). The performance of the brewer's strain, which contained the integrated glucoamylase gene, was superior to that of the laboratory strain with the same gene on a multicopy plasmid. This difference probably reflects plasmid instability with the concomitant loss of the introduced glucoamylase gene. Neither the laboratory strain nor the brewer's strain of *S. cerevisiae* was able to utilize soluble starch unless the strain was transformed with the cloned glucoamylase gene. In both the plasmid and integrated forms, the *A. awamori* glucoamylase cDNA was under the control of regulatory signals of *ENO1* from which the 175-bp negative regulatory region had been removed. The plasmid was maintained under selective pressure.

In an effort to produce large amounts of glucoamylase, several copies of the glucoamylase gene were integrated into the chromosomal DNA of the fungus *A. niger*. Surprisingly, there was no correlation between the number of copies of the glucoamylase gene in the chromosomal DNA and the amount of measured enzyme activity. On the other hand, the level of enzyme activity was strongly dependent upon the sites where the genes were inserted. Thus, merely increasing the gene copy number is not sufficient to produce a larger amount of active enzyme.

While most strains of the yeast *S. cerevisiae* encode only an intracellular glucoamylase, which is generally expressed only during sporulation, a few strains encode a secreted glucoamylase. Unfortunately, none of these enzymes contains a starch-binding domain. Thus, while *S. cerevisiae* glucoamylases can hydrolyze soluble starch (dextrins), they are unable to break down the larger molecules of insoluble starch. In an attempt to construct a strain of *S. cerevisiae* that could hydrolyze insoluble starch and therefore be of use in a variety of industrial processes, the coding region of a secreted *S. cerevisiae* glucoamylase gene was fused to a DNA fragment encoding a starch-binding domain from the fungus *A. niger* (Fig. 14.18). When this construct was expressed in *S. cerevisiae*, the presence of the starch-binding domain increased the ability of the enzyme to degrade

TABLE 14.4 Fermentation of soluble starch (25% [wt/vol]) by various yeast strains

Strain	Carbohydrate utilized (%)	Ethanol produced (g/liter)	Ethanol yield (g/g of substrate)
Laboratory	5	<0.1	0
Laboratory + gene on a plasmid	68	75.6	0.41
Brewer's	<1	3.1	0
Brewer's + integrated gene	93	118.2	0.48
S. diastaticus	43	44.2	0.38

Adapted from Cole et al., *Bio/Technology* **6**:417–421, 1988.

FIGURE 14.18 The genetic construct used to produce in *S. cerevisiae* a secreted glucoamylase containing a starch-binding domain (from *A. niger*). The construct is transcribed under the control of the yeast *pGAL* promoter in the direction indicated by the arrow.

insoluble starch by about sixfold. While this system is far from optimized, this simple genetic manipulation is an important initial step in the development of more efficient industrial systems for the production of alcohol from starch.

Low-ethanol wines. In recent years, many wine drinkers have expressed a strong preference for wines that contain only low levels of alcohol. In addition, consumer preferences have also moved to wines with a high flavor intensity that are prepared from fully matured grapes. However, the juice that is obtained from fully matured grapes generally contains a very high sugar concentration, which in turn produces wines with high levels of alcohol. A number of attempts have been made to engineer brewer's yeasts (*S. cerevisiae*) to reduce the ethanol content of the wine that is produced. Although a number of these approaches have successfully lowered the ethanol concentration, they typically cause the accumulation of undesirable side products. Nevertheless, one novel strategy seems to have avoided many of the problems of past efforts. By expressing in *S. cerevisiae* a gene (*noxE*) from the bacterium *Lactococcus lactis* that encodes an H_2O-NADH oxidase (Fig. 14.19), it was possible to significantly alter some of the metabolic fluxes within the yeast cell. Transformed yeast cells that carried this gene within their chromosomal DNA had an intracellular NADH content that was about 75 to 80% lower than that of the native yeast strain and an oxidized nicotinamide adenine dinucleotide (NAD^+) concentration that was 32 to 45% higher. At the same time, the reduced nicotinamide adenine dinucleotide phosphate (NADPH) and oxidized nicotinamide adenine dinucleotide phosphate ($NADP^+$) ratios of the two yeast strains were identical. The transformed yeast showed a 15% decrease in the amount of ethanol produced and, unfortunately, increases of approximately threefold in the amounts of acetaldehyde and acetic acid that were produced, which

FIGURE 14.19 (A) Oxidation of NADH catalyzed by the H_2O-NADH oxidase encoded by the *noxE* gene from the bacterium *L. lactis*; (B) the bacterial *noxE* gene under the transcriptional control of the yeast glyceraldehyde 3-phosphate dehydrogenase gene promoter and the yeast phosphoglycerate kinase transcription terminator. The entire construct was integrated into the yeast chromosomal DNA.

A

$$4NADH + O_2 \xrightarrow{\ noxE\ } 4NAD^+ + 2H_2O$$

B

impair both growth and fermentation, as well as imparting unacceptable flavors to the wine. To overcome these side effects, researchers undertook a systematic study of the growth of this modified yeast strain under a wide range of conditions. It was observed that if oxygen was supplied to the growing cells only during the stationary phase, there was a 7% reduction in the ethanol yield compared to the native strain, without the inhibitory levels of acetaldehyde and acetone being formed. Researchers are now investigating whether the wine that is produced using the above-mentioned yeast strain is suitable for human consumption.

Improving Fructose Production

The enzyme glucose isomerase should really be called xylose/glucose isomerase, because it primarily catalyzes the conversion of the five-carbon sugar D-xylose to D-xylulose, with the conversion of D-glucose to D-fructose being a secondary or side reaction (Fig. 14.20). Kinetically, xylose/glucose isomerase has a lower k_{cat} (catalytic rate constant) and a higher K_m (binding constant) for glucose than for xylose, which means that xylose is bound more tightly to the enzyme than is glucose and that xylose is converted more rapidly to xylulose than glucose is converted to fructose.

Xylose/glucose isomerases are intracellular enzymes and, as such, do not yield the same quantities or purity of product as do the extracellular, or secreted, enzymes that are used in many industrial processes. Most industrial enzymes are used without any extensive purification. An extracellular enzyme preparation generally contains many fewer proteins than an intracellular extract. In addition, the preparation of an intracellular protein extract requires separation of the cells from the growth medium, mechanical disruption of the cells, and removal of cell debris following disruption. These factors lead to higher production costs for xylose/glucose isomerase than for many other industrial enzymes. One way to overcome this problem is to use a batch of xylose/glucose isomerase more than once. This recycling can be achieved by immobilizing the enzyme on a solid support, which both stabilizes the enzyme and facilitates its reuse.

The isomerization of glucose to fructose is a reversible reaction, and the final fructose content is dependent on the reaction temperature. The higher the temperature, the greater the fructose content in the final product. Most commercial processes use conversion temperatures of around 60°C. The enzyme is typically used in an immobilized state that is obtained by cross-linking it to itself with glutaraldehyde and then using it in a continuous process in a packed bed reactor. Under these conditions, a batch of enzyme can be used for approximately 150 to 200 days before it is discarded. Consequently, increasing the temperature optimum for the enzymatic

FIGURE 14.20 Conversion of glucose to fructose, catalyzed by glucose isomerase.

activity and the thermostability of xylose/glucose isomerase is one way to make it more efficient.

The thermophilic bacterium *Thermus thermophilus* produces a xylose/glucose isomerase that not only is active at 95°C, but also is very stable at high temperatures. Therefore, this enzyme is a good candidate for use in industrial processes. Unfortunately, wild-type *T. thermophilus* does not produce large amounts of the enzyme. To circumvent this problem, the *T. thermophilus* xylose/glucose isomerase gene was isolated and expressed in *E. coli* and *Bacillus brevis* under the control of various promoters and ribosome-binding sites (Table 14.5). One of the constructs (the last one listed in Table 14.5) overproduced xylose/glucose isomerase more than 1,000-fold relative to the amount found in the original organism. Therefore, with this construct, high yields of a thermostable xylose/glucose isomerase can be produced for the industrial synthesis of fructose from glucose.

In addition, the substrate specificity of the enzyme can be enhanced. In one series of experiments, site-directed mutagenesis was used to change the nucleotides encoding either one or two amino acids of the xylose/glucose isomerase from the thermophilic organism *Clostridium thermosulfurogenes*. The targeted sites were selected for modification because of other evidence indicating that the corresponding amino acids were involved in substrate binding. Changing the tryptophan at amino acid residue 139 to phenylalanine or the valine at amino acid residue 186 to threonine produces a 1.7- to 2.6-fold increase in the catalytic efficiency (k_{cat}/K_m) of the enzyme toward glucose (Table 14.6). Moreover, these changes cause a two- to sevenfold reduction in the k_{cat}/K_m values of the enzyme toward xylose. When an enzyme has both of these amino acid changes, the k_{cat}/K_m value for glucose increases by 5.7-fold and the k_{cat}/K_m value for xylose decreases by 4.5-fold. The double amino acid modification changes an enzyme that was initially 17 times more reactive with xylose than with glucose to one that is now 1.5 times more reactive with glucose than it is with xylose. The shift in specificity that has been achieved, together with the thermostability of this xylose/glucose isomerase, should make it attractive for use in the industrial conversion of glucose to fructose.

Silage Fermentation

Crops such as grasses, corn, and alfalfa need to be preserved so that they can be used as animal feed many months after the crop is harvested. Traditionally, these crops are preserved by naturally occurring lactic acid bacteria that use

TABLE 14.5 Amounts of *T. thermophilus* xylose/glucose isomerase in different bacteria

Species	Plasmid copy no.	Promoter source	Source of ribosome-binding site	Enzyme activity (units/liter)
T. thermophilus	None	*T. thermophilus*	*T. thermophilus*	20
E. coli	200	*E. coli lac*	*T. thermophilus*	190
E. coli	20	*E. coli tac*	*T. thermophilus*	1,790
E. coli	20	*E. coli tac*	*E. coli*	3,260
E. coli	20	Phage T7 f10	*E. coli*	7,050
B. brevis	20	*B. brevis cwp*	*T. thermophilus*	1,400
B. brevis	20	*B. brevis cwp*	*T. thermophilus*	25,000

Adapted from Dekker et al., *Appl. Microbiol. Biotechnol.* **36:**727–732, 1992.

The first row represents data for the original enzyme-producing strain. All the other strains are transformants carrying the *T. thermophilus* xylose/glucose isomerase gene on a multicopy plasmid.

TABLE 14.6 Catalytic efficiency of wild-type and mutant xylose/glucose isomerases from *C. thermosulfurogenes*

Amino acid change(s)	Catalytic effiency (k_{cat}/K_m) (min⁻¹ mM⁻¹) toward:	
	Glucose	Xylose
None (wild type)	5.8	97.2
Trp-139 → Phe	15	13.6
Val-186 → Thr	9.7	55.4
Trp-139 → Phe, Val-186 → Thr	32.9	21.6

Adapted from Meng et al., *Proc. Natl. Acad. Sci. USA* **88:**4015–4019, 1991.

the crop as a fermentation substrate to produce lactic and acetic acids. The resulting low pH restricts the growth and metabolic activity of other microorganisms and ensures that the crop is preserved. This preservation strategy is called the making of silage. Often, the numbers of lactic acid bacteria that are found on a fresh crop are quite small, so that a bacterial inoculum, typically *Lactobacillus plantarum*, must be added. Unfortunately, these bacterial inoculants are not especially effective when the amount of water-soluble carbohydrates in the fresh crop is insufficient to support both bacterial growth and lactic acid production.

To develop a bacterium that might be effective in silage fermentation, an α-amylase gene from a strain of *Lactobacillus amylovorus* that does not support silage fermentation was spliced into the *L. plantarum* gene for conjugated acid bile hydrolase *(cbh)* and integrated into the chromosomal DNA of a strain of *L. plantarum* (Fig. 14.21). The *cbh* gene is a dispensable gene when the bacterium is grown on silage; it encodes an enzyme that is active only when the bacterium is located in an animal's intestine. This work is an important first step in the development of *L. plantarum* strains that are more effective in the fermentation of silage from crops such as alfalfa, which contain a high level of starch.

Isopropanol Production

In order to decrease our reliance on nonrenewable petroleum products, it may be possible to engineer microorganisms to produce isopropanol from glucose (e.g., derived from starch). Isopropanol may be used directly as a fuel instead of methanol to esterify fats and oils to produce biodiesel, or it may be dehydrated to yield propylene, which is used to synthesize the polymer polypropylene. To engineer *E. coli* to produce isopropanol, the genes that were introduced into *E. coli* were based on the genes encoding the isopropanol biosynthesis pathway that exists in *Clostridium beijerinckii* (an organism that produces only moderate amounts of isopropanol but is difficult to grow and to manipulate genetically). The engineering of *E. coli* to produce isopropanol required the addition of four foreign genes (Fig. 14.22). The initial source of all four genes was *Clostridium acetobutylicum;* however, genes encoding the same activities from several other bacteria were also tested in an effort to obtain a transformed strain of *E. coli* that produced the greatest amount of isopropanol. The best combination of foreign genes encoding enzymes in the isopropanol biosynthesis pathway produced nearly three times as much isopropanol as the best reported strain of *C. beijerinckii,* indicating that this strain has significant potential for use in the industrial production of isopropanol.

FIGURE 14.21 Chromosomal integration of an α-amylase gene into *L. plantarum*. The α-amylase gene is cloned into the *L. amylovorus cbh* gene on an *E. coli–L. plantarum* shuttle vector, which is then used to transform *L. plantarum*. Erythromycin-resistant and α-amylase-positive clones of *L. plantarum* result from a single crossover between the chromosomal and plasmid DNA at the *cbh* locus. After the growth of transformed *L. plantarum* for approximately 30 generations in the absence of selective pressure, intrachromosomal recombination resulted in the excision of the erythromycin resistance (Erm^r) gene, the chromosomal copy of the *cbh* gene, and the plasmid DNA. The final engineered *L. plantarum* carries only an α-amylase gene and no selectable marker genes.

Engineering Yeast Transcription

Conventional mutagenesis and selection have historically been used to improve the useful behavior of a range of microorganisms. Most prominently, from a biotechnological perspective, this approach has been utilized to develop microbial strains that overproduce specific antibiotics. The advantage of the approach is that it does not predetermine which gene(s) will be altered. However, conventional mutagenesis is a slow and tedious process requiring an inordinate amount of testing of mutated strains. Moreover, conventional mutagenesis and selection, or even sequential rounds of random mutagenesis of an isolated DNA fragment, introduce only a limited number of changes at each round of mutagenesis. Unfortunately, sometimes changing a fundamental property of a microorganism may require altering the expression of dozens or even hundreds of genes. While this cannot be achieved using the above-mentioned approaches, the reprogramming of a microorganism may be realized by mutagenizing one of the proteins that is responsible for regulating global transcription of the microorganism.

FIGURE 14.22 Engineering *E. coli* to produce isopropanol; a simplified overview of the biosynthetic pathway. The introduced portion of the pathway is highlighted in yellow. The enzymes involved in this pathway are as follows: several *E. coli* enzymatic steps are required for the conversion of glucose to pyruvate (**A**); pyruvate is converted to acetyl-CoA by an *E. coli* enzyme (**B**); acetyl-CoA acetyltransferase from *C. acetobutylicum* catalyzes the formation of acetoacetyl-CoA (**C**); acetoacetyl-CoA transferase from *E. coli* catalyzes the production of acetoacetate (**D**); acetoacetate decarboxylase from *C. acetobutylicum* catalyzes the synthesis of acetone (**E**); and secondary alcohol dehydrogenase from *C. beijerinckii* produces isopropanol from acetone (**F**).

In order to engineer yeast to more efficiently produce alcohol, it is necessary that the yeast strain be able to tolerate high concentrations of both glucose and ethanol. To achieve this end, it is likely that the expression of a large number of yeast proteins must be altered. Moreover, it is by no means clear which proteins need to have their levels of expression either increased or decreased. Instead, one group of researchers undertook to reprogram a significant portion of yeast metabolism by generating a large number of randomly mutated yeast transcription factor genes. In a small number of cases, the modified transcription factor will alter yeast gene expression in a manner that increases the tolerance of yeast for high levels of both glucose and ethanol. In yeast, 15 different proteins bind to DNA and regulate the promoter specificity of RNA polymerase II. To dramatically modify yeast metabolism (Fig. 14.23), the gene encoding transcription factor *SPT15* was altered by error-prone PCR (see chapter 8). This amplification reaction produces a range of different mutagenized *SPT15* genes. All of the mutagenized *SPT15* genes were cloned onto a plasmid vector and then introduced into wild-type yeast *(S. cerevisiae)* cells. The transformed cells were grown on agar medium in the presence of 6% ethanol and 120 g/liter of glucose. Any transformant that grew better on this medium than the native yeast strain was then more fully characterized. One particular mutant displayed a higher level of cell viability and grew faster than the native yeast strain at ethanol concentrations of between 10 and 20%. When this strain was examined in detail, it was found that the *SPT15* gene had

FIGURE 14.23 Engineering the yeast *S. cerevisiae* to tolerate high levels of glucose and ethanol. The yeast transcription factor *SPT15* gene was mutagenized by error-prone PCR, cloned into a plasmid vector, and used to transform a laboratory yeast strain. The transformants were selected for the ability to grow on medium containing both 6% ethanol and 12% glucose. The portions of the *SPT15* gene shown in red represent the introduced mutations.

three separate mutations, all of which were required for this activity. In addition, when the mutant was transcriptionally profiled (using microarray technology), several hundred genes were found to be differentially regulated compared to the native strain, with the majority of genes being upregulated. Interestingly, a detailed analysis of the genes whose expression was significantly altered did not reveal that a particular pathway or genetic network was primarily responsible for the observed reprogramming. Finally, the yeast strain that was used in these experiments was a standard laboratory strain, so that to incorporate this approach into a commercial process, it will be necessary to repeat the work with an industrial strain of yeast. If successful, this type of genetic manipulation could facilitate the development of strains of yeast that more efficiently convert glucose to ethanol.

Utilization of Cellulose

With an increasing world population and dramatic increases in the standard of living in parts of the developing world, meeting the growing worldwide demand for energy for heating, transportation, and industry has become a major challenge for all countries for the 21st century and beyond. Moreover, in addition to being sustainable, the future energy supply needs to be nonpolluting so that we may realize a reduction in

TABLE 14.7 Typical compositions of various lignocellulosic materials

Raw material	Amount (%) of:		
	Lignin	Cellulose	Hemicellulose
Pine wood	27.8	44.0	26.0
Birch wood	19.5	40.0	39.0
Sugarcane bagasse	18.9	33.4	30.0
Rice straw	12.5	32.1	24.0
Cotton	12.5	32.1	24.0

Adapted from Brown, *Philos. Trans. R. Soc. Lond.* B **300**:305–322, 1983.

greenhouse gas emissions. To this end, many countries around the world have begun to produce large amounts of alternative fuels in an effort to at least partially replace nonrenewable fossil fuels, such as oil and gas. In this regard, a major effort has been directed toward producing bioethanol. At the present time, Brazil produces large amounts of ethanol from the fermentation of sucrose derived from sugarcane, and the United States produces ethanol from corn starch. However, the reduction of greenhouse gases that results from the use of sugar- or starch-based ethanol is not as high as desired, and many socially conscious individuals have criticized the strategy of converting land from the production of food to the production of ethanol/energy. Moreover, sugar- or starch-based ethanol is unlikely to provide more than a small fraction of what we require. In this regard, in 2008, the Chinese government announced that it would not allow any further increase in starch-based ethanol production because of competing uses as food. If the world is going to produce ethanol on a large enough scale to significantly lower our use of fossil fuels, that ethanol will have to be produced from lignocellulosic waste products, such as corn stover, grasses, and wood chips. Thus, there is now, more than ever before, a tremendous amount of both political and scientific activity directed toward trying to produce ethanol from lignocellulosic materials.

Lignocellulosics

The polymers lignin, hemicellulose, and cellulose combine in various proportions to form a "lignocellulosic" structural support system for nearly all terrestrial plants (Table 14.7). This material constitutes a vast biomass that is often a waste product of agriculture, timber processing, and other human activity and needs to be disposed of in a safe and efficient manner or used as a resource. It has been estimated that annually ~10^{11} tons of these polymers is synthesized in the biosphere, with an energy content that is equivalent to around 640 billion tons of oil.

Lignocellulosic materials (cellulosics) have been grouped into three classes.

- Primary cellulosics include plants that are harvested specifically for cellulosic content, structural use, or feed value, e.g., cotton, timber, and hay.
- Agricultural waste cellulosics are the plant materials that remain after harvesting and processing, e.g., straw, corn stovers, rice hulls, sugarcane bagasse, animal manures, and timber residues.
- Municipal waste cellulosics encompass wastepaper and other discarded paper products.

FIGURE 14.24 Schematic representation of lignin structure, showing some of the various possible linkages between the phenylpropane (a C_6 aromatic group attached to a C_3 alkyl chain) units. The phenylpropane units are linked in an unorganized, nonrepeating fashion.

Components of Lignocellulose

Lignin is a three-dimensional, globular, irregular, insoluble, high-molecular-weight (>10,000) polymer made up of phenylpropane subunits with no chains of regular repeating units or any bonds that are easily hydrolyzed either enzymatically or chemically (Fig. 14.24). The lignin polymer molecule

FIGURE 14.25 Structure of a portion of a cellulose chain. Glucose residues are joined head to tail by β-1,4 linkages.

has many different types of chemical linkages between aromatic phenylpropane units. The physical and chemical characteristics of lignin are generally attributed to the last step in lignin biosynthesis, the nonenzymatic free-radical-based joining of the phenylpropane units in a more or less random fashion. In plants, lignin is chemically bonded to hemicellulose and wraps around fibers composed of cellulose. Lignin is responsible for the rigidity of plants and for their resistance to mechanical stress and microbial attack.

Hemicelluloses are short-chain, heterogeneous polymers that contain both hexoses (six-carbon sugars, such as glucose, mannose, and galactose) and pentoses (five-carbon sugars, such as xylose and arabinose). The three major types of hemicelluloses are xylans, which have a backbone of poly-β-1,4-xylan, with side links to arabinose, glucuronic acid, and arabinoglucuronic acid; mannans, which are composed of glucomannans and galactomannans; and arabinogalactans. The origin of the lignocellulosic material usually defines the nature of the hemicelluloses. For example, xylan hemicellulose is particularly common in hardwoods, and glucomannans are characteristic of softwoods.

Cellulose, which is the simplest of the components found in lignocellulosic material, is the most abundant polymer in the biosphere. It is composed of long chains of D-glucose molecules linked in β-1,4 configuration (Fig. 14.25). Both cellulose and starch can be hydrolyzed to glucose, but their structures are very different. Starch is an energy storage molecule in which the glucose residues are linked in a manner that prevents a tightly ordered arrangement of the polymer chains. This open mesh-like structure is easily penetrated by water; as a result, starch is both water soluble and readily hydrolyzable by amylases and glucoamylases. By contrast, cellulose is a plant-supporting structural molecule. The glucose chains in cellulose are arranged in a manner that permits them to pack together in a crystal-like structure that is impervious to water. Consequently, the cellulose polymer is both insoluble and resistant to hydrolysis.

Nevertheless, cellulose is still a form of stored glucose, so it is the component of lignocellulosics that has the most potential for conversion into a variety of useful compounds, such as alcohol. However, before cellulose can be utilized, it must be released from its complex with lignin and hemicellulose. For most lignocellulosic materials, this separation requires treatment with either a strong acid or a strong base or the use of high temperature and pressure. Regardless of how the cellulose is separated from the lignocellulose complex, the energy that is necessary to achieve this adds significantly to the cost of the final product. However, since the annual production of lignocellulosic materials is huge, effective ways of enzymatically degrading cellulose and hemicellulose are being sought. Chemical and enzymatic methods for the selective degradation of lignin also are being investigated, with less success.

Isolation of Prokaryotic Cellulase Genes

A wide range of bacteria and fungi are naturally capable of degrading cellulose through the concerted action of several enzymes that collectively are referred to as cellulase. Aerobic microorganisms typically secrete large amounts of these cellulase enzymes into the medium outside of the cell. On the other hand, in anaerobic microorganisms, cellulase activity is often found as part of a multiprotein complex that is called a cellulosome (Fig. 14.26) that lies on the external surface of the cell (Fig. 14.27). Cellulases

FIGURE 14.26 Schematic representation of a cellulosome protein complex. This complex contains both structural and enzymatically active protein components. The structural components include scaffoldin, a scaffolding protein (shown in yellow) that contains a strong cellulose-binding module (orange), and a number of cohesin molecules (nine are shown). The cohesin molecules act as binding sites (docking sites) for the dockerin proteins (red), which are attached to the catalytic domains (the active enzymatic components, which are shown in green, purple, and blue). Each cellulosome complex is anchored to the microbial cell surface through the cell surface-binding domain (brown).

Polycellulosome
protuberances

Protracted
protuberance

Cellulose

FIGURE 14.27 Interaction of a cellulolytic bacterium with cellulose. The bacterial cell surface has protuberance-like structures that contain multiple copies of the cellulosome (polycellulosome protuberances). On contact with the cellulose substrate, some of the polycellulosome protuberances protract dramatically and deposit their cellulosomes along the surface of the cellulose (detached from the bacterial surface).

consist of multiple copies of several enzymes with different enzymatic activities. including the following.

- Endoglucanase, which hydrolyzes β-1,4 linkages between adjacent glucose molecules within the amorphous (loosely packed) regions of the cellulose polymer, thereby breaking the chain in the middle
- Exoglucanase, which degrades the nicked cellulose chains from their nonreducing ends and produces glucose, cellobiose (two glucose units), and cellotriose (three glucose units)
- Cellobiohydrolase, which is often found in cellulolytic fungi and is a type of exoglucanase that removes units of 10 or more glucose residues from the nonreducing ends of the cellulose molecule
- β-Glucosidase, or cellobiase, which converts cellobiose and cellotriose to glucose

The breakdown of cellulose by microorganisms (either bacteria or fungi) that produce the various components of cellulase (Fig. 14.28) is slow and often incomplete. Therefore, genetic engineering strategies have been used in an attempt to create organisms with more effective cellulase activity. For this purpose, genes coding for the individual enzymatic functions of cellulase activity have been isolated from both prokaryotic and eukaryotic organisms.

Prokaryotic endoglucanase genes have been cloned by the following simple yet effective identification technique.

1. A clone bank of DNA from a cellulolytic prokaryote is constructed in *E. coli,* and the host cells are grown overnight on solid medium containing a selective antibiotic.
2. The colonies are then overlaid with agar containing carboxymethyl cellulose (CMC), a soluble derivative of cellulose, and the petri plates are incubated at 37°C for several hours. During this time, the CMC molecules that are present in the immediate vicinity of a colony that both synthesizes and secretes an endoglucanase are partially digested. Transformants that synthesize but do not secrete the cloned endoglucanase are not able to degrade the substrate, because it is too large to enter the cell.
3. The digested regions of the CMC are visualized by first flooding the petri plate with a solution of the dye Congo red, which is not toxic to the bacteria, followed by a wash with a solution of sodium chloride. Congo red selectively binds to high-molecular-weight cellulose chains and gives a red color; conversely, it binds weakly to low-molecular-weight polysaccharides and produces a yellow hue. The sodium chloride treatment stabilizes the binding of the dye. If a bacterial colony produces a secreted endoglucanase, it will be surrounded by a yellow halo; the background, where the CMC has not been degraded, will be red (Fig. 14.29).

This technique has been successfully used in the isolation of endoglucanase genes from *Streptomyces, Clostridium, Thermoanaerobacter, Thermomonospora, Erwinia, Pseudomonas, Cellvibrio, Ruminococcus, Cellulomonas, Fibrobacter,* and *Bacillus* species.

There is no convenient plate assay for detecting cells with a cloned exoglucanase gene, so immunological screening has been used to pick out the recombinant clones that express exoglucanase. Although this approach

FIGURE 14.28 Enzymatic biodegradation of cellulose. Cellulose hydrolysis begins with the cleavage of β-1,4 linkages within the accessible amorphous regions of the cellulose chains by endo-glucanase(s). This reaction is followed by the removal of oligosaccharides from the partially cleaved cellulose chains by exoglucanase(s) and cellobiohydrolase(s). The degradation of cellulose is completed when the cellobiose and cellotriose are converted to glucose by β-glucosidase.

requires specific antibodies directed against the target protein, the protein does not have to be secreted to be detected. Recombinant cells can be lysed in situ, e.g., by exposure to chloroform vapor, before the cytoplasmic proteins are transferred to a nylon or nitrocellulose membrane for subsequent immunological testing. In these tests, replica plates are used to ensure that viable cells are available for further propagation and use.

Prokaryotic β-glucosidase genes have been isolated by transforming a clone bank from a β-glucosidase-producing microorganism into *E. coli* and then selecting for transformants that can grow on minimal media with cellobiose as the sole carbon source. Alternatively, clones that express β-glucosidase activity can be detected with a chromogenic substrate, such

FIGURE 14.29 Detection of an *E. coli* clone expressing a bacterial endoglucanase gene. The yellow halo indicates the presence of a positive clone that degrades the soluble cellulose (CMC) in the medium in the vicinity of the clone via the secreted endoglucanase.

as 5-bromo-4-chloro-3-indolyl-β-D-glucopyranoside (BCIP), in the plating medium or with MacConkey–cellobiose agar. In both cases, β-glucosidase-positive colonies turn red.

Isolation of Eukaryotic Cellulase Genes

The strategy of DNA hybridization screening of either cDNA or genomic clone banks with a heterologous probe has not been particularly effective for isolating cellulase genes, because the sequences of cellulolytic enzymes from diverse sources are not very similar. To isolate the messenger RNAs (mRNAs) that encode cellulolytic enzymes from fungi or plants, a novel protocol had to be implemented. Unfortunately, these mRNAs usually constitute only a small fraction of the total mRNA population. Therefore, it is often necessary to enrich for the target mRNA or cDNA and to eliminate cDNA clones that do not carry the target sequences. To meet these ends, the technique of "differential hybridization" has been used for the isolation of a number of different induced eukaryotic cellulase genes, as follows (Fig. 14.30).

1. mRNA is isolated both from cells grown without cellulose (i.e., noninduced cells) and from cells grown in the presence of cellulose to enhance the synthesis of cellulase enzymes (i.e., induced cells).
2. Each mRNA population is fractionated on a sucrose gradient, and each fraction is translated in a cell-free system, either rabbit reticulocytes or wheat germ. A cellulose-induced protein(s) is identified, after separation of the cell-free translation products on a polyacrylamide gel, by the presence of unique bands that appear from the induced cells but not from the noninduced cells (Fig. 14.31). This step indicates which mRNA fractions contain messengers that are induced by the addition of cellulose.
3. The mRNA sucrose gradient fractions from cells that direct the synthesis of cellulose-induced proteins and the comparable fractions from the noninduced cells are used separately to program the synthesis of cDNA.
4. The cDNA sample from the induced-cell population is cloned into a plasmid vector, introduced into *E. coli*, replica plated, and then separately screened with labeled cDNA from both the induced and noninduced fractions as hybridization probes. Clones that hybridize only with the cDNA from the induced cells and not with cDNA from the noninduced cells potentially carry cellulose-induced genes and are characterized further.
5. To establish conclusively which of the positive cDNA clones encode cellulase enzymes, the DNA from these clones is introduced into an *E. coli* expression vector and, after *E. coli* is transformed with these constructs, the protein products are detected with antibodies to the enzymes of the cellulase complex.
6. The sequence of each of the positive cDNA clones is determined. In principle, this scheme can be used for the isolation of any induced eukaryotic gene(s).

Manipulation of Cellulase Genes

There are a variety of uses for cloned cellulase genes. In some cases, the cellulose-binding domain encoded by cellulase genes facilitates the purification of recombinant proteins. In other instances, the cellulolytic activity

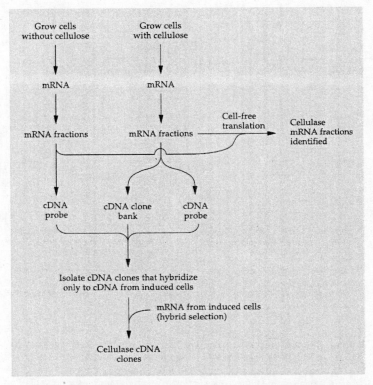

FIGURE 14.30 Differential hybridization for isolating eukaryotic cellulase cDNA clones.

is expressed in organisms that can convert waste cellulose into a commercial product, such as alcohol.

Many cellulase enzymes have three separate domains: a catalytic region; a hinge region that is often rich in proline, serine, or threonine residues; and a cellulose-binding region. The catalytic and binding domains act independently. This separation of functions can be exploited by cloning the DNA sequence that encodes the cellulose-binding domain as part of a fusion gene, where the other portion of the gene encodes a commercial protein. After expression of this fusion protein, it can be purified by passing a crude extract through a column packed with cellulose. Under these conditions, only the fusion protein will bind to the cellulose. Then the fusion protein, in homogeneous form, can be eluted from the column. The commercial protein can be retrieved by removal of the cellulose-binding domain by proteolytic cleavage. This system is similar in principle to immunoaffinity chromatography, except that it should be less expensive than using antibodies.

For convenience, most cellulase genes are initially cloned and expressed in *E. coli*, but other useful microorganisms might be developed by the introduction of cellulase genes. For example, *S. cerevisiae* and *Zymomonas mobilis*, which both efficiently convert simple sugars, such as glucose, into alcohol, have been used as hosts for the expression of cellulase genes. The idea

FIGURE 14.31 Schematic representation of stained polyacrylamide gels of translation products of mRNA fractions, i.e., proteins, following growth of cells either with or without cellulose. The numbers represent the fraction number following sucrose gradient centrifugation of mRNA. The red ovals on the gel without cellulose indicate where bands appear when there is growth in the presence of cellulose.

behind these studies was to test whether the presence of cellulase activity would enable these organisms to convert cellulose directly to alcohol.

In one series of experiments, endoglucanase and exoglucanase genes from the bacterium *Cellulomonas fimi* were each put under the control of an *S. cerevisiae* promoter and signal peptide sequence, subcloned onto the same plasmid vector, and introduced into *S. cerevisiae*. Some transformants secreted about 70% of each activity into the growth medium and were able to degrade the cellulose in filter paper and pretreated wood chips. The rate and extent of hydrolysis of both of these substrates were increased by adding β-glucosidase to the mixture, thereby decreasing the amount of cellobiose that accumulated and preventing end-product (feedback) inhibition of the endoglucanase and exoglucanase activities by cellobiose (Fig. 14.32). The role of β-glucosidase in the cellulolytic process has been examined in more detail. Cellobiose acts as a feedback inhibitor of cellulose hydrolysis, and glucose inhibits cellobiose cleavage. These two regulatory mechanisms may prevent complete enzymatic breakdown of cellulose. Instead of adding β-glucosidase to the medium, a β-glucosidase gene could be cloned into the host cell. To this end, a β-glucosidase gene was isolated from the cellulolytic fungus *Trichoderma reesei*, cloned onto a multiple-copy plasmid, and reintroduced into *T. reesei*. The transformant strain overproduced β-glucosidase activity 5.5-fold, and it degraded microcrystalline cellulose (Avicel), a cellulose derivative, 33% faster than the nontransformed strain. In addition, when a β-glucosidase gene from the yeast *Saccharomycopsis fibuligera* was expressed in *S. cerevisiae*, the transformed strain directed the enzyme to the periplasm. The β-glucosidase-producing *S. cerevisiae* strain was nearly as efficient at utilizing cellobiose to produce ethanol as the nontransformed *S. cerevisiae* strain was at producing alcohol from glucose. Thus, the presence of β-glucosidase genes enhances the enzy-

matic utilization of cellulose and suggests a simple strategy for genetically engineering more effective cellulolytic alcohol-producing microorganisms.

In addition to converting cellulosic wastes into useful materials, endoglucanase genes may have some novel uses. For example, when a winemaking yeast was transformed with an endoglucanase gene under the control of the constitutively expressed yeast actin gene promoter, the wine that was produced had an increased fruity aroma. This improvement was attributed to an increase in the amounts of at least 12 different volatile compounds, including ethyl propionate, 2-butanol, isoamyl acetate, isoamyl alcohol, and isobutyric acid. This type of genetic modification opens the possibility of engineering yeast strains that yield wines with particular desirable characteristics.

The participation of cellulase enzymes in an industrial process for the bioconversion of wastepaper to alcohol has also been examined. Wastepaper was partially digested by the addition of cellulase enzymes at 45°C; then, the released glucose was fermented by *S. cerevisiae* at 37°C. By extrapolation of small-scale results, yields of 400 liters of ethanol per ton of wastepaper were estimated. If all 100 million tons of wastepaper generated annually in North America were converted into ethanol and used as fuel, approximately 16% of the gasoline that is currently being used in North America could be saved.

Designer cellulosomes. Scientists hoping to exploit the activity of microbial cellulosomes to degrade cellulosic waste materials have attempted to manipulate some of the genes involved in the formation of this complex and create designer cellulosomes whose degradative activities are directed toward specific substrates. One of the key ingredients in the assembly and functioning of a cellulosome is the calcium-dependent high affinity (~10^9 M^{-1}) of the cohesin domain of the scaffoldin molecule for the dockerin domain (Fig. 14.26). Unfortunately, within a given species of microorganism, the dockerin domain binds to all of the cohesin domains with the same affinity. Thus, in nature, different catalytic domains attached to the dockerins are randomly incorporated into the cellulosome. However, it is possible, in the laboratory, to engineer cellulosomes that contain certain enzymatic activities designed to facilitate the degradation of specific substrates. In one series of experiments, designer cellulosomes were constructed that were more effective than the free enzymes (i.e., the enzymatic components not assembled into a cellulosome complex) and slightly less effective than native cellulosomes in degrading crystalline cellulose. However, these designer cellulosomes were not especially active at degrading straw (an agricultural waste product). When a xylanase gene was incorporated into the cellulosome complex, the ability of the designer cellulosome to degrade straw, which contains hemicellulose as well as cellulose, increased significantly (Fig. 14.33). Although the designer cellulosomes that have so far been constructed are not yet ready to be used in a commercial process, it is envisioned that these molecules could one day be the central component of a very large industry aimed at efficiently and economically converting cellulosic wastes into useable chemicals.

Zymomonas mobilis

Although industrial fermentations that produce alcohol are performed almost exclusively with *S. cerevisiae*, the bacterium *Z. mobilis* is a potentially useful organism for this purpose. *Zymomonas* is a gram-negative, rod-

FIGURE 14.32 Metabolic control of cellulose hydrolysis. The green arrows indicate cellulose degradation. The red arrows indicate feedback inhibition by a particular metabolite of cellulose degradation. Relief of feedback inhibition may come from overproducing β-glucosidase, thereby decreasing the concentration of cellobiose, and removal of glucose by converting it into other metabolites.

FIGURE 14.33 Digestion of straw by a cellulase-plus-xylanase designer cellulosome complex free cellulase enzyme, a cellulase-based designer cellulosome, and free xylanase enzyme. Although the data are presented as the relative amount of substrate degraded, in this experiment, the substrate was only partially degraded in all cases.

shaped organism that can ferment glucose, fructose, and sucrose and produce a relatively high yield of alcohol (Table 14.8). This high yield of ethanol is probably related to the fact that *Zymomonas* does not proliferate extensively (i.e., produce biomass) during fermentation. Since *Zymomonas* uses less substrate for biomass formation, more is available for ethanol production. In this regard, yeast produces 2 mol of ATP per mol of glucose, whereas *Zymomonas* uses a different pathway and produces only 1 mol of ATP per mol of glucose. Historically, *Zymomonas* has been used in tropical regions as a fermentative agent for the production of alcoholic beverages.

Zymomonas produces alcohol at a much higher rate than does *S. cerevisiae*, even though the organisms are similar in other features (Table 14.8).

TABLE 14.8 Comparison of *Z. mobilis* and *S. cerevisiae* as alcohol producers

Attribute	Value for:	
	Z. mobilis	Yeast
Conversion of sugar to ethanol (%)	96	96
Maximum ethanol concentration (%)	12	12
Ethanol productivity rate (g g^{-1} h^{-1})	5.67	0.67
Volumetric ethanol productivity rate (g liter^{-1} h^{-1})	200	29
Sugar tolerance (%)	>40	>40
pH range for ethanol production	3.5–7.5	2–6.5
Optimum temperature (°C)	25–30	30–38

Adapted from Buchholz et al., *Trends Biotechnol* 5:199–204, 1987.

The ethanol productivity rate was measured under batch fermentation conditions. The volumetric ethanol productivity rate was measured during continuous culture. Both strains yielded the same maximum ethanol concentration (12%) and had the same sugar tolerance (>40%).

However, there are biological and technical constraints that prevent *Zymomonas* from being used more widely for alcohol production. First, it can use only a limited number of carbon substrates for the production of alcohol. Second, broad-host-range cloning vectors and, as a consequence, foreign genes are difficult to maintain in this organism. Third, *Zymomonas* is naturally resistant to many of the more commonly used antibiotics, which precludes using the standard antibiotic resistance marker systems for cloning experiments.

Despite these difficulties, a number of foreign genes have been successfully introduced into and expressed in *Zymomonas*. Many of these experiments have focused on expanding the range of substrates that *Zymomonas* can utilize. For example, genes encoding enzymes that hydrolyze lactose, starch, cellulose, xylose, and cellobiose have all been introduced into *Zymomonas* (Table 14.9). Transformants were able to express all of these genes to some extent. However, in most of these cases, the transformed bacterium was unable to utilize the novel substrate as the sole carbon source.

In early studies directed toward developing strains of *Z. mobilis* that were capable of growth and ethanol production with xylose as a substrate, the bacterium was transformed with genes encoding the xylose utilization enzymes glucose/xylose isomerase and xylulokinase. However, these transformants were limited by their inability to further metabolize the pentoses (xylulose-5-phosphate, ribulose-5-phosphate, and ribose-5-phosphate) that are formed after xylose is assimilated (Fig. 14.34). To remedy this situation, *Z. mobilis* was transformed with a plasmid carrying two synthetic operons, one with two xylose assimilation genes and one with two pentose metabolism genes (Fig. 14.35). The pentose metabolism genes

TABLE 14.9 Some of the heterologous genes expressed in *Z. mobilis*

Enzyme encoded	Enzyme function
α-Amylase	Breakdown of starch to dextrins and glucose
Endo-1,4-β-D-glucanase	Breakdown of cellulose chains
β-D-Glucosidase	Breakdown of cellobiose to glucose
CMC	Breakdown of soluble cellulose
α-D-Galactosidase	Breakdown of raffinose, stachyose, and verbascose into glucose, galactose, sucrose, and fructose
Lac permease	Facilitates transport of lactose into bacterial cells
β-D-Galactosidase	Breakdown of lactose
Glucoamylase	Breakdown of starch and dextrins to glucose
Xylose isomerase	Conversion of xylose to xylulose
Xyulokinase	Conversion of L-xylulose to L-xylulose 5-phosphate
Xylose permease	Facilitates transport of xylose into bacterial cells
Transaldolase	Conversion of sedoheptulose 7-phosphate and D-glyceraldehyde 3-phosphate to yield D-erythrose 4-phosphate and D-fructose phosphate
Phosphomannose isomerase	Conversion of D-mannose 6-phosphate to D-fructose 6-phosphate
L-Arabinose isomerase	Conversion of L-arabinose to L-ribulose
L-Ribulokinase	Conversion of L-ribulose to L-ribulose 5-phosphate
L-Ribulose-phosphate-4-epimerase	Conversion of L-ribulose 5-phosphate to D-xylose 5-phosphate
Transketolase	Conversion of D-xylulose-5-phosphate (1) to sedoheptulose-7-phosphate and glyceraldehyde-3-phosphate and (2) to fructose-6-phosphate and glyceraldehyde-3-phosphate

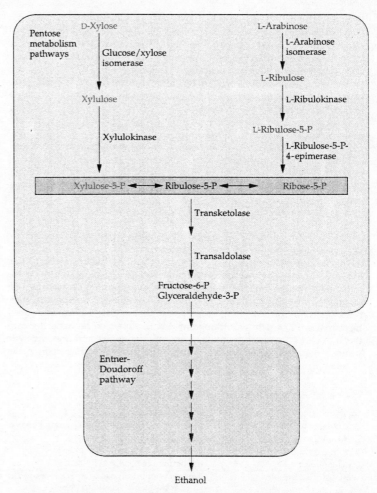

FIGURE 14.34 Schematic representation of the engineered assimilation of either xylose or arabinose by *Z. mobilis* and the engineered conversion of the resultant pentoses (shown in the green box) to ethanol.

encode the enzymes transketolase and transaldolase; both were placed under the control of the *Z. mobilis* enolase promoter. The xylose assimilation genes were placed under the transcriptional control of a strong constitutive promoter from the *Z. mobilis* gene for glyceraldehyde-3-phosphate dehydrogenase. Both constructs were cloned onto an *E. coli–Z. mobilis* shuttle vector, which was then used to transform *Z. mobilis*. As expected, the transformants assimilated xylose and converted the resulting pentoses that formed to fructose-6-phosphate and glyceraldehyde-3-phosphate, which, in turn, were readily converted to ethanol by the Entner-Doudoroff pathway of *Z. mobilis*. Moreover, the transformants grew efficiently on either glucose or xylose, as well as on glucose–xylose mixtures, and con-

FIGURE 14.35 A *Zymomonas–E. coli* shuttle vector carrying one operon with genes encoding enzymes used for xylose assimilation *(xylA* and *xylB)* and another with genes encoding enzymes involved in pentose metabolism *(tktA* and *talB)*. p^{eno}, enolase promoter; p^{gap}, glyceraldehyde-3-phosphate dehydrogenase promoter; *xylA*, xylose isomerase gene; *xylB*, xylulokinase gene; *tktA*, transketolase gene; *talB*, transaldolase gene; Tetr, tetracycline resistance gene; *oriE*, *E. coli* origin of replication. The *Zymomonas* DNA contains a *Zymomonas* origin of replication.

verted xylose to ethanol at high yield. This work demonstrates the feasibility of metabolically engineering *Z. mobilis* as an ethanol producer by using xylose, a waste material produced as a by-product of industrial processes, such as pulp and paper making, as a carbon source.

Xylose is the predominant pentose sugar in hardwoods, while arabinose (Fig. 14.36) is present in large amounts in various agricultural and other herbaceous plants. Some arabinose-containing plants, such as switchgrass, have been considered for use as dedicated energy crops, i.e., plants grown solely for use as sources of energy. Thus, it would be very useful if, in addition to a strain of *Z. mobilis* that can convert xylose to ethanol, an arabinose-fermenting *Z. mobilis* strain were also available. To develop such a strain, the arabinose assimilation genes L-ribulokinase, L-arabinose isomerase, and L-ribulose-5-phosphate-4-epimerase from *E. coli* were isolated and put under the transcriptional control of the constitutive *Z. mobilis* glyceraldehyde-3-phosphate dehydrogenase promoter (Fig. 14.37). Following expression of these genes, transformants produced the pentoses xylulose-5-phosphate, ribulose-5-phosphate, and ribose-5-phosphate. The plasmid used to transform *Z. mobilis* also contained two pentose metabolism genes encoding the enzymes transketolase and transaldolase under the transcriptional control of the constitutive *Z. mobilis* enolase promoter. The expression of these two genes catalyzed the conversion of the above-mentioned pentoses to fructose-6-phosphate and glyceraldehyde-3-phosphate.

The strategy that was used for this work was nearly identical to the strategy that was employed in the development of *Z. mobilis* strains able to utilize xylose as a carbon source. However, for *Z. mobilis* to utilize arabinose as a carbon source, arabinose rather than xylose assimilation genes were used. The metabolites that are produced starting with either xylose or arabinose are converted to ethanol by the Entner-Doudoroff pathway of *Z. mobilis* (Fig. 14.34). Moreover, the xylose- and arabinose-fermenting strains of *Z. mobilis* might be used together in a mixed bacterial culture for the conversion of the major sugars from certain agricultural residues into ethanol. To efficiently and economically convert lignocellulosic wastes to ethanol, it is necessary to convert all of the sugars, the pentoses as well as the hexoses, to ethanol. *Z. mobilis* lacks the pathways needed for the metabolism of mannose and galactose, which constitute a significant fraction of the

FIGURE 14.36 Chemical structures of D-xylose and L-arabinose.

$$\begin{array}{cc}
\text{CHO} & \text{CHO} \\
| & | \\
\text{H}-\text{C}-\text{OH} & \text{HO}-\text{C}-\text{H} \\
| & | \\
\text{HO}-\text{C}-\text{H} & \text{H}-\text{C}-\text{OH} \\
| & | \\
\text{H}-\text{C}-\text{OH} & \text{HO}-\text{C}-\text{H} \\
| & | \\
\text{CH}_2\text{OH} & \text{CH}_2\text{OH} \\
\text{D-Xylose} & \text{L-Arabinose}
\end{array}$$

FIGURE 14.37 A *Zymomonas–E. coli* shuttle vector carrying one operon with genes encoding enzymes used for arabinose assimilation *(araB, araA,* and *araD)* and another with genes encoding enzymes involved in pentose metabolism *(tktA* and *talB)*. *p^{eno}*, enolase promoter; *p^{gap}*, glyceraldehyde-3-phosphate dehydrogenase promoter; *araB*, L-ribulokinase gene; *araA*, L-arabinose isomerase gene; *araD*, L-ribulose-5-phosphate-4-epimerase gene; *tktA*, transketolase gene; *talB*, transaldolase gene; Tet^r, tetracycline resistance gene; *oriE*, *E. coli* origin of replication. The *Zymomonas* DNA contains a *Zymomonas* origin of replication.

hexoses in lignocellulosic material. Whether *Z. mobilis* can be engineered to be the organism of choice as part of a process of this sort is still an open question.

In addition to genetically engineering *Z. mobilis* to efficiently utilize xylose, arabinose, and glucose, researchers have utilized similar genetic approaches in an attempt to modify other microorganisms to utilize sugars derived from lignocellulosic materials to produce ethanol. Most of these efforts have been directed toward modifying *S. cerevisiae*, with some researchers attempting to engineer some strains of *P. putida*.

Instead of genetically engineering *Z. mobilis* to utilize xylose and arabinose and convert them into ethanol, some scientists have engineered *E. coli* to express some *Z. mobilis* genes so that it can produce ethanol. In this case, xylose and arabinose are converted to pyruvate by endogenous *E. coli* enzymes. Workers have mutated different *E. coli* genes to prevent the pyruvate from being converted into other, unwanted metabolites. Instead, the pyruvate is converted to ethanol by the enzymes pyruvate decarboxylase and alcohol dehydrogenase, with the genes for both of these enzymes coming from *Z. mobilis*. This sort of genetic modification has also been used to change the bacterium *Klebsiella oxytoca* into an ethanologenic organism. With both *E. coli* and *K. oxytoca*, the introduction of *Z. mobilis* genes yielded recombinant bacteria that were quite efficient in the laboratory at converting various sugars, both pentoses and hexoses, into alcohol. It now remains to be demonstrated whether any of these bacteria are effective on a large scale with an industrial substrate.

Since several naturally occurring yeast strains can utilize the range of sugars found in lignocellulosic materials, considerable effort has been directed to improving the performance of these strains. However, in contrast to the well-studied laboratory yeast strains, industrial strains are usually diploid or polyploid (and therefore not as easy to engineer), and their genetics are not especially well characterized or understood. Nevertheless, some industrial yeast strains that are able to tolerate the inhibitory compounds found in hydrolyzed lignocellulosic materials and ferment both hexoses and xyloses are being developed, and some researchers believe that within the next few years one or more of these organisms could

FIGURE 14.38 The major components of the *E. coli* formate hydrogen lyase. The purple arrows show the direction of the electron flux and the proteins through which the electrons flow (shown in blue). The Hyc proteins are the components of the formate hydrogen lyase system, which accept electrons from FDH-H (the large subunit of formate dehydrogenase). HycB is the small subunit of formate dehydrogenase and acts as the membrane docking target of FDH-H. HycC and HycD (shown in yellow) are integral membrane proteins and are thought to anchor the rest of the complex. HycE is the large subunit of hydrogenase 3, and HycG is the small subunit of hydrogenase 3. HycF is an electron transport protein.

become the cornerstone of an industrial process to convert lignocellulosic residues into ethanol.

Hydrogen Production

It has been known for some time that formic acid (formate) can be produced inexpensively, often as a by-product of the synthesis of other chemicals, such as acetic acid. Moreover, some types of bacteria are able to convert formate into hydrogen and carbon dioxide via the formate hydrogen lyase system. If the bacterial system that is responsible for hydrogen synthesis could be optimized, it might be possible to develop a practical system for the synthesis of hydrogen from biomass.

The *E. coli* formate hydrogen lyase system consists of a large number of different proteins, including those shown in Fig. 14.38, as well as others that specifically regulate the synthesis and maturation of these proteins. To overproduce the *E. coli* formate hydrogen lyase system and hence the amount of hydrogen, (1) the formate hydrogen lyase repressor gene, *hycA*, was inactivated and (2) the formate hydrogen lyase activator gene, *fhlA*, was overexpressed. These manipulations resulted in the large subunit of formate dehydrogenase (FDH-H) and the large subunit of hydrogenase 3 (HycE) being overexpressed 6.5- and 7.0-fold, respectively, compared to the wild type. These changes resulted in a nearly threefold increase in hydrogen productivity compared to the wild type. Additional enhancement of the amount of hydrogen produced was obtained by employing the engineered *E. coli* cells under anaerobic conditions in a bioreactor at a very high density

(96 g [dry weight] per liter). When the formate concentration was maintained below 25 mM, continuous hydrogen synthesis of 23.6 g of hydrogen per hour per liter was realized. This level of hydrogen production is sufficient for this system to be considered to have significant potential for commercial application.

SUMMARY

Bioremediation is the term that is applied to the use of microorganisms to clear the environment of contaminating substances. Many members of the bacterial genus *Pseudomonas* carry plasmids that encode enzymes capable of degrading aromatic and halogenated organic compounds. In most cases, a single plasmid carries the genes encoding enzymes for a specific degradative pathway. By combining plasmids from different pseudomonad strains within a single host, it is possible to create an organism with multiple degradation capabilities. In addition, by genetic manipulation, the range of substrates degraded by a particular enzymatic pathway can be extended.

Raw biological material is called biomass and is often used as a starting material in industrial processes. The use of milled grain for the production of alcohol or fructose requires a number of enzymatic steps. The enzymes that are used in these processes are often used only once and then discarded. To enhance enzymatic conversions and decrease costs, bacterial genes encoding enzymes that are thermostable, highly efficient catalytically, or tolerant of alcohol have been cloned, characterized, and tested.

To improve the commercial production of alcohol, some workers have genetically transformed the bacterium *Z. mobilis* with genes that allow it to utilize a broad range of compounds as carbon sources. Enzymes that degrade starch can also be used to facilitate the ability of microorganisms, such as *L. plantarum*, to ferment silage.

Often, as a consequence of processing biological material, large amounts of lignocellulose remain. This material generally has been treated as a waste product. However, there is now interest in using lignocellulose as a resource for carbon-containing compounds, especially glucose, that can be used in other processes. Retrieving glucose from lignocellulose is not an easy matter. Lignocellulose is a complex of lignin, hemicellulose, and cellulose; without harsh and expensive pretreatment, it is refractory to enzymatic degradation. Recent research has focused on characterizing the mechanism of breakdown of cellulose to glucose. The genes for endoglucanases, exoglucanases, and β-glucosidases from a variety of organisms have been cloned and characterized, but to date there has been little success in formulating a set of enzymes that efficiently degrades cellulose in vitro on a large scale.

REFERENCES

Alper, H., J. Moxley, E. Nevoigt, G. R. Fink, and G. Stephanopoulos. 2006. Engineering yeast transcription machinery for improved ethanol tolerance and production. *Science* 314:1565–1568.

Barnett, C. C. 1991. Cloning and amplification of the gene encoding an extracellular β-glucosidase from *Trichoderma reesei*: evidence for improved rates of saccharification of cellulosic substrates. *Bio/Technology* 9:562–567.

Bayer, E. A., L. J. W. Shimon, Y. Shoham, and R. Lamed. 1998. Cellulosomes—structure and ultrastructure. *J. Struct. Biol.* 124:221–234.

Béguin, P. 1990. Molecular biology of cellulose degradation. *Annu. Rev. Microbiol.* 44:219–248.

Brown, D. E. 1983. Lignocellulose hydrolysis. *Phil. Trans. R. Soc. Lond. B* 300:305–322.

Buchholz, S. E., M. M. Dooley, and D. E. Eveleigh. 1987. *Zymomonas*—an alcoholic enigma. *Trends Biotechnol.* 5:199–204.

Buchholz, S. E., and D. E. Eveleigh. 1990. Genetic modification of *Zymomonas mobilis*. *Biotechnol. Adv.* 8:547–581.

Chakrabarty, A. M. March 1981. Microorganisms having multiple compatible degradative energy-generating plasmids and preparation thereof. U.S. patent 4,259,444.

Chen, W., and A. Mulchandani. 1998. The use of live biocatalysts for pesticide detoxification. *Trends Biotechnol.* 16:71–76.

Cole, G. E., P. C. McCabe, D. Inlow, D. H. Gelfand, A. Ben-Bassat, and M. A. Innis. 1988. Stable expression of *Aspergillus awamori* glucoamylase in distiller's yeast. *Bio/Technology* 6:417–421.

Cork, D. J., and J. P. Krueger. 1991. Microbial transformation of herbicides and pesticides. *Adv. Appl. Microbiol.* 36:1–66.

Deanda, K., M. Zhang, C. Eddy, and S. Picataggio. 1996. Developing of an arabinose-fermenting *Zymomonas mobilis* strain by metabolic pathway engineering. *Appl. Environ. Microbiol.* 62:4465–4470.

Dekker, K., A. Sugiura, H. Yamagata, K. Sakaguchi, and S. Udaka. 1992. Efficient production of thermostable *Thermus thermophilus* xylose isomerase in *Escherichia coli* and *Bacillus brevis*. *Appl. Microbiol. Biotechnol.* 36:727–732.

Fierobe, H.-P., F. Mingardon, A. Mechaly, A. Bélaïch, M. T. Rinconi, S. Pagès, R. Lamed, C. Tardif, J.-P. Bélaïch, and E. A. Bayer. 2005. Action of designer cellulosomes on homogeneous versus complex substrates. Controlled incorporation of three distinct enzymes into a defined trifunc-

tional scaffoldin. *J. Biol. Chem.* **280**:16325–16334.

Fitzsimons, A., P. Hols, J. Jore, R. J. Leer, M. O'Connell, and J. Delcour. 1994. Development of an amylolytic *Lactobacillus plantarum* silage strain expressing the *Lactobacillus amylovorus* α-amylase gene. *Appl. Environ. Microbiol.* **60**:3529–3535.

Furukawa, K., A. Nishi, T. Watanabe, A. Suyama, and N. Kimura. 1998. Engineering microorganisms capable of efficient degradation of chlorinated environmental pollutants. *Rev. Toxicol.* **2**:179–187.

Ghosal, D., I.-S. You, D. K. Chatterjee, and A. M. Chakrabarty. 1985. Microbial degradation of halogenated compounds. *Science* **228**:135–142.

Hahn-Hägerdal, B., M. Galbe, M. F. Gorwa-Grauslund, G. Lidén, and G. Zacchi. 2006. Bio-ethanol—the fuel of tomorrow from the residues of today. *Trends Biotechnol.* **24**:549–556.

Hahn-Hägerdal, B., K. Kurhumaa, C. Fonseca, I. Spencer-Martins, and M. F. Gorwa-Grauslund. 2007. Towards industrial pentose-fermenting yeast strains. *Appl. Microbiol. Biotechnol.* **74**:937–953.

Hanai, T., S. Atsumi, and J. C. Liao. 2007. Engineering synthetic pathway for isopropanol production in *Escherichia coli. Appl. Environ. Microbiol.* **73**:7814–7818.

Heux, S., R. Cachon, and S. Dequin. 2006. Cofactor engineering in *Saccharomyces cerevisiae*: expression of a H_2O-forming NADH oxidase and impact on redox metabolism. *Metab. Eng.* **8**:303–314.

Heux, S., J.-M. Sablayrolles, R. Cachon, and S. Dequin. 2006. Engineering a *Saccharomyces cerevisiae* wine yeast that exhibits reduced ethanol production during fermentation under controlled microooxygenation conditions. *Appl. Environ. Microbiol.* **72**:5822–5828.

Innis, M. A., M. J. Holland, P. C. McCabe, G. E. Cole, V. P. Wittman, R. Tal, K. W. K. Watt, D. H. Gelfand, J. P. Holland, and J. H. Meade. 1985. Expression, glycosylation and secretion of an *Aspergillus* glucoamylase by *Saccharomyces cerevisiae. Science* **228**:21–26.

Kallio, P., A. Palva, and I. Palva. 1987. Enhancement of α-amylase production by integrating and amplifying the α-amylase gene of *Bacillus amyloliquefaciens* in the genome of *Bacillus subtilis. Appl. Microbiol. Biotechnol.* **27**:64–71.

Kennedy, J. F., V. M. Cabalda, and C. A. White. 1988. Enzymic starch utilization and genetic engineering. *Trends Biotechnol.* **6**:184–189.

Knowles, J., P. Lehtovaara, and T. Teeri. 1987. Cellulase families and their genes. *Trends Biotechnol.* **5**:255–261.

Kolenc, R. J., W. E. Inniss, B. R. Glick, C. W. Robinson, and C. I. Mayfield. 1988. Transfer and expression of mesophilic plasmid-mediated degradative capacity in a psychrotrophic bacterium. *Appl. Environ. Microbiol.* **54**:638–641.

Kumar, V., S. Ramakrishnan, T. T. Teeri, J. K. C. Knowles, and B. S. Hartley. 1992. *Saccharomyces cerevisiae* cells secreting an *Aspergillus niger* β-galactosidase grow on whey permeate. *Bio/Technology* **10**:82–85.

Lamed, R., J. Naimark, E. Morgenstern, and E. A. Bayer. 1987. Specialized cell surface structures in cellulolytic bacteria. *J. Bacteriol.* **169**:3792–3800.

Lange, C. C., L. P. Wackett, K. W. Minton, and M. J. Daly. 1998. Engineering a recombinant *Deinococcus radiodurans* for organopollutant degradation in radioactive mixed waste environments. *Nat. Biotechnol.* **16**:929–933.

Latorre-Garcia, L., A. C. Adam, P. Manzanares, and J. Polaina. 2005. Improving the amylolytic activity of *Saccharomyces cerevisiae* glucoamylase by the addition of a starch binding domain. *J. Biotechnol.* **118**:167–176.

Leonhartsberger, S., I. Korsa, and A. Böck. 2002. The molecular biology of formate metabolism in enterobacteria. *J. Mol. Microbiol. Biotechnol.* **4**:269–276.

Leungsakul, T., G. R. Johnson, and T. K. Wood. 2006. Protein engineering of the 4-methyl-5-nitrocatechol monooxygenase from *Burkholderia* sp. strain DNT for enhanced degradation of nitroaromatics. *Appl. Environ. Microbiol.* **72**:3933–3939.

Lynd, L. R., J. H. Cushman, R. J. Nichols, and C. E. Wyman. 1991. Fuel ethanol from cellulosic biomass. *Science* **251**:1318–1323.

Meng, M., C. Lee, M. Bagdasarian, and J. G. Zeikus. 1991. Switching substrate preference of thermophilic xylose isomerase from D-xylose to D-glucose by redesigning the substrate binding pocket. *Proc. Natl. Acad. Sci. USA* **88**:4015–4019.

Mingardon, F., A. Chanal, A. M. López-Contreras, C. Dray, E. A. Bayer, and H.-P. Fierobe. 2007. Incorporation of fungal cellulases in bacterial minicellulosomes yields viable, synergistically acting cellulolytic complexes. *Appl. Environ. Microbiol.* **73**:3822–3832.

Ohta, K., D. S. Beall, J. P. Mejia, K. T. Shanmugam, and L. O. Ingram. 1991. Genetic improvement of *Escherichia coli* for ethanol production: chromosomal integration of *Zymomonas mobilis* genes encoding pyruvate decarboxylase and alcohol dehydrogenase II. *Appl. Environ. Microbiol.* **57**:893–900.

Panesar, P. S., S. S. Marwaha, and J. F. Kennedy. 2006. *Zymomonas mobilis*: an alternative ethanol producer. *J. Chem. Technol. Biotechnol.* **81**:623–635.

Pérez-González, J. A., R. González, A. Querol, J. Sendra, and D. Ramón. 1993. Construction of a recombinant wine yeast strain expressing β-(1,4)-endoglucanase and its use in microvinification processes. *Appl. Environ. Microbiol.* **59**:2801–2806.

Quax, W. J., N. T. Mrabet, R. G. M. Luiten, P. W. Schuurhuizen, P. Stanssens, and I. Lasters. 1991. Enhancing the thermostability of glucose isomerase by protein engineering. *Bio/Technology* **9**:738–742.

Ramos, J. L., A. Wasserfallen, K. Rose, and K. N. Timmis. 1987. Redesigning metabolic routes: manipulation of TOL plasmid pathway for catabolism of alkylbenzoates. *Science* **235**:593–596.

Richins, R. D., I. Kaneva, A. Mulchandani, and W. Chen. 1997. Biodegradation of organophosphorus pesticides by surface-expressed organophosphorus hydrolase. *Nat. Biotechnol.* **15**:984–987.

Suyama, A., R. Iwakiri, N. Kimura, A. Nishi, K. Nakamura, and K. Furukawa. 1996. Engineering hybrid pseudomonads capable of utilizing a wide range of aromatic hydrocarbons and of efficient degradation of trichloroethylene. *J. Bacteriol.* 178:4039–4046.

Tao, H., R. Gonzalez, A. Martinez, M. Rodriguez, L. O. Ingram, J. F. Preston, and K. T. Shanmugam. 2001. Engineering a homo-ethanol pathway in *Escherichia coli*: increased glycolytic flux and levels of expression of glycolytic genes during xylose fermentation. *J. Bacteriol.* 183:2979–2988.

Timmis, K. N., R. J. Steffan, and R. Unterman. 1994. Designing microorganisms for the treatment of toxic wastes. *Annu. Rev. Microbiol.* 48:525–557.

Van Rooyen, R., B. Hahn-Hägerdal, D. C. La Grange, and W. H. Van Zyl. 2005. Construction of cellulose-growing and fermenting *Saccharomyces cerevisiae* strains. *J. Biotechnol.* 120:284–295.

Verdoes, J. C., A. D. van Diepeningen, P. J. Punt, A. J. M. Debets, A. H. Stouthamer, and C. A. M. J. J. van den Hondel. 1994. Evaluation of molecular and genetic approaches to generate glucoamylase overproducing strains of *Aspergillus niger*. *J. Biotechnol.* 36:165–175.

Wayman, M., S. Chen, and K. Doan. 1992. Bioconversion of waste paper to ethanol. *Process Biochem.* 27:239–245.

Winter, R. B., K.-M. Yen, and B. D. Ensley. 1989. Efficient degradation of trichloroethylene by a recombinant *Escherichia coli*. *Bio/Technology* 7:282–285.

Witholt, B., M.-J. de Smet, J. Kingma, J. B. van Beilen, M. Kok, R. G. Lageveen, and G. Eggink. 1990. Bioconversions of aliphatic compounds by *Pseudomonas oleovorans* in multiphase bioreactors: background and economic potential. *Trends Biotechnol.* 8:46–52.

Wong, W. K. R., C. Curry, R. S. Parekh, S. R. Parekh, M. Wayman,

R. W. Davies, D. G. Kilburn, and N. Skipper. 1988. Wood hydrolysis by *Cellulomonas fimi* endoglucanase and exoglucanase coexpressed as secreted enzymes in *Saccharomyces cerevisiae*. *Bio/Technology* 6:713–719.

Yoshido, A., T. Nishimura, H. Kawaguchi, M. Inui, and H. Yukawa. 2005. Enhanced hydrogen production from formic acid by formate hydrogen lyase-overproducing *Escherichia coli* strains. *Appl. Environ. Microbiol.* 71:6762–6768.

Zhang, M., C. Eddy, K. Deanda, M. Finkelstein, and S. Picataggio. 1995. Metabolic engineering of a pentose metabolism pathway in ethanologenic *Zymomonas mobilis*. *Science* 267:240–243.

Zylstra, G. J., L. P. Wackett, and D. T. Gibson. 1989. Trichloroethylene degradation by *Escherichia coli* containing the cloned *Pseudomonas putida* F1 toluene dioxygenase genes. *Appl. Environ. Microbiol.* 55:3162–3166.

REVIEW QUESTIONS

1. How would you genetically engineer a bacterium to degrade trichloroethylene?

2. Outline a protocol that you would use to clone fungal cellulase genes.

3. Delineate the role of α-amylase and glucoamylase in the industrial production of alcohol. How might genetic manipulation of the genes encoding these enzymes be used to improve this process?

4. What is glucose isomerase? Why is it important? How and why would you modify the gene encoding this enzyme?

5. Elaborate some of the advantages and disadvantages of using *Z. mobilis* instead of *S. cerevisiae* for alcohol production. How would you improve the industrial performance of *Z. mobilis*?

6. How can *Z. mobilis* be engineered to produce ethanol from xylose and arabinose?

7. Starting with a *Pseudomonas* strain that can utilize phenol as its sole carbon source at 0°C, a *Pseudomonas* strain that can degrade anthracene to catechol at 35°C, and a *Pseudomonas* strain that can degrade *p*-toluene to protocatechuate at 35°C, suggest a strategy for developing a strain that can utilize phenol, anthracene, or *p*-toluene as its sole carbon source at 0°C.

8. Explain how a *Pseudomonas* strain that carries plasmid pWWO and does not normally degrade 4-ethylbenzoate can be genetically manipulated to hydrolyze this compound.

9. Suggest schemes for the isolation of prokaryotic endoglucanase and β-glucosidase genes.

10. What is a "superbug"?

11. How can *L. plantarum* be manipulated to improve its ability to ferment silage?

12. How can pesticide-degrading enzymes be expressed on the surface of a bacterium?

13. How would you degrade organic environmental pollutants in the presence of high levels of radioactivity?

14. How would you engineer yeast strains to more efficiently convert glucose into ethanol?

15. How would you expand the substrate range of a strain of *Burkholderia* sp. that normally degrades 2,4-dinitrotoluene?

16. How would you engineer glucoamylase to be more efficient in degrading starch?

17. How would you engineer *E. coli* to produce isopropanol?

18. What is a designer cellulosome? How is it produced?

19. How would you engineer *E. coli* to produce hydrogen gas from formic acid?

15

Plant Growth-Promoting Bacteria

U NDER NATURAL ENVIRONMENTAL CONDITIONS, successful plant growth and development and high crop yields depend on the genetic constitution of the crop species, suitable weather conditions, and soil components, including the availability of nutrients; the absence of growth-inhibitory substances, such as salt; the presence of certain beneficial microorganisms; and the absence of pathogenic ones (called phytopathogens, from *phyto*, meaning plant). Some beneficial indigenous soil bacteria and fungi act directly by providing a plant growth-enhancing product, and others act indirectly. The latter organisms inhibit the growth of pathogenic soil microorganisms, thereby preventing them from hindering plant growth.

The direct promotion of plant growth usually entails providing the plant with a compound that is synthesized by the bacterium, such as fixed nitrogen or a plant hormone. Also, these bacteria can facilitate the uptake by the plant of certain nutrients from the environment. The indirect promotion of plant growth occurs when plant growth-promoting bacteria lessen or prevent the deleterious effects of phytopathogenic organisms, either fungi or bacteria, i.e., they act as biocontrol agents. This activity is called antibiosis, and it either depletes a scarce resource required by the pathogen or produces a compound that impedes the growth of the phytopathogenic organism.

Direct stimulation of plant growth and development by plant growth-promoting bacteria can occur in several different ways. The bacteria can (1) fix atmospheric nitrogen to ammonia that is used by the plant; (2) synthesize siderophores that solubilize and sequester iron from the soil and provide it to plant cells; (3) synthesize phytohormones, such as auxin, cytokinin, or gibberellin, that enhance various stages of plant growth; (4) solubilize minerals, such as phosphorus, that are used by the plant; and (5) synthesize an enzyme that can modulate the level of the plant hormone ethylene. Any particular plant growth-promoting bacterium may utilize one or more of these mechanisms.

Much of the recent genetic research directed at creating microbial strains with augmented plant growth-promoting activity has focused on a few areas of study.

- Engineering of better biocontrol strains of bacteria to decrease the damage to plants from a variety of pathogens. This work is aimed at replacing some of the chemical pesticides that may become environmental pollutants.
- The use of bacteria to lower ethylene levels in plants. These studies are directed toward preventing high levels of ethylene from accumulating in plants and thereby decreasing the damage to the plant from a variety of environmental stresses, including drought, flooding, salt stress, and the presence of pathogens.
- The molecular basis of nitrogen fixation. This topic has been investigated thoroughly to determine whether it is possible to increase the level of microbial nitrogen fixation and consequently lessen the current dependency on chemical fertilizers for crop plants.
- Root nodule formation by symbiotic bacteria. This process has been studied with the aim of producing genetically engineered bacteria that can outcompete naturally occurring symbiotic bacteria.
- Microbial synthesis of iron-sequestering compounds (siderophores). These reactions are being characterized in the hope that it might be possible to produce beneficial strains that prevent the growth of phytopathogenic microorganisms.
- Manipulation of plant growth-promoting bacteria to facilitate phytoremediation (the use of plants to remediate contaminated environments).

Current research in this area mainly deals with plant growth-promoting bacteria rather than fungi. This is at least partly due to the fact that scientists have found it difficult or even impossible to grow many beneficial fungi in culture, so not only is it difficult to manipulate them in the laboratory, it is also extremely difficult to obtain large enough amounts of these organisms for inoculation of crops. In the past, bacterial fertilization had a dubious reputation. During the 1950s in the Soviet Union, more than 10 million hectares (about 39,000 square miles) of farmland were treated with diazotrophic (nitrogen-fixing) bacterial mixtures that consisted primarily of *Azotobacter chroococcum* and *Bacillus megaterium*. In these experiments, about 60% of the time, yields of various crops were increased by 10 to 20%. However, these field trials were poorly designed and not replicable, so many researchers were skeptical about the validity of the work and tended to discount the use of bacterial inoculants as fertilizing agents on a large scale. In recent years, considerable progress has been made toward understanding many of the mechanisms employed by plant growth-promoting bacteria. Thus, there is a much greater likelihood than in the past that results will be predictable and reproducible.

Growth Promotion by Free-Living Bacteria

Plant growth-promoting bacteria include a wide range of bacteria that are free-living or that form a symbiotic relationship with plants, such as *Rhizobium* and *Frankia*. While numerous free-living soil bacteria are considered to be plant growth-promoting bacteria (Table 15.1), not all bacterial

TABLE 15.1 Examples of successful agricultural plant growth stimulation by free-living plant growth-promoting bacteria

Bacterium	Plant(s)	Conditions
Azospirillum brasilense	Guinea grass, millet, sorghum, bean, wheat, barley, fountain grass, Sudan grass, corn, chickpea, fava bean, oat, rice	Field, greenhouse, hydroponic system
Azospirillum irakense	Winter wheat, corn	Field
Azospirillum lipoferum	Millet, sunflower, corn	Field, greenhouse
Azospirillum sp.	Wheat, corn, millet, mustard, rice, sorghum	Field, greenhouse
Azotobacter chroococcum	Barley	Growth chamber
Bacillus amyloliquefaciens	Tomato, pepper	Field
Bacillus cereus	Tomato, pepper	Field
Bacillus polymyxa	Wheat, sugar beet	Field
Bacillus pumilis	Tomato, pepper	Field
Bacillus subtilis	Tomato, pepper, peanut, onion	Field, growth chamber
Bacillus sp.	Sorghum, wheat	Field
Burkholderia vietnamiensis	Rice	Field
Enterobacter cloacae	Tomato, pepper, mung bean	Greenhouse
Pseudomonas cepacia	Winter wheat	Field, growth chamber
Pseudomonas chlororaphis	Spring wheat	Field, laboratory
Pseudomonas fluorescens	Winter wheat, potato, tomato, cucumber, blueberry	Field, greenhouse, growth chamber
Pseudomonas putida	Winter wheat, potato, canola, cucumber, lettuce, tomato, barley, oat	Field, greenhouse, growth chamber
Pseudomonas syringae	Bean	Greenhouse
Pseudomonas sp.	Canola, potato, rice, lettuce, cucumber, tomato, corn	Field, greenhouse, growth chamber, hydroponic system

strains of a particular genus and species have identical metabolic capabilities. Thus, for example, some *Pseudomonas putida* strains actively promote plant growth, while others have no measurable effect on plants.

The major applications of bacteria for improving plant growth include agriculture, horticulture, forestry, and environmental restoration (phytoremediation). In the past 20 years or so, based on a better understanding of the mechanisms employed by these bacteria and following a large number of successful laboratory and field studies, an increasing number of plant growth-promoting bacteria have been commercialized.

The mechanism most commonly invoked to explain the various effects of plant growth-promoting bacteria on plants is the production of phytohormones. Research in this area has focused on the role of a class of phytohormones called auxins. The most common and best-characterized auxin is indole-3-acetic acid (IAA), which stimulates in plants both rapid responses, such as increases in cell elongation, and long-term effects, such as increases in cell division and differentiation. Since both plants and plant growth-promoting bacteria can synthesize auxin, it is difficult for researchers to distinguish between plant responses that result from bacterial auxin synthesis and those that result from plant auxin synthesis. This uncertainty notwithstanding, there is considerable evidence to suggest that many plant growth-promoting bacteria facilitate plant growth by altering the hormonal balance within a plant.

In the early 1990s, it was discovered that many plant growth-promoting bacteria contain an enzyme that can modulate levels of the plant hormone ethylene. This enzyme, 1-aminocyclopropane-1-carboxylate

FIGURE 15.1 Cleavage of ACC to α-ketobutyrate and ammonia by ACC deaminase.

(ACC) deaminase, cleaves ACC, which is the immediate biosynthetic precursor of ethylene in plants (Fig. 15.1). As depicted in Fig. 15.2, the bacterium binds to seed coats or plant roots and then sequesters and cleaves ACC. As a result, the level of ethylene in the developing (or stressed) plant is lowered. In many plants, ethylene stimulates germination and breaks the

FIGURE 15.2 Schematic representation of the mechanisms by which an ACC deaminase-containing plant growth-promoting bacterium bound to either a seed or a plant root lowers the ethylene concentration and thereby prevents ethylene inhibition of root elongation. The arrows indicate chemical or physical steps in the mechanism, and the symbol ⊥ indicates inhibition of root elongation by ethylene. IAA is synthesized and secreted by a plant growth-promoting bacterium that is bound to the surface of either the seed or the root of a developing plant. After being taken up by the plant, together with the IAA from the plant, the bacterial IAA can stimulate either plant cell proliferation and elongation or the activity of the enzyme ACC synthase, which converts S-adenosylmethionine (AdoMet) to ACC. A significant portion of the ACC is exuded from plant roots or seeds, along with other small molecules normally present in seed or root exudates; taken up by the bacterium; and hydrolyzed by the enzyme ACC deaminase to ammonia and α-ketobutyrate (α-KB). This uptake and cleavage of ACC decreases the amount of ACC outside the plant. To maintain the equilibrium between internal and external ACC, the plant exudes more ACC. Consequently, the concentration of ACC, and therefore ethylene, in the plant is lowered. Adapted from Glick et al., *J. Theor. Biol.* **190:**63–68, 1998.

dormancy of the seeds; however, if the level of ethylene remains high after germination, a problem that is especially acute when plants are under stress, root elongation is inhibited. Thus, the ACC deaminase that is provided by a plant growth-promoting bacterium prevents the inhibition of root elongation (Fig. 15.3), and consequently, the plant produces longer roots during early development, resulting in a healthier and larger plant. In addition, many plant growth-promoting bacteria synthesize IAA. The IAA that is produced by the bacterium and taken up by the plant that is not used to promote plant cell elongation or proliferation stimulates the transcription of the enzyme ACC synthase in the plant. A greater amount of ACC synthase causes an increase in the level of ACC, eventually resulting in an increase in the ethylene concentration. When ACC deaminase activity is present, it prevents the buildup of ACC, even in the presence of high levels of IAA, so that the ethylene level does not become elevated to the point where plant growth is impaired.

In general, nitrogen fixation by free-living plant growth-promoting bacteria probably makes only a minor contribution to the growth of a plant. In fact, not all plant growth-promoting bacteria are diazotrophic, and many of those that are diazotrophic fix only limited amounts of nitrogen.

A number of plants use bacterial iron–siderophore complexes to obtain iron from the soil. Without this mechanism, plant growth in many soils would be severely limited, as iron is an essential plant nutrient. However, while bacterial siderophores undoubtedly contribute to the nutrition, and hence to the growth, of plants, in many instances this effect is small.

There is some controversy regarding the mechanism that plant growth-promoting bacteria use to facilitate the uptake of minerals such as phosphorus by a plant. On one hand, the increased mineral uptake in plants treated with plant growth-promoting bacteria may reflect a better-developed root system and an overall healthier plant. On the other hand, experiments with *Azospirillum* have shown that this organism enhances mineral uptake by secreting organic acids that can solubilize and bind some minerals.

FIGURE 15.3 Effect of treating canola seeds with ACC deaminase-containing plant growth-promoting bacteria on root ACC content **(A)** and root length **(B)**, following growth of the plant for 4.5 days after the seeds were sown. The seeds were treated with $MgSO_4$ as a control, the ACC deaminase-containing bacterium *P. putida* GR12-2, or the chemical ethylene inhibitor 1-aminovinylglycine (AVG). The error bars indicate standard errors.

MILESTONE

A Model for the Lowering of Plant Ethylene Concentrations by Plant Growth-Promoting Bacteria
B. R. GLICK, D. M. PENROSE, and J. LI
J. Theor. Biol. **190**:63–68, 1998

In addition to the profound influence that ethylene has on normal plant growth and development, it is a stress hormone whose synthesis is increased when a plant is subjected to any one of a variety of environmental stresses. These stresses include mechanical trauma, pathogen infection, extremes of temperature, drought, flooding, salt, and the presence of environmental contaminants. Following periods of stress, the ethylene that is produced by the plant often exacerbates the effects of the stress. This can lead to plant senescence or death. Any chemical or biological treatment that lowers the amount of ethylene that is produced by a plant as a consequence of an environmental stress should therefore also decrease some of the resulting damage to the plant.

It has been known for many years that certain strains of bacteria can promote the growth of plants. At the time that this article was published, many of the mechanisms involved in the promotion of plant growth by bacteria had apparently been elucidated. However, there did not seem to be any one mechanism that could reliably and reproducibly promote the growth of a wide variety of plants under a range of different conditions. This was in spite of the fact that some strains of *Rhizobium,* some biocontrol strains, and some *Azospirillum* strains had been commercialized, albeit to a limited extent.

In this article, Glick and coworkers developed a conceptual framework to explain a number of empirical observations that their laboratory had reported beginning in 1994. In its simplest terms, the model that they elaborated suggested that some plant growth-promoting bacteria that were bound to plant tissues could act as a sink for some of the ACC that was produced by the plant in response to various types of stress. Since ACC is the immediate precursor of ethylene in all higher plants, the model predicted that lowering ACC levels before it could be converted to ethylene would limit some of the deleterious effects of a particular stressor on a plant. The model was tested in a growth chamber, then in a greenhouse, and eventually in field experiments. It was found that plant growth-promoting bacteria that contained active ACC deaminase could significantly decrease the inhibition of growth and damage to plants following exposure to either high salt levels, the presence of metals or organic contaminants, phytopathogens, flooding, or drought. Moreover, workers in many different laboratories around the world have found that this approach works well with a wide range of plants, including canola, tomato, lettuce, soybean, mung bean, Indian mustard, various grasses, wheat, pea, corn, and cotton. Thus, by either selecting or engineering plant growth-promoting bacteria to express ACC deaminase, the productivity of a range of crop plants can be improved dramatically.

As a better understanding of the mechanisms used by plant growth-promoting bacteria emerges, it will become possible to genetically engineer improved organisms that can stimulate the growth of a wide range of plants in a variety of environments.

Decreasing Plant Stress

In addition to its effect on seed germination and root elongation, ethylene mediates a wide range of plant responses and developmental steps. Ethylene is involved in tissue differentiation, formation of root and shoot primordia, lateral bud development, flowering initiation, anthocyanin synthesis, flower opening and senescence, fruit ripening and degreening, production of volatile organic compounds that are responsible for aroma formation in fruits, storage product hydrolysis, leaf and fruit abscission, and the response of plants to biotic and abiotic stress. In some processes, ethylene is stimulatory, while in others it is inhibitory.

The term "stress ethylene" describes the increase in ethylene biosynthesis associated with biological and environmental stresses and pathogen attack. The increased level of ethylene formed in response to trauma

inflicted by chemicals, temperature extremes, water stress, ultraviolet light, insect damage, disease, and mechanical wounding can be both the cause of some of the symptoms of stress (e.g., onset of wilting and increased senescence) and the inducer of responses that will enhance the survival of the plant under adverse conditions. Often, a small burst of ethylene is synthesized by plants within a few hours after an environmental stress. This low level of ethylene acts as a trigger to initiate the biosynthesis of a number of plant defense proteins. Subsequently, some 2 to 4 days after the onset of the stress, the plant produces a much larger burst of ethylene. It is this second peak of ethylene synthesis that is responsible for attenuating the deleterious effect(s) of the stress (Fig. 15.4).

While chemicals have been successfully used to control ethylene levels in plants, many of them are either expensive or potentially harmful to the environment. Consequently, ACC deaminase-containing plant growth-promoting bacteria have been tested to determine whether they could be used as an environmentally safe method for lowering plant ethylene levels.

Flooding is a common abiotic stress that affects many plants, often several times during the same growing season. Plant roots suffer a lack of oxygen as a consequence of flooding; this, in turn, causes deleterious effects, such as wilting (epinasty), inhibition of leaf chlorophyll synthesis (chlorosis), cell death (necrosis), and reduced fruit yield. Many plants respond to flooding by activating the transcription, in root cells, of some of the genes that code for isozymes of ACC synthase, the enzyme that converts the compound S-adenosylmethionine into ACC. This eventually results in an increase in the amount of ACC inside plant roots. However, since ACC oxidase cannot catalyze ethylene synthesis in the absence of oxygen, ACC is transported from the anaerobic environment of flooded roots into the aerobic shoots, where it is converted to ethylene (Fig. 15.5). The ethylene in the shoots causes plants to wilt, to lose biomass, and eventually (if the ethylene remains elevated for a prolonged time) to senesce and die. Treatment of tomato plants with ACC deaminase-containing plant growth-promoting bacteria significantly decreases the damage suffered by these plants due to stress ethylene brought on as a consequence of flooding (Fig. 15.6). These ACC deaminase-containing plant growth-promoting bacteria can act as a sink for ACC, lowering the level of ethylene that can be formed in the shoots and thereby protecting the tomato plants from a portion of the damage caused by flooding.

In addition to protecting plants from flooding damage, ACC deaminase-containing plant growth-promoting bacteria can also significantly decrease the damage to plants that is caused by drought, temperature extremes, high concentrations of salt, and a variety of environmental contaminants. For example, in greenhouse experiments, tomato plants treated with *Achromobacter piechaudii* ARV8, which contains ACC deaminase, were able to grow better in the presence of 86 mM salt (which is usually inhibitory to plant growth) than were tomato plants grown without the added bacterium in either the presence or the absence of salt (Fig. 15.7). This bacterium, which was isolated from a soil sample from the Arava region of the Negev desert in Israel, significantly lowered the level of stress ethylene produced by tomato plants in the presence of salt. More recently, several groups have shown that this approach can facilitate the growth of a range of crops in saline soils in the field, a problem that is endemic to about 25% of the world's arable land.

FIGURE 15.4 Time course of plant ethylene synthesis following environmental stress or fungal pathogen infection.

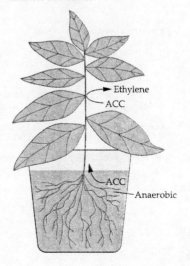

FIGURE 15.5 Schematic representation of a flooded potted plant, where the ACC that is produced in the roots as a consequence of the stress is unable to be converted to ethylene because of the absence of oxygen. The ACC is subsequently transported to the shoots, where oxygen is plentiful, and converted to ethylene, causing epinasty and loss of biomass.

FIGURE 15.6 Effect of ACC deaminase-containing plant growth-promoting bacteria on flooded tomato plants. **(A and B)** Fifty-five-day-old tomato plants were either grown for an additional 9 days (A) or flooded for 9 days before the dry weight of the leaves and shoots was determined (B). **(C)** The amount of ethylene produced by 55-day-old tomato plant leaf stems (petioles) following 9 days of flooding was also measured. ACC deaminase activity is present in *Enterobacter cloacae* CAL2 and *P. putida* UW4, and in another *P. putida* strain transformed with the plasmid pRK415ACC, which carries a bacterial ACC deaminase gene. *P. putida* strain pRK415 has no ACC deaminase activity. The error bars indicate standard errors; the standard errors in panel C were negligible. Nonflooded plants produce approximately 0.07 pmol of ethylene g^{-1} s^{-1}, regardless of the presence or absence of bacteria. Adapted from Grichko and Glick, *Plant Physiol. Biochem.* **39**:11–17, 2001.

Increasing Phosphorus Availability

While a number of plant growth-promoting bacteria can synthesize and secrete organic acids that can dissolve inorganic phosphate in the environment, these organisms can rarely break down phytate, the complex compound (inositol hexaphosphate) that is the major chemical form of phosphorus within cereal grains and oilseeds. Several plants can produce phytases, enzymes that degrade phytate. However, the activity of these

FIGURE 15.7 (A) The ACC deaminase-containing bacterium *A. piechaudii* ARV8 (green) increases the tolerance of tomato plants for salt compared to plants grown without the bacterium (red). **(B)** Treatment of tomato plants with salt causes an increase in the synthesis of stress ethylene. Ethylene production in the presence of salt is partially inhibited by *A. piechaudii* ARV8. The error bars indicate standard errors.

enzymes in plant roots is generally low, so these plants cannot efficiently utilize the phytate that is found in the soil. A gene encoding the enzyme phytase was isolated from the fungus *Aspergillus fumigatus*. This gene was inserted, using a transposon, into the chromosomal DNA of a strain of the bacterium *Bacillus mucilaginosus*, which can dissolve phosphorus from calcium phosphate. The transformed bacterial strain can express and secrete active phytase. In greenhouse experiments, this transformed bacterium was found to be superior to the wild-type strain in providing phosphorus to tobacco plants cultivated in its presence (Table 15.2). Importantly, the stimulation of plant growth that was observed in greenhouse experiments

TABLE 15.2 Growth of tobacco plants for 90 days in pots in the greenhouse with different treatments

Characteristic	Soil with no added bacteria	Soil plus wild-type bacterium	Soil plus transformed bacterium
Plant height (cm)	17.4	21.4	24.7
Plant dry weight (mg)	1,297	1,685	1,870
Leaf P content ($\mu g/g$)	710	732	800

was also evident in the field, where the yield of tobacco plants increased by 19%. Notwithstanding these results, it may be some time before this work is commercialized because of political concerns about the use of genetically engineered bacteria in the environment.

Biocontrol of Pathogens

Phytopathogens are an ongoing and serious agricultural problem that can reduce crop yields by 25 to 100%. This is an enormous loss of productivity. Currently, phytopathogen damage to crops is generally dealt with by the use of chemical agents, although other treatments have also been employed. For most bacterial diseases, plants may be symptomless for prolonged periods before changes in environmental conditions which favor the proliferation of the bacteria cause a rapid outbreak of disease. Under these conditions, severe damage can occur and destroy an entire crop. These field epidemics are difficult and costly to control.

Many of the chemicals that are used to control phytopathogens are hazardous to animals and humans, and they persist and accumulate in natural ecosystems. It is therefore desirable to replace these chemical agents with biological control agents that are more "friendly" to the environment. One approach for the control of phytopathogens is the development of transgenic plants that are resistant to one or more of them (see chapter 18). Alternatively, some plant growth-promoting bacteria can act as biocontrol agents to suppress or prevent phytopathogen damage, and a number of these biocontrol bacteria have been commercialized (Table 15.3). Plant growth-promoting bacteria can produce a variety of substances that limit damage to plants by phytopathogens. They include siderophores, antibiotics, other small molecules, and a variety of enzymes. This approach is still at an early stage of development but appears to have considerable potential. However, the ultimate utility of a strategy based on a particular mechanism can be assessed only under field conditions.

Siderophores

Iron is one of the most abundant minerals on Earth and is an essential requirement for living organisms. However, iron in the soil is unavailable for direct assimilation by microorganisms because ferric iron, or Fe(III), which is the predominant form in nature, is only sparingly soluble, i.e., its solubility is about 10^{-18} M at pH 7.4. This amount of soluble iron is much too small to support microbial growth. Consequently, to survive in this environment, soil microorganisms synthesize and secrete low-molecular-mass (~400- to 1,000-dalton) iron-binding molecules known as siderophores (Fig. 15.8). Siderophores bind Fe(III) with a very high affinity (dissociation constant $[K_d] = 10^{-20}$ to 10^{-50} M) and transport it back to cell

FIGURE 15.8 A six-coordinate iron–siderophore complex. Three bidentate functional groups on a siderophore molecule bind with ferric iron.

TABLE 15.3 Some commercially available biocontrol plant growth-promoting bacteria

Bacterium	Pathogen or disease	Crop(s)
Agrobacterium radiobacter	Crown gall disease caused by *A. tumefaciens*	Fruit trees, nut trees, and ornamental nursery stock
Azotobacter brasilense	Root rot and damping-off	Turf, forage crops, corn
Bacillus subtilis	*Rhizoctonia solani, Pythium* spp., *Fusarium* spp., *Alternaria* spp., and *Aspergillus* spp. that attack roots; also various seedling pathogens	Cotton, legumes, barley, tomato, rice
Bacillus amyloliquefaciens	*Fusarium* spp., *Rhizoctonia* spp.	Herbs, spices, vegetables, tree seedlings, ornamentals
Bacillus pumilis	Powdery mildew, downy mildew, *Fusarium* spp., *Phytophthora* spp., *Rhizoctonia* spp., *Sclerotinia* spp.	Fruits and vegetables, oak, maple, stored seeds
Burkholderia cepacia	*Fusarium* spp., *Pythium* spp., nematodes	Vegetables
Burkholderia cepacia	*Rhizoctonia* spp., *Fusarium* spp., *Pythium* spp., nematodes	Alfalfa, barley, beans, clover, corn, cotton, peas, grain sorghum, vegetables, wheat
Paenibacillus polymyxa	Damping-off, powdery mildew	Cucumber
Pseudomonas chlororaphis	*Fusarium*, leaf stripe, leaf spot, net blotch, spot blotch	Barley, oat
Pseudomonas fluorescens	Frost, *Erwinia amylovora, Pseudomonas tolassii*	Almond, apple, cherry, mushrooms, peach, pear, potato, strawberry, tomato
Pseudomonas syringae	*Botrytis cinerea, Penicillium* spp., *Mucor piriformis, Geotrichum candidum*	Citrus and pome fruit, potatoes
Streptomyces griseoviridis	*Fusarium* spp., *Alternaria brassicola, Phomopsis* spp., *Botrytis* spp., *Pythium* spp., and *Phytophthora* spp.	Field, ornamental, and vegetable crops
Streptomyces lydicus	Control of root rot and damping-off caused by *Fusarium, Rhizoctonia, Pythium, Phytophthora, Sclerotinia, Postia,* and *Verticillium;* also suppresses foliar diseases caused by *Botrytis*	Useful for protection of cuttings of a variety of plants; also used with turfgrass
Mixture of *B. subtilis, P. polymyxa, Bacillus circulans,* and *B. amyloliquefaciens*	A range of fungal damping-off diseases	Especially useful in hydroponic gardens

surface receptors, where it is taken into the cell. Once inside a cell, the iron is released and is then available to support microbial growth.

Plant growth-promoting bacteria can prevent the proliferation of fungal phytopathogens by producing siderophores that bind most of the Fe(III) in the area around the plant root (the rhizosphere). The resulting lack of iron prevents fungal pathogens from proliferating in the immediate vicinity. Fungal phytopathogens also synthesize siderophores, but these generally have a much lower affinity for iron than do the siderophores produced by plant growth-promoting bacteria. In effect, the plant growth-promoting bacteria outcompete fungal phytopathogens for available iron.

Unlike microbial phytopathogens, plants are not generally harmed by the localized depletion of iron in the soil caused by plant growth-promoting bacteria. Most plants can grow at much lower iron concentrations than microorganisms. In addition, some studies have shown that iron that has been sequestered by bacterial siderophores is taken up from the soil by the plant, to its benefit.

FIGURE 15.9 Iron-binding groups of microbial siderophores.

Because the sequestering of iron by a siderophore-producing bacterium can simultaneously prevent the proliferation of a number of different phytopathogenic microorganisms, siderophore genes are being examined to determine whether they can be used to create more effective biocontrol inoculants.

Siderophores generally have three functional, or iron-binding, groups connected by a flexible backbone, often a peptide. Each functional group usually presents two atoms of oxygen or, less commonly, two nitrogen atoms, that bind iron. In chemical terms, the functional groups are bidentate. Trivalent ferric iron can accommodate three of these groups to form a six-coordinate complex (Fig. 15.8). With some exceptions, the functional groups on microbial siderophores are either hydroxamates or catecholates (Fig. 15.9). Different combinations of functional groups may be present on a single siderophore. Other functional groups include carboxylate moieties, such as citrate, and ethylenediamine (Fig. 15.9). In general, hydroxamate-type siderophores are typical of fungi, and catecholates, which bind iron more tightly than hydroxamates, are common in bacterial siderophores. Plant siderophores, on the other hand, are linear hydroxy- and amino-substituted iminocarboxylic acids, such as mugineic acid and avenic acid.

One bacterial siderophore, called pseudobactin (Fig. 15.10), has been estimated to bind to Fe(III) with an affinity constant of approximately 10^{25} liters mol^{-1}. All fluorescent pseudomonads, so named because they produce a siderophore that fluoresces when excited by ultraviolet light, syn-

FIGURE 15.10 Structure of the siderophore called pseudobactin from *Pseudomonas* sp. strain B10. One molecule of Fe(III) is bound to the siderophore.

thesize structurally related siderophores that differ mainly in the number and configuration of the amino acids in the peptide chain that makes up the backbone.

The synthesis and regulation of pseudobactin in the plant growth-promoting bacterium *P. putida* WCS358 has been examined in detail. Mutagenesis was used to generate a set of 28 mutants that were defective for siderophore production. Two criteria were used for identifying the siderophore-deficient mutants: (1) lack of fluorescence under ultraviolet light and (2) inability to grow in the presence of bipyridyl, a molecule that sequesters most of the iron in the growth medium. When most of the iron is unavailable, only a cell that produces siderophores can grow.

A clone bank of *P. putida* WCS358 DNA was constructed in the broad-host-range cosmid vector pLAFR1 and was introduced by conjugation into each of the 28 siderophore mutants (Fig. 15.11). All of the resultant transformants were tested by complementation for restoration of fluorescence and/or the ability to grow in the presence of bipyridyl. Thirteen separate complementing cosmid clones, with an average insert size of 26 kilobase pairs (kb), were identified. After detailed analyses, these clones were found to represent at least five separate gene clusters.

One of these gene clusters has been studied further. It has a length of 33.5 kb and contains five transcriptional units with at least seven separate genes. Thus, like nitrogen fixation and nodulation, siderophore biosynthesis

FIGURE 15.11 Cloning genes involved in siderophore biosynthesis. The clone bank is constructed using the broad-host-range cosmid pLAFR1. The cells that have mutations in one of the genes involved in siderophore biosynthesis are unable to grow on medium containing bipyridyl, which sequesters all of the free iron in the medium. Cells with mutations in genes involved in siderophore biosynthesis are selected from the replica plate that does not contain bipyridyl. Transformants that can grow in the presence of bipyridyl are able to complement the mutation in one of the siderophore biosynthesis genes.

TABLE 15.4 Effect of additional copies of the *rpoD* gene that encodes ρ⁷⁰ from *P. fluorescens* CHA0 on the ability of the bacterium to prevent damage to cucumber roots caused by the pathogenic fungus *P. ultimum*

Plant growth-promoting bacterium added	Average root fresh weight (mg)	
	Without *P. ultimum*	With *P. ultimum*
None	382	44
P. fluorescens CHA0	386	177
P. fluorescens CHA0 with vector	365	146
P. fluorescens CHA0 with vector and *rpoD* gene	371	335

Adapted from Schnider et al., *J. Bacteriol.* **177**:5387–5392, 1995.

In the absence of the plant growth-promoting bacterium *P. fluorescens* CHA0, the pathogen *P. ultimum* dramatically inhibits root growth. The presence of the *rpoD* gene on the plasmid vector enhanced the activity of the plant growth-promoting bacterium. Plants were grown for 2 weeks before their roots were measured.

is a complex process. Since each siderophore is encoded by a number of different genes, genetically engineering bacteria to produce modified siderophores is not a simple matter. However, there may be other ways to improve the effectiveness of plant growth-promoting bacteria as biocontrol agents. For example, it may be possible to extend the range of iron–siderophore complexes that one bacterial strain can utilize so that a genetically altered plant growth-promoting biocontrol bacterial strain could take up and use siderophores synthesized by other soil microorganisms, thereby giving it a competitive advantage. This was done by cloning the genes for iron–siderophore receptors from one plant growth-promoting control bacterium and introducing them into other strains.

Antibiotics

One of the most effective mechanisms by which a plant growth-promoting bacterium can prevent phytopathogen proliferation is the synthesis of antibiotics. For example, the antibiotics synthesized by biocontrol pseudomonads include agrocin 84, agrocin 434, 2,4-diacetylphloroglucinol, herbicolin, oomycin, phenazines, pyoluteorin, and pyrrolnitrin.

The biocontrol activity of a plant growth-promoting bacterium may be improved by providing it with genes that encode the biosynthesis of antibiotics that are normally produced by other bacteria. In this way, the range of phytopathogens that a single biocontrol bacterium can suppress can be extended. Moreover, by limiting the growth of other soil microorganisms, antibiotic-secreting plant growth-promoting bacteria should facilitate their own proliferation, since they will have fewer competitors for limited nutritional resources. In addition, genetic manipulation can be used to increase the amount of antibiotic that a bacterium synthesizes.

The production of a number of antifungal metabolites that are produced by pseudomonads appears to be controlled by a protein that acts as a global transcriptional regulator; therefore, it should be possible to enhance antibiotic production by modifying this global regulation. For example, antibiotic production was enhanced after *Pseudomonas fluorescens* CHA0 was transformed with a vector carrying the gene encoding the housekeeping RNA polymerase sigma-70 (σ⁷⁰). The modified strain was more effective at protecting cucumber plants against a root disease caused by the fungus *Pythium ultimum* (Table 15.4).

A single copy of the operon carrying all seven of the genes that encode the biosynthesis of the antibiotic phenazine-1-carboxylic acid (i.e., *phzAB-CDEFG*) was inserted into the chromosomal DNA of a plant growth-promoting bacterial strain of *P. fluorescens* (Fig. 15.12). The wild-type version of this bacterium, which does not synthesize phenazine-1-carboxylic acid, acts as a biocontrol agent against some fungal diseases. As indicated by a much larger zone of clearance of the fungal pathogen *P. ultimum* on solid medium, the engineered bacterium has a higher level of biocontrol activity than the wild type (Fig. 15.13). Also, the phenazine-1-carboxylic acid-producing bacterium prevented *P. ultimum*-caused damping-off disease in pea plants in soil. This work demonstrates the efficacy of this approach under greenhouse conditions; however, it remains to be demonstrated whether this altered bacterium is effective in the field.

FIGURE 15.12 Chromosomal insertion of the antibiotic phenazine-1-carboxylic acid operon *(phz)* into a biocontrol strain of *P. fluorescens*. The regulatory genes that normally control the expression of the seven biosynthetic genes were removed, and the entire operon was placed under the control of the *tac* promoter *(p^{tac})*. Since *P. fluorescens* does not utilize lactose as a carbon source, it does not encode the *lac* repressor, and in the absence of the *lac* repressor, any genes under the control of the *tac* promoter are expressed constitutively. The operon, under the control of the *tac* promoter, was inserted into a derivative of transposon Tn5 adjacent to a kanamycin resistance gene (not shown) on a plasmid. Tn5 facilitates integration of DNA into the chromosome of the host cell. Transconjugants in which the chromosomal insertion had not inactivated any important bacterial functions were tested for their effectiveness as biocontrol strains. The Tn5 derivative is designed so that it does not easily pass from the biocontrol strain to other bacteria in the environment.

No bacterium

P. ultimum lawn

Wild-type
bacterium

Engineered
bacterium

Zone of clearance
around bacterial
colony

FIGURE 15.13 Effect of transforming a strain of *P. fluorescens* with genes expressing the antibiotic phenazine-1-carboxylic acid biosynthetic pathway on the ability of the bacterium to prevent the growth of the fungal pathogen *P. ultimum* on solid medium. The antifungal activity of the bacterium is proportional to the area of the zone of clearance around the center of the petri plate to which the bacterium is added.

At present, there is still only one commercially available genetically engineered biocontrol bacterial strain. A modified version of *Agrobacterium radiobacter* K84 has been marketed, first in Australia in 1989, and more recently all over the world, as a means of controlling crown gall disease, which is caused by the bacterium *Agrobacterium tumefaciens*. This disease affects almond trees and stone fruit trees, such as peach trees. The antibiotic agrocin 84, which is produced by *A. radiobacter*, is toxic to *A. tumefaciens*. However, agrocin 84-resistant strains of *A. tumefaciens* can develop if the plasmid carrying the genes for the biosynthesis of agrocin 84 is accidentally transferred from *A. radiobacter*. To avoid this possibility, the region of DNA responsible for plasmid transfer was removed from the agrocin 84 plasmid, pAgK84 (Fig. 15.14). As a result of this deletion, the *A. radiobacter* strain retains the capacity to act as a biocontrol agent, but it can no longer transfer the plasmid to pathogenic agrobacteria.

Enzymes

Some plant growth-promoting bacteria produce enzymes, such as chitinase, β-1,3-glucanase, protease, and lipase, that can degrade fungal cell walls and cause the fungal cells to lyse (Fig. 15.15). In one study, the incidence of plant disease caused by the phytopathogenic fungi *Rhizoctonia solani*, *Sclerotium rolfsii*, and *P. ultimum* was reduced by using a β-1,3-glucanase-producing strain of *Burkholderia cepacia*. In another study, the antifungal activities of three different strains of the plant growth-promoting bacterium *Enterobacter agglomerans* were attributed to a complex of four separate polypeptides that act together to degrade the chitin in fungal cell walls. When tested, these bacteria significantly decreased the damage to cotton plants following infection with *R. solani*. Moreover, Tn5 mutants of *E. agglomerans* that were deficient in chitinase activity were unable to protect plants against damage caused by the fungal pathogen, indicating that the chitinase was the active element.

Many of the bacterial enzymes that can lyse fungal cells, including chitinases and β-glucanases, are encoded by a single gene. It should therefore be straightforward to isolate these genes and transfer them to plant growth-promoting bacteria to construct strains that produce fungus-degrading enzymes. In one series of experiments, a chitinase gene was isolated from the bacterium *Serratia marcescens* and then transferred into *Trichoderma harzianum* and *Rhizobium meliloti* cells. In both cases, the transformed microorganisms produced chitinase and displayed increased antifungal activity. When the *S. marcescens* chitinase gene was introduced into a strain of *P. fluorescens* that directly promotes plant growth, the transformant also stably expressed and secreted active chitinase and effectively controlled the phytopathogen *R. solani*.

Ice Nucleation and Antifreeze Proteins

One of the ways in which some pathogenic leaf bacteria, such as *Pseudomonas syringae*, damage plants is by synthesizing ice nucleation proteins. These proteins, which are produced at low temperatures, are present on the surface of the bacterium and act as sites that facilitate the formation of ice crystals at freezing temperatures. As the ice crystals grow, they can pierce the plant cells and cause irreparable damage. The bacteria benefit from this damage by gaining direct access to the nutrients from the lysed plant cells. In the absence of ice nucleation proteins on the leaf surface, a

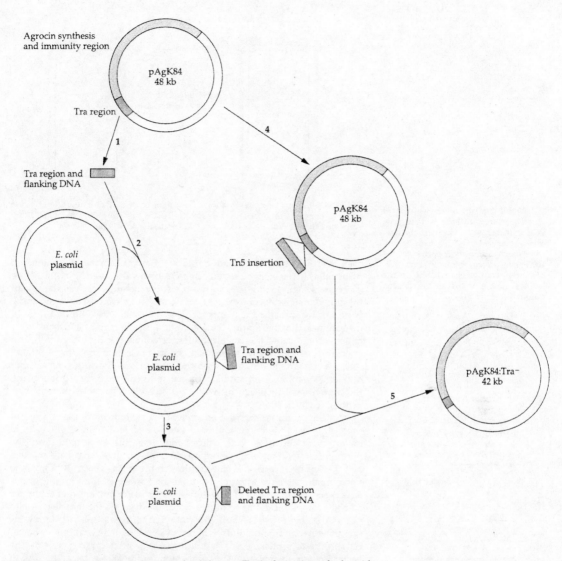

FIGURE 15.14 Construction of a transfer-deficient (Tra⁻) derivative of plasmid pAgK84 from *A. radiobacter*, which encodes both synthesis of and immunity to the antibiotic agrocin 84. Based on knowledge of the restriction enzyme map of pAgK84, a DNA fragment containing the transfer (Tra) region, together with some of the flanking DNA, is isolated **(1)** and spliced into an *E. coli* plasmid vector **(2)**. By restriction enzyme digestion, approximately 80% of the Tra region and some of the flanking DNA (a total of about 6 kb) is deleted from the cloned DNA containing the Tra sequence **(3)**. Homologous recombination of the *E. coli* plasmid containing the deleted Tra region with plasmid pAgK84, in which transposon Tn5, which carries a kanamycin resistance gene, has been inserted into the Tra region, is performed **(4)**. This results in some derivatives of pAgK84 in which a portion of the Tra region of the plasmid has been deleted **(5)**. The resultant Tra⁻ mutant of pAgK84 can no longer be conjugationally transferred to other agrobacteria, although it is still able to synthesize and provide immunity to agrocin 84. None of the DNA fragments is shown to scale.

615

FIGURE 15.15 Schematic representation of a fungal cell wall being degraded by one or more enzymes produced by a biocontrol plant growth-promoting bacterium. Following the breakdown of the fungal cell wall, the cell is readily lysed.

FIGURE 15.16 Strategy for the isolation of a *Pseudomonas* antifreeze protein gene. PCR primers based on the partial amino acid sequence of the isolated protein were used to amplify a portion of the antifreeze protein gene. Inverse PCR primers were designed based on the DNA sequence of the amplified gene fragment.

Purified antifreeze protein

Partially digest the antifreeze protein with trypsin, and sequence the peptides

Design PCR primers

Amplify part of the antifreeze protein gene by PCR, determine the DNA sequence, clone it, and design inverse PCR primers

Inverse PCR

brief overnight frost would not damage the plant because the water in a plant cell must usually be several degrees below the freezing point before ice crystals begin to form (i.e., it must be supercooled). One way to prevent freezing damage caused by *P. syringae* to susceptible crops, such as strawberries, is by spraying the plants, prior to the frost, with a mutant form of the ice-nucleating bacterium. Such a mutant, which may be constructed by either recombinant DNA manipulation or conventional mutagenesis and selection, lacks the ability to produce the ice nucleation protein, and therefore, ice crystals are not formed on the leaf surface. If a sufficient number of these "ice-minus" mutant bacteria are sprayed onto a susceptible plant, the mutant will displace the wild-type (ice-plus) bacteria, thereby preventing ice nucleation.

An important facet of the effectiveness of a biocontrol plant growth-promoting bacterium is its ability to persist and proliferate in the natural environment. In areas such as Canada, Scandinavia, Russia, and the northern United States, these organisms must survive long, cold winters and then grow at cool soil temperatures in the spring (~5 to 10°C). While microorganisms have a variety of adaptive strategies for thriving under adverse conditions, it may be possible to engineer organisms that are better able to deal with cold temperatures. Some soil bacteria that are also able to promote plant growth can both grow at 5°C and secrete antifreeze proteins into the surrounding medium when grown at low temperatures. A bacterial antifreeze protein regulates the formation of ice crystals outside the bacterium and thereby provides protection for the bacterium in the soil. In the presence of bacterial antifreeze protein, ice crystals still form, but their size is limited. In the absence of antifreeze proteins, ice crystals can grow to a large size and eventually puncture the bacterial cell wall and membrane, causing cell lysis. Ice crystals do not form inside the bacterium to any great extent. This is because at low temperatures bacteria decrease their volume by pumping some of their water from inside to outside the cell.

Recently, the gene for a bacterial antifreeze protein was isolated and characterized (Fig. 15.16). The strategy that was used to isolate this gene included purifying the protein, digesting it into small peptides with the proteolytic enzyme trypsin, determining the amino acid sequences of several of these peptides, and using those amino acid sequences to design polymerase chain reaction (PCR) primers for a portion of the antifreeze

MILESTONE

Cloning of *Rhizobium meliloti* Nodulation Genes by Direct Complementation of Nod⁻ Mutants

S. R. LONG, W. J. BUIKEMA, and F. M. AUSUBEL
Nature 298:485–488, 1982

The isolation of a gene, when its basic features are unknown and there is no heterologous probe or antibody available, can be a daunting task. In these instances, it is often necessary to devise an innovative selection scheme. The selection scheme may be based on immunological detection of the target protein, determination of the activity of the target protein, DNA hybridization with an oligonucleotide probe whose sequence is deduced from the partial amino acid sequence of the purified target protein, or mutant complementation. Often, after a gene that encodes a particular function has been isolated, similar genes from other organisms can be isolated by using the first gene as a heterologous DNA hybridization probe. This approach depends on nucleotide sequence similarity between the probe and the target gene. This strategy generally works well for genes that are evolutionarily conserved, such as those that encode proteins involved in the process of nitrogen fixation, but it works poorly for many other genes, including those that encode proteins that degrade cellulose.

When Long and her coworkers set out to isolate and characterize the nodulation genes from *R. meliloti*, nodulation genes had never been isolated. Very little was known about how many genes were involved in this process or what products they might encode. As a starting point, these workers isolated and characterized several nodulation-defective mutants of *R. meliloti*. However, these studies had not given them any clue to the functions of these genes. Therefore, they set about selecting nodulation genes that could complement their nodulation-defective *R. meliloti* mutants. This work was further complicated by the fact that, at that time, clone banks were almost always constructed and maintained in *E. coli*. Therefore, to facilitate the assembly of the *R. meliloti* clone bank and its subsequent transfer to nodulation-defective mutant strains of *R. meliloti*, the researchers first constructed a broad-host-range cosmid vector in which there were large DNA fragments, with an average size of approximately 23 kb, that could be stably maintained in a number of different gram-negative bacteria. The large size of the DNA on the cosmid increased the likelihood that other genes involved in nodulation would be on the same DNA fragment as the complementing DNA sequence. After the cosmids had been transferred by conjugation to *R. meliloti*, the transformed bacteria were tested for their ability to nodulate alfalfa plants. In previous experiments, it had been found that even one nodulation-proficient bacterium in the presence of 10^4 defective ones could successfully nodulate alfalfa plants. Bacteria with cosmids carrying a complementing gene were isolated directly from the nodules.

In summary, these researchers were the first to isolate nodulation genes. They devised a clever and effective selection scheme. The broad-host-range cosmid vector that they developed has since been used many times by a large number of other researchers.

protein gene. Following the sequence determination of the PCR-amplified DNA, inverse PCR (Fig. 15.16) was used to obtain the remaining portion of the gene. It should be possible to transfer this gene to various strains of plant growth-promoting bacteria to create strains that can persist and proliferate at cold temperatures. Although there is currently no evidence to link antifreeze activity with the mechanism that bacteria use to function at low temperatures, it will be interesting to examine experimentally whether antifreeze protein activity is part of the adaptive strategy used by some bacteria for cold, as well as freezing, tolerance.

Ethylene

Fungal pathogens not only directly inhibit plant growth, they also cause the plant to synthesize stress ethylene, which causes some of the damage sustained by plants infected with fungal phytopathogens. For example, it is well known that exogenous ethylene often increases the severity of a fungal infection, whereas ethylene synthesis inhibitors significantly decrease the severity of a fungal infection.

TABLE 15.5 Reduction in the severity of damage (damping off) of cucumber caused by *P. ultimum*

Treatment	Seed germination rate (%)	Shoot fresh weight (g)	Root fresh weight (g)
None	100	3.48	2.85
P. ultimum	31	0.69	0.21
CHA0 + *P. ultimum*	79	2.11	0.95
CHA0/ACC + *P. ultimum*	87	2.27	1.27

Adapted from Wang et al., *Can. J. Microbiol.* **46:**898–907, 2000.

CHA0, the biocontrol bacterium *P. fluorescens* CHA0; CHA0/ACC, the biocontrol bacterium *P. fluorescens* CHA0 transformed with the ACC deaminase gene from *E. cloacae* UW4; UW4, *E. cloacae* UW4. The expression of a foreign ACC deaminase gene in *P. fluorescens* CHA0 results in an increase in the number of cucumber seeds that germinate in the presence of the fungal pathogen, as well as an increase in the fresh weight of both shoots and roots of the resulting plants.

As mentioned earlier, stress ethylene that is synthesized in response to fungal pathogen infection is produced in two peaks, a small one that occurs within a few hours after fungal infection and a much larger peak that occurs several days after fungal infection (Fig. 15.4). The first peak turns on the transcription of genes that encode proteins that protect plants against the pathogen, while the second peak is deleterious to the plant. Ideally, it would appear to be advantageous to allow the plant to synthesize the first, but not the second, peak of ethylene in response to a fungal pathogen. This is readily achieved using ACC deaminase-containing plant growth-promoting bacteria, since high-level expression of ACC deaminase does not occur until several hours after the appearance of increased amounts of ACC. Thus, these bacteria do not alter the first ethylene peak but significantly decrease the magnitude of the second peak.

A biocontrol bacterial strain, *P. fluorescens* CHA0, was transformed with the *P. putida* UW4 ACC deaminase gene, and the effect of this manipulation on the damage to cucumbers caused by *P. ultimum* was assessed. The ACC deaminase-containing biocontrol bacterial strain was more effective in lessening the damage than the wild-type biocontrol strain that did not possess the enzyme. Not only did plants inoculated with the ACC deaminase-transformed strains have greater root and shoot biomass than those treated with the wild-type biocontrol strain, but also the number of seeds that germinated in pathogen-containing soil was larger (Table 15.5). In addition, the ACC deaminase-transformed biocontrol strain reduced the extent of soft rot of potato slices, caused by the bacterial pathogen *Erwinia carotovora* subsp. *carotovora*, in sealed plastic bags by 50% compared with the wild-type biocontrol strain (Table 15.6). In effect, ACC deaminase acts synergistically with other mechanisms of biocontrol, such as the production of antibiotics or antifungal enzymes, to prevent phytopathogens from damaging plants.

Root Colonization

Depending upon the mechanism that a particular biocontrol bacterium uses to thwart the damage to plants caused by pathogenic microorganisms, it can be advantageous for the biocontrol strain to bind as tightly as possible to the plant root. One way to improve root colonization by biocontrol bacteria entails overexpressing the bacterial *sss* gene. This gene is normally thought to play a role in DNA rearrangements that regulate the transcrip-

tion of a gene(s) involved in the biosynthesis of cell surface components. When the *sss* gene was introduced on a plasmid into two strains of *P. fluorescens*, one that was normally a poor root colonizer and the other a good root colonizer, colonization of tomato roots was increased by approximately 28- and 12-fold, respectively. This work is an important first step in engineering more effective strains of biocontrol bacteria.

Nitrogen Fixation

Nitrogen gas (N_2), which makes up approximately 80% (by volume) of the air that we breathe, cannot be used directly by plants or animals to synthesize essential nitrogen-containing biomolecules, such as amino acids and nucleotides. Rather, it must first be converted (fixed) into ammonia. This conversion requires a high input of energy because the triple bond of N_2 ($N \equiv N$) is extremely stable. The energy for the biological fixation of nitrogen comes from the hydrolysis of large amounts of ATP. Similarly, the chemical (industrial) conversion of N_2 to ammonia uses a considerable amount of energy in the form of high temperature and pressure.

More than 100 million tons of fixed nitrogen is needed annually to sustain global food production. Synthetic (chemically produced) fertilizers account for about half of this nitrogen supply, and most of the remainder is derived from diazotrophic bacteria. No eukaryote is known to fix nitrogen. Chemical fertilizers have helped considerably in increasing crop yields, but their continual use has led to pollution problems as a result of runoff and to depletion of the nutrient reserves in the soil. Moreover, their cost has been rising steadily. These factors have provided an incentive for developing alternative sources of fixed nitrogen, including the development of diazotrophic microorganisms as "bacterial fertilizers."

A wide range of bacteria can fix nitrogen, and a number of them have potential as crop fertilizers. However, until a bacterial fertilizer has been shown conclusively to be as effective as a chemical formulation, there will be reluctance to change current practices, especially in those countries where the cost of chemical fertilizer is not significant relative to the value of the crop. For example, soybeans, which constitute the second largest crop in the United States in terms of both cash value and total acres planted, form a beneficial symbiotic relationship with the bacterium *Bradyrhizobium japonicum*. In this symbiosis, the bacteria provide the plant with fixed

TABLE 15.6 Effect of *P. fluorescens* CHA0 and CHA0/ACC on soft rot of potatoes by *E. carotovora* subsp. *carotovora*

Treatment	Weight of rotted potatoes (g/slice)
None	15.6
CHA0	14.5
CHA0/ACC	7.5

Adapted from Wang et al., *Can. J. Microbiol.* **46**:898–907, 2000.

For definitions of abbreviations, see Table 14.9. While the biocontrol strain *P. fluorescens* CHA0 does not significantly alter the extent of damage to potatoes due to the bacterial pathogen, expression of ACC deaminase lowers the level of stress ethylene and decreases the damage to the potatoes by approximately 50%. The total weight of each potato slice was approximately 20 g.

nitrogen and, in turn, receive photosynthetically fixed carbon from the plant. When plants are inoculated with specific strains of *B. japonicum*, the final yield of plant material can be increased by 25 to 50%, and the inoculated plants no longer require the addition of chemically fixed nitrogen. Although approximately 40% of the world's soybean crop is produced in just a few locales in the United States and agricultural practices tend to be similar throughout these locales, at present, only a small fraction of this crop is treated with *B. japonicum*. Most of these farmers continue to depend on the naturally occurring strains of *B. japonicum* in the soil and chemical fertilizers.

The most important microorganisms that are currently used agriculturally to improve the nitrogen content of plants include a range of rhizobial genera and species (Table 15.7). These bacteria are gram negative, flagellated, and rod shaped, and they form symbiotic relationships with legumes. Generally, each rhizobial species is specific for a limited number of plants and will not interact with plants other than its natural hosts (Table 15.7).

As part of their life cycle, rhizobial bacteria invade plant root cells and initiate a complex series of developmental changes that lead to the forma-

TABLE 15.7 Plant specificities of various rhizobial species

Bacterial species	Host plant(s)
Azorhizobium caulinodans	West African legume (*Sesbania rostrata*)
Bradyrhizobium elkanii	Soybean (*Glycine max*), black-eyed pea (*Vigna unguiculata* subsp. *dekindtiana*), mung bean (*Vigna radiata*)
Bradyrhizobium japonicum	Soybean (*G. max*)
Mesorhizobium amorphae	Desert false indigo (*Amorpha fruticosa*)
Mesorhizobium ciceri	Chickpea (*Cicer arietinum*)
Mesorhizobium chacoense	White carob tree (*Prosopis alba*)
Mesorhizobium huakuii	Chinese milk vetch (*Astragalus sinicus*)
Mesorhizobium loti	Lotus (*Lotus japonicus*)
Mesorhizobium mediterraneum	Chickpea (*C. arietinum*)
Mesorhizobium tianshanense	7 Legume species
Rhizobium sp. strain NGR234	>100 Tropical legume species
Rhizobium etli	Kidney bean (*Phaseolus vulgaris*), mung bean (*V. radiata*)
R. etli bv. mimosae	Mimosa (*Mimosa affinis*)
Rhizobium galegae	Goat's rue (*Galega officinalis, Galega orientalis*)
Rhizobium gallicum	Common bean (*P. vulgaris*)
Rhizobium huautlense	Danglepod (*Sesbania herbacea*)
Rhizobium leguminosarum bv. phaseoli	Kidney bean, mung bean
R. leguminosarum bv. trifolii	Clover (*Trifolium* spp.)
R. leguminosarum bv. viciae	Pea (*Pisum sativum*)
Rhizobium sullae	Sweetvetch (*Hedysarum coronarium*)
Rhizobium tropici	Mimosoid trees (*Leucaena* spp.) and some tropical legume trees (*Macroptilium* spp.)
Sinorhizobium fredii	Soybean (*G. max*)
Sinorhizobium meliloti	Alfalfa (*Medicago sativa*)
Sinorhizobium morelense	White popinac (*Leucaena leucocephala*)

tion of a root nodule. Inside the root nodule, the bacteria proliferate and persist in a form that has no cell wall. The bacteria within the nodules fix atmospheric nitrogen by means of the enzyme nitrogenase. The structural and biochemical interactions between a symbiotic rhizobacterium and a host plant are quite intricate and mutually beneficial. Inside a nodule, nitrogenase is protected from the toxic effects of atmospheric oxygen in two ways. First, oxygen does not readily diffuse into a nodule. Second, the oxygen content within a nodule is regulated by the protein leghemoglobin. The heme moiety of this oxygen-binding protein is synthesized by the bacterium, and the globin portion of the molecule is encoded by a plant gene. The plant also provides the bacterium with photosynthetically fixed carbon, which the bacterium requires for growth. For its part, the plant benefits from this symbiotic relationship by receiving fixed nitrogen from the bacterium.

Nitrogenase

The renewed interest in diazotrophs as biological fertilizers overlapped the development of techniques for gene isolation and manipulation and provided the impetus for studying the biochemical and molecular biological aspects of nitrogen fixation. Initially, scientists believed that these studies would lead to the development of improved nitrogen-fixing organisms that would enhance crop yields. Some researchers even went so far as to suggest that bacterial genes for nitrogen fixation might be introduced directly into plants to enable them to fix their own nitrogen. Although this overly optimistic prediction has not materialized, a detailed understanding of the process of nitrogen fixation has emerged. And with this understanding, the possibility of improving the nitrogen-fixing activity of some diazotrophs by genetic manipulation is a little closer to becoming a reality.

Components of Nitrogenase

All known nitrogenases have two oxygen-sensitive components. Component I is a complex of two identical α-protein subunits (approximately 50,000 daltons each), two identical β-protein subunits (approximately 60,000 daltons each), 24 molecules of iron, 2 molecules of molybdenum, and an iron–molybdenum cofactor, often called FeMoCo (Fig. 15.17). Component II has two α-protein subunits (approximately 32,000 daltons each), which are not the same as the α-protein subunits of component I, and a number of associated iron molecules. The catalysis of nitrogen to ammonia requires the combination of components I and II, a complex of magnesium and ATP, and a source of reducing equivalents (reaction 1; the upward-pointing arrow indicates a gas and P_i is inorganic phosphate).

$$N_2 + 8H^+ + 8e^- + 16MgATP \rightarrow 2NH_3 + H_2\uparrow + 16MgADP + 16P_i \quad (1)$$

In addition to fixing nitrogen, the nitrogenase can reduce the gas acetylene to ethylene (reaction 2).

$$H{-}C{\equiv}C{-}H + 2H^+ \rightarrow H_2{=}C{=}C{=}H_2 \quad (2)$$

The measurement by gas chromatography of ethylene production as a function of time provides a convenient assay for nitrogenase activity. This assay can be performed with intact cells in solution (Fig. 15.18), bacteria associated with plant roots, crude cell extracts, or highly purified enzyme preparations.

FIGURE 15.17 Structure of the iron–molybdenum cofactor bound to a molecule of dinitrogen (N_2).

Component I catalyzes the actual reduction of N_2, and component II donates electrons to component I. Both components are extremely sensitive to oxygen and can be rapidly and irreversibly inactivated when the oxygen concentration is too high. In addition to components I and II, the activity of a complete, functional nitrogenase depends on 15 to 20 additional accessory proteins. The roles of most of the accessory proteins have been delineated and include the transfer of electrons to component II and the biosynthesis of the iron–molybdenum cofactor that is a part of component I.

Genetic Engineering of the Nitrogenase Gene Cluster

Nitrogen fixation is a very complicated process requiring the concerted actions of a large number of different proteins. Therefore, it was not realistic to expect either that an intact single DNA fragment containing all the genetic information for nitrogen fixation could be readily cloned from a diazotrophic microorganism and transferred into a nondiazotrophic organism or that a recipient organism could maintain the physiological conditions needed for nitrogenase activity. Consequently, the most direct way to isolate the genes involved in nitrogen fixation (*nif* genes) was to identify and characterize those clones of a wild-type library that restore nitrogen fixation to various mutants of the original organism. This process is called genetic complementation.

The first *nif* genes identified by complementation were isolated from clone banks of the diazotroph *Klebsiella pneumoniae*. This well-studied organism is found in soil and water, as well as in the human intestine. The isolation protocol comprises the following steps (Fig. 15.19).

1. *K. pneumoniae* cells are treated with a dose of a mutagenic agent that allows approximately 0.1 to 1.0% of the cells to survive. Some of the mutagenized cells are able to grow on a minimal medium containing a source of fixed nitrogen, such as NH_4Cl, but do not grow in the absence of fixed nitrogen. These cells are likely to have a mutation in a *nif* gene and are designated Nif⁻.
2. A clone bank that consists of chromosomal DNA from wild-type (Nif⁺) *K. pneumoniae* cells is constructed in a broad-host-range plasmid expression vector and maintained in *Escherichia coli*.
3. The Nif⁻ *K. pneumoniae* cells are conjugated with the *E. coli* cells that carry the clone bank on a plasmid shuttle vector.

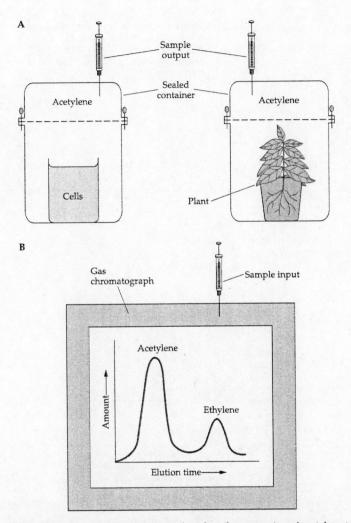

FIGURE 15.18 Assay for nitrogenase activity based on the conversion of acetylene to ethylene. **(A)** The source of the nitrogenase enzyme, for example, bacteria growing in culture, bacteria associated with plant roots, or a purified enzyme preparation (not shown), is placed in a sealed container under an atmosphere of acetylene. **(B)** Samples are periodically withdrawn from the sealed container, and the levels of acetylene and ethylene are measured by gas chromatography. The extent of nitrogenase activity is proportional to the amount of ethylene produced.

4. The transformed *K. pneumoniae* cells are selected for the acquisition of the Nif⁺ phenotype by plating them onto a minimal medium that does not contain a source of fixed nitrogen. The only cells that grow under these conditions are Nif⁻ *K. pneumoniae* cells containing a plasmid encoding and expressing the protein that is either missing or nonfunctional in the Nif⁻ mutant.

FIGURE 15.19 Procedure for isolating *nif* genes by genetic complementation. A clone bank that was constructed with Nif⁺ *K. pneumoniae* DNA is used to complement a Nif⁻ *K. pneumoniae* strain. Transformants are selected for growth on minimal medium that does not contain fixed nitrogen.

The DNA fragment in the plasmid that complements the Nif⁻ chromosomal mutation contains a *nif* gene that can be characterized more thoroughly and used to isolate other *nif* genes.

FIGURE 15.20 Partial restriction endonuclease digestion of the region of the chromosomal DNA encoding *nif* genes. The *nif* gene that was isolated by genetic complementation is used as a DNA hybridization probe (red). The probe and the DNA fragments from the partial digest are ordered as they would be in the chromosomal DNA. Colony hybridization of a clone bank consisting of the illustrated fragments, using the probe shown, would be expected to yield clones containing plasmids with fragments C and D. Using fragments C and D separately as probes to screen the same clone bank would be expected to yield clones containing plasmids with fragments B and E, respectively. Eventually, in this way, a large contiguous section of the host chromosome is isolated as a set of overlapping clones.

Two approaches have been used to isolate other genes that are involved in the nitrogen fixation process. First, the *K. pneumoniae* clone bank has been used to complement a series of independently derived Nif⁻ mutants, increasing the likelihood that in each case a different *nif* gene will be isolated. Second, isolated *nif* genes have been used as DNA hybridization probes, which have then been used to screen a *K. pneumoniae* chromosomal DNA clone bank that carries large (7- to 10-kb) inserts (Fig. 15.20). The premise behind the latter scheme is based on the observation that in prokaryotic organisms many of the genes involved in one pathway are clustered on the chromosomal DNA and are often arranged in operons. Thus, DNA hybridization enables investigators to identify clones containing additional *nif* genes that are adjacent to the sequence initially isolated.

As a result of a considerable amount of research, the entire set of *nif* genes from *K. pneumoniae* has been isolated and characterized. These genes are arranged in a single cluster that occupies approximately 24 kb of the bacterial genome (Fig. 15.21). The cluster contains seven separate operons that together encode 20 distinct proteins (Table 15.8). All of the *nif* genes must be transcribed and translated in a concerted fashion, under the regulatory control of the *nifA* and *nifL* genes, to produce a functional nitrogenase. The NifA protein is a positive regulatory factor. It turns on the transcription of all of the *nif* operons except its own by binding to a specific DNA sequence (5′-TGT-N$_{10}$-ACA-3′) that is part of each promoter of each *nif* operon. There is a site on the DNA approximately 80 to 150 nucleotides upstream of each transcriptional start site where the NifA protein binds.

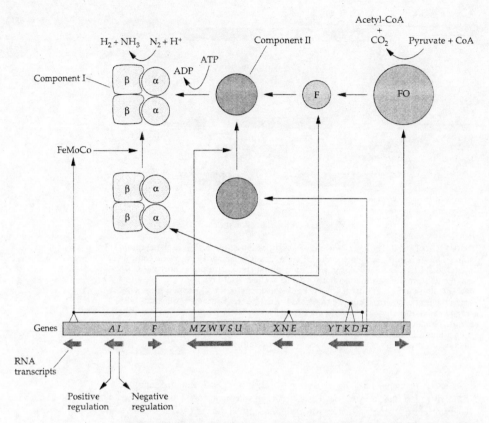

FIGURE 15.21 Arrangement of the genes in the *K. pneumoniae nif* gene cluster and some of the functions that they encode. The *nif* genes are represented by italic uppercase letters; each red arrow below sets of these letters denotes a specific *nif* operon and the direction of its transcription. The arrows pointing up and away from the gene designations show how some of the various gene products participate in nitrogen fixation. F, flavodoxin molecule; FO, pyruvate–flavodoxin oxidoreductase; FeMoCo, the iron–molybdenum cofactor; CoA, coenzyme A.

The DNA-bound NifA protein then interacts with a specific transcription initiation protein called sigma-54 (σ^{54}) before transcription from the *nif* promoter is initiated. The NifL protein is a negative regulatory factor. In the presence of either oxygen or high levels of fixed nitrogen, it acts as an antagonist of the NifA protein and, as a result, turns off the transcription of all other *nif* genes.

The bacterium *K. pneumoniae* does not make a major contribution to the overall global biological fixation of nitrogen. Therefore, to genetically engineer nitrogen fixation in soil bacteria that are more important in promoting plant growth, other *nif* genes have been cloned and characterized. To do this, the *nif* genes from *K. pneumoniae* have been used as DNA hybridization probes to isolate *nif* genes from clone banks of other diazotrophic microorganisms. Most diazotrophic organisms have a similar array of genes

encoding their nitrogen-fixing apparatus, and the DNA sequences of these genes do not vary much from one organism to another.

It may be possible to increase the amount of nitrogen fixed by diazotrophic organisms by manipulating the *nifA* and *nifL* genes. After researchers genetically engineered extra copies of the *nifA* gene into a *Sinorhizobium meliloti* strain, alfalfa plants that were inoculated with this transformant grew larger and produced more biomass than plants that were treated with the nontransformed strain. Similarly, it may be possible to engineer the *nifL* gene so that the NifL protein, the negative regulator, is less sensitive to the presence of fixed nitrogen. With this kind of deregulation, an organism would fix more nitrogen for its plant partner. However, not all nitrogen-fixing organisms have a NifL protein, so this sort of manipulation may be limited to only certain bacterial strains. In some organisms, the essential regions of NifL are part of NifA. Moreover, increasing the amount of nitrogen that an organism can fix also increases the amount of energy, usually in the form of fixed carbon, that is needed to power its metabolism. Consequently, an engineered microorganism that can fix a higher than normal level of nitrogen may lose its effectiveness as a plant growth-promoting agent because of a diminished growth rate.

Because of the complexity of nitrogen fixation by microorganisms, the simple addition of one or two *nif* genes will not confer on a nondiazotrophic recipient cell the ability to fix nitrogen. Moreover, genetic modification of plants with the entire 24-kb *nif* gene cluster would not be effective because the normal level of oxygen in the host cell would inactivate nitrogenase, and if this level were reduced, the host plant cell would probably die. In addition, the engineering of nitrogen fixation in plant cells requires resolving major, if not insurmountable, transcriptional, translational, and regulatory problems. For example, it is difficult to conceive how the regulation of nitrogen fixation could be achieved, since there are no plant promoters that respond to the NifA protein. Consequently, *nif* genes would not be turned on in such a transgenic plant. Each of the *nif* genes would also have to be under the control of separate promoters because plant cells cannot process multigene transcripts. The introduction of a functional nitrogen fixation capability into plants is therefore extremely unlikely.

TABLE 15.8 *K. pneumoniae* genes involved in nitrogen fixation and the functions of the proteins that they encode

nif gene	Function
D	Nitrogenase component I α subunit
K	Nitrogenase component I β subunit
H	Nitrogenase component II
F	Flavodoxin
J	Pyruvate:flavodoxin oxidoreductase
Q, B, N, E, V	FeMoCo synthesis
M	Processing of dinitrogenase reductase
A	Positive activator
L	Negative regulator
S	Maturation of component I
W, Z, T, Y, U, X	Other, less well-defined functions

FIGURE 15.22 Schematic representation of the partitioning of rhizobial intracellular glucose between glycogen synthesis and respiration. A mutation in the gene for glycogen synthase prevents glycogen from being synthesized, so that all of the glucose enters the tricarboxylic acid (TCA) cycle. In this cycle, the acetyl group of acetyl coenzyme A (CoA) is enzymatically degraded to form carbon dioxide and hydrogen. The hydrogen (or the corresponding electrons) is fed into the electron transport chain, and a large portion of the energy released is conserved by the phosphorylation of ADP to ATP. The ATP is then available to "power" a large number of energy-requiring metabolic processes, including nitrogen fixation.

Engineering Improved Nitrogen Fixation

Engineering oxygen levels. The concentration of oxygen is a critical factor in determining the amount of nitrogen that is fixed by a rhizobial strain. On one hand, oxygen is inhibitory to nitrogenase and is a negative regulator of *nif* gene expression. On the other hand, oxygen is required for bacteroid respiration. This conundrum can be resolved by the introduction of leghe-

moglobin, which binds free oxygen tightly (Fig. 15.23) so that both the transcription of *nif* genes and the functioning of nitrogenase can proceed unimpaired. In fact, the addition of exogenous leghemoglobin to isolated bacteroids results in a dramatic increase in nitrogenase activity. Thus, it is possible to engineer more efficient strains of *Rhizobium* by overproducing leghemoglobin. Alternatively, since the globin portion of leghemoglobin is produced by the plant, it may be more efficient to transform rhizobial strains with genes encoding a bacterial equivalent of leghemoglobin.

Following the transformation of a strain of *Rhizobium etli* with a broad-host-range plasmid carrying the *Vitreoscilla* sp. (a gram-negative aerobic or microaerophilic bacterium) hemoglobin gene at low levels of dissolved oxygen (0.25 to 1.0%) in the growth medium, the rhizobial cells had a two- to threefold-higher respiratory rate than the nontransformed strain. These data suggest that free-living *R. etli* with a *Vitreoscilla* sp. hemoglobin gene may have a competitive advantage over nontransformed rhizobial strains in soil (which usually has a low level of oxygen). As has been observed in the laboratory for numerous other free-living bacteria, the hemoglobin-containing strain can grow to a greater extent because it is able to sequester oxygen and provide it to the reactions, where it is necessary for bacterial metabolism (nitrogenase activity is at its peak at this time).

In greenhouse experiments, when bean plants were inoculated with either nontransformed or hemoglobin-containing *R. etli*, the plants inoculated with the hemoglobin-containing strain had approximately 68% more nitrogenase activity. This difference in nitrogenase activity leads to a 25 to 30% increase in leaf nitrogen content at 40 to 50 days after infection and a 16% increase in the nitrogen content of the seeds that are produced. Thus, the expression of a bacterial hemoglobin gene may be advantageous to *Rhizobium* bacteria both when they are free-living and when they are in bacteroids as part of a symbiotic relationship with their host plant.

Modulating *nifH* and poly-β-hydroxybutyrate. In Mexico, most of the bean plants (the second most important crop in Mexico) are nodulated by *R. etli.*

FIGURE 15.23 **(A)** *R. etli* cells engineered to express a *Vitreoscilla* sp. hemoglobin gene bind low levels of dissolved oxygen, either from solution or from the soil. **(B)** The *Vitreoscilla* sp. hemoglobin protein binding to dissolved oxygen.

Leghemoglobin molecule
with four subunits

The most common strain of *R. etli* encodes three copies of the nitrogenase reductase (*nifH*) gene, each under the transcriptional control of a separate promoter. To increase the amount of nitrogenase, the strongest of the three *nifH* promoters (i.e., *PnifHc*) was coupled to the *nifHcDK* operon, which encodes the nitrogenase structural genes (where *nifHc* is one of the three *nifH* genes in this bacterium). The *nifHc* promoter is typically induced during nodule development. The *PnifHc–nifHcDK* construct was cloned into a broad-host-range plasmid and introduced into the wild-type strain of *R. etli*. The net result of this genetic manipulation was a significant increase in nitrogenase activity, plant dry weight, seed yield, and the nitrogen content of the seeds (Table 15.9). Moreover, this genetic manipulation worked as well or better when the *PnifHc–nifHcDK* construct was introduced into the large Sym plasmid from *R. etli* that contains all of the genetic information for nodulation and nitrogen fixation.

Biological nitrogen fixation requires a large amount of energy in the form of ATP. Thus, any mutation or genetic manipulation that increases the flux of carbon sources consumed by a bacterium through the citric acid cycle should be beneficial for nitrogen fixation (Fig. 15.22 and 15.24). This is because metabolism of glucose via the citric acid cycle results in the production of ATP. Consistent with this principle, it was observed that expression of the *PnifHc–nifHcDK* construct in a poly-β-hydroxybutyrate-negative strain of *R. etli* enhanced plant growth to an even greater extent than when this construct was expressed in a wild-type poly-β-hydroxybutyrate-positive strain. Finally, since no foreign genes were introduced into *R. etli*, the scientists who constructed these strains hope that the regulatory bodies in their country will view the manipulated strains as benign and approve them for widespread environmental use.

Hydrogenase

An undesirable side reaction of nitrogen fixation is the reduction of H^+ to H_2 (hydrogen gas) by nitrogenase. Energy in the form of ATP is wasted on the production of hydrogen, which is eventually lost to the atmosphere. Because of this side reaction, only 40 to 60% of the electron flux through the nitrogenase system is transferred to N_2, thereby significantly lowering the overall efficiency of the nitrogen-fixing process. Theoretically, if H_2 could be recycled to H^+, the extent of energy loss could be diminished and the nitrogen-fixing process would become more efficient. It is probably impossible to prevent this side reaction directly, because it is a consequence of the chemistry of the active site of the nitrogenase; hence,

TABLE 15.9 Symbiotic performance of genetically modified strains of *R. etli* in concert with common beans (*Phaseolus vulgaris*)

Bacterial strain	Nitrogenase activity (μmol of ethylene/h/g of nodule)	Plant dry wt (g/plant)	Seed yield (g/plant)	Seed N content (mg of N/g of seed)
Wild type	64.5	0.54	1.43	33.9
Wild type + extra *nifHDK*	72.7	0.66	1.56	41.4
Wild type + *nifHc*	77.3	0.75	1.73	31.2
Wild type + *PnifHc-nifHcDK*	108.2	0.81	2.50	43.6

Adapted from Peralta et al., *Appl. Environ. Microbiol.* 70:3272–3281, 2004.

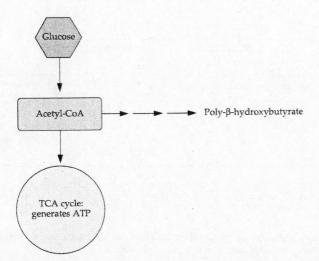

FIGURE 15.24 Conversion of glucose to acetyl coenzyme A (CoA), which can either enter the tricarboxylic acid (TCA) cycle, with the concomitant production of ATP, or be converted into the carbon storage polymer poly-β-hydroxybutyrate.

blocking the side reaction by altering nitrogenase would concomitantly inhibit nitrogenase activity.

Hydrogen Metabolism

In the mid-1970s, it was discovered that some strains of *B. japonicum* could use hydrogen as an energy source for growth under microaerophilic (low-oxygen-concentration) conditions. These strains have an enzyme called hydrogenase that is able to take up H_2 from the atmosphere and convert it into H^+ (Fig. 15.25). Experiments were undertaken to test whether the presence of hydrogenase in *B. japonicum* had an impact on the growth of soybean plants. Plants inoculated with strains that produce hydrogenase (Hup$^+$) had more biomass and nitrogen than plants that were treated with non-hydrogenase-producing (Hup$^-$) strains, despite higher levels of nitrogenase activity in the Hup$^-$ strains (Table 15.10). From this and similar experiments, it was concluded that the presence of a hydrogen uptake system in a symbiotic diazotroph, such as *B. japonicum*, improves its ability to stimulate plant growth, presumably by binding and then recycling the hydrogen gas that is formed inside the nodule by the action of nitrogenase (Fig. 15.25). Within the nodule, the contribution of atmospheric hydrogen is negligible.

Although it is clearly beneficial to the plant to obtain its nitrogen from a symbiotic diazotroph that has a hydrogen uptake system, this trait is not common in naturally occurring rhizobial strains. In one study, it was found that the majority of naturally occurring *Rhizobium* and *Bradyrhizobium* strains examined were Hup$^-$ (Table 15.11). In that study, the data were based on a small number of strains for each species except *B. japonicum*, for which over 1,400 strains were assayed. The conclusion that can be drawn

FIGURE 15.25 Recycling of the hydrogen gas that is produced as a by-product of nitrogen fixation. Hydrogen is generated by nitrogenase at the expense of ATP, but by using this pathway, the hydrogen can be recaptured by hydrogenase.

from this work is that commercial Hup⁻ rhizobial strains are prime candidates for transformation to a Hup⁺ phenotype.

Genetic Engineering of Hydrogenase Genes

Although a considerable amount of effort has been directed over the past 30 years or so toward studying hydrogenases from both diazotrophic and nondiazotrophic microorganisms, an in-depth understanding of the structures and functions of these enzymes remains elusive. Many organisms have more than one hydrogenase, and many hydrogenases consist of more than a single polypeptide chain. Some hydrogenases are active only in the uptake of hydrogen from the atmosphere, whereas others, depending on the conditions, can also synthesize hydrogen. One result of this complexity is that the conversion of a Hup⁻ strain of *Rhizobium* into a Hup⁺ strain may not be readily achieved by the introduction of just any hydrogenase gene. Rather, the introduced gene(s) must encode all of the enzyme's subunits and must be able to interact with the appropriate electron transport molecule within the host organism.

The most common strategy for isolating hydrogenase genes has been genetic complementation. The first hydrogenase gene to be isolated was

TABLE 15.10 Relative enzyme activities and growth-stimulating performance of a parental Hup⁺ *B. japonicum* strain (SR) and three Hup⁻ mutants (SR1, SR2, and SR3)

B. japonicum strain	Relative nitrogenase activity	Relative hydrogenase activity	Relative plant dry weight	Relative nitrogen content
SR	1.00	1.00	1.00	1.00
SR1	1.27	0.01	0.81	0.93
SR2	1.13	0.01	0.74	0.91
SR3	1.23	0.01	0.65	0.85

Adapted from Albrecht et al., *Science* **203**:1255–1257, 1979.

Nitrogenase activity was assessed by monitoring the amount of acetylene that was reduced to ethylene as a function of time. Hydrogenase activity was measured by means of a hydrogen electrode. Plant dry weight included the weights of both the leaf material and root material. The nitrogen content was calculated as the fraction of the dry weight of the plant that was nitrogen. All values have been normalized relative to the parental strain.

TABLE 15.11 Percentages of native *Rhizobium, Sinorhizobium,* and *Bradyrhizobium* strains that have functional hydrogen uptake systems (Hup⁺)

Bacterium	Hup⁺ strains (%)
Rhizobium leguminosarum bv. leguminosarum	9.3
Rhizobium leguminosarum bv. trifolii	0
Rhizobium leguminosarum bv. phaseoli	0
Sinorhizobium meliloti	21
Bradyrhizobium japonicum	21
Bradyrhizobium sp.	91

Adapted from Evans et al., *Annu. Rev. Microbiol.* **41**:335–361, 1987.

the gene for an *E. coli* membrane-bound hydrogenase, and it was selected by complementation of an *E. coli* mutant that did not express this activity.

After the work with *E. coli,* hydrogenase *(hup)* genes from *B. japonicum* were isolated from a clone bank of wild-type DNA constructed in the broad-host-range cosmid vector pLAFR1 by complementation of *B. japonicum* Hup⁻ mutants. The presence of a hydrogenase that takes up hydrogen from the atmosphere in the complemented Hup⁻ mutant strains was indicated by the ability of the active hydrogenase to reduce the dye methylene blue in a hydrogen atmosphere. More detailed studies of the *B. japonicum hup* genes showed that they were organized into at least two, and possibly three, transcriptional units covering approximately 20 kb of the genome and including 18 separate genes. Subsequent work on the *hup* genes from *Rhizobium leguminosarum* has indicated that these genes are similar in both DNA sequence and gene organization to the *hup* genes from *B. japonicum*. Thus, the isolated *hup* genes from *B. japonicum* may be used as DNA hybridization probes to select homologous genes from a clone bank of *R. leguminosarum*.

Following the isolation of *R. leguminosarum hup* genes, and despite the complexity of this system, it has been possible to use cosmid vectors to transfer a complete set of uptake hydrogenase genes from a Hup⁺ strain of *R. leguminosarum* to a Hup⁻ strain (Table 15.12). Plants treated with *R. leguminosarum* that had been transformed to Hup⁺ grew larger and contained more nitrogen than the plants inoculated with the Hup⁻ parental strain (Table 15.12). Although hydrogenase genes have not received as much attention as *nif* genes, this simple gene transfer experiment is a convincing demonstration of the use of genetic manipulation to improve the ability of a diazotroph to stimulate plant growth.

More recently, one group of scientists modified the *hup* gene promoter in *R. leguminosarum* and in the process engineered a more efficient rhizobial

TABLE 15.12 Plant growth and nitrogen assimilation after the introduction of *hup* genes into a Hup⁻ strain of *R. leguminosarum*

Bacterial phenotype	Relative plant dry weight	Relative nitrogen amount	Relative leaf area	Relative nitrogen concentration
Hup⁻	1.00	1.00	1.00	1.00
Hup⁺	1.35	1.52	1.53	1.15

Adapted from Brewin and Johnston, U.S. patent 4,567,146, January 1986.
The data have been normalized relative to the Hup⁻ parental strain.

strain. In *R. leguminosarum*, 18 genes are associated with hydrogenase activity. There are 11 *hup* genes (Fig. 15.26) responsible for the structural components of the hydrogenase, the processing of the enzyme, and electron transport. There are also seven *hyp* (hydrogenase pleitropic) genes, which are involved in processing the nickel that is part of the active center of the enzyme. The *hup* promoter is dependent on the NifA protein (which is also required to activate the synthesis of *nif* genes), so that *hup* genes are expressed only within bacteroids. On the other hand, the *hyp* genes are transcriptionally regulated by an FnrN-dependent promoter, which is turned on by low levels of oxygen. Thus, the *hyp* genes are expressed both in bacteroids and microaerobically. By modifying the chromosomal DNA of *R. leguminosarum* and exchanging the *hup* promoter for an FnrN-dependent promoter (Fig. 15.26), a derivative of the original bacterium with an increased level of hydrogenase was created (Table 15.13). The engineered *R. leguminosarum* strain displayed a twofold increase in hydrogenase activity compared to the wild type, and no discernible amount of hydrogen gas was produced as a by-product of nitrogen fixation. This is expected to make this strain of *R. leguminosarum* much more effective at promoting plant growth and increasing plant nitrogen content. Moreover, regardless of whether nickel was added to the system, the amount of hydrogen evolved from nitrogen-fixing nodules was extremely low, indicating that virtually all of the hydrogen produced by nitrogenase was recycled. The reason that nickel was added to this system is that in many soils, the availability of nickel limits hydrogenase activity. In some soils, the level of nickel is so low that even if a naturally occurring strain contains hydrogenase genes, the hydrogenase activity may be so low as to be ineffectual. On

FIGURE 15.26 Replacement of the NifA-dependent *R. leguminosarum hup* promoter with an FnrN-dependent promoter. The *R. leguminosarum hyp* gene cluster is already under the transcriptional control of an FnrN-dependent promoter.

TABLE 15.13 Biological activities of wild-type and engineered (replacing the *hup* promoter with an FnrN-dependent promoter) strains of *R. leguminosarum*

Strain	Bacteroid hydrogenase activity (nmol of H_2/h/mg of protein)		Nodule H_2 evolution (mmol/H_2/g [fresh weight] of nodule)	
	-Ni	+Ni	-Ni	+Ni
Wild type	1,080	2,930	2.13	<0.25
Engineered strain	2,210	5,060	0.34	<0.25

Adapted from Brito et al., *Appl. Environ. Microbiol.* **68:**2461–2467, 2002, and Ureta et al., *Appl. Environ. Microbiol.* **71:**7603–7606, 2005.

the other hand, when the engineered *R. leguminosarum* was tested with various field soils, hydrogenase overproduction invariably overcame the limitation of low nickel levels, with the net result that the amount of fixed nitrogen, and hence plant productivity, was greater.

Nodulation

Competition among Nodulating Organisms

A major goal of agricultural biotechnology research is the development, by genetic manipulation, of *Rhizobium* strains that can increase plant productivity more effectively than naturally occurring strains. Many commercial inoculant strains that have been developed by mutation and selection to be superior nitrogen fixers are not very effective at establishing nodules on host plant roots when placed in competition with *Rhizobium* strains that are already present in the soil. Conversely, although many of the strains that are indigenous to the soil are highly successful in establishing nodules in competitive situations, they are not especially efficient at nitrogen fixation. Therefore, to make use of the commercial inoculant strains, either the nodulation capability of these strains must be enhanced or indigenous rhizobial strains must be inhibited.

Studies were undertaken to determine the genetic basis of this "competitiveness" with the aim of adding these particular genes to the strains that are used as inoculants. The nature of the competitive advantage of soil rhizobial species is not known, but it was reasoned that the indigenous bacteria might be more efficient at nodulation and, as a consequence, might prevent an inoculated strain from becoming established and forming its own nodules.

Genetic Engineering of Nodulation Genes

When scientists first attempted to isolate nodulation (*nod*) genes, the absence of any specific information about the biochemical or genetic basis of nodulation meant that a strategy had to be devised for the identification of the genes. Therefore, once again, genetic complementation was used. Nodulation-defective (Nod⁻) mutants of *S. meliloti* were transformed with a clone bank of wild-type chromosomal DNA from *S. meliloti*, and those colonies that had acquired the ability to nodulate alfalfa roots were isolated (Fig. 15.27). More specifically, the steps of the procedure were as follows.

1. A clone bank of wild-type (Nod⁺) *S. meliloti* was constructed by partial digestion of *R. meliloti* DNA with EcoRI and insertion into

the unique EcoRI site of the broad-host-range cosmid pLAFR1, which can carry up to 40 kb of cloned DNA.

2. The clone bank was packaged into bacteriophage λ, introduced into *E. coli*, and subsequently transferred to Nod⁻ mutants of *S. meliloti* by conjugation. The vector carries a tetracycline resistance gene that can be used as a selectable marker in both *E. coli* and *S. meliloti*.

3. After conjugation, suspensions of 200 to 300 transformed *S. meliloti* cells were tested for the ability to nodulate sterile alfalfa plants, with the expectation that only those transformants that carried and expressed a gene that complemented the nodulation defect in the *S. meliloti* host would produce nodules.

4. The bacteria that formed nodules on the test plants were recovered from within the nodules. These bacteria were then grown in culture and used to retrieve the vector carrying the complementing gene. The specific portion of the large insert DNA that carried the complementing gene was then subcloned onto another plasmid vector and analyzed further.

5. Once a single nodulation gene was identified, it was used as a DNA hybridization probe to identify adjacent regions of *S. meliloti* chromosomal DNA in a genomic library (Fig. 15.20).

The complete repertoire of nodulation genes from *S. meliloti* has been characterized. Detailed biochemical and genetic studies have revealed that nodulation and its regulation are complex processes that require the functioning of a large number of genes (Table 15.14). Some of the nodulation genes are highly conserved (common) among nodulating microorganisms, and others are species specific. The *nod* genes are grouped into three separate classes: common genes, host-specific genes, and the regulatory *nodD* gene. Thus, for example, the *nodABC* genes are common to all *Rhizobium* species and are structurally interchangeable. In most species, the *nodABC* genes are found on a single operon.

A number of events are now known to occur during nodulation. First, the *nodD* gene product, which is constitutively expressed, recognizes and binds to a flavonoid molecule, which is excreted by the roots of the potential host plants. Flavonoids are a class of plant phenolic molecules with a basic structure that consists of 15 carbons arranged as two aromatic rings connected by a 3-carbon bridge. They perform a number of different functions for the plant, such as pigmentation and defense against fungi or insects. The binding of flavonoids to the NodD gene product is one of the major determinants of rhizobial host specificity, because each rhizobial species recognizes only a limited number of flavonoid structures and each plant species produces its own specific set of flavonoid molecules (Table 15.15). In a limited number of instances, other small organic molecules, such as aldonic acids and betaines, that are exuded by plant roots or germinating seeds and are present in large amounts can interact with the NodD protein. Some strains, such as *R. leguminosarum* biovar (bv.) trifolii, have a very narrow host range, responding to only a few kinds of flavonoids, while others, such as *Rhizobium* sp. strain NGR234, have a very broad host range and respond to a much larger number of different flavonoids.

The binding of a flavonoid molecule activates the NodD gene product, presumably causing it to undergo a conformational change, and enables the flavonoid–NodD complex to attach to a nodulation promoter element

cos EcoRI

pLAFR1

Nod⁺ *S. meliloti* DNA

EcoRI partial digest

DNA (~40-kb pieces)

Ligate

Package into λ heads and tails

Infect
E. coli

Nod⁻ *S. meliloti*

Conjugate

Inoculate alfalfa

No nodules Nodules

Isolate and
culture

nod⁺ *nod⁻*

Nod⁺ *S. meliloti*
transformants

FIGURE 15.27 Procedure for the isolation of *S. meliloti* nodulation genes. The DNA from wild-type *S. meliloti* is cloned into the broad-host-range cosmid pLAFR1, packaged into bacteriophage λ, and introduced into *E. coli*. The clone bank is then transferred from *E. coli* to a Nod⁻ *R. meliloti* strain by conjugation. Alfalfa plants are inoculated with transformed Nod⁻ *S. meliloti*. Those plants that develop root nodules have been infected with Nod⁺ *S. meliloti* cells that presumably carry a complementing nodulation gene inserted into the cosmid vector. The transformed Nod⁺ *S. meliloti* cells can be isolated directly from the root nodules.

TABLE 15.14 Some *Rhizobium* nodulation gene products and their probable functions

Nod protein	Probable function
NodA	Common; cytoplasmic membrane; with NodB, stimulates cell division
NodB	Common; cytoplasmic membrane; with NodA, stimulates cell division
NodC	Common; outer membrane; chitin synthase
NodD	Common; positive transcriptional regulator; constitutive
NodE	Cytoplasmic membrane; β-ketoacyl synthase
NodF	Cytoplasmic; acyl carrier protein
NodG	Host-specific gene; dehydrogenase
NodH	Host-specific gene; sulfotransferase
NodIJ	Common; cytoplasmic membrane; capsular polysaccharide secretion
NodK	Affects onset of nodulation in some bradyrhizobia
NodL	Cytoplasmic membrane; acetyltransferase
NodM	D-Glucosamine synthetase
NodN	Unknown
NodO	Secreted, hemolysin
NodP	With NodQ; ATP sulfurylase
NodQ	With NodP; ATP sulfurylase
NodS	Methyltransferase
NodT	Outer membrane; secretion
NodU	Unknown
NodX	Cultivar specificity

Where biochemical or genetic evidence for the function of a particular protein is lacking, a possible function is assigned based on homology of the amino acid sequence to a protein of known sequence. Different rhizobial strains contain different subsets of these proteins. "Common" genes perform the same function in all species of rhizobia.

called a *nod* box. This promoter element is located upstream from all the nodulation genes except the *nodD* gene, and it activates the transcription of these genes.

The *nodABC* genes encode proteins that cause the plant root hair tips to swell and curl, an effect that is recognized as the initial step in the infection of the plant root by the bacterium. The bacteria synthesize an oligosaccha-

TABLE 15.15 Some legumes and the *nodD* gene inducers that they produce

Legume	Compound
Lupin (*Lupinus albus*)	Erythronic acid, tetronic acid
Alfalfa (*Medicago sativa*)	Stachydrine, trigonelline, luteolin, chrysoeriol, 4,4'-dihydroxy-2'-methoxychalcone, liquiritigenin, 7,4'-dihydroxyflavone
Clover (*Trifolium repens*)	7,4'-Dihydroxyflavone, geraldone, 4'-hydroxy-7-methoxyflavone
Common bean (*Phaseolus vulgaris*)	Delphinidin, kaempferol, malvidin, myricetin, petunidin, quercetin, eriodictyol, genistein, naringenin
Pea (*Pisum sativa*)	Apigenin, eriodictyol
Soybean (*Glycine max*)	Daidzein, genistein, coumesterol
Vetch (*Vicia sativa* subsp. *nigra*)	3,5,7,3'-Tetrahydroxy-4'-methoxyflavanone, 7,3'-dihydroxy-4'-methoxyflavanone, naringenin, 4,4'-dihydroxy-2'-methoxychalcone, liquiritigenin, 7,4'-dihydroxy-3'-methoxyflavanone, 5,7,4'-trihydroxy-3'-methoxyflavanone, 5,7,3'-trihydroxy-4'-methoxyflavanone naringenin

The inducers are released by either roots or germinating seeds.

ride Nod factor that is modified by the NodH gene product and perhaps also by the NodQ and NodP gene products. This factor (Fig. 15.28) elicits in the plant a host-specific response that includes root hair curling and deformation and is essential for *Rhizobium* to induce nodules. After the initial change in the root morphology, the bacterium attaches to the root hair. Next, the bacterial cell penetrates the plant cell through an infection thread. Finally, depending on the bacterial strain, up to approximately 20 additional *nod* gene products are synthesized. These proteins, together with some plant-encoded proteins, contribute to the formation of the nodule.

DNA sequencing and computer analysis revealed that in a slow-growing variant of a *Bradyrhizobium* sp., the region of the DNA between the *nodD* and *nodABC* genes contained an open reading frame that the fast-growing form lacked. This open reading frame was designated *nodK*. When plants were inoculated with a *Bradyrhizobium* sp. that had a mutagenized *nodK* gene (NodK⁻) and were compared with those treated with the wild-type strain (NodK⁺), the onset of nodulation in the NodK⁻ strain-treated plants was 5 days earlier, the nodulation number was doubled, and there was a 120% enhancement of plant yield.

To date, despite the fact that *nod* genes from several different rhizobial strains have been isolated and characterized, no simple genetic means has been devised for using *nod* genes to enable inoculated strains of *Rhizobium* to outcompete indigenous strains. Nevertheless, host specificity can be altered by the transfer of a *nodD* gene from a broad-specificity rhizobial strain to one with narrow specificity.

It has become clear that the process of nodulation is quite complicated. Thus, considerable additional effort will be required before it is possible to further enhance the competitiveness of rhizobial strains by genetic engineering.

FIGURE 15.28 Proposed structure of a typical Nod factor, NodRm-1. This compound elicits a host-specific plant response that includes root curling and deformation.

Nodulation and Ethylene

Ethylene is often produced by plants following the initial stages of infection (eventually leading to nodule formation) by rhizobia. This small rise in the plant ethylene level is generally localized to a portion of the root and can inhibit, and therefore limit, subsequent rhizobial infection and nodulation. One way in which some strains of *Rhizobium* naturally increase the number of nodules that they can form on the roots of a host legume is to limit the rise in ethylene that occurs following the initial infection. Different *Rhizobium* species decrease ethylene levels either by synthesizing a small molecule called rhizobitoxin that chemically inhibits ACC synthase, one of the ethylene biosynthetic enzymes, or by producing ACC deaminase and removing some of the ACC before it can be converted to ethylene. The result of lowering the local level of ethylene is that both the number of nodules and the biomass of the plant are increased by 25 to 40%. Assays of isolated rhizobia indicate that in the field approximately 1 to 10% of rhizobial strains possess ACC deaminase. It should therefore be possible to increase the nodulation efficiency of *Rhizobium* strains that lack ACC deaminase by genetically engineering these strains with isolated *Rhizobium* ACC deaminase genes (and their regulatory regions). In fact, insertion of a single copy of an ACC deaminase gene from *R. leguminosarum* bv. viciae into the chromosomal DNA of a strain of *S. meliloti* that lacked this enzyme dramatically increased both the nodule numbers and biomass of host alfalfa plants (Fig. 15.29). While genetically engineered strains of *Rhizobium* may not be acceptable for use in the field in all jurisdictions at this time, as a result of this work, several commercial inoculant producers are already screening their more recently isolated *Rhizobium* strains for active ACC deaminase.

FIGURE 15.29 Increased ability of *S. meliloti* transformed with an ACC deaminase gene (and its regulatory region) to nodulate alfalfa (pink bars) and to promote plant growth (purple bars).

Phytoremediation

Scientists are currently trying to develop new and improved methods to deal with both inorganic and organic environmental contaminants. However, most of these procedures are either very expensive or not especially effective. One recently developed method of environmental cleanup is called phytoremediation. This procedure uses plants to remove or sequester hazardous substances from the environment or to destroy them. Phytoremediation of metals and other inorganic compounds may take one of several forms: phytoextraction, the absorption and concentration of metals from the soil into the roots and shoots of the plant; rhizofiltration, the use of plant roots to remove metals from effluents; or phytostabilization, the use of plants to reduce the spread of metals in the environment. Phytoremediation of organic compounds may occur by phytostabilization, i.e., reducing the spread of the organic material in the environment; phytostimulation, the stimulation of microbial biodegradation in the rhizosphere, the area around the roots of plants; or phytotransformation, the absorption and degradation of contaminants by the plant.

Following the testing of a large number of different plants, several plants that can naturally accumulate large amounts of metal have been identified and are being used to a limited extent for the phytoremediation of metals in the environment. These plants are called hyperaccumulators and are often found growing in soils with elevated metal concentrations. Unfortunately, plants that grow in the presence of very high concentrations of metals, even hyperaccumulating plants, are quite small. Depending upon the amount of metal at a particular site, it could take 15 to 20 years to completely remediate that site, even with hyperaccumulating plants. This is a time frame that is usually considered to be too long for practical application.

A number of different types of plants, such as many common grasses, as well as corn (maize), wheat, soybean, peas, and beans, are effective at stimulating the degradation of organic molecules in the rhizosphere. Typically, these plants all have extensive and fibrous root systems which form an extended rhizosphere. In addition to the biodegradation that takes place in the rhizosphere, several varieties of plants and trees can take up and degrade some organic contaminants. For example, plants with phytotransformation activity may contain nitroreductases, which are useful for degrading the explosive TNT (trinitrotoluene) and other nitroaromatics; dehalogenases for the degradation of chlorinated solvents and pesticides; and laccases that can degrade anilines, such as triaminotoluene.

Engineering Strains That Facilitate Growth

Although using plants for remediation of persistent organic contaminants has advantages over other methods, many limitations exist for the large-scale application of this technology. For example, many plant species are sensitive to contaminants, so they grow slowly, and it is necessary to establish sufficient biomass for meaningful soil remediation. In addition, in most contaminated soils, the number of microorganisms is depressed, so that there are not enough bacteria either to facilitate contaminant degradation or to support plant growth. To remedy this situation, both degradative and plant growth-promoting bacteria may be added to the plant rhizosphere. Phytoremediation (i.e., degradation of organic compounds in the presence of plants) alone is not much faster than bioremediation (i.e., where biodeg-

radation of the organics is due to the activities of microorganisms independent of plants). On the other hand, cultivating plants together with plant growth-promoting bacteria allows the plants to germinate to a much greater extent and then to accumulate a larger amount of biomass in the presence of an environmental contaminant (Fig. 15.30). Typically, plant growth-promoting bacteria alleviate a portion of the stress imposed upon a plant by the presence of organic contaminants, and healthier plants are more efficient at breaking down organic contaminants.

In one study, plant growth-promoting bacteria that facilitate the phytoremediation of polycyclic aromatic hydrocarbons were developed and tested. Polycyclic aromatic hydrocarbons in the environment are of concern because of their toxic, mutagenic, and carcinogenic properties. The strain *Pseudomonas asplenii* AC, isolated from polycyclic aromatic hydrocarbon-contaminated soil, has plant growth-promoting activity, most likely due to its synthesis of indoleacetic acid. This strain was engineered to be more efficient at reducing stress in plants by transforming it with a bacterial gene for the enzyme ACC deaminase (and its regulatory region). The engineered strain was designated *P. asplenii* AC-1. The ability of the wild-type and transformed strains, as well as the transformed strain encapsulated in an alginate matrix (alginate is a biodegradable carbohydrate-based polymer), to promote the growth of canola plants grown in the greenhouse in soil containing polycyclic aromatic hydrocarbons was tested. In the presence of high levels of polycyclic aromatic hydrocarbons, the growth of canola plants was dramatically reduced. When strain AC was added to canola seeds, plant growth improved somewhat. Moreover, addition of strain AC-1, either in suspension or alginate encapsulated, dramatically improved plant growth (Fig. 15.31). These results suggest that plant growth in the

FIGURE 15.30 Growth of Kentucky bluegrass with (+) or without (−) plant growth-promoting bacteria (PGPB) in the presence of increasing amounts of polycyclic aromatic hydrocarbons. In every instance, the plants attain a significantly greater amount of biomass when plant growth-promoting bacteria are added to the seeds before they are planted.

FIGURE 15.31 Canola root (brown) and shoot (green) biomass after 25 days of growth in soil containing 6 g of polycyclic aromatic hydrocarbons per kg. Adapted from Reed and Glick, *Can. J. Microbiol.* **51**:1061–1069, 2005.

presence of polycyclic aromatic hydrocarbons was facilitated by both bacterial indoleacetic acid and ACC deaminase. In addition, several factors may favor the alginate-encapsulated inoculant. As the alginate matrix dissolves, the encapsulated bacteria are released steadily over time, potentially allowing greater bacterial colonization of the plant roots, especially in the presence of polycyclic aromatic hydrocarbons, which can limit bacterial growth and persistence. Alginate encapsulation has also been reported to increase plasmid stability, which is important because the ACC deaminase gene was introduced into strain AC-1 on a broad-host-range plasmid. While these results are preliminary, they indicate that this approach may be useful in the cleanup of contaminated field sites.

Engineering Degradative Plasmids

In addition to engineering bacterial strains to facilitate plant growth in the presence of stressful contaminants, it is also possible to develop plant growth-promoting bacteria that can degrade some contaminants. In one study, scientists engineered a plant growth-promoting strain of *P. fluorescens* to be able to degrade 2,4-dinitrotoluene (Fig. 15.32). The compound 2,4-dinitrotoluene, which is an intermediate in the synthesis of both polyurethane and various explosives, is a problem pollutant. Its presence in the environment is widespread, and it is both toxic and carcinogenic. Several species of *Burkholderia* carry plasmids that encode enzymes that can break down 2,4-dinitrotoluene. However, some species of *Burkholderia* have been found to be either plant pathogens or opportunistic human pathogens, so that there has been reluctance to deliberately release any *Burkholderia* strains, even seemingly harmless ones, into the environment. Instead, using three minitransposons, all of the genes necessary for the complete degradation of 2,4-dinitrotoluene were introduced into the chromosomal DNA of a plant growth-promoting strain of *P. fluorescens*. In liquid culture,

FIGURE 15.32 Pathway for 2,4-dintrotoluene (2,4-DNT) degradation. The enzymes involved in this pathway include DntA, 2,4-dinitrotoluene dioxygenase; DntB, 4-methyl-5-nitrocathecol (4M5NC) monooxygenase; DntC, 2-hydroxy-5-methylquinone (2H5MQ) reductase; DntD, 2,4,5-trihydroxytoluene (2,4,5-THT) oxygenase; DntG, 2,4-dihydroxy-5-methyl-6-oxo-2,4-hexadienoic acid (DMOHA) isomerase/4-hydroxy-2-keto-5-methyl-6-oxo-3-hexenoate hydrolase; and DntE, coenzyme A-dependent methylmalonate semialdehyde (CoASH) dehydrogenase.

the engineered *P. fluorescens* strain completely degraded toxic levels of 2,4-dinitrotoluene at both 28 and 10°C. Following inoculation of plant seeds, a much greater fraction of the seedlings survived in contaminated soil when the engineered rather than the wild-type *P. fluorescens* strain was used (Table 15.16).

Engineering Bacterial Endophytes

Some bacteria that normally bind to and proliferate on the roots of plants (rhizosphere bacteria) contain biodegradative plasmids that encode the enzymes for the complete breakdown of various organic contaminants (see chapter 13). However, the rhizosphere (the area around plant roots) is not always the environment that is most conducive to the degradation of these compounds. This is because when bacteria are attached to the root surface they are affected by soil pH, temperature, water content, and chemical composition, as well as the presence of amoebae, fungi, and other bacteria. Since many plants readily take up a wide range of organic compounds, it might be advantageous if the contaminant-degrading bacteria were localized within the plant roots rather than on the root surface (bacteria that can proliferate within plant tissues are called endophytes). To achieve this, one group of workers transferred, by conjugation, a plasmid containing biodegradative genes encoding enzymes that degrade toluene from a bacterium

TABLE 15.16 Survival of plant seedlings 14 days after being planted in the presence of DNT

Presence of DNT	Added bacterial strain	Seedling survival (%)
–	None	65
+	None	4
+	Wild type	11
+	Engineered	42

The seeds were inoculated with the indicated bacterium before being planted. –, absent; +, present.

that binds only to root surfaces to an endophytic bacterium that can colonize the interior tissue of the plant root but does not normally degrade toluene (Fig. 15.33). The endophyte that cannot degrade toluene, the surface-colonizing bacterium that can degrade toluene, and the transconjugant endophyte that can degrade toluene were tested for the ability to

FIGURE 15.33 Conjugal transfer of a plasmid carrying toluene degradation genes from a root surface-colonizing bacterium (yellow) to a soil endophytic bacterium (green). In the presence of 3-week-old lupine plants, the resultant transconjugant is able to completely degrade toluene that is added to the soil.

Bacterium with a degradative plasmid that proliferates on root surfaces

Bacterium without a plasmid that proliferates within roots

Transconjugant bacterium with a degradative plasmid that proliferates within roots

FIGURE 15.34 Schematic representation of a plant growth-promoting bacterium bound to a plant root. In the presence of large amounts of metal (such as nickel [Ni^{2+}]) in the environment, the plant has difficulty acquiring a sufficient amount of iron (Fe^{3+}) from the soil. However, the siderophore that is secreted by the bound bacterium has a very high affinity for iron, forming an iron–siderophore complex that can be taken up by the plant. Once inside the plant, the bacterial siderophore is cleaved, and the iron that is released is utilized in plant metabolic reactions.

degrade toluene in the presence of 3-week-old lupine plants. When either no bacterium or the endophyte that could not degrade toluene was present, the toluene remained intact and was toxic to the plants. The surface-colonizing bacterium that could degrade toluene removed some of the toluene from the soil and allowed the plant to grow to a limited extent. On the other hand, the transconjugant toluene-degrading endophytic strain completely degraded the toluene and protected its host against toluene toxicity. Given the fact that there is still widespread reluctance to deliberately release genetically engineered bacteria into the environment in many jurisdictions, transconjugants carrying naturally occurring biodegradative pathways may be advantageous in that they are not necessarily considered to be genetically modified bacteria.

Metals in the Environment

While plants grown in metal-contaminated soils can withstand some of the effects of high concentrations of metals within their tissues, two features of most plants result in a decrease in plant growth and viability. That is, in the presence of high levels of metals, most plants (1) synthesize stress ethylene and (2) become severely iron depleted. However, plant growth-promoting bacteria can relieve some of the effects of metals on plants. First, ACC deaminase-containing plant growth-promoting bacteria decrease the level of stress ethylene in a plant growing in soil that contains high levels of metal. Second, plants can take up and utilize complexes between bacterial siderophores and iron. In metal-contaminated soils, plants are generally unable to obtain enough iron because iron uptake is inhibited by the metal contaminant(s). Plant siderophores bind to iron with a much lower affinity

FIGURE 15.35 Effect of adding the wild-type plant growth-promoting bacterium *Kluyvera ascorbata* SUD165 (WT) or a siderophore-overproducing mutant of the bacterium, *K. ascorbata* SUD165/26 (mutant), on plant dry weight and chlorophyll concentration in the presence of nickel (Ni). The error bars indicate standard errors.

than bacterial siderophores, so plants are often unable to accumulate a sufficient amount of iron unless bacterial siderophores are present (Fig. 15.34).

Some metal-resistant bacterial strains promote plant growth in the presence of inhibitory levels of nickel, lead, or zinc and are therefore an effective adjunct to plants in phytoremediation studies. In one instance, a mutation that caused the overproduction of a bacterial siderophore was selected. When the wild-type bacterium and the siderophore-overproducing mutant were tested in the laboratory, the siderophore-overproducing mutant stimulated plant growth significantly more than the wild-type bacterium (Fig. 15.35). When the siderophore-overproducing mutant was tested in the field with the plant Indian mustard (*Brassica juncea*) in soil that had been contaminated with nickel over a period of many years, both the number of seeds that germinated in the nickel-contaminated soil and the size that the plants were able to attain were increased by 50 to 100%. Overall, there was a two- to fourfold increase in the amount of nickel removed from the soil by the addition of the mutant compared with the wild-type bacterium. On the other hand, the presence of the mutant bacterium had no measurable influence on the amount of nickel accumulated per milligram (dry weight) in either plant roots or shoots. Therefore, the bacterial plant growth-promoting effect in the presence of nickel is attributable to the increase in the amount of plant material and the number of plants.

Phytoremediation is still at an early stage of development and currently accounts for only a very small fraction of the total amount spent each year for the remediation of hazardous sites. However, the world remediation market, estimated in 2001 to be $25 billion to $30 billion, is expected to grow to nearly $100 billion by around 2010, and it is estimated that phytoremediation could account for up to 10% of this market.

At present, the largest number of sites being remediated contain organic contaminants, because organics are easier and less expensive than metals to remediate. However, the removal of metal contaminants from the environment is expected to receive more attention in the future.

SUMMARY

Many soil microorganisms have the ability to stimulate the growth of plants. With an eye to diminishing dependency on chemical fertilizers, the molecular mechanisms by which bacteria promote plant growth have been examined. Plant growth promotion may be achieved directly by the ability of the bacteria to fix nitrogen, sequester iron, facilitate phosphorus uptake, produce phytohormones that trigger responses in a growing plant, or enzymatically reduce potentially inhibitory levels of the plant hormone ethylene. Some soil bacteria can also stimulate plant growth indirectly by inhibiting the growth of phytopathogenic microorganisms.

Recently, considerable effort has been devoted to understanding and productively utilizing the ability of plant growth-promoting bacteria to facilitate plant growth by lowering plant ethylene levels. This occurs as a consequence of the action of the enzyme ACC deaminase, which breaks down ACC, the immediate precursor of ethylene in all higher plants.

Plants often respond to a variety of different environmental stresses by synthesizing ethylene, which can trigger a stress/senescence response in the plant. The increased level of ethylene synthesized in response to trauma inflicted by chemicals, temperature extremes, water stress, ultraviolet light, insect predation, disease, and mechanical wounding can be both the cause of some symptoms of stress and the inducer of responses that enhance the survival of the plant under adverse conditions. This seemingly paradoxical situation is explained by the presence of two bursts of ethylene synthesis following the stress. The first, small peak activates the synthesis of plant defense proteins, while the much larger peak of ethylene, which is synthesized later, can exacerbate the impact of the stressor.

The enzyme ACC deaminase, when present in plant growth-promoting bacteria, can act to modulate the level of ethylene in a plant and thereby decrease the deleterious effects of a variety of stressors. Bacteria that contain ACC deaminase activity can significantly decrease the inhibition of plant growth that is observed in the presence of high salt levels, phytopathogens, flooding, or drought. These bacteria can also be used as an adjunct in phytoremediation (environmental cleanup using plants) strategies that are designed to remove metals or organic contaminants from the environment.

Of the plant growth-promoting bacteria that have been studied in detail and are currently used in agricultural practice, much of the research has focused on rhizobial bacteria. These organisms form a complex, obligatory symbiotic relationship with specific plants.

The molecular basis of nitrogen fixation has been examined extensively. Nitrogenase, the nitrogen-fixing enzyme, has been characterized in detail. Molecular genetic studies have established that bacterial nitrogen fixation is a complex process that requires seven operons, with a total of 20 different proteins, that are coordinately regulated. This complexity has so far frustrated attempts to create plants that can fix nitrogen and has prevented transfer of the ability to fix nitrogen to other bacteria.

The amount of nitrogen that can be fixed by a rhizobial strain may be increased by genetic engineering of genes that indirectly affect nitrogen fixation. For example, nitrogen fixation may be increased either by inhibiting the synthesis of rhizobial glycogen, by modulating the level of oxygen within the bacterial cell, or by preventing rhizobial synthesis of the polymer poly-β-hydroxybutyrate, which normally acts as a carbon storage compound.

As part of the action of nitrogenase, hydrogen gas (H_2) is generated at the expense of ATP. Some *Rhizobium* strains possess the enzyme hydrogenase, which is able to recycle H_2 in vivo to H^+, an activity that increases the efficiency of nitrogen fixation. When strains are defective in hydrogenase activity, the ability to fix nitrogen and promote plant growth is diminished. With this in mind, hydrogenase genes have been cloned into strains of rhizobial bacteria that form symbiotic relationships with crop plants. Genetic engineering of hydrogenase genes can produce rhizobial strains with an enhanced ability to fix nitrogen.

Part of the interaction between symbiotic rhizobial strains and plants is the formation of nodules on the roots of plants that are the sites of bacterial nitrogen fixation. It has been reasoned that enhancing nodulation by genetic engineering will enable inoculated rhizobial strains to be more effective competitors for sites on the roots of target plants than indigenous strains. However, studies to date have shown that the genetic basis of nodulation is complex, involving a number of different genes, so that at present there is no simple way to manipulate this process genetically.

The indirect promotion of plant growth occurs when plant growth-promoting bacteria decrease or prevent the damage that is caused by either fungal or bacterial phytopathogens. The bacteria that act in this way are referred to as biocontrol bacterial strains. Some of the substances produced by biocontrol bacteria, such as siderophores, antibiotics, other small molecules, and various enzymes that can lyse fungal cell walls, help to limit the damage to plants by phytopathogens. The activity of biocontrol bacteria may be augmented by engineering these strains to be better root colonizers, more efficient at lowering plant ethylene levels, and more active producers of antibiotics or enzymes.

REFERENCES

Adams, M. W. W., L. E. Mortenson, and J. S. Chen. 1981. Hydrogenase. *Biochim. Biophys. Acta* **594:**105–176.

Albrecht, S. L., R. J. Maier, F. J. Hanus, S. A. Russell, D. W. Emerich, and H. J. Evans. 1979. Hydrogenase in *Rhizobium japonicum* increases nitrogen fixation by nodulated soybeans. *Science* **203:**1255–1257.

Arp, D. J. 1990. H_2 cycling in N_2 fixation: past, present, and future outlook, p. 67–76. *In* P. M. Gresshoff, L. E. Roth, G. Stacey, and W. E. Newton (ed.), *Nitrogen Fixation: Achievements and Objectives.* Chapman & Hall, New York, NY.

Barac, T., S. Taghavi, B. Borremans, A. Provoost, L. Oeyen, J. V. Colpaert, J. Vangronsveld, and D. van der Lelie. 2004. Engineered endophytic bacteria improve phytoremediation of water-soluble, volatile, organic pollutants. *Nat. Biotechnol.* **22:**583–588.

Bar-Ness, E., Y. Chen, Y. Hadar, H. Marschner, and V. Römheld. 1991. Siderophores of *Pseudomonas putida* as an iron source for dicot and monocot plants, p. 271–281. *In* Y. Chen and Y. Hadar (ed.), *Iron Nutrition and Interactions in Plants.* Kluwer Academic Publishers, Dordrecht, The Netherlands.

Brewin, N. J., and A. W. B. Johnston. January 1986. Synthetic plasmid and bacteria containing it. U.S. patent 4,567,146.

Brito, B., J. M. Palacios, J. Imperial, and T. Ruiz-Argüeso. 2002. Engineering the *Rhizobium leguminosarum* bv. viciae hydrogenase system for expression in free-living microaerobic cells and increased hydrogenase activity. *Appl. Environ. Microbiol.* **68:**2461-2467.

Burd, G. I., D. G. Dixon, and B. R. Glick. 1998. A plant growth promoting bacterium that decreases nickel toxicity in plant seedlings. *Appl. Environ. Microbiol.* **64:**3663–3668.

Burd, G. I., D. G. Dixon, and B. R. Glick. 2000. Plant growth-promoting bacteria that decrease heavy metal toxicity in plants. *Can. J. Microbiol.* **46:**237–245.

Cantrell, M. A., R. A. Haugland, and H. J. Evans. 1983. Construction of a *Rhizobium japonicum* gene bank and use in isolation of a hydrogen uptake gene. *Proc. Natl. Acad. Sci. USA* **80:**181–185.

Cheng, Z., E. Park, and B. R. Glick. 2007. 1-Aminocyclopropane-1-carboxylate (ACC) deaminase from *Pseudomonas putida* UW4 facilitates the growth of canola in the presence of salt. *Can. J. Microbiol.* **53:**912–918.

Chet, I., and J. Inbar. 1994. Biological control of fungal pathogens. *Appl. Biochem. Biotechnol.* **48:**37–43.

Crosa, J. H. 1989. Genetics and molecular biology of siderophore-mediated iron transport in bacteria. *Microbiol. Rev.* **53:**517–530.

Dekkers, L. C., I. H. M. Mulders, C. C. Phoelich, T. F. C. Chin-A-Woeng, A. H. M. Wijfjes, and B. J. J. Lugtenberg. 2000. The *sss* colonization gene of the tomato-*Fusarium oxysporum* f. sp. *radicis-lycopersici* biocontrol strain *Pseudomonas fluorescens* WCS365 can improve root colonization of other wild-type *Pseudomonas* spp. bacteria. *Mol. Plant-Microbe Interact.* **13:**1177–1183.

Evans, H. J., A. R. Harker, H. Papen, S. A. Russell, F. J. Hanus, and M. Zuber. 1987. Physiology, biochemistry, and genetics of the uptake hydrogenase in rhizobia. *Annu. Rev. Microbiol.* **41:**335–361.

Fischer, H.-M. 1994. Genetic regulation of nitrogen fixation in rhizobia. *Microbiol. Rev.* **58:**352–386.

Glick, B. R. 1995. The enhancement of plant growth by free-living bacteria. *Can. J. Microbiol.* **41:**109–117.

Glick, B. R. 2004. Teamwork in phytoremediation. *Nat. Biotechnol.* **22:**526–527.

Glick, B. R., C. L. Patten, G. Holguin, and D. M. Penrose. 1999. *Biochemical and Genetic Mechanisms Used by Plant Growth Promoting Bacteria.* Imperial College Press, London, United Kingdom.

Glick, B. R., C. B. Jacobson, M. M. K. Schwarze, and J. J. Pasternak. 1994. 1-Aminocyclopropane-1-carboxylic acid deaminase mutants of the plant growth-promoting rhizobacterium *Pseudomonas putida* GR12-2 do not stimulate canola root elongation. *Can. J. Microbiol.* **40:**911–915.

Glick, B. R., D. M. Penrose, and J. Li. 1998. A model for the lowering of plant ethylene concentrations by plant growth-promoting bacteria. *J. Theor. Biol.* **190:**63–68.

Glick, B. R., J. Zeisler, A. M. Banaszuk, J. D. Friesen, and W. G. Martin. 1981. The identification and partial characterization of a plasmid containing the gene for the membrane-associated hydrogenase from *E. coli. Gene* **15:**201–206.

Gresshoff, P. M., L. E. Roth, G. Stacey, and W. E. Newton (ed.). 1990. *Nitrogen Fixation: Achievements and Objectives.* Chapman & Hall, New York, NY.

Grichko, V. P., and B. R. Glick. 2001. Ethylene and flooding stress in plants. *Plant Physiol. Biochem.* **39:**1–9.

Grichko, V. P., and B. R. Glick. 2001. Amelioration of flooding stress by ACC deaminase-containing plant growth-promoting bacteria. *Plant Physiol. Biochem.* **39:**11–17.

Hennecke, H. 1990. Nitrogen fixation genes involved in the *Bradyrhizobium japonicum*-soybean symbiosis. *FEBS Lett.* **268:**422–426.

Higashi, S. 1993. (*Brady)Rhizobium*-plant communications involved in infection and nodulation. *J. Plant Res.* **106:**201–211.

Huang, X.-D., Y. El-Alawi, D. M. Penrose, B. R. Glick, and B. M. Greenberg. 2004. Responses of plants to creosote during phytoremediation and their significance for remediation processes. *Environ. Pollut.* **130:**453–463.

Huang, X.-D., Y. El-Alawi, J. Gurska, B. R. Glick, and B. M. Greenberg. 2005. A multi-process phytoremedia-

tion system for decontamination of persistent total petroleum hydrocarbons (TPHs) from soils. *Microchem. J.* **81**:139–147.

Jones, D. A., M. H. Ryder, B. G. Clare, S. K. Farrand, and A. Kerr. 1988. Construction of a Tra⁻ deletion mutant of pAgK84 to safeguard the biological control of crown gall. *Mol. Gen. Genet.* **212**:207–214.

Kloepper, J. W., R. Lifshitz, and M. N. Schroth. 1988. *Pseudomonas* inoculants to benefit plant production. *ISI Atlas Sci. Anim. Plant Sci.* **1**:60–64.

Layva, A., J. M. Palacios, T. Mozo, and T. Ruiz-Argüeso. 1987. Cloning and characterization of hydrogen uptake genes from *Rhizobium leguminosarum. J. Bacteriol.* **169**:4929–4934.

Lerouge, P., P. Roche, C. Faucher, F. Maillet, G. Truchet, J. C. Promé, and J. Dénarié. 1990. Symbiotic host-specificity of *Rhizobium meliloti* is determined by a sulphated and acylated oligosaccharide signal. *Nature* **344**:781–784.

Li, X., S. H. Yang, X. C. Yu, Z. X. Jin, W. D. Li, L. Li, and M. G. Li. 2005. Construction of transgenic *Bacillus mucilaginosus* strain with improved phytase secretion. *J. Appl. Microbiol.* **99**:878–884.

Li, X., Z. Wu, W. D. Li, R. Yan, L. Li, J. Li, Y. Li, and M. G. Li. 2007. Growth promoting effect of a transgenic *Bacillus mucilaginosus* on tobacco planting. *Appl. Microbiol. Biotechnol.* **74**:1120-1125.

Long, S. R., W. J. Buikema, and F. M. Ausubel. 1982. Cloning of *Rhizobium meliloti* nodulation genes by direct complementation of Nod⁻ mutants. *Nature* **298**:485–488.

Lynch, J. M. 1990. Beneficial interactions between microorganisms and roots. *Biotechnol. Adv.* **8**:335–346.

Ma, W., S. B. Sebestianova, J. Sebestian, G. I. Burd, F. C. Guinel, and B. R. Glick. 2003. Prevalence of 1-aminocyclopropane-1-carboxylate deaminase in *Rhizobium* spp. *Antonie van Leeuwenhoek* **83**:285–291.

Ma, W., T. C. Charles, and B. R. Glick. 2004. Expression of an exogenous 1-aminocyclopropane-1-carboxylate deaminase gene in *Sinorhizobium meliloti* increases its ability to nodulate alfalfa. *Appl. Environ. Microbiol.*

70:5891–5897.

Maier, R. J., and E. W. Triplett. 1996. Toward more productive, efficient, and competitive nitrogen-fixing symbiotic bacteria. *Crit. Rev. Plant Sci.* **15**:191–234.

Marroquí, S., A. Zorreguieta, C. Santamaría, F. Temprano, M. Soberón, M. Megías, and J. A. Downie. 2001. Enhanced symbiotic performance by *Rhizobium tropici* glycogen synthase mutants. *J. Bacteriol.* **183**:854–864.

Marugg, J. D., M. van Spanje, W. P. M. Hoekstra, B. Schippers, and P. J. Weisbeek. 1985. Isolation and analysis of genes involved in siderophore biosynthesis in plant-growth-stimulating *Pseudomonas putida* WCS358. *J. Bacteriol.* **164**:563–570.

Marugg, J. D., H. B. Nielander, A. J. G. Horrevoets, I. van Megen, I. van Genderen, and P. J. Weisbeek. 1988. Genetic organization and transcriptional analysis of a major gene cluster involved in siderophore biosynthesis in *Pseudomonas putida* WCS358. *J. Bacteriol.* **170**:1812–1819.

Mayak, S., T. Tirosh, and B. R. Glick. 2004. Plant growth-promoting bacteria that confer resistance in tomato to salt stress. *Plant Physiol. Biochem.* **42**:565–572.

Monti, M. R., A. M. Smania, G. Fabro, M. E. Alvarez, and C. E. Argaraña. 2005. Engineering *Pseudomonas fluorescens* for biodegradation of 2,4-dinitrotoluene. *Appl. Environ. Microbiol.* **71**:8864–8872.

Morris, R. O. 1986. Genes specifying auxin and cytokinin biosynthesis in phytopathogens. *Annu. Rev. Plant Physiol.* **37**:509–538.

Muryoi, N., H. Kawahara, H. Obata, M. Griffith, and B. R. Glick. 2004. Cloning and expression of *afpA*, a gene encoding an antifreeze protein from the arctic plant growth-promoting rhizobacterium *Pseudomonas putida* GR12-2. *J. Bacteriol.* **186**:5661-5671.

Mylona, P., K. Pawlowski, and T. Bisseling. 1995. Symbiotic nitrogen fixation. *Plant Cell* **7**:869–885.

Nap, J.-P., and T. Bisseling. 1990. Developmental biology of a plant-prokaryote symbiosis: the legume root nodule. *Science* **250**:948–954.

Neilands, J. B., and S. A. Leong. 1986. Siderophores in relation to plant growth and disease. *Annu. Rev. Plant Physiol.* **37**:187–208.

O'Sullivan, D. J., and F. O'Gara. 1992. Traits of fluorescent *Pseudomonas* spp. involved in suppression of plant root pathogens. *Microbiol. Rev.* **56**:662–676.

Paau, A. S. 1991. Improvement of *Rhizobium* inoculants by mutation, genetic engineering, and formulation. *Biotechnol. Adv.* **9**:173–184.

Patten, C. L., and B. R. Glick. 1996. Bacterial biosynthesis of indole-3-acetic acid. *Can. J. Microbiol.* **42**:207–220.

Patten, C. L., and B. R. Glick. 2002. The role of bacterial indoleacetic acid in the development of the host plant root system. *Appl. Environ. Microbiol.* **68**:3795–3801.

Peralta, H., Y. Mora, E. Salazar, S. Encarnación, R. Palacios, and J. Mora. 2004. Engineering the *nifH* promoter region and abolishing poly-β-hydroxybutyrate accumulation in *Rhizobium etli* enhance nitrogen fixation in symbiosis with *Phaseolus vulgaris. Appl. Environ. Microbiol.* **70**:3272-3281.

Peters, J. W., K. Fisher, and D. R. Dean. 1995. Nitrogenase structure and function: a biochemical-genetic perspective. *Annu. Rev. Microbiol.* **49**:335–366.

Ramírez, M., B. Valderrama, R. Arrendondo-Peter, M. Soberón, J. Mora, and G. Hernández. 1999. *Rhizobium etli* genetically engineered for the heterologous expression of *Vitreoscilla* sp. hemoglobin: effects on free-living and symbiosis. *Mol. Plant-Microbe Interact.* **12**:1008–1015.

Reed, M. L. E., and B. R. Glick. 2004. Applications of free living plant growth-promoting rhizobacteria. *Antonie van Leeuwenhoek* **86**:1–25.

Reed, M. L. E., and B. R. Glick. 2005. Growth of canola (*Brassica napus*) in the presence of plant growth-promoting bacteria and either copper or polycyclic aromatic hydrocarbons. *Can. J. Microbiol.* **51**:1061–1069.

Rossen, L., E. O. Davis, and A. W. B. Johnston. 1987. Plant-induced expression of *Rhizobium* genes involved in host specificity and early stages of nodulation. *Trends Biol. Sci.* **12**:430–433.

Schnider, U., C. Keel, C. Blumer, J. Troxler, G. Défago, and D. Haas. 1995. Amplification of the housekeeping sigma factor in *Pseudomonas fluorescens* CHA0 enhances antibiotic production and improves biocontrol abilities. *J. Bacteriol.* **177**:5387–5392.

Spaink, H. 2000. Root nodulation and infection factors produced by rhizobial bacteria. *Annu. Rev. Microbiol.* **54**:257–288.

Spaink, H. P., C. A. Wijffelman, E. Pees, R. J. H. Okker, and B. J. J. Lugtenberg. 1987. *Rhizobium* nodulation gene *nodD* as a determinant of host specificity. *Nature* **328**:337–340.

Sprent, J. I. 1986. Benefits of *Rhizobium* to agriculture. *Trends Biotechnol.* **4**:124–129.

Stacey, G. 1995. *Bradyrhizobium japonicum* nodulation genetics. *FEMS Microbiol. Lett.* **127**:1–9.

Sun, X., M. Griffith, J. J. Pasternak, and B. R. Glick. 1995. Low temperature growth, freezing survival and production of antifreeze protein by the plant growth-promoting rhizobacterium *Pseudomonas putida* GR12-2. *Can. J. Microbiol.* **41**:776–784.

Timms-Wilson, T. M., R. J. Ellis, A. Renwick, D. J. Rhodes, D. V. Mavrodi, D. M. Weller, L. S. Thomashow, and M. J. Bailey. 2000. Chromosomal insertion of phenazine-1-carboxylic acid biosynthetic pathway enhances efficacy of damping-off disease control by *Pseudomonas fluorescens*. *Mol. Plant-Microbe Interact.* **13**:1293–1300.

Ureta, A.-C., J. Imperial, T. Ruiz-Argüeso, and J. M. Palacios. 2005. *Rhizobium leguminosarum* biovar viciae symbiotic hydrogenase activity and processing are limited by the level of nickel in agricultural soils. *Appl. Environ. Microbiol.* **71**:7603–7606.

van Rhijn, P., and J. Vanderleyden. 1995. The *Rhizobium*-plant symbiosis. *Microbiol. Rev.* **59**:124–142.

Wang, C., E. Knill, B. R. Glick, and G. Défago. 2000. Effect of transferring 1-aminocyclopropane-1-carboxylic acid (ACC) deaminase genes into *Pseudomonas fluorescens* strain CHA0 and its *gacA* derivative CHA96 on their growth-promoting and disease-suppressive capacities. *Can. J. Microbiol.* **46**:898–907.

REVIEW QUESTIONS

1. Starting with a strain of *Bradyrhizobium japonicum* that can fix nitrogen and form a symbiotic relationship with soybean roots, and assuming that you do not have a DNA hybridization probe for *nod* genes, outline a scheme that you would use for isolating the cluster of nodulation genes from this organism.

2. How does glycogen synthesis affect the ability of a strain of *Rhizobium* to fix nitrogen?

3. How would you engineer a rhizobial strain to have a lower internal level of free oxygen? How might this affect the bacterium in the free-living state? As a bacteroid?

4. What is hydrogenase? How could it be used to improve the yield of alfalfa?

5. Suggest a strategy that you might employ to isolate all of the genes involved in nitrogen fixation from *Azotobacter vinelandii*, assuming that you do not have *nif* genes from other microorganisms to use as hybridization probes.

6. What might be the consequences of mutagenizing either *nifA* or *nifL* with respect to the amount of nitrogen that an organism can fix?

7. Discuss whether it is possible to genetically engineer plants to fix nitrogen.

8. What are siderophores? How could genetic manipulation of siderophore genes enable bacteria to enhance plant growth?

9. Suggest a scheme for isolating siderophore biosynthesis genes.

10. What are the advantages of microbial fertilizers over chemical fertilizers?

11. How do ACC deaminase-containing plant growth-promoting bacteria facilitate plant growth?

12. What is phytoremediation? How do plant growth-promoting bacteria affect phytoremediation?

13. How can *A. radiobacter* be engineered to be a more effective biocontrol agent?

14. Which enzymes secreted by plant growth-promoting bacteria contribute to their ability to act as biocontrol agents? How do these enzymes contribute to biocontrol?

15. How does poly-β-hydroxybutyrate affect the ability of a strain of *Rhizobium* to fix nitrogen?

16. How might endophytic bacteria be useful as part of a phytoremediation strategy?

17. Assuming that you do not have a DNA hybridization probe available, how would you isolate a bacterial antifreeze protein gene?

18. What strategies can be employed to increase the effectiveness of biocontrol bacterial strains?

19. What mechanisms do free-living plant growth-promoting bacteria use to facilitate plant growth?

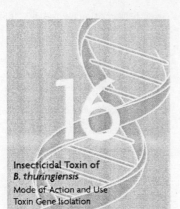

Microbial Insecticides

O F ALL CLASSES OF ORGANISMS, insects have the largest number of described species (more than 750,000). Insects negatively affect humans in a variety of ways: they cause massive crop damage, and they act as vectors of both human and animal diseases. During the 1940s, a number of chemical insecticides were developed as a means of controlling the proliferation of noxious insect populations. One of these was the chlorinated hydrocarbon DDT (dichlorodiphenyltrichloroethane), which had originally been synthesized in the 1870s but was not recognized as an insecticide until the late 1930s. DDT proved to be exceptionally effective in killing and controlling many species of pests. Chlorinated hydrocarbons such as DDT function by attacking the nervous system and muscle tissue of insects. Later, other chlorinated hydrocarbons, such as dieldrin, aldrin, chlordane, lindane, and toxophene, were synthesized and applied on a massive scale against crop pests and insects that carry infectious agents.

Organophosphates, another class of chemical insecticides that includes malathion, parathion, and diazinon, were initially developed as chemical warfare agents. Now they are used to control insect populations by inhibiting the enzyme acetylcholinesterase, which hydrolyzes the nerve transmitter acetylcholine, thereby disrupting the functioning of motor neurons and neurons in the brain of the insect.

By the early 1960s, over 100 million acres of U.S. agricultural land was being treated annually with chemical insecticides. At about that time, researchers realized that chlorinated hydrocarbon insecticides, to a large extent, and organophosphate insecticides, to a lesser extent, had dramatic and immediate side effects and long-term and indirect effects on animals, ecosystems, and humans. Chlorinated hydrocarbons, exemplified by DDT, were found to persist in the environment for more than 20 years and to accumulate in increasing concentrations through food chains. This bioaccumulation in fatty tissues had a significant biological impact on many organisms. For example, in North America, many species of birds, including peregrine falcons, sparrow hawks, bald eagles, brown pelicans, and double-crested cormorants, underwent severe population declines.

During the 1950s, as the targeted insect pest populations became increasingly resistant to treatment with many chemical insecticides, higher concentrations of the insecticides were applied to control the pests. In addition, chemical insecticides were found to lack specificity; consequently, beneficial insects were killed along with those that were considered to be pests. In fact, in some instances, the natural enemies of the insect pest species were killed off more efficiently than the target organisms, with the bizarre result that pesticide treatment led to greater numbers of the insects.

Given all the drawbacks associated with the use of chemical insecticides, alternative means of controlling harmful insects have been sought. Using insecticides that are produced naturally by either microorganisms or plants was an obvious choice. On the positive side, these compounds are usually highly specific for a target insect species, biodegradable, and slow to select for resistance. But, on the negative side, their low potency and high cost of production limit their use for a variety of applications. Recombinant DNA technology provides an opportunity to overcome many of these negative attributes. In particular, the insecticidal activities of the bacterium *Bacillus thuringiensis* and insect baculovirus systems have been developed into safe, specific, and effective insecticides.

The worldwide market for pesticides is enormous: currently more than $30 billion per year and growing rapidly. Although biopesticides, mostly *B. thuringiensis*, make up only about 1% of this total, much of the expected growth in this field is likely to involve biopesticides.

Insecticidal Toxin of *B. thuringiensis*

Mode of Action and Use

A microbial insecticide can be a microbially produced toxic substance that kills an insect species or an organism that has the ability to fatally infect a specific target insect. The most studied, most effective, and most often utilized microbial insecticides are the toxins synthesized by *B. thuringiensis*. This bacterium comprises a large number of strains and subspecies, each of which produces a different toxin that can kill specific insects—there are more than 150 different subspecies of *B. thuringiensis* (Table 16.1). For

TABLE 16.1 Some properties of the insecticidal toxins from various strains of *B. thuringiensis*

B. thuringiensis strain or subspecies	Protoxin size (kDa)	Target insects	Serotype
berliner	130–140	Lepidoptera	1
kurstaki KTO, HD-1	130–140	Lepidoptera	3
entomocidus 6.01	130–140	Lepidoptera	6
aizawai 7.29	130–140	Lepidoptera	7
aizawai IC 1	135	Lepidoptera, Diptera	7
kurstaki HD-1	71	Lepidoptera, Diptera	3
tenebrionis (*san diego*)	66–73	Coleoptera	8
morrisoni PG14	125–145	Diptera	8
israelensis	68	Diptera	14

Adapted from Lereclus et al., p. 37–69, in Entwistle et al. (ed.), *Bacillus thuringiensis, an Enviromental Biopesticide: Theory and Practice* (John Wiley & Sons, Chichester, United Kingdom, 1993).

example, *B. thuringiensis* subsp. *kurstaki* is toxic to lepidopteran larvae, including those of moths, butterflies, and skippers; cabbage worms; and spruce budworms. *B. thuringiensis* subsp. *israelensis* kills diptera, such as mosquitoes and blackflies. *B. thuringiensis* subsp. *tenebrionis* (also known as *B. thuringiensis* subsp. *san diego*) is effective against coleoptera (beetles), such as the potato beetle and the boll weevil. In addition, some subspecies of *B. thuringiensis* produce insecticidal toxins that are directed against hymenoptera (sawflies, wasps, bees, and ants), orthoptera (grasshoppers, crickets, and locusts), and mallophaga (lice).

The insecticidal activity (toxin) of *B. thuringiensis* subsp. *kurstaki* (first discovered in 1911) and other strains is contained within a very large structure called a parasporal crystal, which is synthesized during bacterial sporulation. Although no significant role on behalf of the bacterium has been attributed to the parasporal crystal structure, by synthesizing the crystal, the bacterium is "providing for its future" in that a dead insect provides sufficient nutrients to allow germination of the dormant spore. The parasporal crystal contains approximately 20 to 30% of the dry weight of a sporulated culture and usually consists mainly of protein (~95%) and a small amount of carbohydrate (~5%). About 150 different parasporal crystal proteins (Cry proteins) are known. The crystal is an aggregate of protein that can generally be dissociated by mild alkali treatment into subunits. The subunits can be further dissociated in vitro by treatment with β-mercaptoethanol, which reduces disulfide linkages (Fig. 16.1).

The insecticidal toxins from the *B. thuringiensis* strains were previously grouped into four major classes—CryI, CryII, CryIII, and CryIV—based on the insecticidal activity of the toxin. These proteins were further organized into subclasses (A, B, C, etc.) and subgroups (a, b, c, etc.). In the past few years, as increasing numbers of *B. thuringiensis* strains were isolated and their genes were characterized, it became clear that the original classification was unable to accommodate many of the newly discovered *B. thuringiensis* toxin genes. Therefore, a new system of *B. thuringiensis* gene classification was introduced.

In the current classification scheme (established in 1998), *B. thuringiensis* insecticidal (Cry) proteins are assigned designations based on their degree of evolutionary divergence, as estimated by certain mathematical algorithms. This scheme is readily visualized by constructing a phylogenetic tree based on the amino acid sequences of *B. thuringiensis* toxin proteins, i.e., Cry proteins (Fig. 16.2). Basically, the amino acid sequences of the proteins are compared, and if the proteins are identical, then they are 100% homologous. If only 50% of the amino acids are the same, then the proteins have 50% identity. The relationship among a set of protein sequences can be deduced and represented as a branched tree. The nodes (branch points) of the tree represent points of divergence. For the classification of the *B. thuringiensis* Cry proteins, a four-part naming system was devised. Demarcations, set at 95, 78, and 45% homology, show the boundaries that define the different nomenclature ranks. The name that is given to a particular toxin depends on the location of the node where the toxin protein sequence enters the tree relative to these set boundaries. A toxin that joins the tree to the left of the leftmost boundary is assigned a new primary rank (an Arabic numeral), one that joins the tree between the central and left boundaries is assigned a new secondary rank (an uppercase letter), one that joins the tree between the central and the right boundaries is assigned a new tertiary rank (a lowercase letter), and one that joins to the right of the

FIGURE 16.1 Schematic representation of a *B. thuringiensis* parasporal crystal composed of Cry1 protoxin protein. Each 250-kDa protein subunit of the parasporal crystal contains two 130-kDa polypeptides. (Molecular masses determined by polyacrylamide gel electrophoresis are approximations and do not always provide exact multiples.) Conversion of the 130-kDa protoxin into an active 68-kDa toxin requires the combination of a slightly alkaline pH (7.5 to 8) and the action of a specific protease(s), both of which are found in the insect gut. The activated toxin binds to protein receptors on the surface of the gut epithelial cell membrane.

FIGURE 16.2 Schematic representation of a portion of the phylogenetic tree of *B. thuringiensis* insecticidal (Cry) proteins. The different background colors delineate the different levels of nomenclature ranks. Cry1 and Cry7 share less than 45% identity, Cry1A and Cry1F are between 45% and 78% identical, and Cry1Ab and Cry1Ae are between 78% and 95% identical. Adapted from Crickmore et al., *Microbiol. Mol. Biol. Rev.* **62:**807–813, 1998.

rightmost boundary is assigned a new quaternary rank (an Arabic numeral). For example, Cry proteins that are less than 45% homologous are given a number (e.g., Cry1 and Cry7) and are assigned to the primary rank. Cry proteins that are 45 to 78% identical to proteins of the primary rank are further designated with an uppercase letter (e.g., Cry1A and Cry1F). The complete Cry protein tree consists of the positions of all Cry proteins. This classification system is utilized throughout this chapter, even when referring to work that was published prior to the development of this system.

The parasporal crystal does not usually contain the active form of the insecticide. Rather, once the crystal has been solubilized, the protein that is released is generally a protoxin, a precursor of the active toxin. The protoxin of many of the Cry toxins that are directed against lepidoptera has a molecular mass of approximately 130 kilodaltons (kDa) (Fig. 16.1). When a parasporal crystal is ingested by a target insect, the protoxin is activated within its gut by the combination of alkaline pH (7.5 to 8.0) and specific digestive proteases, which convert the protoxin into an active toxin with a molecular mass of approximately 68 kDa (Fig. 16.1). In its active form, the toxic protein inserts itself into the membranes of the gut epithelial cells of the insect and creates an ion channel, which leads to an excessive loss of cellular ATP (Fig. 16.3). About 15 minutes after this ion channel forms, cellular metabolism ceases; the insect stops feeding within a few hours, becomes dehydrated, and eventually dies (in about 2 to 5 days). Because the conversion of the protoxin to the active toxin requires both alkaline pH and the presence of specific proteases, it is extremely unlikely that nontarget species, such as humans and farm animals, will be affected.

The mode of action of *B. thuringiensis* toxins imposes certain constraints on its application. To kill an insect pest, *B. thuringiensis* parasporal crystals must be ingested. Contact of the bacterium or the insecticidal toxin with the surface of the target organism has no effect on it. The requirement that the

FIGURE 16.3 Insertion of the *B. thuringiensis* toxin into the membrane of an insect gut epithelial cell. The toxin forms an ion channel between the cell cytoplasm and the external environment.

insecticide be ingested, in part, limits the susceptibility of nontarget insects and other animals to the insecticide. *B. thuringiensis* is generally applied by spraying, so it is usually formulated with insect attractants to increase the probability that the target insect will ingest the toxin. However, insects that bore into plants or attack plant roots are less likely to ingest a *B. thuringiensis* toxin that has been sprayed on a host plant, so other strategies have been devised to control such pests. One approach is to create transgenic plants that carry and express a *B. thuringiensis* toxin gene so that they are protected from infestation throughout the growing season (see chapter 18).

It was recently discovered for gypsy moths (and suggested to possibly be the case for other insects, as well) that the *B. thuringiensis* toxin does not kill the larvae by itself as previously thought. Rather, bacteria that are part of the insect's gut microbial community are required for toxicity to the insect. Elimination of the insect's gut bacteria by oral administration of antibiotics abolished *B. thuringiensis* insecticidal activity, and reintroduction of an *Enterobacter* sp. that is normally part of the insect's gut microbial community restored this activity. The data indicate that the *B. thuringiensis* toxin enables the enteric bacteria to reach the insect hemocoel by permeabilizing the gut epithelium. In this way, the insect is killed much more rapidly than might otherwise be expected. The discovery that *B. thuringiensis* insecticidal activity depends on insect enteric bacteria should not have any significant effect on the efficacy or use of *B. thuringiensis*-based insecticides. However, this information may be important in the design and execution of some laboratory experiments intended to better understand the functioning of *B. thuringiensis* insecticidal strains and to facilitate the development of improved biological insecticides.

A limiting feature of the action of the *B. thuringiensis* toxin is that it can kill a susceptible insect only during a specific developmental stage. Therefore, the toxin must be applied when the pest population is at a particular stage in its life cycle (generally the larval stage). The other major impediment to more widespread application of *B. thuringiensis* subsp. *kurstaki* is that it costs from 1.5 to 3 times as much as chemical insecticides. The limitations and the cost notwithstanding, several subspecies of *B. thuringiensis* have been approved for use and have rapidly gained widespread acceptance (Table 16.2).

B. thuringiensis subsp. *kurstaki* was first discovered in 1901, although its commercial potential was largely ignored until 1951. Within recent decades, however, *B. thuringiensis* subsp. *kurstaki* has become the major means of

TABLE 16.2 Some subspecies of *B. thuringiensis* that have been approved for use in the field and some of their targets

B. thuringiensis subspecies	Targets
aizawai	Fruits and nuts, berries, peppers, tomato, root crops, tobacco, beans, corn, cotton, cabbage, eggplant, melons, cucumber, cauliflower, broccoli, ornamentals
kurstaki	Berries, fruits, nuts, melons, cucumber, squash, eggplant, tomato, broccoli, cabbage, kale, mustard, parsley, spinach, turnip, lettuce, stored grain, stored crop seed, ornamentals, cotton, celery, peanut, sugar beet, tobacco, avocado, onion, carrot, forestry products, grape, canola, sorghum, wheat, forage crops, corn, sunflower, root crops, cranberry
israelensis	Mosquito breeding habitat, including rice fields, ponds, pastures, ditches, salt marshes, tidal water, sewage lagoons, lakes; ornamental and nursery plants; mushrooms (*Agaricus bisporus*)
tenebrionis	Eggplant, tomato, potato, ornamentals

controlling the spruce budworm in Canada. In 1979, approximately 1% of the forest area in Canada that was treated with an insecticide to combat the spruce budworm (about 2 million hectares, or 8,000 square miles) was sprayed with *B. thuringiensis* subsp. *kurstaki*. The remainder of the treated forests were sprayed with chemical insecticides. By 1986, the use of *B. thuringiensis* subsp. *kurstaki* had increased dramatically. It was used to treat approximately 74% of the forests sprayed in that year for spruce budworm. In other countries, *B. thuringiensis* subsp. *kurstaki* has been used against tent caterpillars, gypsy moths, cabbage worms, cabbage loopers, and tobacco hornworms.

For the biological control (biocontrol) of insect pests, *B. thuringiensis* subsp. *kurstaki* is typically applied by spraying approximately 1.3×10^8 to 2.6×10^8 spores per square foot (1 square foot is equivalent to 0.093 m^2) of the target area. Administration of the spores is timed to coincide with the peak of the larval population of the target organism, because the parasporal crystals, being sensitive to sunlight, are short-lived in the environment. Under simulated conditions, sunlight degrades over 60% of the tryptophan residues of the parasporal crystal within a 24-hour period, thereby rendering the protein inactive. Depending on the amount of sunlight present, parasporal crystals may persist in the environment for as little as a day or as long as a month. The lack of persistence of the insecticidal protoxin in the natural environment means that natural selection of resistant insects is highly unlikely.

Toxin Gene Isolation

To develop *B. thuringiensis*-based insecticides that have greater potencies and broader host ranges, it is necessary to isolate and characterize the protoxin gene(s). For the initial isolation of insecticidal protoxin genes, the first step was to determine whether the toxin genes are located on a plasmid or on the chromosomal DNA. To test for plasmid-borne toxin genes, the source *B. thuringiensis* strain was conjugated with a strain that lacks insecticidal activity. If the latter strain acquired the ability to synthesize the insecticidal toxin, then the toxin gene(s) was most likely present on a plasmid, because the transfer of chromosomal DNA during conjugation is a rare event.

The procedure for isolating a protoxin-encoding DNA sequence is a familiar one. *B. thuringiensis* cells are grown in laboratory culture and lysed. The total cellular DNA is isolated and separated into plasmid and chromosomal DNA fractions by cesium chloride (CsCl) gradient centrifugation. When the protoxin gene is part of the genome, a clone bank is constructed from the chromosomal DNA. When the toxin gene(s) is plasmid encoded, the plasmid DNA can be further fractionated by sucrose gradient centrifugation, which separates different plasmids according to their sizes and enriches for the DNA that serves as the starting material for the isolation of a protoxin gene(s) (Fig. 16.4).

B. thuringiensis subsp. *kurstaki* contains an insecticidal protoxin gene on one of seven different plasmids that are approximately 2.0, 7.4, 7.8, 8.2, 14.4, 45, and 71 kilobase pairs (kb) in length. To determine which *B. thuringiensis* subsp. *kurstaki* plasmid carries the protoxin gene, following sucrose gradient centrifugation, the plasmid DNA sample is divided into three fractions that contain, respectively, the small (2.0-kb), medium-sized

FIGURE 16.4 Procedure for the isolation and partial enrichment of plasmid DNA fractions from a microorganism with a number of different plasmids, one of which encodes an insecticidal protoxin. OD_{260}, optical density at 260 nm.

(7.4-, 7.8-, 8.2-, and 14.4-kb), and large (45- and 71-kb) plasmids. The fraction with the small plasmid is discarded, because the plasmid is too small to encode a protein equivalent to the 130-kDa protoxin. A protein of this size requires at least 4.0 kb of coding DNA. The medium and large plasmid fractions are each partially digested with the restriction enzyme Sau3AI and then ligated into the BamHI site of plasmid pBR322. In the original experiments, these clone banks were transformed into *Escherichia coli*, and then the colonies were screened immunologically (see chapter 3) by the following procedure to detect clones that expressed a Cry protein and therefore carried a *cry* gene.

1. Colonies were transferred from agar plates to a nitrocellulose membrane.
2. The transferred colonies were lysed with organic solvents.
3. All available sites on the membrane to which primary and secondary antibodies could potentially bind (nonspecifically) were blocked by treating the membrane with bovine serum albumin (which bound to the nonspecific sites and prevented antibodies from binding to those sites).
4. The bovine serum albumin-treated membranes were treated with rabbit antiserum that contained antibodies against the insecticidal toxin. The antibodies bound only to the insecticidal toxin and not to any nonspecific sites on the membrane.
5. The membranes were washed to remove unbound antibodies and then treated with ^{125}I-labeled *Staphylococcus aureus* protein A, which bound only to the Fc portion of the bound antibodies and not to any nonspecific sites on the membrane.
6. Spots on the membrane corresponding to colonies that actively synthesized the insecticidal toxin were visualized by autoradiography.

The isolated protoxin gene was then used as a DNA hybridization probe to localize the *cry* gene to the 71-kb plasmid of *B. thuringiensis* subsp. *kurstaki*. Similar cloning and screening procedures have been used to isolate other *B. thuringiensis* toxin genes. However, given the current knowledge regarding sequence similarity among *B. thuringiensis* protoxin genes, the cloning and screening of these genes are more easily achieved by using polymerase chain reaction (PCR) and DNA hybridization techniques.

Engineering of *B. thuringiensis* Toxin Genes

Once the isolation and sequencing of a toxin gene were accomplished, the complete amino acid sequence was determined. Comparisons of amino acid sequences from other *B. thuringiensis* toxin proteins showed that a common toxic domain exists in these strains. Moreover, a subcloned segment of the complete protein-coding sequence produced a truncated protein that retained full insecticidal activity. Thus, an intact protoxin gene, a portion of one, or a chemically synthesized coding sequence can be used for further genetic manipulation.

Synthesis during Vegetative Growth

Under normal conditions, most *B. thuringiensis* protoxin proteins are synthesized only during the sporulation phase of growth. In other words, only a portion of the growth cycle of the organism is devoted to parasporal

crystal production. It might therefore be advantageous, in terms of increased yield and decreased production time, to have the toxin gene transcribed and translated during vegetative growth. Furthermore, production of the insecticidal toxin during vegetative growth would permit the toxin to be synthesized by a continuous fermentation process, potentially significantly decreasing the cost of producing it. Continuous fermentations are carried out with smaller-scale—and therefore less expensive—bioreactors and downstream processing equipment than conventional batch fermentations. (See chapter 17 for additional details.)

During the sporulation of *B. thuringiensis,* a specific transcription initiation factor (sigma factor) interacts with the promoters of genes that are active only within this phase of the bacterial life cycle. This factor turns on the transcription of the messenger RNAs (mRNAs) that are unique to sporulation. In fact, when a *B. thuringiensis* toxin gene with its sporulation-specific promoter was cloned and expressed in *Bacillus subtilis, Bacillus megaterium,* or *B. thuringiensis,* gene transcription occurred only during

FIGURE 16.5 Procedure for subcloning the *B. thuringiensis* subsp. *kurstaki* insecticidal toxin gene so that it is expressed constitutively under the control of the promoter of the tetracycline resistance (Tetr) gene (p^{tet}). The isolated *B. thuringiensis* toxin gene is removed from its promoter by digestion of the isolated DNA fragment with restriction enzymes RE1 and RE2. It is spliced by T4 DNA ligase into the plasmid vector downstream from p^{tet} in place of the tetracycline resistance gene, which has been removed by digestion with restriction enzymes RE1 and RE2.

sporulation. Thus, to express a *B. thuringiensis* insecticidal toxin during vegetative growth, it is necessary to place the toxin-producing gene(s) under the control of a promoter that is active during vegetative growth.

When a DNA fragment containing a toxin gene that lacked its native promoter was cloned into a plasmid under the control of a continuously active, constitutive promoter from a tetracycline resistance gene that had been originally isolated from a *Bacillus cereus* plasmid and reintroduced into *B. thuringiensis*, active toxin protein was produced continuously throughout the growth cycle, including both the vegetative and sporulation phases (Fig. 16.5). In addition, when the construct was used to transform a sporulation-defective mutant of *B. thuringiensis*, toxin synthesis occurred in the absence of sporulation. Under these conditions, toxin synthesis is more efficient than in wild-type cells, i.e., the final yield of protein is greater in the transformed cells, and less time and substrate are required to produce the toxin. A refinement of this system might entail integration of this vegetatively expressed toxin gene into the chromosomal DNA of the sporulation-defective *B. thuringiensis* host. This manipulation would ensure that the insecticidal toxin gene is not lost because of plasmid instability during a continuous fermentation process.

FIGURE 16.6 Construction of a strain of *B. thuringiensis* with greater potency and UV resistance. The C-terminal third of the *cry1Ab* gene was spliced together with the N-terminal two-thirds of the *cry1C* gene, all under the control of the *cry3Aa* promoter (p^{cry3Aa}), and then integrated into the chromosomal DNA of a sporulation-minus strain of *B. thuringiensis*. Adapted from Sanchis et al., *Appl. Environ. Microbiol.* 65:4032–4039, 1999.

Unlike that of most other *B. thuringiensis* toxin protein *(cry)* genes, the expression of *cry3A* is normally controlled by a vegetative promoter, rather than by a sporulation-specific promoter. The *cry3A* gene encodes a toxin that is directed against coleopteran larvae. When a mutant strain of *B. thuringiensis* that was unable to form spores was transformed with a plasmid carrying a cloned *cry3A* gene, the insecticidal toxin was both overproduced and stabilized in comparison to when this protein was produced in the wild-type strain. This result suggests that other *cry* genes that are normally expressed only during sporulation could be placed under the control of the *cry3A* promoter and overproduced by expressing these constructs in a sporulation-defective *B. thuringiensis* mutant.

In one experiment, a chimeric *cry1C–cry1Ab* gene was constructed, placed under the transcriptional control of the vegetative *cry3A* promoter, and then integrated into the chromosomal DNA of a nonsporulating derivative of *B. thuringiensis* subsp. *kurstaki* (Fig. 16.6). The chimeric *cry1C–cry1Ab* gene consisted of approximately 2.2 kb of DNA from the *cry1C* gene and 1.3 kb of DNA from the *cry1Ab* gene. Although the mature toxin that is produced following proteolytic cleavage of the hybrid protoxin is identical to the toxin that is produced from the *cry1C* gene, this toxin was found to be considerably more active than Cry1C (Table 16.3). Thus, depending upon the insect tested, Cry1C–Cry1Ab was 3 to 34 times more active than Cry1C. This seemingly strange result probably occurs because of the increased stability to proteolytic digestion of the Cry1Ab portion of the hybrid protoxin protein, which is removed upon activation of the protoxin. The nonsporulating *B. thuringiensis* host strain had a disrupted *sigK* gene, which encodes the sigma factor σ^{28}, which is required for sporulation-specific transcription. Other workers have created nonsporulating *B. thuringiensis* strains by inserting modified protoxin genes into the late-stage sporulation gene $spoV_{Bt}$. Since the chimeric protoxin Cry1C–Cry1Ab was encapsulated with the bacterial cells, the protein was considerably more resistant to the degradative effect of ultraviolet (UV) light, which rapidly inactivates the protoxin that is normally secreted outside of the bacterial cell during sporulation. In addition to increased potency and greater UV resistance, the environmental persistence of the nonsporulating mutant was significantly decreased compared with that of the sporulating wild-type strain. This may actually be an advantage, since it is less likely that the nonsporulating mutant will transfer any of its DNA to other organisms in the environment.

Broadening the Spectrum of Target Insects

Because many crops are attacked by more than one insect species, it would be advantageous, if feasible, to create microbial insecticides that are effective

TABLE 16.3 Activities of Cry1C and a chimeric Cry1C-Cry1Ab toxin against three insect species

Insect species	LC$_{50}$ of Cry1C (ng)	LC$_{50}$ of Cry1C-Cry1Ab (ng)
Spodoptera littoralis	378	103
Plutella xylostella	174	4.6
Ostrinia nubilalis	3,200	822

The LC$_{50}$ values reflect the amount of insecticidal toxin (in nanograms) required to kill half of the insect population being tested under a defined set of conditions. The smaller the LC$_{50}$, the more potent the toxin.

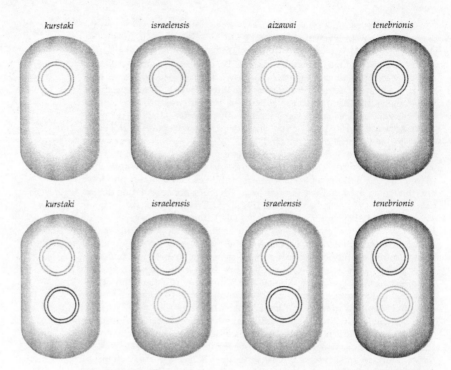

FIGURE 16.7 Naturally occurring and transformed subspecies of *B. thuringiensis*. The oval shape represents a bacterium, while the circle represents an insecticide-encoding plasmid. The plasmids are colored the same as the bacterium in which the toxin gene originated.

against a broad spectrum of target insects. Such a broad-specificity molecule could be obtained (1) by transferring the gene for a particular toxin, e.g., one against diptera, into a *B. thuringiensis* strain that normally synthesizes a different species-specific toxin, e.g., one against coleoptera; (2) by fusing portions of two different species-specific toxin genes to one another so that a unique dual-acting toxin (hybrid toxin) is produced; or (3) by modifying the portion of the insecticidal toxin that is responsible for binding to insect gut epithelial cell receptors.

Transferring *cry* genes. To test whether the spectrum of target insect pests could be widened, the insecticidal toxin genes from *B. thuringiensis* subsp. *aizawai* and *tenebrionis* were cloned into shuttle vectors that could be maintained in both *B. thuringiensis* and *E. coli*. These genetic constructs were then introduced by electroporation into *B. thuringiensis* subsp. *kurstaki*, *israelensis*, and *tenebrionis* (Fig. 16.7), and all the transformed strains were tested for toxicity to three different insect species.

In each case, the toxicity of the native host toxin protein(s) was maintained, and in most cases, the introduced toxin gene also expressed an active toxin with the same specificity as the toxin produced by the source bacterium (Table 16.4). In addition, and surprisingly, when the *B. thuringiensis*

subsp. *tenebrionis* toxin gene was introduced into *B. thuringiensis* subsp. *israelensis,* the resultant transformant was somewhat toxic to *Pieris brassicae,* the cabbage white butterfly, against which neither of the gene products alone has insecticidal activity.

In many instances, introduced plasmid vectors carrying isolated *cry* genes are unstable in *B. thuringiensis.* Often, in the absence of selective pressure, all or a portion of these plasmids are lost. The problem of plasmid instability with introduced genes was overcome by integrating cloned *cry* genes into the chromosomal DNA of the host cell. One group of researchers attempted to broaden the insect specificity of a strain of *B. thuringiensis* subsp. *kurstaki,* which normally carries five different insecticidal toxin genes, *cry1Aa, cry1Ab, cry1Ac, cry2Aa,* and *cry2Ab.* While the products of these *cry* genes are active against a variety of lepidopteran species, they are not effective against *Spodoptera* spp. Therefore, a *cry1Ca* gene, which is normally found only in *B. thuringiensis* subsp. *aizawai* and *entomocidus,* was introduced into the chromosomal DNA of the *B. thuringiensis* subsp. *kurstaki* host strain. The transformed *B. thuringiensis* subsp. *kurstaki* strain showed a sixfold increase in its ability to kill *Spodoptera exigua* (beet armyworm) larvae.

Modifying the loop regions of domain II. The toxic moiety of many Cry proteins is composed of three separate domains. Domain II is involved in the specific binding of the toxin to protein receptors that are found on the surfaces of insect midgut epithelial cells, although domain III may also play a role in receptor binding. Following binding, a portion of domain I, in the N-terminal region of the toxin, inserts into the membrane. It is believed that the interaction of portions of domain I from several toxin molecules interact to make up the pore. Domain III, which is located at the C-terminal end of the toxin molecule, is also thought to be involved in pore function.

Modification of *cry* genes to increase the binding of the Cry protein to receptors generally leads to an increase in insecticidal activity. In particular,

TABLE 16.4 Toxicities of naturally occurring and transformed subspecies of *B. thuringiensis* against the insects *Pieris brassicae* (cabbage white butterfly), *Aedes aegypti* (mosquito), and *Phaedon cochleariae* (beetle)

Source of toxin		Toxicity to:		
Host DNA	**Introduced DNA**	**Pieris**	**Aedes**	**Phaedon**
aizawai	None	++	+	−
israelensis	None	−	++	−
israelensis	*aizawai*	++	++	−
israelensis	*tenebrionis*	+	++	++
kurstaki	None	++	+	−
kurstaki	*tenebrionis*	++	+	++
tenebrionis	None	−	−	++
tenebrionis	*aizawai*	++	+	+

Adapted from Crickmore et al., *Biochem. J.* **270**:133–136, 1990.

In these experiments, the toxicity was graded as follows: ++, 0 to 5% of the leaf was consumed (for *Phaedon* and *Pieris*) or 100% mortality occurred within 1 hour (*Aedes*); +, 5 to 50% of the leaf was consumed (*Phaedon* and *Pieris*) or 50 to 100% mortality occurred within 24 hours (*Aedes*); −, 50% of the leaf was consumed (*Phaedon* and *Pieris*) or no mortality occurred within 24 hours (*Aedes*). The test plant was either cabbage leaf (for *Pieris*) or turnip leaf (for *Phaedon*).

Loop 2 ———— Loop 1

FIGURE 16.8 Schematic representation of the three-dimensional structure of the Cry19Aa protein, highlighting loops 1 and 2, which were modified to alter the insecticide's specificity. Adapted from Abdullah and Dean, *Appl. Environ. Microbiol.* **70**:3769–3771, 2004, with permission.

modification of domain II is an effective means of increasing Cry toxicity to particular insects. In one series of experiments, researchers modified the insect specificity of Cry19Aa. This was done by directed mutagenesis of the *cry19Aa* gene, replacing a nucleotide sequence that encoded the amino acids Ser–Tyr–Trp–Thr in loop 1 of domain II with a sequence encoding Tyr–Gln–Asp–Leu–Arg and deleting a sequence in loop 2 encoding Tyr–Pro–Trp–Gly–Asp (Fig. 16.8). The decisions regarding which sequences to alter were based on computer models comparing the three-dimensional structure of Cry19Aa with the structure of Cry4Ba. These changes—alterations of both loop 1 and loop 2 were required—yielded a modified Cry19Aa protein whose insecticidal activity against the mosquito *Aedes aegypti* was increased more than 42,000-fold while its activity against other insects was essentially unchanged. This work suggests that it may be possible to rationally engineer various Cry toxins to have desired activities by manipulating specific amino acid sequences within the protein loops. However, even if the genetic manipulations are successful and designer-engineered Cry proteins are attainable, it remains to be seen whether the general public and the regulatory authorities in various countries will embrace this technology, which would include releasing genetically manipulated bacteria into the environment.

Improving Delivery of a Mosquitocidal Toxin

The *B. thuringiensis* subsp. *israelensis* insecticidal protein is highly toxic when ingested by mosquito larvae. Since 1982, it has been used successfully worldwide to control mosquitoes and blackflies. However, the parasporal crystal of this species sinks rapidly after it is sprayed on water, which effectively removes it from the feeding area of mosquito larvae and dramatically decreases its efficacy as a mosquitocide. To overcome this shortcoming, several approaches have been attempted. Currently, *B. thuringiensis* subsp.

israelensis insecticidal protein is available as granules or as slow-release rings or brickettes, which float on the surface of water. Another solution is to introduce the insecticidal toxin gene into organisms that are common food sources for mosquito larvae. Good candidate organisms for this purpose include *Synechocystis* and *Synechococcus* spp., which are photosynthetic cyanobacteria that proliferate near the water surface, where there is sufficient light for their growth and where mosquito larvae are normally found. Another organism with the potential to be a host for the expression of foreign insecticidal toxin genes is *Caulobacter crescentus*, an aquatic bacterium that generally is widely distributed throughout aquatic environments where mosquito larvae feed. The toxin gene from *B. thuringiensis* subsp. *israelensis* was introduced into and expressed in these organisms. In laboratory trials, the insecticidal toxin that was produced by either transformed cyanobacteria or *C. crescentus* was toxic to mosquito larvae. However, in field trials, transformed cyanobacteria or *C. crescentus* expressing *B. thuringiensis* insecticidal toxin genes had poor viability, and the cloned genes were expressed at a low level.

A possible alternative host for the expression of mosquitocidal *cry* genes is *Asticcacaulis excentricus*, a gram-negative aerobic bacterium that is found in aqueous environments near the surface of the water. In a series of experiments, *A. excentricus* was transformed with a broad-host-range plasmid vector that carried the genes for mosquitocidal toxin proteins produced by a strain of *Bacillus sphaericus* (a bacterium similar to *B. thuringiensis*) under the control of the *tac1* promoter, which is a variant of the *tac* promoter. This transformant produced insecticidal toxin proteins of 51 and 42 kDa and was almost as toxic to *Anopheles* and *Culex* mosquito larvae as the naturally occurring high-toxicity strains of *B. sphaericus*. However, unlike *B. sphaericus*, *A. excentricus* does not sink when it is sprayed onto

MILESTONE

Cloning and Expression of the *Bacillus thuringiensis* Crystal Protein Gene in *Escherichia coli*

H. E. SCHNEPF and H. R. WHITELEY
Proc. Natl. Acad. Sci. USA **78**:2893–2897, 1981

Although it had been well known for a long time that the parasporal crystal that is produced by *B. thuringiensis* contained insecticidal activity, it took scientists many years before the conditions for solubilizing the crystal were discovered and the insecticidal protein toxin was isolated in a pure form. Moreover, although some *B. thuringiensis* mutants that were defective in the synthesis of the parasporal crystal were known, protocols for the genetic transformation of *B. thuringiensis* were not well developed. Therefore, when Schnepf and Whiteley decided to isolate *B. thuringiensis* insecticidal toxin protein genes, they were limited to screening *E. coli* transformants carrying *B. thuringiensis* DNA either immunologically, using antibodies directed against the whole crystal, or by the insecticidal activity of extracts of the transformants. Since evidence at the time suggested that the insecticidal toxin was probably plasmid encoded, clone banks were constructed from fractionated plasmid preparations with the idea of significantly enriching the clone banks for the presence of insecticidal toxin genes. Moreover, despite some concerns that antibodies against the whole (*B. thuringiensis*-produced and glycosylated) crystal protein might not interact with (*E. coli*-produced and nonglycosylated) crystal protein subunits in solution, this did not turn out to be a problem. Finally, extracts of the particulate fraction of *E. coli* transformants carrying the *B. thuringiensis* insecticidal toxin gene were found to be toxic to susceptible insects. This first cloning of a *B. thuringiensis* insecticidal toxin gene made it clear to workers in this field that these genes could be isolated in a straightforward manner and provided an impetus for increased activity both in the search for new strains of *B. thuringiensis* and in studies of the biochemistry of the insecticidal toxin.

ponds infested with mosquito larvae. Moreover, *A. excentricus* is inexpensive to produce, as it can be grown on much simpler media than either *B. sphaericus* or *B. thuringiensis*. It does not have a high level of protease activity, so the insecticidal toxin is not readily degraded. It is well adapted to environments such as those near the surface of standing water that are exposed to relatively high levels of UV light. Thus, *A. excentricus* cells should not be as sensitive to inactivation by UV light as those of either *B. sphaericus* or *B. thuringiensis*. However, to use a genetically engineered strain of *A. excentricus* to control mosquito populations in the environment, it will be necessary to integrate the insecticidal toxin genes into the chromosomal DNA without any antibiotic resistance genes.

Protecting Plant Roots

Insects that attack the roots of plants are not affected by *B. thuringiensis*-based insecticides that are sprayed onto leaves and shoots. However, it is possible to introduce the toxin gene from a *B. thuringiensis* strain into a bacterial species that colonizes the region adjacent to plant roots (the rhizosphere). The engineered bacteria could be introduced into the soil, where they would synthesize the insecticidal toxin and release it into the area immediately surrounding the plant roots, thereby conferring protection against root-attacking insects. In addition, as long as the engineered bacteria were able to persist in the soil, they would continue to synthesize the insecticidal toxin, thus obviating the need for repeated spraying of either biological or chemical insecticides. This approach has been tested on a small scale. The gene for the *B. thuringiensis* subsp. *kurstaki* insecticidal toxin was integrated into the chromosomal DNA of a strain of *P. fluorescens* that colonizes corn (maize) roots. The integration of the toxin gene was achieved as follows (Fig. 16.9).

1. A transposon Tn5 element that had been cloned into a plasmid was genetically modified by altering portions of its left and right borders and deleting its transposase gene. Such an altered Tn5 element cannot be excised from the plasmid, even by exogenous transposase, because the left and right borders are not are recognized by the transposase.
2. An isolated *B. thuringiensis* subsp. *kurstaki* insecticidal toxin gene was spliced into the middle of the altered Tn5 element on the plasmid and placed under the control of a constitutive promoter.
3. A wild-type Tn5 element was transposed into the chromosome of the root-colonizing strain of *P. fluorescens*.
4. The plasmid carrying the altered Tn5 element with the inserted toxin gene was introduced into *P. fluorescens* carrying the integrated wild-type Tn5 element.
5. Homologous recombination by means of a double crossover between the nontransposable Tn5 element on the plasmid that carried the toxin gene and the chromosomally integrated wild-type Tn5 led to the integration of the altered Tn5 with the toxin gene into the chromosomal DNA, with the concomitant loss of the wild-type Tn5 element.

In this form, the toxin gene is unlikely to be lost either during large-scale laboratory growth or after release of the engineered microorganism into the environment. Also, the probability of transfer of the toxin gene to

FIGURE 16.9 Procedure for the development of a genetically engineered *P. fluorescens* strain that carries a copy of the *B. thuringiensis* insecticidal toxin gene integrated into its chromosomal DNA. The *B. thuringiensis* insecticidal toxin gene is cloned into an excision-defective variant of Tn5 on a plasmid. This construct is introduced into a *P. fluorescens* strain containing a wild-type Tn5 sequence that has been integrated into its chromosomal DNA. By homologous recombination, the excision-defective Tn5 element carrying the *B. thuringiensis* insecticidal toxin gene becomes integrated into the *P. fluorescens* chromosome.

other microorganisms in the environment is very low. Laboratory trials showed that the engineered *P. fluorescens* was toxic to tobacco hornworm larvae. However, the ability of this genetically manipulated microorganism to minimize root damage from insect predation remains to be tested in the greenhouse and in open-field trials.

In other laboratories, various *B. thuringiensis* insecticidal toxin genes have been introduced into the chromosomal DNA of a number of different microorganisms. For example, the *cry1Ac* genes were introduced into a strain of *P. fluorescens* and found to protect sugarcane plants against the sugarcane borer, *Eldana saccharina*. Also, when this gene was used to

transform *Clavibacter xyli* subsp. *cynodontis*, a bacterium that normally inhabits the xylem of Bermuda grass, the bacterium protected corn plants from damage caused by the European corn borer, *Ostrinia nubilalis*.

Protoxin Processing

Occasionally, during the proteolytic processing of the protoxin to the active toxin, the insect midgut proteases continue to cleave the toxin protein and thereby render it inactive (Fig. 16.10). This degradation process occurred when the 63-kDa Cry2Aa1 protoxin was treated with the midgut juices of the gypsy moth *(Lymantria dispar)*. The midgut juices, which contained the protoxin-processing protease, first cleaved the protoxin on the C-terminal side of Tyr49, producing the active 58-kDa Cry2Aa1 toxin. However, continued incubation of the toxin with the midgut enzymes resulted in the cleavage of the toxin on the C-terminal side of Leu144. This second cleavage inactivated the toxin, producing an inactive 49-kDa protein, dramatically reducing its effectiveness. To ascertain that this result was not an artifact, researchers radiolabeled the Cry2Aa1 protoxin and showed that this excessive cleavage also occurred in vivo. To try to prevent the production of the inactive form of the toxin, the protoxin gene was altered in five different ways by site-directed mutagenesis. The amino acid residue in position 144 of the protoxin was changed from leucine to aspartic acid, alanine, glycine, histidine, or valine. All of the mutant proteins yielded a higher level of active toxin than the native form, and with the exception of the leucine-to-histidine change, the active mutant toxin proteins were no longer cleaved to an inactive form.

Since the C-terminal half of many *B. thuringiensis* insecticidal protoxins is not toxic to insects, it would be advantageous if that half of the protein could be eliminated. Then, the cellular resources that had previously gone into synthesizing the C-terminal half of the protoxin might be used to synthesize more of the active toxin, thereby increasing the amount of toxin that a bacterium might produce. Unfortunately, when such truncated *cry1* genes

FIGURE 16.10 Activation and subsequent cleavage of *B. thuringiensis* Cry2Aa1 protoxin by *L. dispar* midgut enzymes. Activation occurs by cleavage of the protoxin on the C-terminal side of Tyr49. Toxin inactivation occurs when the protein is cleaved on the C-terminal side of Leu144. When Leu144 is changed to one of several different amino acids, the toxin is both active and resistant to further proteolytic cleavage.

FIGURE 16.11 A genetic construct that produces a high level of stable truncated Cry1C protein. This construct includes the promoter from a *cyt1A* gene (*p^cyt1A*), a ribosome-binding site (RBS) from *cry3A* that stabilizes mRNA, a *cry3A* gene transcription terminator region (TT), a gene from the *cry11A* operon encoding a 20-kDa chaperone-like protein that stabilizes the structure of the Cry1C protein, and a gene from the *cry2A* operon encoding a 29-kDa protein that facilitates protoxin crystal formation. Each of the last two genes has its own promoter, ribosome-binding site, and transcription termination site (not shown).

were expressed in *B. thuringiensis*, the toxin yields were low and crystals did not form. To remedy this situation, several genetic elements that were known to enhance the synthesis and crystallization of "naturally truncated" Cry proteins were tested both separately and together in order to improve the stability and yield of truncated Cry1C (Fig. 16.11). The construct that significantly increased both the stability and yield of truncated Cry1C protein, with the truncated protein now forming crystals within sporulated cells, contained a number of different genetic elements, including the gene for a 20-kDa chaperone-like protein and a 29-kDa protein that facilitated protoxin crystal formation.

Preventing the Development of Resistance

When *B. thuringiensis* subsp. *kurstaki* is used as an insecticide in a controlled environment where there is no sunlight to rapidly break down the protoxin, e.g., when stored grain is treated to protect it against insect predation, resistant target insects develop within a few generations. This inherited resistance is typically due to an alteration in a midgut membrane protein that normally acts as a receptor for the *B. thuringiensis* subsp. *kurstaki* toxin. Resistant insects accumulate because the protoxin persists under these conditions and selects for resistant individuals. The lesson here is that the simplest way to avoid selecting for insects that are resistant to *B. thuringiensis* subsp. *kurstaki* in the absence of sunlight is to limit the use of this bacterium to field applications. However, extensive annual use, even under natural conditions, may result in a level of persistence high enough to allow selection to occur. Certainly, as larger quantities of *B. thuringiensis* are used over a wider geographical area, the probability that resistant strains of insects will be selected will increase. Various ways to avert this problem are being examined. These strategies, which may be utilized either with *B. thuringiensis* that is sprayed or with transgenic plants expressing the insecticidal toxin, include the following.

1. The use of two or more *B. thuringiensis* insecticidal toxins at the same time. Provided that the toxins bind to different receptors, it is extremely unlikely that an insect will develop resistance to both toxins at the same time. When this approach is used in transgenic plants, it is often called "gene pyramiding."
2. Application of a *B. thuringiensis* insecticidal toxin along with traditional chemical insecticides. The idea here is that almost no insect survives these two very different treatments, and resistance does not develop to either. Transgenic plants that produce a

B. thuringiensis insecticidal toxin are commonly treated with chemical insecticides. However, the number of chemical insecticide treatments is significantly reduced when the plants produce a *B. thuringiensis* insecticidal toxin. In Florida, nontransgenic corn plants often require as many as 10 sprayings of chemical insecticides per growing season. Plants that produce a *B. thuringiensis* insecticidal toxin are more likely to be sprayed with chemical insecticides only about three or four times a season.

3. Application of a *B. thuringiensis* insecticidal toxin at the same time as another biologically based insecticidal protein (typically isolated from plants; see chapter 18). Again, it is extremely unlikely that the target insects will survive both types of insecticides.

4. The use of two *B. thuringiensis* insecticidal toxins, one of which has had its toxin gene modified so that it binds to a different receptor than the other toxin.

5. The use of refugia (small tracts of land where the crop is not treated with the microbial insecticide). Approximately 20% of a crop is not sprayed with *B. thuringiensis* (or 20% is nontransgenic, with the remaining 80% of the plants being transgenic and producing a *B. thuringiensis* insecticidal toxin). The wild-type insects can proliferate in the absence of the *B. thuringiensis* insecticidal toxin, and only (a very small number of) mutant insects that are resistant to the high levels of *B. thuringiensis* insecticidal toxin survive in the presence of the toxin. Upon mating, the small number of resistant insects will all mate with sensitive insects, so that the next generation will contain mostly homozygous sensitive insects and a small number of heterozygous sensitive insects. This strategy assumes that resistance to the *B. thuringiensis* insecticidal toxin is inherited as a recessive trait. This approach has been used in the field for a number of years, with all of the available evidence indicating that little to no resistance to any *B. thuringiensis* insecticidal toxins has developed.

As noted above, fusion of the coding portions of the active regions of two different toxin genes is another way of generating a novel protein with extended toxicity. This idea has been examined in laboratory experiments. When a series of lepidopteran-specific hybrid toxins were constructed, some of them were more toxic than the products of either of the contributing genes by themselves, and in one case, a hybrid protein had acquired a totally new biological activity.

Generally, resistance to *B. thuringiensis* insecticidal toxins is the consequence of a mutation(s) that alters an insect midgut receptor protein(s) so that it no longer binds to the Cry protein. However, if a toxin gene were engineered so that the toxin bound to more than one midgut cell surface protein, then resistance might be less likely to arise, since it would require alterations to several proteins.

The insecticidal proteins Cry1Ca and Cry1Ea are both toxic to lepidoptera but have different species specificities. Cry1Ca is active against *S. exigua, Mamestra brassicae,* and *Manduca sexta,* while Cry1Ea is active only against *M. sexta.* In one experiment, hybrid Cry1Ca–Cry1Ea proteins were constructed and tested for their toxicities to different insect species, as well as for their abilities to bind to different receptors (Fig. 16.12). The hybrid toxin G27, which contained domain III from Cry1Ca, was toxic to *S. exigua*

	Domain I	Domain II	Domain III	Toxic to *S. exigua*	Competes for Cry1C site	Competes for Cry1E site
Cry1C				+	+	−
Cry1E				−	−	+
G27				+	−	+
F26				−	+	−

FIGURE 16.12 Toxicities and binding specificities of Cry1Ca, Cry1Ea, and hybrid toxins G27 and F26. A toxin–receptor-binding assay was used to determine binding specificities. Unlabeled Cry1Ca or Cry1Ea was added to a complex of the *S. exigua* midgut receptor protein and radiolabeled toxin, and the extent of binding of the radiolabeled toxin was determined. Adapted from Bosch et al., *Bio/Technology* 12:915–918, 1994.

larvae even though it bound to the Cry1Ea receptor but not to the Cry1Ca receptor (Fig. 16.13). Conversely, the hybrid toxin F26 was not toxic to *S. exigua* larvae even though it bound to the Cry1Ca receptor. Since the Cry1Ca and G27 proteins bind to different insect midgut receptors (although both are toxic to *S. exigua*), either simultaneous or alternating treatments of *S. exigua* with these two *B. thuringiensis* insecticidal toxins might limit the development of strains that are resistant to the toxins. Resistance to both Cry1C and G27 would require mutations in two separate midgut proteins.

B. thuringiensis subsp. israelensis thwarts insect resistance. In contrast to what has been observed with other strains of *B. thuringiensis*, no instances of field resistance of mosquitoes to *B. thuringiensis* subsp. *israelensis* have ever been reported, and only low levels of resistance have been observed in laboratory studies. This lack of insect resistance may reflect the fact that, in addition to synthesizing at least three different Cry proteins—Cry4A, Cry4B, and Cry11A—*B. thuringiensis* subsp. *israelensis* also produces Cyt1A, a highly hydrophobic endotoxin that is not at all homologous to any of the Cry proteins and appears to have a completely different mode of action. While Cry proteins bind to glycoproteins on the insect midgut epithelial membrane, the primary affinity of Cyt1A is the lipid component of the membrane, especially the unsaturated fatty acids. Cyt1A acts synergistically with the Cry proteins, and its presence may explain why mosquitoes do not develop resistance to the Cry proteins. In one series of experiments, using purified insecticidal proteins, it was demonstrated that with the addition of the Cyt1A protein, insects that had become resistant to Cry4A, Cry4B, and Cry11A (all of which are encoded by *B. thuringiensis* subsp. *israelensis*) were killed when they were treated with *B. thuringiensis* subsp. *israelensis*. Recent experiments suggest that, following the binding of Cyt1A to the midgut epithelial membrane, the protein can act as a receptor for some of the Cry proteins encoded by *B. thuringiensis* subsp.

FIGURE 16.13 Schematic representation of Cry1C binding to the Cry1C receptor and hybrid G27 binding to the Cry1E receptor. For Cry1C, CI, CII, and CIII indicate that these domains all originate from Cry1C. For G27, EII and EIII indicate that these domains are from Cry1E.

israelensis. The reason that *B. thuringiensis* subsp. *israelensis* is a highly effective insect pathogenic bacterium may be because the strain not only carries several insecticidal proteins, but also contains a protein that acts as the receptor for these insecticidal proteins. It is therefore extremely unlikely that any target insect will be able to develop resistance to *B. thuringiensis* subsp. *israelensis*. To capitalize on the advantage that the Cyt1A protein provides to *B. thuringiensis* subsp. *israelensis*, genes for Cyt1A and Cry1Ac (which is typically found in *B. thuringiensis* subsp. *kurstaki* strains and targets lepidopteran larvae) were used to transform a strain of *B. thuringiensis* (Fig. 16.14). The combination of these two proteins in one strain was highly toxic to the diamondback moth (*Plutella xylostella*), a lepidopteran species. On the other hand, strains that expressed one or the other of these proteins, but not both, required extremely high levels of the proteins before any toxicity could be detected. These results suggest, in this case, that Cyt1A (which usually targets diptera) is uncharacteristically behaving as a receptor for Cry1Ac (a lepidopteran toxin). It will be exciting to ascertain whether this synergism can be extended to other Cry proteins combined with Cyt1A.

Other strategies that have been proposed as a means of avoiding the development of insects that are resistant to *B. thuringiensis* insecticidal toxins include alternating the strain of *B. thuringiensis* that is employed from one season to the next, alternating *B. thuringiensis* treatment with the use of chemical or other biological insecticides, or applying mixtures of different strains of *B. thuringiensis*.

Improved Biocontrol

Insects such the sugarcane borer (*E. saccharina*) that attack the internal regions of plants such as sugar cane are not affected by *B. thuringiensis*-based insecticides that are sprayed onto leaves and shoots. However, it is possible to introduce the toxin gene from a *B. thuringiensis* strain into a bacterium that colonizes either plant roots or interior surfaces. In these instances, the insecticidal toxin is delivered to the part of the plant that is normally attacked by the insect.

FIGURE 16.14 Schematic representation of an engineered strain of *B. thuringiensis* encoding both Cyt1A (which is from *B. thuringiensis* subsp. *israelensis* and becomes the membrane-bound receptor) and Cry1A (the lepidopteran-specific insecticidal toxin) proteins.

In one series of experiments, researchers genetically engineered two different *P. fluorescens* strains that, when fed to *E. saccharina* larvae, acted synergistically in limiting the proliferation of the insect. One *P. fluorescens* strain was engineered to express the *cry1Ac7* gene under the transcriptional control of the *tac* promoter, with the entire construct integrated into the host chromosomal DNA. The other *P. fluorescens* strain was engineered to

TABLE 16.5 Synergistic effects of *P. fluorescens* expressing Cry1Ac7 toxin and *P. fluorescens* expressing chitinase on sugarcane borer larvae

Concentration (mg/g of diet)		Insect mortality (%)	
Toxin-producing strain	Chitinase-producing strain	Day 2	Day 5
0	0	5.5	7.6
0.3	0	12.5	33.8
3.0	0	30.8	42.7
0	0.3	8.2	20
0	30.0	21.8	42.7
0.3	0.3	39.3	55.7
0.3	30.0	37.5	68.3

Adapted from Downing et al., *Appl. Environ. Microbiol.* **66**:2804–2810, 2000.

Day 2 and Day 5 indicate the number of days after the treatment was started.

FIGURE 16.15 Location of α-chymotrypsin recognition and cut site within domain I of Cry3A and mCry3A. The letters represent the amino acid residues located between α-helices 3 and 4.

express a chitinase gene, originally isolated from the bacterium *Serratia marcescens,* also under the control of the *tac* promoter and integrated into the host chromosomal DNA. The chitinase is believed to cause perforations in the chitin-containing peritrophic membrane of the insect larvae, thereby lysing the membrane and killing the larvae, as well as increasing the accessibility of the midgut membranes to the *B. thuringiensis* insecticidal toxin. In laboratory tests, each of these *P. fluorescens* strains separately was toxic to *E. saccharina* larvae (Table 16.5). Moreover, when the two *P. fluorescens* strains were used together, there was significant synergism between the treatments so that low levels of both strains yielded a high level of insect mortality. Ideally a bacterial endophyte that can colonize the interior surfaces of the plant, rather than a surface-colonizing bacterial strain, would be preferred as a host strain, and of course, the efficacy of any construct must be demonstrated in the field, as well as in the laboratory.

Other workers have reported that the expression of a chitinase gene in a mosquitocidal strain of *B. sphaericus* (which is similar to *B. thuringiensis* subsp. *israelensis*) yielded a recombinant strain that was ~4,300 times more toxic than the wild type against a strain of the mosquito *Culex quinquefasciatus* that is considered to be resistant to the wild-type strain. The higher toxicity of the chitinase-expressing strain is thought to reflect the fact that chitinase digestion facilitates the interaction between the insecticidal toxin and its target cells.

While the Cry3A protein is an effective insecticide against the Colorado potato beetle *(Leptinotarsa decemlineata)*, it shows very little activity against the western corn rootworm *(Diabrotica undecempunctata howardi)*. Researchers speculated that the low level of activity against the western corn rootworm might reflect the fact that in this insect, proteolytic cleavage of the precursor form of the toxin is not sufficient for biological activity. That is, processing of Cry3A by the protease chymotrypsin might be necessary to increase the solubility and functional binding of the insecticide to the insect brush border membrane. It was found that the normal Cry3A chymotrypsin cleavage site (Fig. 16.15) was not efficiently cleaved in vitro. However, when a new enzyme recognition site for chymotrypsin was introduced into Cry3A (near the existing site), cleavage of the modified protein (mCry3A) by chymotrypsin increased substantially, and the protein solubility and insecticidal activity of the protein against the western corn rootworm, both in vitro and in vivo, also increased. Before a strain of *B. thuringiensis* that carries a gene for this modified Cry3A can be used in the environment, it will be necessary to elaborate its complete insect specificity and to ascertain (first in the laboratory) that this small modification in the structure of

TABLE 16.6 Some insect pests that are currently controlled with baculoviruses

Pest	Common name	Crop
Anticarsia gemmatalis	Velvetbean caterpillar	Soybean
Chrysomela scripta	Cottonwood leaf beetle	Trees
Cydia pomonella	Codling moth	Apple, walnut
Heliothis sp.	Cotton bollworm	Cotton, sorghum
Lymantria dispar	Gypsy moth	Deciduous trees
Mamestra brassicae	Cabbage moth	Vegetables
Neodiprion sertifer	European pine sawfly	Pine
Oryctes rhinoceros	Rhinoceros beetle	Coconut
Spodoptera exigua	Beet armyworm	Vegetables, flowers
Spodoptera littoralis	Egyptian cotton leaf worm	Cotton
Trichoplusia ni	Cabbage looper	Brassicas

Cry3A has not inadvertently generated any toxic activities against humans or other animals.

Activated Cry toxins bind to specific proteins (cadherins) on the surfaces of the microvilli of the insect midgut epithelial cells. Binding of toxin monomers to cadherins, which are transmembrane glycoproteins containing 12 cadherin repeating domains and one membrane-proximal extracellular domain (Fig. 16.16), facilitates the development of a multimeric form of the toxin monomers and formation of a pore in the membrane. Loss of cadherin or mutation of cadherin genes is generally associated with resistance to *B. thuringiensis*. A fragment of a cadherin protein containing the 12 repeating units and the membrane-proximal extracellular domain was mixed with Cry1A and fed to insect larvae. It was expected that the cadherin protein fragment would block the binding of the Cry1A protein to the midgut epithelial cells. Instead, its addition dramatically enhanced the Cry1A-induced insect mortality. The cadherin peptide fragment may first bind to microvilli and then attract Cry1A molecules, thereby increasing the probability of the toxin interacting with the bona fide receptor. It is thought that this approach, that is, the simultaneous application of Cry proteins and a peptide containing a portion of the receptor protein, will overcome or significantly delay the development of insect resistance by increasing Cry protein insect toxicity.

Baculoviruses as Biocontrol Agents

Mode of Action

Baculoviruses are rod-shaped double-stranded DNA viruses that can infect and kill a large number of different invertebrate organisms. Subgroups of this viral family are pathogenic to several orders of insects, including the Lepidoptera, Hymenoptera, Diptera, Neuroptera, Trichoptera, Coleoptera, and Homoptera. In nature, some of these baculoviruses are important for the control of certain pest insects, and several have been registered for use as biological insecticides. Baculoviruses were used in North America against forest pests, such as the spruce sawfly *(Neodiprion sertifer)*, starting in the 1930s and ending with the advent of chemical pesticides in the 1960s. Baculoviruses continue to be used on a limited basis—approximately 0.1% of the money spent on pest control is directed toward baculoviruses—mostly by the forestry industry in an effort to control the gypsy moth, *L. dispar* (Table 16.6). It has been estimated that the costs associated with the development, production, and use of baculoviruses in developing countries

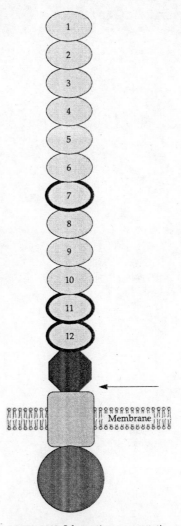

FIGURE 16.16 Schematic representation of a cadherin protein molecule embedded in a midgut epithelial membrane. Twelve cadherin domains are labeled. Domains 7, 11, and 12, which are highlighted, have been implicated as binding sites for Cry proteins. The purple region represents the membrane-proximal extracellular domain; the transmembrane domain is shown in light blue; and the cytoplasmic domain is shown in red. The arrow indicates the junction between the membrane-proximal extracellular domain and the transmembrane domain. The cadherin peptide analogue includes the 12 cadherin domains and the membrane-proximal extracellular domain.

are much less than in industrialized countries. This is due to lower material and labor costs in developing countries, as well as to the smaller size of farms in some countries, lower levels of agricultural mechanization, and less expensive registration procedures. Nevertheless, even in the more developed countries of the world, the costs of the development and registration of a naturally occurring baculovirus are much less than the costs for a chemical insecticide. However, because baculoviruses have a high degree of host specificity, it is necessary to develop a large number of different baculoviruses to deal with different insect pests, whereas a single chemical pesticide might control all of them.

The vast majority of baculoviruses used as biological control agents are members of the genus *Nucleopolyhedrovirus,* and all subsequent discussion of baculoviruses refers to viruses from this genus. A baculovirus particle consists of a cylindrical nucleocapsid that surrounds the viral DNA. Often, in the nucleus of an infected cell, baculovirus particles are embedded in a crystalline protein matrix called an occlusion body. The occlusion body, or polyhedron, is largely composed of the protein polyhedrin. When an infected insect dies, millions of polyhedra are released. Upon ingestion by an insect, the polyhedra move to the midgut, where the alkaline environment facilitates the dissolution of the polyhedrin protein coat, releasing infectious nucleocapsids. The nucleocapsids are taken up by the insect midgut cells and then migrate through the cytoplasm to the nucleus, where the nucleocapsid is removed. After viral replication, which takes place in the nucleus, and nucleocapsid assembly, some nucleocapsids are released by budding through the plasma membranes of infected cells into the circulatory system of the insect. Consequently, the infection spreads to other cells throughout the insect. It usually takes about 10 rounds of viral replication, or about 5 to 9 days, for the insect to die. At that stage, about 25% of the dry weight of the insect consists of polyhedra.

A positive feature of using baculoviruses as biocontrol agents is that they generally have limited host ranges and do not affect nontarget organisms. However, this means that any particular baculovirus can be used to control only a limited number of insect pests. Since baculoviruses coevolved with their insect hosts over thousands of years, they are well adapted to avoid the insect's defense mechanisms, and resistance to these viruses develops only rarely, and much less frequently than resistance to *B. thuringiensis.*

Control of the European spruce sawfly *(Gilipinia hercyniae)* population in eastern Canada is the best example of insect control by a baculovirus. European sawfly populations were reduced to below economic threshold levels by 1943 and remain under control today. Ironically, the reason why some baculoviruses are not used commercially is related to the effectiveness of the virus. If a virus is effective at preventing proliferation of a particular insect species, the virus has to be applied only once every year or so, making it difficult for the industry to justify the high registration costs. Farmers and growers prefer to use a single insecticidal agent that can control many different insect pests rather than a number of different insecticides, so if baculoviruses are to be used more extensively, their limited host range needs to be expanded.

It has been known for some time that when insect cells are infected with two different strains of baculovirus at the same time, new variant viruses with slightly different specificities can form after the two starting viruses have replicated. These new viruses are the product of homologous

recombination between the two starting viruses. Detailed analysis of this phenomenon revealed that a region of DNA that is only 79 base pairs (bp) long and located within the p143 helicase gene was sufficient to permit homologous recombination between different baculoviruses. More importantly, this 79-bp DNA segment may be responsible for the host ranges of different baculoviruses. Therefore, alteration of some of the nucleotides within this 79-bp DNA segment may allow researchers to generate baculoviruses with modified (expanded) insect specificities.

Genetic Engineering for Improved Biocontrol

Baculoviruses are relatively slow in killing target insects. Depending on conditions, it can take from a few days to several weeks before the viral infection leads to the host's death. To remedy this ineffectiveness, several attempts have been made to enhance the virulence of baculoviruses by introducing foreign genes that either severely impair or kill the targeted insect species (Table 16.7). One approach has been to use a gene that disrupts the normal life cycle of the insect when it is expressed within the host insect cells.

During insect development, a reduction in the level of juvenile hormone in larvae initiates metamorphosis into pupae and leads to a cessation of larval feeding. The reduction in the juvenile hormone level is due to an increase in the amount of juvenile hormone esterase, an enzyme that converts the biologically active methyl ester form of juvenile hormone into an inactive acid form. Inhibition of juvenile hormone esterase activity leads to an in vivo accumulation of active juvenile hormone, so the larvae remain in the feeding stage longer, continue to grow, and eventually become giant larvae. Therefore, researchers reasoned that an experimentally induced increase in the supply of juvenile hormone esterase should lower the endogenous level of active juvenile hormone and cause a premature cessation of feeding. Basically, their premise was that shortening the duration of larval feeding would curtail the extent of crop damage.

To test this idea, the investigators first had to clone and express the gene for juvenile hormone esterase. This task was achieved by purifying the enzyme from the tobacco budworm (*Heliothis virescens*), determining its amino acid sequence, synthesizing a DNA oligomer that corresponds to a portion of the esterase amino acid sequence, and then using this oligomer as a hybridization probe. The coding sequence for juvenile hormone esterase was isolated from an *H. virescens* complementary DNA (cDNA) library and inserted into the genome of a baculovirus under the control of baculovirus transcription signals. When the cabbage looper (*Trichoplusia ni*)

TABLE 16.7 Some genes that have been introduced into the baculovirus genome to increase insecticidal activity

Gene	Effect on host insect of introduced gene
Diuretic hormone	Reduced hemolymph volume
Juvenile hormone esterase	Feeding cessation
B. thuringiensis toxin	Feeding cessation
Scorpion toxin	Paralysis
Mite toxin	Paralysis
Wasp toxin	Premature melanization, low weight gain

FIGURE 16.17 Survival of *T. ni* larvae after treatment of cabbage leaves with either wild-type or recombinant baculovirus expressing a scorpion neurotoxin gene. The control cabbage plants were treated only with insect larvae. The lower the percentage of live larvae recovered, the greater the killing of the larvae and the more effective the treatment. Plants were treated with baculovirus only once at the start of the experiment.

at the first larval instar stage was treated with this genetically modified baculovirus, the amount of juvenile hormone in the insect was reduced by the cloned juvenile hormone esterase, and larval feeding and growth were dramatically curtailed relative to feeding and growth by the control larvae that were treated with native baculovirus.

The usefulness of this approach for enhancing baculoviruses as general biocontrol agents has been questioned, because the reduction in larval feeding that is attributable to the effect of juvenile hormone esterase is confined to the first larval instar. Other stages of development are much less sensitive to this treatment. A baculovirus engineered to express juvenile hormone esterase would have to be applied when the majority of the target insect population was in its first larval instar stage, which, under natural conditions, is difficult to achieve.

Another approach for enhancing the effectiveness of baculoviruses as a pesticide is to incorporate into the viral genome an insect-specific toxin gene that, when expressed during the viral infection cycle, will yield a potent insect toxin. The gene that encodes the insect-specific neurotoxin produced by the North African fat-tailed scorpion (*Androctonus australis* Hector) was cloned into a baculovirus strain, and the genetically engineered virus was tested as a biological insecticide. This neurotoxin, which does not have any effect on mice, disrupts the flow of sodium ions in the neurons of targeted insects and eventually leads to paralysis and death. Laboratory-raised insects that were infected with a baculovirus carrying the scorpion neurotoxin gene caused 50% less damage to the leaves of test plants than did insects that had been treated with wild-type baculovirus.

When the cDNA for the toxin from the Israeli yellow scorpion (*Leiurus quinquestriatus hebraeus*) was cloned and introduced into the baculovirus *Autographa californica* multiple nuclear polyhedrosis virus, the time that it took to kill 50% of the insect larvae that were tested was reduced from 120 to 78 h. Moreover, 120 h after infection, the insect larvae treated with recombinant virus gained only one-third as much weight as larvae treated

with wild-type virus. Thus, this engineered baculovirus not only hastened the demise of the infected insect larvae, it also significantly decreased the ability of the insects to damage plants. Subsequent experiments have taken this system a step further. Researchers have studied the effects of different scorpion toxins, either separately or two at a time. They assessed whether either a combination of excitatory and depressant or alpha and depressant scorpion toxins would improve the efficacy of *A. californica* nuclear polyhedrosis virus, over a virus expressing only a single toxin, toward three different insect larvae. The best result was achieved by combined expression of the excitatory toxin and the depressant toxin. Under these conditions, the "effective time to paralysis" of *H. virescens* neonates was reduced to slightly less than 47 h. Additional improvements to this system have come from placing the scorpion toxin(s) under the transcriptional control of the *p-PCm* promoter, which contains the human cytomegalovirus minimal (*CMVm*) promoter ligated in *cis* with the polyhedrin upstream (*pu*) sequence. This results in a high level of expression of foreign genes at an early infection stage of the baculovirus.

Recently, a genetically engineered *A. californica* nuclear polyhedrosis virus that expresses the insect-specific neurotoxin from *Androctonus australis* was tested under field conditions. Interestingly, the modified baculovirus was even more effective in the field than in the laboratory studies that demonstrated a 25 to 50% reduction in the time it took to kill the insect pest *T. ni* (Fig. 16.17). In the field, the genetically engineered baculovirus killed the insect pests faster, decreased the damage to cabbage plants, and reduced the secondary cycle of infection (infections caused by the next generation of the virus) compared to the wild-type virus.

No matter how effective a particular genetically engineered baculovirus may be in small-scale experiments, a major hurdle to more widespread use is the difficulty and cost of propagating such viruses. Baculoviruses are obligate parasites; therefore, they must be grown either in living whole organisms or in insect cell culture. In more developed countries, the cost of baculovirus preparations, whether or not the virus has been genetically engineered, is not currently competitive with that of chemical insecticides. However, biological insecticides may become more appealing when the adverse environmental impact of chemical insecticides is factored into the cost-benefit analysis.

SUMMARY

Microbial insecticides are currently being developed as environmentally friendly biological substitutes for chemical pesticides. A number of subspecies of the bacterium *B. thuringiensis* produce a protoxin as part of a parasporal crystal that, after ingestion, kills specific insects. The transition from insecticidal protoxin to toxin occurs in the gut of the target insect and is mediated by the pH and digestive proteases in the gut. The death of the insect is the consequence of the formation of membrane channels in the gut cells, which allow ATP to escape and in turn lead to decreased cellular metabolism, cessation of feeding, dehydration, and eventually death. The *B. thuringiensis* toxins are highly specific for a limited number of insect species, nontoxic to nontarget species, and biodegradable. Consequently, they are unlikely to cause significant biological selection for resistant forms under normal conditions. These attributes make these biological insecticides effective agents for controlling insect damage to certain crops and preventing the proliferation of insects that act as vectors of human diseases.

The genes (*cry*) for various *B. thuringiensis* toxins have been cloned and characterized. By expressing a *B. thuringiensis cry* gene in a nonsporulating *Bacillus* strain, production of the insecticidal protein was achieved during vegetative growth, bypassing the need for parasporal crystal formation.

To expand the specificity of a *B. thuringiensis* toxin to other pest insects, toxin genes from different subspecies were cloned into plasmids and introduced into another *B. thuringiensis* strain, either on a broad-host-range plasmid or by integration into the chromosomal DNA of the host cell. In addition to expressing the toxicity of the original strain, the bacteria with

two different toxin genes sometimes showed an effect against a nontarget insect pest. In one study, it was found that modification of domain II of the Cry protein is an effective means of increasing its toxicity to particular insects. Similarly, a fusion protein consisting of two toxin domains from different B. thuringiensis toxin genes was constructed by genetic manipulation, and the fusion protein retained both toxic activities. In another study, the receptor-binding domain of one insecticidal toxin was combined with the toxin domain of another. It is thought that insect resistance is less likely to develop when such hybrid toxins are used. In addition, the simultaneous application of Cry proteins and a peptide containing a portion of the host Cry receptor protein increases Cry protein insect toxicity, another strategy that can be used to overcome or significantly delay the development of insect resistance to Cry proteins. A further strategy that can both improve biocontrol activity and serve to limit the development of B. thuringiensis-resistant insects is the use of B. thuringiensis toxins together with other insecticidal proteins, such as chitinase or the B. thuringiensis subsp. israelensis Cyt1A protein.

To ensure that B. thuringiensis spraying for the control of mosquitoes is effective, the B. thuringiensis toxin genes have been cloned into various microorganisms that live near the surfaces of ponds and are eaten by mosquito larvae. This strategy appears to be an effective means of delivering the B. thuringiensis toxin to the targeted insect. Also, rhizosphere bacteria that have been engineered with B. thuringiensis toxin genes lessen the damage caused by insects that attack the roots of plants.

Baculoviruses are pathogenic to many different species of insects, but each strain of baculovirus is specific to a small number of insect species. Although baculoviruses kill their host organisms, the process is usually considered to be too slow to be effective for controlling insects that attack crop plants. However, when certain genes are cloned into different strains of baculovirus, the virus can act as a delivery system for a gene that produces an insecticidal protein during the viral life cycle. Several tests of this strategy have been successful in laboratory trials. In addition, when a gene for a neurotoxin that kills insects was cloned into a baculovirus, the construct was effective in field trials.

REFERENCES

Abdullah, M. A. F., O. Alzate, M. Mohammad, R. J. McNall, M. J. Adang, and D. H. Dean. 2003. Introduction of Culex toxicity into Bacillus thuringiensis Cry4Ba by protein engineering. Appl. Environ. Microbiol. 69:5343–5353.

Abdullah, M. A. F., and D. H. Dean. 2004. Enhancement of Cry19Aa mosquitocidal activity against Aedes aegypti by mutations in the putative loop regions of domain II. Appl. Environ. Microbiol. 70:3769–3771.

Ananda Kumar, P., R. P. Sharma, and V. S. Malik. 1996. The insecticidal proteins of Bacillus thuringiensis. Adv. Appl. Microbiol. 42:1–43.

Aronson, A. I., and Y. Shai. 2001. Why Bacillus thuringiensis insecticidal toxins are so effective: unique features of their mode of action. FEMS Microbiol. Lett. 195:1–8.

Audtho, M., A. P. Valatis, O. Alzate, and D. H. Dean. 1999. Production of chymotrypsin-resistant Bacillus thuringiensis Cry2Aa1 δ-endotoxin by protein engineering. Appl. Environ. Microbiol. 65:4601–4605.

Baum, J. A., and T. Malvar. 1995. Regulation of insecticidal crystal protein production in Bacillus thuringiensis. Mol. Microbiol. 18:1–12.

Bosch, D., B. Schipper, H. van der Kleij, R. A. de Maagd, and W. J. Stiekema. 1994. Recombinant Bacillus thuringiensis crystal proteins with new properties: possibilities for resistance management. Bio/Technology 12:915–918.

Bravo, A., S. S. Gill, and M. Soberón. 2007. Mode of action of Bacillus thuringiensis Cry and Cyt toxins and their potential for insect control. Toxicon 49:423–435.

Broderick, N. A., K. F. Raffa, and J. Handelsman. 2006. Midgut bacteria required for Bacillus thuringiensis insecticidal activity. Proc. Natl. Acad. Sci. USA 103:15196–15199.

Cai, Y., J. Yan, X. Hu, B. Han, and Z. Yuan. 2007. Improving the insecticidal activity against resistant Culex quinquefasciatus mosquitoes by expression of chitinase gene chiAC of Bacillus sphaericus. Appl. Environ. Microbiol. 73:7744–7746.

Calogero, S., A. M. Albertini, C. Fogher, R. Marzari, and A. Galizzi. 1989. Expression of a cloned Bacillus thuringiensis delta-endotoxin gene in Bacillus subtilis. Appl. Environ. Microbiol. 55:446–453.

Caramori, T., A. M. Albertini, and A. Galizzi. 1991. In vivo generation of hybrids between two Bacillus thuringiensis insect-toxin-encoding genes. Gene 98:37–44.

Cerda, H., and M. G. Paoletti. 2004. Genetic engineering with Bacillus thuringiensis and conventional approaches for insect resistance in crops. Crit. Rev. Plant Sci. 23:317–323.

Chejanovsky, N., N. Zilberberg, H. Rivkin, E. Zlotkin, and M. Guervitz. 1995. Functional expression of an alpha anti-insect scorpion neurotoxin in insect cells and lepidopterous larvae. FEBS Lett. 376:181–184.

Chen, J., G. Hua, J. L. Jurat-Fuentes, M. A. Abdullah, and M. J. Adang. 2007. Synergism of Bacillus thuringiensis toxins by a fragment of a toxin-binding cadherin. Proc. Natl. Acad. Sci. USA 104:13901–13906.

Cory, J. S., M. L. Hirst, T. Williams, R. S. Hails, D. Goulson, B. M. Green, T. M. Carty, R. D. Possee, P. J. Cayley, and D. H. L. Bishop. 1994. Field trial of a genetically improved baculovirus insecticide. Nature 370:138–140.

Crickmore, N., C. Nicholls, D. J. Earp, T. C. Hodgman, and D. J. Ellar. 1990. The construction of Bacillus thuringiensis strains expressing novel entomocidal δ-endotoxin combinations. Biochem. J. 270:133–136.

Crickmore, N., D. R. Zeigler, J. Fewitelson, E. Schnepf, J. Van Rie, D. Lereclus, J. Baum, and D. H. Dean. 1998. Revision of the nomenclature for the *Bacillus thuringiensis* pesticidal crystal protein. *Microbiol. Mol. Biol. Rev.* **62**:807–813.

Croizier, G., L. Croizier, O. Argaud, and D. Poudevigne. 1994. Extension of *Autographa californica* nuclear polyhedrosis virus host range by interspecific replacement of a short DNA sequence in the p143 helicase gene. *Proc. Natl. Acad. Sci. USA* **91**:48–52.

De Maagd, R. A., A. Bravo, and N. Crickmore. 2001. How *Bacillus thuringiensis* has evolved specific toxins to colonize the insect. *Trends Genet.* **17**:193–199.

Downing, K. J., G. Leslie, and J. A. Thomson. 2000. Biocontrol of the sugarcane borer *Eldana saccharina* by expression of the *Bacillus thuringiensis cry1Ac7* and *Serratia marcescens chiA* genes in sugarcane-associated bacteria. *Appl. Environ. Microbiol.* **66**:2804–2810.

Ferré, J., M. D. Real, J. Van Rie, S. Jansens, and M. Peferoen. 1991. Resistance to the *Bacillus thuringiensis* bioinsecticide in a field population of *Plutella xylostella* is due to a change in a midgut membrane receptor. *Proc. Natl. Acad. Sci. USA* **88**:5119–5123.

Ge, A. Z., N. I. Shivarova, and D. H. Dean. 1989. Location of the *Bombyx mori* specificity domain on a *Bacillus thuringiensis* δ-endotoxin protein. *Proc. Natl. Acad. Sci. USA* **86**:4037–4041.

Gelernter, W., and G. E. Schwab. 1993. Transgenic bacteria, viruses, algae and other microorganisms as *Bacillus thuringiensis* toxin delivery systems, p. 89–104. *In* P. F. Entwistle, J. S. Cory, M. J. Bailey, and S. Higgs (ed.), *Bacillus thuringiensis, an Environmental Biopesticide: Theory and Practice*. John Wiley & Sons, Chichester, United Kingdom.

Hammock, B. D., B. C. Bonning, R. D. Possee, T. N. Hanzlik, and S. Maeda. 1990. Expression and effects of the juvenile hormone esterase in a baculovirus vector. *Nature* **344**:458–461.

Held, G. A., L. A. Bulla, E. Ferrari, J. Hoch, A. I. Aronson, and S. A. Minnich. 1982. Cloning and localization of the lepidopteran protoxin gene of *Bacillus thuringiensis* subsp. *kurstaki. Proc. Natl. Acad. Sci. USA* **79**:6065–6069.

Herrera, G., S. J. Snyman, and J. A. Thomson. 1994. Construction of a bio-insecticidal strain of *Pseudomonas fluorescens* active against the sugarcane borer, *Eldana saccharina. Appl. Environ. Microbiol.* **60**:682–690.

Kalman, S., K. L. Kiehne, N. Cooper, M. S. Reynoso, and T. Yamamoto. 1995. Enhanced production of insecticidal proteins in *Bacillus thuringiensis* strains carrying an additional crystal protein gene in their chromosomes. *Appl. Environ. Microbiol.* **61**:3063–3068.

Lampel, J. S., G. L. Canter, M. B. Dimock, J. L. Kelly, J. J. Anderson, B. B. Uratani, J. S. Foulke, Jr., and J. T. Turner. 1994. Integrative cloning, expression, and stability of the *cryIA(c)* gene from *Bacillus thuringiensis* subsp. *kurstaki* in a recombinant strain of *Clavibacter xyli* subsp. *cynodontis. Appl. Environ. Microbiol.* **60**:501–508.

Lereclus, D., H. Agaisse, M. Gominet, and J. Chaufaux. 1995. Overproduction of encapsulated insecticidal crystal proteins in a *Bacillus thuringiensis spo0A* mutant. *Bio/Technology* **13**:67–71.

Lereclus, D., A. Delécuse, and M. M. Lecadet. 1993. Diversity of *Bacillus thuringiensis* toxins and genes, p. 37–69. *In* P. F. Entwistle, J. S. Cory, M. J. Bailey, and S. Higgs (ed.), *Bacillus thuringiensis, an Environmental Biopesticide: Theory and Practice*. John Wiley & Sons, Chichester, United Kingdom.

Liu, J. T., M. J. Sui, D. D. Ji, I. H. Wu, C. C. Chou, and C. C. Chen. 1993. Protection from ultraviolet radiation by melanin of mosquitocidal activity of *Bacillus thuringiensis* var. *israelensis. J. Invertebr. Pathol.* **62**:131–136.

Liu, J. W., W. H. Yap, T. Thanabalu, and A. G. Porter. 1996. Efficient synthesis of mosquitocidal toxins in *Asticcacaulis excentricus* demonstrates potential of gram-negative bacteria in mosquito control. *Nat. Biotechnol.* **14**:343–347.

Maeda, S. 1995. Further development of recombinant baculovirus insecticides. *Curr. Opin. Biotechnol.* **6**:313–319.

McCutchen, B. F., P. V. Choudary, R. Crenshaw, D. Maddox, S. G. Kamita, N. Palekar, S. Volrath, E. Fowler, B. D. Hammock, and S. Maeda. 1991. Development of a recombinant baculovirus expressing an insect-selective neurotoxin: potential for pest control.

Bio/Technology **9**:848–852.

Mettus, A. M., and A. Macaluso. 1990. Expression of *Bacillus thuringiensis* δ-endotoxin genes during vegetative growth. *Appl. Environ. Microbiol.* **56**:1128–1134.

Murphy, R. C., and E. S. Stevens. 1991. Cloning and expression of the *crylVD* gene of *Bacillus thuringiensis* subsp. *israelensis* in the cyanobacterium *Agmenellum quadruplicatum* PR-6 and its resulting larvicidal activity. *Appl. Environ. Microbiol.* **58**:1650–1655.

Obukowicz, M. G., F. J. Perlak, K. Kusano-Kretzmer, E. J. Mayer, S. L. Bolten, and L. S. Watrud. 1986. Tn5-mediated integration of the delta-endotoxin gene from *Bacillus thuringiensis* into the chromosome of root-colonizing pseudomonads. *J. Bacteriol.* **168**:982–989.

Obukowicz, M. G., F. J. Perlak, K. Kusano-Kretzmer, E. J. Mayer, and L. S. Watrud. 1986. Integration of the delta-endotoxin gene of *Bacillus thuringiensis* into the chromosome of root-colonizing strains of pseudomonads using Tn5. *Gene* **45**:327–331.

Perez, C., L. F. Fernandez, J. Sun, J. L. Folch, S. S. Gill, M. Soberón, and A. Bravo. 2005. *Bacillus thuringiensis* subsp. *israelensis* Cyt1Aa synergizes Cry11Aa toxin by functioning as a membrane-bound receptor. *Proc. Natl. Acad. Sci. USA* **102**:18303–18308.

Priest, F. G. 1992. Biological control of mosquitoes and other biting flies by *Bacillus sphaericus* and *Bacillus thuringiensis. J. Appl. Bacteriol.* **72**:357–369.

Regev, A., H. Rivkin, B. Inceoglu, E. Gershburg, B. D. Hammock, M. Gurevitz, and N. Chejanovsky. 2003. Further enhancement of baculovirus insecticidal efficacy with scorpion toxins that interact cooperatively. *FEBS Lett.* **537**:106–110.

Sanchis, V., M. Gohar, J. Chaufaux, O. Arantes, A. Meier, H. Agaisse, J. Cayley, and D. Lereclus. 1999. Development and field performance of a broad-spectrum nonviable asporogenic recombinant strain of *Bacillus thuringiensis* with greater potency and UV resistance. *Appl. Environ. Microbiol.* **65**:4032–4039.

Sayyed, A. H., N. Crickmore, and D. J. Wright. 2001. Cyt1Aa from *Bacillus thuringiensis* subsp. *israelensis* is toxic to the diamondback moth, *Plutella*

xylostella, and synergizes the activity of Cry1Ac towards a resistant strain. *Appl. Environ. Microbiol.* 67:5859–5861.

Schnepf, E., N. Crickmore, J. Van Rie, D. Lereclus, J. Baum, J. Feitelson, D. R. Zeiger, and D. H. Dean. 1998. *Bacillus thuringiensis* and its pesticidal crystal proteins. *Microbiol. Mol. Biol. Rev.* 62:775–806.

Schnepf, H. E., and H. R. Whiteley. 1981. Cloning and expression of the *Bacillus thuringiensis* crystal protein gene in *Escherichia coli*. *Proc. Natl. Acad. Sci. USA* 78:2893–2897.

Stewart, L. M. D., M. Hirst, M. L. Ferber, A. T. Merryweather, P. J. Cayley, and R. D. Possee. 1991. Construction of an improved baculovirus insecticide containing an insect-specific toxin gene. *Nature* 352:85–88.

Thanabalu, T., J. Hindley, S. Brenner, C. Oei, and C. Berry. 1992. Expression of the mosquitocidal toxins of *Bacillus sphaericus* and *Bacillus thuringiensis* subsp. *israelensis* by recombinant *Caulobacter crescentus*, a vehicle for biological control of aquatic insect larvae. *Appl. Environ. Microbiol.* 58:905–910.

Thiery, I., L. Nicholas, R. Rippka, and N. Tandeau de Marsac. 1991. Selection of cyanobacteria isolated from mosquito breeding sites as a potential food source for mosquito larvae. *Appl. Environ. Microbiol.* 57:1354–1359.

Tomalski, M. D., and L. K. Miller. 1991. Insect paralysis by baculovirus-mediated expression of a mite neurotoxin gene. *Nature* 352:82–84.

Tuan, S.-J., R. F. Hou, C.-F. Lee, and Y.-C. Chao. 2007. High level production of polyhedra in a scorpion toxin containing recombinant baculovirus for better control of insect pests. *Bot. Stud.* 48:273–281.

Walters, F. S., C. M. Stacy, M. K. Lee, N. Palekar, and J. S. Chen. 2008. An engineered chymotrypsin/cathepsin G site in domain I renders *Bacillus thuringiensis* Cry3A active against western corn rootworm larvae. *Appl. Environ. Microbiol.* 74:367–374.

Whalon, M. E. and B. A. Wingerd. 2003. Bt: mode of action and use. *Arch. Insect Biochem. Physiol.* 54:200–211.

Wirth, M. C., G. P. Georghiou, and B. A. Federici. 1997. CytA enables CryIV

endotoxins of *Bacillus thuringiensis* to overcome high levels of CryIV resistance in the mosquito, *Culex quinquefasciatus*. *Proc. Natl. Acad. Sci. USA* 94:10536–10540.

Wood, H. A., and R. R. Granados. 1991. Genetically engineered baculoviruses as agents for pest control. *Annu. Rev. Microbiol.* 45:69–87.

Xu, Y., M. Nagai, M. Bagdasarian, T. W. Smith, and E. D. Walker. 2001. Expression of the p20 gene from *Bacillus thuringiensis* H-14 increases Cry11A toxin production and enhances mosquito-larvicidal activity in recombinant gram-negative bacteria. *Appl. Environ. Microbiol.* 67:3010–3015.

Yamamoto, T., S. Kalman, G. Powell, N. Cooper, and D. Cerf. 1998. Environmental release of genetically engineered *Bacillus thuringiensis*. *Rev. Toxicol.* 2:157–166.

Yap, W. H., T. Thanabalu, and A. G. Porter. 1994. Expression of mosquito-cidal toxin genes in a gas-vacuolated strain of *Ancylobacter aquaticus*. *Appl. Environ. Microbiol.* 60:4199–4202.

REVIEW QUESTIONS

1. What are the advantages of biological insecticides over chemical insecticides?

2. Draw a simple phylogenetic tree that shows the relationship among Cry1Aa, Cry1Ab, Cry1Ba, Cry1Bb, Cry2Aa, and Cry2Ab.

3. Why is the *B. thuringiensis* toxin not toxic to humans?

4. Outline a strategy that you would use to isolate an insecticidal protoxin gene from *B. thuringiensis* subsp. *israelensis*. How would you use this gene in a practical way?

5. How would you determine whether a particular insecticidal protoxin gene is present on a plasmid or part of the chromosome of a *B. thuringiensis* strain?

6. How would you use genetic engineering to improve the usefulness of a particular *B. thuringiensis* protoxin?

7. If a *cry1C–cry1Ab* fusion gene encoding an insecticidal protoxin consists of approximately 2,200 bp of DNA from the *cry1C* gene and 1,300 bp of DNA from the *cry1Ab* gene, what is the advantage of synthesizing this fusion protoxin compared with the *cry1C* protoxin?

8. How can insect gut enzymes be limited to processing the

B. thuringiensis insecticidal protoxin to the active toxin without degrading the toxin?

9. How would you engineer a Cry protein to lessen or avoid the development of insect resistance to this toxin?

10. Why is the bacterium *A. excentricus* an attractive host organism for the expression of *B. thuringiensis* insecticidal toxin genes?

11. How can the species range of an insecticidal *B. thuringiensis* strain be extended?

12. What is a truncated *B. thuringiensis* insecticidal protoxin?

13. Why is it unlikely that insects will ever develop resistance to *B. thuringiensis* subsp. *israelensis* strains?

14. What are cadherins, and how can they be used to enhance the toxicity of a particular Cry protein?

15. How would you improve the insecticidal properties of baculoviruses?

16. How might it be possible to expand the range of insects that are infected by a particular baculovirus?

17

Large-Scale Production of Proteins from Recombinant Microorganisms

T HE PRODUCTION OF COMMERCIAL PRODUCTS that are synthesized by genetically engineered microorganisms requires the partnership of two kinds of experts. Molecular biologists are responsible for isolating, characterizing, modifying, and creating effectively expressed genes in microorganisms that can be used for industrial production, and biochemical engineers ensure that the genetically engineered form of a microorganism can be grown in large quantities under conditions that give optimal product yields. In the early days of molecular biotechnology, biologists naively thought that scale-up was simply a matter of multiplication; i.e., they believed that whatever conditions were found to be effective on a small scale would be equally effective on a large scale and that to achieve this it was merely necessary to use a larger reaction vessel with a correspondingly larger volume of medium.

This simplistic view is far from reality. For example, good growth of aerobic microorganisms can usually be achieved in a standard 200-mL laboratory flask that is aerated with a mixer driven by a 300-watt motor. If the system were directly scaled up, a single 10,000-liter container would require a mixer with a 15-megawatt motor. Such a motor would be as large as a house, and the heat generated during stirring would boil the microorganisms. Although biochemical engineers may quibble about some aspects of this specific example, they all know that the industrial production of microorganisms is not merely a multiplication of bench scale conditions. For a start, increasing the size of the reaction vessel (bioreactor, or fermenter) is required for the large-scale growth of microorganisms, because it would be impractical to set up 50,000 individual culture flasks, each containing 200 mL, to obtain 10,000 liters of cell suspension.

A number of parameters must be precisely regulated to obtain maximum yields from either small (1- to 10-liter) or large (>1,000-liter) bioreactors. These parameters include the temperature, pH, rate and nature of mixing of the growing cells, and, with aerobic organisms, oxygen demand. Moreover, the optimal conditions generally change with each 10-fold increase in the volume of a bioreactor.

There are also other technical considerations. The design of the bioreactor is important. It should ensure adequate sterility and provide appropriate levels of containment of genetically engineered microorganisms. The reactor should also include probes that permit the accurate and continuous on-line monitoring of as many critical reaction parameters as possible so that adjustments can be made rapidly and easily throughout the course of the fermentation reaction (i.e., the growth of the microorganism). In addition, because sterilization may alter the composition of the medium (e.g., by destroying vitamins), it is important to ascertain that the medium composition is still optimal for maximal microbial growth following sterilization.

Generally, large-scale fermentation and product purification are stepwise processes (Fig. 17.1). A typical procedure begins with formulation and sterilization of the growth medium and sterilization of the fermentation equipment. The cells are grown first as a stock culture (5 to 10 mL), then in

FIGURE 17.1 Generalized scheme for a large-scale fermentation process. The commercial product is usually in either the cell or cell-free fraction, but not in both; consequently, one or the other of these fractions will be processed further (+) or discarded (–).

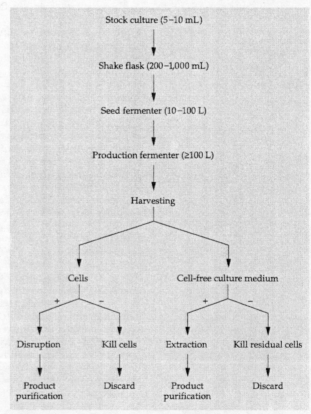

a shake flask (200 to 1,000 mL), and then in a seed fermenter (10 to 100 liters). Finally, the production fermenter (1,000 to 100,000 liters) is inoculated. After the fermentation step is completed, the cells are separated from the culture fluid by either centrifugation or filtration. If the product is intracellular, the cells are disrupted, the cell debris is removed, and the product is recovered from the debris-free fluid. If the product is extracellular, it is purified from the cell-free culture medium.

Principles of Microbial Growth

Microorganisms can be grown in batch, fed-batch, or continuous culture (Fig. 17.2). In batch fermentation, the sterile growth medium is inoculated with the appropriate microorganisms, and the fermentation proceeds without the addition of fresh growth medium. In fed-batch fermentation, nutrients are added incrementally at various times during the fermentation reaction; no growth medium is removed until the end of the process. In the continuous fermentation process, fresh growth medium is added continuously during fermentation, but there is also concomitant removal of an equal volume of spent medium containing suspended microorganisms. For each type of fermentation, oxygen (which is usually provided in the form of sterile air), an antifoaming agent, and, if required, acid or base are injected into the bioreactor as needed.

Batch Fermentation

During a batch fermentation, the composition of the culture medium, the concentration of microorganisms (biomass concentration), the internal chemical composition of the microorganisms, and the amount of either target protein or metabolite all change as a consequence of the state of cell growth, cellular metabolism, and availability of nutrients. Under these conditions, six typical phases of growth are usually observed: lag phase, acceleration phase, logarithmic (log) or exponential phase, deceleration phase, stationary phase, and death phase (Fig. 17.3).

Typically, there is no immediate increase in the numbers of cells after the inoculation into sterilized growth medium. This initial period is called

FIGURE 17.2 Schematic representation of the time course (progress curves) of cell concentration (mass) and substrate concentration in batch **(A)**, fed-batch **(B)**, and continuous **(C)** fermentations.

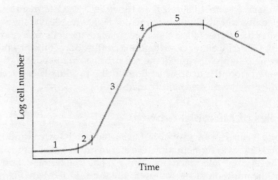

FIGURE 17.3 Pattern of microbial cell growth in a batch fermenter. The six phases of the growth cycle are (1) lag, (2) acceleration, (3) log (exponential), (4) deceleration, (5) stationary, and (6) death.

the lag phase. During the lag period, the microbial cells adapt to the new environmental conditions. The cells may have to adjust to a different pH or to a new level of available nutrients. As part of an adaptive response, previously unexpressed metabolic pathways may be induced. A lag phase generally occurs whenever the cells of the inoculum are derived from a culture that has stopped growing (i.e., has entered stationary phase) because of substrate limitation or product inhibition. These cells need time to reset their metabolic systems to adjust to the new medium. The length of the lag phase corresponds to how long the inoculated cells were in stationary phase and the extent to which the previous growth medium of the starting cells differed from the new, fresh culture medium. Conversely, when the inoculum is a cell culture from a growing cell population in log phase, a discernible lag phase may not occur and growth may begin immediately. Following the lag phase, the brief period when the rate of cell growth increases until log-phase growth is attained is called the acceleration phase.

During the log phase of growth, the cell mass undergoes several cell doublings and the specific growth rate of the culture remains constant. With excess substrate (nutrient supply) and no inhibition of growth by a compound that is present in the growth medium, the specific growth rate is independent of the substrate concentration. These changes and other related steps can be represented in mathematical form, making it possible for biochemical engineers to precisely model and then more easily scale up microbial cell growth. In this case, the rate of increase of the cell biomass with time, dX/dt, is the product of the specific growth rate, μ, and the biomass concentration, X:

$$dX/dt = \mu X$$

Similarly, the rate of increase of the cell number, dN/dt, is the product of the specific growth rate, μ, and the cell number, N:

$$dN/dt = \mu N$$

The specific growth rate, μ, is a function of the concentration of the limiting substrate (i.e., the carbon or nitrogen source), S; the maximum specific

growth rate, μ_{max}; and a substrate-specific constant, K_s. Both S and K_s are expressed in terms of concentration, e.g., in either grams or moles per liter:

$$\mu = \mu_{max}S/(K_s + S)$$

Sometimes, scientists refer to the doubling or generation time, t, of a culture rather than to its specific growth rate, μ, where $t = \ln 2/\mu$. The generation time of a culture is the length of time that it takes, under defined conditions, for the number of cells or the cell biomass to double. For the microorganisms that are commonly grown in culture, the value of μ_{max} varies from about 2.1 to 0.086 h^{-1} (reciprocal hours), which corresponds to doubling times of approximately 20 minutes to 8 hours.

When there is an excess of substrate (i.e., when $S >> K_s$), then $\mu = \mu_{max}$ and the maximal rate of log-phase growth of the culture occurs. In practice, the value of K_s is often so low that substrate levels equivalent to K_s are rarely encountered during log-phase growth. For example, for *Escherichia coli*, while the K_s for glucose is approximately 1 mg/liter, the initial glucose level is usually around 10,000 mg/liter. However, as the culture nears the end of the log phase, the concentration of the remaining substrate, S, is depleted and may even fall below the value of K_s. Under conditions where $S < K_s$, the microorganisms rapidly enter the deceleration phase. However, because of the large cell population at the end of the log phase, the substrate may be so rapidly assimilated that the deceleration phase is short-lived and not observable.

After either the depletion of a critical growth substance, such as the carbon source, from the medium or the accumulation of metabolic end products that inhibit growth, the increase in cell mass eventually ceases and the cells enter the stationary phase. During this phase, although the amount of biomass remains constant, cellular metabolism often changes dramatically; in some instances, compounds (secondary metabolites) that are of considerable commercial interest are synthesized. For example, antibiotics are usually produced during the stationary phase of the microbial growth cycle. The duration of the stationary phase depends on the particular organism and the conditions of growth.

In the death phase, the energy reserves of the cell are virtually exhausted, and metabolic activity ceases. For most commercial processes, the fermentation reaction is halted and the cells are harvested before the death phase begins.

Fed-Batch Fermentation

In fed-batch fermentations, substrate is added in increments at various times throughout the course of the reaction. These additions prolong both the log and stationary phases, thereby increasing the biomass and the amount of synthesis of stationary-phase metabolites, such as antibiotics. However, microorganisms in stationary phase often produce proteolytic enzymes (proteases), and these enzymes can degrade proteins synthesized by a genetically engineered microorganism. Therefore, when proteins are produced from a recombinant microorganism, it is important that the fermentation reaction not be allowed to reach this part of the growth cycle. Because it is often difficult to measure the substrate concentration directly during the fermentation reaction, other indicators that are correlated with the consumption of substrate, such as the production of organic acids,

MILESTONE

**Expression of Intracellular Hemoglobin Improves
Protein Synthesis in Oxygen-Limited *Escherichia coli***
C. KHOSLA, J. E. CURTIS, J. DEMODENA, U. RINAS, and J. E. BAILEY
Bio/Technology 8:849–853, 1990

Because of the low solubility of oxygen in water, the growth of aerobic bacteria often becomes limited by the amount of dissolved oxygen in the fermentation broth. This problem is especially acute at high cell densities or when fermentations are performed on a large scale. To address this problem, chemical engineers have attempted to increase the rate of transfer of introduced oxygen to the liquid of the growth medium. Their approaches have included (1) sparging the growth medium with pure oxygen rather than with air; (2) introducing the air (or oxygen) under pressure; (3) adding chemicals, such as perfluorocarbons, to the fermentation broth to increase the solubility of oxygen; and (4) modifying the configuration of the fermentation vessel to optimize the aeration or agitation of the fermentation broth. While all of these solutions to the "oxygen problem" are somewhat effective, they are subject to a threshold effect beyond which it is impossible to introduce a sufficient amount of oxygen to improve the final yield of the fermentation.

As an alternative to these "hardware" solutions, Bailey and coworkers designed a biological system in which the host organism was modified so that it would be more efficient at using the low levels of oxygen that are normally present in the growth medium. They cloned a gene encoding a hemoglobin-like molecule from the gram-negative bacterium *Vitreoscilla* and introduced it into several different recombinant bacteria. The introduced bacterial hemoglobin bound oxygen from the environment and created a higher level of available oxygen within the cells, which resulted in an increase in growth and foreign-gene expression. This approach provided a clever biological solution to what at first glance seemed to be an almost insurmountable engineering problem.

changes in the pH, or the production of CO_2, can be used to estimate when additional substrate is needed. Generally, fed-batch fermentations require more monitoring and greater control than batch fermentations and are therefore used to a lesser extent. However, since they may be advantageous in the development of systems for the production of proteins from recombinant microorganisms, they are becoming increasingly popular.

The periodic addition of substrate to a growing microbial culture prolongs the log phase of growth and delays the onset of the stationary phase, which initiates cellular stress responses, the production of proteases, and other metabolic changes that affect the yield of a recombinant protein. Nevertheless, with continued cell growth, an increasing amount of the incoming substrate is needed for maintenance of the host cell metabolism. This means that fewer cellular resources are used for the synthesis of the recombinant protein or commercial metabolite(s). To ensure that the synthesis and stability of a recombinant protein are not impaired, increasing amounts of nutrients must be added to the growing culture. This may be done by carefully monitoring the fermentation reaction and adding substrates (carbon and nitrogen sources, together with trace elements) in increasing amounts as they are needed. Depending upon the particular microorganism, its genetic background, and the nature of the recombinant protein, a fed-batch fermentation strategy can increase the yield from 25% to more than 1,000% compared with batch fermentation.

Fed-batch processes are not limited to microbial cells but are also used with mammalian and insect cells in culture. This is important because (1) these cell culture systems are increasingly being used for the production of human therapeutic proteins, and (2) in the absence of fed-batch strategies, animal cells in batch culture are not very efficient in producing foreign proteins.

Continuous Fermentation

In a continuous fermentation, a steady-state condition, where $dX/dt = 0$, is attained when the total number of cells and the total volume in the bioreactor remain constant. In other words, under these conditions, the loss of cells due to outflow (product removal) is exactly balanced by the gain in new cells by growth (division). In more formal terms, for a continuous steady-state fermentation process, the dilution rate, D, is defined as the volumetric flow rate, F, divided by the constant liquid volume, V, in the bioreactor:

$$D = F/V$$

where D is equal to the specific growth rate, μ:

$$D = (dX/dt)(1/X) = \mu$$

To obtain hydrodynamically stable continuous cultures, the specific growth rate, μ, of the culture must be lower than the maximum attainable specific growth rate, μ_{max}. In practice, this condition is achieved by adjusting a pump that controls the volumetric flow rate, F, while keeping the volume of the culture within the bioreactor, V, constant.

The fundamental objective of industrial fermentations is to minimize costs and maximize yields. This goal can be achieved by developing the most efficient mode of fermentation for each particular process. Although the commercial use of continuous fermentation processes is typically limited to production of single-cell protein, antibiotics, and organic solvents, primarily because of the greater experience that scientists have with growing cells in batch mode, the cost of producing a specific amount of cell biomass by continuous culture is potentially much lower than producing the same amount by batch fermentation. The following factors account for the savings.

- Continuous fermentations use smaller bioreactors than batch fermentations to produce the same amount of product.
- After a large-scale batch fermentation is completed, large-scale equipment is needed for cell harvesting, cell breakage, and subsequent downstream processing (purification) of the protein or metabolite product that is produced by the microorganism. Continuously grown cells, however, are produced "a little bit at a time," so that the equipment required for cell harvesting, cell breakage, and downstream processing can be much smaller.
- Continuous fermentation, by definition, avoids the "down time" between batch runs, during which the bioreactor is prepared for reuse. A common hindrance to efficient industrial fermentation is the loss of productivity due to the down time of the bioreactor for repairs, cleaning, or sterilization. Continuous fermentations have less down time, because a single reaction can be maintained for a much longer period.
- The physiological state of the cells during continuous fermentation is more uniform, so that yields of product are more consistent. In batch fermentations, small differences in the timing of cell harvest, which coincides with the mid- to late log phase of growth, can lead to significant physiological differences.

Despite its merits, continuous fermentation has potential drawbacks that must be addressed before its use becomes more widespread.

- The duration of a continuous fermentation can be 500 to 1,000 hours, and therefore, some cells might lose recombinant plasmid constructs. Cells that lack plasmids usually have a smaller energy burden and divide faster than do plasmid-containing microorganisms, so that yields may decline with time because fewer cells are synthesizing the product protein. Integration of the cloned gene into the genome of the host organism avoids this problem.

- Maintenance of sterile conditions on an industrial scale for long periods is difficult. Furthermore, continuous processes need sterile backup equipment, a requirement that can greatly increase capital costs.

- The composition of culture medium that is used for industrial fermentations is not subject to the same level of quality assurance as that accorded laboratory medium components and therefore may vary from batch to batch. This variation can alter the physiology of the cells and decrease productivity.

Because batch fermentation has a proven history of reliability, there is reluctance to switch to another type of fermentation system, even though a continuous mode of operation is generally regarded as the most efficient fermentation strategy. Nevertheless, a number of researchers have recently developed, on the scale of a laboratory (up to 10 liters) or pilot plant (up to 1,000 liters), both continuous and fed-batch processes for the production of proteins from recombinant microorganisms. Therefore, it is probably only a matter of time before the use of continuous and fed-batch fermentations becomes more widespread in industry.

Maximizing the Efficiency of the Fermentation Process

Regardless of the type of fermentation process that is used to grow cells, it is necessary to monitor and control culture parameters, such as the dissolved oxygen concentration, pH, temperature, and degree of mixing. Changes in any one of these parameters can have a dramatic effect on the yield of cells and the stability of the protein product.

Optimal growth of *E. coli* cells and many other microorganisms that are used as hosts for cloned genes usually requires large amounts of dissolved oxygen. The maximal oxygen demand in a fermentation, Q_{max}, is dependent on the cell mass, X; the maximal specific growth rate, μ_{max}; and the growth yield based on oxygen consumed, Y_{O_2}, where

$$Q_{max} = X\mu_{max}/Y_{O_2}$$

Because oxygen is only sparingly soluble in water (0.0084 gram/liter at 25°C), it must be supplied continuously—generally in the form of sterilized air—to a growing bacterial culture. However, the introduction of air into a bioreactor produces bubbles, and if the bubbles are too large, the rate of transfer of oxygen to the cells is insufficient to support optimal growth. Thus, fermenter design should include provision for monitoring the dissolved-oxygen level of the culture, providing oxygen to the culture, and adequately mixing the culture to efficiently disperse the bubbles.

Most microorganisms grow optimally between pH 5.5 and 8.5. However, during growth in a bioreactor, cellular metabolites are released into the growth medium, a process that can change the pH of the medium. Therefore, the pH of the medium must be monitored and either acid or base must be added as needed to maintain a constant pH. Of course, the added acid or base must be well mixed into the fermentation broth so that the pH of the growth medium is the same throughout the entire reaction vessel.

Maintenance of the correct temperature is essential for the success of a fermentation reaction. Microorganisms grown at a temperature below the optimum grow slowly and have a reduced rate of cellular production (productivity). On the other hand, if the growth temperature is too high—but not lethal—there may be premature induction of the expression of the target protein, if it is under the control of a temperature-sensitive repressor, or induction of a heat shock (stress) response, which will produce cellular proteases that lower the yield of the protein product.

Adequate mixing of a microbial culture is essential for many aspects of a fermentation, including assurance of an adequate supply of nutrients to the cells and prevention of the accumulation of any toxic metabolic by-products in local, poorly mixed regions of the bioreactor. Effective mixing is relatively easily attained with small-scale cultures, but it is one of the major problems when the scale of fermentation is increased.

Agitation of the fermentation broth also affects other factors, such as the rate of transfer of oxygen from the gas bubbles to the liquid medium and then from the medium to the cells, efficient heat transfer, accurate measurement of specific metabolites in the culture fluid, and efficient dispersion of added solutions, such as acids, bases, nutrients, or antifoaming agents. On these grounds, it might be concluded that the more mixing there is, the better the growth. However, excessive agitation of a fermentation broth can cause hydromechanical stress (shear), which damages larger microbial or mammalian cells, and a temperature increase, which may also decrease cell viability. Thus, a balance must be struck between the need to provide thorough mixing and the need to avoid damage to the cells.

There is an additional consideration for scaled-up fermentations that has nothing to do with the technical aspects of the process but depends instead on whether a genetically engineered microorganism is being used. In most countries, specific rules and regulations must be followed when genetically engineered microorganisms are grown on a large scale. Although most recombinant microorganisms are not hazardous, it is nevertheless important to ensure that they are not inadvertently released into the environment. Therefore, fail-safe systems are used to prevent accidental spills of live recombinant organisms and to contain them if they occur. Furthermore, all recombinant microorganisms must be treated by an approved procedure to render them nonviable before they are discharged from the production facility. The spent culture medium must also be treated to ensure that it does not contain viable organisms and that its disposal does not create an environmental problem.

High-Density Cell Cultures

A major objective of fermentation is to maximize the volumetric productivity, i.e., to obtain the largest amount of product in a given volume in as

short a time as possible. High cell densities are absolutely necessary for high productivity. Generally, when foreign proteins are produced by recombinant *E. coli,* the greater the final cell density, the greater the amount of product that is formed. In practice, cell concentrations of more than 50 (and in a few cases more than 150) grams (dry weight) of cells per liter of culture have been obtained with fed-batch cultures of recombinant *E. coli.* The dry weight of *E. coli* cells is approximately 20 to 25% of the wet weight.

One way to achieve a high density of *E. coli* cells is to optimize the growth medium. Some nutrients, including carbon and nitrogen sources, can inhibit cell growth if they are present at too high a concentration. Glucose is inhibitory above 50 grams per liter, ammonia is inhibitory above 3 grams per liter, iron is inhibitory above 1.15 grams per liter, magnesium is inhibitory above 8.7 grams per liter, phosphorus is inhibitory above 10 grams per liter, and zinc is inhibitory above 0.038 gram per liter. Therefore, merely increasing the amount of nutrients in the growth medium in batch culture does not necessarily yield a high cell density. In addition, since the nutrients in complex media, such as peptone or yeast extract, can vary from one batch of medium to another, fermentations that use complex media are not always reproducible.

Acetate, which can be inhibitory to cell growth, is produced by *E. coli* both when the cells are grown under oxygen-limiting conditions and in the presence of excess glucose. The acetate problem can be minimized by using glycerol instead of glucose as a carbon source, lowering the culture temperature, or using an *E. coli* strain that has been genetically engineered to shunt acetate into less toxic compounds (see below).

Oxygen may also become limited in high-density cell cultures. To overcome this problem, the rate of introduction of air (sparging), the agitation rate, or both can be increased. Also, pure oxygen rather than air, which is only approximately 20% oxygen, can be introduced into growing cell cultures. Cells can also be grown under pressure to increase the solubility of oxygen, which increases the rate of transfer of oxygen to the cells in the aqueous growth medium. Alternatively, expression in host cells of the *Vitreoscilla* hemoglobin gene in a number of different organisms has been shown to significantly increase the uptake of oxygen by growing cells and to thereby increase the amount of product formed (see chapter 6). For example, *Vitreoscilla* hemoglobin can enhance growth and heterologous protein production in *E. coli,* improve enzyme production in *Bacillus subtilis,* increase erythromycin production by *Saccharopolyspora erythraea,* improve the rate of degradation of benzoic acid by *Xanthomonas maltophilia,* and enhance the production of cephalosporin C by *Acremonium chrysogenum.*

High-density cell cultures are most readily attained in fed-batch cultures. The addition of nutrients following the depletion of some of the original nutrients may be constant, stepwise, or exponential. With constant-rate feeding, nutrients are added at the same rate throughout the fermentation. However, under these conditions, the specific growth rate continually declines. With stepwise feeding, increasing amounts of nutrients are added at higher cell concentrations. In this case, the specific growth rate decline is largely compensated for. With exponential feeding, nutrients are added at an exponential rate, with the result that a constant specific growth rate can be achieved. It is possible to automate the fed-batch addition of nutrients based on measuring the concentration of a growth-limiting substrate, such as glucose, in the culture medium during the fermentation process.

Increasing Plasmid Stability

The loss of plasmids during the large-scale growth of recombinant *E. coli* cells is a major industrial problem. Plasmid loss often limits the yield of plasmid-encoded recombinant proteins, especially when cells are grown in continuous culture. Plasmid instability in bacterial cultures is typically a consequence of the unequal distribution of plasmids to daughter cells during growth and cell division. Generally, once cells have lost a plasmid, they grow faster, with the result that cells lacking plasmids eventually dominate the culture. One approach to avoid this problem is to include an antibiotic resistance gene on the plasmid being used and then add that antibiotic to the culture medium. In addition to the obvious economic cost of the antibiotic, especially when dealing with large-scale cultures, disposal of spent growth medium is a potential environmental hazard in that both the antibiotic and antibiotic resistance genes may be released into the environment. One way to get around this problem is to delete an essential gene from the chromosomal DNA of the host bacterium and at the same time place this gene on the plasmid that is being stabilized. As a result, only plasmid-carrying cells can grow, making the bacterial strain totally dependent upon maintenance of the plasmid. In one example, the essential gene that was used encoded translation initiation factor 1 (Fig. 17.4). The target gene was placed under the transcriptional control of the strong and IPTG (isopropyl-β-D-thiogalactopyranoside)-inducible p^{trc} promoter.

FIGURE 17.4 Schematic representation of a bacterial cell in which the essential protein synthesis initiator factor 1 gene *(infA)* was deleted from the chromosome and included on a plasmid. The target gene is under the transcriptional control of the strong Trc promoter *(p^{trc})* that is controlled by the *lac* repressor encoded by *lacI^q*, which overproduces the protein.

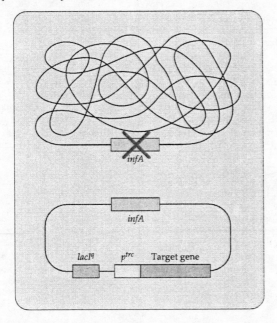

With this system, selection that utilizes antibiotics is no longer necessary, thereby decreasing both the cost and the environmental risk associated with large-scale fermentation.

Quiescent *E. coli* Cells

While it is possible to achieve high levels of foreign-gene expression in *E. coli* and other bacterial host cells, it is difficult to engineer recombinant bacteria to produce large amounts of a foreign protein and, at the same time, to grow to a high cell density. This is because a recombinant bacterial cell partitions its resources between production of the foreign protein and cell growth. It would be advantageous to be able to first grow cells to a high density and then to shift the allocation of available resources from growth to foreign-protein production. With this in mind, one group of workers engineered a quiescent cell expression system in which a plasmid-encoded protein is expressed in nongrowing but metabolically active cells. The quiescent state is established by the overexpression of Rcd, a regulatory protein, in an *hns* mutant *E. coli* host cell. The *hns* gene codes for a histone-like nucleoid-structuring protein. Cultures of the *hns* mutant of *E. coli* in which the *rcd* gene is induced gradually cease synthesizing host proteins but continue synthesizing plasmid-encoded foreign proteins for many hours after induction. In one study that utilized this system, the *rcd* gene was placed under the transcriptional control of the p^R promoter while the recombinant protein gene (encoding a single-chain antibody variable fragment [scFv]) was controlled by the p^L promoter (Fig. 17.5). The activities of both the p^R and p^L promoters are repressed by a temperature-sensitive cI repressor protein; in this system, the gene for this protein is encoded in the host chromosomal DNA. When cells are grown at 30°C, the cI repressor prevents transcription from both p^R and p^L. When the temperature is shifted to 42°C, the temperature-sensitive cI repressor protein is inactivated, and transcription can proceed from both p^R and p^L (see chapter 6). The temperature shift therefore causes the cells to become quiescent and at the same time to synthesize the recombinant scFv protein. In this particular case, the scFv protein contained a leader peptide that directed ~90% of the protein to be secreted into the growth medium. As shown in Table 17.1, in both batch and fed-batch modes, the quiescent cells produce less biomass and secrete considerably more of the scFv protein into the growth medium than do control *E. coli* host cells engineered to express scFv under the control of the p^L promoter. Understanding the commercial potential of this unique system, the scientists who developed this approach have applied for a patent to protect their intellectual property rights.

Protein Secretion

High-level cytoplasmic expression in *E. coli* of many different foreign proteins results in the formation of inclusion bodies consisting of insoluble improperly folded protein. Even when the foreign protein is soluble, purifying it from a cytoplasmic extract can be a major undertaking. In addition, sometimes proteins that are secreted into the growth medium are produced at a much higher level than when they are expressed in the cytoplasm. While these considerations make only a small difference in laboratory-scale experiments, they are of critical importance when foreign proteins are produced on a large scale.

FIGURE 17.5 Synthesis of a single-chain antibody fragment (scFv) in "quiescent *E. coli* cells." At 30°C, the *cI* repressor, encoded by *cI857* (inserted into the chromosomal DNA), binds to the operators of the *p*R and *p*L promoters and prevents transcription of the plasmid-encoded *scFv* and *rcd* genes. At 42°C, the temperature-sensitive *cI* repressor is inactivated so that transcription directed by the *p*R and *p*L promoters proceeds. Turning on the *p*R promoter causes the Rcd protein to be synthesized, thereby causing the cells to become quiescent. At the same time, turning on the *p*L promoter activates transcription of the gene encoding scFv. When the *rcd* gene is induced, a mutant of the *hns* gene causes the cessation of host cell protein synthesis.

TABLE 17.1 Cell growth and foreign protein (scFv) secreted into the growth medium for *E. coli* cells with induced quiescence compared to control (wild-type) cells

Cell type	Batch culture		Fed-batch culture	
	Cell growth (optical density at 600 nm)	scFv secreted (mg/liter)	Cell growth (optical density at 600 nm)	scFv secreted (mg/liter)
Quiescent	3.5	37	20	150
Control	20	13	80	35

One group of investigators observed that expression levels were quite low when they expressed several different foreign proteins, i.e., human granulocyte-macrophage colony-stimulating factor, α-interferon 2b (IFN-α2b), or scFv, under the transcriptional control of the strong $p^m/xylS$ promoter/regulator system. The yields of human granulocyte-macrophage colony-stimulating factor and scFv, but not IFN-α2b, increased dramatically when the genes encoding these proteins were fused to a translocation signal sequence (Fig. 17.6). Interestingly, different translocation signal sequences were optimally effective with each of the proteins tested. To obtain a high level of expression of IFN-α2b, before assembling the construct, it was necessary to chemically synthesize the gene in order to eliminate the use of codons that are rarely used in *E. coli*. While the use of translocation signal sequences significantly stimulated the levels of expression of these three human proteins, depending on the protein and the translocation signal sequence, from 20 to 50% of the protein that was produced was found to be in an insoluble form. In order for this system to be used routinely for the large-scale production of human proteins in *E. coli*, a strategy that minimizes the extent of insoluble protein formation needs to be developed.

Reducing Acetate

It is often difficult to achieve high levels of foreign-gene expression and a high cell density at the same time because of the accumulation of harmful waste products, especially acetate, which inhibits both cell growth and protein production and also wastes carbon and energy resources. One strategy to reduce the inhibitory effects of acetate is to remove the acetate from the culture during the course of the fermentation. This may be achieved by several different methods, including continuous dialysis and the use of macroporous ion-exchange resins. However, these methods tend to remove nutrients that are necessary for cell growth along with the acetate.

Since acetate is often associated with the use of glucose as a carbon source, lower levels of acetate, and hence higher yields of protein, are generally obtained when fructose or mannose is used as a carbon source. Another strategy for reducing acetate accumulation in rich medium without impairing cell growth entails decreasing the glucose uptake rate of the cells by adding methyl α-glucoside, a glucose analogue, to the growing cells. The same effect has also been achieved by using an *E. coli* host cell that contained a mutation in *ptsG*, a gene encoding enzyme II in the glucose phosphotransferase system. In a comparison of batch cultures of wild-type and *ptsG* mutant *E. coli* cells in rich medium, with both carrying a plasmid expressing β-galactosidase activity, the wild-type cells attained a density of approximately 10 grams (dry weight) per liter, while the mutant cells attained more

FIGURE 17.6 Engineering proteins for high-level expression following high-cell-density growth. **(A)** A target protein gene is placed under the transcriptional control of the strong and inducible (in this case by m-toluic acid) p^m promoter. **(B)** The target gene is fused to any one of several different secretion signal sequences. **(C)** Rare codons are removed from protein coding sequences that are not well expressed by chemically synthesizing the entire gene. GM-CSF, granulocyte-macrophage colony-stimulating factor; IFN, IFN-α2b.

than 15 grams (dry weight) per liter. At the same time, the mutant cells synthesized about 25% more β-galactosidase per gram (dry weight) of cells than the wild-type cells did. Overall, the $ptsG$ mutant cells synthesized nearly twice as much β-galactosidase as did the wild-type cells.

Since it is often much easier and quicker to alter a particular host cell by genetic transformation than by mutagenesis and selection, alternative means of reducing acetate production in cells were developed. One of these methods includes introducing a gene (from *B. subtilis*) encoding the enzyme acetolactate synthase into *E. coli* host cells. This enzyme catalyzes the formation of acetolactate from pyruvate, thereby decreasing the flux through acetyl coenzyme A to acetate (Fig. 17.7). In practice, the acetolactate synthase genes are introduced into the cell on one plasmid, while the target gene (encoding the protein that is to be overexpressed in *E. coli*) is introduced on a second plasmid from a separate incompatibility group. The cells that were transformed with the acetolactate synthase genes produced 75% less acetate than the nontransformed cells and instead synthesized acetoin, which is approximately 50-fold less toxic to cells than acetate. The protein yield was also doubled.

An alternative strategy to converting acetate to acetoin is to redirect carbon flow to the tricarboxylic acid (TCA) cycle (citric acid cycle, or Krebs

FIGURE 17.7 Schematic representation of the pathways for glucose metabolism in an *E. coli* strain that has been transformed with a plasmid carrying the genes for the protein subunits of acetolactate synthase (ALS). Note that the conversion of glucose to biomass is a multistep process. CoA, coenzyme A.

cycle). This is necessary because recombinant protein production decreases carbon flow in the TCA cycle as a consequence of the withdrawal of the intermediates that serve as protein precursor biochemicals. In one study, workers overexpressed the gene for the enzyme phosphoenolpyruvate carboxylase, which converts phosphoenolpyruvate to oxaloacetate, with the result that they obtained a 17% increase in the specific growth rate of the *E. coli* cells and a 44% decrease in acetate production. Unfortunately, overexpressing this enzyme also decreases the amount of glucose uptake by the bacterial cells and diminishes the growth rate. As an alternative approach to replenishing the TCA cycle, another group of researchers transformed *E. coli* host cells with the gene for the enzyme pyruvate carboxylase, which converts pyruvate directly to oxaloacetate (Fig. 17.8). Since *E. coli* does not normally contain pyruvate carboxylase, the gene was isolated from a strain of the gram-negative bacterium *Rhizobium etli*. With the introduction of pyruvate carboxylase, acetate levels were decreased, the cell yield was increased, and the amount of foreign protein synthesized was increased (Table 17.2). This result reflects the fact that the addition of pyruvate carboxylase allows *E. coli* cells to use the available carbon more efficiently, directing it away from acetate toward biomass and protein formation. Although it has not been tested extensively, it is thought that this strategy may be a generally effective method for increasing the level of expression of foreign proteins produced in *E. coli* host cells.

Similar to the strategy discussed above, the TCA cycle may also be replenished by converting aspartate to fumarate (Fig. 17.8). To do this, *E. coli* host cells were transformed with the gene for L-aspartate ammonia lyase

FIGURE 17.8 Replenishment of the TCA cycle in *E. coli* by the introduction of a gene from *R. etli* encoding pyruvate carboxylase. This avoids the conversion of pyruvate to acetate. The TCA cycle may also be replenished by the introduction of a gene encoding aspartase, converting aspartate in the medium to fumarate. Note that the conversion of glucose to biomass is a multistep process. CoA, coenzyme A.

(aspartase) under the control of the strong *tac* promoter on a stable low-copy-number plasmid. Aspartase activity is induced by the addition of IPTG at the mid- to late log phase of growth. The target recombinant protein is introduced on a separate plasmid. Using this system in minimal medium containing aspartate, the production of different recombinant proteins could be increased up to fivefold, with 30 to 40% more biomass production.

Bioreactors

A cursory examination of the biochemical engineering literature may give the impression that there are a limitless number of bioreactor designs. However, closer inspection reveals that virtually all of these designs fall into three fundamental classes:

- Stirred-tank reactors (STRs), which have internal mechanical agitation (Fig. 17.9A)
- Bubble columns, which rely on the introduction of air or another gas (sparging) for agitation (Fig. 17.9B)

- Airlift reactors, which have either an internal (Fig. 17.9C) or an external (Fig. 17.9D) loop; the mixing and circulation of the culture fluid in these reactors are the results of the motion of an introduced gas (usually air), which causes density differences within the different parts of the bioreactor.

The traditional, and by far the most commonly used, bioreactor is the STR. This type of bioreactor has several advantages over other bioreactor configurations.

- It has highly flexible operating conditions.
- It is readily available commercially.
- It provides efficient gas transfer to the growing microbial cells, or, in the words of fermentation engineers, the volumetric mass transfer coefficient, k_La, of STRs is high.
- It has been used extensively by fermentation engineers and microbiologists for growing a variety of microorganisms.

In an STR, gas, usually air, is added to the culture medium under pressure through a device called a sparger, which can be either a ring with many small holes or a tube with a single orifice. Although sparging rings generate smaller bubbles and consequently create better initial gas distribution, sparging tubes are often preferred in many small-scale applications (<20 liters) because they are less likely to become plugged. Thorough dispersion of the gas within the bioreactor requires one or more impellers (agitators) in addition to the sparger. Mechanical agitation of the culture medium by the impellers breaks larger bubbles into smaller ones, disperses the bubbles throughout the medium, and enhances the residence time of the bubbles in the bioreactor. At high levels of agitation, the mean size of the bubbles in large bioreactors is essentially independent of the size of the holes in the sparger. The type of impeller, its rotational speed, and the physicochemical properties of the liquid phase are important factors that give rise to efficient gas dispersion. In large bioreactors, however, if the initial gas distribution from the sparger is not uniform across the tank, even vigorous agitation may not create a homogeneous gas environment.

Because of the corrosive or abrasive nature of many culture media and sterilization procedures, STRs are usually constructed from stainless steel or glass. The glass units are usually limited to laboratory-scale bioreactors that have a capacity of <50 liters.

One limitation on the size of a bioreactor is the ability of the system to efficiently remove heat that is generated as a consequence of either the metabolism of the growing cells or the energy input by agitation. Too much heat raises the temperature and alters the physiological state of the cells,

TABLE 17.2 Relative acetate levels, cell yields, and foreign-protein activities from *E. coli* cells transformed with an *R. etli* pyruvate carboxylase gene

E. coli strain	Acetate concentration	Cell yield	Foreign-protein activity
− Pyruvate carboxylase	1.0	1.0	1.0
+ Pyruvate carboxylase	0.43	1.41	1.68

Adapted from March et al., *Appl. Environ. Microbiol.* **68**:5620–5624, 2002.

The foreign protein was β-galactosidase, whose activity is relatively easy to quantify. The data have been normalized to the values for the *E. coli* strain without (−) pyruvate carboxylase.

FIGURE 17.9 Simplified examples of bioreactor configurations. **(A)** STR; **(B)** bubble column; **(C)** internal-loop airlift reactor with a central draft tube; **(D)** external-loop airlift reactor. The arrows within the bioreactors indicate the direction of flow of the culture medium.

and decreases the product yield. Heat can be removed by using a cooling jacket around the reaction vessel or by internal coils. Although internal cooling coils are more effective than jackets in keeping the fermentation reaction close to the desired temperature, they can become fouled (coated) with microorganisms, which prevents cooling, and they sometimes interfere with the proper agitation of the fermentation broth.

Contamination of a fermentation with fungi or bacteria is usually disastrous. Therefore, bioreactors are designed so that they can be sterilized, usually with pressurized steam. There should be no internal dead spaces or surfaces that escape contact with the steam during sterilization. All seals, probes, and valves also must be readily steam sterilizable. When a bioreactor is designed, a trade-off is often made between a full set of ports for probes, which enables monitoring of the fermentation parameters, and fewer ports, which makes the maintenance of sterility easier.

The high level of agitation of the culture medium during a fermentation reaction often causes considerable foaming. Excessive foam can wet

the filter at the port through which the introduced air exits the bioreactor, thereby both decreasing the air flow and providing a potential pathway for the entry of contaminating cells. Either chemical antifoaming agents or mechanical foam breakers can be used to control foaming. However, the chemical agents can diminish the extent of microbial growth by preventing oxygen transfer or, in some cases, by inhibiting cellular enzymes. Furthermore, if an antifoaming compound is not removed before downstream processing, it can contaminate the final product. Foaming can also be controlled by providing sufficient "head space" within the bioreactor, i.e., space above the liquid in which the bubbles can dissipate. In practice, then, the "working volume," or actual volume of the culture, in an STR is typically only about 75% of the total volume of the bioreactor.

Many of the considerations that apply to STRs also apply to pneumatic reactors, such as bubble columns and airlift bioreactors. Thus, for example, sterility, constant pH, and constant temperature are key components of any fermentation, regardless of the precise configuration of the bioreactor.

The configurations of bubble columns and airlift bioreactors give them some distinct advantages over STRs. These pneumatic reactors are more energy efficient than STRs because agitation is provided by the injection of a stream of air—or another gas if anaerobic microorganisms are being grown—rather than by a mechanical stirrer. Also, with the elimination of the mixer shaft in these units, there is one less potential site of entry for contaminating organisms.

Pneumatic reactors generate a lower-shear environment than do STRs. Also, in airlift reactors, the shear stress is more evenly distributed throughout the vessel than in STRs. The reduction of shear forces is important for the following reasons.

- Genetically engineered microorganisms are often more susceptible to lysis when exposed to shear stress than are unmodified organisms, because the extra metabolic burden of synthesizing a foreign protein often causes genetically engineered microorganisms to form weakened cell walls.
- A frequent cellular response to the shear forces is decreased synthesis of all cellular proteins, including the recombinant protein.
- Shear stress can alter the physical and chemical properties of the cells so that the downstream processing steps become more difficult to perform. For example, the fermentation conditions can inadvertently increase the amount of surface polysaccharides that a microorganism produces and, as a consequence, can change the conditions for effective harvesting and lysis of these cells, making it more difficult to purify the target protein.

In bubble columns, the air is introduced under high pressure near the bottom, but the smaller bubbles coalesce into larger ones as they rise through the column, leading to uneven gas distribution. In addition, the use of high-pressure air tends to cause excessive foaming of the medium. These disadvantages restrict the flexibility or effective range of operating conditions, as well as the potential size of bubble columns.

Airlift bioreactors, however, can be readily adapted for either pilot plant or large-scale fermentation processes. In an airlift reactor, the gas is introduced into the bottom of a vertical channel (riser). Both the gas and liquid flow up the riser until they reach an open space at the top (gas–liquid separator), where the gas is at least partially disengaged from the liquid. The

degassed liquid, which is denser than the gassed liquid, descends in a separate vertical channel (downcomer) and moves along the base of the reactor until it reaches the bottom of the riser. In this way, the culture fluid and cells are continuously being circulated around the bioreactor.

There are two main types of airlift bioreactors: those that have a single container with internal baffles that create interior liquid circulation channels (internal-loop reactors) (Fig. 17.9C) and those that have an external loop so that the culture liquid circulates through separate, independent channels (external-loop reactors) (Fig. 17.9D). Internal-loop airlift reactors are simple in design, but once they are constructed, both the volume and the circulation rate are fixed for all fermentation processes. In contrast, the external loop of external-loop airlift reactors can be easily changed or modified, e.g., by altering its volume, to suit the requirements of different fermentations.

Airlift bioreactors are generally more efficient than bubble columns, especially for denser or more viscous suspensions of microorganisms. In airlift reactors, mixing is generally better, and bubble coalescence is not as big a problem as it is in bubble columns. In extremely large airlift fermenters, such as the 1,500,000-liter fermenter built by Imperial Chemical Industries, Ltd., in England for the production of single-cell protein, it takes a considerable amount of time for a cell to complete a full cycle through the reactor. To prevent the cells from becoming substrate depleted while they are traversing the bioreactor, there are multiple injection points for the introduction of substrate along the length of the unit.

Typical Large-Scale Fermentation Systems

When recombinant microorganisms are used to overproduce protein products, such as pharmaceuticals like insulin, cells are typically grown to mid- to late log phase of the growth cycle so that the target protein levels will be optimal. On the other hand, when recombinant microorganisms are used as "factories" to synthesize useful metabolites, such as antibiotics, host cells are commonly grown to the deceleration or stationary phase, where the synthesis of secondary metabolites is often optimal. Clearly, these sorts of differences must be considered when a large-scale fermentation process is being developed.

For maximal protein production, it is generally preferable to use cloned genes that are under the control of strong promoters that can be regulated. Initially, it was thought that constitutive expression of a cloned gene would be sufficient to obtain reasonable quantities of the product. However, experience has shown that continuous transcription and translation of a cloned gene drains energy from essential cell functions and slows cell growth. With an inducible system, the expression of a cloned gene can be confined to a specific period in the growth cycle of the microorganism. On these grounds, for optimal protein production, the process should consist of two separate stages. First, the cells are grown under optimum conditions to a relatively high cell density. Second, depending on the nature of the promoter that drives the cloned gene, transcription is induced either by shifting the temperature or by adding a chemical inducer, such as IPTG, to the medium.

A two-stage system is not easy to implement in a large bioreactor (>100 liters) because it is technically very difficult either to raise the temperature quickly, typically from 30 to 42°C, or to ensure that the chemical inducer is

rapidly and evenly mixed in a large vessel. Moreover, many chemical inducers, such as IPTG, are too expensive to be used on a large scale. However, as discussed below, this problem can be overcome by using two connected bioreactors (two-stage fermentation) so that the cells are grown in the first vessel and the induction is carried out in the second. Under these conditions, growth and induction are separately optimized, thereby increasing the overall amount of product formed per unit of time (productivity) of the fermentation.

Two-Stage Fermentation in Tandem Airlift Reactors

E. coli NM989, which carries the gene encoding the enzyme T4 DNA ligase under the transcriptional control of the p^L promoter and a temperature-sensitive *c*I repressor, was grown and induced in a two-stage airlift bioreactor. In this bacterial strain, the T4 DNA ligase gene was integrated in the chromosomal DNA, a location obviating any potential problems of plasmid instability that might occur during extended fermentation. The growth stage was carried out at 30°C in an external-loop airlift bioreactor that had a 10-liter working volume. The T4 DNA ligase gene was not expressed under these conditions. A second external-loop airlift bioreactor, with a working volume of approximately 5 liters at 42°C, was used for the induction stage (Fig. 17.10). The two bioreactors were linked by a transfer tube with a pump that controlled the continuous flow of cell suspension from the growth stage bioreactor (first) into the induction stage vessel (second). In addition, cells suspended in culture medium were removed from the induction stage bioreactor at a specific rate and prepared for downstream processing.

The maximal specific growth rate (μ_{max}) of the microbial culture was approximately 0.66 reciprocal hour in the first bioreactor and 0.54 reciprocal hour in the second. These values correspond to cell doubling times of 63 and 77 minutes, respectively. Fresh medium was continuously added at a rate of 2 liters per hour to the growth stage fermenter, and cell suspension (effluent) was simultaneously removed from the induction stage fermenter at the same rate. As a consequence of the liquid volumes of the two bioreactors, an average cell spent about 5 hours in the growth stage bioreactor and 2 hours in the induction stage bioreactor. The different residence times in the two phases of this fermentation process were necessary to optimize the number of cells produced and the yield and stability of the T4 DNA ligase. Generally, residence times can be altered as required by adjusting the relative working volumes in the two fermenters of a two-stage system and by adjusting the volumetric rate of input of nutrients into the first bioreactor.

The double-external-loop design of the airlift fermenter (Fig. 17.10) used in this work facilitated the adjustment of the working volumes of the two fermenters relative to one another. It also added versatility to the system, so that it was possible to obtain a variety of different growth conditions for different populations of recombinant cells. For T4 DNA ligase production, the best results were obtained when approximately 33 mL of cell suspension was transferred every minute from the growth stage bioreactor to the induction stage bioreactor. Because this amount of cell suspension was equivalent to only 0.67% of the volume of the induction stage bioreactor, the incoming cells underwent a virtually instantaneous temperature shift from 30 to 42°C. Nutrients in a concentrated form were added at a specific rate to the induction stage bioreactor throughout the

FIGURE 17.10 Two-stage airlift reactor used for the temperature-dependent induction of a protein product. Cells from the growth stage (left) fermenter, which is at 30°C, are pumped into the induction stage fermenter (right), which is at 42°C. Each bioreactor has a double external loop that is fitted with valves. By changing the valve settings, working volumes best suited for different fermentations can be created.

fermentation to keep the cells in this bioreactor in log phase. This action prevented the T4 DNA ligase from being degraded by the proteolytic enzymes that are normally synthesized during the deceleration and stationary phases.

With this continuous two-stage bioreactor, induced *E. coli* NM989 can be grown to a density of approximately 4 grams (dry weight) of cells per liter of culture. After induction, about 4% of the cell protein is T4 DNA ligase, an amount that corresponds to approximately 25,000 units of enzyme activity per gram (dry weight). This process can produce approximately 100,000 units of enzyme activity per liter of culture, or about 4,800,000 units per day. Assuming that it is possible to recover about 20% of the initial activity following purification of the enzyme and that the enzyme sells for about $0.25 per unit, then the final yield of purified

enzyme in 1 day will be worth about $240,000. Although these calculations do not consider all of the costs that go into the production of protein from a genetically engineered microorganism, it is clear that for highly valued products, small to moderate-size continuous fermentation systems can generate significant returns on the initial capital investment.

Two-Stage Fermentation in a Single Stirred-Tank Reactor

The tripartite fusion protein AGβ-Gal, which is used for immunological assays, was produced on a large scale in a single STR. The gene encoding AGβ-Gal was constructed by recombinant DNA techniques and encodes the five immunoglobulin G-binding regions of *Staphylococcus aureus* protein A, two immunoglobulin G-binding regions from *Streptococcus* sp. strain G148 protein G, and β-galactosidase from *E. coli*. The synthetic AGβ-Gal gene was placed under the control of the bacteriophage λ p^R promoter, which is regulated in the same manner as the p^L promoter; cloned into a plasmid that carries the gene for ampicillin resistance; and introduced by transformation into *E. coli*. The strain with the AGβ-Gal plasmid carries a second plasmid that has the genes for a temperature-sensitive *c*I repressor protein and a kanamycin resistance gene.

A 5-liter volume of these cells was grown in an STR at 30°C in the presence of both ampicillin and kanamycin—to provide selective pressure for the retention of both plasmids—and then used to initiate growth without antibiotics at 30°C in a 45-liter STR. The cell suspension in the 45-liter fermenter in turn served as an inoculum for a 600-liter STR, where the cells were grown at 30°C without antibiotics (Fig. 17.11). In general, to keep the cost of the process to a minimum, antibiotics are not added to large-scale microbial cultures. When the cell density in the 600-liter bioreactor reached the equivalent of about 4 grams (dry weight) per liter of growth medium, the temperature was shifted from 30 to 40°C to induce the expression of the AGβ-Gal protein. Under these conditions, it takes about 1 hour to reach 40°C. A temperature of 40°C rather than 42°C was chosen because the lower temperature was found to yield the same level of AGβ-Gal protein while allowing the cells to grow for a longer time. In other words, the low-temperature (40°C) conditions yielded a larger amount of protein product.

The specific activity of the AGβ-Gal protein increased for 2 hours after the initiation of the induction and then decreased. This decrease in activity was probably due to the synthesis of proteases by cells that had entered the deceleration and stationary phases of the growth cycle. In addition, 50% of the cells had lost their plasmids after growth for 4 hours at 40°C. These problems notwithstanding, after 4 hours at 40°C, the AGβ-Gal protein was approximately 20% of the dry weight of the total biomass. Considering the very high yield of the target protein that was produced by this strategy, it is probably not necessary to integrate the genes for the AGβ-Gal protein and the *c*I repressor into the chromosomal DNA of the *E. coli* host cell in an effort to increase the final yield.

Batch versus Fed-Batch Fermentation

In some instances, a simple fed-batch strategy can be used to produce both a high cell density and a high level of expression of a target protein (Fig. 17.12). For example, a plasmid carrying a gene encoding a hybrid protein that includes the insulin B peptide under the control of the *E. coli trp* promoter was introduced into a *trp*-minus mutant strain of *E. coli* that cannot

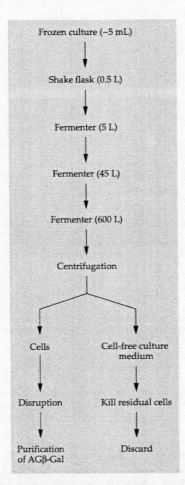

FIGURE 17.11 Scheme for the large-scale production of the protein AGβ-Gal. The volumes in parentheses indicate how much culture medium was used at each step of the process. The culture medium occupied about 60 to 75% of the total volume of each of the bioreactors (fermenters).

synthesize tryptophan, and the transformant was grown in media containing various amounts of tryptophan. At high levels of tryptophan, the synthesis of the target protein was repressed. However, after consumption of the tryptophan in the medium by the growing cells, synthesis of the target protein was induced. With this system, the addition of tryptophan to the medium resulted, in batch cultures, in increases in the amounts of both biomass and target protein produced. However, fed-batch fermentation was more effective than batch fermentation with or without added tryptophan (Table 17.3).

In another experiment, IFN-γ was produced in *E. coli*. Expression of the IFN-γ gene was controlled by the p^L promoter regulated by the tempera-

FIGURE 17.12 Schematic representation of the amount of foreign protein produced as a function of time by recombinant *E. coli* following induction (arrow) in the mid-log phase of growth. Prior to induction, no foreign protein is synthesized. After induction in batch mode, in the absence of additional nutrients, the cells soon enter stationary phase and synthesize proteases that degrade the foreign protein product. After induction in fed-batch mode, the added nutrients ensure that the cells remain in log phase for an extended time and do not produce any proteases until 1.5 to 2 hours later than the cells in batch mode; therefore, the foreign protein is more stable and is easier to recover. In addition, the provision of nutrients in fed-batch mode makes it less likely that plasmids carrying foreign genes will be lost than in batch mode. The time represents the number of hours from the start of the fermentation.

ture-sensitive *c*I repressor. Cells that contained this construct on a plasmid were grown in either batch or fed-batch mode (with both stepwise and constant-rate medium-feeding strategies). In the fed-batch mode, the addition of growth medium was carried out simultaneously with the temperature induction of the p^L promoter in the late exponential growth phase. Use of the fed-batch mode resulted in a significant increase in the length of the cell growth phase following induction. This fed-batch strategy enabled researchers studying this system to achieve a cell biomass that was 5-fold higher and a final IFN-γ concentration that was 23-fold higher than they were able to achieve in batch culture.

Another group studied the fermentation conditions that yielded the optimum expression of a monoclonal antibody (Fab) fragment directed

TABLE 17.3 Comparison of batch and fed-batch fermentations for the production of a fusion protein including the insulin B peptide

Product	Yield in fermentation system:		
	Batch	Batch + Trp	Fed batch
Biomass (g [DW]/liter)	6.7	12	20
Fusion protein ÷ total protein (%)	4.6	7.9	11
Total amount of fusion protein (g/liter)	0.17	0.53	1.21
Plasmid-bearing cells (%)	86	62	90

Adapted from Gosset et al., *Appl. Microbiol. Biotechnol.* **39**:541–546, 1993. DW, dry wieght. In the "Batch + Trp" fermentation, 0.1 g of tryptophan was added. In the fed-batch fermentation, 0.1 g of tryptophan was added every 2 hours, for a total of five times during the course of the 10-hour fermentation. A larger amount of tryptophan added to the batch fermentation did not increase the amount of either biomass or target protein produced.

against tetanus toxoid under the transcriptional control of the *E. coli lac* promoter. The plasmid construct included signal sequences that were inserted immediately upstream of the antibody (light and heavy) genes to target the antibody fragments to the *E. coli* periplasm. In this case, inexpensive lactose, rather than the considerably more expensive IPTG, could be used to induce the expression of the monoclonal antibody fragment gene, provided that the host strain of *E. coli* was Lac$^+$ and therefore able to take up lactose from the medium and convert it to glucose and galactose. In fact, allolactose, an isomer of D-lactose (and not D-lactose itself), is the actual inducer of the *E. coli lac* operon and is formed only if the host strain of *E. coli* contains a small amount of β-galactosidase (see chapter 6). An important facet of these experiments is that lactose not only acts as an inducer, but also is metabolized, providing an additional carbon source for the Fab-producing *E. coli* cells, thereby supporting both cell growth and product accumulation (Fig. 17.13). Again, in these experiments, fed-batch fermentation was clearly superior to batch fermentation, yielding both a larger amount of cell biomass and a greater concentration of Fab fragment.

Fed-batch fermentation strategies have also been successfully employed in the production of nonprotein products, such as poly(3-hydroxybutyrate) and poly(3-hydroxybutyrate-co-3-hydroxyvalerate), biopolymers with plastic-like properties (see chapter 13). In this case, the *E. coli* host cells carried a plasmid that contained polyhydroxyalkanoate biosynthesis genes from the bacterium *Alcaligenes latus*. By using an inexpensive growth medium, such as whey (a waste by-product of cheese making that consists mainly of lactose), to produce these polymers, it is hoped that a commercially viable product can be produced on a large scale.

Another group reported that instead of a single introduction of lactose in a fed-batch fermentation, to produce active protein fragments of human apolipoprotein(a), a strategy that employed continuous induction with lactose beneficially influenced the expression of the target protein. With a 75-liter fermenter, using lactose as the sole feed was not efficient for cell growth, presumably because the host strain of *E. coli* was unable to metabolize galactose. However, with a 1:50 ratio of lactose to glycerol, the target protein reached 16% of the total cellular protein. It remains to be seen whether continuous lactose induction will benefit the expression of proteins other than human apolipoprotein(a) and to what extent this process can be scaled up.

Harvesting Microbial Cells

The first step in the process of purification of a product that is synthesized during microbial fermentation is the separation of the cells from the culture medium. Recombinant and native microbial cells can both be harvested with the same type of equipment. However, as a consequence of physiological changes, such as alterations in cell size and the production of extracellular polysaccharides, conditions that have been established for nontransformed cells may not be optimal for recombinant cells expressing a foreign protein.

For large volumes, either high-speed centrifugation, which is the current method of choice, or membrane microfiltration is used to separate cells from the growth medium. High-speed semicontinuous centrifuges have been specifically designed for the harvesting of microbial cells. The cell suspension is continuously fed into a running centrifuge, and the cells are

concentrated within it while the clarified medium is collected in an external container. When the centrifuge chamber is full of packed cells, the run is stopped and the cells are removed. The need to stop and then restart the procedure periodically, especially when large volumes are being processed, can be a major inconvenience. Furthermore, the cost of both the equipment and the power to run it, the release of the microorganisms into the air as aerosols during the harvesting procedure, and the difficulty in removing all the microbial cells from the spent medium also limit the use of this separation procedure.

Membrane filtration is an alternative method of separating the cells from the culture medium. Unfortunately, with traditional (dead-end) filtration, the microbial cells accumulate on the surface of the polymeric mem-

FIGURE 17.13 Induced recombinant protein production with batch and fed-batch *E. coli* cells grown to late logarithmic phase. The cells were either not induced, induced with 0.05 mM IPTG, or induced with 2.0 grams of lactose per liter. **(A)** In batch culture, the cells that were induced with lactose, which acts as both an inducer and a growth substrate, grew to a significantly greater extent than either the noninduced or the IPTG-induced cells. With fed-batch cells, the lesser extent of growth of induced versus noninduced cells probably reflects the resources that the induced cells direct to the synthesis of the Fab antibody fragment. **(B)** Under both batch and fed-batch conditions, more of the Fab antibody fragment was produced when the cells were induced with lactose than with IPTG. Fab antibody fragment synthesis in the absence of inducer represents incomplete repression of the *lac* promoter.

A

Cell suspension

Cells

Membrane

Cell-free culture medium

B

Cells

Cell
suspension

Cell
concentrate

Membrane

Cell-free culture medium

FIGURE 17.14 Membrane filtration systems for concentrating microbial cells. **(A)** Dead-end filtration; **(B)** cross-flow filtration. The arrows within each unit show the direction of the liquid flow.

brane filter. Consequently, the flow rate of spent medium through the membrane decreases rapidly (Fig. 17.14A). Increasing the pressure on the membrane enhances the flow for a short time; however, the cells still accumulate on the surface of the membrane and may even form a more compact and less permeable layer as a result of the pressure.

An alternative filtration technique entails passing the cell suspension at a high speed across the surface of the membrane (cross-flow filtration) (Fig. 17.14B). Under these conditions, only a very small fraction of the

circulating liquid actually goes through the membrane in any one pass. The remaining cell suspension acts to sweep the membrane clean of accumulated cells, so that the rate of liquid flow through the membrane does not decrease as rapidly as it does in dead-end filtration. In both dead-end and cross-flow filtration, the average pore size of the membranes is 0.2 to 0.45 μm. After many cycles in a cross-flow filtration system, almost all of the culture medium will have passed through the membrane. The use of cross-flow filtration is generally limited to laboratory-scale operations. Most industrial-scale operations still rely on centrifugation.

The next step in the purification process depends on both the nature and the location of the product. If the final product is a protein and it is in the culture medium, the medium is concentrated, often by ultrafiltration, and the target protein is purified by column chromatography or other standard procedures. If the product is a low-molecular-weight compound in the culture medium, it can be purified by the appropriate extraction procedures. Finally, if the product is in the cellular fraction, the cells must be disrupted (lysed) before the steps leading to product purification are initiated.

Disrupting Microbial Cells

A large number of chemical, biological, and physical methods have been developed for disrupting microbial cells. All of these procedures represent a compromise, because they must be vigorous enough to break the microbial cell walls yet gentle enough to ensure that the protein product is not denatured. There is no single set of conditions for cell wall lysis because the cell walls of diverse microbial species are composed of different polymers.

- In gram-positive bacteria, the cell wall is external to the cytoplasmic membrane and consists of a thick peptidoglycan layer of N-acetylglucosamine and N-acetylmuraminic acid residues cross-linked by oligopeptides.
- The cell wall of gram-negative bacteria has an outer membrane, a thin peptidoglycan layer, and a cytoplasmic membrane.
- The yeast cell wall is composed of a thick layer of partially phosphorylated mannans and β-glucan.

Cell wall composition and strength depend on culture conditions, the cellular growth rate, the phase of the growth cycle when the cells are harvested, how the concentrated cells are stored, and whether the isolated microorganism was expressing a cloned gene. All of these factors affect the cells' susceptibility to disruption.

The chemical methods that disrupt microbial cell walls include treatment with alkali, organic solvents, or detergents. If the protein product is stable at pH values from about 10.5 to 12.5, then bacterial cell lysis can easily be carried out on a large scale at low cost. For example, recombinant human growth hormone is efficiently released from E. coli by treatment with sodium hydroxide at pH 11. Few, if any, viable cells remain after alkali treatment, which obviates concerns about the inadvertent release of a genetically engineered microorganism from a production facility. Treatment with an organic solvent is a simple and inexpensive way to disrupt cells and has been used for the isolation of enzymes from yeasts. However, preliminary tests must be run to make sure that the proposed treatment does not denature the target protein. Detergents permeabilize bacterial cells by solubilizing cell membranes and membrane proteins. As a consequence of

this activity, holes are formed, and proteins and other molecules are released from the cells. Unfortunately, detergents are expensive, frequently denature the protein product, and are often retained as contaminants throughout the purification process.

The major biological method for disrupting microbial cells is enzymatic lysis. For example, the cell walls of gram-positive bacteria are readily hydrolyzed by the enzyme lysozyme, which is isolated from egg whites; the cell walls of gram-negative bacteria are hydrolyzed by lysozyme and the metal-chelating agent ethylenediaminetetraacetic acid (EDTA); and the cell walls of yeasts are hydrolyzed by combinations of one or more of the following enzymes: β-1,3-glucanase, β-1,6-glucanase, mannanase, and chitinase. Enzymatic treatments are highly specific, and the conditions for lysis are mild. Currently, cost considerations limit the use of enzymes as cell lysis agents. However, the use of genetically engineered microorganisms for large-scale production of the enzymes that attack cell walls should make them less expensive.

Microbial cells can be physically disrupted either by nonmechanical methods, which include osmotic shock and repeated cycles of freezing and thawing, or by mechanical procedures, such as sonication, wet milling, high-pressure homogenization, and impingement. Generally, after treatment by a nonmechanical method, many of the cells remain intact. In contrast, mechanical disruption is highly efficient, which makes it the preferred choice. A sonicator that generates high-pressure sound waves that cause cell disruption by shear and cavitation (production of internal holes) is generally useful for small volumes.

Wet milling is quite commonly used for disrupting large quantities of cells (Fig. 17.15A). A concentrated cell suspension is pumped into the chamber of a high-speed agitator bead mill that is filled with an inert abrasive material, such as small glass beads (<1 mm in diameter) and is fitted with a central shaft that has a number of attached blades. When the device is turned on and the blades are put in motion, most of the cell disruption occurs as a consequence of the shear forces generated by the high-speed motion of the glass beads. Optimized cell disruption depends on both the number and configuration of the agitator disks, the agitator speed, the size of the glass beads, the number of glass beads, the cell concentration, the geometry of the grinding chamber, and the temperature. Bead mills have been successfully used to disrupt a wide range of different kinds of

FIGURE 17.15 Schematic representation of three methods of mechanical cell disruption of microbial cells. **(A)** Wet milling; **(B)** high-pressure homogenization; **(C)** impingement.

FIGURE 17.16 Schematic representation of large-scale ultrafiltration dialysis of a protein solution. The solution from the feed tank is pumped across the ultrafiltration membrane, with only a small fraction of the solution actually passing through the membrane and the rest being used to sweep the membrane clean of protein. The volume that passes through the membrane is matched by an equal volume of buffer added to the system. A membrane with a nominal molecular mass cutoff below the size of the target protein is used. For example, a 10-kDa cutoff membrane might be used to retain a 30-kDa protein while removing salt from the solution. Following dialysis, the target protein is found, in a dilute solution, in the feed tank. This solution may be concentrated by ultrafiltration using an identical setup except that no buffer tank is used. The arrows indicate the direction of liquid flow. The relative volume of permeate (liquid that passes through the membrane) compared with the retentate (retained liquid) is controlled by adjusting the permeate and retentate valves; this helps to keep the membrane relatively free of protein that might otherwise clog its pores.

microbial cell types and can readily break recombinant, as well as nonrecombinant, cells.

In the high-pressure homogenization process (Fig. 17.15B), concentrated cells are pumped into a valve assembly under high pressure, and the pressure is then rapidly decreased, causing the cells to lyse. This process can be customized for different microorganisms and protein products by changing the operating pressure, the design of the valve, the temperature of the cell suspension, or the number of times the cell mass is treated.

Impingement (Fig. 17.15C) is a cell disruption procedure in which a high-velocity stream of suspended cells under pressure hits either a stationary surface or a second fluid stream of suspended cells. The forces that are created at the point of contact disrupt the cells. With a device called a Microfluidizer, for example, two parallel streams of *E. coli* cells in suspension are directed toward one another. With this device, a high percentage of the cells are disrupted by a single passage through the unit. However, additional passages may be required for complete breakage of other cell types. Unlike high-pressure homogenizers and high-speed agitator bead mills, which generally require highly concentrated cell suspensions, this device can be used to disrupt cells in either dilute or concentrated preparations. The activities of cellular proteins are not significantly impaired by the technique. When the cell suspension is pretreated with low levels of lysozyme and then disrupted in the Microfluidizer at much lower than normal pressure and fluid velocity, the activities of labile proteins, which might be otherwise inactivated by the high pressure, are retained.

Downstream Processing

After cell disruption, cell debris is removed by either low-speed, high-capacity centrifugation or membrane microfiltration. The protein product is precipitated from the crude lysate, the clarified lysate, or the cell-free culture medium with organic solvents (alcohol or acetone) or ammonium sulfate. Under these conditions, the target protein is usually enriched approximately two- to fivefold. Unfortunately, the cost of the precipitant can add significantly to the cost of the process. Alternatively, the crude protein mixtures are concentrated and fractionated by cross-flow ultrafiltration through membranes that have a smaller average pore size than those used for either cell concentration or debris removal (Fig. 17.14B). This approach can be used with volumes ranging from 1 liter to several thousand liters and can be performed continuously, which means that large-volume systems are not required. Depending on the size and properties of the target protein, this method can yield 10- to 100-fold enrichment.

On a large scale, it is impractical to remove small molecules, such as salts or organic solvents, from protein solutions by conventional laboratory procedures. Consequently, the same apparatus that is used to concentrate proteins by ultrafiltration has been developed for the large-scale dialysis of proteins (Fig. 17.16). In addition, by using two different-size membranes,

FIGURE 17.17 Schematic representation of large-scale protein purification using ultrafiltration membranes. In the example shown, two membranes are used sequentially, a 100-kDa cutoff membrane and a 10-kDa cutoff membrane, in order to purify a 30-kDa protein. The solution, which contains a protein mixture, is pumped through the 100-kDa cutoff membrane, with the larger proteins being retained and the smaller proteins, including the 30-kDa target protein, passing through the membrane. This protein solution is next pumped through a 10-kDa cutoff membrane, with the 30-kDa target protein being retained. The arrows indicate the direction of the liquid flow. The symbols are identical to those found in Fig. 17.16.

large volumes of target proteins with different molecular masses may be fractionated by ultrafiltration (Fig. 17.17).

The required degree of purity of the final protein product depends on its end use. In some cases, such as enzymes for use with laundry detergent, crude preparations are satisfactory, but for other products, such as pharmaceutical proteins, additional purification procedures are required.

A number of proteins that are overproduced intracellularly are confined to insoluble particles (inclusion bodies) within the bacterium. After disruption, such inclusion bodies can be readily separated from the bulk of the remaining cell components. Initially, researchers found it difficult to solubilize inclusion bodies without irreversibly denaturing the protein, but protocols have now been devised to renature the proteins found in inclusion bodies. Of course, these additional steps increase the cost of the purification process.

Protein Solubilization

In some instances, overexpression of a target protein can result in the production of both soluble and insoluble forms, which complicates the purification process. For example, when human insulin-like growth factor I (IGF-I), a 7.6-kilodalton (kDa) peptide, was expressed in *E. coli* cells, approximately 90% of the recombinant protein was localized in the *E. coli* periplasm (soluble and insoluble) and about 10% was found in the external medium (soluble). To recover both forms of IGF-I from the periplasm, high concentrations of urea and dithiothreitol at alkaline pH were added to solubilize the insoluble forms of the peptide in situ. This treatment kills but does not lyse the cells. Consequently, the cytoplasmic proteins remain within the cells. The solubilization procedure produces a highly viscous solution, which precludes removing the cells and cell debris by centrifugation. Instead, an aqueous two-phase liquid extraction procedure that separates soluble and insoluble materials was developed for this purpose. Both

FIGURE 17.18 Schematic representation of a process for the continuous thermal lysis of *E. coli* cells for the large-scale preparation of purified plasmid DNA.

the in situ solubilization and aqueous two-phase liquid extraction procedure are highly efficient; 80 to 95% of the IGF-I is recovered from 10-, 100-, or 1,000-liter fermentations by these methods.

Large-Scale Production of Plasmid DNA

Gene therapy and genetic immunization protocols are being tested in a large number of clinical trials. Many of these trials require plasmids as vectors to deliver the remedial DNA to the patient. As these procedures become more routine and are extended to many more patients, it will be necessary to produce plasmid DNA, initially in the 5- to 20-kilobase size range, on a large scale and in a highly purified form, i.e., pharmaceutical grade.

A number of factors, including the choice of a host strain, such as *E. coli* K-12, that is safe and well characterized; growth conditions; defined medium; and the purification process that removes all of the undesired genomic DNA, RNA, proteins, lipids, and lipopolysaccharides, need to be considered for the large-scale production of plasmid DNA. Generally, to ensure that the plasmid DNA will be stable, a host strain should produce only low levels of nucleases. In addition, the presence of antibiotics in the culture medium should be avoided, since it is difficult to remove all traces of an antibiotic from the final preparation. For DNA isolation, the current method of choice for cell breakage is the alkaline-lysis procedure—treatment with 0.2 M NaOH and 1% sodium dodecyl sulfate—which breaks cells without disrupting plasmid DNA. The lysis solution must be added so that mixing is sufficient to lyse all of the cells and local pH extremes are avoided while the shear that is generated by the mixing does not damage the plasmid DNA. After cell lysis, the precipitates formed, which contain cell debris, denatured proteins, and nucleic acids, must be removed. This is most commonly done by centrifugation using fixed-angle rotors, a process which is difficult to scale up. After removal of the precipitated material, plasmid purification is best achieved by anion-exchange chromatography, followed by size exclusion (gel filtration) chromatography. In the industrial production of many recombinant proteins, high-pressure homogenizers are used to continuously disrupt cells. However, the use of such homogenizers typically results in the degradation of a large portion of the plasmid DNA as a consequence of the severe shear stress generated during cell breakage. To work out a process for the large-scale preparation of plasmid DNA, one group of researchers developed and optimized a unique continuous thermal-lysis protocol. In this procedure, cells were harvested after high-cell-density batch culture, filtered to remove most of the growth medium, and resuspended in lysis buffer containing lysozyme. After incubation at 37°C and gentle stirring for 20 minutes, the cells were heated to 70°C for 20 seconds and then filtered to remove the cell debris (Fig. 17.18). Using this procedure, researchers have reported obtaining 100 mg of high-quality plasmid DNA, free of contaminating chromosomal DNA, per liter of high-cell-density cell culture. The use of lysozyme is the most expensive component of this process. Nevertheless, as a consequence of the high plasmid yield, the avoidance of time-consuming and expensive centrifugation steps, the short processing time—17 liters of *E. coli* cells can be processed in ~45 minutes—and the ease with which the process can be scaled up, this approach is likely to provide a highly effective means of preparing large amounts of highly purified plasmid DNA.

SUMMARY

The large-scale production of genetically engineered organisms in industrial-size bioreactors (>1,000 liters) is not achieved merely by extrapolating directly from laboratory growth conditions (0.1 to 1.0 liter). The temperature, pH, rate and nature of mixing, oxygen demand for aerobic organisms, and nutrient levels must be taken into consideration when large bioreactors are being designed.

Microbial fermentations can be performed in several different ways. In batch fermentation, an inoculum of cells is added to fresh medium, and the fermentation is allowed to proceed without supplementation until the maximum amount of the target product is synthesized. Under these conditions, the cell culture passes through six phases of growth: lag, acceleration, log, deceleration, stationary, and death. Protein production is optimal during the log phase, whereas peak production of many low-molecular-weight products occurs during the stationary phase. It is important to monitor batch fermentations closely to ensure that the cells are harvested at the appropriate time. In fed-batch fermentation, growth medium is added at various intervals, usually to prolong the log phase of the fermentation process. Continuous fermentation entails adding fresh growth medium throughout the course of the fermentation and simultaneously removing cells and spent medium.

Each of these fermentation systems has disadvantages and advantages for large-scale production of recombinant products. Although continuous fermentation is still a relatively untried industrial process, the approach has some inherent benefits, making it likely that its use will become more widespread in the future.

One way to increase the amount of a recombinant protein is to grow transformants to as high a cell density as possible. The best way to obtain high-density cell cultures is to use a fed-batch fermentation strategy. Fed-batch fermentation has been directly compared with batch fermentation for the production of several different proteins, and in all cases examined, fed-batch fermentation has resulted in a higher yield of the target protein.

To obtain the largest amount of product in a given volume, it is helpful to attain high cell densities, to avoid the loss of the recombinant plasmid, to utilize E. coli cells that can become quiescent during foreign-gene expression, to secrete the foreign protein into the growth medium, and to avoid the formation of acetate in the medium.

There are three basic bioreactor configurations: STRs, bubble columns, and airlift reactors. Currently, STRs are used most frequently in industry, but interest in airlift bioreactors is increasing. In STRs, mixing is achieved by mechanical agitation. In airlift reactors, both aeration and mixing are performed by a gas, usually air, that is introduced through a sparger at the bottom of the vessel, with either internal baffles or external loops causing the fluid to circulate within the vessel. Bubble columns are similar to airlift reactors but lack the design features that cause the culture medium to circulate in the vessel. The problems of maintaining sterility, pH, temperature, and other fermentation parameters are overcome in different ways depending on the design of the bioreactor. Two-stage fermentation processes with either tandem airlift reactors or a single STR have been successfully used for the production of recombinant proteins.

When the product is present within the cells, the cells can be harvested by either centrifugation or cross-flow filtration and lysed chemically, enzymatically, or mechanically. The preferred forms of mechanical cell lysis include wet milling, high-pressure homogenization, and impingement. The product is then fractionated from the cell lysate. Ultrafiltration has been found to be an effective method for large-scale dialysis, concentration, and initial fractionation of proteins produced by recombinant organisms.

Scientists have begun to establish procedures for the large-scale isolation of plasmid DNA. These procedures must take into account the host cell and its growth and metabolism, plasmid size, cell lysis methods, and the complete removal of a number of potentially contaminating cell components.

REFERENCES

Aristidou, A. A., K. Y. San, and G. N. Bennett. 1995. Metabolic engineering of *Escherichia coli* to enhance recombinant protein production through acetate reduction. *Biotechnol. Prog.* **11:**475–478.

Bailey, J. E., and D. F. Olis. 1977. *Biochemical Engineering Fundamentals.* McGraw-Hill Book Co., New York, NY.

Charles, M. 1985. Fermentation scale-up: problems and possibilities. *Trends Biotechnol.* **3:**134–139.

Choi, J.-I., and S. Y. Lee. 1999. High-level production of poly(3-hydroxybutyrate-co-3-hydroxyvalerate) by fed-batch culture of recombinant *Escherichia coli. Appl. Environ. Microbiol.* **65:**4363–4368.

Datar, R. 1986. Economics of primary separation steps in relation to fermentation and genetic engineering. *Process Biochem.* **21:**19–26.

Donovan, R. S., C. W. Robinson, and B. R. Glick. 2000. Optimizing the expression of a monoclonal antibody fragment under the transcriptional control of the *Escherichia coli lac* promoter. *Can. J. Microbiol.* **46:**532–541.

Eiteman, M. A., and E. Altman. 2006. Overcoming acetate in *Escherichia coli* recombinant protein fermentations. *Trends Biotechnol.* **24:**530–536.

Engler, C. R. 1985. Disruption of microbial cells, p. 305–324. *In* C. L. Cooney, A. E. Humphrey, and M. Moo-Young (ed.), *Comprehensive Biotechnology,* vol. 2. Pergamon Press, Oxford, United Kingdom.

Giorgio, R. J., and J. J. Wu. 1986. Design of large scale containment facilities for recombinant DNA fermentations. *Trends Biotechnol.* 4:60–65.

Gosset, G., R. de Anda, N. Cruz, A. Martínez, R. Quintero, and F. Bolivar. 1993. Recombinant protein production in cultures of an *Escherichia coli* trp2 strain. *Appl. Microbiol. Biotechnol.* 39:541–546.

Grund, G., C. W. Robinson, and B. R. Glick. 1991. Cross-flow ultrafiltration of proteins, p. 69–83. *In* M. D. White, S. Reuveny, and A. Shafferman (ed.), *Biologicals from Recombinant Microorganisms and Animal Cells: Production and Recovery.* Verlag Chemie, Weinheim, Germany.

Hägg, P., J. Wa de Pohl, F. Abdulkarim, and L. A. Isakson. 2004. A host/plasmid system that is not dependent on antibiotics and antibiotic resistance genes for stable plasmid maintenance in *Escherichia coli. J. Biotechnol.* 111:17–30.

Hart, R. A., P. M. Lester, D. H. Reifsnyder, J. R. Ogez, and S. E. Builder. 1994. Large scale, in situ isolation of periplasmic IGF-I from *E. coli. Bio/Technology* 12:113–117.

Khosla, C., J. E. Curtis, J. DeModena, U. Rinas, and J. E. Bailey. 1990. Expression of intracellular hemoglobin improves protein synthesis in oxygen-limited *Escherichia coli. Bio/Technology* 8:849–853.

Kroner, K. H. 1986. Cross-flow filtration in the downstream processing of enzymes: current status. *Biotechnol. Forum* 3:20–31.

Kroner, K. H., H. Nissinen, and H. Zeigler. 1987. Improved dynamic filtration of microbial suspensions. *Bio/Technology* 5:921–926.

Lee, S. Y. 1996. High cell-density culture of *Escherichia coli. Trends Biotechnol.* 14:98–105.

Levy, M. S., R. D. O'Kennedy, P. Ayazi-Shamlou, and P. Dunnill. 2000. Biochemical engineering approaches to the challenges of producing pure plasmid DNA. *Trends Biotechnol.* 18:296–305.

Lim, H.-K., and K.-H. Jung. 1998. Improvement of heterologous protein productivity by controlling postinduction specific growth rate in recombinant *Escherichia coli* under control of

the *p*L promoter. *Biotechnol. Prog.* 14:548–553.

Lim, H.-K., S.-G. Kim, K.-H. Jung and J.-H. Seo. 2004. Production of the kringle fragments of human apolipoprotein(a) by continuous lactose induction strategy. *J. Biotechnol.* 108:271–278.

March, J. C., M. A. Eiteman, and E. Altman. 2002. Expression of an anaplerotic enzyme, pyruvate carboxylase, improves recombinant protein production in *Escherichia coli. Appl. Environ. Microbiol.* 68:5620–5624.

McKillip, E. R., A. S. Giles, M. H. Levner, P. P. Hung, and R. N. Hjorth. 1991. Bioreactors for large-scale t-PA production. *Bio/Technology* 9:805–812.

Mendoza-Vega, O., C. Hebert, and S. W. Brown. 1994. Production of recombinant hirudin by high cell density fed-batch cultivations of a *Saccharomyces cerevisiae* strain: physiological considerations during the bioprocess design. *J. Biotechnol.* 32:249–259.

Merchuk, J. C. 1990. Why use airlift bioreactors? *Trends Biotechnol.* 8:66–71.

Mukherjee, K. J., D. C. D. Rowe, N. A. Watkins, and D. K. Summers. 2004. Studies of single-chain antibody expression in quiescent *Escherichia coli. Appl. Environ. Microbiol.* 70:3005–3012.

Park, T. H., J.-H. Seo, and H. C. Lim. 1991. Two-stage fermentation with bacteriophage λ as an expression vector in *Escherichia coli. Biotechnol. Bioeng.* 37:297–302.

Paulson, D. J., R. L. Wilson, and D. D. Spatz. 1984. Cross-flow membrane technology and its applications. *Food Technol.* December 1984:77–87.

Prazeres, D. M. F., G. N. M. Ferreira, G. A. Monteiro, C. L. Cooney, and J. M. S. Cabral. 1999. Large-scale production of pharmaceutical-grade plasmid DNA for gene therapy: problems and bottlenecks. *Trends Biotechnol.* 17:169–174.

Ramírez, D. M., and W. E. Bentley. 1995. Fed-batch feeding and induction policies that improve foreign protein synthesis and stability by avoiding stress response. *Biotechnol. Bioeng.* 47:596–608.

Reuss, M. 1995. Stirred tank bioreactors, p. 207–255. *In* J. A. Asenjo and J. Merchuk (ed.), *Bioreactor System*

Design. Marcel Dekker, Inc., New York, NY.

Riesenberg, D., and R. Guthke. 1999. High-cell-density cultivation of microorganisms. *Appl. Microbiol. Biotechnol.* 51:422–430.

Robinson, D. K., C. P. Chan, C. Yu Ip, P. K. Tsai, J. Tung, T. C. Seamans, A. B. Lenny, D. K. Lee, J. Irwin, and M. Silberklang. 1994. Characterization of a recombinant antibody produced in the course of a high yield fed-batch process. *Biotechnol. Bioeng.* 44:727–735.

Rowe, D. C. D., and D. K. Summers. 1999. The quiescent-cell expression system for protein synthesis in *Escherichia coli. Appl. Environ. Microbiol.* 65:2710–2715.

Sauer, T., C. W. Robinson, and B. R. Glick. 1989. Disruption of native and recombinant *Escherichia coli* in a high-pressure homogenizer. *Biotechnol. Bioeng.* 33:1330–1342.

Sayadi, S., M. Nasri, F. Berry, J. N. Barbotin, and D. Thomas. 1987. Effect of temperature on the stability of plasmid pTG201 and productivity of *xylE* gene product in recombinant *Escherichia coli*: development of a two-stage chemostat with free and immobilized cells. *J. Gen. Microbiol.* 133:1901–1908.

Schleef, M. 1999. Issues for large-scale DNA manufacturing, p. 443–470. *In* H. J. Rehm and G. Reed (ed.), *Biotechnology: a Multi-Volume Comprehensive Treatise,* vol. 5a. *Recombinant Proteins, Monoclonal Antibodies, and Therapeutic Genes.* Wiley-VCH, New York, NY.

Schügerl, K., and A. Lübbert. 1995. Pneumatically agitated bioreactors, p. 257–303. *In* J. A. Asenjo and J. Merchuk (ed.), *Bioreactor System Design.* Marcel Dekker, Inc., New York, NY.

Schütte, H., and M.-R. Kula. 1990. Pilot- and process-scale techniques for cell disruption. *Biotechnol. Appl. Biochem.* 12:599–620.

Seigel, R., and D. D. Y. Ryu. 1985. Kinetic study of instability of recombinant plasmid pPLc23trpAl in *E. coli* using two-stage continuous culture system. *Biotechnol. Bioeng.* 27:28–33.

Siegel, M. H., H. Hallaille, and J. C. Merchuk. 1988. Air-lift reactors: design, operation, and applications. *Adv. Biotechnol. Processes* 7:79–124.

Sletta, H., A. Tøndervik, S. Hakvåg, T. E. Vee Aune, A. Nedal, R. Aune, G. Evensen, S. Valla, T. E. Ellingsen, and T. Brautaset. 2007. The presence of N-terminal secretion signals leads to strong stimulation of the total expression levels of three tested medically important proteins during high-cell-density cultivations of *Escherichia coli*. *Appl. Environ. Microbiol.* **73**:906–912.

Strandberg, L., L. Andersson, and S.-O. Enfors. 1994. The use of fed batch cultivation for achieving high cell densities in the production of a recombinant protein in *Escherichia coli*. *FEMS Microbiol. Rev.* **14**:53–56.

Strandberg, L., K. Köhler, and S.-O. Enfors. 1991. Large-scale fermentation and purification of a recombinant protein from *Escherichia coli*. *Process Biochem.* **26**:225–234.

Strathman, H. 1985. Membranes and membrane processes in biotechnology. *Trends Biotechnol.* **3**:112–118.

Tanny, G. B., D. Mirelman, and T. Pistole. 1980. Improved filtration techniques for concentrating and harvesting bacteria. *Appl. Environ. Microbiol.* **40**:269–273.

Tutunjian, R. S. 1985. Scale-up considerations for membrane processes. *Bio/Technology* **3**:615–626.

Van Brunt, J. 1985. Scale-up: the next hurdle. *Bio/Technology* **3**:419–424.

Van Brunt, J. 1986. Fermentation economics. *Bio/Technology* **4**:395–401.

Wang, Z. W., Y. Chen, and Y.-P. Chao. 2006. Enhancement of recombinant protein production in *Escherichia coli* by coproduction of aspartase. *J. Biotechnol.* **124**:403–411.

White, M. D., B. R. Glick, and C. W. Robinson. 1995. Bacterial, yeast and fungal cultures: the effect of microorganism type and culture characteristics on bioreactor design and operation, p. 47–87. *In* J. A. Asenjo and J. Merchuk (ed.), *Bioreactor System Design*. Marcel Dekker, Inc., New York, NY.

Whitney, G. D., B. R. Glick, and C. W. Robinson. 1989. Induction of T4 DNA ligase in a recombinant strain of *Escherichia coli*. *Biotechnol. Bioeng.* **33**:991–998.

Yamane, T. 1995. Bioreactor operation modes, p. 479–509. *In* J. A. Asenjo and J. Merchuk (ed.), *Bioreactor System Design*. Marcel Dekker, Inc., New York, NY.

Zhu, K., H. Jin, Y. Ma, Z. Ren, C. Xiao, Z. He, F. Zhang, Q. Zhu, and B. Wang. 2005. A continuous thermal lysis procedure for the large-scale preparation of plasmid DNA. *J. Biotechnol.* **118**:257–264.

REVIEW QUESTIONS

1. What are the differences between batch, fed-batch, and continuous fermentations?

2. How has fed-batch fermentation been used to improve the production of the insulin B peptide, IFN-γ, and Fab fragment?

3. What parameters must be monitored and controlled in an optimized fermentation process?

4. What is the effect of a recombinant plasmid on the growth of microbial cells?

5. How does the mixing of a growing microbial culture affect the transfer of oxygen from the growth medium to the cells?

6. What are the advantages of a high cell density during a large-scale fermentation? What conditions lead to a high cell density during a large-scale fermentation?

7. What strategies can be employed to prevent acetate inhibition of the growth of recombinant *E. coli* strains?

8. What are the relative advantages and disadvantages of using an STR or an airlift fermenter?

9. Compare the growth and induction of a recombinant microbial culture using (1) two reactors in tandem and (2) a single reactor.

10. What is downstream processing?

11. What strategy would you use to purify a recombinant protein that is secreted into the growth medium?

12. What are the advantages and disadvantages of large-scale mechanical lysis of cells compared to chemical lysis?

13. How are cells mechanically disrupted using (1) wet milling, (2) high-pressure homogenization, and (3) impingement?

14. How are microbial cells concentrated after the fermentation stage of a biotechnological process? What are the advantages and disadvantages of these procedures?

15. How are large volumes of protein solutions partially purified using ultrafiltration?

16. How can the activity of an insoluble recombinant protein be recovered?

17. What factors should be considered for the large-scale isolation of plasmid DNA?

18. How can "quiescent *E. coli* cells" be engineered to produce large amounts of foreign protein?

19. What strategy would you use to ensure that a plasmid encoding a target protein is not lost during the large-scale growth of a recombinant bacterium?

20. What are some of the advantages of secreting a recombinant protein into the growth medium?

III MOLECULAR BIOTECHNOLOGY OF EUKARYOTIC SYSTEMS

IN THE PAST, HIGH-YIELDING STRAINS of many different crop plants and farm animals have been successfully developed by selective cross-breeding. This time-consuming process has been superseded in part by the development of methods for the genetic engineering of higher organisms. Now, genes that contribute to specific traits can be introduced into plants and animals and then passed on from one generation to the next. How these transgenic plants and animals are formed and what sorts of traits are being manipulated are examined in part III.

A number of transgenic plants have been engineered to be able to overcome a variety of biotic and abiotic stresses, including insect predation, viral infection, herbicides, pathogenic fungi and bacteria, oxidative stress, salt stress, and drought. Transgenic plants that have a significantly improved nutritional content, produce fruit or vegetables with enhanced taste or appearance, or produce flowers with altered pigmentation have been created. In addition, some transgenic plants have been used to facilitate environmental cleanup (phytoremediation) while others have been used as living bioreactors in the production of a range of foreign proteins, including many therapeutic agents. Transgenesis of animals has included studies of cattle, sheep, goats, birds, and fish, all based on the principles that have been established for creating transgenic mice. Some of these transgenic animals have been developed to produce therapeutic proteins in their milk or eggs.

This page intentionally left blank

18

Genetic Engineering of Plants: Methodology

ONSIDERABLE EFFORT HAS GONE INTO DEVELOPING VARIETIES of plants that produce increased yields and have enhanced nutritional value. Although much of this endeavor has been directed toward the three major grains—corn (maize), wheat, and rice—successful breeding programs for other food plants and horticultural species have also been established. Recombinant DNA technology, which has been used extensively with microbial systems, is also an important tool for the direct genetic manipulation of plants. There are a number of effective DNA delivery systems and expression vectors that work with a range of plant cells. Furthermore, most plant cells are totipotent—meaning that an entire plant can be regenerated from a single plant cell—so fertile plants that carry an introduced gene(s) in all cells (i.e., transgenic plants) can be produced from genetically engineered cells. If the transgenic plant flowers and produces viable seed, the desired trait is passed on to successive generations.

There are three major reasons for developing transgenic plants. First, the addition of a gene(s) often improves the agricultural, horticultural, or ornamental value of a crop plant. Second, transgenic plants can act as living bioreactors for the inexpensive production of economically important proteins or metabolites. Third, plant genetic transformation (transgenesis) provides a powerful means for studying the actions of genes during development and other biological processes.

Some of the genetically determined traits that can be introduced into plants by a single gene or, possibly, a small cluster of genes are insecticidal activity, protection against viral infection, resistance to herbicides, protection against pathogenic fungi and bacteria, delay of senescence, tolerance of environmental stresses, altered flower pigmentation, improved nutritional quality of seed proteins, increased postharvest shelf life, and self-incompatibility. In addition, transgenic plants can be made to produce a variety of useful compounds, including therapeutic agents, polymers, and diagnostic tools, such as antibody fragments. Alternatively, they can be engineered to synthesize viral antigenic determinants and, after ingestion, can be used as edible vaccines. To date, over 150 different plant species have been genetically transformed, including many crop and forest species,

Is the Debate over Genetically Modified Foods Effectively Over?

Rice is the most important crop in the world. In 2004, China, the world's largest producer of rice, announced a ramping up of efforts to commercialize genetically modified rice. India, the second-largest producer of rice, was quick to follow suit. With the two largest rice producers in the world (with ~40% of the world's population) switching to genetically modified rice, the rest of the world will eventually have little choice but to accept genetically modified foods.

From 1996 to 2007, the global area devoted to transgenic crops has increased from 1.7 million to 114 million hectares (ha). In 2007, the major producers of transgenic plants were the United States (57.7 million ha planted), Argentina (19.1 million ha), Brazil (15.0 million ha), Canada (7.0 million ha), India (6.2 million ha), China (3.8 million ha), Paraguay (2.6 million ha), and South Africa (1.8 million ha). Major transgenic crops worldwide include (in order of number of hectares planted) soybean, corn, cotton, canola, rice, squash, papaya, alfalfa, wheat, and eggplant. The major traits that have been introduced into plants include herbicide tolerance and insect resistance.

In 2002, the Food and Agriculture Organization of the United Nations endorsed the development and use of genetically modified crops. According to researcher Florence Wambugu of Nairobi, Kenya, "The African continent urgently needs agricultural biotechnology, including transgenic crops, in order to improve food production. Famine provides critics with an opportunity to promote an antibiotech message that only results in millions of people, who urgently need food, starving to death." Wambugu urged the public to recognize the difference in needs between Europe and Africa. Europe, with a population that is under control, has surplus food and does not experience hunger, whereas Africa, in contrast, experiences mass starvation and death. By mid-2008, South Africa was the only country in Africa to have approved the commercial use of genetically modified crops.

in over 50 countries worldwide. Plant biotechnology is having an enormous impact on plant-breeding programs because it significantly decreases the 10 to 15 years that it takes to develop a new variety using traditional plant-breeding techniques.

By mid-2008, researchers had reported the complete DNA sequences of hundreds of microorganisms and dozens of animals, but only three plants: *Arabidopsis thaliana*, rice, and poplar. At that time, the genome sequencing of several other plants, including corn, soybean, canola, tomato, cotton, potato, cassava, sorghum, grape, and peach, had been initiated. While the study of plant genes and genomes clearly lags behind studies of animals, it is gaining momentum, so that within the next 5 to 10 years, a wealth of information, with an enormous impact on plant biotechnology, is expected to become available.

Despite all of the progress that has been made in the development of transgenic plants for a wide variety of purposes, a vocal minority of individuals in North America and a larger number in Europe still oppose the use of this technology. Nevertheless, with each succeeding year since the mid-1990s, the use of transgenic crops has continued to increase both in absolute terms and in the number of countries using this technology (Box 18.1). It is expected that in the not too distant future, the majority of agricultural crops worldwide will be transgenic.

Plant Transformation with the Ti Plasmid of *A. tumefaciens*

The gram-negative soil bacterium *Agrobacterium tumefaciens* is a phytopathogen that, as a normal part of its life cycle, genetically transforms plant cells. This genetic transformation leads to the formation of crown gall tumors, which interfere with the normal growth of an infected plant (Fig.

18.1). This agronomically important disease affects only dicotyledonous plants (dicots), including grapes, stone fruit trees (e.g., peaches), and roses.

Crown gall formation is the consequence of the transfer, integration, and expression of genes of a specific segment of bacterial plasmid DNA—called the T-DNA (transferred DNA)—into the plant cell genome. The T-DNA is actually part of the "tumor-inducing" (Ti) plasmid that is carried by most strains of *A. tumefaciens*. Depending on the Ti plasmid, the length of the T-DNA region can vary from approximately 10 to 30 kilobase pairs (kb). Strains of *A. tumefaciens* that do not possess a Ti plasmid cannot induce crown gall tumors.

The initial step in the infection process is the attachment of *A. tumefaciens* to a plant cell at the site of an open wound, often at the base of the stem, i.e., the crown, of the plant. After the initial attachment step, *A. tumefaciens* produces a network of cellulose fibrils that bind the bacterium tightly to the plant cell surface. Originally, it was thought that *A. tumefaciens* infected wounded plants because the physical barrier of the cell wall had been breached by injury, thereby facilitating entry of the bacterium. However, it is now recognized that these bacteria respond to certain plant phenolic compounds, such as acetosyringone and hydroxyacetosyringone (Fig. 18.2), which are excreted by susceptible wounded plants. These wound response compounds resemble some of the products of phenylpropanoid metabolism, which is the major plant pathway for the synthesis of plant secondary metabolites, such as lignins and flavonoids. These small molecules (i.e., acetosyringone and hydroxysyringone) act to induce the virulence *(vir)* genes that are carried on the Ti plasmid (Fig. 18.3).

The *vir* genes are located on a 35-kb region of the Ti plasmid that lies outside of the T-DNA region. There are 25 *vir* genes arranged in seven operons on the plasmid. The products of the *vir* genes are essential for the transfer and integration of the T-DNA region into the genome of a plant cell.

After a Ti plasmid-carrying cell of *A. tumefaciens* attaches to a host plant cell and the *vir* genes are induced, the T-DNA is transferred by a process that is similar to plasmid transfer from donor to recipient cells during bacterial conjugation. In this model, the T-DNA is transferred as a linear, single-stranded molecule from the Ti plasmid, enters the plant cell, and eventually becomes integrated into the plant chromosomal DNA.

The formation of the single-stranded form of T-DNA is initiated by strand-specific cutting, by an enzyme encoded by one of the *vir* genes, at both borders of the intact T-DNA region. The 5' end of the single-stranded T-DNA carries the right-border sequence, and the left-border sequence is at the 3' end. The integration of the T-DNA into the plant genome depends on specific sequences that are located at the right border of the T-DNA. This border contains a repeating unit that consists of 25 base pairs (bp) (Fig. 18.4). Although the left border contains a similar 25-bp repeat (Fig. 18.4), deletion studies have shown that this region is not involved in the integration process.

During the insertion of the T-DNA into the plant chromosomal DNA, short deletions of the plant DNA are often produced at the junction between the T-DNA and the plant chromosomal DNA. In addition, while the insertion of the T-DNA into the plant DNA occurs at random sites, the T-DNA borders exhibit some homology with the plant DNA at the site of insertion.

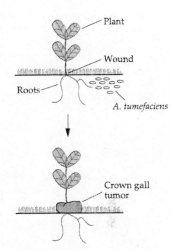

FIGURE 18.1 Infection of a plant with *A. tumefaciens* and formation of a crown gall.

FIGURE 18.2 Structures of the plant molecules acetosyringone and hydroxyacetosyringone. These compounds are released in response to wounding and can induce the *vir* genes of the Ti plasmid.

Acetosyringone

Hydroxyacetosyringone

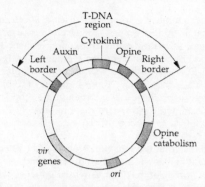

FIGURE 18.3 Schematic representation of a Ti plasmid. The T-DNA is defined by its left and right borders and includes genes for the biosynthesis of auxin, cytokinin, and an opine; these genes are transcribed and translated only in plant cells. Outside of the T-DNA region, there is a cluster of *vir* genes, a gene(s) that encodes an enzyme(s) for opine catabolism, and an origin of DNA replication *(ori)* that permits the plasmid to be stably maintained in *A. tumefaciens*. None of these features is drawn to scale.

Most of the genes that are located within the T-DNA region are activated only after the T-DNA is inserted into the plant genome. This reflects the fact that these are essentially plant genes, which cannot be expressed in bacteria because of the differences in transcriptional and translational regulatory sequences between the two types of organisms. The products of these genes are responsible for crown gall formation. The T-DNA region includes the genes *iaaM* and *iaaH*. This pair of genes encodes enzymes that synthesize the plant hormone auxin (indoleacetic acid). Specifically, *iaaM* codes for the enzyme tryptophan 2-monooxygenase, which converts tryptophan to indole 3-acetamide, and *iaaH* encodes indole 3-acetamide hydrolase, which converts indole 3-acetamide to indoleacetic acid (Fig. 18.5A). In addition, the T-DNA region carries the *tmr* gene (also known as *ipt*), which encodes isopentenyltransferase. This enzyme adds an isopentenyl side chain to 5'-AMP to form isopentenyladenosine 5'-phosphate, the first committed step in the synthesis of the cytokinin isopentenyladenine (Fig. 18.5B). Hydroxylation of these two molecules by plant enzymes generates the cytokinins called transzeatin and transribosylzeatin, respectively. Both auxin and the cytokinins regulate plant cell growth and development. In excess, they can cause the plant to develop tumorous growths, such as crown galls.

In addition to auxin and cytokinin biosynthesis genes, the T-DNA region from each specific Ti plasmid carries a gene for the synthesis of a molecule called an opine. Opines are unique and unusual condensation products of either an amino acid and a keto acid or an amino acid and a

FIGURE 18.4 Conserved bases on the right and left borders of the T-DNA of Ti plasmids. N indicates any one of the four nucleotides, i.e., there is no sequence conservation at these positions.

Right 5'-TGNCAGGATATATNNNNNNGTNANN-3'

Left 5'-TGGCAGGATATATNNNNNNTGTAAAN-3'

A

Tryptophan

Indole-3-acetamide

Indoleacetic acid

B

IPP

5′-AMP

IPA

FIGURE 18.5 Biosynthesis of auxin and cytokinin by the enzymes encoded by the T-DNA genes of the Ti plasmid of *A. tumefaciens*. **(A)** The auxin pathway involves the conversion of tryptophan to indole 3-acetamide by tryptophan monooxygenase and then indole 3-acetamide to indoleacetic acid by indole-3-acetamide hydrolase. **(B)** The cytokinin synthesis reaction entails the attachment of an isopentenyl moiety from isopentenyl diphosphate (IPP) to 5′-AMP by the enzyme isopentenyltransferase to form isopentenyl adenosine monophosphate (IPA).

sugar. For example, the condensation product of arginine and pyruvic acid is called octopine, arginine with α-ketoglutaraldehyde is nopaline, and agropine is a bicyclic sugar derivative of glutamic acid (Fig. 18.6). The opines are synthesized within the crown gall and then secreted. They can

FIGURE 18.6 Chemical structures of three opines: octopine, nopaline, and agropine.

be used as a carbon source, and sometimes also as a nitrogen source, by any *A. tumefaciens* cell that carries a Ti plasmid-borne gene for the catabolism of that particular opine (Fig. 18.3). The opine catabolism gene(s) is on the Ti plasmid and is not part of the T-DNA region. All other soil microorganisms that have been tested are incapable of utilizing opines as a carbon source. Thus, a unique set of mechanisms has evolved whereby each strain of *A. tumefaciens* genetically engineers plant cells to be biological factories for the production of a carbon compound that it alone is able to use.

Ti Plasmid-Derived Vector Systems

The simplest way to exploit the ability of the Ti plasmid to genetically transform plants would be to insert a desired DNA sequence into the T-DNA region and then use the Ti plasmid and *A. tumefaciens* to deliver and insert this gene(s) into the genome of a susceptible plant cell. However, although the Ti plasmids are effective as natural vectors, they have several serious limitations as routine cloning vectors.

- The production of phytohormones by transformed cells growing in culture prevents them from being regenerated into mature plants. Therefore, the auxin and cytokinin genes must be removed from any Ti plasmid-derived cloning vector.

- A gene encoding opine synthesis is not useful to a transgenic plant and may lower the final plant yield by diverting plant resources into opine production. Therefore, the opine synthesis gene should be removed.
- Ti plasmids are large (approximately 200 to 800 kb). For recombinant DNA experiments, however, a much smaller version is preferred, so large segments of DNA that are not essential for a cloning vector must be removed.
- Because the Ti plasmid does not replicate in *Escherichia coli,* the convenience of perpetuating and manipulating Ti plasmids carrying inserted DNA sequences in that bacterium is not available.
- Transfer of the T-DNA, which begins from the right border, does not always end at the left border. Rather, vector DNA sequences past the left border are often transferred, although the transfer of these sequences is not often tested for.

To overcome these constraints, recombinant DNA technology was used to create a number of Ti plasmid-based vectors. These vectors are similarly organized and contain the following components.

- A selectable marker gene, such as neomycin phosphotransferase, that confers kanamycin resistance on transformed plant cells. Because the neomycin phosphotransferase gene, as well as many of the other marker genes used in plant transformation, is prokaryotic in origin, it is necessary to put it under the control of plant (eukaryotic) transcriptional regulation signals, including both a promoter and a termination–polyadenylation sequence, to ensure that it is efficiently expressed in transformed plant cells.
- An origin of DNA replication that allows the plasmid to replicate in *E. coli.* In some vectors, an origin of replication that functions in *A. tumefaciens* has also been added.
- The right border sequence of the T-DNA region. This region is absolutely required for T-DNA integration into plant cell DNA, although most cloning vectors include both a right and a left border sequence.
- A polylinker (multiple cloning site) to facilitate insertion of the cloned gene into the region between T-DNA border sequences.
- A "killer" gene encoding a toxin downstream from the left border to prevent unwanted vector DNA past the left border from being incorporated into transgenic plants. If this incorporation occurs, and the killer gene is present, the transformed cells will not survive.

Because these cloning vectors lack *vir* genes, they cannot by themselves effect the transfer and integration of the T-DNA region into recipient plant cells. Two different approaches have been used to achieve these ends. In one approach, a binary vector system is used (Fig. 18.7A). The binary cloning vector contains either *E. coli* and *A. tumefaciens* origins of DNA replication, i.e., an *E. coli–A. tumefaciens* shuttle vector, or a single broad-host-range origin of DNA replication. In either case, no *vir* genes are present on a binary cloning vector. All the cloning steps are carried out in *E. coli* before the vector is introduced into *A. tumefaciens*. The recipient *A. tumefaciens* strain carries a modified (defective, or disarmed) Ti plasmid that contains a complete set of *vir* genes but lacks portions, or all, of the

FIGURE 18.7 Two Ti plasmid-derived cloning vector systems. **(A)** The binary cloning vector has origins of DNA replication (*ori*) for both *E. coli* and *A. tumefaciens* (or a broad-host-range origin), a selectable marker gene that can be used in either *E. coli* or *A. tumefaciens*, and both a target gene and a plant selectable marker gene inserted between the T-DNA left and right borders. **(B)** The cointegrate cloning vector (top) carries only an *E. coli* origin of replication and cannot exist autonomously within *A. tumefaciens*. It also contains a selectable marker that can be used in either *E. coli* or *A. tumefaciens*, a T-DNA right border, a plant selectable marker (reporter) gene, a target gene, and a sequence of Ti plasmid DNA that is homologous to a segment on the disarmed Ti plasmid. The disarmed Ti plasmid (middle) contains the T-DNA left border, the *vir* gene cluster, and an *A. tumefaciens ori*. Following recombination between the cointegrate cloning vector and the disarmed Ti plasmid, the final recombinant plasmid (bottom) has the T-DNA left and right borders bracketing the cloned and plant reporter genes.

T-DNA region, so that this T-DNA cannot be transferred. With this system, the defective Ti plasmid synthesizes the *vir* gene products that mobilize the T-DNA region of the binary cloning vector. By providing the proteins encoded by the *vir* genes, the defective Ti plasmid acts as a helper plasmid, enabling the T-DNA from the binary cloning vector to be inserted into the plant chromosomal DNA. Since transfer of the T-DNA is initiated from the right border, the selectable marker, which will eventually be used to detect the presence of the T-DNA inserted into the plant chromosomal DNA, is usually placed next to the left border. If the selectable marker were adjacent to the right border, transfer of only a small portion of the T-DNA would yield plants that contained the selectable marker but not the gene of interest. A few binary vectors have been designed to include two plant selectable markers, one adjacent to the right border and the other adjacent to the left border.

In the second approach, called the cointegrate vector system, the cloning (cointegrate) vector has a plant selectable marker gene, the target gene, the right border, an *E. coli* origin of DNA replication, and a bacterial selectable marker gene. The cointegrate vector recombines with a modified (disarmed) Ti plasmid that lacks both the tumor-producing genes and the right border of the T-DNA within *A. tumefaciens*, and the entire cloning vector becomes integrated into the disarmed Ti plasmid to form a recombinant Ti plasmid (Fig. 18.7B). The cointegrate cloning vector and the disarmed helper Ti plasmid both carry homologous DNA sequences that provide a shared site for in vivo homologous recombination; normally these sequences lie inside the T-DNA region. Following recombination, the cloning vector becomes part of the disarmed Ti plasmid, which provides the *vir* genes necessary for the transfer of the T-DNA to the host plant cells. The only way that this cloning vector can be maintained in *A. tumefaciens* is as part of a cointegrate structure. In this cointegrated configuration the genetically engineered T-DNA region can be transferred to plant cells.

A practical problem that arises when using binary vectors is that their relatively large size (usually >10 kb) often makes it difficult and inconvenient to manipulate them in vitro. In addition, larger plasmids tend to have fewer unique restriction sites for cloning purposes. For these reasons, it is advantageous to develop and use smaller binary vectors. Based on the DNA sequence of a commonly used binary vector, pBIN19, it was predicted that more than half of the DNA could be deleted and the vector would still be completely functional. Thus, instead of the 11.8-kb size of the original vector, a 3.5-kb mini-binary vector (pCB301) was constructed (Fig. 18.8). This minivector, which can be used to clone DNA fragments to be transferred into the plant genome, cannot be introduced into *A. tumefaciens* by conjugation because certain regions of DNA required for conjugal transfer have been deleted. However, electroporation can be used as an alternative means. To facilitate the use of the minivector, a number of derivatives of pCB301 were constructed. For example, a *bar* gene, together with a plant promoter and transcription termination region, encoding the enzyme phosphinothricin acetyltransferase was inserted into the multiple cloning site so that transformants expressing this gene would be easily selected. Adjacent to the *bar* gene but in the opposite orientation is an expression cassette which includes a 35S promoter, a DNA sequence to target the protein for expression in either chloroplasts or mitochondria, a translational enhancer element (not shown in Fig. 18.8) that increases the level of expression of the protein encoded by the cloned gene, a portion of the multiple cloning site,

FIGURE 18.8 The mini-binary vector pCB301 system. *oriV*, part of the origin of replication; *npt*, neomycin phosphotransferase gene; *trfA*, part of the origin of replication; RB, right border of T-DNA; MCS, multiple cloning site; LB, left border of T-DNA; P$_{35S}$, 35S constitutive promoter from cauliflower mosaic virus; TP, targeting protein sequence; T$_{35S}$, transcription termination sequence from the cauliflower mosaic virus 35S gene; *bar*, gene for phosphinothricin acetyltransferase. By varying the DNA sequence of the TP, the protein encoded by the introduced gene may be targeted to either the mitochondria or chloroplast. Adapted from Xiang et al., *Plant Mol. Biol.* **40:**711–717, 1999.

and a transcription termination sequence (Fig. 18.8). These derivatives of the minivector pCB301 are flexible and easy to use and contain a variety of unique restriction enzyme sites in the multiple cloning site. After the target gene has been cloned into the multiple cloning site, the final construct is introduced into *A. tumefaciens* by electroporation.

In many instances it may be advantageous to transform plants with several foreign genes, for example, genes that encode an entire biochemical pathway. While this is not yet commonly done, it is nevertheless possible to introduce a large amount of foreign DNA into plants. Although the transformation efficiency is low, plants have been successfully transformed with large DNA fragments ranging from 30 to 150 kb.

Although *A. tumefaciens*-mediated gene transfer systems are effective in several species, monocotyledonous plants (monocots), including the world's major cereal crops (rice, wheat, and corn), are not readily transformed by *A. tumefaciens*. However, by refining and carefully controlling conditions, protocols have been devised for the transformation of corn and rice by *A. tumefaciens* carrying Ti plasmid vectors. For example, immature corn embryos were immersed in an *A. tumefaciens* cell suspension for a few minutes and then incubated for several days at room temperature in the absence of selective pressure. The embryos were then transferred to a medium with a selective antibiotic that allowed only transformed plant cells to grow. These cells were maintained in the dark for a few weeks. Finally, the mass of transformed plant cells was transferred to a different growth medium that contained plant hormones to stimulate differentiation and incubated in the light, which permitted regeneration of whole transgenic plants. Many of the early plant transformation experiments were conducted with limited-host-range strains of *Agrobacterium*. However, more recently, broad-host-range strains that infect most plants have been tested and found to be effective, so many of the plant species that previously appeared to be refractory to transformation by *A. tumefaciens* can now be transformed. Thus, when setting out to transform a new plant species, it is necessary to determine which *Agrobacterium* strain and Ti plasmid are best suited to that particular plant. In addition, modification of the tissue culture conditions by the inclusion of antioxidants during transfor-

mation of grape, rice, corn, or soybean has been found to increase the transformation frequencies of those plant cells.

A systematic examination of the conditions that are used in *Agrobacterium*-mediated plant transformation revealed that ethylene significantly decreased the transfer of genes to plant genomes. Ethylene is produced as a consequence of *Agrobacterium* infection of plants. To remedy this, a bacterial gene encoding aminocyclopropane-1-carboxylate (ACC) deaminase, which when expressed can lower plant ethylene levels (see chapter 15), was introduced into an *A. tumefaciens* strain that is utilized to introduce foreign DNA into plants. When melon cotyledon segments were genetically transformed using the *A. tumefaciens* strain expressing ACC deaminase, the transformation frequency of the plants (as judged by the level of introduced marker enzyme activity) increased significantly (Fig. 18.9). Although this innovation has yet to be tested with other plants, it is hoped that the introduction of this ethylene-lowering gene will increase the transformation frequencies for a wide range of different plants.

Physical Methods of Transferring Genes to Plants

When the difficulties in transforming some plant species first became apparent, a number of procedures that could act as alternatives to transformation by *A. tumefaciens* were developed (Table 18.1). A number of these methods require the removal of the plant cell wall to form protoplasts. Plant protoplasts can be maintained in culture as independently growing cells, or with a specific culture medium, new cell walls can be formed and whole plants can be regenerated. In addition, transformation methods that introduce cloned genes into a small number of cells of a plant tissue from which whole plants can be formed, thereby bypassing the need for regeneration from a protoplast, have been developed. At present, most researchers

FIGURE 18.9 Effect of lowering ethylene levels on the transformation of melon cotyledons. Following transformation, the activity of the marker enzyme β-glucuronidase was measured. Treatments: 1, no *A. tumefaciens*; 2, *A. tumefaciens* carrying the marker gene on a Ti plasmid; 3, *A. tumefaciens* carrying the marker gene on a Ti plasmid with aminoethoxyvinylglycine (AVG), a chemical inhibitor of ethylene synthesis, added to the system; 4, *A. tumefaciens* carrying the marker gene on a Ti plasmid and an ACC deaminase gene on a separate plasmid.

TABLE 18.1 Plant cell DNA-delivery methods

Method	Comment
Ti plasmid-mediated gene transfer	An excellent and highly effective system that is limited to a few kinds of plants
Microprojectile bombardment	Used with a wide range of plants and tissues; easy and inexpensive
Viral vectors	Not an effective way to deliver DNA to plant cells
Direct gene transfer into plant protoplasts	Can be used only with plant cell protoplasts that can be regenerated into viable plants
Microinjection	Has limited usefulness because only one cell can be injected at a time; requires the services of a highly skilled individual
Electroporation	Generally limited to plant cell protoplasts that can be regenerated into viable plants
Liposome fusion	Can be used only with plant cell protoplasts that can be regenerated into viable plants

favor the use of either Ti plasmid-based vectors or microprojectile bombardment to deliver DNA into plant cells. A very large number of different plants have been genetically transformed with these various techniques (Table 18.2).

Microprojectile Bombardment

Microprojectile bombardment, also called biolistics, is the most important alternative to Ti plasmid DNA delivery systems for plants. Spherical gold or tungsten particles (approximately 0.4 to 1.2 µm in diameter, or about the size of some bacterial cells) are coated with DNA that has been precipitated with $CaCl_2$, spermidine, or polyethylene glycol. The coated particles are accelerated to high speed (300 to 600 meters/second) with a special apparatus called a particle gun (or gene gun). The original version of the gene gun used a small amount of gunpowder to provide the propelling force. The device that is currently used employs high-pressure helium as the source of particle propulsion (Fig. 18.10). The projectiles can penetrate plant cell walls and membranes; however, the particle density used does not significantly damage the cells. The extent of particle penetration into the target plant cells may be controlled by varying the intensity of the explosive burst, altering the distance that the particles must travel before reaching the target cells, or using different-size particles.

Once inside a cell, the DNA is removed from the particles and, in some cells, integrates into the plant DNA. Microprojectile bombardment can be

TABLE 18.2 Plants that have been genetically transformed

Alfalfa	Carnation	Kiwi fruit	Papaya	Potato	Sunflower
Apple	Carrot	Lettuce	Pea	Red fescue	Sweet potato
Arabidopsis	Corn (maize)	Licorice	Peanut	Rice	Tall fescue
Asparagus	Cotton	Lily	Pear	Rye	Tobacco
Banana	Cranberry	Lotus	Pearl millet	Sorghum	Tomato
Barley	Cucumber	Norway spruce	Peony	Soybean	Wheat
Bean	Eggplant	Oat	Petunia	Strawberry	White spruce
Cabbage	Flax	Orchard grass	Plantain	Sugar beet	
Canola	Grape	Orchid	Poplar	Sugarcane	

used to introduce foreign DNA into plant cell suspensions, callus cultures, meristematic tissues, immature embryos, protocorms, coleoptiles, and pollen in a wide range of different plants, including monocots and conifers, plants that are less susceptible to *Agrobacterium*-mediated DNA transfer (Table 18.3). Furthermore, this method has also been used to deliver genes into chloroplasts and mitochondria, thereby opening up the possibility of introducing exogenous (foreign) genes into these organelles.

Typically, plasmid DNA dissolved in buffer is precipitated onto the surfaces of the microprojectiles. Using this procedure, it is possible to increase the transformation frequency by increasing the amount of plasmid DNA; however, too much plasmid DNA can be inhibitory. It is estimated that there are approximately 10,000 transformed cells formed per bombardment. With this technique, cells that appear to be transformed, based on the expression of a marker gene, often only transiently express the introduced DNA. Unless the DNA becomes incorporated into the genome of the plant, the foreign DNA will be degraded eventually.

The configuration of the vector that is used for biolistic delivery of foreign genes to plants influences both the integration and expression of those genes. For example, transformation is more efficient when linear rather than circular DNA is used. Moreover, large plasmids (>10 kb), in contrast to small ones, may become fragmented during microprojectile bombardment and therefore produce lower levels of foreign-gene expression. However, large segments of DNA may be introduced into plants

FIGURE 18.10 Schematic representation of a microprojectile bombardment apparatus. When the helium pressure builds up to a certain point, the plastic rupture disk bursts, and the released gas accelerates the flying disk with the DNA-coated gold particles on its lower side. The gold particles pass the stopping screen, which holds back the flying disk, and penetrate the cells of the sterile leaf.

TABLE 18.3 Transgenic plants formed by microprojectile bombardment of various plant cells

Plant(s)	Cell source(s)
Corn	Embryonic cell suspension, immature zygotic embryos
Rice	Immature zygotic embryos, embryogenic callus
Barley	Cell suspension, immature zygotic embryos
Wheat	Immature zygotic embryos
Turfgrass	Embryogenic callus
Rye	Meristems
Sorghum	Immature zygotic embryos
Pearl millet	Immature zygotic embryos
Orchid	Protocorms
Banana and plantain	Embryonic cell suspension
Poplar	Callus
Norway and white spruce	Somatic embryos
Pea	Zygotic embryos
Cucumber	Embryogenic callus
Sweet potato	Callus
Cranberry	In vitro-derived stem sections
Peony and lily	Pollen
Alfalfa	Embryogenic callus
Bean	Zygotic embryos
Cotton	Zygotic embryos
Grape	Embryonic cell suspension
Peanut	Embryogenic callus
Tobacco	Pollen

Adapted from Southgate et al., *Biotechnol. Adv.* 13:631–651, 1995.

using yeast artificial chromosomes (YACs) (see chapter 7). The YACs were engineered to contain plant selectable markers, as well as yeast selectable markers, which were already present on the YAC vector (Fig. 18.11). As a test system, various amounts of DNA from the fungus *Cochliobolus heterostrophus* were cloned so that the total size of the engineered YAC ranged from 80 to 550 kb. Following biolistic transfer of the engineered YACs with fungal DNA to plant (tobacco) cells, a number of transformants resistant to the antibiotic kanamycin were isolated. These transformed plant cells were then tested for the presence of the second plant selectable marker gene (encoding resistance to the antibiotic hygromycin), which was located on the other arm of the YAC vector. The presence of both plant selectable marker genes in transformed plant cells indicated that the entire YAC, along with all of the inserted foreign DNA, was probably transferred. DNA hybridization experiments revealed that YACs up to 150 kb in total size have a good chance of being transferred to plant cells and that the transferred DNA can be stably integrated into the plant cell. Thus, the production of transgenic plants that contain several foreign genes is feasible; eventually, entire biosynthetic pathways may be introduced into plant cells.

Chloroplast Engineering

While the vast majority of plant genes are found as part of the nuclear DNA, both the chloroplast and mitochondrion contain genes that encode a number of important and unique functions. However, not all of the proteins that are present in these organelles are encoded by organellar DNA. Some chloroplast and mitochondrion proteins are encoded in the nuclear DNA, synthesized in the cell's cytoplasm, and then, by a special mechanism, imported into the appropriate organelle. Accordingly, there are two ways that a specific foreign protein can be introduced into the chloroplast or mitochondrion. In one way, a fusion gene encoding the foreign protein and additional amino acids that direct the transport of the protein to the organelle can be inserted into the nuclear chromosomal DNA, and after synthesis, the recombinant protein can be transported into the targeted organelle. In the other way, the gene for the foreign protein can be inserted directly into either the chloroplast or mitochondrial DNA.

Most higher plants have approximately 50 to 100 chloroplasts per leaf cell, and each chloroplast has about 10 to 100 copies of the chloroplast DNA genome. Stable genetic transformation of chloroplasts in order to modify chloroplast functioning or to produce foreign proteins requires insertion of the foreign DNA into the chloroplast genome rather than into the much

FIGURE 18.11 Schematic representation of a YAC vector used to transfer large pieces of DNA to plant genomes. TEL, telomere; SM, selectable marker; CEN, centromere. The various elements are not drawn to scale; the foreign DNA, especially, is much larger than shown. Each of the plant selectable marker genes contains its own promoter and transcription terminator (not shown). The plant selectable markers are a hygromycin resistance gene and a kanamycin resistance gene. Adapted from Mullen et al., *Mol. Breed.* 4:449–457, 1998.

MILESTONE

Regeneration of Normal and Fertile Plants That Express Octopine Synthase from Tobacco Crown Galls after Deletion of Tumour-Controlling Functions

H. DE GREVE, J. LEEMANS, J. P. HERNALSTEENS, L. THIA-TOONG, M. DE BEUCKELEER, L. WILLMITZER, L. OTTEN, M. VAN MONTAGU, and J. SCHELL
Nature 300:752–755, 1982

An efficient vector system is essential for the routine construction of transgenic plants. Most of the early efforts to develop such a vector focused on the Ti plasmid of the soil bacterium *A. tumefaciens* because, following infection of susceptible dicots, a portion of the Ti plasmid (the T-DNA) is inserted directly into the chromosomal DNA of the host plant cells. However, infection of plants with the native Ti plasmid results in the formation of a crown gall tumor that interferes with the normal growth of the plant. Therefore, before the Ti plasmid could be used as a vector to transform plants, crown gall tumor formation had to be prevented.

By studying the mRNAs that were transcribed from intact and modified T-DNAs, Schell and his colleagues determined that the tumor-inducing genes were a part of the T-DNA. Therefore, a modified T-DNA in which the tumor-inducing genes were deleted was constructed. This modified T-DNA was then introduced by homologous recombination into the Ti plasmid. Such a "disarmed" Ti plasmid could be introduced into plant cells and transfer its T-DNA into their chromosomal DNA. Under these conditions, the modified T-DNA was stably maintained in the plant genome, and importantly, no crown gall tumors were formed. The next logical step in the development of this system was the cloning of foreign marker and target genes into the T-DNA so that they could also be transferred to the chromosomal DNA of the host plant. This vector system utilizing the Ti plasmid has become the system of choice for creating transgenic plants and has been used successfully in thousands of laboratories around the world.

larger chromosomal DNA. (Plant chromosomal DNA is generally around 10^4 to 10^5 times larger than chloroplast DNA.) Moreover, the foreign DNA needs to be present in all of the approximately 10^3 to 10^4 chloroplast DNA genomes per leaf cell.

Foreign DNA is typically introduced by microprojectile bombardment into the chloroplast genome on a plasmid vector with both the (usually nonselectable) foreign DNA and a selectable marker, such as an antibiotic resistance gene, flanked by specific chloroplast DNA sequences (Fig. 18.12). Homologous recombination is the normal mode of DNA integration into the chloroplast genome.

Some chloroplast genes are transcribed by chloroplast-encoded RNA polymerase plus a nucleus-encoded RNA polymerase sigma factor, while others are transcribed solely by a nucleus-encoded RNA polymerase. The promoter sequences that are recognized by these two different RNA polymerases are completely different. At present, it is not known how the use of one or the other type of promoter sequence affects the expression of the downstream genes. The efficient expression of foreign genes in the chloroplast requires not only the use of an appropriate promoter sequence, but also the presence of the correct sequences in the 5′ and 3′ untranslated regions of the messenger RNA (mRNA). Many biotechnological applications have focused on the strong sigma-70-type ribosomal RNA (rRNA) promoter, which is recognized by the chloroplast-encoded RNA polymerase. This promoter is fused at the DNA level with chloroplast translational control sequences, followed by the gene of interest and a 3′ chloroplast untranslated region containing a stem-and-loop structure, which may act as a transcription termination signal (Fig. 18.13). Any nucleus-encoded proteins that are synthesized outside of the chloroplast contain a transit peptide that is removed as the protein is imported into the chloroplast.

FIGURE 18.12 Plasmid vector used for integrating a foreign gene and a marker gene into the chloroplast genome. Regulatory sequences are not shown. Homologous recombination can occur between chloroplast DNA sequences on the vector and the chloroplast genome. Spcr, spectinomycin resistance.

Chloroplast DNA is inherited in a non-Mendelian fashion. In most angiosperm plants, it is maintained in egg cells, but not sperm (pollen) cells, and is therefore transmitted uniparentally by the female. Thus, pollen cannot transmit the contents of the chloroplast genome to the zygote. This has practical importance, since this trait could prevent the spread of foreign genes, localized in the chloroplast, through pollen to neighboring plants, thereby addressing one of the concerns of critics of the genetic engineering of plants.

An important component of a successful chloroplast transformation system is the availability of suitable selectable marker and reporter genes that facilitate selection and analysis of cells with transgenic chloroplasts. A number of selectable marker genes are currently available for monitoring chloroplast transformation (Table 18.4). Most transformed chloroplasts are selected by resistance to spectinomycin, streptomycin, or kanamycin, all of which inhibit protein synthesis on prokaryotic-type ribosomes. These antibiotics inhibit greening, faster proliferation, and shoot formation. However, plant cells with transformed chloroplasts that express the genes conferring resistance to the antibiotic are readily identified in the presence of (otherwise) inhibitory antibiotics by their greening, faster proliferation, and shoot formation. Since only one, or at most a few, of the chloroplasts actually incorporates the foreign DNA, repeated rounds of growth on selective antibiotics are often required so that the chloroplast population becomes enriched and eventually dominated by the transformants. Eventually, all chloroplast genomes that do not carry the transgenic DNA with its selectable marker gene are lost.

The chloroplast genome is an attractive location for engineering any gene that, as a consequence of the multiple copies of the chloroplast DNA, might benefit from high levels of expression. For example, active human somatotropin accumulated to 7% of the total soluble protein in tobacco chloroplasts. In addition, most chloroplast-borne genes are organized into operons and produce polycistronic mRNAs. This should make it easier to

FIGURE 18.13 Organization of an engineered chloroplast gene transcription cassette. UTR, untranslated region.

| Promoter | 5′ UTR | Gene of interest | 3′ UTR |

TABLE 18.4 Some foreign genes that have been used as selectable markers and reporters of transgenic chloroplasts

Gene	Gene product	Function
aadA	Aminoglycoside 3′-adenylyltransferase	Positive selection (spectinomycin and streptomycin resistance)
nptII	Neomycin phosphotransferase	Positive selection (kanamycin resistance)
uidA	β-Glucuronidase	Reporter gene
gfp	Green fluorescent protein	Reporter gene
codA	Cytosine deaminase	Negative selection (5-fluorocytosine sensitivity)

Adapted from Hager and Bock, *Appl. Microbiol. Biotechnol.* **54:**302–310, 2000.

engineer plants with transgenic chloroplasts that express several genes that are regulated together as part of a new metabolic pathway than to coordinately express several genes under the control of different promoters that have been introduced into a plant's chromosomal DNA.

Chloroplasts belong to a group of plant organelles called plastids, which contain approximately 120 to 180 kb of circular double-stranded DNA bounded by a double membrane. Plastids include amyloplasts, which contain starch grains; chloroplasts, which contain chlorophyll; elaioplasts, which contain oil; and chromoplasts, which contain other pigments. While photosynthetic tissues, such as green leaves, contain chloroplasts, other tissues contain other types of plastids. For example, tomato fruit contains a large number of chromoplasts. Thus, in much the same way that foreign DNA may be expressed as a part of the chloroplast genome, it can also be targeted for expression in the chromoplast.

Researchers can transform tomato plastids and obtain high-level expression of foreign proteins both in green leaves and in tomato fruit. One of the advantages of this system is that transgenic tomatoes expressing high levels of certain foreign proteins (which are normally found as part of an animal or human pathogen) may be used as edible vaccines (see chapter 20).

Use of Reporter Genes in Transformed Plant Cells

It is essential to be able to detect the foreign DNA that has been integrated into plant genomic DNA so that those cells that have been transformed can be identified; this requires the use of a selectable marker. Furthermore, in studies of plant transcriptional regulatory signals and the functioning of these signals in specific plant tissues (such as leaves, roots, and flowers), it is often important to be able to quantify the level of expression of a gene with a readily identified product. Quantification and other applications require the use of reporter genes that encode an activity that can be assayed. To these ends, a number of different genes have been tested as reporters for transformation, including genes that can be used as dominant selectable markers and genes whose proteins produce a detectable response to a specific assay (Table 18.5). Many of these reporter genes are from bacteria and have been equipped with plant-specific regulatory sequences for expression in plant cells. Dominant-marker selection provides a direct means of obtaining only transformed cells in culture. For example, in the presence of the antibiotic kanamycin, only plant cells with a functional neomycin phosphotransferase gene can grow.

TABLE 18.5 Plant cell reporter and selectable marker gene systems

Enzyme activity	Selectable marker	Reporter gene
Neomycin phosphotransferase	Yes	Yes
Hygromycin phosphotransferase	Yes	Yes
Dihydrofolate reductase	Yes	Yes
Chloramphenicol acetyltransferase	Yes	Yes
Gentamicin acetyltransferase	Yes	Yes
Nopaline synthase	No	Yes
Octopine synthase	No	Yes
β-Glucuronidase	No	Yes
Streptomycin phosphotransferase	Yes	Yes
Bleomycin resistance	Yes	No
Firefly luciferase	No	Yes
Bacterial luciferase	No	Yes
Threonine dehydratase	Yes	Yes
Metallothionein II	Yes	Yes
enol-Pyruvylshikimate-3-phosphate synthase	Yes	No
Phosphinothricin acetyltransferase	Yes	Yes
β-Galactosidase	No	Yes
Blasticidin S deaminase	Yes	Yes
Acetolactate synthase	Yes	No
Bromoxynil nitrilase	Yes	No
Green fluorescent protein	No	Yes

Adapted from Walden and Schell, *Eur. J. Biochem.* **192**:563–576, 1990, and Gruber and Crosby, p. 89–119, in B. R. Glick and J. E. Thompson (ed.), *Methods in Plant Molecular Biology and Biotechnology* (CRC Press, Boca Raton, FL, 1993).

The desired outcome of a particular experiment often dictates which reporter gene will be used. Clearly, when the expression of a reporter gene interferes with normal plant functions, it cannot be used. Moreover, the presence of some reporter genes and their products may taint a commercial product. In this context, it is best to remove the reporter gene once transformants with the desired traits have been selected, especially in crop plants.

Some reporter gene products, e.g., β-D-glucuronidase (GUS), both firefly and bacterial luciferases, and green fluorescent protein (GFP), can be detected in situ in intact plant tissues. One of the most popular of these systems is the *E. coli* GUS gene. The GUS gene encodes a stable enzyme that is not normally present in plants and that catalyzes the cleavage of a range of β-D-glucuronides. The GUS activity in transformed plant tissues can be localized by the presence of a blue color that is formed after the hydrolysis of the uncolored substrate 5-bromo-4-chloro-3-indolyl β-D-glucuronic acid. Alternatively, GUS activity in plant extracts can be quantitatively and sensitively assayed by a fluorometric analysis that involves the hydrolysis of the substrate 4-methylumbelliferyl β-D-glucuronide to form a fluorescent product.

GFP is an ideal in vivo marker for monitoring transgenic plants because it fluoresces green when excited with either ultraviolet or blue light and does not require the addition of any substrates or cofactors. Normally, wild-type plants (which do not contain the gene for GFP) fluoresce reddish purple when they are excited by ultraviolet or blue light. Moreover, derivatives of the gene that encodes the GFP protein that have different spectral

properties and increased levels of fluorescence have been constructed. Importantly, the expression of GFP has no effect on the survival and growth of transformed plants under field conditions.

Manipulation of Gene Expression in Plants

When genetic transformation of plants became routine, research efforts were directed toward introducing a wide range of plant and bacterial genes in plant cells. The transformed plants were assayed for the production of the foreign protein and studied physiologically to assess how the presence of an additional protein affected the whole plant. Many of these early experiments utilized promoters that were expressed constitutively in a range of plant cells. More recently, many additional plant promoters have been isolated and characterized and used to express foreign proteins in specific cells at certain times during the growth and development of the plant. For example, instead of the strong constitutive 35S promoter from cauliflower mosaic virus, which is expressed in all plant tissues and throughout the life of the plant, researchers have used the promoter for the small subunit of the photosynthetic enzyme ribulosebisphosphate carboxylase, which is active only in photosynthetic tissues, such as leaves. Similarly, plant promoters active only in specific tissues, such as roots or flowers, or only during periods of environmental stress—e.g., the pathogenesis-related promoters—have been used to control the expression of some foreign genes.

Isolation and Use of Different Promoters

In order to minimize any deleterious effects on plant growth from the expression of foreign genes, it is necessary to regulate the expression of introduced genes, spatially and temporally, and the amount of the foreign protein that is produced. While a major factor in the initiation of transcription in plants is the binding of RNA polymerase II to the promoter sequence, other factors affect this process. Much of the specificity of transcription in plants is controlled by sequence-specific transcription factors and/or enhancer-binding proteins (Fig. 18.14). Enhancer elements are regions on the DNA that bind to enhancer-binding proteins, which interact with transcription factors and RNA polymerase to maximize the level of transcription from a particular promoter. Enhancer sequences may be located several thousand base pairs from the promoter sequence, although they are typically much closer. Enhancer sequences are generally considered to be important determinants of the tissue and temporal specificity of gene expression. While the importance of promoter and enhancer sequences has been recognized, a thorough understanding of how these and other elements regulate plant gene expression is still at an early stage. Despite the complexity of this system, there have been several successful experiments in which "designer promoters" were created.

Specialized vectors, called promoter-tagging (labeling) vectors, have been used to isolate plant promoters from several plant species. This approach relies on the *Agrobacterium*-mediated Ti plasmid transformation system. Briefly, a promoterless reporter gene is placed next to the right border of a Ti plasmid vector. After transfer of the T-DNA into a plant chromosome, the reporter gene from the vector is inserted randomly into the plant DNA (Fig. 18.15A). If the T-DNA is inserted immediately downstream of the promoter region of a functional gene, transcription of the reporter

FIGURE 18.14 Schematic representation of a plant RNA transcription complex including RNA polymerase II binding to the TATA box (an essential portion of a eukaryotic promoter), various transcription factors bound to the polymerase, and an enhancer-binding protein bound to an enhancer element on the DNA, which is located at some distance from the promoter sequence.

gene occurs. For example, with the neomycin phosphotransferase *(npt)* gene as a reporter, its expression is detected by selecting kanamycin-resistant transformants. However, with this method, only constitutive promoters will be selected. Thus, it is difficult to identify (tag) a promoter that is active only during a certain developmental stage or that is induced by a specific environmental factor because insertion downstream from this type of promoter will be selected against using kanamycin. To overcome this problem, a two-gene selectable marker system was devised. In this case, a hygromycin resistance gene is placed under the control of a constitutive promoter next to a promoterless reporter gene within the T-DNA (Fig. 18.15B). After hygromycin-resistant transformants are selected, the transformants can be checked by an enzyme assay that measures neomycin phosphotransferase activity under different conditions for expression to identify potentially useful plant promoters. With this strategy, 5 to 30% of the transformed plant cells have the reporter gene under the control of an active promoter.

The cauliflower mosaic virus 35S promoter is frequently used as a strong promoter in plant systems, although the level of expression of a foreign protein under the control of this promoter is often lower than desired. To address this problem, it is necessary to test different promoter–gene constructs in plants to see if more effective promoters can be found. In addition to the promoter, several other elements may enhance foreign-gene expression. As indicated above, these include enhancer sequences that are typically found from one to several hundred nucleotides upstream

A

Plant DNA — | — T-DNA —

P → RB *npt* TT

B

Plant DNA — | — T-DNA —

P → RB *npt* TT P Hyg^r gene TT

FIGURE 18.15 Using a promoterless reporter gene to isolate a plant promoter. **(A)** A promoterless neomycin phosphotransferase *(npt)* reporter gene is placed downstream from a right-border (RB) sequence of the T-DNA. After transfer of the T-DNA into the plant chromosomal DNA, if the T-DNA is inserted near the promoter (P) region of a functional plant gene that is oriented in the same direction as *npt,* transcription occurs. The expression of *npt* is detected by selecting for kanamycin-resistant transformants. **(B)** To ensure that transformed cells are selected, a hygromycin resistance (Hyg^r) gene, under the control of a constitutive promoter (P), is placed downstream from the promoterless reporter gene within the T-DNA. Both the *npt* and Hyg^r genes are equipped with transcription terminator (TT) regions.

of the promoter sequence, introns that may stabilize mRNA, and transcription terminator sequences.

In one series of experiments, DNA constructs that contained all or some of the following elements were tested: the 35S promoter, the nopaline synthase gene transcription terminator, from one to seven tandemly repeated enhancer elements, and a DNA sequence from tobacco mosaic virus called Ω (omega) that increases gene expression at the translational level (Fig. 18.16). The most active construct contained seven enhancer elements and directed a much higher level of foreign-gene expression in both transgenic tobacco and rice plants than the 35S promoter alone (Table 18.6). The expression levels of foreign genes from these promoter constructs were quite variable in transgenic plants. This variation is thought to be due to the site within the plant genome where the T-DNA is inserted. Nevertheless, this work shows that it is possible to engineer promoters that are much stronger than the naturally occurring 35S promoter. With this approach, it should be possible to engineer promoters that are tissue specific, developmentally regulated, and strong.

Gene Targeting

In bacteria, and to a lesser extent in animal cells, it is relatively straightforward to alter the genomic DNA of an organism by homologous recombination between the native form of the target DNA in the genome and a

FIGURE 18.16 Example of a composite promoter assembled from a variety of different elements, including enhancer elements (only one is shown; however, the most active composite promoter contained seven), a 35S promoter, a 5′ untranslated region (UTR) containing an Ω sequence, the gene of interest, and a 3′ UTR containing a transcriptional terminator sequence.

Enhancer Promoter 5′ UTR Gene of interest 3′ UTR

TABLE 18.6 Testing promoter constructs in transgenic plants

Plant	Average gene expression		Maximum gene expression	
	35S promoter	Composite promoter	35S promoter	Composite promoter
Tobacco	1.0	2.8	2.8	18.3
Rice	1.0	14.4	7.2	47.1

Adapted from Mitsuhara et al., *Plant Cell Physiol.* 37:49–59, 1996.

E. coli β-glucuronidase was the reporter gene. Enzyme activities were normalized to the average value per plant when the gene was under the control of the 35S promoter. The actual values in tobacco are approximately 30-fold higher than the values in rice. The composite promoter included the 35S promoter, the nopaline synthase gene transcription terminator, seven tandemly repeated enhancer elements, and the tobacco mosaic virus Ω sequence. Average gene expression is the mean value of a number of different transgenic plants. Maximum gene expression is the highest value observed in any transgenic plant with that promoter.

modified form of the target DNA, usually on a plasmid vector (see chapter 6). Using similar techniques, the targeted alteration of plant cell genes occurs quite infrequently. However, based on successful experiments in which genomic changes were introduced into animal cells, researchers have used RNA–DNA chimeric molecules—actually, the RNA is 2'-*O*-methyl RNA—to stably change the genomic DNA of plant cells (Fig. 18.17). These chimeric oligonucleotides are designed to have one or more bases that do not pair with the endogenous plant DNA sequence. Following the delivery of a chimeric oligonucleotide into a plant cell by microprojectile bombardment, it is thought that DNA repair enzymes recognize the mismatches between the targeted gene and a large molar excess of the chimeric oligonucleotide. During the repair process, the altered DNA is incorporated into the plant genome. The changed chromosomal DNA can be readily detected phenotypically if the mutation that is created is dominantly or codominantly expressed. This is because plants are diploid, with two copies of each gene, and this procedure typically changes only one of those copies. In addition to changing one or two bases in the sequence of a plant gene, this technique may also be used to modify plant DNA through the site-specific insertion or deletion of a single base.

Gene targeting is extremely inefficient in plants, where the frequency of random DNA integration into the plant genome generally exceeds that of homologous integration by 3 or 4 orders of magnitude. Moreover, because the transformation frequency in plants is often around 1 to 5%, the number of seeds or plant cell cultures that must be screened to detect a single homologous-integration event is around 10^4 to 10^6. However, in

FIGURE 18.17 Example of a chimeric oligonucleotide used to change the nucleotide sequence of plant DNA. The 2'-*O*-methyl RNA residues are shown in lowercase red letters. The DNA residues are shown in uppercase letters. The codon that was targeted for change is shown in blue. In this case, a CCA codon (which encodes the amino acid proline) that is part of a tobacco acetolactate synthase (ALS) gene was changed to CAA—this is the complementary sequence of the 3'-GTT-5' sequence shown in blue—which encodes glutamine. Plants with the mutated gene may be selected for by their resistance to the toxic effects of sulfonylurea herbicides, which normally target the ALS enzyme.

plants that have been engineered to overexpress the *RAD54* gene from the yeast *Saccharomyces cerevisiae*, the gene-targeting frequency of subsequently introduced cloned genes increases by up to 2 orders of magnitude (Fig. 18.18). The yeast *RAD54* gene promotes integration of homologous introduced DNA into the plant genomic DNA. Transgenic plants that express *RAD54* to a high level are readily selected on the basis of their resistance to high levels of γ-irradiation that are lethal to nontransformed plants. This resistance occurs as a consequence of the increased recombination repair efficiency conferred by *RAD54*. Initial experiments with plants that overexpress *RAD54* utilized a GFP gene, whose product is easily detected, that was inserted in frame in the middle of the target gene. However, in experiments in which the gene of interest is not marked by GFP, it may be necessary to screen large numbers of transformants to find the target gene with the desired modification. Nevertheless, the use of *RAD54*-transgenic plants dramatically increases the probability of targeting specific changes in plant genes. The *RAD54* gene may be deleted from the plant genome, prior to the agricultural use of the modified plant, by traditional genetic crosses with the wild-type plant, selecting for plants that contain the desired altered gene but not the *RAD54* gene.

Consumers and regulators in a number of countries have expressed serious concerns about the commercialization of transgenic plants. However, modification of an existing plant gene, which is generally not considered to be genetic engineering, should allow some specifically altered plants to more rapidly reach the marketplace in those countries. The targeted stable modification of plant genomes is conceptually similar to conventional mutagenesis and selection procedures, and with this approach, no foreign DNA is introduced into the plant.

Targeted Alterations in Plant RNA

To modify the phenotypes of plants, researchers have directed their efforts toward the downregulation of the expression of certain plant genes. This inhibition of mRNA expression can be achieved by the expression of an additional copy of a gene (using a mechanism originally called cosuppression and currently thought to involve RNA interference), addition of an antisense version of a gene, or the use of ribozymes, small RNA molecules with the ability to act as sequence-specific endoribonucleases (for a discus-

FIGURE 18.18 Constructs used in gene targeting. **(A)** The construct used to introduce the *RAD54* gene includes a left border (LB) and right border (RB), a glufosinate (a herbicide) resistance gene with appropriate regulatory signals (BASTA) for selection, and the *S. cerevisiae RAD54* gene under the control of the cauliflower mosaic virus 35S promoter (P_{35S}) and transcription termination (TT) signals. **(B)** The construct containing the target gene and its regulatory signals.

sion of RNA interference, antisense RNA, and ribozymes, see chapter 11). When they are present in a cell, ribozymes are able to recognize and cleave one specific mRNA of the many that are present in that cell, thereby decreasing the amount of protein that is encoded by that mRNA. In one experiment, a number of potential ribozyme cleavage sites were identified in the corn stearoyl-acyl carrier protein (ACP) Δ9 desaturase mRNA sequence, and then 20 different hammerhead ribozymes were synthesized and tested. Genes for the three most effective ribozymes were fused to the open reading frame of a functional plant structural gene to enhance ribozyme stability, and then each of the constructs was used to generate transgenic plants. A few of the transgenic plants demonstrated a reduction in stearoyl-ACP Δ9 desaturase mRNA and protein levels and an increase in the plant's stearate content (Fig. 18.19). The oil from plants that have a high stearic acid content is used in cooking and to make margarine. In order to inhibit translation, it is not sufficient for a ribozyme to merely base pair with mRNA. The biological activity of the ribozyme is dependent on its cleaving the target mRNA.

Facilitating Protein Purification

Transgenic plants have some advantages over bacteria as expression systems for foreign proteins. For example, transgenic bacteria are typically grown in expensive bioreactors under precisely defined conditions and require highly skilled personnel to oversee the entire growth process. On the other hand, it is generally thought that plants may be grown in the field by somewhat less highly skilled individuals at a much lower cost and in more or less unlimited quantities. Thus, one of the main advantages of expressing a foreign protein in a transgenic plant is that it is relatively inexpensive to grow plants on a large scale.

With both plants and bacteria, following growth, the organisms must be harvested and processed before the recombinant protein can be purified. Protocols for the purification of proteins from transgenic bacteria are well established, and many proteins produced by bacteria are in the marketplace. However, transgenic plants produce a much lower level of foreign proteins; therefore, for commercial production of a range of protein products, the purification of target proteins produced by transgenic plants requires special strategies and approaches.

Oleosins. A novel way to facilitate recombinant plant protein purification is to fuse the foreign protein to plant oleosins. Oleosins, or oil body proteins, are found in the seeds of a wide range of plants. These proteins are quite hydrophobic and are mostly embedded within small oil droplets (0.6 to 2 μm in diameter) called plant oil bodies, thus stabilizing the oil bodies

FIGURE 18.19 Modification of fatty acid biosynthesis in maize. The conversion of stearic to oleic acid is blocked by the action of the added ribozyme on the mRNA encoding stearoyl-ACP Δ9 desaturase, and stearic acid accumulates. The numbers to the left of the colons indicate the numbers of carbon atoms in the fatty acid, and the numbers to the right of the colons indicate the numbers of C=C bonds, which are formed by the activity of desaturases. CoA, coenzyme A.

as discrete organelles. However, the N- and C-terminal regions of oleosins are more hydrophilic than the rest of the protein and are exposed to the aqueous environment. It is therefore possible to engineer fusions between oleosins and water-soluble proteins at the DNA level (Fig. 18.20), with the expectation that the fusion protein will be targeted to plant oil bodies, making it relatively easy to purify. In this case, the water-soluble target protein will not be embedded in the oil body but rather will be exposed to the aqueous environment. Since it is relatively easy to purify oil bodies from plant seeds, the purification of the recombinant protein is simplified. A cleavable linker is included between the oleosin and the target protein so that the recombinant protein can be recovered by cleavage of the fusion protein. Expression in seeds is particularly attractive, as proteins accumulate stably and seeds can be stored without deterioration prior to being processed. This system has the potential to significantly lower the costs of purifying target proteins produced in plants.

Rhizosecretion. Harvesting the variety of protein products that can be produced in transgenic plants can be difficult, since they are generally localized within plant cells that must be disrupted before their purification. Moreover, since the cost of purifying a recombinant protein can be as much as 90% of the total cost of producing that protein, if plants are going to be used as bioreactors for protein production, it is essential that purification costs be kept to a minimum. One way around this problem is to engineer plants to secrete foreign proteins through the roots in a process that has been called "rhizosecretion." If a plant engineered for rhizosecretion is grown hydroponically, the protein will be secreted directly into the culture medium (Fig. 18.21).

Normally, roots secrete large amounts of small molecules, such as sugars and amino acids; however, they secrete only low levels of relatively few proteins. These small organic molecules, including mainly amino acids and sugars, are first secreted to the root intercellular space (apoplast) before they are exuded by the roots. In one series of experiments, three different proteins—xylanase from the thermophilic bacterium *Clostridium thermocellum*, GFP from the jellyfish *Aequorea victoria*, and human placental secreted alkaline phosphatase—were tested to determine whether they could be engineered for secretion through the roots. The three proteins were directed to the root apoplast using three different secretion signals (Fig. 18.22). Each protein was efficiently exuded by the roots of transgenic tobacco plants, as long as the genetic construct contained a DNA fragment encoding a signal peptide, even one that was not of plant origin, placed upstream (at the 5' end) of the gene whose protein was targeted for secretion. Both the 35S promoter, which is expressed in all plant cell types, and the *mas2'* promoter, which is preferentially expressed in roots, directed the synthesis of a significant amount of the target protein in root tissue. With the 35S promoter, the foreign protein could also be recovered from the guttation fluid (i.e., leaf exudate). However, given the ease of collecting root as opposed to leaf exudate, this approach appears to have the most promise at the present time.

Glycosylation. A large number of mammalian proteins, including many potentially therapeutic molecules, are glycosylated (i.e., they contain specific sugars attached to the hydroxyl group of either serine or threonine or the amide group of asparagine). While the addition of glycans (polysaccharides) containing high levels of mannose at specific asparagine residues

FIGURE 18.20 Schematic representation of a fusion protein including oleosin and a water-soluble target protein embedded in a plant seed oil body. The N- and C-terminal ends of the oleosin and the target protein are hydrophilic and are therefore found in the aqueous environment.

FIGURE 18.21 Schematic representation of a plant in hydroponic culture secreting proteins and small molecules (red arrows) into the medium. The arrows at the inlet and outlet ports indicate the direction of flow of added nutrient solutions. The proteins secreted by the roots are concentrated and harvested from the hydroponic medium and then purified.

FIGURE 18.22 DNA constructs of proteins engineered for secretion into the apoplast in tobacco. **(A)** A truncated xylanase *(xyl-t)* gene from *C. thermocellum* is transcriptionally controlled by the cauliflower mosaic virus 35S promoter (P_{35S}) and targeted to the apoplast by a tobacco proteinase inhibitor signal peptide (SP_{pri}). **(B)** A GFP *(gfp)* gene from *A. victoria* controlled by the strong modified *Agrobacterium* mannopine synthase promoter ($p^{mas2'}$) that is preferentially active in plant roots and targeted to the apoplast by a *Nicotiana plumbaginifolia* (another type of tobacco) calreticulin proteinase inhibitor signal peptide (SP_{cal}). **(C)** A truncated human alkaline phosphatase *(alk)* gene controlled by the strong modified *Agrobacterium* mannopine synthase promoter ($p^{mas2'}$) that is preferentially active in plant roots and targeted to the apoplast by the human alkaline phosphatase signal peptide (SP_{alk}).

on proteins is initially identical in mammalian and plant cells, trimming of the sugar residues generates complex N-glycans with very different structures and properties in the two different types of organisms. Although differences in glycosylation may not directly alter the activity of a protein, other properties, such as folding, stability, solubility, susceptibility to proteases, blood clearance rate, and antigenicity, can be affected profoundly.

To avoid some of the problems that result from the incorrect glycosylation of mammalian proteins that are produced in plant cells, it is possible to modify the plant so that it does not add "problematic" carbohydrate residues. For example, when the aquatic plant *Lemna minor* was engineered to produce light and heavy chains that are part of a human monoclonal antibody, the plant was simultaneously transformed with an RNA interference construct (see chapter 11) that specifically inhibited the expression of the plant enzymes α-1,3-fucosyltransferase and β-1,2-xylosyltransferase. The antibodies that were produced by these transgenic plants contained a single major N-glycan species without any plant-specific N-glycan residues (Fig. 18.23). While these truncated glycan side chains are not identical to the glycans that are produced when a human monoclonal antibody is synthesized in Chinese hamster ovary (CHO) cells in culture, they share the same core molecules. When human monoclonal antibodies produced in genetically modified plants were tested, they displayed better antibody-dependent cell-mediated cytotoxicity and effector cell receptor-binding activities than antibodies that were produced in CHO cells. Thus, with this system, it may be possible to produce a wide range of mammalian proteins in which the glycan side chains no longer limit the use of the final protein. In addition, it should be much less expensive to produce mammalian proteins in transgenic plants than in mammalian cell culture.

Production of Marker-Free Transgenic Plants

Usually, at the same time that a foreign gene is introduced into plants, a selectable marker gene is also introduced. Although none of these genes or their products have been shown to have an adverse effect on human,

FIGURE 18.23 Structures of the N-glycan side chains found on proteins synthesized by CHO cells, the native form of the aquatic plant *L. minor,* or a genetically modified form of *L. minor.*

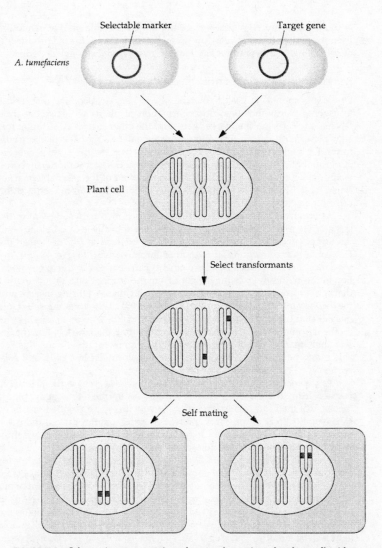

FIGURE 18.24 Schematic representation of cotransformation of a plant cell with two separate DNAs. One DNA carries a selectable marker, while the other carries the target gene. On average, more than half of the transformed plants have both of these genes, but at separate sites on the chromosome. Several rounds of self-mating allow the segregation of the marker and target genes into different plants.

animal, or environmental safety, their inclusion in transgenic plants has raised some concerns. For example, it is possible that the products of some marker genes might be either toxic or allergenic. Also, the antibiotic resistance genes that are used as selectable markers might be transferred to pathogenic soil microorganisms. Moreover, the presence of a selectable marker makes it technically more difficult to transform a transgenic plant

with additional foreign genes, since the same selectable marker cannot be used more than once. To allay these concerns, strategies for the production of transgenic plants without any marker genes have been developed.

Removing Marker Genes from Nuclear DNA

One experimental approach that has been used to produce markerless transgenic plants includes cotransformation of plants with two separate DNAs, one carrying the marker gene and the other carrying the target foreign gene. With cotransformation, approximately 30 to 80% of the transformed plants contain both genes. However, since the two genes are integrated at different sites on the chromosomal DNA, traditional breeding techniques can be used to rid the transgenic plant of the selectable marker (Fig. 18.24). Thus, the two genes are separated by chromosome segregation during a few rounds of matings.

Alternatively, a selectable marker gene is cloned between plant transposable elements (Ds elements) and inserted into the T-DNA along with the target gene and a transposase gene that excises the DNA between the Ds elements and integrates it at another chromosomal site (Fig. 18.25). Any sequence that is between two Ds elements can be mobilized to a new location in the genome—excising the gene from the original location—provided that the appropriate transposase enzyme is available. During insertion of the T-DNA into the host plant DNA, about 90% of the time the selectable marker that is between the two Ds elements will be moved to another site on the chromosomal DNA. About half of the time the new location for the selectable marker will be far away from the original location. Thus, a selectable marker gene can be used to identify transformed plant cells, and subsequently, it can be removed by breeding.

Any procedure that uses sexual crossing to segregate the selectable marker from the gene of interest cannot be applied to woody plants (because of their long generation times), vegetatively propagated plants, or sterile plants. In addition, if several related genes are introduced, and these genes are unlinked, they may segregate independently and consequently be lost in subsequent generations. One simple way around this problem is to utilize DNA sequences that flank the selectable marker and mark it for eventual removal from the genome (Fig. 18.26). In this way, the selectable marker and flanking sequences are only transiently present as a component of the transgenic plant. For example, if the selectable marker gene is fused to a recombinase gene and flanked by sequences that are recognized by the recombinase, both from the yeast *Zygosaccharomyces rouxii*, the selectable gene will be initially expressed. However, the recombinase is also expressed and mediates excision of the region between its recognition sites, thus removing both the selectable marker and recombinase genes after growth

FIGURE 18.25 Schematic representation of a T-DNA-based selectable marker gene excision system. Following integration of the T-DNA into the plant chromosomal DNA, the transposase can excise the selectable marker gene and insert it into a different chromosomal location. LB, the T-DNA left border; RB, the T-DNA right border. The promoter and transcription termination sequences of the genes are not shown.

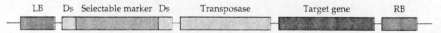

| LB | Ds | Selectable marker | Ds | Transposase | Target gene | RB |

FIGURE 18.26 Schematic representation of a DNA construct for generating marker-free transgenic plants. RB and LB are the right and left borders of the T-DNA, respectively. After transformation, selection of transformed cells, and growth in culture, recombinase cleaves the DNA at the recombination sites, and the selectable marker and recombinase genes are lost. Transgenic plants are formed from the cells without the selectable marker gene.

in culture for several months (Fig. 18.26). In this case, transformed plant cells are selected immediately following transformation, characterized to ascertain whether they contain and express the target gene, and then grown in culture until the selectable marker has been excised. In addition, several similar excision systems that result in the removal of the selectable marker have been developed. Importantly, regardless of the details, it is no longer necessary to produce transgenic plants that retain antibiotic resistance genes or other undesirable selectable markers.

Most transgenic plants are selected using any one of a small number of antibiotic or herbicide resistance genes. An alternative to utilizing these genes includes expressing the D-amino acid oxidase *(DAO)* gene from the yeast *Rhodotorula gracilis* in transgenic plants. This enzyme catalyzes the deamination of several D-amino acids that might otherwise become inhibitory to plant growth. Thus, for example, nontransgenic plants (which lack this enzyme) are inhibited in the presence of D-alanine despite the fact that they can grow normally in the presence of D-isoleucine (Fig. 18.27). On the other hand, plants that have been transformed to express the *DAO* gene grow normally in the presence of D-alanine but are inhibited by D-isoleucine. An innovative way to utilize this selection would involve cotransforming plants with two separate DNAs, one with the *DAO* gene and the other with the target gene (with the expectation that the cotransformation frequency will be on the order of 30% to 80%). Alternatively, the *DAO* gene flanked by Ds elements (Fig. 18.25) and a target gene may be inserted into the same T-DNA. In either case, the *DAO* gene and the target gene will be located far away from one another so that sexual crossing (breeding) may be used to segregate the target gene from the *DAO* gene. The initial transformants with both genes are selected following growth on D-alanine. Following sexual crossing, the segregated transformants that have lost the *DAO* gene are selected following growth on D-isoleucine. The selected transformants are then assayed for the presence of the target gene. A significant fraction of the plants that lose the *DAO* gene nevertheless retain the target gene. Despite the elegance of this negative/positive selection system, its efficacy in producing marker-free plants remains to be demonstrated.

Removing Marker Genes from Chloroplast DNA

The promise of high levels of foreign-gene expression, as well as the possibility of expressing several related genes under the control of the same promoter, has resulted in an increasing number of foreign genes being introduced into plant chloroplast DNA. One way to remove marker genes

A Wild type

D-Alanine ──────▶ Growth inhibition

D-Isoleucine ──────▶ Normal growth

B *DAO* transformed

D-Alanine ──────▶ Normal growth

D-Isoleucine ──────▶ Growth inhibition

C Mix of wild type
and transformants
with *DAO* gene

D-Alanine ──────▶ Transformants grow well, but the wild type does not

1. Breeding
2. D-Isoleucine ──────▶

Transformants with the *DAO* gene do not grow well. Those without the *DAO* gene grow well but need to be tested for the target gene.

FIGURE 18.27 A possible positive-negative selection scheme for marker-free transformed plants. **(A)** Wild-type plants that lack D-amino acid oxidase (DAO) are inhibited by growth on D-alanine but not D-isoleucine. **(B)** *DAO*-transformed plants are inhibited by growth on D-isoleucine but not D-alanine. **(C)** Plants are cotransformed with one DNA carrying the *DAO* gene as a selectable marker and a separate DNA fragment with the target gene and then grown on medium containing D-alanine. Only transformants carrying the *DAO* gene will proliferate under these conditions, and most (>50%) of those transformants will also carry the target gene integrated at a separate site on the plant chromosome. Following breeding, plants that proliferate on medium containing D-isoleucine (because they no longer contain the *DAO* gene) are tested for the presence of the target gene. Adapted from Scheid, *Nat. Biotechnol.* **22:**398–399, 2004.

from chloroplast DNA is to introduce the foreign genes as part of a genetic construct that includes a selectable bacterial gene, e.g., *aadA,* which confers resistance to the antibiotics spectinomycin and streptomycin. This marker gene is flanked by directly repeating DNA sequences (in this case 174 bp); following cell growth in the absence of selective pressure, the selectable gene will be excised by homologous recombination between the 174-bp sequences (Fig. 18.28).

An alternative approach is to develop selectable markers that do not encode antibiotic resistance or any other undesirable trait. One possible selectable marker of this type is the spinach gene for the enzyme betaine aldehyde dehydrogenase. This enzyme, which is present in the chloro-

FIGURE 18.28 Schematic representation of a selectable marker gene excision system for transformed chloroplasts. Following introduction into chloroplasts, the chloroplast (Cp) DNA sequences on the plasmid direct the integration of the foreign gene into the chloroplast genome by homologous recombination. Transformants are selected by their resistance to spectinomycin. Then, transformants are grown without antibiotics, and the selectable marker gene is lost as a result of homologous recombination between the 174-bp repeat elements. The promoters, transcription termination regions, and ribosome-binding sites of both genes are not shown.

plasts of a limited number of plants, converts the toxic betaine aldehyde to the nontoxic glycine betaine. In addition, glycine betaine acts as an osmo-protectant, conferring some measure of salt or drought resistance. When resistance to betaine aldehyde was used to select transgenic plants, the transformation efficiency was approximately 25-fold higher than when transformants were selected with spectinomycin. The use of this approach should facilitate the chloroplast transformation of many important crops, including cereals that are naturally resistant to spectinomycin.

SUMMARY

Plants are genetically engineered by (1) introducing a gene into plant cells that are growing in culture, (2) selecting transformed cells, and then (3) regenerating a fertile plant. Strains of the soil bacterium *A. tumefaciens* can genetically engineer plants naturally. In this system, after responding to chemical signals from a surface wound, *A. tumefaciens* makes contact with an exposed plant cell membrane. A series of steps then occurs that results in the transfer of a segment (T-DNA) of a plasmid (Ti plasmid) from the bacterium into the nucleus of the plant cell. The T-DNA region becomes integrated into the plant genome, and subsequently, the genes on the T-DNA region are expressed. The T-DNA region contains genes that encode enzymes for the production of phytohormones. These compounds cause the plant cells to enlarge and proliferate. Also, the plant cell becomes a factory for the production of an opine that is encoded by a T-DNA gene that can be catabolized only by *A. tumefaciens* with a specific Ti plasmid. Thus, *A. tumefaciens* has evolved a mechanism that converts a plant cell into a production center for a carbon and nitrogen source (opine) for its exclusive use.

The *A. tumefaciens*–Ti plasmid system has been modified for use as a delivery mechanism for cloned genes to some plant cells. In these vector systems, the phytohormone and opine metabolism genes have been removed from the T-DNA region, and the modified T-DNA sequence has been cloned into a plasmid that can exist stably in *E. coli*. A cloned gene that is inserted into this T-DNA region is part of the DNA that is transferred into the nucleus of a recipient plant cell. To achieve this transfer, *A. tumefaciens* is used as a delivery system. In one system, the shuttle vector with the T-DNA-cloned gene segment is introduced into an *A. tumefaciens* strain that carries a compatible plasmid with genes that are essential for transferring a T-DNA region into a plant cell (*vir* genes). In addition to this binary vector system, a cointegrate system has been designed so that, after the introduction of the shuttle vector carrying the target gene into *A. tumefaciens*, it recombines with the *vir* gene-containing, disarmed Ti plasmid to give a single plasmid that has both *vir* gene functions and the T-DNA-cloned gene segment.

The *A. tumefaciens* T-DNA region has been used to produce a large number of transgenic plants. Unfortunately, this system is not effective with all plants. However, microprojectile bombardment (biolistics) has been an effective procedure for delivering DNA to a wider range of plant cells. Moreover, foreign DNA up to 150 kb in size that is cloned in YACs can be transferred to plant cells using a biolistic procedure. This transferred DNA can be stably integrated into the genome of the plant cells.

Different plant promoters that are active only in specific plant tissues, or only at certain times during the life of the

plant, are identified by the acquisition of expression of a promoterless reporter gene after it has integrated into plant chromosomal DNA. Methods for the insertion of the foreign gene directly into either the chloroplast or mitochondrial DNA and protocols to make targeted changes to existing genes within the genomic DNA of plant cells have been developed. In addition, techniques have been devised to decrease the amount of a specific mRNA in a plant cell and thereby downregulate the expression of that gene. To facilitate the purification of foreign proteins that are produced in plants, it is possible to fuse a target gene to an oleosin gene so that the fusion protein that is produced is localized in seed oil bodies. A technique called rhizosecretion can be employed to secrete the foreign protein along with other root exudates. To increase the usefulness of plants as production systems for mammalian proteins, it is possible to modify the glycosylation patterns of foreign proteins synthesized in plants to avoid problematic carbohydrate moieties. Finally, experimental protocols that remove marker genes from transgenic plants have been developed.

REFERENCES

Beetham, P. R., P. B. Kipp, X. L. Sawycky, C. J. Arntzen, and G. D. May. 1999. A tool for functional plant genomics: chimeric RNA/DNA oligonucleotides cause in vivo gene-specific mutations. *Proc. Natl. Acad. Sci. USA* 96:8774–8778.

Borisjuk, N. V., L. G. Borisjuk, S. Logendra, F. Petersen, Y. Gleba, and I. Raskin. 1999. Production of recombinant proteins in plant root exudates. *Nat. Biotechnol.* 17:466–469.

Capuano, F., F. Beaudoin, J. A. Napier, and P. R. Shewry. 2007. Properties and exploitation of oleosins. *Biotechnol. Adv.* 25:203–206.

Chiu, W.-L., Y. Niwa, W. Zeng, T. Hirano, H. Kobayashi, and J. Sheen. 1996. Engineered GFP as a vital reporter in plants. *Curr. Biol.* 6:325–330.

Christou, P. 1992. Genetic transformation of crop plants using microprojectile bombardment. *Plant J.* 2:275–281.

Cox, K. M., J. D. Sterling, J. T. Regan, J. R. Gasdaska, K. K. Frantz, C. G. Peele, A. Black, D. Passmore, C. Moldovan-Loomis, M. Srinivasan, S. Cuison, P. M. Cardarelli, and L. F. Dickey. 2006. Glycan optimization of a human monoclonal antibody in the aquatic plant *Lemna minor*. *Nat. Biotechnol.* 24:1591–1597.

Dale, E. C., and D. Ow. 1991. Gene transfer with subsequent removal of the selection gene from the host genome. *Proc. Natl. Acad. Sci. USA* 88:10558–10562.

Daniell, H., P. O. Wiebe, and A. Fernandez-San Millan. 2001. Antibiotic-free chloroplast genetic engineering—an environmentally friendly approach. *Trends Plant Sci.* 6:237–239.

Darbani, B., A. Eimanifar, C. N.

Stewart, Jr., and W. N. Camargo. 2007. Methods to produce marker-free transgenic plants. *Biotechnol. J.* 2:83–90.

De Greve, H., J. Leemans, J. P. Hernalsteens, L. Thia-Toong, M. De Beuckeleer, L. Willmitzer, L. Otten, M. Van Montagu, and J. Schell. 1982. Regeneration of normal and fertile plants that express octopine synthase from tobacco crown galls after deletion of tumour-controlling functions. *Nature* 300:752–755.

Erikson, O., M. Hertzberg, and T. Näsholm. 2004. A conditional marker gene allowing both positive and negative selection in plants. *Nat. Biotechnol.* 22:455–458.

Gelvin, S. B. 2003. Agrobacterium-mediated plant transformation: the biology behind the "gene-jockeying" tool. *Microbiol. Mol. Biol. Rev.* 67:16–37.

Goldsbrough, A. P., C. N. Lastrella, and J. I. Yoder. 1993. Transposition mediated re-positioning and subsequent elimination of marker genes from transgenic tomato. *Bio/Technology* 11:1286–1292.

Gruber, M. Y., and W. L. Crosby. 1993. Vectors for plant transformation, p. 89–119. *In* B. R. Glick and J. E. Thompson (ed.), *Methods in Plant Molecular Biology and Biotechnology.* CRC Press, Boca Raton, FL.

Hadi, M. Z., M. D. McMullen, and J. J. Finer. 1996. Transformation of 12 different plasmids into soybean via particle bombardment. *Plant Cell Rep.* 15:500–505.

Hager, M., and R. Bock. 2000. Enslaved bacteria as new hope for plant biotechnologists. *Appl. Microbiol. Biotechnol.* 54:302–310.

Halfter, U., P. C. Morris, and L. Willmitzer. 1992. Gene targeting in

Arabidopsis thaliana. Mol. Gen. Genet. 231:186–193.

Heifetz, P. B., and A. M. Tuttle. 2001. Protein expression in plastids. *Curr. Opin. Plant Biol.* 4:157–161.

Heim, R., and R. Y. Tsien. 1996. Engineering green fluorescent proteins for improved brightness, longer wavelengths and fluorescence resonance energy transfer. *Curr. Biol.* 6:178–182.

Iamtham, S., and A. Day. 2000. Removal of antibiotic resistance genes from transgenic tobacco plastids. *Nat. Biotechnol.* 18:1172–1176.

Ishida, Y., H. Saito, S. Ohta, Y. Hiei, T. Komari, and T. Kumashiro. 1996. High efficiency transformation of maize (*Zea mays* L.) mediated by *Agrobacterium tumefaciens*. *Nat. Biotechnol.* 14:745–750.

Jefferson, R. A., T. A. Kavanagh, and M. W. Bevan. 1987. GUS fusions: β-glucuronidase as a sensitive and versatile gene fusion marker in higher plants. *EMBO J.* 6:3901–3907.

Klein, T. M., E. D. Wolf, R. Wu, and J. C. Sanford. 1987. High-velocity microprojectiles for delivering nucleic acids into living cells. *Nature* 327:70–73.

Komarnytsky, S., N. V. Borisjuk, L. G. Borisjuk, M. Z. Alam, and I. Raskin. 2000. Production of recombinant proteins in tobacco guttation fluid. *Plant Physiol.* 124:927–933.

Krüger-Lebus, S., and I. Potrykus. 1987. A simple and efficient method for direct gene transfer to *Petunia hybridia* without electroporation. *Plant Mol. Biol. Rep.* 5:289–294.

Lee, W. S., J. T. C. Tzen, J. C. Kridl, S. E. Radke, and A. H. C. Huang. 1991. Maize oleosin is correctly targeted to seed oil bodies in *Brassica*

napus transformed with the maize oleosin gene. *Proc. Natl. Acad. Sci. USA* 88:6181–6185.

Merlo, A. O., N. Cowen, T. Delate, B. Edington, O. Folkerts, N. Hopkins, C. Lemieux, T. Skokut, K. Smith, A. Woosley, Y. Yang, S. Young, and M. Zwick. 1998. Ribozymes targeted to stearoyl-ACP Δ9 desaturase mRNA produce heritable increases of stearic acid in transgenic maize leaves. *Plant Cell* 10:1603–1621.

Maliga, P. 2004. Plasmid transformation in higher plants. *Annu. Rev. Plant Biol.* 55:289–313.

Miki, B. L., and S. McHugh. 2004. Selectable marker genes in transgenic plants: applications, alternatives and biosafety. *J. Biotechnol.* 107:193–232.

Mitsuhara, I., M. Ugaki, H. Hirochika, M. Ohshima, T. Murakami, Y. Gotoh, Y. Katayose, S. Nakamura, R. Honkura, S. Nishimiya, K. Ueno, A. Mochizuki, H. Tanimoto, H. Tsugawa, Y. Otsuki, and Y. Ohashi. 1996. Efficient promoter cassettes for enhanced expression of foreign genes in dicotyledonous and monocotyledonous plants. *Plant Cell Physiol.* 37:49–59.

Mullen, J., G. Adam, A. Blowers, and E. Earle. 1998. Biolistic transfer of large DNA fragments to tobacco cells using YACs retrofitted for plant transformation. *Mol. Breed.* 4:449–457.

Nonaka, S., M. Sugawara, K. Minamisawa, K. Yuhashi, and H. Ezura. 2008. 1-Aminocyclopropane-1-carboxylate deaminase enhances *Agrobacterium tumefaciens*-mediated gene transfer into plant cells. *Appl. Environ. Microbiol.* 74:2526–2528.

Ow, D. W., K. V. Wood, M. DeLuca, J. R. de Wet, D. R. Helinski, and S. H. Howell. 1986. Transient and stable expression of the firefly luciferase gene in plant cells and transgenic plants. *Science* 234:856–859.

Paszkowski, J., M. Baur, A. Bogucki, and I. Potrykus. 1988. Gene targeting in plants. *EMBO J.* 7:4021–4026.

Pauls, K. P. 1995. Plant biotechnology for crop improvement. *Biotechnol. Adv.* 13:673–693.

Potenza, C., L. Aleman, and C. Sengupta-Gopalan. 2004. Targeting transgene expression in research, agricultural, and environmental applications: promoters used in plant transformation. *In Vitro Cell Dev. Biol-Plant* 40:1–22.

Potrykus, I. 1990. Gene transfer to cereals: an assessment. *Bio/Technology* 8:535–542.

Potrykus, I. 1991. Gene transfer to plants: assessment of published approaches and results. *Annu. Rev. Plant Physiol.* 42:205–225.

Ruf, A., M. Hermann, I. J. Berger, H. Carrer, and R. Bock. 2001. Stable genetic transformation of tomato plastids and expression of foreign protein in fruit. *Nat. Biotechnol.* 19:870–875.

Scheid, O. M. 2004. Either/or selection markers for plant transformation. *Nat. Biotechnol.* 22:398–399.

Shaked, H., C. Melamed-Bessudo, and A. A. Levy. 2005. High-frequency gene targeting in *Arabidopsis* plants expressing the yeast *RAD54* gene. *Proc. Natl. Acad. Sci. USA* 102:12265–12269.

Southgate, E. M., M. R. Davey, J. B. Power, and R. Marchant. 1995. Factors affecting the genetic engineering of plants by microprojectile bombardment. *Biotechnol. Adv.* 13:631–651.

Sugita, K., E. Matsunaga, and H. Ebinuma. 1999. Effective selection system for generating marker-free transgenic plants independent of sexual crossing. *Plant Cell Rep.* 18:941–947.

Vain, P., J. de Buyser, V. Bui Trang, R. Haicour, and Y. Henry. 1995. Foreign delivery into monocotyledonous species. *Biotechnol. Adv.* 13:653–671.

Walden, R., and J. Schell. 1990. Techniques in plant molecular biology—progress and problems. *Eur. J. Biochem.* 192:563–576.

Walden, R., and R. Wingender. 1995. Gene-transfer and plant-regeneration techniques. *Trends Biotechnol.* 13:324–331.

Xiang, C., P. Han, I. Lutziger, K. Wang, and D. J. Oliver. 1999. A mini binary vector series for plant transformation. *Plant Mol. Biol.* 40:711–717.

Yoder, J. I., and A. P. Goldsbrough. 1994. Transformation systems for generating marker-free transgenic plants. *Bio/Technology* 12:263–267.

Zambryski, P. 1988. Basic processes underlying *Agrobacterium*-mediated DNA transfer to plant cells. *Annu. Rev. Genet.* 22:1–30.

Zambryski, P., J. Tempe, and J. Schell. 1989. Transfer and function of T-DNA genes from *Agrobacterium* Ti and Ri plasmids in plants. *Cell* 56:193–201.

Zhu, T., K. Mettenburg, D. J. Peterson, L. Tagliani, and C. L. Baszczynski. 2000. Engineering herbicide-resistant maize using chimeric RNA/DNA oligonucleotides. *Nat. Biotechnol.* 18:555–558.

Zhu, T., D. J. Peterson, L. Tagliani, G. St. Clair, C. L. Baszczynski, and B. Bowen. 1999. Targeted manipulation of maize genes in vivo using chimeric RNA/DNA oligonucleotides. *Proc. Natl. Acad. Sci. USA* 96:8768–8777.

REVIEW QUESTIONS

1. Why is the Ti plasmid from *A. tumefaciens* well suited for developing a vector to transfer foreign genes into plant chromosomal DNA?

2. How do (1) binary and (2) cointegrate Ti plasmid-based vector systems for plant transformation differ from one another?

3. What are reporter genes, and how are they used when plant cells are transformed?

4. How are plants transformed by microprojectile bombardment?

5. Describe how you would isolate a root-specific plant promoter.

6. How is foreign DNA targeted for integration into chloroplast DNA?

7. How would you produce a transgenic plant that does not contain a marker gene?

8. How would you ensure that a foreign gene that has been inserted into the chloroplast is expressed at a high level?

9. How can RNA–DNA chimeric molecules be used to introduce targeted alterations to plant genomic DNA?

10. How would you downregulate the expression of a plant gene?

11. What is the advantage of introducing foreign genes into chloroplast rather than nuclear DNA?

12. What is rhizosecretion? Why is it useful? How can it be engineered?

13. How can chromosomal marker genes be removed without using sexual crossing to segregate the selectable marker from the gene of interest?

14. Describe a strategy that could be used to remove antibiotic-resistant marker genes from chloroplast DNA.

15. Suggest a strategy that would facilitate the large-scale purification of soluble proteins, such as antibody fragments, in plants.

16. How do enhancer sequences facilitate plant gene expression?

17. How can oleosins be used to facilitate the purification of a target protein synthesized in a transgenic plant?

18. How would you modify the glycosylation pattern of a mammalian protein produced in plants?

19. How would you use the yeast *DAO* gene to select transgenic plants that contain only the introduced target gene and no selectable marker gene?

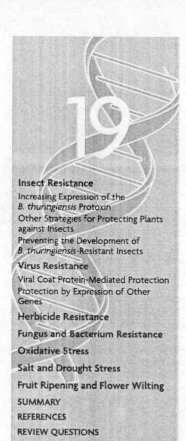

19

Engineering Plants To Overcome Biotic and Abiotic Stress

T HE PRINCIPAL OBJECTIVE OF PLANT BIOTECHNOLOGY is to create new varieties of cultivated plants (cultivars). The majority of the initial studies of transgenic plants have focused on developing strains that give better yields. Genes that confer resistance to insects, viruses, herbicides, environmental stress, and senescence have been incorporated into various plants. A considerable amount of this work has been commercialized and has been the subject of much public scrutiny and discussion. Some of this work is discussed below.

Insect Resistance

The genetic engineering of crop plants to produce functional insecticides makes it possible to develop crops that are intrinsically resistant to insect predators and do not need to be sprayed (often six to eight times during a growing season) with costly and potentially hazardous chemical pesticides. It has been estimated that in 2007 the amount spent on chemical insecticides worldwide was approximately $15 billion to $20 billion. The cost of maintaining such genetically engineered insect-resistant crops is lower than that for nonresistant crops. Moreover, biological insecticides are usually highly specific for a limited number of insect species, and they are generally considered to be nonhazardous to humans and other higher animals. In addition, by reducing the damage to plants from insect predation, a corresponding decrease in the damage to plants from a number of fungal diseases should result, since many pathogenic fungi often invade a plant either together with or as a consequence of insect infection.

Several different strategies have been used to confer resistance to insect predators. One approach involves a gene for an insecticidal protoxin produced by one of several subspecies of the bacterium *Bacillus thuringiensis* (see chapter 16). Other common strategies use genes for plant proteins, such as α-amylase inhibitors, protease inhibitors, and lectins, that have been shown to be effective against a wide variety of insects. After an insect ingests one of these inhibitors, it is not able to digest food (i.e., plants)

because the inhibitor interferes with the hydrolysis of starch or plant proteins. Thus, the insect will feed less and eventually die.

Increasing Expression of the *B. thuringiensis* Protoxin

B. thuringiensis protoxin does not persist in the environment, nor is it hazardous to mammals. Thus, it is a safe means of protecting plants. It is both simpler and less costly to express the genes for *B. thuringiensis* toxins in plants than to spray *B. thuringiensis* preparations onto the surface of the plant. This mode of insecticidal-toxin delivery limits the environmental distribution of the toxin and avoids problems associated with spraying *B. thuringiensis* preparations, such as limited environmental stability and the timing of the toxin application.

The scientific challenge in utilizing the *B. thuringiensis* protoxin is to create a transgenic plant that expresses and synthesizes a functional form of this prokaryotic insecticide at sufficient levels to prevent damage by insect predation. In initial experiments, the *B. thuringiensis* subsp. *kurstaki* insecticidal-protein genes, *cry1Aa*, *cry1Ab*, and *cry1Ac*, were not particularly well expressed in plants (Table 19.1). This is problematic, because high levels of expression of these insect control proteins are needed in order to produce commercially viable insect-resistant plants. To raise the level of the expressed protein, scientists truncated the gene so that only the N-terminal portion of the insecticidal protoxin—the part of the protoxin that contains the toxin (see chapter 16)—was produced and inserted a strong plant promoter to direct gene expression. Under these conditions, there was a significant increase in the level of insecticidal toxin produced, affording transgenic plants some protection against damage from insect predation.

The minimum sequence that encoded toxin activity had to be determined. To this end, the amino acid sequences of protoxins from various strains of *B. thuringiensis* were compared to determine whether there is a common insecticidal (toxin) domain. This analysis showed that the N-terminal portion of the protoxin molecule is highly conserved (~98%) and the C-terminal region is more variable (~45% conserved). Further work showed that all of the insecticidal-toxin activity resides within the first 646

TABLE 19.1 Expression of some *B. thuringiensis* insecticidal toxin genes in transgenic plants

Plant(s)	Gene	% Expression	Insecticidal
Tobacco	*cry1Ab*, full	0.0001–0.0005	No
Tobacco	*cry1Ab*, truncated	0.003–0.012	Yes
Tobacco	*cry1Aa*, full	Not detected	No
Tobacco	*cry1Aa*, truncated	0.00125	Yes
Tobacco	*cry1Ac*, truncated	<0.014	Yes
Tomato	*cry1Ab*, truncated	0.0001	Yes
Cotton	*cry1Ab*, truncated, WT	<0.002	No
Cotton	*cry1Ab*, truncated, PM	0.05–0.1	Yes
Tomato, tobacco	*cry1Ab*, truncated, WT	0.002	Yes
Tomato, tobacco	*cry1Ab*, truncated, PM	0.002–0.2	Yes
Tomato, tobacco	*cry1Ab*, truncated, FM	0.3	Yes

Adapted from Ely, p 105–124, *in* Entwistle et al. (ed)., *Bacillus thuringiensis, an Environmental Biopesticide: Theory and Practice* (John Wiley & Sons, Chichester, United Kingdom, 1993).

Terms and abbreviations: full, the complete protoxin gene; truncated, a shortened version of the protoxin gene; WT, wild-type codons; PM, partially modified codons; FM, fully modified codons.

FIGURE 19.1 Cointegrate cloning vector carrying a *B. thuringiensis* (Bt) insecticidal-toxin gene. The toxin gene is under the control of the strong, constitutive 35S promoter (P_{35S}) from cauliflower mosaic virus and the nopaline synthase transcription terminator–polyadenylation site (*t*NOS). The vector has an *E. coli* origin of DNA replication (*ori*) and an Spcr gene, which allow the vector to be maintained and selected in *E. coli* cells; a T-DNA right border; a plant selectable marker gene; and a region of DNA that is homologous to DNA in the disarmed Ti plasmid, for integrating the two plasmids. The neomycin phosphotransferase gene (*NPT*), which acts as a plant reporter gene, is under the transcriptional control of nopaline synthase gene sequences (*p*NOS and *t*NOS) and is used to select for kanamycin-resistant transformed plant cells.

amino acids from the N terminus of the 1,156-amino-acid protoxin. When the segment of the protoxin gene that encodes the highly conserved amino acid sequence was cloned and expressed in bacteria, the shortened protein was as active as the native (protoxin) form in protecting plants against lepidopteran insects in laboratory trials.

Transgenic tomato plants with a truncated *B. thuringiensis* protoxin gene were produced to test whether the shortened protoxin would be able to protect the plants from damage by various insect pests. The shortened version of the protoxin gene was put under the transcriptional control of the strong constitutive 35S promoter from cauliflower mosaic virus and the nopaline synthase transcription termination–polyadenylation site and was then cloned into the T-DNA (transferred DNA) region of a cointegrate-type Ti plasmid vector (Fig. 19.1). The vector contained a spectinomycin resistance (Spcr) gene that allowed it to be selected in either *Escherichia coli* or *Agrobacterium tumefaciens*, an *E. coli* origin of DNA replication, and a neomycin phosphotransferase gene that was under the control of the nopaline synthase promoter and transcription termination–polyadenylation sites and enabled the selection of transformed plant cells in the presence of kanamycin. In addition, the cointegrate cloning vector had the right border of the T-DNA from a nopaline Ti plasmid and a segment of the octopine Ti plasmid that provides a region of homology for cointegrate formation by homologous recombination with a disarmed Ti plasmid. The plasmid was constructed and manipulated in *E. coli* before it was transferred by conjugation to a strain of *A. tumefaciens* that contained a disarmed Ti plasmid. After recombination in *A. tumefaciens*, the short form of the protoxin gene was transferred to the chromosomal DNA of tomato plants.

In both greenhouse and field trials, transgenic tomato plants that expressed the short form of the protoxin were protected to some degree against damage caused by tobacco hornworms (*Manduca sexta*), tomato

fruitworms *(Heliothis zea)*, and tomato pinworms *(Keiferia lycopersicella)*. The extent of the protection was not the same for each of the insects, nor was it complete. The transgenic plants were protected to some extent from damage caused by tobacco hornworms and tomato fruitworms and to a lesser degree from damage by tomato pinworms. A combination of a low dose of chemical insecticide and production of the protoxin by the plants increased the level of protection afforded by the protoxin.

In an effort to dramatically increase the level of expression, an isolated insecticidal-toxin gene was modified by site-directed mutagenesis to change any DNA sequences that could inhibit efficient transcription or translation in a plant host (Table 19.1). This "partially" modified gene had a nucleotide sequence that was 96.5% unchanged from that of the wild-type gene and encoded the identical insecticidal-toxin protein. Transgenic plants that expressed this partially modified sequence produced a 10-fold-higher level of insecticidal-toxin protein than did plants that were transformed with the wild-type gene. Subsequently, a "fully" modified version of the insecticidal-toxin gene was designed and chemically synthesized. This fully modified gene contained codons more commonly used by plants, as opposed to those favored by gram-positive bacteria, such as *B. thuringiensis*. This gene was also modified to eliminate any potential messenger RNA (mRNA) secondary structure or chance plant polyadenylation sequences that might decrease gene expression. After modification, it had a G+C content of 49% (the wild-type gene is 37% G+C) and a nucleotide sequence that was only 78.9% identical to that of the wild-type gene.

Transgenic plants that were transformed with this highly modified synthetic protoxin gene had an approximately 100-fold-higher level of toxin protein than did plants transformed with the wild-type gene.

MILESTONE

Light-Inducible and Chloroplast-Associated Expression of a Chimaeric Gene Introduced into *Nicotiana tabacum* Using a Ti Plasmid Vector

L. HERRERA-ESTRELLA, G. VAN DEN BROECK, R. MAENHAUT, M. VAN MONTAGU, J. SCHELL, M. TIMKO, and A. CASHMORE
Nature 310:115–120, 1984

After researchers had established the Ti plasmid system as an effective means of transforming many different plants, their attention turned to the development of procedures for the expression of foreign genes in plants. Initially, most of the genes that were introduced into plant cells were under the transcriptional control of either the relatively strong constitutive 35S promoter from cauliflower mosaic virus or the nearly as strong constitutive promoter for the nopaline synthase gene that is encoded within some T-DNAs. However, the development of plants with useful new and modified traits often requires that a specific protein be expressed only in certain tissues, e.g., leaves or roots, or only at certain times in the life of the plant, e.g., during early seedling development, fruit formation, or high-temperature stress. As a first step toward the development of plants that expressed foreign genes in a tissue-specific or time-specific manner, Herrera-Estrella et al. constructed a chimeric gene that included the 5'-flanking region from the pea gene for the small subunit of ribulose bisphosphate carboxylase containing transcriptional regulatory sequences, the coding region of a bacterial chloramphenicol acetyltransferase gene as an easily selectable gene, and the 3'-flanking region from the nopaline synthase gene containing signals both for termination of transcription and for polyadenylation of the mRNA. Normally the gene for the small subunit of ribulose bisphosphate carboxylase is expressed only in green or photosynthetic tissue; as expected, the chloramphenicol acetyltransferase gene under the regulatory control of this DNA sequence was also expressed only in photosynthetic tissues. This work provided one of the first demonstrations that, despite their complexity, plant promoters could direct the transcription of heterologous proteins accurately and with tissue specificity. Since this study was done, researchers have used a wide range of plant promoters to direct tissue- and development-specific heterologous gene expression in transgenic plants.

FIGURE 19.2 Site on the chloroplast genome where a foreign gene encoding the *B. thuringiensis* Cry2Aa2 protoxin is integrated by homologous recombination. The genes *rbcL* and *accD* are both present in a single copy per chloroplast genome. The intergenic region between these two genes, which is the site of insertion of the foreign genes, is smaller than it appears in this representation. The *aadA* gene (encoding spectinomycin and streptomycin resistances) and the *cry2Aa2* gene are both under the transcriptional control of the constitutive chloroplast *rrn* promoter and transcription terminator (TT), and each contains its own ribosomal binding site. Integration of foreign DNA into the intergenic spacer region prevents insertion of a foreign gene from interfering with the expression of any endogenous chloroplast genes. Adapted from Kota et al., *Proc. Natl. Acad. Sci. USA* **96**:1840–1845, 1999.

Moreover, this higher level of insecticidal-toxin synthesis was directly correlated with increased insecticidal activity.

In another approach to increasing the expression of the protoxin, one group of researchers expressed the fully modified protoxin gene under the control of the promoter for the gene that codes for the small subunit of the plant enzyme ribulose bisphosphate carboxylase and downstream from the chloroplast transit peptide sequence of this enzyme, so that the overproduced protoxin became localized within the chloroplast. This strategy led to a very high level of expression (nearly 1% of the total leaf protein) of the insecticidal protoxin. Other researchers have introduced an insecticidal-protoxin gene directly into the chloroplast DNA of the host plant. The *B. thuringiensis* protoxin gene was integrated into a specific site on the chloroplast DNA by constructing a vector that contained the protoxin gene flanked by two single-copy chloroplast genes (Fig. 19.2). Integration of the introduced genes occurs by homologous recombination. Once integrated into the chloroplast DNA, a protoxin gene under the transcriptional control of a strong chloroplast promoter may be expressed at high levels, so the protoxin may compose as much as 2 to 3% of the total soluble protein in the leaf, yielding a very high level of insecticidal activity. In addition, even this level of foreign-protein expression could be dramatically increased (by 10- to 20-fold) by coexpressing (as part of the same operon that was introduced into the chloroplast DNA) a *B. thuringiensis* gene that encodes a chaperonin protein that facilitates the correct folding of the insecticidal-protein protoxin.

Integration of the *B. thuringiensis* protoxin gene into chloroplast DNA has a number of potential advantages over inserting it into the chromosomal

DNA. First, the protoxin gene does not have to be modified, because the chloroplast transcriptional and translational apparatuses are typically prokaryotic. Second, because there are many chloroplasts per cell and many copies of chloroplast DNA per chloroplast, the protoxin gene is present in multiple copies and therefore is more likely to be expressed at a high level. Third, in most plants, chloroplasts are transmitted only through the egg and not through pollen, which means that plants receive all of their chloroplast DNA from their female parent. Consequently, there is no risk of unwanted transfer of the protoxin gene to other plants in the environment by pollen. The disadvantage of expressing the *B. thuringiensis* protoxin in chloroplasts is that insects that attack stems or fruit will not encounter the protoxin, since these tissues do not have any chloroplasts.

To date, some form of the gene for the protoxin has been introduced and expressed in a wide variety of plant species, including alfalfa, apple, broccoli, cabbage, canola, corn (maize), cotton, cranberry, eggplant, grape, hawthorn, juneberry, peanut, pear, poplar, potato, rice, rutabaga, soybean, spruce, sugar cane, tobacco, tomato, walnut, white clover, and white spruce. Following several seasons of successful field trials, these transgenic plants were approved for commercial release in the United States, Canada, and Argentina, and large-scale growth of the plants in the field began in 1996. Although insect populations still have to be monitored to keep track of the frequency of resistant organisms, the use of crops expressing *B. thuringiensis* insecticidal proteins has already exceeded the length of time that it typically takes for resistance to arise in insects to conventional pesticides. A number of transgenic plants that express an insecticidal toxin or protoxin are currently being used commercially—it is estimated that worldwide, in 2007, farmers planted approximately 40 million hectares of transgenic *B. thuringiensis* insecticidal-protein-containing crops. This technology has more than lived up to the hopes and expectations of scientists. Notwithstanding the initial concerns about the technology, especially in Europe, this approach to crop protection has gained widespread acceptance throughout much of the world.

Other Strategies for Protecting Plants against Insects

No single *B. thuringiensis* protoxin is effective against a broad range of insect species. This may limit the overall usefulness of these protoxins. However, plants have evolved general insect defense mechanisms that are sufficient for plant survival but not always effective enough to keep the damage to a level that would be acceptable for crop plants. For example, some plants produce protease inhibitors that, when ingested, prevent the feeding insect from hydrolyzing plant proteins, thereby effectively starving the predator insect. Consequently, it seemed reasonable to isolate a plant gene for a protease inhibitor, add a strong promoter, and create transgenic crop plants that produce sufficiently high levels of the protease inhibitor to reduce damage from insect predation.

Protease inhibitors. In one study, researchers isolated a clone that encodes cowpea trypsin inhibitor from a complementary DNA (cDNA) clone bank by using a chemically synthesized DNA probe based on the amino acid sequence of the cowpea trypsin inhibitor protein. The full-length cDNA was subcloned onto a Ti plasmid binary cloning vector (Fig. 19.3) and introduced into a strain of *A. tumefaciens* carrying a disarmed Ti plasmid that

FIGURE 19.3 Binary cloning vector carrying a cowpea trypsin inhibitor gene. The vector contains a broad-host-range origin of DNA replication *(ori)* and a kanamycin resistance (Kanr) gene, which function in both *E. coli* and *A. tumefaciens*. Between the T-DNA left and right borders, there are (1) a neomycin phosphotransferase gene *(NPT)* under the transcriptional control of nopaline synthase signals *(pNOS* and *tNOS)*, which enables kanamycin-resistant transformed plant cells to be selected, and (2) the cowpea trypsin inhibitor gene, which is under the control of the 35S promoter (P$_{35S}$) from cauliflower mosaic virus and the transcription terminator–polyadenylation region from the nopaline synthase gene *(tNOS)*.

| Pin2 5' end | Act1 intron | Pin2 gene | Pin2 3' end | P₃₅ₛ 5' end | bar gene | nos 3' end |

FIGURE 19.4 Plasmid vector carrying the potato proteinase inhibitor II gene *(Pin2)*. 5' end, the region of DNA preceding the gene; 3' end, the region of DNA following the gene; *Act1* intron, the first intron from the rice actin 1 gene; P_{35S} 5' end, the 35S promoter from cauliflower mosaic virus; *bar* gene, the bacterial phosphinothricin acetyltransferase gene; *nos* 3' end, the region of DNA following the nopaline synthase gene. The *bar* gene serves as a selectable marker for transgenic plants, conferring resistance to the herbicide Basta (ammonium glufosinate).

contained active *vir* genes. Following *A. tumefaciens* infection of tobacco leaf disks with this vector, cells that incorporated the cloned DNA were selected for growth on kanamycin, and transgenic plants were regenerated. The damage caused by *Heliothis virescens* (tobacco budworm) larvae to transgenic plants that expressed more than 2 mg of cowpea trypsin inhibitor per mg of protein was significantly less than the damage inflicted on nontransformed plants.

Cowpea seeds that contain approximately 2 mg of inhibitor per mg of plant protein are not toxic to either animals or humans. However, if the amount of protease inhibitor produced by a transgenic plant is determined to be a potential hazard, then it is possible to limit the expression of the protease inhibitor to the plant tissues that the major insect pests prefer but that are not used as food by humans or animals. In other words, a cloned protease inhibitor gene could be active in the leaves and roots of a plant but not in the commercially valuable fruit.

Introduction of the potato proteinase inhibitor II gene provides rice plants with protection against the pink stem borer *(Sesamia inferens)*, a major insect pest of rice. Infestation of rice plants by pink stem borers causes severe damage to the plants, often resulting in a hollow stem and dead panicles with no seeds. A plasmid carrying the potato proteinase inhibitor II gene under the control of its own promoter and transcription termination region was constructed. The plasmid also contained the first intron from the rice actin gene inserted between the promoter and the potato proteinase inhibitor II coding region (Fig. 19.4). This construct was introduced into rice suspension cells by microprojectile bombardment, and transgenic plants were generated. When pink stem borer larvae were artificially applied, 70 to 100% of the wild-type plants were severely damaged by insect predation, while only 15 to 20% of the transgenic plants were damaged. Since plant proteinase inhibitors are common components of both human and animal food and are readily inactivated by cooking, their introduction into new crops can be regarded as safe.

Another strategy that is designed to increase the effectiveness of relatively low levels of *B. thuringiensis* insecticidal-toxin activity entails combining the toxin with a serine protease inhibitor. In laboratory trials, investigators found that when the amount of purified *B. thuringiensis* insecticidal toxin that causes minimal insect mortality was mixed with a low concentration of protease inhibitor, the insecticidal activity of the mixture was 20-fold greater than that of the *B. thuringiensis* protoxin alone. To test whether this scheme would function in transgenic plants, a DNA fragment

that encoded a fusion protein consisting of both a protease inhibitor and a truncated toxin was constructed. Transgenic tobacco plants that produced small amounts of this fusion protein were protected from insect attack.

α-Amylase inhibitor. Another way of imparting insect resistance to susceptible plants entails using a gene that encodes an α-amylase inhibitor. The cowpea weevil *(Callosobruchus maculatus)* and the azuki bean weevil *(Callosobruchus chinensis)* are seed-feeding beetles that cause considerable economic loss of these legume crops, especially in developing countries. When larvae of these insects are fed a diet that includes the common bean *(Phaseolus vulgaris)*, insect growth is inhibited. This growth inhibition is attributable to the presence of an α-amylase inhibitor in the seed proteins of the common bean. Accordingly, the gene for the α-amylase inhibitor from the common bean was isolated, placed under the transcriptional control of the strong seed-specific promoter for the bean phytohemagglutinin gene, and used to transform pea plants *(Pisum sativum)*. Peas are usually quite susceptible to damage by both cowpea weevils and azuki bean weevils. However, transgenic pea plants that expressed the α-amylase inhibitor were resistant to both of these insects. The level of resistance to cowpea weevils was found to be proportional to the amount of α-amylase inhibitor that the transgenic plant produced (Fig. 19.5).

Cholesterol oxidase. Another approach to developing insect-resistant transgenic plants makes use of a bacterial cholesterol oxidase gene. Cholesterol oxidase, which is present in a range of different bacterial genera, catalyzes the oxidation of 3-hydroxysteroids to ketosteroids and hydrogen peroxide. This enzyme is commonly used in assays to determine the levels of cholesterol in human serum. Low levels of the enzyme have a high level of insecticidal activity against larvae of the boll weevil *(Anthonomus grandis grandis)* (Fig. 19.6), a common and economically important insect (Coleoptera) pest of cotton, and have lower levels of activity against some lepidopteran pests. Cholesterol oxidase probably acts by disrupting the insect's midgut epithelial membrane, thus killing the insect. A cholesterol oxidase gene encoding a protein with a molecular mass of approximately 55,000 daltons

FIGURE 19.5 Mortality of cowpea weevil larvae reared on transgenic pea plants that produce different amounts of α-amylase inhibitor.

with a length of 504 amino acids plus a leader peptide of approximately 5,000 daltons (43 amino acids) was isolated from a strain of *Streptomyces* and cloned into a vector under the control of a plant virus (figwort mosaic virus) promoter and a termination sequence from the 3′ region of the *A. tumefaciens* nopaline synthase gene. When this construct was introduced into tobacco cell protoplasts, the transformed cells actively expressed the cholesterol oxidase. When the gene is introduced into cotton plants on a commercial scale, either by itself or in combination with genes for other biological insecticides, it should be an effective means of protecting plants against damage from insect predation.

Vegetative insecticidal toxins. In addition to the well-characterized Cry insecticidal toxins—over 350 of which have been identified—*B. thuringiensis* produces a secreted insecticidal protein during its vegetative growth stage. To date, two major groups of vegetative insecticidal proteins (Vip) have been identified. One group consists of the proteins Vip1 and Vip2, which are not toxic to lepidoptera, and Vip3, which targets several major lepidopteran pests. The less-well-characterized Vip proteins may act synergistically with Cry proteins to kill their target insects, providing a double-barreled approach to insect toxicity, so that it is extremely difficult for susceptible insects to develop resistance. It would therefore be advantageous if transgenic plants expressing both Cry and Vip proteins could be created. As a first step, researchers shuffled the two major domains of two Vip3 proteins, Vip3Ac1 and VipAa1 (Fig. 19.7). One of the hybrid Vip3 proteins (i.e., Vip3AcAa) displayed the highest activity of the four proteins against fall armyworms, cotton bollworms, and silkworms. Moreover, only the Vip3AcAa construct was toxic to a strain of cabbage looper that was resistant to the well-characterized *B. thuringiensis* insecticidal protein Cry1Ac. The chimeric toxin Vip3AcAa enriches the diversity of Vip toxins that can be used together with conventional Cry proteins to generate transgenic plants that are highly unlikely to select for resistant insects.

Other proteins. The activities of several other proteins have been utilized in an effort to protect plants from insect predation. For example, some

FIGURE 19.6 Effect of increasing amounts of cholesterol oxidase on the mortality of boll weevil larvae. ppm, parts per million. Adapted from Corbin et al., *Appl. Environ. Microbiol.* **60:**4239–4244, 1994.

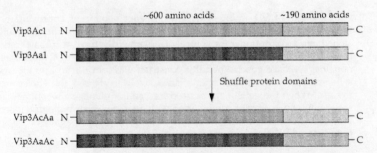

FIGURE 19.7 Generation of two hybrid insecticidal proteins constructed by domain shuffling. The approximate sizes of the amino- and carboxy-terminal fragments are indicated. The hybrid protein Vip3AcAa was found to have the greatest level of insecticidal activity with the insect larvae tested.

lectins, i.e., carbohydrate-binding proteins found in the seeds and storage tissues of a variety of plant species, are toxic to certain species of insects. While many plant lectins are toxic to mammals as well as insects, the lectin from the snowdrop plant *(Galanthus nivalis)* is toxic only to insects. With this in mind, the snowdrop lectin gene has been introduced into approximately a dozen different plants, with the result that plants that expressed this protein were damaged by aphids to a lesser extent than nontransformed plants. However, although the snowdrop lectin significantly lowered the amount of leaf material eaten, insect mortality was only slightly increased.

When the gene encoding the enzyme tryptophan decarboxylase from periwinkle *(Catharanthus roseus)* is expressed in tobacco, the plants are protected from damage by the whitefly *(Bemisia tabaci)*. While the precise mechanism of this protection is unknown, it has been suggested that the tryptamine that is produced by this enzyme, following the decarboxylation of tryptophan, is used in the production of insect-inhibiting plant alkaloids.

The gram-negative bacterium *Photorhabdus luminescens* produces a 283-kilodalton protein, toxin A, that is highly toxic to a variety of insects. When this protein was expressed in transgenic *Arabidopsis thaliana* (Box 19.1) plants in amounts of ≥700 ng/mg of extractable plant protein, it was found to be highly toxic to the tobacco hornworm, as well as the southern corn rootworm, with insect mortality typically 100%.

Finally, transgenic corn plants that express avidin—a glycoprotein isolated from chicken eggs that binds the coenzyme biotin with extremely high affinity—caused biotin deficiency that led to stunted growth and death in a number of different insect species. Importantly, the levels of avidin that are toxic to insects are not toxic to mice, suggesting that protecting plants with an avidin transgene is not necessarily a problem for humans.

RNA interference. The ingestion or microinjection of double-stranded RNA into some worms and insects has been used to silence genes in these organisms. This gene silencing works through the generation of RNA interference (RNAi) (see chapter 11). In one study, when 290 different double-stranded RNAs thought to encode essential or important functions were

fed (one at a time) at a low level to larvae of the western corn rootworm (*Diabrotica virgifera* LeConte), growth was significantly inhibited with 67 of the RNAs. Fourteen of the double-stranded RNAs had 50% lethal concentrations of ≤5.2 ng/cm². Based on these results, transgenic corn expressing one of the double-stranded RNAs, targeting the transcript for vacuolar ATPase, was constructed (Fig. 19.8). The transgenic plants were protected against the western corn rootworm to an extent comparable to the protection afforded by a *B. thuringiensis* transgene. The demonstration that it is possible to produce RNAi in coleoptera following oral delivery of double-stranded RNA is an important first step in the development of a completely novel approach to developing a wide range of insect-resistant plants, including resistance to some insects that are refractory to the *B. thuringiensis* insecticidal toxin.

In a variation on the above-mentioned strategy, another group of researchers first identified the mechanism that the cotton bollworm uses to protect itself against the compound gossypol, which is produced by cotton plants to prevent insect predation. Gossypol is a yellow polyphenolic aldehyde that permeates cells and acts as an inhibitor of several of the insect's dehydrogenase enzymes. It has been used as a male oral contraceptive in China, possesses antimalarial properties, and may have anticancer properties. The cotton bollworm protects itself from the toxic effects of gossypol by inactivating the gossypol with the enzyme cytochrome P450 monooxygenase. Thus, transgenic plants were constructed to synthesize an RNAi molecule that would silence the insect's gene for the cytochrome P450 monooxygenase. By preventing the expression of cytochrome P450 monooxygenase, the insect was exposed to the full toxic effects of the plant-produced gossypol, so that it was either killed or at least debilitated, and the damage to the plant was limited (Fig. 19.9). Plants produce a myriad of allelochemicals to protect themselves against insects, and many insects have developed strategies to overcome the toxic effects of these compounds. Therefore, the mechanisms utilized by insects to overcome the toxicity of the plant-produced compounds are attractive targets for developing insect-resistant plants in the future.

BOX 19.1

Arabidopsis thaliana

Arabidopsis thaliana (thale cress) is a small weed in the same family (Brassicaceae) as canola, mustard, and broccoli. It is native to Europe, Asia, and northwestern Africa. *A. thaliana* is popular with scientists as a model organism in plant biology and genetic studies. It has one of the smallest genomes—at 7×10^7 bp, it is similar to the size of the yeast genome, which is approximately 1.5×10^7 bp—of any flowering plant, which makes it readily amenable to molecular genetic studies. The small size of its genome has made *A. thaliana* useful for the generation and selection of mutants, and it was the first plant genome to be sequenced, in 2000.

The plant's small size and short life cycle are also advantageous for research. Laboratory strains of *A. thaliana* take about 6 weeks from germination to mature seed. The small size of the plant is convenient for cultivation in limited space, and it produces many seeds—an individual plant can produce several thousand seeds.

Plant transformation in *Arabidopsis* is straightforward and has become a routine procedure in many laboratories, using *A. tumefaciens* to transfer DNA to the plant genome. The current *Arabidopsis* transformation protocol, termed "floral dip," involves dipping a flower into a solution containing *Agrobacterium*, the DNA of interest, and a detergent. This method avoids the need for tissue culture or plant regeneration. The idea is that some of the *Agrobacterium* cells will transfer their T-DNA containing the target DNA into the reproductive tissue of the plant. As a consequence of the above-mentioned traits, and the relative complexity of most other plants, *Arabidopsis* has become the *E. coli* of the plant world.

Coleoptera larvae

Larval cDNA library

Test dsRNAs and select

Corn
P35S hsp70 intron V-ATPase A Wheat hsp17
3' UTR

Transform corn plants

Test transgenic corn for resistance to western corn rootworm

FIGURE 19.8 Use of RNAi to protect plants against insect predation. The double-stranded RNAs (dsRNAs) were produced using a commercial in vitro transcription system developed for this purpose. A number of double-stranded RNAs from essential insect genes were tested for the ability to elicit RNAi and inhibit insect larval proliferation. One of the most effective double-stranded RNAs, which encodes a portion of an ATPase gene, was spliced into a Ti plasmid vector and used to transform corn plants. The transformants with the highest levels of resistance to the western corn rootworm were selected. UTR, untranslated region.

Preventing the Development of *B. thuringiensis*-Resistant Insects

There is little doubt that insects have the genetic potential to develop resistance to *B. thuringiensis* insecticidal toxins, and the more that *B. thuringiensis* insecticidal toxins are used, the greater the likelihood that populations of target insects will accumulate resistant individuals. Experimental strategies have been devised to prevent transgenic plants that express the *B. thuringiensis* protoxin gene from acting as selection agents for resistant insects. In one approach, the expression of the insecticidal toxin in transgenic plants was limited to a short period. The gene for the *B. thuringiensis* protoxin was cloned downstream of the promoter of a gene from tobacco called the pathogenesis-related protein 1a (PR-1a) gene. The expression of the PR-1a gene is part of a natural defense mechanism that combats pathogens. The PR-1a gene is normally induced by any one of a variety of pathogenic organisms or by chemicals, such as salicylic acid and polyacrylic acid. When transgenic plants with the *B. thuringiensis* protoxin gene under the control of the PR-1a promoter were treated with a chemical inducer, they synthesized detectable levels of insecticidal toxin within 1 day of application, which protected the plants against insect attack. Therefore, it is conceivable that the protoxin could be induced by the administration of an inexpensive and safe chemical inducer only when it is required during the

growing season, e.g., when insect larvae are feeding. Such periodic production should lower the selection pressure for resistant insects.

One approach that might increase the insecticidal effectiveness of *B. thuringiensis* expressed in transgenic plants and also decrease the development of insect resistance is to fuse the bacterial insecticidal gene with another protein that increases the binding of the insecticide to the target intestinal cellular receptor. With this in mind, a fusion protein consisting of an N-terminal *B. thuringiensis* insecticidal toxin and a C-terminal peptide consisting of the nontoxic B-chain of the protein ricin was constructed. Ricin is a protein toxin that is extracted from castor beans. It consists of an A-chain of 267 amino acids that contains the toxin activity and a B-chain of 262 amino acids that is catalytically inactive but serves to mediate entry of the complex into the cytosol. The *B. thuringiensis* insecticidal toxin binds to a receptor located within the membrane of the insect midgut (Fig. 19.10). Normally, since each insecticidal toxin interacts with a single receptor, the loss or modification of the receptor leads to resistance to the insecticidal toxin. However, since the ricin B-chain binds with very high affinity to *N*-acetylgalactosamine residues (which are adjacent to the *B. thuringiensis* insecticidal-toxin receptor), the fusion protein has two separate and independent means by which it is targeted to the receptor. With this fusion protein, it becomes extremely unlikely that both targeting mechanisms will cease to be effective at the same time. It has been suggested that this approach may be most effective in field situations where it is difficult or

FIGURE 19.9 Use of RNAi to inhibit the synthesis of a P450 monooxygenase enzyme that inactivates the plant secondary metabolite gossypol. **(A)** In wild-type plants, the P450 monooxygenase inactivates the gossypol, the plant is defenseless, and the insect can severely damage the plant. **(B)** In transgenic plants that produce an RNAi that directs the degradation of the P450 monooxygenase mRNA, the gossypol synthesized by the plant is able to prevent the insect from severely damaging the plant.

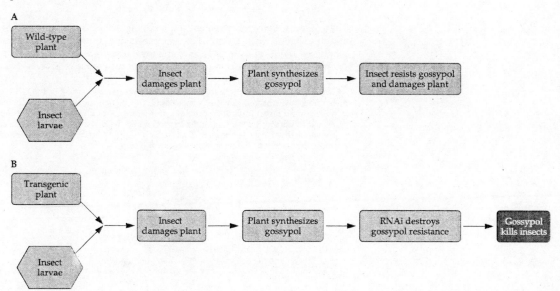

impossible to implement a spatial-refuge (refugium) strategy (such as for transgenic rice).

A number of additional strategies designed to prevent the development of insects that are resistant to the *B. thuringiensis* insecticidal toxin have been devised. They include the following.

- Using spatial-refuge strategies. In this approach, a certain fraction of each farmer's land, generally around 20%, is planted with a non-transgenic crop, while the remainder of the land is planted with a transgenic version of the same crop expressing a high level of the *B. thuringiensis* insecticidal toxin. The idea behind this strategy is that the very small number of insects that are able to survive on the transgenic insecticidal crop—a high dose of toxin kills 99.9% of susceptible insects—will mate with the much larger number of toxin-sensitive insects from the nontransgenic crop. Thus, the gene for resistance is effectively diluted—a high dose of the toxin kills 99% of the heterozygotes—and the pest population remains sensitive to the insecticide.

- Using two or more different *B. thuringiensis* insecticidal toxins (sometimes called gene stacking) or fusing portions of the active regions of two different toxin genes to generate novel hybrid protein insecticidal toxins (Box 19.2; also see chapter 16). This approach assumes that resistance to two control methods is much less likely to develop simultaneously. This approach has been found to be effective in the field when it is combined with spatial refugia.

- Transforming plants with both a *B. thuringiensis* insecticidal-toxin gene and another form of biological insecticide (e.g., an α-amylase inhibitor gene). This also assumes that resistance to two control methods is much less likely to develop simultaneously.

- Spraying low levels of chemical insecticides at the same time that transgenic plants expressing a *B. thuringiensis* insecticidal-toxin gene are used. This also assumes that resistance to two control methods is much less likely to develop simultaneously.

The insect resistance management strategies that have been used up to now appear to have been successful. For example, in one large study, researchers monitored the level of resistance of the pink bollworm (*Pectinophora gossypiella*) to *B. thuringiensis* in cotton fields over the course of 8 years, from

FIGURE 19.10 Schematic representation of a hybrid protein consisting of the Cry1Ac insecticidal-toxin protein (at the N terminus), the B-chain of ricin (at the C terminus), and an insect midgut insecticidal-protein receptor. The Cry protein recognizes and binds to the insect midgut receptor, while the B-chain of ricin acts as an *N*-acetygalactosamine-specific lectin that binds very tightly to these residues, which are located adjacent to the receptor. Bt, *B. thuringiensis*.

BOX 19.2

Managing Insect Resistance to *B. thuringiensis* by Gene Stacking

Although various strains of *B. thuringiensis* produce hundreds of different bacterial insecticidal proteins, transgenic field crops engineered to produce these proteins have utilized only a few types of insecticidal toxin. This has led to concerns that the expression of a single toxin throughout the growing season could result in insects evolving resistance to the toxin's effects. One of the strategies that has been employed to prevent or delay the development of insect resistance to *B. thuringiensis* insecticidal toxins includes trans-

forming plants with two unrelated *B. thuringiensis* insecticidal-toxin genes. Recent data indicate that gene stacking (also called gene pyramiding) of two genes encoding proteins with different modes of action significantly delays the development of insect resistance to these insecticidal toxins.

Bollgard II is a strain of genetically engineered cotton that was developed by the Monsanto Corporation to produce both the Cry2Ab2 and Cry1Ac insecticidal proteins. This strain was produced by retransformation of the previously commercialized Bollgard cotton, which produces only the Cry1Ac insecticidal protein. The commercial use of Bollgard cotton began in 1996, and by 2003, it had been

grown globally on more than 32 million acres with the benefits of reduced insecticide use, improved control of target insect pests, increased yield, and reduced production costs accruing to farmers. The two insecticidal proteins produced by Bollgard II provide protection against several major lepidopteran pests of cotton, including the cotton bollworm, tobacco budworm, pink bollworm, and armyworm. In addition to an expanded insecticidal range, Bollgard II is expected to significantly delay (or prevent) the development of insect resistance in the field. Nevertheless, the use of Bollgard II requires the concomitant employment of refugia.

1997 to 2004. They found that the frequency of resistance did not change over this period and attributed this result to the use of refugia, the recessive inheritance of the resistance, the fact that the resistance that developed was incomplete, and the fitness costs associated with the development of insect resistance. It is nevertheless essential that new strategies to prevent the development of insect resistance continue to be developed. The amount of land that is devoted to the growth of transgenic crops that express a *B. thuringiensis* insecticidal toxin continues to increase rapidly worldwide. The types of crops that have been engineered to express a *B. thuringiensis* insecticidal toxin are also continuing to expand. Thus, a responsible approach dictates that we continue to be careful and vigilant in avoiding the development of insect resistance so as not to waste this resource.

Virus Resistance

Plant viruses often cause considerable crop damage and significantly reduce yields. Therefore, in the absence of effective chemical treatments, plant breeders have attempted to transfer naturally occurring virus resistance genes from one plant strain (cultivar) to another. However, resistant cultivars often revert to virus sensitivity, and resistance to one virus does not necessarily confer resistance to other, similar viruses. Natural virus resistance can be achieved in different ways: viral transmission can be blocked, establishment of the virus can be prevented, or viral symptoms can be bypassed or resisted. Genetic engineering has been used to develop nonconventional types of virus-resistant transgenic plants.

Viral Coat Protein-Mediated Protection

When transgenic plants express the gene for a coat protein (which usually is the most abundant protein of a virus particle) of a virus that normally infects those plants, the ability of the virus to subsequently infect the plants and spread systemically is often greatly diminished. For a long time, the

precise mechanism by which the presence of coat protein genes inhibits viral proliferation was not understood; however, it is now thought that it likely works through the generation of RNAi. Moreover, the antiviral effect occurs early in the viral replication cycle and, as a result, prevents any significant amount of viral synthesis. This feature is an advantage because it decreases the probability of selecting for spontaneous viral mutants that can overcome this resistance and replicate in the presence of viral coat protein. The viral coat protein gene approach has been used to confer tolerance for a number of different plant viruses (Table 19.2). With this approach, researchers have developed virus-resistant transgenic plants for a number of different crops. Although complete protection is not usually achieved, high levels of virus resistance have been reported. In addition, a coat protein gene from one virus sometimes provides tolerance for a broad spectrum of unrelated viruses. The utility of this strategy is supported by the observation that transgenic plants that encode viral coat proteins do as well in field trials as in the laboratory studies.

In both eukaryotes and prokaryotes, an RNA molecule that is complementary to a normal gene transcript (mRNA) is called antisense RNA. The mRNA, being translatable, is considered to be a sense RNA. The presence of antisense RNA can decrease the synthesis of the gene product by forming a duplex molecule with the normal sense mRNA, thereby preventing it from being translated. The antisense RNA–mRNA duplex is also rapidly degraded, a response that diminishes the amount of that particular mRNA in the cell. Theoretically, it should be possible to prevent plant viruses from

TABLE 19.2 Some transgenic plants engineered to have viral coat protein-mediated protection against viral infection

Viral source of coat protein	Transgenic plant(s)
Alfalfa mosaic virus	Alfalfa, tobacco, tomato
Arabis mosaic virus	Tobacco
Beet necrotic yellow vein virus	Sugar beet
Cucumber mosaic virus	Cucumber, tobacco
Cymbidium ringspot virus	Tobacco
Grapevine chrome mosaic virus	Tobacco
Maize dwarf mosaic virus	Sweet corn
Papaya ringspot virus	Papaya, tobacco
Plum pox virus	Tobacco
Potato aucuba mosaic virus	Tobacco
Potato leafroll virus	Potato
Potato virus S	Potato
Potato virus X	Potato, tobacco
Potato virus Y	Potato, tobacco
Rice stripe virus	Rice
Soybean mosaic virus	Tobacco
Tobacco etch virus	Tobacco
Tobacco mosaic virus	Tobacco, tomato
Tomato mosaic virus	Tomato
Tomato rattle virus	Tobacco
Tomato streak virus	Tobacco
Tomato spotted wilt virus	Tobacco
Watermelon mosaic virus 2	Tobacco
Zucchini yellow mosaic virus	Muskmelon, tobacco

FIGURE 19.11 Procedure for introducing CuMV coat protein cDNA into plant cells. RNA4, which encodes the coat protein, is isolated from a viral RNA preparation and used as the template for the synthesis of double-stranded cDNA. Linkers are added to the cDNA preparation, and the cDNAs are cloned into an *E. coli* plasmid vector. A full-length cDNA clone is identified, excised from the *E. coli* vector, and subcloned into a Ti plasmid cloning vector between the 35S promoter from cauliflower mosaic virus (P_{35S}) and the transcription terminator from the gene for the small subunit of ribulose bisphosphate carboxylase (*t*RBC). This cloning step creates two orientations for the RNA4 cDNA. In one case, the RNA that is transcribed is translated into coat protein (sense RNA), and in the other case, the transcribed RNA is complementary to the mRNA for the coat protein (antisense RNA).

replicating and subsequently damaging plant tissues by creating transgenic plants that synthesize antisense RNA that is complementary to viral coat protein mRNA.

In one of many studies, the efficacies of the viral coat protein gene and antisense RNA approaches were compared by cloning the cDNA for the coat protein of cucumber mosaic virus (CuMV) into tobacco plants in two orientations (sense and antisense; one orientation per plant) and then testing transgenic plants for sensitivity to viral infection (Fig. 19.11). The genome of CuMV consists of three separate single-stranded pieces of RNA, each coding for a specific viral protein. In vivo, one of these pieces, RNA3, is processed to remove a portion of its sequence, thereby generating RNA4, which encodes the viral coat protein. To create transgenic plants that either produced normal mRNA and expressed the viral coat protein or produced its antisense RNA, the following steps were carried out:

1. Isolation of RNA4
2. In vitro enzymatic conversion of RNA4 into a double-stranded cDNA
3. Addition of linkers onto the cDNA
4. Insertion of the full-length cDNA sequences into cloning vectors in both orientations, with each oriented sequence under the control of the 35S promoter sequence from cauliflower mosaic virus and the termination-regulatory sequences from the plant gene for the small subunit of ribulose bisphosphate carboxylase
5. Formation of separate transgenic plants carrying the cDNA sequence in one of the two possible orientations

The Ti plasmid binary vector system was used to transfer both protein-producing sense and antisense RNA-producing cDNA sequences to separate tobacco cells, from which transgenic plants were regenerated (Fig. 19.12). The transgenic tobacco plants that expressed the CuMV coat protein were protected from viral-particle accumulation and did not show symptoms of viral infection, regardless of whether the inoculum of the challenge

FIGURE 19.12 Ti plasmid binary cloning vectors containing either the protein-producing sense **(A)** or the RNA-producing antisense **(B)** orientation of the CuMV coat protein cDNA. Each cDNA sequence is under the control of the 35S promoter (P_{35S}) from cauliflower mosaic virus and the transcription terminator–polyadenylation site (tRBC) from the gene for the small subunit of ribulose bisphosphate carboxylase. The vector also contains a neomycin phosphotransferase (NPT) gene under the control of nopaline synthase transcription signals (pNOS and tNOS), an Spcr gene, a T-DNA right-border sequence, a T-DNA left-border sequence, and a broad-host-range origin of DNA replication (ori). The protein-producing sense (+) orientation is shown by the A→Z arrow, and the RNA-producing antisense (−) orientation is shown by the Z→A arrow.

virus was high or low, whereas the antisense orientation construct protected transgenic plants only against low viral doses.

Several groups of scientists have constructed transgenic plants that synthesize antisense RNA copies of viral coat protein genes and tested whether these plants can withstand a viral challenge. In all instances, the plants were protected against the invading virus only when low concentrations of the virus were used. At high concentrations, the plants were damaged by the virus. In addition, antisense RNA copies of viral coat protein genes generally afforded a much lower level of protection to transgenic plants than did sense versions of the viral coat protein genes. Although the antisense RNA approach may not be an effective means of creating virus-resistant plants, it may be possible to use small interfering RNA (double-stranded RNAs about 21 nucleotides long) to protect plants against invading viruses. In this case, the interfering RNA would act to target specific mRNAs (e.g., mRNAs encoding viral coat proteins) for nuclease digestion.

Often field crops are exposed to several different viruses, any one of which may damage the plant and lower the final yield. Ideally, transgenic plants should be resistant to more than one virus. With this in mind, Ti plasmid binary vectors expressing one or more coat protein genes for CuMV, zucchini yellow mosaic virus, and watermelon mosaic virus 2 were used to transform yellow crookneck squash *(Cucurbita pepo)* plants (Fig. 19.13). Transgenic plants that contained the coat protein genes from all three viruses were resistant to damage by all three viruses under laboratory conditions. Initially, transgenic plants expressing coat protein genes for zucchini yellow mosaic virus and watermelon mosaic virus 2 were tested under field conditions by using aphids, which are small insects that naturally transmit these viruses to developing plants. The transgenic plants that expressed both coat protein genes were completely resistant to infection when the two viruses were transmitted at the same time (Fig. 19.14). On the other hand, while transgenic plants expressing only one of the two viral coat proteins were

FIGURE 19.13 (A) A T-DNA construct with a neomycin phosphotransferase (NPT II) gene as a selectable marker, a β-glucuronidase (GUS) gene as a reporter gene, two copies of the coat protein gene from watermelon mosaic virus 2 (WMV 2), and the coat protein gene from CuMV. The left and right borders of the T-DNA are indicated by LB and RB, respectively. (B) Similar to panel A without CuMV and GUS, with one copy of WMV 2, and with the coat protein gene from zucchini yellow mosaic virus (ZYMV). (C) Same as panel B with the addition of CuMV. All of the genes in these constructs include both promoters and transcription terminator regions.

FIGURE 19.14 Disease frequencies in transgenic and nontransformed (wild-type) yellow crookneck squash in the field. Aphids were used to transmit a mixture of zucchini yellow mosaic virus (ZYMV) and watermelon mosaic virus 2 (WMV) to the squash plants. Adapted from Fuchs and Gonsalves, *Bio/Technology* **13**:1466–1473, 1995.

delayed in succumbing to the viruses in comparison with the nontransformed control plants, all of these plants eventually developed severe symptoms of viral disease, making them unfit for sale to consumers.

More recently, transgenic squash plants that express viral coat protein genes for zucchini yellow mosaic virus, watermelon mosaic virus 2, and CuMV have been tested in the field. Following the demonstration that they effectively protected plants against disease caused by any or all of these viruses, these transgenic squash plants were made commercially available. The increase in plant yield resulting from virus protection depends upon which viruses the plants are challenged with, how great the viral pressure is, and the time of the growing season. Despite these many variables, one study estimated that transgenic squash with resistance to these three viruses, subjected to severe viral pressure, could produce as much as a 50-fold increase in marketable squash over nontransgenic varieties. Clearly, using more than one viral coat protein gene is an effective strategy that should be useful in developing a range of transgenic plants that are resistant to all of the major viruses that normally inhibit their growth and development. However, it must be borne in mind that in order to satisfy the variety of consumer tastes, there are a large number of squash varieties, all of which are potentially susceptible to these viruses, and with this approach, all of them would have to be genetically engineered in a similar manner. In addition, those transgenic lines that are resistant to three different viruses are still susceptible to papaya ringspot virus type W, so "complete" viral protection of summer squash will require the introduction of the viral coat protein for this virus, as well.

The phenomenon of using a plant-encoded viral gene to disrupt the virus life cycle and thereby confer resistance to the virus is sometimes called homology-dependent gene silencing (formerly called cosuppression). In homology-dependent gene silencing, the addition of new copies of a gene to the genome inhibits expression of both the introduced gene and the previously present endogenous copies or, in the case of viral genes, those genes that are synthesized after infection. In fact, in some cases, the

plant's own defense mechanisms may include the possibility of homology-dependent gene silencing.

Perhaps the most successful employment of the viral coat protein strategy to prevent damage from a plant virus is the use of the coat protein of papaya ringspot virus to protect papaya plants against the virus. In fact, these transgenic papaya plants are widely credited with saving the Hawaiian papaya industry (Box 19.3).

Protection by Expression of Other Genes

RNase III. Engineered resistance to plant viruses—generally as a result of expressing a viral coat protein or other viral gene in the transgenic plant—is usually an effective strategy only against closely related viruses. Since there are a large number of different viruses that could potentially infect a crop, it would be advantageous if plants could be engineered to be resistant to a broad spectrum of viruses. To do this, a strain of wheat was engineered to express the *E. coli* gene *(rnc)* for ribonuclease (RNase) III, an enzyme that cleaves only double-stranded RNA; most plant viruses have double-stranded RNA as their genetic material. When tested, transgenic plants that expressed the *rnc* gene were resistant to several different RNA plant viruses. Unfortunately, plants that expressed this gene were often stunted and did not develop normally. This was probably a result of the interaction between the plant RNA and the enzyme. To overcome this problem, a mutant of RNase III was used. The mutant enzyme was still able to bind stoichiometrically to double-stranded RNA, but it no longer cleaved this

BOX 19.3

Saving the Hawaiian Papaya Industry

Papaya (*Carica papaya*) is an important tropical fruit crop grown in Brazil, India, Mexico, and Thailand (as well as several other tropical countries) and in Hawaii. It is valued as a healthy food because it is rich in vitamins C and A and because it contains large amounts of the proteolytic enzyme papain, which is potentially an aid to the digestion of proteins. The tree is relatively easy to grow from seeds, and the first fruit can be harvested a few months after the seeds are sown. Thereafter, fruit is produced continuously on a year-round basis.

Papaya ringspot virus (PRSV) is a potyvirus that is transmitted by aphids. In addition to papaya, the virus also infects a number of cucurbits (e.g., squash, watermelon, and cucumber). The viral RNA genome consists of approximately 10,000 nucleotides, which exist as a single

strand. The genome is monocistronic, so it is expressed as a single large polypeptide that is subsequently processed into several different functional proteins. When PRSV was discovered to be present on the Hawaiian island of Oahu in the late 1950s, the papaya industry was moved over the course of several years to the area of Puna on the island of Hawaii (sometimes called the Big Island). However, by the 1970s, PRSV was also detected in Puna.

Subsequently, a team of scientists, headed by Dennis Gonsalves, developed (from the commercial cultivar called Sunset) a line of transgenic papaya (called 55-1) which expressed the coat protein gene of PRSV. At the time that this work was undertaken, papaya had not been genetically transformed, and thus, the coat protein was introduced by microprojectile bombardment. The homozygous (for the coat protein gene) version of this strain (now called UH SunUP) was

shown to be highly resistant to PRSV under field conditions. The UH SunUP strain was then crossed with the nontransgenic Kapoho strain (which is the dominant strain of papaya grown in Hawaii) to create a hybrid strain called UH Rainbow. Importantly, while both the transgenic and nontransgenic papaya strains could be infected with PRSV, the transgenic strains have remained resistant to the virus for up to (at least) 3 years.

The main markets for Hawaiian papaya are the mainland United States, Canada, and Japan. These transgenic plants have been approved for use in the United States and Canada, and it is expected that they will receive Japanese regulatory approval shortly. The success with papaya demonstrates that the approach of using coat protein-mediating protection may be both a safe and an efficacious way to develop protection from virus for a range of crops.

substrate (Fig. 19.15). The mutant gene *(rnc70)* was introduced into wheat, under the control of a corn ubiquitin gene promoter (Fig. 19.16), by microprojectile bombardment. Transgenic plants that expressed mutant RNase III developed normally and exhibited a high level of resistance to infection by barley stripe mosaic virus. In this instance, binding of the mutant RNase III to replicating barley stripe mosaic virus prevented viral replication. In addition to being useful with RNA viruses, this approach should be an effective strategy for eliminating viroid infection of plants. Viroids are disease-causing agents with a circular single-stranded RNA genome that contains double-stranded regions formed by intrastrand base pairing. Plant viroids are difficult to control because they do not encode any proteins; therefore, the viroid nucleic acid must be targeted.

Pokeweed antiviral protein. In addition to "immunizing" plants against damage from viruses by expressing viral proteins in the plant cells, protection can be conferred by antiviral plant proteins. For example, pokeweed *(Phytolacca americana)* has three antiviral proteins in its cell wall: pokeweed antiviral protein (PAP), which is found in spring leaves; PAPII, which is found in summer leaves; and PAP-S, which appears in seeds. Although they are only 40% identical at the protein level, and antibodies directed against PAP do not react with PAPII, they employ similar modes of action. Both PAP and PAPII are ribosome-inactivating proteins that remove a specific adenine residue from the large ribosomal RNA of the 60S subunit of eukaryotic ribosomes. When pokeweed plants are infected with viruses, either PAP or PAPII is synthesized, depending on the season, and the ribosomes in the infected cells are inactivated. Based on their mode of action, PAP and PAPII are good candidates for developing transgenic plants that are resistant to a broad spectrum of plant viruses.

After a cDNA encoding PAP was isolated, it was introduced, under the transcriptional control of the 35S promoter, into tobacco and potato plants with binary Ti plasmid vectors. Transformants that expressed a high level of PAP (>10 ng/mg of protein) had a stunted and mottled appearance and were sterile. On the other hand, plants with a lower level of PAP (1 to 5 ng/mg of protein) were normal in appearance and fertile. Thus, above a certain level, PAP interferes with normal cellular functioning. In transgenic plants

FIGURE 19.15 Binding of the native form **(A)** and the mutant form **(B)** of *E. coli* RNase III to double-stranded RNA. The native form of the enzyme cleaves the RNA, while the mutant form does not.

No digestion

| *Ubi* promoter | *Ubi* exon | *Ubi* intron | *rnc*70 gene | TT |

FIGURE 19.16 A portion of the genetic construct used to transform wheat plants with the gene for the mutant form of *E. coli* RNase III *(rnc70)*. The construct includes the corn ubiquitin gene *(Ubi)* promoter, the first exon and intron in front of a mutant form of *E. coli* RNase III, and a transcription terminator (TT) region from a nopaline synthase gene.

expressing PAP, the major effect of the antiviral protein was to reduce the number of lesions in virus-infected plants. When transgenic tobacco and potato plants expressing low levels of PAP were challenged with either potato virus X or Y, they developed significantly fewer lesions on their leaves than nontransformed control plants.

Transgenic plants that contained the cDNA for PAPII expressed the protein at a much higher level than that observed for PAP (up to 250 ng/ mg of protein). Plants with >150 ng of PAPII per mg of protein had chlorotic lesions, while those with 10 to 100 ng of PAPII per mg of protein were normal. Transgenic plants that expressed the lower level of PAPII and were otherwise normal were resistant to tobacco mosaic virus, potato virus X, and the fungal pathogen *Rhizoctonia solani*. While this gene is highly effective in the laboratory, it remains to be seen how it will function under field conditions.

Single-chain antibodies. One way to protect plants against viral infection is to engineer the plants to produce antibodies that are directed against the invading viruses. This was done, with some success, by expressing single-chain Fv antibodies directed against tobacco mosaic virus in tobacco plants. However, as a consequence of the variability between coat proteins from different viruses, this strategy is not useful for providing broad-range resistance against several different viruses.

The majority of plant viruses are RNA viruses, and many of them contain positive-stranded RNA as the genetic material. These viruses all encode RNA-dependent RNA polymerases that are essential for their replication. Thus, a single-chain Fv antibody that recognizes epitopes that are common to the RNA-dependent RNA polymerases from several different viruses should be an effective means of inhibiting the replication of all of these viruses, thereby making transgenic plants that express these single-chain Fv antibodies resistant to these viruses (Fig. 19.17). That is because the antibody fragment can bind to RNA polymerases and thereby block their activities. In addition, since even in virus-infected cells RNA-dependent RNA polymerases are found in only low concentrations, a high level of antibody expression is not required. When two phage display libraries were screened against purified denatured fragments of the RNA-dependent RNA polymerase of tomato bushy stunt virus, the three single-chain Fv antibodies that displayed the highest affinity were isolated and characterized. A cDNA encoding one of these single-chain Fv antibodies was expressed in *Nicotiana benthamiana* (a close relative of tobacco, native to Australia). The resultant transgenic plants were significantly protected against tomato bushy stunt virus and cucumber necrosis virus and partially resistant to turnip crinkle virus and red clover necrotic virus. In addition, the single-chain Fv antibody directed against tomato bushy stunt virus bound to the RNA-dependent RNA polymerase of hepatitis C virus, which is much more distantly related.

vRNA

FIGURE 19.17 Schematic representation of the inhibition of tomato bushy stunt virus RNA-dependent RNA polymerase by a single-chain Fv antibody. Tomato bushy stunt virus has a genome of 4,775 nucleotides that encodes five separate proteins, one of which is the viral RNA-dependent RNA polymerase.

This work represents an important first step in using a simple and straightforward strategy to develop transgenic plants that are resistant to a wide range of different viruses.

Micro-RNAs. One approach to developing plants that are resistant to a range of different viruses might include engineering the plants to produce micro-RNAs (miRNAs) that interfere with viral replication by targeting the viral RNA (or the viral mRNA) for degradation. In a recent series of experiments, starting with a 273-nucleotide precursor of a naturally occurring plant miRNA, scientists used PCR to replace a small portion of the existing sequence so that the precursor could be processed to yield a 20- to 24-nucleotide-long miRNA that was complementary to viral RNA (Fig. 19.18). The newly synthesized artificial miRNA (amiRNA) became part of an RNA-induced silencing complex (see chapter 11) in which the viral RNA (mRNA) was specifically bound and cleaved. It is also possible to clone two or more different pre-amiRNAs in tandem—this was done using turnip yellow mosaic virus and turnip mosaic virus—so that plants transformed with this construct become resistant to two separate viruses. This approach can be made even more effective by targeting more than one portion of each viral RNA using several pre-amiRNAs. Despite its intriguing possibilities, this system still requires a considerable amount of development before it is shown to be effective under field conditions.

Herbicide Resistance

A significant fraction of global crop production is lost through weed infestation every year, despite the expenditure of $10 billion on more than 100 different chemical herbicides. In addition, many herbicides do not discriminate weeds from crop plants; others must be applied early, before the weeds

FIGURE 19.18 Use of amiRNAs to provide protection against viruses. The 273-nucle-otide-long precursor (labeled pre-mR159a) of a naturally occurring miRNA, which is 20 to 24 nucleotides long, is cloned, and then PCR is used to alter a portion of the pre-miRNA sequence. The modified amiRNA sequence is cloned into a binary vector under the control of the 35S promoter, which is then used to transform *Arabidopsis* plants that now produce a pre-amiRNA that, when it is processed, targets a specific viral RNA for cleavage. Adapted from Niv et al., *Nat. Biotechnol.* **24**:1420–1428, 2006.

take hold; and some persist in the environment. The creation of herbicide-resistant crop plants is one way to overcome some of these drawbacks.

A number of different biological manipulations that would cause a crop plant to be herbicide resistant can be envisioned.

1. Inhibit uptake of the herbicide.
2. Overproduce the herbicide-sensitive target protein so that enough of it remains available for cellular functions despite the presence of the herbicide.
3. Introduce a bacterial or fungal gene that produces a protein that is not sensitive to the herbicide but performs the same function as the plant (herbicide-sensitive) protein.
4. Reduce the ability of a herbicide-sensitive target protein to bind to a herbicide.
5. Endow plants with the capability to metabolically inactivate the herbicide.

A number of these strategies have been implemented to produce herbicide-resistant transgenic plants (Table 19.3). This approach has been so successful that more than 75% of the transgenic crops that are currently planted world-wide have been engineered to be herbicide resistant. By far, the most widely

TABLE 19.3 Some examples of gene-based herbicide resistance

Herbicide(s)	Mode of development of herbicide resistance
Triazines	Resistance is due to an alteration in the *psbA* gene, which codes for the target of this herbicide, chloroplast protein D-1.
Sulfonylureas	Genes encoding resistant versions of the enzyme acetolactate synthetase have been introduced into poplar, canola, flax, and rice.
Imidazolinones	Strains with resistant versions of the enzyme acetolactate synthetase have been selected in tissue culture.
Aryloxphenoxypropionates, cyclohexanediones	These herbicides inhibit the enzyme acetyl coenzyme A carboxylase. Resistance, selected in tissue culture, is due either to an altered enzyme that is not herbicide sensitive or to the degradation of the herbicide.
Glyphosate	Resistance is from overproduction of EPSPS, the target of this herbicide. Resistance has been engineered by transforming soybean with the gene for a glyphosate-resistant EPSPS and tobacco with a glyphosate oxidoreductase gene, which encodes an enzyme that degrades glyphosate.
Bromoxynil	Resistance to this photosystem II inhibitor has been created by transforming tobacco and cotton plants with a bacterial nitrilase gene, which encodes an enzyme that degrades this herbicide.
Phenoxycarboxylic acids (e.g., 2,4-D and 2,4,5-T)	Resistant cotton and tobacco plants have been created by transformation with the *tfdA* gene from *Alcaligenes*, which encodes a dioxygenase that degrades this herbicide.
Glufosinate (phosphinothricin)	Over 20 different plants have been transformed with either the *bar* gene from *Streptomyces hygroscopicus* or the *pat* gene from *S. viridochromogenes*. The phosphinothricin acetyltransferase that these genes encode detoxifies this herbicide.
Cyanamide	Resistant tobacco plants were produced when a cyanamide hydratase gene from the fungus *Myrothecium verrucaria* was introduced. The enzyme encoded by this gene converts cyanamide to urea.
Dalapon	Tobacco plants transformed with a dehalogenase gene from *Pseudomonas putida* can detoxify this herbicide.

used herbicide is glyphosate, which is considered to be safe, cheap, effective, and "environmentally friendly" because it is readily degraded to nontoxic compounds in the soil. Glyphosate, trademarked as Roundup by the Monsanto Corporation, inhibits a key enzyme in the shikimate pathway, 5-enolpyruvylshikimate-3-phosphate synthase (EPSPS), that plays an important role in the synthesis of aromatic amino acids in both bacteria and plants. Plants resistant to this herbicide have been developed by putting an EPSPS-encoding gene from a glyphosate-resistant strain of *E. coli* under the control of plant promoter and transcription termination–polyadenylation sequences and cloning the construct into plant cells. Transgenic soybean,

corn, canola, tobacco, petunia, tomato, potato, and cotton plants that produce an amount of the resistant *E. coli* EPSPS sufficient to replace the inhibited plant enzyme are resistant to the effects of glyphosate. Thus, in these cases, the crop plant would not be affected by glyphosate treatment, whereas the weeds would be. Crops that have been engineered to be resistant to glyphosate by this approach are said to be "Roundup ready."

Notwithstanding the many years of successful use of glyphosate and Roundup-ready plants, two important factors are now changing people's thinking about this approach. In the first instance, the herbicide patent has now expired and other companies are very actively pursuing the development of plants that are resistant to glyphosate using other approaches. Secondly, there is a realization that worldwide agriculture has become too dependent upon a single herbicide and that alternative strategies need to be developed.

To find an enzyme that can inactivate glyphosate, one group of researchers assayed a collection of several hundred *Bacillus* sp. strains for the ability to acetylate glyphosate (Fig. 19.19). The assay was based on the ability to measure N-acetylglyphosate in the supernatant of permeabilized cells (Fig. 19.20). The three strains (all *Bacillus licheniformis*) that had the highest level of glyphosate N-acetyltransferase activity were isolated, and

FIGURE 19.19 N-acetylation of the herbicide glyphosate by the bacterial enzyme glyphosate N-acetyltransferase. CoASH, coenzyme A.

FIGURE 19.20 Overview of a scheme to isolate a bacterial enzyme with a sufficient level of glyphosate N-acetyltransferase activity to allow it to be used to engineer plants so that they are resistant to high levels of glyphosate.

the enzymes were characterized. In all cases, these strains exhibited only a very low level of enzyme activity. Subsequently, the genes from each of the three selected strains encoding glyphosate *N*-acetyltransferase activity were isolated. These genes were then shuffled (see chapter 8) numerous times, each time selecting the strain with glyphosate *N*-acetyltransferase with the highest level of activity. In fact, following 11 iterations of DNA shuffling, the enzyme catalytic efficiency (see chapter 8) improved by nearly 10,000-fold. Interestingly, while the modified enzyme still functions as a glyphosate *N*-acetyltransferase, after so many rounds of modification, the amino acid sequence of the modified enzyme is only 76 to 79% identical to the amino acid sequences of the parental enzymes. Finally, the modified glyphosate *N*-acetyltransferase gene was introduced into *Arabidopsis*, tobacco, and corn plants. The transgenic plants, which expressed the enzyme in the plant cytosol and were both morphologically normal and fertile, were tolerant of approximately six times the dose of glyphosate that killed the parental nontransformed plants. This work is an important first step in developing plants that can act as an alternative to Roundup-ready plants. However, the efficacy of this approach remains to be proven in the field.

The herbicide dicamba has been used since the 1960s to control a wide range of broadleaf weeds. When it is applied to dicotyledonous plants, dicamba acts by mimicking the effects of high levels of the plant hormone indole-3-acetic acid and binding to indole-3-acetic acid receptors, which are essential for normal growth and development of the plant. The herbicide is widely used, relatively inexpensive, and environmentally friendly in that it does not persist in soils and has no toxicity to humans or other animals. Moreover, the widespread use of the herbicide has not led to the development of any dicamba-resistant weeds. Researchers have therefore sought to develop crop plants that are resistant to dicamba. To do this, a dicamba monooxygenase gene was expressed in *Arabidopsis*, tomato, and tobacco

FIGURE 19.21 (A) Conversion of dicamba to 3,6-dichlorosalicylic acid by dicamba monooxygenase. (B) The genetic construct used to express the dicamba monooxygenase gene within the chloroplasts of transgenic plants. The promoter was from peanut chlorotic streak virus, the enhancer was from tomato etch virus, the transit peptide was from the small subunit of pea ribulose 1,6-bisphosphate carboxylase, the diooxygenase gene was from the soil bacterium *P. maltophilia*, and the terminator sequence was from the small subunit of pea ribulose 1,6-bisphosphate carboxylase. Adapted from Behrens et al., *Science* **316**:1185–1188, 2007.

plants (all as test systems). The dicamba monooxygenase is part of the three-component enzyme dicamba O-demethylase, from the bacterium *Pseudomonas maltophilia*, that converts dicamba to 3,6-dichlorosalicylic acid, a compound without any appreciable herbicidal activity (Fig. 19.21). In transgenic plants, only dicamba monooxygenase is needed for the inactivation of the herbicide, since the enzyme can be targeted to the chloroplast, where there is a ready source of reduced ferredoxin (the product of the other two genes in the dicamba O-demethylase complex). The reduced ferredoxin supplies electrons for the monooxygenase reaction. As expected, transgenic plants expressing dicamba monooxygenase are resistant to high levels of the herbicide when grown in both the greenhouse and the field. It is speculated that it may be possible to "stack" plants with genes encoding both glyphosate and dicamba resistance so that farmers can either alternate the use of the two herbicides or else apply them at the same time. In this way, it is anticipated that unwanted weeds are unlikely to develop resistance to both herbicides, while the transgenic crop plant is uninhibited by the herbicide.

Resistance due to inactivation of bromoxynil (3,5-dibromo-4-hydroxybenzonitrile), a herbicide that acts by inhibiting photosynthesis, has been achieved for some plants. In this case, resistant plants were created by the introduction of a bacterial gene that encodes the enzyme nitrilase, which can inactivate bromoxynil before the herbicide can act (Fig. 19.22). The gene for nitrilase was isolated from the soil bacterium *Klebsiella ozaenae* and placed under the control of the light-regulated promoter from the small subunit of the enzyme ribulose bisphosphate carboxylase before it was transferred to tobacco plants. As expected, the transgenic plants expressed nitrilase activity in their shoots and leaves, but not in their roots, and were resistant to the toxic effects of the herbicide.

Fungus and Bacterium Resistance

Extensive damage and loss of crop productivity are caused by phytopathogenic fungi. It has been estimated that one fungal disease of one major crop, i.e., fungal rice blast, a disease that affects rice plants, costs farmers in Southeast Asia, Japan, and the Philippines more than $5 billion per year. At present, the major way of controlling the damage and losses to crop plants that result from fungal infection is through the use of chemical agents that may persist and accumulate in the environment and that are subsequently hazardous to animals or humans. It would therefore be beneficial if a

FIGURE 19.22 Detoxification of the herbicide bromoxynil by the enzyme nitrilase from *K. ozaenae*.

Pathogen infection

↓

Salicylic acid
2-O-β-D-Glucoside → Salicylic acid

↓

Induction of
pathogenesis-related proteins

↓

Fungal and bacterial pathogen resistance

FIGURE 19.23 Overview of systemic acquired resistance in plants. After infection of a plant by a pathogenic fungus or bacterium (shown in blue), the inactive storage compound salicylic acid 2-O-β-D-glucoside is converted to salicylic acid and/or salicylic acid is synthesized. The salicylic acid activates or induces the *NPR1* gene, whose protein product acts as a "master" regulatory protein to turn on the expression of the PR proteins, which have enzyme activities directed against various pathogenic organisms.

simple, inexpensive, effective, and environmentally friendly nonchemical means of preventing fungal damage to crop plants could be found.

Plants often respond to fungal or bacterial pathogen invasion or other environmental stresses by converting a conjugated storage form of salicylic acid (salicylic acid 2-O-β-D-glycoside) to salicylic acid, which induces a broad systemic defense response in the plant. This "systemic acquired resistance" to pathogens extends to plant tissues that are far from the site of the initial infection and may last for weeks to months. It results from the synthesis of a group of proteins called pathogenesis-related (PR) proteins (Fig. 19.23). The PR proteins include β-1,3-glucanases, chitinases, thaumatin-like proteins (thaumatin is a small, very sweet protein), and protease inhibitors that protect the plant-invading pathogens. To develop plants resistant to fungal pathogens, researchers have attempted to utilize parts of the systemic acquired resistance system. For example, transgenic plants that constitutively express high levels of one or more PR proteins, such as chitinase, which can hydrolyze the β-1,4 linkages of the N-acetyl-D-

FIGURE 19.24 Plasmid vector containing a rice chitinase gene cassette and a hygromycin resistance gene cassette (in both cases including transcriptional regulatory sequences) used to transform rice protoplasts. Rice cell protoplasts were transformed by polyethylene glycol treatment in the presence of this plasmid. Transformed cells were selected for their resistance to hygromycin. Later, they were tested for the presence of chitinase genes by Southern hybridization and for chitinase by Western blot analysis; then, they were used to regenerate transgenic plants.

Hygromycin resistance cassette Chitinase gene cassette

glucosamine polymer chitin, a major component of many fungal cell walls, have been engineered (Fig. 19.24).

The *NPR1* gene from the plant *A. thaliana* encodes a "master" regulatory protein that controls the expression of the PR proteins, and it can be activated or induced by the addition of salicylic acid. In *A. thaliana*, overexpression of the *NPR1* gene can lead to the generation of broad-spectrum disease resistance against both fungal and bacterial pathogens. Moreover, scientists have observed that overproduction of this "master switch" is an effective strategy in several plants other than *A. thaliana*, including rice, sugar beet, apple, and corn.

Another approach to engineering plants with broad-spectrum disease resistance involves overproducing salicylic acid. Theoretically, this can be done by transforming plants with bacterial genes that encode the enzymes isochorismate synthase and isochorismate pyruvate lyase, which catalyze salicylate synthesis (Fig. 19.25). Salicylate is synthesized from chorismate, which is produced in large amounts in the chloroplast and is also an intermediate in the biosynthesis of the amino acid tryptophan. The two bacterial genes for salicylate synthesis were fused to chloroplast-targeting sequences from the gene for the small subunit of ribulose bisphosphate carboxylase— the small subunit of ribulose bisphosphate carboxylase is encoded within the nuclear DNA, but following its synthesis, this protein is transmitted to the chloroplast (Fig. 19.26). The result of this genetic manipulation was that when both of these enzymes were localized in the (tobacco) plant chloroplast, salicylic acid was produced constitutively. Consequently, the plants constitutively expressed a number of PR proteins. The plants appeared normal but exhibited enhanced resistance to both viral and fungal pathogens. Since it is not necessarily advantageous to the plant to constitutively express PR proteins, there is some question as to how effective this strategy of conferring protection against a broad range of pathogens will be in the field.

Transgenic plants that have been engineered to constitutively express chitinase under the control of the cauliflower mosaic virus 35S promoter include rice, tobacco, and canola. Transgenic plants that expressed chitinase were more resistant to damage by fungal pathogens than control plants, even though the control plants synthesized their own PR proteins in response to the fungal infection. Presumably, this resistance reflects the higher level of chitinase expressed by the transgenic plants than by non-

FIGURE 19.25 Use of bacterial enzymes to convert plant chloroplast chorismate to salicylate.

| P_{35S} | CTS | ICS gene | TT | P_{35S} | CTS | IPL gene | TT |

FIGURE 19.26 Construct used to transform plants so that they constitutively overproduce salicylate. P_{35S}, the 35S promoter from cauliflower mosaic virus; CTS, chloroplast targeting sequence; ICS, isochorismate synthase; TT, transcription termination region; IPL, isochorismate pyruvate lyase.

transformed plants. In addition, while transgenic plants constitutively expressing chitinase were resistant to fungal pathogens, binding of the beneficial root fungus *Glomus mosseae* to the plant roots was not affected. This was probably a consequence of a difference in the cell wall compositions of different fungi. Importantly, a transgenic plant constitutively expressing chitinase has been found to be effective at resisting fungal damage under field conditions. In a variation on the strategy described above, a cDNA encoding chitinase from the biocontrol fungus *Trichoderma harzianum* was isolated and introduced, under the control of the 35S promoter, into tobacco and potato plants. As expected, these transgenic plants were resistant to both soil-borne fungal pathogens (primarily affecting roots) and foliar fungal pathogens (primarily affecting shoots and leaves). In sum, the overexpression of some PR-like proteins, such as chitinase, appears to be an effective strategy for protecting plants against damage from pathogenic fungi.

Pathogenic fungi belonging to the genus *Fusarium* are the causative agents of some of the most costly and devastating plant diseases in the world. Therefore, a strategy that targeted various *Fusarium* spp. would be quite important for agriculture worldwide. A number of different antimicrobial peptides (which can disrupt the cell membrane) and the enzyme chitinase (mentioned above) are inhibitory to the growth of *Fusarium* spp. However, these biological approaches (regardless of how they are administered) are not as effective as spraying plants with chemical fungicides. To overcome this limitation, workers have fused the genes (cDNAs) for two different antimicrobial peptides (one from the radish *Raphanus sativus* and one from the mold *Aspergillus giganteus*) and a chitinase (from wheat) to a single-chain Fv antibody that binds to a *Fusarium* cell wall protein (Fig. 19.27). Although the single-chain Fv antibody was originally selected from a library constructed from chickens that had been immunized with

FIGURE 19.27 Schematic representation of three different anti-fungal fusion proteins. Each protein includes a single-chain Fv antibody that binds to a *Fusarium* sp. cell wall protein and an antifungal peptide/protein directed against either the cell membrane or the chitin component of the cell wall. Adapted from Bohlmann, *Nat. Biotechnol.* **22**:682–683, 2004.

Fusarium graminearum, the selected antibody cross-reacted with cell wall antigens from nine different species and subspecies of *Fusarium.* Constructs encoding the three fusion proteins were used to transform *A. thaliana,* and the transgenic plants were tested for resistance to infection and growth inhibition by *Fusarium oxysporum.* When either the selected single-chain Fv antibody or any one of the three antipathogenic peptides/proteins was expressed in transgenic plants, it endowed the plants with a low to moderate level of resistance to damage by the pathogen (Table 19.4). However, all three of the antibody-peptide/protein fusions conferred a high level of resistance to the pathogen, suggesting, in each case, that the two components of the fusion protein were acting synergistically. This is an interesting and potentially quite useful approach that merits further development.

The annual worldwide losses to farmers from potato diseases caused by the pathogenic soil bacterium *Erwinia carotovora* are approximately $100 million. Moreover, potato breeders have not identified any resistance traits that can be bred into commercial cultivars. To address this problem, transgenic potato plants that actively express bacteriophage T4 lysozyme were developed. The lysozyme was targeted for secretion into the apoplast (the intercellular spaces inside the plant but outside the plant cells) in potato plants, since this is the part of the plant where *E. carotovora* enters and spreads. More specifically, the T4 lysozyme gene was fused to the barley α-amylase signal peptide coding sequence and placed under the transcriptional control of the cauliflower mosaic virus 35S promoter, transcription terminator, and polyadenylation site. Although the T4 lysozyme gene was under the control of this strong promoter, only a very low level of lysozyme was synthesized, perhaps reflecting differences in codon usage between a bacteriophage gene and the potato genome. This result notwithstanding, under laboratory and greenhouse conditions, transgenic plants with this construct were significantly protected from damage by high levels of *E. carotovora.* Since much lower levels of the pathogen than were used in these laboratory experiments are present in the field, this type of genetic construct should provide a high level of protection under natural conditions. To avoid killing plant-beneficial bacteria in the vicinity of the roots, researchers have employed hen egg lysozyme instead of T4 lysozyme because it is more specific for various phytopathogenic *Erwinia* spp. Moreover, researchers have found this strategy to be useful for protecting

TABLE 19.4 Resistance of transgenic *A. thaliana* to the phytopathogen *F. oxysporum*

Transgene	Disease index (%)
None (wild type)	100
Fv antibody	55
Peptide 1	50
Peptide 2	60
Chitinase	52
Antibody–peptide 1 fusion	10
Antibody–peptide 2 fusion	0
Antibody–chitinase fusion	5

Adapted from Peschen et al., *Nat. Biotechnol.* **22:**732–738, 2004.

The extent of disease was assessed 2 weeks after infection with *F. oxysporum.* A disease index of 100% indicates that all of the plants are dead, 50% indicates that the average plant has disease symptoms but is alive, and 0% indicates that all plants are disease free.

many different plants, including potato, rice, tomato, and tobacco, from various bacterial pathogens. Finally, in addressing the concern that proteins that are present in the apoplast of root cells may be exuded from the roots (see chapter 18) and kill plant growth-promoting bacteria, as well as pathogenic bacteria, researchers have noted that the endogenous rhizosphere microbial community (containing many beneficial bacteria) was essentially unchanged when a lysozyme transgene was expressed. Despite this apparent success, it remains to be determined whether this sort of genetic manipulation, which functions well in the laboratory, will be useful in the field.

Oxidative Stress

Unlike many animals, plants cannot physically avoid adverse environmental conditions, such as high levels of light, ultraviolet (UV) irradiation, heat, high salt concentrations, or drought, so physiological strategies have evolved to cope with these stresses. At the molecular level, one of the undesirable consequences of physiological stress is the production of oxygen radicals. Thus, investigators reasoned that if they could create plants that were able to tolerate increased levels of oxygen radicals, these plants should also be able to withstand various forms of environmental stress.

A variety of biotic stresses, including salt, freezing, and drought, as well as exposure to pollutants, stimulate the formation of reactive oxygen species in plant cells. These toxic molecules damage membranes, membrane-bound structures, and macromolecules, including proteins and nucleic acids, especially in the mitochondria and chloroplast, resulting in oxidative stress. A common type of potentially damaging oxygen radical is the superoxide anion. Within a cell under oxidative stress, the enzyme superoxide dismutase detoxifies superoxide anion by converting it to hydrogen peroxide, which in turn is broken down to water by various cellular peroxidases or catalases (Fig. 19.28). In one study, tobacco plants that were transformed with a superoxide dismutase gene that was under the control of the 35S promoter from cauliflower mosaic virus had reduced oxygen radical damage under stress conditions compared with control plants.

Plants have several different isoforms of the enzyme superoxide dismutase. The Cu/Zn superoxide dismutases are found primarily in chloroplasts and to a lesser extent in the cytosol. The Mn superoxide dismutase is located in the mitochondria, and some plants also have an Fe form of superoxide dismutase. Transgenic tobacco plants that carried the cDNA for a chloroplast-localized Cu/Zn superoxide dismutase under the control of the 35S promoter from cauliflower mosaic virus were much more resistant to high-light damage than nontransformed plants. When they were tested, the transgenic plants retained 94% of their photosynthetic activity under

FIGURE 19.28 Conversion of superoxide anion to hydrogen peroxide and then to water and oxygen.

$$O_2^- \xrightarrow[\text{Superoxide dismutase}]{O_2} H_2O_2 \xrightarrow[\text{Catalase}]{} H_2O + O_2$$

$$\begin{array}{ccc}
& & \gamma\text{-Glu-Cys-Gly} \\
& & | \\
\gamma\text{-Glu-Cys-Gly} & \xrightarrow{\text{Glutathione peroxidase}} & S \\
| & & | \\
SH & & S \\
& & | \\
& & \gamma\text{-Glu-Cys-Gly}
\end{array}$$

Glutathione (GSH) Oxidized glutathione
(GSSG)

$$R-O-OH \xrightarrow{\text{Glutathione peroxidase}} R-OH$$

Organic peroxide Organic alcohol

FIGURE 19.29 Oxidation of glutathione to oxidized glutathione and simultaneous reduction of an organic peroxide to an organic alcohol, catalyzed by glutathione peroxidase. γ-Glu, glutamic acid residue linked to the next amino acid through the gamma carboxyl group rather than through the alpha amino group, as in a usual peptide linkage; Cys, cysteine; Gly, glycine.

conditions in which nontransformed plants lost all of their activity. In another experiment, transgenic plants with cloned Mn superoxide dismutase targeted to their chloroplasts were three- to fourfold less sensitive to oxidative damage caused by ozone than nontransformed plants.

Oxidative stress may also be reduced if the level of oxidized glutathione within a plant is increased. Glutathione peroxidase catalyzes the conversion of glutathione to oxidized glutathione by reacting with organic peroxides and reducing them to organic alcohols (Fig. 19.29). To test this idea, a tobacco cDNA encoding an enzyme with both glutathione S-transferase and glutathione peroxidase activities was isolated. Transgenic tobacco plants that expressed glutathione peroxidase were created using the isolated cDNA under the control of the 35S promoter, and the construct was introduced into plants with a binary Ti plasmid system. The transformed plants had approximately twice the level of enzyme activity found in nontransformed plants. Seedlings of these transgenic plants grew significantly faster than control seedlings when exposed to either chilling or salt stress. The efficacy of this system remains to be demonstrated in the field.

Salt and Drought Stress

Many plants live in environments where growth is severely impaired by either drought or high salinity. With increasing dependence on irrigation in agriculture and more frequent salting of icy and snowy roads in the winter, increased soil salinity has become a common problem worldwide. Approximately one-third of the world's irrigated land has become unsuitable for growing crops because of contamination with high levels of salt. Irrigation typically increases the amount of salt present in soil. To survive under these conditions, many plants synthesize low-molecular-weight nontoxic compounds collectively called osmoprotectants. These compounds facilitate both water uptake and retention and also protect and stabilize cellular macromolecules from damage by high salt levels. Some well-known osmoprotectants are sugars, alcohols, the amino acid proline,

$$CH_3$$
$$|$$
$$CH_3\text{-}N\text{-}CH_2CH_2OH$$
$$|$$
$$CH_3$$

$$\downarrow CMO$$

$$CH_3$$
$$|$$
$$CH_3\text{-}N\text{-}CH_2CHO$$
$$|$$
$$CH_3$$

$$\downarrow BADH$$

$$CH_3$$
$$|$$
$$CH_3\text{-}N\text{-}CH_2COO^-$$
$$|$$
$$CH_3$$

FIGURE 19.30 Conversion of choline to glycine betaine. CMO, choline monooxygenase; BADH, betaine aldehyde dehydrogenase.

and quaternary ammonium compounds. To create more salt-tolerant plants, scientists have tried to engineer an increase in the cellular accumulation of the following osmoprotectants: trehalose, proline, D-ononitol, mannitol, sorbitol, glycine betaine, and 3-dimethylsulfoniopropionate.

The quaternary ammonium compound betaine is a highly effective osmolyte that accumulates in some plants during periods of water stress or high salinity. However, several important crops, including potatoes, rice, and tomatoes, do not accumulate betaine. Thus, the introduction of betaine-biosynthetic enzymes into these plants might enable them to withstand water stress and/or high salinity. Betaine is synthesized from choline in two steps in both plants and bacteria (Fig. 19.30). In plants, such as spinach, choline is converted to betaine aldehyde by the enzyme choline monooxygenase and then to betaine by betaine aldehyde dehydrogenase. In bacteria, such as *E. coli*, both steps of betaine biosynthesis are catalyzed by the same enzyme, choline dehydrogenase. To create a more salt-tolerant tobacco, plant cells were transformed with a Ti plasmid vector carrying the *E. coli betA* gene, which encodes choline dehydrogenase, under the control of the cauliflower mosaic virus 35S promoter. In laboratory tests, tobacco plants expressing this gene were up to 80% more tolerant of a high (300 mM) salt concentration than were nontransformed tobacco plants. While it may be possible to improve the osmoprotection afforded by the *E. coli betA* gene by using a plant tissue-specific promoter to direct the expression of the gene, this experiment is an important step in the development of plants that are more tolerant of high levels of salt.

It is also possible to increase the trehalose (Fig. 19.31) concentration in plants (where trehalose is a natural alpha-linked disaccharide formed by an α or α-1 bond between two α-glucose units) and thereby protect the plants against inhibition by high levels of salt in the soil. To do this, rice plants were transformed, using a binary vector, with one of two different DNA constructs (Fig. 19.32). In *E. coli*, trehalose-6-phosphate is first formed from uridine diphosphate (UDP)-glucose and glucose-6-phosphate, and then the trehalose-6-phosphate is converted to trehalose. A fusion of the genes encoding the two enzymes that normally catalyze the two steps in the biosynthesis of trehalose in *E. coli* was constructed so that a single protein contained both activities. This simplifies the transformation of plants in that only one target gene needs to be introduced and ensures that the two enzyme activities necessary for the synthesis of trehalose are present at identical levels. In one genetic construct, the fusion protein gene is under the transcriptional control of an abscisic acid-inducible promoter and is expressed in the cytosol. In the other construct, it is under the control of the promoter for the small subunit of ribulose bisphosphate carboxylase, and the fusion protein is expressed in plant chloroplasts. In transgenic rice

FIGURE 19.31 Structure of trehalose.

A

B

FIGURE 19.32 Two genetic constructs used to engineer rice plants to synthesize trehalose to protect them against growth inhibition by high salt levels. The fusion protein is under the control of an abscisic acid (ABA)-inducible promoter where ABA synthesis increases in the presence of salt **(A)** or the promoter from the small subunit of ribulose bisphosphate carboxylase **(B)**. In panel B, the transit peptide facilitates the localization of the fusion protein in the chloroplasts. RB, right border; LB, left border; UTR, untranslated region.

plants that contain either DNA construct, the level of trehalose is 3 to 10 times higher than in nontransformed rice plants in the presence of salt. Moreover, the biomass of the transgenic plants is four to six times that of the nontransformed plants in the presence of salt. Thus, by increasing the amount of trehalose that a plant synthesizes, the plant acquires increased tolerance for moderate levels of salt in the environment.

Researchers have engineered the plant *A. thaliana* to be salt tolerant by sequestering sodium ions in the large intracellular vacuole (Fig. 19.33). The strategy consisted of overproducing the endogenous *A. thaliana* gene encoding an Na^+/H^+ antiport protein. The Na^+/H^+ antiport protein transports Na^+ into the vacuole using the electrochemical gradient of protons generated by vacuolar H^+-translocating enzymes. When tested, the transgenic plants that overproduced the Na^+/H^+ antiport protein thrived in soil that was watered with a solution of 200 mM salt. This approach to the manipulation of salt stress in plants is effective with corn, canola, cotton, rice, tobacco, and tomato plants, as well as with *A. thaliana*. In transgenic tomato plants, the salt is localized in the leaves, and therefore, the transgenic tomato fruits do not accumulate salt and are quite normal in all respects, including taste. In addition to Na^+ toxicity, plants that live in saline environments have to contend with water loss caused by osmotic stress. By concentrating the salt in the plant's large vacuole, water that is free of salt should be driven into the plant cells, resulting in plants that use water more efficiently. This system has been quite successful in greenhouse trials and in the limited number of field trials where it has been tested. It provides researchers with the potential, especially in combination with other approaches, such as the overproduction of certain osmolytes, to engineer a wide range of salt-tolerant crop plants that can be grown on marginal land or possibly watered with seawater or other salt-containing water.

Many of the strategies that have been used to engineer plants to become more salt tolerant are also effective at making the plant drought tolerant; however, some strategies are specific for one stress or the other. In fact, a very large number of different genes have been employed in attempts to create drought-tolerant transgenic plants. These approaches have included introducing genes encoding overproduction of various osmolytes (e.g., trehalose, proline, glycine betaine, and polyamines), plant stress proteins (e.g., chaperones and heat shock proteins), reactive-oxygen-scavenging proteins

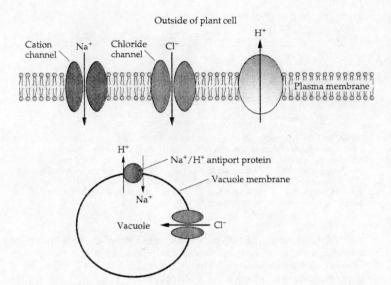

FIGURE 19.33 Schematic representation of ion transport in the plant *A. thaliana* showing the Na⁺ ions being sequestered in the large vacuole.

(e.g., superoxide dismutases), hormone biosynthesis and catabolism proteins (e.g., affecting cellular levels of abscisic acid, cytokinin, and ethylene), transcription factors that turn on the synthesis of a host of other proteins, and signaling proteins that activate the synthesis of other proteins.

One group of researchers reasoned that in order to increase the tolerance of plants for drought, it is necessary to delay the onset of drought-induced senescence during the drought episode. Moreover, by suppressing this response, plants would be more likely to resume normal growth when water became available. Of course, it is necessary to keep in mind that regardless of their genetic makeup, plants cannot exist for indefinite periods in the absence of water. Prior to this work, it had been observed that leaf senescence could be delayed in transgenic plants expressing a foreign gene encoding isopentenyltransferase, an enzyme that catalyzes the rate-limiting step in cytokinin biosynthesis. Therefore, tobacco plants were transformed to express isopentenyltransferase under the control of a *SARK* (senescence-associated protein kinase gene) promoter (Fig. 19.34). This regulatable promoter is induced during late maturation and decreased during the development of senescence. When these transgenic tobacco plants were watered with only 30% of the amount of water used under normal conditions, the suppression of leaf senescence resulted in a four- to fivefold-higher level of biomass in the transgenic versus the nontransformed plants. This result suggests that it may be possible to get irrigated crops to grow normally with only one-third the amount of water that is usually used.

Fruit Ripening and Flower Wilting

A major problem in fruit marketing is premature ripening and softening during transport. These changes are part of the natural aging (senescence)

FIGURE 19.34 Overview of how overexpressing cytokinin protects plants against drought. P_{SARK} is a senescence-induced promoter. The *IPT* gene encodes isopentenyltransferase, which catalyzes the rate-limiting step in cytokinin biosynthesis.

process of the fruit. Some of the genes that are induced during ripening encode the enzymes cellulase and polygalacturonase. It has been postulated that by interfering with the expression of one or more of these genes, the ripening process might be delayed. This interference could be achieved by creating transgenic plants with antisense or sense (cosuppression) RNA-producing versions of these genes. In fact, when an antisense RNA-producing gene for polygalacturonase was introduced into tomato plants, a $1.3 billion-a-year crop in the United States, both polygalacturonase mRNA and enzymatic activity were reduced by 90%. The lowering of polygalacturonase production inhibited fruit ripening in tomatoes, permitting the tomatoes to ripen on the vine instead of being harvested while they were still green. These tomatoes were claimed to have a long shelf life while retaining the flavor of the tomato. This genetically engineered tomato is known as the Flavr Savr (pronounced "flavor saver") tomato. On 18 May 1994, the U.S. Food and Drug Administration ruled that the Flavr Savr tomato was as safe for human consumption as tomatoes that were bred by conventional means, and because Flavr Savr tomatoes were essentially the same as other tomatoes, special labeling was not required.

The plant growth regulator ethylene induces the expression of a number of genes that are involved in fruit ripening and senescence and in flower wilting. It is synthesized from methionine by way of the intermediate compounds S-adenosylmethionine and 1-aminocyclopropane-1-carboxylic acid (ACC) (Fig. 19.35). Treatment of plants with chemical compounds that block ethylene production delays fruit ripening, senescence, and flower wilting. Thus, premature fruit ripening and flower wilting might be prevented by inhibiting the synthesis of ethylene. This can be achieved by blocking several different steps in the ethylene biosynthesis pathway (Fig. 19.35). For

FIGURE 19.35 Centrality of ACC in the synthesis of ethylene. M-ACC, 1-(malonylamino)-cyclopropane-1-carboxylic acid; G-ACC, 1-(γ-L-glutamylamino) cyclopropane-1-carboxylic acid.

example, transgenic plants that have been engineered to contain antisense RNA versions of S-adenosylmethionine synthetase, ACC synthase, or ACC oxidase have much lower than normal levels of ethylene. Similarly, the amount of ACC, and hence the amount of ethylene, that can be synthesized may be decreased by increasing the activity of either malonyl ACC transferase or glutamyl ACC transferase, thereby converting ACC into one of these dead-end storage compounds (Fig. 19.35), or by transforming plants

FIGURE 19.36 Inhibition of ethylene biosynthesis by genetic manipulation. Normally, ACC is synthesized from S-adenosylmethionine by the enzyme ACC synthase, and then ACC oxidase converts ACC to ethylene. Ethylene synthesis may be inhibited in transgenic plants either by an antisense mRNA version of ACC synthase; by ACC oxidase, which inhibits the synthesis of these enzymes; or by the enzyme ACC deaminase, which competes with ACC oxidase for the available ACC, producing ammonia and α-ketobutyrate rather than ethylene.

S-Adenosylmethionine

$$CH_3 - S - CH_2 - CH_2 - C - NH_2$$

with Adenosine on the S, COOH and H on the central C.

ACC synthase

ACC

$$\underset{H_2C - CH_2}{\overset{NH_3^+ \quad COO^-}{C}}$$

ACC deaminase \longrightarrow $NH_3 + CH_3 - CH_2 - C - COOH$ (with =O)

α-Ketobutyrate

ACC oxidase $\longrightarrow CO_2 + NH_3 + HCOOH$

$$CH_2 = CH_2$$

Ethylene

with the bacterial enzyme ACC deaminase, which converts ACC to α-ketobutyrate (Fig. 19.36). Each of these genetic manipulations results in a decreased level of ethylene and thereby extends the storage life of fruit and flowers.

By screening a large number of soil bacteria for the ability to utilize ACC as a sole source of nitrogen, strains that degrade ACC were identified. From one of these strains, the gene for the enzyme ACC deaminase was isolated based on the ability of transformed *E. coli* strains that expressed this gene to grow on minimal medium containing ACC. This gene was subcloned, put under the control of the 35S promoter from cauliflower mosaic virus, and expressed in tomato plants. The transgenic plants synthesized a much lower level of ethylene than did normal plants, and the fruit of the transgenic plants had a significantly longer shelf life. These bioengineered changes result in fewer losses due to spoilage because of the much lower levels of ethylene. Similar results have been observed with transgenic cantaloupes that have lowered ethylene levels. This strategy to delay fruit ripening is effective with a range of different fruits.

In another experiment, researchers isolated an 850-base-pair (bp) DNA fragment that corresponded to a portion of the cDNA for ACC oxidase from the tropical plant torenia (*Torenia fournieri* Lind.)—the complete cDNA is about 1 kilobase pair. The cDNA fragment was cloned in both the sense and antisense orientations into a binary vector and then used to transform torenia. In wild-type plants, the flowers lasted an average of 2.0 days before they wilted; transgenic plants with the ACC oxidase cDNA fragment in the antisense orientation lasted 2.7 days—a small but significant difference— and transgenic plants with the ACC oxidase cDNA fragment in the sense orientation lasted around 4.4 days. With both types of transgenic plants, not only did the flowers last longer, but also more flowers bloomed per stem than with the wild-type plant, yielding a more aesthetically pleasing plant.

In the future, a large number of plants will be engineered to have lower ethylene levels, primarily so that fruit ripening and flower wilting, or abscission, are inhibited. Fruits that are likely to be the targets of such genetic manipulation include melons, pineapples, and bananas; targeted flowers might include roses, carnations, tulips, chrysanthemums, and orchids.

SUMMARY

By using a variety of techniques (see chapter 18), it has become relatively straightforward to transform plants with foreign genes. Plants have been engineered to be resistant to a range of environmental stresses, including insects, viruses, herbicides, pathogens, and oxidative and salt stress.

Several different strategies have been used to confer resistance against insect predators, including introducing a gene encoding an insecticidal protoxin produced by one of several subspecies of *B. thuringiensis;* plant proteins, such as α-amylase inhibitors, lectins, or protease inhibitors; or other bacterial insecticidal proteins.

Transgenic plants expressing the gene for a viral coat protein are protected against infection by that virus. They may also be protected against damage from infective viruses by expression of other genes, such as an *E. coli* gene for RNase III,

pokeweed antiviral proteins, and single-chain antibodies directed against various viruses.

To permit crop plants to proliferate in the presence of weeds, many plants have been engineered to be resistant to one or more "environmentally friendly" herbicides. This approach has become enormously successful and is the basis for the largest number of transgenic plants that are used in the field.

To develop plants resistant to fungal and bacterial pathogens, several approaches have been tested. For example, transgenic plants have been engineered to express high levels of chitinase or lysozyme or to overproduce PR proteins.

Different foreign proteins protect plants against different stresses. Superoxide dismutase and oxidized glutathione protect plants against oxidative stress, betaine overproduction

and compartmentalization into the vacuole are effective against salt stress, and lowering plant ethylene levels has an impact on many different types of stress.

In sum, numerous transgenic plants with altered properties and contents have been successfully produced and tested in the laboratory and in some cases in the field. More and more genetically engineered plants have entered the marketplace, and it is likely that transgenic plants will become an integral part of agricultural and horticultural practice.

REFERENCES

Ahrenholtz, I., K. Harms, J. de Vries, and W. Wackernagel. 2000. Increased killing of *Bacillus subtilis* on the hair roots of transgenic T4 lysozyme-producing potatoes. *Appl. Environ. Microbiol.* 66:1862–1865.

Aida, R., T. Yoshida, K. Ichimura, R. Goto, and M. Shibata. 1998. Extension of flower longevity in transgenic torenia plants incorporating ACC oxidase transgene. *Plant Sci.* 138:91–101.

Anderson, E. J., D. M. Stark, R. S. Nelson, N. E. Tumer, and R. N. Beachy. 1989. Transgenic plants that express the coat protein gene of TMV or A1MV interfere with disease development of non-related viruses. *Phytopathology* 12:1284–1290.

Apse, M. P., G. S. Aharon, W. A. Snedden, and E. Blumwald. 1999. Salt tolerance conferred by overexpression of a vacuolar Na⁺/H⁺ antiport in *Arabidopsis*. *Science* 285:1256–1258.

Bates, S. L., J.-Z. Zhao, R. T. Roush, and A. M. Shelton. 2005. Insect resistance management in GM crops: past, present and future. *Nat. Biotechnol.* 23:57–61.

Baum, J. A., T. Bogaert, W. Clinton, G. R. Heck, P. Feldmann, O. Ilagan, S. Johnson, G. Plaetinck, T. Munyikwa, M. Pleau, T. Vaughn, and J. Roberts. 2007. Control of coleopteran insect pests through RNA interference. *Nat. Biotechnol.* 25:1322–1326.

Beachy, R. N., S. Loesch-Fries, and N. E. Tumer. 1990. Coat protein-mediated resistance against virus infection. *Annu. Rev. Phytopathol.* 28:451–474.

Behrens, M. R., N. Mutlu, S. Chakraborty, R. Dumitru, W. Z. Jiang, B. J. LaVallee, P. L. Herman, T. E. Clemente, and D. P. Weeks. 2007. Dicamba resistance: enlarging and preserving biotechnology-based weed management strategies. *Science* 316:1185–1188.

Bohlmann, H. 2004. The best of both worlds in plant protection. *Nat. Biotechnol.* 22:682–683.

Boonrod, K.-J., D. Galetzka, P. D. Nagy, U. Conrad, and G. Krczal. 2004. Single-chain antibodies against a plant viral RNA-dependent RNA polymerase confer virus resistance. *Nat. Biotechnol.* 22:856–862.

Boulter, D., A. M. R. Gatehouse, and V. Hilder. 1989. Use of cowpea trypsin inhibitor (CpTI) to protect plants against insect predation. *Biotechnol. Adv.* 7:489–498.

Cao, H., X. Li, and X. Dong. 1998. Generation of broad-spectrum disease resistance by overexpression of an essential regulatory gene in systemic acquired resistance. *Proc. Natl. Acad. Sci. USA* 95:6531–6536.

Castle, L. A., D. L. Siehl, R. Gorton, P. A. Patten, Y. H. Chen, S. Bertain, H.-J. Cho, N. Duck, J. Wong, D. Liu, and M. W. Lassner. 2004. Discovery and directed evolution of a glyphosate tolerance gene. *Science* 304:1151–1154.

Comai, L., D. Facciotti, W. R. Hiatt, G. Thompson, R. E. Rose, and D. M. Stalker. 1985. Expression in plants of a mutant *aroA* gene from *Salmonella typhimurium* confers tolerance to glyphosate. *Nature* 317:741–744.

Corbin, D. R., J. T. Greenplate, E. Y. Wong, and J. Purcell. 1994. Cloning of an insecticidal cholesterol oxidase gene and its expression in bacteria and in plant protoplasts. *Appl. Environ. Microbiol.* 60:4239–4244.

Cuozzo, M., K. M. O'Connell, W. Kaniewski, R.-X. Fang, N.-H. Chua, and N. E. Tumer. 1988. Viral protection in transgenic tobacco plants expressing the cucumber mosaic virus coat protein or its antisense RNA. *Bio/Technology* 6:549–557.

De Cosa, B., W. Moar, S.-B. Lee, M. Miller, and H. Daniell. 2001. Overexpression of the *Bt cry2Aa2* operon in chloroplasts leads to formation of insecticidal crystals. *Nat. Biotechnol.* 19:71–74.

Dekker, J., and S. O. Duke. 1995. Herbicide-resistant field crops. *Adv.*

Agron. 54:69–116.

Delannay, X., B. J. LaVallee, R. K. Proksch, R. L. Fuchs, S. R. Sims, J. T. Greenplate, P. G. Marrone, R. B. Dodson, J. J. Augustine, J. G. Layton, and D. A. Fischhoff. 1989. Field performance of transgenic tomato plants expressing the *Bacillus thuringiensis* var. *kurstaki* insect control protein. *Bio/Technology* 7:1265–1269.

De Maagd, R. A., D. Bosch, and W. Stiekema. 1999. *Bacillus thuringiensis* toxin-mediated insect resistance in plants. *Trends Plant Sci.* 4:8–13.

Duan, X., X. Li, Q. Xue, M. Abo-El-Saad, D. Xu, and R. Wu. 1996. Transgenic rice plants harboring an introduced potato proteinase inhibitor II gene are insect resistant. *Nat. Biotechnol.* 14:494–498.

Düring, K., P. Porsch, M. Fladung, and H. Lörz. 1993. Transgenic potato plants resistant to the phytopathogenic bacterium *Erwinia carotovora*. *Plant J.* 3:587–598.

Ely, S. 1993. The engineering of plants to express *Bacillus thuringiensis* δ-endotoxins, p. 105–124. *In* P. F. Entwistle, J. S. Cory, M. J. Bailey, and S. Higgs (ed.), *Bacillus thuringiensis, an Environmental Biopesticide: Theory and Practice.* John Wiley & Sons, Chichester, United Kingdom.

Estruch, J. J., N. B. Carozzi, N. Desai, N. B. Duck, G. W. Warren, and M. G. Koziel. 1997. Transgenic plants: an emerging approach to pest control. *Nat. Biotechnol.* 15:137–141.

Fang, J., X. Xu, P. Wang, J. Z. Zhao, A. M. Shelton, J. Cheng, M.-G. Feng, and Z. Shen. 2007. Characterization of chimeric *Bacillus thuringiensis* Vip3 toxins. *Appl. Environ. Microbiol.* 73:956–961.

Ferry, N., M. G. Edwards, J. Gatehouse, T. Capell, P. Christou, and A. M. R. Gatehouse. 2006. Transgenic plants for insect pest control: a forward looking scientific perspective. *Transgen. Res.* 15:13–19.

Fitch, M. M. M., R. M. Manshardt, D. Gonsalves, J. L. Slightom, and J. C. Sanford. 1992. Virus resistant papaya plants derived from tissues bombarded with the coat protein gene of papaya ringspot virus. *Bio/Technology* 10:1466–1472.

Fitchen, J. H., and R. N. Beachy. 1993. Genetically engineering protection against viruses in transgenic plants. *Annu. Rev. Microbiol.* 47:739–763.

Fuchs, M., and D. Gonsalves. 1995. Resistance of transgenic hybrid squash ZW-20 expressing the coat protein genes of zucchini yellow mosaic virus and watermelon mosaic virus 2 to mixed infections by both potyviruses. *Bio/Technology* 13:1466–1473.

Garg, A. K., J.-K. Kim, T. G. Owens, A. P. Ranwala, Y. D. Choi, L. V. Kochian, and R. J. Wu. 2002. Trehalose accumulation in rice plants confers high tolerance levels to different abiotic stresses. *Proc. Natl. Acad. Sci. USA* 99:15898–15903.

Gonsalves, D. 1998. Control of papaya ringspot virus in papaya: a case study. *Annu. Rev. Phytopathol.* 36:415–437.

Grison, R., B. Grezes-Besset, M. Schneider, N. Lucante, L. Olsen, J.-J. Leguay, and A. Toppan. 1996. Field tolerance to fungal pathogens of *Brassica napus* constitutively expressing a chimeric chitinase gene. *Nat. Biotechnol.* 14:643–646.

Halpin, C. 2005. Gene stacking in transgenic plants—the challenge for 21st century plant biotechnology. *Plant Biotechnol. J.* 3:141–155.

Herrera-Estrella, L., G. Van den Broeck, R. Maenhaut, M. Van Montagu, J. Schell, M. Timko, and A. Cashmore. 1984. Light-inducible and chloroplast-associated expression of a chimaeric gene introduced into *Nicotiana tabacum* using a Ti plasmid vector. *Nature* 310:115–120.

Johnson, R., J. Narvaez, G. An, and C. Ryan. 1989. Expression of protease inhibitors I and II in transgenic tobacco plants: effects on natural defense against *Manduca sexta* larvae. *Proc. Natl. Acad. Sci. USA* 86:9871–9875.

Jongedijk, E., A. A. J. M. de Schutter, T. Stolte, P. J. M. van den Elzen, and B. J. C. Cornelissen. 1992. Increased resistance to potato virus X and preservation of cultivar properties in trans-genic potato under field conditions. *Bio/Technology* 10:422–429.

Jouanin, L., M. Bonadé-Bottino, C. Girard, G. Morrot, and M. Giband. 1998. Transgenic plants for insect resistance. *Plant Sci.* 131:1–11.

Kota, M., H. Daniell, S. Varma, S. F. Garczynski, F. Gould, and W. J. Moar. 1999. Overexpression of the *Bacillus thuringiensis* (Bt) Cry2Aa2 protein in chloroplasts confers resistance to plants against susceptible and Bt-resistant insects. *Proc. Natl. Acad. Sci. USA* 96:1840–1845.

Lin, W., C. S. Anuratha, K. Datta, I. Potrykus, S. Muthukrishnan, and S. K. Datta. 1995. Genetic engineering of rice for resistance to sheath blight. *Bio/Technology* 13:686–691.

Lodge, J. K., W. K. Kaniewski, and N. E. Tumer. 1993. Broad-spectrum virus resistance in transgenic plants expressing pokeweed antiviral protein. *Proc. Natl. Acad. Sci. USA* 90:7089–7093.

MacIntosh, S. C., G. M. Kishore, F. J. Perlak, P. G. Marrone, T. B. Stone, S. R. Sims, and R. L. Fuchs. 1990. Potentiation of *Bacillus thuringiensis* insecticidal activity by serine protease inhibitors. *J. Agric. Food Chem.* 38:1145–1152.

Mao, Y.-B., W.-J. Cai, J.-W. Wang, G.-J. Hong, X.-Y. Tao, L.-J. Wang, Y.-P. Huang, and X.-Y. Chen. 2007. Silencing a cotton bollworm P450 monooxygenase gene by plant-mediated RNAi impairs larval tolerance of gossypol. *Nat. Biotechnol.* 25:1307–1313.

Mehlo, L., D. Gahakwa, P. T. Nghia, T. Capell, J. A. Gatehouse, A. M. R. Gatehouse, and P. Christou. 2005. An alternative strategy for sustainable pest resistance in genetically enhanced crops. *Proc. Natl. Acad. Sci. USA* 102:7812–7816.

Niu, Q.-W., S.-S. Lin, J. L. Reyes, K.-C. Chen, H.-W. Wu, S.-D. Yeh, and N.-H. Chua. 2006. Expression of artificial microRNAs in transgenic *Arabidopsis thaliana* confers virus resistance. *Nat. Biotechnol.* 24:1420–1428.

Osusky, M., G. Zhou, L. Osuska, R. E. Hancock, W. W. Kay, and S. Misra. 2000. Transgenic plants expressing cationic peptide chimeras exhibit broad-spectrum resistance to phytopathogens. *Nat. Biotechnol.* 18:1162–1166.

Peñarrubia, L., R. Kim, J. Giovannoni, S.-H. Kim, and R. L. Fischer. 1992. Production of the sweet protein monellin in transgenic plants. *Bio/Technology* 10:561–564.

Perlak, F. J., R. L. Fuchs, D. A. Dean, S. L. McPherson, and D. A. Fischhoff. 1991. Modification of the coding sequence enhances plant expression of insect control protein genes. *Proc. Natl. Acad. Sci. USA* 88:3324–3328.

Peschen, D., H.-P. Li, R. Fischer, F. Kreuzaler, and Y.-C. Liao. 2004. Fusion proteins comprising a *Fusarium*-specific antibody linked to antifungal peptides protect plants against a fungal pathogen. *Nat. Biotechnol.* 22:732–738.

Quinn, J. P. 1990. Evolving strategies for the genetic engineering of herbicide resistance in plants. *Biotechnol. Adv.* 8:321–333.

Rivero, R. M., M. Kojima, A. Gepstein, H. Sakakibara, R. Mittler, S. Gepstein, and E. Blumwald. 2007. Delayed leaf senescence induces extreme drought tolerance in a flowering plant. *Proc. Natl. Acad. Sci. USA* 104:19631–19636.

Ryan, C. A. 1990. Protease inhibitors in plants: genes for improving defenses against insect and pathogens. *Annu. Rev. Phytopathol.* 28:425–449.

Schuler, T. H., G. M. Poppy, B. R. Kerry, and I. Denholm. 1998. Insect-resistant transgenic plants. *Trends Biotechnol.* 16:168–175.

Service, R. F. 2007. A growing threat down on the farm. *Science* 316:1114–1117.

Shade, R. E., H. E. Schroeder, J. J. Pueyo, L. M. Tabe, L. L. Murdock, T. J. V. Higgins, and M. J. Chrispeels. 1994. Transgenic pea seeds expressing the α-amylase inhibitor of the common bean are resistant to bruchid beetles. *Bio/Technology* 12:793–796.

Shah, D. M., C. M. T. Rommens, and R. N. Beachy. 1995. Resistance to diseases and insects in transgenic plants: progress and applications to agriculture. *Trends Biotechnol.* 13:362–368.

Tabashnik, B. E., T. J. Dennehy, and Y. Carrière. 2005. Delayed resistance to transgenic cotton in pink bollworm. *Proc. Natl. Acad. Sci. USA* 43:15389–15393.

Tricoli, D. M., K. J. Carney, P. F. Russell, J. R. McMaster, D. W. Groff, K. C. Hadden, P. T. Himmel, J. P. Hubbard, M. L. Boeshore, and H. D. Quemada. 1995. Field evaluation of transgenic squash containing single or multiple virus coat protein gene constructs for resistance to cucumber mosaic virus, watermelon mosaic virus 2, and zucchini yellow mosaic virus. *Bio/Technology* **13**:1458–1465.

Tu, J., G. Zhang, K. Datta, C. Xu, Y. He, Q. Zhang, G. S. Khush, and S. K. Datta. 2000. Field performance of transgenic elite commercial hybrid rice expressing *Bacillus thuringiensis* δ-endotoxin. *Nat. Biotechnol.* **18**:1101–1104.

Umezawa, T., M. Fujita, Y. Fujita, K. Yamaguchi-Shinozaki, and K. Shinozaki. 2006. Engineering drought tolerance in plants: discovering and tailoring genes to unlock the future. *Curr. Opin. Biotechnol.* **17**:113–122.

Verberne, M. C., R. Verpoorte, J. F. Bol, J. Mercado-Blanco, and H. J. M. Linthorst. 2000. Overproduction of salicylic acid in plants by bacterial transgenes enhances pathogen resistance. *Nat. Biotechnol.* **18**:779–783.

Vierheilig, H., M. Alt, J.-M. Neuhaus, T. Boller, and A. Wiemken. 1993. Colonization of transgenic *Nicotiana sylvestris* plants, expressing different forms of *Nicotiana tabacum* chitinase, by the root pathogen *Rhizoctonia solani* and by the mycorrhizal symbiont *Glomus mosseae*. *Mol. Plant-Microbe Interact.* **6**:261–264.

Wang, P., O. Zoubenko, and N. E. Tumer. 1998. Reduced toxicity and broad spectrum resistance to viral and fungal infection in transgenic plants expressing pokeweed antiviral protein II. *Plant Mol. Biol.* **38**:957–964.

Yamaguchi, T., and E. Blumwald. 2005. Developing salt-tolerant crop plants: challenges and opportunities. *Trends Plant Sci.* **10**:615–620.

Zhang, H.-X. and E. Blumwald. 2001. Transgenic salt-tolerant tomato plants accumulate salt in foliage but not in fruit. *Nat. Biotechnol.* **19**:765–768.

Zhang, L., R. French, W. G. Langenberg, and A. Mitra. 2001. Accumulation of barley stripe mosaic virus is significantly reduced in transgenic wheat plants expressing a bacterial ribonuclease. *Transgen. Res.* **10**:13–19.

Zhao, J.-Z., J. Cao, Y. Li, H. L. Collins, R. T. Roush, E. D. Earle, and A. M. Shelton. 2003. Transgenic plants expressing two *Bacillus thuringiensis* toxins delay insect resistance evolution. *Nat. Biotechnol.* **21**:1493–1497.

Zhu, Q., E. A. Maher, S. Masoud, R. A. Dixon, and C. J. Lamb. 1994. Enhanced protection against fungal attack by constitutive co-expression of chitinase and glucanase genes in transgenic tobacco. *Bio/Technology* **12**:807–812.

REVIEW QUESTIONS

1. A local crop is being ravaged by a nonenveloped virus with a single-stranded RNA genome (8,000 nucleotides long). The virus and its RNA can be readily isolated. In addition, you have antibodies against all four of the proteins encoded within the viral genome. Describe a strategy that you could use to protect the crop against this viral infection and prevent subsequent damage.

2. Suggest several different strategies for developing insect-resistant plants.

3. How can protease inhibitors, α-amylase inhibitor, cholesterol oxidase, Vip proteins, and ricin each protect a plant against damage from insect predation?

4. How can RNAi be used to protect plants against damage from insect predation?

5. Suggest a couple of strategies for simultaneously protecting a plant against damage from several different viruses.

6. How can RNAi be used to protect plants against damage from plant viruses?

7. What general strategies can be employed in genetically engineering plants to be resistant to herbicides?

8. Suggest two different strategies for engineering plants that are resistant to the herbicide glyphosate. Why is this important?

9. How can crop plants be engineered to be resistant to the herbicide dicamba?

10. How can plants be engineered to resist damage from pathogenic soil fungi?

11. How can plants be genetically engineered to be resistant to pathogenic bacteria?

12. How can single-chain Fv antibodies be engineered to protect plants against fungal pathogens?

13. How can a plant's systematic acquired resistance response be engineered to confer resistance to a broad spectrum of both fungal and bacterial pathogens?

14. What is the effect of increasing the level of oxidized glutathione within a plant? How would you genetically manipulate a plant to do this?

15. Suggest several strategies that could be used to engineer plants that are resistant to growth inhibition by salt and by drought.

16. You have been asked by an avocado grower to find a way to genetically engineer his crop to prevent it from ripening during shipping. What experimental approaches would you consider?

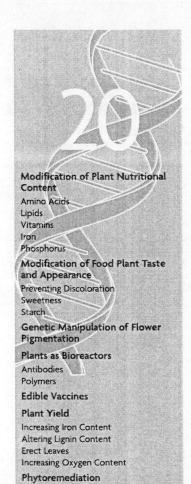

Engineering Plant Quality and Proteins

Modification of Plant Nutritional Content

OVER THE YEARS, agronomists and plant breeders have been extremely successful in optimizing the useful properties (e.g., protein or oil content) and increasing the productivity (yield) of a large number of crop plants. However, traditional breeding approaches to crop improvement are both difficult and slow, and they are intrinsically limited by the existing genetic content of cross-breeding strains. Conversely, the use of genetic engineering techniques allows scientists both to dramatically speed up the process of developing plants with improved characteristics and to introduce traits that would otherwise be impossible to develop by traditional techniques. For example, on a laboratory scale, genetic engineering has been used to improve (1) the nutritional quality of several different plants, including corn (maize) and pea, by modification of the amino acid content of some of their seed storage proteins; (2) the fatty acid compositions of both edible and nonedible oil-producing crops; and (3) the taste of fruits and vegetables by the introduction of monellin, a sweet-tasting protein.

Amino Acids

Seed storage proteins, which are used as sources of both carbon and nitrogen during seed germination, contain a limited number of amino acids, which are organized into repeating peptide units. Often, the nutritional value of these proteins is deficient because they lack one or more of the amino acids, usually lysine or methionine, that are essential for human health. The amino acid composition of the seed storage proteins can be altered to a limited extent by breeding programs, but genetic engineering strategies can also be used.

The bulk of the lupine, a grain legume, that is produced annually in Australia (>800,000 tons) is used to feed cattle, pigs, and chickens. Unfortunately, like most other grain legumes, lupine is deficient in methionine and cysteine. Therefore, lupine feed is supplemented with methionine. To provide animals with more nutritious feed without methionine

803

| LB | TT | *uidA* | P$_{35S}$ | TT | *ssa* | P$_{vic}$ | P$_{35S}$ | *bar* | TT | RB |

FIGURE 20.1 Schematic representation of the T-DNA construct used to transform lupines to increase the methionine content. The arrows indicate the direction of transcription. LB, left border; P$_{35S}$, the 35S promoter from cauliflower mosaic virus; *uidA*, a bacterial gene encoding β-glucuronidase; TT, transcription termination region, including a polyadenylation site; *ssa*, the sunflower seed albumin gene; P$_{vic}$, the promoter from the pea vicilin gene; *bar*, a bacterial gene that confers resistance to the herbicide phosphinothricin, which is used as a selectable marker; RB, right border.

supplementation, lupines were engineered to express sunflower seed albumin, which is both stable in the rumen and unusually rich in the sulfur-containing amino acids methionine and cysteine (Fig. 20.1). Sunflower seed albumin escapes microbial breakdown in the rumen and is therefore available for digestion and absorption in the lower gastrointestinal tract. The transgenic lupine plants that expressed sunflower seed albumin were used as an animal feed, and, as expected, rats that received transgenic lupines as their sole nitrogen source made significantly greater weight gains than did rats fed nontransgenic lupines, comparable to what would be expected if a nontransgenic lupine diet had been supplemented with pure methionine.

FIGURE 20.2 Schematic representation of the biosynthetic pathway for amino acids derived from aspartic acid. Not all of the steps and intermediates are shown. Feedback inhibition is shown by the dashed lines. DHDPS, dihydrodipicolinic acid synthase; AK, aspartokinase.

| LB | $P_{v5'}$ | cts-*dapA* | $T_{v3'}$ | $P_{v5'}$ | cts-*lysCM4* | $T_{v3'}$ | RB |

FIGURE 20.3 Schematic representation of a Ti plasmid vector used to transform soybean and canola with genes that modify their lysine contents. $P_{v5'}$, the promoter from the bean β-phaseolin gene; $T_{v3'}$, the transcription termination region from the bean β-phaseolin gene; cts, the coding region for the chloroplast transit peptide from the small subunit of ribulose bisphosphate carboxylase; *dapA*, a gene from *Corynebacterium* that encodes a lysine-insensitive DHDPS; *lysCM4*, a mutant version of the *E. coli lysC* gene that encodes a lysine-insensitive AK. The left and right borders of the T-DNA are indicated by LB and RB, respectively.

One novel way to increase the lysine content of seeds is to increase the production of lysine in transgenic plants by deregulating the lysine biosynthetic pathway. The amino acids lysine, threonine, methionine, and isoleucine are all derived from aspartic acid (Fig. 20.2). The first step in the conversion of aspartic acid to lysine is phosphorylation of the aspartic acid by aspartokinase (AK) to produce β-aspartyl phosphate. The condensation of aspartic β-semialdehyde with pyruvic acid to form 2,3-dihydrodipicolinic acid, which is catalyzed by dihydrodipicolinic acid synthase (DHDPS), is the first reaction in the pathway that is committed to lysine biosynthesis. Both AK and DHDPS are feedback inhibited by lysine. Thus, to overproduce lysine, it is necessary to abolish the feedback inhibition of these two enzymes. This was accomplished by cloning naturally lysine feedback-insensitive genes for DHDPS and AK from *Corynebacterium* and *Escherichia coli*, respectively; fusing each of these genes to a chloroplast transit peptide (to ensure that the two proteins are localized in seed plastids); placing each gene under the control of a seed-specific promoter; and then introducing the two genes on a Ti plasmid binary vector into canola and soybean plants (Fig. 20.3). Transgenic canola and soybean plants had more than a 100-fold increase in the free lysine in their seeds, with an overall doubling of the total seed lysine content in canola and a fivefold increase in the total lysine content in soybean.

Currently, when corn is used as an animal feed, it must be supplemented with soybean meal, purified lysine, or both. In the future, it may be possible to replace the use of expensive lysine with inexpensive transgenic soybean meal from soybean plants that overproduce lysine. Moreover, it may eventually be possible, by using the approach that has been successful with soybean, to engineer corn to overproduce lysine. High-lysine corn would be more nutritious for both animals and humans.

Lipids

It has been estimated that annual global plant oil production will be worth around $70 billion by 2010. More than 90% of this production is for human consumption in margarines, shortenings, salad oils, and frying oils. Together, soybean, palm, canola (rapeseed), and sunflower account for approximately 80% of worldwide plant oil production. For the most part, these oils consist of palmitic, stearic, oleic, linoleic, and linolenic acids (Table 20.1). In addition, some vegetable oils contain fatty acids with conjugated double bonds. This is in contrast to the more usual case in which

TABLE 20.1 Some important plant fatty acids

Common name	Abbreviation
Caprylic acid	$C_{8:0}$
Capric acid	$C_{10:0}$
Lauric acid	$C_{12:0}$
Myristic acid	$C_{14:0}$
Palmitic acid	$C_{16:0}$
Stearic acid	$C_{18:0}$
Petroselinic acid	$\Delta 6C_{18:1}$
Oleic acid	$\Delta 9C_{18:1}$
Linoleic acid	$\Delta 9,12C_{18:2}$
Linolenic acid	$\Delta 9,12,15C_{18:3}$
Ricinoleic acid	$12OH\Delta 9C_{18:1}$
Erucic acid	$\Delta 13C_{22:1}$

The first number after the C denotes the number of carbon atoms; the number after the colon is the degree of unsaturation, i.e., the number of C=C bonds; a Δ followed by a number indicates the position of the first carbon atom that is involved in the C=C bond; a number followed by an OH indicates the position on the chain of a hydroxyl group. All C=C bonds are *cis*. The numbering system for fatty acids begins with the carboxyl group as 1.

the typical polyunsaturated fatty acid of plant seed oils contains double bonds that are separated by methylene (—CH$_2$—) groups. The presence of conjugated double bonds increases the rate of oxidation compared with polyunsaturated fatty acids, with methylene-interrupted double bonds making them well suited for use as drying agents in paints and inks because they require less oxygen for the polymerization reactions that occur during the drying process. In an effort to eat healthier foods, consumers have become concerned about the nutritional content of various edible oils. As can be seen in Table 20.2, the fatty acid content of edible oils can vary dramatically. Moreover, it is deemed desirable to have as low a level as possible of saturated fats, a high level of oleic acid (which lowers the undesirable low-density lipoproteins, or LDLs, without affecting the desirable high-density lipoproteins, or HDLs), and as high a level as possible of omega-3 fatty acids.

TABLE 20.2 Dietary fats present in various oils

Oil	Saturated fat (%)	Polyunsaturated fat (%)	Monounsaturated fat (oleic acid) (%)	Omega-3 fatty acids (%)
Canola	7	21	61	11
Safflower	10	76	14	Trace
Sunflower	12	71	16	1
Corn	13	57	29	1
Olive	15	9	75	1
Soybean	15	54	23	8
Peanut	19	33	48	Trace
Cottonseed	27	54	19	Trace
Palm	51	10	39	Trace
Butterfat	66	3	28	1
Coconut	91	2	7	None

Canola oil is considered to be one of the healthiest and most nutritious edible oils. In 1989, canola oil received an award from the American Health Foundation as the Health Product of the Year. Canola is derived from rapeseed (which may contain up to 40% erucic acid); however, following more than 40 years of conventional breeding, by definition, canola (for *Canada oil low* erucic *acid*) contains less than 1% erucic acid (several reports have associated erucic acid with various cancers and heart ailments) and a maximum of 18 μmol of all glucosinolates (secondary metabolites responsible for the bitter or sharp taste of many common foods, such as mustard and horseradish) per gram in whole seed. Notwithstanding the enormous success that has been achieved in developing canola by conventional breeding, it is currently possible, by genetic engineering, to rapidly modify a number of genetic traits to continue to improve canola. For example, approximately 90% of the Canadian canola crop has been engineered to be herbicide resistant. In addition, some varieties of canola have been engineered to be insect resistant, and it is currently feasible to change the degree of unsaturation, i.e., the number of carbon–carbon double bonds, and to modify the chain lengths of fatty acids in canola plants by genetic manipulation. A number of transgenic varieties of canola, each producing a different modified oil, have been created (Table 20.3). Each transgenic variety contains one additional gene. For example, the production of shortening, margarine, and confectionery goods requires large amounts of stearate. One variety of transgenic canola contains an antisense copy of a *Brassica* stearate desaturase gene, which inhibits the expression of the normal canola gene and leads to the accumulation of stearic acid rather than the desaturation of stearic acid to oleic acid. Progress on the production of transgenic canola varieties with modified seed oil properties has been both rapid and impressive.

The omega-3 and omega-6 fatty acids are precursors for many prostaglandins and are therefore directly responsible for regulating a number of important human metabolic functions. Until now, the major source for these important fatty acids has been marine and fish oils. However, for a variety of reasons, including the fact that global fish resources have declined dramatically in recent years, researchers have turned their attention to genetically engineering plants to produce safe, affordable, and renewable alternatives to the traditional sources. Given the fact that plants can synthesize linoleic and α-linolenic acid, C-18 precursors of the long-chain omega-3 and omega-6 fatty acids, it may be possible to engineer

TABLE 20.3 Transgenic canola varieties with modified seed lipid contents

Seed product	Commercial use(s)
40% Stearic acid	Margarine, cocoa butter
40% Lauric acid	Detergents
60% Lauric acid	Detergents
80% Oleic acid	Food, lubricants, inks
Petroselinic	Polymers, detergents
"Jojoba" wax	Cosmetics, lubricants
40% Myristate	Detergents, soaps, personal care items
90% Erucic acid	Polymers, cosmetics, inks, pharmaceuticals
Ricinoleic acid	Lubricants, plasticizers, cosmetics, pharmaceuticals

Adapted from Murphy, *Trends Biotechnol.* **14**:206–213, 1996.

plants to transform linoleic and α-linolenic acids into long-chain omega-3 and omega-6 fatty acids. In fact, when *Arabidopsis thaliana* plants were transformed (in three separates stages) with three additional genes, the linoleic and α-linolenic acids were converted to arachadonic and eicosapentaenoic acids, respectively (Fig. 20.4). The three introduced genes included a Δ9-specific elongase from the marine microalga *Isochrysis galbana*, a Δ8-desaturase from the protist *Euglena gracilis*, and a Δ5-desaturase from the fungus *Mortierella alpina*. Despite the fact that the engineered plants contained higher than normal levels of arachidonic acid and eicosapentaenoic acid, i.e., 7% and 3%, respectively, in their leaf tissue, plant growth and development were normal. Thus, it is possible to engineer pathways in plants for the production of long-chain polyunsaturated fatty acids that are vital for human health. It is now necessary to engineer this pathway so that the three introduced genes are expressed in a seed-specific manner in an oilseed crop, such as soybean or canola.

Vitamins

Vitamin E. A substantial body of evidence indicates that dietary supplementation with the lipid-soluble antioxidant vitamin E (400 international units, or approximately 250 mg, of [*R,R,R*]-α-tocopherol daily) results in a decreased risk for cardiovascular disease and cancer, assists in immune function, and prevents or slows a number of degenerative diseases in humans. The oils that are extracted from seeds have a relatively high level

FIGURE 20.4 Overview of the conversion of linoleic acid to arachidonic acid and linolenic acid to eicosapentaenoic acid in transgenic *A. thaliana* expressing three foreign genes (all under the control of the cauliflower mosaic virus 35S promoter). IgASE1, Δ9-specific fatty acid elongase from *I. galbana*; EuΔ8, Δ8-desaturase from *E. gracilis*; MortΔ5, Δ5-desaturase from *M. alpina*.

Linoleic acid ($C_{18:2}$) to arachidonic acid ($C_{20:3}$) Linolenic acid ($C_{18:2}$) to eicosapentaenoic acid ($C_{20:4}$)

FIGURE 20.5 Conversion of γ-tocopherol to α-tocopherol by the enzyme γ-tocopherol methyltransferase.

of total tocopherols, but in most cases, only a very small fraction is α-tocopherol. Moreover, even in those instances where the fraction of α-tocopherol is large, e.g., sunflower oil, to obtain a sufficient amount of vitamin E to confer the above-mentioned health benefits, it would be necessary for an individual to consume nearly 400 g of oil daily. An alternative approach to this problem is to engineer plants to produce a greater percentage of α-tocopherol than γ-tocopherol by transforming plants with a gene encoding the enzyme γ-tocopherol methyltransferase, which catalyzes the addition of a methyl group to γ-tocopherol (Fig. 20.5). However, since a suitable γ-tocopherol methyltransferase gene was not available, a strategy for its isolation had to be devised (Fig. 20.6). One of the genes in the α-tocopherol biosynthetic pathway had previously been cloned from the plant *A. thaliana*. However, at the time, it was not possible to isoate the other genes in the pathway. This gene encodes the enzyme *p*-hydroxyphenylpyruvate dioxygenase (HPPDase). A computer comparison of the sequence of the HPPDase gene with the complete DNA sequence of the cyanobacterium *Synechocystis* sp. strain PCC6803 revealed the presence of an open reading frame that encoded a protein of the expected size that was 35% identical to the amino acid sequence of the *Arabidopsis*-encoded protein. The *Synechocystis* putative HPPDase gene was found within a 10-gene operon thought to encode all of the enzymes involved in the synthesis of α-tocopherol. One of the other genes within this operon encoded a protein whose predicted amino acid sequence was similar to those of several known plant Δ-(24)-sterol-C-methyltransferases. This enzyme has *S*-adenosylmethionine-binding domains, and *S*-adenosylmethionine donates the methyl group to γ-tocopherol during the conversion to α-tocopherol. In addition, the gene had an N-terminal bacterial signal sequence. When the cyanobacterial gene was cloned and expressed in *E. coli*, the recombinant protein catalyzed the methylation of γ-tocopherol to α-tocopherol. The DNA sequence of the *Synechocystis* γ-tocopherol methyl-

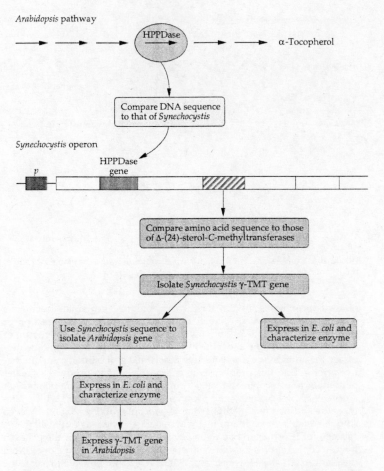

Arabidopsis pathway

HPPDase

α-Tocopherol

Compare DNA sequence
to that of *Synechocystis*

Synechocystis operon

HPPDase
gene

p

Compare amino acid sequence to those
of Δ-(24)-sterol-*C*-methyltransferases

Isolate *Synechocystis* γ-TMT gene

Use *Synechocystis* sequence to
isolate *Arabidopsis* gene

Express in *E. coli* and
characterize enzyme

Express in *E. coli* and
characterize enzyme

Express γ-TMT gene
in *Arabidopsis*

FIGURE 20.6 Schematic overview of the isolation of the *A. thaliana* cDNA encoding the enzyme γ-tocopherol methyltransferase (γ-TMT) and its use to engineer *A. thaliana* to overproduce the enzyme. HPPDase, *p*-hydroxyphenylpyruvate dioxygenase.

transferase gene was then compared with DNA sequences that were normally expressed in *Arabidopsis*, and one *Arabidopsis* gene that showed 66% homology to the bacterial protein at the amino acid level was identified, cloned, and expressed in *E. coli*. This recombinant protein converted γ-tocopherol to α-tocopherol. The *Arabidopsis* γ-tocopherol methyltransferase gene under the transcriptional control of a seed-specific promoter from carrots was then used to transform *Arabidopsis* plants. The α-tocopherol levels of these transgenic plants were significantly higher than they were in the nontransformed plants. Based on this model system, with the introduction of additional genetic manipulations (which increase the flux through the pathway), these results have been extended to corn embryos and soybean seeds, significantly increasing the nutritional value of the oils

produced by these plants. Despite the progress that has been made, transgenic crops that produce higher levels of vitamin E are not yet sufficiently optimized for them to be commercialized.

Vitamin A. Although rice (*Oryza sativa*) is the staple food of approximately half of the world's population, it is a poor source of several nutrients and vitamins, including vitamin A. About 124 million children worldwide are deficient in vitamin A; this deficiency leads to 1 million to 2 million deaths per year and is a leading cause of vision impairment, including night blindness and total blindness. One way to address the myriad of health problems that result from vitamin A deficiency would be to engineer rice to produce the vitamin A precursor provitamin A (β-carotene). Mammals synthesize vitamin A from β-carotene, which is a common carotenoid pigment normally found in plant photosynthetic membranes. In the year 2000, an international group of scientists reported using *Agrobacterium*-mediated transformation to introduce the entire β-carotene biosynthetic pathway into rice (Fig. 20.7). The phytoene synthase and phytoene desaturase genes were introduced on a construct that did not contain any selectable marker. The lycopene β-cyclase gene was part of a separate construct that contained a selectable marker. The frequency of insertion of all three genes into the rice genome and their subsequent expression were quite high. Thus, the engineered rice produces β-carotene, which, after ingestion, is converted to vitamin A. At the time, it was thought that this strategy would facilitate the eventual development of transgenic strains of rice that not only produced high levels of β-carotene but also no longer contained any antibiotic resistance marker genes (removed as described in chapter 18). The transgenic rice that produces β-carotene has a yellow or golden color and has been called "golden rice" by the scientists involved in its development. Unfortunately, the initial version of golden rice, now called golden rice 1, synthesized only 1.6 µg of β-carotene per gram of rice, so that individuals would have had to consume around 3 kg of golden rice 1 each day to reach the recommended minimal daily requirement of vitamin A. However, in 2005, scientists reported replacing the daffodil phytoene synthase gene (Fig. 20.7) with a similar gene from corn that produces an enzyme with a higher level of activity, resulting in a variety called golden rice 2 that produces a 23-fold-higher level of β-carotene than golden rice 1. Moreover, in contrast to vitamin A, there are no harmful effects when individuals consume excess amounts of dietary β-carotene. The research that culminated in the development of golden rice was funded by several nonprofit agencies, and the companies that hold the patents on the technologies that made this work possible have agreed to forgo their usual royalties. Therefore, the rice is expected to be freely available to farmers in the world's poorest countries.

One of the problems for the more widespread use of golden rice 2 in Asia has been a general mistrust of genetically modified foods by some consumers. In addition, both golden rice 1 and golden rice 2 were produced from subspecies *japonica* cultivars of rice, which are popular with scientists but do not do well in the field in Asia. To remedy this situation, researchers are currently introducing the traits from golden rice 1 and golden rice 2 into the more popular subspecies *indica* varieties of rice by traditional genetic crossing of the *indica* strains with the engineered *japonica* cultivars. As of mid-2008, the first field trial of an *indica* variety of golden rice was taking place at the International Rice Research Institute in the Philippines. It is

FIGURE 20.7 Biosynthesis of β-carotene in rice and vitamin A in humans. The daffodil phytoene synthase gene (*psy*) was controlled by a promoter from the rice seed storage protein glutelin. The phytoene desaturase (*crt*) gene was from the bacterium *Erwinia uredovora* and was controlled by the 35S promoter. The lycopene β-cyclase (*lcy*) gene originated from daffodil and was controlled by the rice glutelin promoter. All three genes were fused to transit peptides so that the proteins that they encoded would be transported into the plastid. GGPP, geranylgeranyl pyrophosphate.

hoped, following successful field trials, that golden rice can finally start fulfilling its promise.

Folate. Tetrahydrofolate, or vitamin B9, is an essential micronutrient that is a necessary component of human diets. While the recommended daily intake of this vitamin is only 400 μg, the diets of many individuals in developing countries are chronically deficient in tetrahydrofolate. Tetrahydrofolate deficiency can result in severe birth defects, anemia, and neural tube defects. For approximately 3 billion people, most of them in developing countries, rice provides around 80% of the daily caloric intake; however, rice is a poor source of tetrahydrofolate, as well as many other micronutri-

FIGURE 20.8 (A) Structure of tetrahydrofolate. **(B)** Major steps in the pathway leading to the synthesis of tetrahydrofolate and tetrahydrofolate polyglutamates in rice. A portion of the molecule is synthesized in the chloroplast and a portion in the cytosol, and the molecule is assembled in the mitochondria. Two enzymatic steps (marked by asterisks) that represent rate-limiting steps in the biosynthetic pathway were engineered by the addition of foreign genes to increase the flux through the pathway.

FIGURE 20.9 The T-DNA construct used to transform rice and produce ferritin in the seeds. The arrows indicate the direction of transcription. LB, left border; TT, transcription termination region; *bar,* the bacterial phosphinothricin acetyltransferase gene; P_{35S}, 35S promoter from cauliflower mosaic virus; P_{gluB}, the promoter from the rice seed storage protein glutelin; *fer,* the soybean ferritin-encoding cDNA; RB, right border.

ents. To increase the nutritive value of rice, the pathway for the production of tetrahydrofolate and tetrahydrofolate polyglutamates may be genetically manipulated.

Folates are tripartite molecules; that is, they consist of three separate parts, including pteridine, *p*-aminobenzoic acid, and one or more glutamate molecules (Fig. 20.8A). In plants, the pteridine precursors are synthesized from GTP in the cytosol, *p*-aminobenzoic acid is synthesized from chorismate in the chloroplasts, and then both the pteridine precursor and *p*-aminobenzoic acid are imported into the mitochondria, where the final molecule is assembled and modified (Fig. 20.8B). To express high levels of folate in rice, the first genes in each of the chloroplastic and cytosolic pathways, starting from chorismate and GTP, respectively, were introduced from *A. thaliana* so that the two enzymes from these genes were overexpressed (Fig. 20.8B). In one transgenic line, the level of tetrahydrofolate was approximately 100 times the level found in nontransgenic rice plants, which was more than sufficient to meet the recommended daily dietary amount of this vitamin. In another study by a different research group, similar genetic manipulations led to the enhancement of the level of the vitamin in transgenic tomatoes.

Iron

The World Health Organization has estimated that iron deficiency affects approximately 30% of the world's population and is especially problematic where vegetable-based diets are the primary food source. Although a number of crops are rich in iron, absorption of this iron is often prevented by the phytic acid that is present in many of the plants. As a first step toward developing food crops with sufficient levels of iron to prevent iron deficiency anemia, scientists engineered rice plants to express the soybean protein ferritin (Fig. 20.9). Ferritin is an iron storage protein that is found in animals, plants, and bacteria and carries up to 4,500 iron atoms in its central cavity, which is formed from the interaction of 24 monomeric ferritin subunits. The soybean ferritin complementary DNA (cDNA) was cloned into a binary vector under the transcriptional control of the rice seed storage protein glutelin promoter (Fig. 20.9), and the entire construct was introduced into plants by electroporation. In this case, soybean ferritin was expressed in the seeds of rice plants and not in any other tissues. As a result, the iron content of rice seeds per gram (dry weight) of tissue was increased to approximately 2.5 times the original value while the iron content of leaves, stems, and roots did not change to any significant extent. Based on a typical daily adult portion of 150 grams of rice, the transgenic ferritin rice provides approximately 30 to 50% of the recommended daily adult requirement of iron.

While overproducing ferritin is an important first step in engineering plants to provide additional dietary iron, it is also necessary to ensure that the additional iron can be absorbed efficiently. To do this, rice plants were transformed with three different genes. First, to increase the iron content, the rice plants were transformed with a ferritin-encoding cDNA from green beans (*Phaseolus vulgaris*). Then, to improve the bioavailability of the introduced iron, plants were transformed separately with cDNAs encoding phytase (phytate is an inhibitor of iron absorption that can be removed by microbial phytase) and metallothionein (a family of cysteine-rich, low-molecular-weight proteins that bind metals through the thiol groups of cysteine residues) from the fungus *Aspergillus fumigatus* and from rice, respectively. To limit the expression of these genes to rice grains, their expression was controlled by an endosperm-specific promoter (Fig. 20.10). Each of the three different transgenic plants that were engineered produced the protein encoded by its transgene. Before these strains are crossed to generate a plant that can express all three of these transgenes, a more heat-stable version of the phytase is required, since cooking the rice resulted in the inactivation of around 90% of the phytase. Nevertheless, because obtaining sufficient dietary iron is so important to such a large number of people in the world, these preliminary results are exciting and promise to eventually have an enormous impact on the health of millions of people.

Phosphorus

Most of the phosphorus in cereals and legumes is found in the form of phytate (phytic acid, or inositol hexaphosphate). Phytate cannot be digested by nonruminant animals (or by humans), so the unabsorbed phytate passes through the gastrointestinal tract and elevates the amount of phosphorus

FIGURE 20.10 Genetic constructs used to transform rice and produce ferritin (**A**), metallothionein (**B**), and phytase (**C**) in seeds. The arrows indicate the direction of transcription. To ensure that phytase would be secreted into the apoplast, *phyA* in construct C was fused to DNA encoding the signal peptide for a barley β-glucanase gene (not shown). Constructs A and B were introduced into rice plants by *A. tumefaciens*-mediated transformation, and construct C was transferred by microprojectile-mediated transformation. LB, left border; TT, transcription termination region; *hpt*, the *E. coli* hygromycin phosphotransferase gene; P_{35S}, 35S promoter from cauliflower mosaic virus; P_{gluB}, the promoter from the rice seed storage protein glutelin; *fer*, a cDNA encoding green bean ferritin; *mth*, a cDNA encoding rice metallothionein; *phyA*, an *A. fumigatus* cDNA encoding phytase; RB, right border.

in manure. The excretion of high levels of phosphorus can sometimes lead to environmental problems, such as eutrophication (excessive plant and algal growth and decay). To increase the nutritional value of crops such as soybean and corn to nonruminant animals, such as poultry, swine, and fish, animal feed is generally supplemented either with phosphorus derived from rock phosphate or with phytase, which degrades phytate after it is ingested. Unfortunately, such supplementation is expensive, adding significantly to the cost of producing these animals. However, beginning in the early 1990s, several low-phytate mutants were isolated in corn, barley, rice, wheat, and soybean. In these mutants, an enzyme involved in one of the many steps in the conversion of glucose-6-phosphate to phytate (Fig. 20.11) was typically altered so that the amount of phytate in the seed was often reduced by 50 to 90%. Moreover, the reduction in phytate was generally accompanied by an increase in inorganic phosphate that maintained the total seed phosphorus level. The problem with this strategy is that the systemic reduction of phytate often has negative effects on the whole plant, resulting in decreases in seed germination, emergence, stress tolerance, and seed filling. Therefore, as an alternative to limiting the synthesis of phytate, one group of researchers constructed mutants of corn and soybean that were defective in the transport of phytate to seeds by silencing the ATP-binding cassette (ABC) transporter in a seed-specific manner (Fig. 20.11). The seeds of these plants had approximately 10 to 20% of the normal level of phytate with a commensurate increase in the level of inorganic phosphate. Moreover, the phytate levels in the rest of the plant were essentially unchanged. While these transgenic plants still need to be tested for their efficacy as animal feed, this approach promises to be important from both agricultural and environmental perspectives.

Modification of Food Plant Taste and Appearance

Preventing Discoloration

The postharvest discoloration of fruits and vegetables is a considerable problem for the food industry. A lack of acceptance of discolored foods by

FIGURE 20.11 Schematic representation of the biosynthesis of phytic acid, by six separate enzyme-catalyzed reactions, from glucose-6-phosphate and the subsequent storage of the phytic acid in protein storage vacuoles.

Glucose-6-phosphate

Phytic acid
(inositol hexaphosphate)

$P = PH_2O_3$

ABC transporter

Phytate salts in
storage vacuoles

consumers has been dealt with by the food industry through the use of additives in a wide range of foods. However, the safety of some of these food additives, in particular sulfites, has been questioned.

The enzymes that are thought to be responsible for the initial step in the discoloration of fruits and vegetables, the oxidation of monophenols and o-diphenols to o-quinones, are polyphenol oxidases. These nucleus-encoded enzymes with a molecular weight of around 59,000 are localized in chloroplast and mitochondrial membranes.

The contention that inhibition of the enzyme polyphenol oxidase would decrease the extent of discoloration has been tested with transgenic potatoes carrying a number of different polyphenol oxidase cDNA constructs. Vectors were constructed with either the full-length or partial potato polyphenol oxidase cDNA in either the sense or antisense orientation under the control of the cauliflower mosaic virus 35S promoter, the granule-bound starch synthase promoter, or the patatin type I promoter (Fig. 20.12). The last two promoters are specific for the potato tuber. The two commercial varieties of potato that were transformed with these constructs are considered to have a good level of intrinsic resistance to black spot (enzymatic discoloration), so any increase in black spot resistance by genetic manipulation would be greater than what could be attained by traditional breeding techniques. Transgenic plants with the polyphenol oxidase cDNA constructs were deliberately bruised, and then the extent of black spot damage was assessed. Most of the transgenic potato plants with an antisense version of the polyphenol oxidase gene under the control of either the cauliflower mosaic virus 35S promoter or the granule-bound starch synthase promoter were significantly more resistant to black spot than the nontransformed potatoes. The patatin promoter, which may not be fully active in potato tubers, did not prevent polyphenol oxidase accumulation. The sense constructs all synthesized increased amounts of polyphenol oxidase and showed larger amounts of black spot than nontransformed control plants. It is hoped that these and similar antisense constructs will

FIGURE 20.12 Sense and antisense polyphenol oxidase gene constructs. Transcription of either the sense or antisense cDNA is separately under the control of the cauliflower mosaic virus 35S promoter (P_{35S}), the granule-bound starch synthase promoter (P_{GBSS}), or the patatin type I promoter ($P_{patatin}$) with the nopaline synthase transcription terminator region (tNOS). RB and LB, right and left borders of the T-DNA, respectively. Adapted from Bachem et al., *Bio/Technology* **12**:1101–1105, 1994.

reduce enzymatic discoloration in a wide range of commercially important plants.

Sweetness

Even though a fruit or vegetable may have high nutritional value, if it is not tasty, humans usually will not eat it. Although palatability of food can be achieved by adding salt, sugar, flavors, or other ingredients during preparation, it would be advantageous to the food industry if certain foods could be made intrinsically more appetizing.

Monellin, a protein that is found in the fruit of an African plant with the unlikely name of serendipity (*Dioscoreophyllum cumminsii* Diels), is approximately 3,000 times sweeter than sucrose on a weight basis. This feature makes monellin a candidate as a sugar substitute, with the added bonus that, because it is a protein, it would not have the same metabolic impact as sugar.

Monellin is a dimer with an A chain of 45 amino acid residues and a B chain of 50 residues; the chains are held together by weak noncovalent bonds. Unfortunately, the fact that monellin is composed of two separate polypeptide chains limits its usefulness as a sweetener because it is readily dissociated (denatured) and consequently loses its sweetness when it is either heated during cooking or exposed to acid (e.g., lemon juice or vinegar). Also, the need to clone and express two separate genes in a coordinated manner complicates efforts to produce the protein in either transgenic plants or microorganisms. To circumvent this problem, a monellin gene that encodes both the A and B chains as a single peptide was chemically synthesized (Fig. 20.13). The fusion protein was produced in transgenic tomato and lettuce plants. Two different promoters were used to express the monellin fusion protein gene. In the experiment with tomatoes, expression was directed by the tomato fruit-specific promoter E8, which is activated at the onset of fruit ripening. The construct for the lettuce experiment was under the control of the 35S promoter from cauliflower mosaic virus. Each construct used the transcription termination–polyadenylation site from a Ti plasmid nopaline synthase gene. In each case, the synthetic monellin gene was introduced into plant cells by *A. tumefaciens* infection, using the Ti plasmid cointegrate vector system. Monellin was detected in ripe and partially ripe tomatoes and in lettuce leaves, but not in green tomatoes. The monellin level in tomatoes could also be elevated by a burst of the plant hormone ethylene. This strategy for sweetening plants without sugar or chemical additives would be applicable to a wide range of fruits and vegetables.

In addition to monellin, several other sweet proteins have been reported (Table 20.4). The genes for some of these proteins have been isolated and characterized. Given the demand for low-calorie sweeteners, as well as the interest in healthy and natural food products, it is likely that many different plants will be genetically engineered to produce proteins to increase their sweetness.

Fructans are naturally occurring polymers of fructose that are not usually degraded in the human digestive tract. However, some beneficial bacteria in the human intestinal tract can utilize fructans. Small fructans, i.e., up to five monosaccharide units, have a sweet taste and can be used as a natural low-calorie sweetener instead of sucrose. Fructans are generally produced from sucrose by fungal invertases on a large scale in an expensive

FIGURE 20.13 Schematic representation of heat treatment of monellin (**A**) and modified monellin (**B**).

TABLE 20.4 Properties of some sweet-tasting proteins

Protein	Plant source	Sweetness factor (weight basis)	Molecular mass (kDa)	No. of amino acids	Active form
Thaumatin	*Thaumatococcus daniellii* Benth	3,000	22.2	207	Monomer
Monellin	*Dioscoreophyllum cumminsii* Diels	3,000	10.7	45 (A chain), 50 (B chain)	AB dimer
Mabinlin	*Capparis masakai* Levl	100	12.4	33 (A chain), 72 (B chain)	AB dimer
Pentadin	*Pentadiplandra brazzeana* Baillon	500	12.0	ND	ND
Brazzein	*Pentadiplandra brazzeana* Baillon	2,000	6.5	54	Monomer
Curculin	*Curculigo latifolia*	550	24.9	114	A_2 dimer
Miraculin	*Richadella dulcifica*	ND	98.4	191	A_4 tetramer

ND, not determined; kDa, kilodaltons.

process, or they are extracted from the roots of chicory plants or Jerusalem artichoke tubers. To develop an inexpensive means of producing fructans, researchers engineered sugar beet plants to convert the sucrose that they normally store in the vacuoles of taproot parenchyma cells into fructans. This was done by transforming sugar beets with a genetic construct that contained the 1-sucrose:sucrose fructosyl transferase cDNA from Jerusalem artichokes under the transcriptional control of the 35S promoter. To transform sugar beets, the genetic construct was introduced into protoplasts in the presence of 20% polyethylene glycol. The transgenic sugar beets accumulated fructan up to 40% of the taproot dry weight. The mixture of fructans that was produced by the transgenic sugar beet plants is essentially the same as the fructans that are produced enzymatically. Biologically produced fructan may be an attractive alternative to the current industrial process and can be sold as either a nondigestible sweetener or as a health component that improves the intestinal flora.

Starch

The starch that is found in most crop plants, such as potato, consists of 20 to 30% (straight-chain) amylose and 70 to 80% (branched-chain) amylopectin. The ratio of amylose to amylopectin has a large influence on the physical and chemical properties of the starch. For many industrial applications, it would be useful to have starch that is highly enriched in either amylose or amylopectin (Fig. 20.14). Starch is normally synthesized in a stepwise process (Fig. 20.15). The enzyme ADP-glucose pyrophosphorylase catalyzes the transfer of ADP (from ATP) to glucose-1-phosphate to form ADP-glucose. The enzyme starch synthase catalyzes the transfer of glucose from ADP-glucose to the nonreducing end of a preexisting glucan chain, which is a short version of an amylose chain, by means of an α-1,4 linkage. Branching can occur, catalyzed by starch-branching enzyme, when two glucan chains are joined by an α-1,6 linkage. To generate potatoes with a high percentage of amylose and a corresponding low percentage of amylopectin, plants were transformed by using *A. tumefaciens* with antisense versions of the starch-branching enzyme under the transcriptional control of the 35S promoter. In transgenic lines that exhibited only approximately 1% of the normal amount of the starch-branching enzyme activity, the fraction of amylose increased from around 28% to 60 to 89% of the starch content. This is an initial step toward developing potatoes with unique starch

A

B

FIGURE 20.14 (A) A portion of an amylose chain with only α-1,4 linkages; (B) a portion of an amylopectin chain with α-1,4 and α-1,6 linkages.

compositions that may be used either for food or as a source of unusual starches with unique industrial properties.

The freezing and thawing that are common in the development and use of frozen foods often lead to unwanted changes in the texture of the starch component, making the product less attractive to consumers. Under these conditions, the starch can separate into a solid phase and a liquid phase, a process known as syneresis. The long, unbranched amylose chains have a much greater tendency to form separate phases following freezing and thawing than the shorter, branched amylopectin chains. One approach to creating a starch that could withstand freezing and thawing would be to modify the starch structure by decreasing the synthesis of amylose chains. This was achieved by transforming potatoes with antisense versions of three different starch synthase genes (Fig. 20.15). This reduced the expression of each of these genes to very low levels and resulted in a dramatic decrease in the amount of amylose and, at the same time, in the length of the amylopectin chains. These modified potatoes are currently being thoroughly tested to ensure that a variety of physical and chemical properties are unaltered so that they can be used in the production of frozen foods.

Since starch is both inexpensive and very abundant, it is used in a number of industrial processes as a thickener, a gelling agent, or an adhesive. In addition, it is a substrate for the production of high-fructose syrups and ethanol (see chapter 14). The production of high-fructose syrups requires the starch to be degraded, usually at high temperature, by the enzyme α-amylase and then treated, also at high temperature, with glucose

FIGURE 20.15 The major reactions in the biosynthesis of starch.

isomerase, which converts the glucose (released from the starch that was degraded by α-amylase) into fructose. The enzymes that catalyze these reactions account for a major portion of the cost of the industrial conversion of starch into fructose. Therefore, reducing the cost of the enzymes makes the overall process more attractive. With this in mind, researchers constructed a bifunctional enzyme containing the essential regions of both α-amylase and glucose isomerase, using the polymerase chain reaction (PCR) to fuse together the genes for these enzymes (Fig. 20.16). Of course, care was taken to ensure that the chimeric gene retained the correct reading frames of the two genes. When the bifunctional enzyme was synthesized in *E. coli,* both α-amylase and glucose isomerase activities were found, and both activities were identical to that found in the thermotolerant source organisms. The chimeric gene was introduced into potato plants under the transcriptional control of the granule-bound-starch synthase promoter. Biochemical analysis performed on transgenic potatoes, after treatment at 65°C (the optimal temperature for the α-amylase), revealed a 3.9-fold and a 14.7-fold increase compared with nontransgenic potatoes in the concentrations of glucose and fructose, respectively. At 25°C, the glucose and fructose concentrations were the same in transgenic and nontransgenic potatoes. Thus, both enzymes function optimally at high temperatures and only very little or not at all at low temperatures. This work indicates that it is technically feasible to engineer potatoes to produce their own α-amylase and glucose isomerase and that the enzyme that is produced can then be used directly, without the need for any purification, in a process directed toward producing fructose.

For many of the applications that employ plants containing high levels of starch, it would be desirable to be able to significantly increase the amount of starch produced by each plant. While it may be possible to manipulate the genes for some of the enzymes involved in the biosynthesis of starch, another approach to increasing the starch yield would be to increase the supply of ATP so that the flux through the first reaction of starch biosynthesis is increased (Fig. 20.15). This may be done by decreasing the level of the enzyme adenylate kinase, which catalyzes the interconversion of ATP and AMP into ADP (Fig. 20.17). To do this, a genetic construct encoding a plastid version of adenylate kinase in an antisense orientation was used to transform potato plants. In the resulting transgenic plants, the

α-Amylase gene

Glucose isomerase gene

PCR
Insert into vector

PCR
Insert into vector

Digestion by NsiI and SacI
Ligation

FIGURE 20.16 Construction of an α-amylase–glucose isomerase fusion gene. The α-amylase and glucose isomerase genes were from *Bacillus stearothermophilus* and *Thermus thermophilus*, respectively. The portions of the PCR primers that do not match the target genes are designed to retain both genes in the same reading frame and to include appropriate restriction endonuclease sites. Adapted from Beaujean et al., *Biotechnol. Bioeng.* **70:**9–16, 2000.

activity of adenylate kinase decreased significantly in leaves and tubers and dramatically in chloroplasts (Table 20.5). Moreover, the transgenic plants showed an altered pattern of activity of the enzymes involved in the biosynthesis of starch and, most importantly, a significant increase in both the yield of potato tubers and the amount of starch in each potato tuber. This manipulation opens up the possibility of modifying other starch-containing plants in a similar manner.

Genetic Manipulation of Flower Pigmentation

The worldwide value of the flower industry, at the consumer level, is around $150 billion. This includes the value of cut flowers as well as pot and bedding plants. The main areas of both flower production and consumption are the United States, Europe, and, to a lesser extent, Japan and China. In addition, several countries, including Colombia, Ecuador, Ethiopia, Israel, Kenya, Morocco, and Turkey, are major producers but not major consumers of flowers.

FIGURE 20.17 Regulation of adenylate pools by the action of the enzyme adenylate kinase.

$$\text{ATP} + \text{AMP} \xrightleftharpoons[\text{}]{\text{Adenylate kinase}} 2\,\text{ADP}$$

TABLE 20.5 Comparison of nontransformed potatoes with potatoes transformed with an antisense version of adenylate kinase

Trait or activity	Nontransformed	Transgenic
Leaf adenylate kinase activity (μmol/g [FW]/min)	21.3	14.4
Chloroplast adenylate kinase activity (μmol/g [FW]/min)	12.4	5.6
Tuber adenylate kinase activity (μmol/g [FW]/min)	15.2	9.7
AGPase activity (μmol/g [FW]/min)	519	717
Soluble starch synthase activity (μmol/g [FW]/min)	143	109
Branching enzyme activity (μmol/g [FW]/min)	6,921	7,841
Total tuber yield (g)	867	1,596
Starch (g/plant)	106	224

FW, fresh weight; AGPase, ADP-glucose pyrophosphorylase.

The most important cut-flower crops are roses, carnations, tulips, lilies, gerberas, and chrysanthemums. Genetic transformation protocols have been worked out for most of the major commercial flower-producing plants. For example, transgenic chrysanthemums with both sense and antisense constructs of the chrysanthemum chalcone synthase cDNA have been produced. Chalcone synthase catalyzes the first step in anthocyanin biosynthesis (Fig. 20.18). Both the sense and the antisense cDNAs can suppress chalcone synthase gene expression in transgenic plants and produce white flowers instead of the normal pink. Sense suppression, which is also called cosuppression, occurs when an additional copy of an endogenous gene prevents the accumulation of the messenger RNA (mRNA) from the endogenous gene, typically through the production of interfering RNA. On the other hand, the antisense chalcone synthase RNA should block translation of endogenous chalcone synthase mRNA.

The sense and antisense constructs were placed under the control of the cauliflower mosaic virus 35S promoter on a binary Ti plasmid vector and then introduced into plant cells. Three of the 133 sense transformants and three of the 83 antisense transformants produced white flowers, which indicated that endogenous chalcone synthase gene expression and, as a consequence, anthocyanin synthesis had been suppressed. The white-flowering plants were propagated vegetatively through cuttings, and approximately 90 to 98% of the plants continued to produce white flowers when planted in the field.

The flower industry is continually attempting to improve flower appearance and postharvest lifetime. By traditional breeding techniques, over the years it has been possible to create thousands of new varieties that differ from one another in color, shape, and plant architecture. However, traditional plant breeding is a slow and painstaking procedure that is limited by the gene pool of a particular species; thus, for example, no one has been able to breed a blue rose. As an alternative to traditional breeding techniques, uniquely colored flowers can be developed by manipulating the genes for enzymes in the anthocyanin biosynthesis pathway. Anthocyanins, which are a class of flavonoids, are the most common type

FIGURE 20.18 Biosynthesis of anthocyanins. CoA, coenzyme A; CHS, chalcone synthase; CHI, chalcone isomerase; F3H, flavonone 3-hydroxylase; F3'H, flavonoid 3'-hydroxyase; F3'5'H, flavonoid 3',5'-hydroxylase; DFR, dihydroflavonol 4-reductase; 3GT, UDP-glucose:flavonoid 3-O-glucosyltransferase. Petunia DFR can convert dihydroquercetin to cyanidin-3-glucoside and can convert dihydromyricetin to blue delphinidin-3-glucoside. In addition to these conversions, corn DFR can convert dihydrokaempferol to pelargonidin-3-glucoside.

of flower pigment and are the major constituent in orange, red, violet, and blue flowers. They are synthesized from the amino acid phenylalanine by a series of enzyme-catalyzed reactions. The color of the flower is determined by the chemical side chain substitutions of different chemical structures, with the cyanidin derivatives producing more red and the delphinidin derivatives producing more blue (Fig. 20.18). Moreover, plants sometimes contain both flavonoids and carotenoids, and it is the combination of the two that produces the wide range of colors seen in nature.

While the petunia enzyme dihydroflavonol 4-reductase can convert colorless dihydroquercetin to red cyanidin-3-glucoside and colorless dihydromyricetin to blue delphinidin-3-glucoside, it cannot use colorless dihydrokaempferol as a substrate (Fig. 20.18). However, when petunias were transformed with a dihydroflavonol 4-reductase gene from corn, the flowers of the transgenic plants were brick red-orange. This unique color, which had never been seen before in petunias, was due to the production of pelargonidin-3-glucoside by the transgenic plants. Moreover, following laboratory manipulation of transgenic flower pigmentation and subsequent field testing, in 1996, the company Florigene introduced Moondust, a mauve carnation, into the marketplace, followed by Moonshadow, a violet carnation, in 1998. Conventional breeding had failed to produce these flowers with hues in the mauve–blue–violet range because they lacked the ability to produce the blue pigment, delphinidin. Four additional varieties of carnations that feature different tones of violet and blue have been added. To date, over 75 million of these flowers have been sold worldwide.

By mid-2009, several uniquely colored transgenic roses were undergoing field trials and were expected to be available to consumers around 2010. More than two dozen field tests with new designer plants have been permitted. Among them are light-blue torenias, bronze-colored forsythia, and yellow petunias.

In one recent study, the production of anthocyanin pigment 1 *(Pap1)* *Myb* transcription factor from the plant *A. thaliana* was stably introduced into petunia plants *(Petunia hybrida)*. This transcription factor is known to regulate the production of nonvolatile phenylpropanoids, including anthocyanins, Surprisingly, in addition to an increase in pigmentation, *Pap1*-transgenic petunia flowers demonstrated a very large increase in the production of volatile phenylpropanoid–benzenoid compounds. This coordinated regulation of petunia flower color and scent production by *Pap1* provides a clear advantage for plant survival in terms of attracting pollinator insects. In addition, this work suggests a strategy to create flowers with both novel colors and enhanced scents.

The carotenoid astaxanthin, which provides the characteristic pink color to salmon, trout, and shrimp, is synthesized by marine bacteria and microalgae and then passed on to fish through the food chain. More important, astaxanthin protects salmon and trout eggs from damage by UV radiation and improves the survival and growth rate of juveniles. Most likely, these properties of astaxanthin are related to its function as a powerful antioxidant. However, when fish are grown in aquaculture, they are separated from the natural food chain and astaxanthin must be added to their feed in order to impart the typical pink color to their flesh. Currently, astaxanthin is chemically synthesized and accounts for approximately 15% of the total cost of salmon farming.

To produce astaxanthin biologically, one group of researchers first cloned a cDNA encoding the enzyme β-carotene ketolase (β-C-4 oxygenase) from the unicellular green alga *Haematococcus pluvialis*. When this cDNA was expressed in tobacco plants that contain β-carotene and the gene for β-carotene hydroxylase, astaxanthin was synthesized. By appropriate genetic manipulation, astaxanthin has been synthesized in tobacco flowers. The cDNA for the algal β-carotene ketolase was fused to DNA encoding a chloroplast transit peptide and used to transform tobacco plants. To limit the expression of astaxanthin to flowers and fruits, the

pds promoter	β-Glucuronidase activity, relative units			
	Leaves	Sepals	Petals	Ovaries
Full length 5′ — 3′	1	3.4	42.3	21.4
Deletion 1 5′ — 3′	0.53	2.1	17.1	186.1
Deletion 2 5′ — 3′	0.05	0	0	0

FIGURE 20.19 Activity of the β-glucuronidase reporter protein directed by the *pds* promoter and two of its deletion derivatives. The full-length promoter is approximately 1.0 kb, the deletion 1 derivative is 0.7 kb, and the deletion 2 derivative is 0.44 kb. All deletions are from the 5′ end of the DNA promoter fragment.

cDNA for the algal β-carotene ketolase was fused to the promoter of the tomato *pds* gene, which is active primarily in tomato reproductive tissues. To increase the expression of the cDNA for the algal β-carotene ketolase, the DNA fragment carrying the *pds* promoter was modified by deleting portions of its DNA sequence and then fused to a β-glucuronidase gene (Fig. 20.19). The construct, which had a 305-bp deletion from the 5′ terminus of the *pds* promoter, showed a decrease in β-glucuronidase activity in leaves, sepals, and petals and a very large increase in activity in flower ovaries (nectaries). To obtain maximal gene expression in ovaries, the 305-bp deleted *pds* promoter was placed upstream of the cDNA for the algal β-carotene ketolase (Fig. 20.20A). The net result of all of these genetic manipulations was that, once the introduced transferred DNA (T-DNA) had been inserted into the plant genomic DNA, the algal β-carotene ketolase, together with a transit peptide, was inserted through the chromoplast membrane, with the transit peptide being removed in the process. Once inside the chromoplast, the algal β-carotene ketolase worked in concert with the endogenous β-carotene hydroxylase to convert the β-carotene to astaxanthin, which accumulated in the flower nectaries (Fig. 20.20B). The advantage to producing astaxanthin in plants rather than bacteria or other microorganisms is that plants can store large amounts of carotenoids inside cells in lipid vesicles within the plastids. Thus, plants can accumulate 10- to 50-fold-higher concentrations of carotenoids than microorganisms, whose membranes are damaged by high concentrations of carotenoids. These manipulations have the potential to dramatically lower the cost of the astaxanthin that is used in salmon farming.

Plants as Bioreactors

Plants are easy to grow and can generate considerable biomass. With these features in mind, research has been carried out to determine whether transgenic plants can be used for the production of commercial proteins and chemicals. Unlike recombinant bacteria, which are grown in large bioreactors, a process that requires highly trained personnel and expensive equipment, crops can be produced relatively inexpensively by less-skilled workers (Table 20.6). In addition, when proteins that are intended for

FIGURE 20.20 **(A)** Schematic representation of the genetic construct used to overproduce astaxanthin in tobacco flowers. The activity of the tomato *pds* gene deletion 1 promoter is shown in Fig. 20.19. The β-carotene ketolase gene is from the green alga *H. pluvialis*. The chloroplast transit peptide ensures that the protein will be expressed in the chromoplast. **(B)** The conversion of β-carotene to astaxanthin.

human use are produced in transgenic plants, there is a significantly reduced risk of mammalian virus contamination in comparison to proteins that are produced in animal cells grown in culture. Ultimately, the biggest hurdle to overcome in the production of foreign proteins in plants is the purification of the product of a transgene from the mass of plant tissue. On a laboratory scale, plants have been used to produce monoclonal antibodies and antibody fragments; the polymer polyhydroxybutyrate, which can be used to make a biodegradable plastic-like material; and a number of potential therapeutic agents (Table 20.7) and vaccine antigens (Table 20.8).

TABLE 20.6 Comparison of recombinant protein production in plants and other systems

Parameter	Bacteria	Yeast	Mammalian cell culture	Transgenic plants
Glycosylation	None	Incorrect	Correct	Generally correct
Assembles multimeric proteins	Limited	Limited	Limited	Yes
Production costs	Medium	Medium	High	Low
Protein-folding accuracy	Low	Medium	High	High
Protein yield	High	High	Medium	Medium
Scale-up costs	High	High	High	Low
Time required	Low	Low	High	Medium
Skill level required for growth	Medium	Medium	High	Low

TABLE 20.7 Some of the therapeutic agents produced in transgenic plants

Protein	Plant(s)	Application(s)
Human protein C	Tobacco	Anticoagulant
Human hirudin variant 2	Tobacco, canola, Ethiopian mustard	Anticoagulant
Human granulocyte–macrophage colony-stimulating factor	Tobacco	Neutropenia
Human erythropoietin	Tobacco	Anemia
Human enkephalins	Thale cress, canola	Antihyperanalgesic by opiate activity
Human epidermal growth factor	Tobacco	Wound repair, control of cell proliferation
Human α-interferon	Rice, turnip	Hepatitis C and B
Human serum albumin	Potato, tobacco	Liver cirrhosis
Human hemoglobin	Tobacco	Blood substitute
Human homotrimeric collagen I	Tobacco	Collagen synthesis
Human α1-antitrypsin	Rice	Cystic fibrosis, liver disease, hemorrhage
Human growth hormone	Tobacco	Dwarfism, wound healing
Human aprotinin	Corn	Trypsin inhibitor for transplantation surgery
Angiotensin-1-converting enzyme	Tobacco, tomato	Hypertension
α-Tricosanthin	Tobacco	HIV therapy
Glucocerebrosidase	Tobacco	Gaucher disease
Human muscarinic cholinergic receptors	Tobacco	Central and peripheral nervous system
Human interleukin-2 and interleukin-4	Tobacco	Immunotherapy
Human placental alkaline phosphatase	Tobacco	Children with achonodroplasia or cretinism
Human insulin	Safflower	Diabetes
Trout growth factor	Tobacco	Fish growth
Lipase	Corn	Cystic fibrosis
Lactoferrin	Rice	Diarrhea

HIV, human immunodeficiency virus.

Antibodies

The production of antibodies and antibody fragments in transgenic plants has several potential advantages over their synthesis in recombinant microbial cells (Table 20.6). For example, transformation of plants generally results in the stable integration of the foreign DNA into the plant genome, while most microorganisms are transformed with plasmids that can be lost during a prolonged or large-scale fermentation. In addition, the processing and assembly of foreign proteins in plants are similar to those in animal cells, whereas bacteria do not readily process, assemble, or posttranslationally modify eukaryotic proteins. Moreover, plants are inexpensive to grow on a large scale, and their production is not limited by fermentation capability—it is estimated that it costs approximately $5,000 per gram to produce antibodies from hybridoma cells in culture, $1,000 per gram to produce antibodies from transgenic bacteria, and $10 to $100 per gram to produce antibodies from transgenic plants. However, since most harvested plant tissues cannot usually be stored for long periods, foreign proteins might be produced in seeds, where they will be stable for long periods under ambient conditions. To date, a large number of antibodies, including immunoglobulin G (IgG), IgM, single-chain Fv fragments, and Fab fragments, have been produced in plants (Table 20.9). Some of these plant-produced antibodies (sometimes called plantibodies) have been purified and used for diagnostic and therapeutic purposes, and others have been

TABLE 20.8 Some recombinant vaccine antigens expressed in plants

Vaccine antigen	Plant(s) or vector
Hepatitis virus B surface proteins	Tobacco, potato, yellow lupin, lettuce
Malaria parasite antigen	Virus
Rabies virus glycoprotein	Tomato
Human rhinovirus 14 and human immunodeficiency virus (HIV) epitopes	Virus
E. coli heat-labile enterotoxin	Tobacco, potato
Norwalk virus capsid protein	Tobacco, potato
Diabetes-associated autoantigen	Tobacco, potato, carrot
Mink enteritis virus epitope	Virus
Rabies and HIV epitopes	Virus
Foot and mouth disease VP1 structural protein	Arabidopsis, alfalfa
Cholera toxin B subunit	Potato
Human insulin–cholera toxin B subunit fusion protein	Potato
Human cytomegalovirus glycoprotein B	Tobacco
Dental caries (S. mutans)	Tobacco
Respiratory syncytial virus	Tomato

Note that in some cases the antigen was cloned into a transient-expression system, such as a plant virus (usually tobacco mosaic virus), that could be sprayed onto the leaves of a variety of different plants and begin producing protein within 2 weeks.

TABLE 20.9 Some antibodies and antibody fragments that have been produced in plants

Host plant	Antigen
Tobacco	Phosphonate ester
Tobacco	(4-Hydroxy-3-nitrophenyl)acetyl
Tobacco	Phytochrome
Tobacco	Artichoke mottled crinkle virus
Tobacco	Human creatine kinase
Tobacco	Streptococcus mutans cell surface antigen SA I/II
Tobacco	Fungal cutinase
Tobacco	Oxazolone
Tobacco	Abscisic acid
Tobacco	Cell surface protein from mouse B-cell lymphoma
Tobacco	Human carcinoembryonic antigen
Tobacco	Tobacco mosaic virus
Tobacco	Gibberellin
Tobacco	Beet necrotic yellow vein virus coat protein
Tobacco	Stolbur phytoplasma membrane protein
Tobacco	Root rot nematode surface glycoprotein
Petunia	Dihydrofolate reductase
Soybean	Herpes simplex virus
Pea	Abscisic acid
Pea	Human cancer cell surface antigen
Tobacco	substance P (neuropeptide)
Tobacco	CD40 (cell surface protein)
Tobacco	38C13 mouse B-cell lymphoma
Alfalfa	Human IgG

used to protect the plant against certain pathogenic agents, such as viruses. In a small number of instances, plant-produced antibodies are being tested in clinical trials to determine whether they are essentially equivalent to antibodies produced in other host cells.

The effective industrial-scale production of antibodies synthesized by plants has until recently been hampered by a very low yield, typically in the range of 1 to 10 μg/g of fresh biomass. Moreover, with conventional transgenic plant technology, it is estimated that it takes about 2 years from the beginning of the cloning process to produce gram quantities of antibody. The use of transient-expression systems can significantly speed up this process, but it is still problematic to coordinate the synthesis and assembly of the two different polypeptides that are integral components of antibody molecules. Moreover, traditional transient-expression systems are limited by the low infectivity of the viral vectors, especially those carrying medium-size to large inserts. It is also necessary to ensure that transient-expression systems based on viral vectors do not spread to plants other than the intended host. This is typically done by using mutant plant viruses that are unable to produce capsid (coat) proteins and therefore cannot form functional viral particles. However, these systems generally produce only very low levels of active antibody. Fortunately, an alternative transient-expression system has been developed. This expression system involves coinfection of plant cells with two separate plant virus vectors, one based on tobacco mosaic virus and the other on potato virus X, so that the two vectors do not compete with one another but rather can coexist within the same cell. These vectors coreplicate within the plant with each vector expressing a different antibody chain, i.e., one expresses the light chain and the other expresses the heavy chain (Fig. 20.21). This system has been used to increase the amount of IgG antibody that is typically synthesized by a plant transient-expression system by about 100-fold, so that it is possible to produce up to 0.5 mg of assembled IgG antibody per gram of fresh leaf biomass. At this high level of expression, it is possible to grow transgenic plants that produce specific IgG molecules in small areas indoors in controlled greenhouses, thereby avoiding environmental concerns regarding the inadvertent "escape" of antibody-producing plants. The potential of this technology provided the incentive for the sale of the company where it was originally developed to a larger company that hopes to open a clinical-grade manufacturing plant with the objective of beginning clinical trials of the antibodies produced.

FIGURE 20.21 Schematic representation of a portion of the viral vectors used to produce full-size IgG antibodies in plants. In each case, the viral replicase and movement protein (MP) are cloned together with the gene (cDNA) for either a light chain (LC) or a heavy chain (HC). Each antibody gene is controlled by a promoter, a signal peptide (to ensure secretion), and a transcription termination region from the appropriate virus, none of which are shown. The viruses used included tobacco mosaic virus (TMV) and potato virus X (PVX). In both cases, the viruses were unable to replicate because of the absence of the viral coat protein. Recombinant viruses were introduced into plants as part of the T-DNA that is transferred during A. tumefaciens infection.

Polymers

It is costly to produce the polymer poly(3-hydroxybutyric acid), which is used in the synthesis of biodegradable plastics, by bacterial fermentation. Consequently, research has been conducted to determine if the polymer could be produced at a lower cost in plants. In bacteria, such as *Alcaligenes eutrophus*, poly(3-hydroxybutyric acid) is synthesized from acetyl coenzyme A in three steps catalyzed by three enzymes (see Fig. 13.36). The genes that encode these enzymes are organized on a single operon. Since plants are unable to process the transcript of an operon with more than one gene, each of the three genes was isolated and cloned separately into a plasmid. The genes were targeted to the chloroplast of the plant *A. thaliana* because previous experiments had demonstrated that cytoplasmic synthesis produced only low levels of the polymer, and the transgenic plants were highly stunted. Moreover, chloroplasts can accumulate high levels of starch, another biological polymer, so it was thought that they would similarly be able to accumulate large amounts of poly(3-hydroxybutyric acid). Unlike highly valued proteins that are used as therapeutics or specialty chemicals, biological polymers need to be produced at high levels in plants for production to be economically feasible.

Each of the three poly(3-hydroxybutyric acid) biosynthesis genes was fused to a DNA fragment that encodes the chloroplast transit peptide of the small subunit of pea ribulose bisphosphate carboxylase and was placed under the transcriptional control of the cauliflower mosaic virus 35S promoter. Separate plants were transformed with each construct with Ti plasmid binary vectors. Two transgenic plants, each with a different foreign gene in its genomic DNA, were crossed to form a transgenic plant with two foreign genes. Then the double-gene-transgenic plant was crossed with a transgenic plant that carried the third foreign gene, and a transgenic plant carrying all three of the bacterial poly(3-hydroxybutyric acid) biosynthesis genes was selected. Mature leaves of some of the triple-gene-transgenic plants produced more than 1 mg of poly(3-hydroxybutyric acid) per gram (fresh weight) of leaf. Unfortunately, *A. thaliana* plants that produced very high levels of poly(3-hydroxybutyric acid) were severely stunted. Nevertheless, this work is a first step in the development of plants that produce large amounts of poly(3-hydroxybutyric acid). However, to realize the commercial potential of this system, these polymers will have to be produced in plants other than *A. thaliana* so that there will be a much greater amount of plant biomass produced.

Edible Vaccines

Although considerable progress has been made in recent years in the development of new vaccines, in many countries, either the vaccine itself is too expensive to be used on a large scale or there is a lack of physical infrastructure (e.g., roads and refrigeration) that makes it impossible to disseminate the vaccine. Commercial vaccines are expensive to produce and package and require trained personnel to administer injections. Clearly, it would be advantageous if vaccines could be delivered inexpensively on a broad scale in an edible form, e.g., as part of a fruit or vegetable. When vaccines are taken orally, they can directly stimulate the immune system (Fig. 20.22). An edible vaccine, in contrast to traditional vaccines, would not require elaborate production facilities, purification, sterilization, packaging, or special-

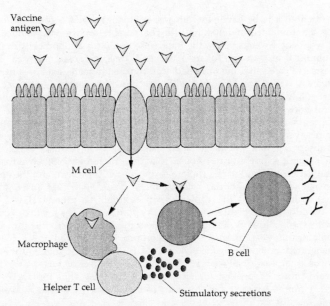

FIGURE 20.22 Schematic representation of how an edible vaccine generates an immune response against an antigen from an infectious agent. The ingested antigen, which is expressed as part of a plant, binds to and is taken up by M cells present in the lining of the intestine and is then passed to other cells in the immune system, including macrophages and B cells. The macrophages display portions of the antigen to the helper T cells, which in turn respond by secreting small molecules that activate B cells to synthesize and release antibodies that can neutralize the antigen.

ized delivery systems. Moreover, unlike many currently utilized recombinant protein expression systems, plants glycosylate proteins, a factor that may contribute to the immunogenicity and stability of a target protein. Much of the work on edible vaccines that has been reported so far utilizes potatoes as the delivery vehicle. Potatoes were originally chosen for this work because they were easy to manipulate. However, potatoes were never intended to be the vaccine delivery plant; they require cooking to make them palatable, and cooking destroys (inactivates) most protein antigens. Plants that are being considered for the delivery of edible vaccines include bananas (although banana trees require several years to mature), tomatoes (although tomatoes spoil readily), lettuce, carrots, peanuts, and corn (mainly for "vaccinating" animals).

Cholera is an infectious diarrheal disease caused by the enterotoxin produced by the gram-negative bacterium *Vibrio cholerae* (see chapter 12). Globally, there are more than 5 million cases and 200,000 deaths from cholera each year. To test whether it might be possible to develop an edible vaccine against *V. cholerae*, potato plants were transformed, using *A. tumefaciens*, with the cholera toxin subunit B gene. Cholera toxin subunit B binds to an intestinal receptor; subunit A contains the toxin activity. One gram of transgenic potato produced approximately 30 µg of subunit B. After the transgenic potatoes were cooked in boiling water until they were

soft enough to be edible by humans, approximately 50% of the subunit B protein remained undenatured. The cooked potatoes were fed to mice once a week for 4 weeks before the mice were tested for antibodies against the subunit B protein and for resistance to *V. cholerae*-caused diarrhea. These tests indicated that the mice had acquired a significant level of protection against *V. cholerae*. Moreover, although mucosal antibody titers declined gradually after the last immunization, they were rapidly restored after an oral boost (an additional feeding) of transgenic potato. In an interesting variation of the strategy outlined above, the cholera toxin subunit B and A2 genes were each fused to different antigen genes and then used to generate transgenic potato plants. To create these two fusion proteins, a 22-amino-acid epitope from murine (mouse) rotavirus enterotoxin NSP4 was fused to the C-terminal end of the cholera toxin subunit B protein, and the enterotoxigenic *E. coli* fimbrial colonization factor CFA/I was fused to the N-terminal end of the cholera toxin subunit A2 protein (Fig. 20.23). Normally, the A2 peptide links the A1 peptide, which has the toxic activity, with the subunit B peptide, which has the binding activity. Transgenic potatoes that expressed the two fusion proteins were fed to mice, which generated antibodies against cholera toxin subunit B protein, murine rotavirus enterotoxin NSP4, and *E. coli* fimbrial colonization factor CFA/I and were protected against rotavirus-caused diarrhea. This approach holds great promise for the development of inexpensive and readily available vaccines for a wide range of diseases.

It has been estimated that Shiga toxin-producing strains of *E. coli* cause approximately 100,000 cases of hemorrhagic colitis a year. About 6% of those infections produce severe complications, including kidney failure. Similar to cholera toxin, the Shiga toxin contains one A subunit, which encodes the catalytic, or toxin, activity, per five B subunits, which act (together) to bind to cellular surface receptors. To develop an oral vaccine against type 2 Shiga toxin (type 2 is responsible for the most severe disease in humans), the genes for a genetically inactivated version of the Shiga toxin A and B peptides were both cloned and expressed in tobacco cells (Fig. 20.24). To test the ability of transformed tobacco plants that synthesized the modified Shiga toxin to protect mice against the toxin, scientists infected mice with Shiga toxin-producing strains of *E. coli*. Before the introduction of the Shiga toxin-producing bacteria, some of the mice were fed leaves from transgenic tobacco plants expressing the inactivated Shiga toxin once a week for 4 weeks, while other mice were untreated. One week after the introduction of the toxic *E. coli* strain, all of the mice that were not fed the antigen-producing tobacco had died. By contrast, 2 weeks after treatment with the toxic *E. coli* strain, all of the orally vaccinated mice were still alive. This experiment serves as a proof of the concept that oral administration of the inactivated Shiga toxin is a highly effective means of protecting animals against Shiga toxin-producing *E. coli*. Of course, for a human oral vaccine, a more suitable host plant, such as tomato or banana, would be desirable.

Plant Yield

In nearly every instance where plants are utilized, it is desirable to optimize the yield of the plant or its components. Theoretically, increases in plant yield may be achieved in a number of ways. For example, preliminary studies directed toward introducing the C_4 pathway of photosynthesis in

FIGURE 20.23 Schematic representation of the association of two components of an engineered vaccine. The cholera toxin B subunit is synthesized as a fusion protein to the rotavirus peptide, the cholera toxin A2 subunit is fused to the enterotoxigenic *E. coli* fimbrial colonization factor, and the cholera toxin B and A2 peptides are noncovalently attached to one another. Both fusion proteins are made in transgenic potatoes and combine to form a cholera toxin-like protein, as shown.

Cholera toxin B subunit

Cholera toxin A2 peptide

Rotavirus peptide

E. coli fimbrial colonization factor

FIGURE 20.24 Schematic representation of Shiga toxin A and B subunits encoded in a bacterial operon (*stxA* and *stxB* genes, respectively) under the control of a single promoter and transcription terminator. These two genes were subsequently isolated and modified, first to inactivate the A subunit and then to eliminate sequences on both genes that might adversely affect their transcription in plant cells. The modified genes were inserted between the left and right borders (LB and RB) of the T-DNA of a binary Ti plasmid-based vector, each under the control of a separate cauliflower mosaic virus 35S promoter. The T-DNA also contained a gene encoding kanamycin resistance under the control of its own promoter. The transcription terminator sequences of the three genes contained within the T-DNA are not shown for the sake of simplicity. The final construct was used to transform tobacco plants.

plants that normally use the C_3 pathway have been reported; plants have been engineered to take up iron from the soil more efficiently; the supply of oxygen to plant cells has been enhanced, thereby increasing the rate of plant growth; and the lignin content of some trees has been decreased, making it easier to isolate the cellulose. The work of increasing plant yields is still in its infancy. Nevertheless, based on what has been achieved to date, the various strategies are likely to be fruitful.

Increasing Iron Content

Plant growth is often limited by the availability of iron. Despite the abundance of this element on the earth's surface, plants have difficulty obtaining enough iron to support their growth, because the iron in soil, especially in alkaline soil, is largely present as insoluble ferric hydroxides, which cannot be readily transported into cells. To solve this problem, bacteria, fungi, and plants secrete small, specialized iron-binding molecules, called siderophores, that scavenge iron. Once bound, the now soluble iron–siderophore complex is taken up by specific receptors on the surfaces of these organisms; after reduction to the ferrous state, the iron is released from the siderophore.

FIGURE 20.25 Overview of the biosynthesis of the mugineic acid family of phytosiderophores.

Siderophores are low-molecular-weight molecules, usually less than 1 kilodalton, with three functional, or iron-binding, groups connected by a flexible backbone. Each functional group presents two atoms of either oxygen or (less commonly) nitrogen that bind to iron. In chemical terms, the functional groups are bidentate, and trivalent ferric iron can accommodate three of these groups to form a six-coordinate complex (see Fig. 15.8). The functional groups of microbial siderophores are usually either hydroxamates or catecholates. Other functional groups include carboxylate moieties (such as citrate) and ethylenediamine. Plant siderophores, on the other hand, are linear hydroxy- and amino-substituted iminocarboxylic acids, such as mugineic acid and avenic acid.

Since rice plants secrete only very small amounts of mugineic acid and are highly susceptible to growth inhibition from iron deficiency, it was reasoned that increasing the amount of mugineic acid should enable the plant to take up more iron and hence increase the yield of the plant. Mugineic acid is synthesized in several steps from the amino acid L-methionine (Fig. 20.25). To increase the amount of mugineic acid, rice plants were transformed (using *Agrobacterium*) with an 11-kb fragment of barley genomic DNA containing two *naat* genes, *naat-A* and *naat-B*, encoding the subunits of the enzyme nicotianamine aminotransferase. Both of these genes were under the transcriptional control of their native promoters. In the resulting transgenic rice plants, the pattern of expression of the two proteins was the same as in barley: expression in roots was very low in the presence of high levels of iron and was high in the presence of low levels of iron. After 16 weeks of growth in an alkaline soil, the shoot dry weight and grain yield of the transgenic plants were more than four times those of the nontransgenic plants, an enormous difference in yield. Hopefully, this spectacular gain will be realized in the field as well as under controlled laboratory conditions.

Altering Lignin Content

After cellulose, lignin is the second most abundant organic compound on Earth. Depending on the species of tree, it accounts for approximately 15 to 35% of the dry weight of wood. While lignin is important in the mechanical support of trees and in their defense against pathogens, it is a major impediment in obtaining the cellulose that is needed by the pulp and paper industry—releasing cellulose requires harsh physical and chemical treatment. In the United States, over 80 million tons of wood pulp is produced annually. This process, which removes nearly 30 million tons of lignin from wood, consumes enormous amounts of energy and chemicals. In addition, high levels of lignin decrease the nutritional value of forage crops that are used for cattle feed.

Lignin is synthesized by the oxidative polymerization of one of three hydroxycinnamyl alcohols: *p*-coumaryl, coniferyl, or sinapyl alcohol. In one approach to reduce the level of lignin produced by quaking aspen trees (*Populus tremuloides*) and to make it easier to harvest the cellulose, one of the steps in the biosynthesis of lignin was altered. The enzyme 4-coumarate:coenzyme A ligase catalyzes the conversion of 4-coumarate to 4-coumarate:coenzyme A. The latter compound is a precursor of both flavonoids and lignin (Fig. 20.26). Moreover, there are two isoforms of the enzyme 4-coumarate:coenzyme A ligase. One isoform is expressed in the epidermis of stems and leaves and is probably involved in flavonoid biosynthesis. The other isoform is expressed in differentiating xylem and

Phenylalanine

Cinnamate

COOH

4-Coumarate:coenzyme A ligase

OH

4-Coumarate

CO-SCoA

Flavonoids

OH

Lignin

4-Coumaroyl CoA

Nonlignin cell
wall phenolics

FIGURE 20.26 Role of 4-coumarate:coenzyme A (CoA) ligase in lignin biosynthesis.

presumably functions mainly in lignin biosynthesis. The gene for the iso-
form expressed in xylem was isolated, and an antisense version of the gene
was placed under the transcriptional control of the 35S promoter and intro-
duced into aspen by *A. tumefaciens*-mediated transformation. Transformed
aspen trees exhibited up to a 45% decrease in lignin content and, at the
same time, as much as a 15% increase in cellulose. In addition, the trans-
genic trees were about 25% larger and had thicker stems and larger leaves
than the nontransgenic trees. The altered lignin and cellulose content of the
transgenic aspen should make it easier to extract cellulose during pulp and
paper manufacture.

Recently, a considerable amount of effort has been directed toward
finding ways to efficiently utilize plants to produce renewable biofuels.
Some of this research has focused on converting materials such as corn
stover, wheat straw, grasses, and wood by-products to glucose and then to
ethanol. However, with all of these compounds, it is necessary to pretreat
the substrate under harsh conditions to remove the lignin and make the cel-
lulose and hemicellulose more accessible to hydrolytic enzymes. These
pretreatment steps are generally costly in terms of materials and energy, and
often the harsh conditions employed make it much more difficult to enzy-
matically digest the cellulose. However, by reducing the lignin content of
plant tissues, it may be possible to employ mild pretreatment or even no
pretreatment prior to enzymatic digestion (Fig. 20.27). In fact, by con-
structing transgenic alfalfa plants that contained an antisense version of the
gene for the enzyme skimiate hydroxycinnamoyl transferase, which cata-
lyzes one of the steps in the biosynthesis of lignin, it was possible to reduce
the lignin content of the plant by about 50 to 70%. Interestingly, the trans-
genic plants that had the lowest lignin content also had the highest carbo-
hydrate levels, suggesting that the plant has somehow compensated for the
reduction in lignin. Moreover, when the lignin levels are low, the cell wall
carbohydrates are more accessible to cellulose- and hemicellulose-degrading

FIGURE 20.27 Schematic representation of native **(A)** and transgenic **(B)** plant cell walls treated to partially break down their structure and make the hemicellulose and cellulose components more accessible to enzymatic digestion. Lignin is shown in black, cellulose in blue, and hemicellulose in red.

enzymes. Importantly, since the biochemical steps that lead to the synthesis of lignin are highly conserved across the plant kingdom, it may be possible to apply this approach to a variety of plants so that, for example, corn may be engineered to continue to be a food source for both animals and humans while the parts of the corn plant that are not consumed may be converted into biofuels.

Erect Leaves

Conventional varieties of wheat and rice allocate a considerable amount of their resources to the growth of vegetative tissues. On the other hand, semidwarf varieties, developed by the conventional breeding strategies that were part of the "green revolution," allocate more of their resources to grain. In addition, semidwarf varieties are more resistant to damage from wind and rain and produce much less residual (waste) biomass. However, to feed an ever-increasing world population, it is necessary to engineer plants to produce even higher grain yields. One way to do this is to develop dwarf strains of rice and wheat that accumulate even less vegetative material and put more resources into increasing the grain yield. Scientists have approached this problem by using genetic engineering to manipulate the levels of some plant hormones, most notably gibberellins and brassinosteroids.

Brassinosteroids include more than 40 different plant polyhydroxy-lated sterol derivatives. They affect a variety of plant processes, typically at low concentrations, including cell elongation, vascular development, and stress tolerance. By genetically engineering rice plants to have a decreased level of brassinosteroids, scientists were able to increase the grain yield when the crop was planted at a high density.

The rate-limiting step in the synthesis of brassinosteroids is the hydroxylation of carbon 22 (Fig. 20.28). In rice, the hydroxylation of C-22 is controlled by two differentially regulated genes. One gene, called *OsDWARF4L1*, contributes primarily to brassinosteroid synthesis in shoots. The other gene, *OsDWARF4*, primarily controls brassinosteroid synthesis for leaf inclination (Fig. 20.29). Initially, a collection of transposon mutants of rice was screened for an "erect-leaf" phenotype, i.e., plants in which the leaves did not lean over but stood more or less straight up. One of the mutants that was selected was characterized in detail and found to have a mutation in the *OsDWARF4* gene. Mutation of the other C-22 hydroxyla-tion gene or mutation of both genes yielded smaller plants that did not exhibit the erect-leaf phenotype. Since the mutation that conferred the erect-leaf phenotype on plants was created by transposon mutagenesis, it was relatively easy to isolate, and subsequently characterize, the trans-poson-labeled gene. Importantly, when plants that showed the erect-leaf phenotype were planted at a high density, they produced about 20% more rice than wild-type plants planted at the same density. This increase was attributed to the reduced shading (and hence the greater amount of photo-synthesis) of the lower leaves in the mutant (erect-leaf) plants. Having identified the gene whose activity is critical to increasing rice yield, it should now be possible to attenuate the activity of that gene using either antisense constructs or RNA interference. Moreover, it is expected that any approach that works in rice should be equally effective in other plants.

Increasing Oxygen Content

Oxygen is an essential substrate for plant respiratory metabolism, and in fact, the amount of available oxygen may limit a number of plant biochem-ical reactions. Since it is impractical to increase the external oxygen supply

FIGURE 20.28 Chemical structure of brassinolide, with an arrow pointing to the position of C-22.

Strain	Genotype	Phenotype
Wild-type rice	OsDWARF4 OsDWARF4L1	100% size Leaves not erect
Mutant rice 1	OsD✗ARF4 OsDWARF4L1	95% size Leaves erect
Mutant rice 2	OsDWARF4 OsDW✗RF4L1	~60% size Leaves not erect
Mutant rice 1-2	OsD✗ARF4 OsDW✗RF4L1	~10% size Leaves not erect

FIGURE 20.29 Wild-type and mutant strains of rice with altered DWARF4 genes.

to the plant, one way to increase the oxygen concentration inside a plant is to provide the plant with a protein that can sequester oxygen and provide it where it is needed.

The gram-negative bacterium *Vitreoscilla* produces a dimeric hemoglobin that binds oxygen tightly and allows the bacterium to proliferate under oxygen-limited conditions. The gene encoding this hemoglobin has been isolated and expressed in a variety of bacteria, increasing the growth rate, the final cell density, and the yield of cloned foreign genes. When the *Vitreoscilla* hemoglobin under the transcriptional control of the 35S promoter was introduced into tobacco by *A. tumefaciens*-mediated gene transfer, transgenic plants produced 80 to 100% more dry weight than nontransgenic plants, seed germination time was reduced from 6 to 8 days to 3 to 4 days, and transgenic plants contained approximately 35% more chlorophyll and 34% more nicotine than nontransgenic plants. It is thought that the *Vitreoscilla* hemoglobin increases the availability of oxygen and/or energy in the cell. For example, the synthesis of 1 mol of chlorophyll from glutamate requires 4 mol of oxygen and 2 mol of ATP. Similarly, the last step in the synthesis of nicotine, the conversion of nicotinic acid and N-methyl-Δ'-pyrrolinium salt to nicotine, is catalyzed by the oxygen-dependent enzyme nicotine synthase (Fig. 20.30). While this sort of genetic manipulation raises more questions than it answers, the possibility of increasing plant yield by manipulating the oxygen concentration is quite exciting.

Phytoremediation

Phytoremediation is defined as the use of plants to remove, destroy, or sequester hazardous substances from the environment. Phytoremediation of metals and other inorganic compounds may take one of several forms:

FIGURE 20.30 The last step in the biosynthesis of nicotine.

Nicotinic acid N-Methyl-Δ'-pyrrolinium salt Nicotine

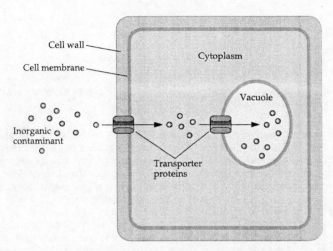

FIGURE 20.31 Uptake of inorganic pollutants into plant cell vacuoles.

phytoextraction, the absorption and concentration of metals from the soil into the plant; rhizofiltration, the use of plant roots to remove metals from effluents; phytostabilization, the use of plants to reduce the spread of metals in the environment; or phytovolatilization, the uptake and release into the atmosphere of volatile materials, such as mercury- or arsenic-containing compounds. A number of plants that can naturally accumulate large amounts of metal have been identified. These plants are called hyperaccumulators. Unfortunately, in the presence of very high concentrations of metals, even hyperaccumulating plants attain only a small size. That is, high concentrations of metals are inhibitory to the growth of plants, even those plants that are capable of hyperaccumulating metals. Depending upon the amount of metal at a particular site and the type of soil at that site, it could take many years to completely remove the metal from the soil and remediate the site, even with hyperaccumulating plants. Since this is too slow for practical application, scientists have undertaken to engineer plants for more efficient metal phytoremediation.

In general, plants sequester toxic pollutants in places where the toxicants can do the least harm to plant cellular processes. Thus, pollutants are typically accumulated in vacuoles or cell walls. The uptake and accumulation in leaves of inorganic contaminants without toxic effects are desirable properties for phytoextraction. To this end, plants can be engineered to have higher levels of transporters involved in the uptake of inorganic pollutants from the xylem into the leaf symplast and from the cytosol into vacuoles.

To engineer plants that can accumulate greater amounts of lead and cadmium, toxic metals that contaminate a wide range of environments, the yeast gene *YCF1* was used to transform *A. thaliana* plants. The yeast YCF protein is a member of the ABC transporter family of proteins and, when it is expressed in *A. thaliana*, detoxifies metals, which are taken up by the plant by transporting them to plant cell vacuoles (Fig. 20.31). Despite the fact that the YCF protein is expressed at a relatively low level in transgenic plants—the protein cannot be detected by immunological assays of plant

$$R-CH_2-Hg^+ \; + \; H^+ \; \xrightarrow{\text{MerB}} \; R-CH_3 \; + \; Hg(\text{II})$$

$$Hg(\text{II}) \; \xrightarrow{\text{MerA}} \; Hg(0)$$

FIGURE 20.32 Detoxification of organomercural compounds by bacterial organomercural lyase (MerB) and mercuric ion reductase (MerA).

cellular extracts—it can nevertheless effectively sequester metals into the vacuoles. Transgenic plants grown in the presence of high levels of either lead or cadmium have nearly four times as much metal in their vacuoles and about twice as much metal overall throughout the plant as nontransformed plants. This model system is an important first step in developing transgenic plants, such as poplar trees, that can remove metals from contaminated soils.

Organic forms of mercury (Hg), especially methyl mercury, are highly toxic to both plants and animals. In plants, these compounds inhibit electron transport and photosynthesis; both are chloroplast functions. At the present time, there are no simple and inexpensive procedures for removing mercury from the environment. However, it is possible to engineer plants with bacterial genes that encode enzymes that can detoxify organic forms of mercury. Mercury-resistant bacteria detoxify organomercurals by producing two enzymes: organomercural lyase, which catalyzes the conversion of the organomercural to the less toxic inorganic species, Hg(II), and mercuric ion reductase, which catalyzes the reduction of Hg(II) to the volatile and less reactive elemental form, Hg(0) (Fig. 20.32). The enzymes are encoded by the *merB* and *merA* genes, respectively, of the plasmid-borne mercury resistance *(mer)* operon. Expressing the *mer* genes in plants by transformation of the nuclear genome provides some protection against the toxic effects of mercury. However, the operon containing both genes may be expressed in tobacco chloroplasts (in a single transformation event), obviating concerns about positioning effects, codon usage, or transmission

FIGURE 20.33 Transgenic tobacco plants engineered to express *mer* genes in their chloroplasts produce more biomass than nontransgenic tobacco plants in the presence of increasing amounts of mercury.

of the foreign genes to other plants via pollen. Moreover, chloroplast expression of the *mer* genes leads to a high level of protein expression and partially protects the plant from inhibition of electron transport and photosynthesis (Fig. 20.33). Having demonstrated the efficacy of this approach with tobacco, it may be useful to fine tune the system to increase the ability of plants to detoxify mercury. Also, it may be advantageous to introduce the *mer* operon into other plants with more extensive root systems that are better suited to take up mercury from the soil.

Phytoremediation of organic compounds may occur by phytostabilization; by phytostimulation, the stimulation of microbial biodegradation around the roots of plants; or by phytotransformation, the absorption and degradation of organic contaminants by the plant. A number of different types of plants are effective at stimulating the degradation of organic molecules in the rhizosphere (i.e., around the plant roots). Typically, these plants, including many common grasses, as well as crop species, have extensive and fibrous roots, which form an extended rhizosphere. In addition, several varieties of trees can take up and degrade some organic contaminants. Plants with phytotransformation activity may contain nitroreductases, which are useful for degrading TNT (trinitrotoluene) and other nitroaromatics; dehalogenases for the degradation of chlorinated solvents and pesticides; and laccases that can degrade anilines, such as triaminotoluene. However, there is less incentive to engineer plants to be more efficient degraders of organic compounds, since (1) many plants can already do this effectively and (2) selecting and/or engineering soil microbes that live in the vicinity of plant roots may provide a simpler means to the same end.

SUMMARY

The expression of foreign genes in plants makes it possible to produce a wide range of new plant varieties. Plants with new flower colors have been developed; the nutritional content of crops has been enhanced; discoloration of potatoes has been prevented by genetic manipulation; the sweetness of some plants has been augmented; plants have been developed to act as factories for the large-scale production of important foreign proteins, such as antibodies and therapeutics; and plant yield has been increased by increasing the iron and oxygen content, by modulating the lignin content, and by modifying the response of the plant to brassinosteroids. Also, plants have been utilized as components of phytoremediation protocols designed to remove contaminating metals and organic compounds from the environment.

Plant nutritional content may be improved in a variety of ways. The amino acid content (specifically methionine and lysine) can be increased, the lipid composition can be modified to suit the intended end use of the oil, pathways for the synthesis of vitamin E and the precursor to vitamin A have been engineered, and plants with increased levels of available iron have been created.

As bioreactors, plants can produce, on a laboratory scale, monoclonal antibodies and antibody fragments; the polymer polyhydroxybutyrate, which can be used to make a biodegradable plastic-like material; and a number of potential therapeutic agents. Finally, transgenic plants have also been used as edible vaccines, an approach that could result in a wide range of new and inexpensive vaccines.

REFERENCES

Arakawa, T., D. K. X. Chong, and W. H. R. Langridge. 1998. Efficacy of a food plant-based oral cholera toxin B subunit vaccine. *Nat. Biotechnol.* 16:292–297.

Ayub, R., M. Guis, M. Ben Amor, L.

Gillot, J.-P. Roustan, A. Latché, M. Bouzayen, and J.-C. Pech. 1996. Expression of ACC oxidase antisense gene inhibits ripening of cantaloupe melon fruits. *Nat. Biotechnol.* 14:862–866.

Bachem, C. W. B., G.-J. Speckmann, P. C. G. van der Linde, F. T. M. Verheggen, M. D. Hunt, J. C. Steffens, and M. Zabeau. 1994. Antisense expression of polyphenol oxidase genes inhibits enzymatic

browning in potato tubers. *Bio/Technology* 12:1101–1105.

Beaujean, A., C. Ducrocq-Assaf, R. S. Sangwan, G. Lilius, L. Bülow, and B. S. Sangwan-Norreel. 2000. Engineering direct fructose production in processed potato tubers by expressing a bifunctional alpha-amylase/glucose isomerase gene complex. *Biotechnol. Bioeng.* 70:9–16.

Bowler, C., L. Slooten, S. Vandenbranden, R. De Rycke, J. Botterman, C. Sybesma, M. Van Montagu, and D. Inzé. 1991. Manganese superoxide dismutase can reduce cellular damage mediated by oxygen radicals in transgenic plants. *EMBO J.* 10:1723–1732.

Chandler, S., and Y. Tanaka. 2007. Genetic modification in floriculture. *Crit. Rev. Plant Sci.* 26:169–197.

Chapple, C., M. Ladisch, and R. Meilan. 2007. Loosening lignin's grip on biofuel production. *Nat. Biotechnol.* 25:746–748.

Chen, F., and R. A. Dixon. 2007. Lignin modification improves fermentable sugar yields for biofuel production. *Nat. Biotechnol.* 25:759–761.

Courtney-Gutterson, N., C. Napoli, C. Lemieux, A. Morgan, E. Firoozabady, and K. E. P. Robinson. 1994. Modification of flower color in florist's chrysanthemum: production of a white-flowering variety through molecular genetics. *Bio/Technology* 12:268–271.

DellaPenna, D. 2005. Progress in the dissection and manipulation of vitamin E synthesis. *Trends Plant Sci.* 10:574–579.

Diaz de la Garza, R. I., J. F. Gregory III, and A. D. Hanson. 2007. Folate biofortification of tomato fruit. *Proc. Natl. Acad. Sci. USA* 104:4218–4222.

Falco, S. C., T. Guida, M. Locke, J. Mauvais, C. Sanders, R. T. Ward, and P. Webber. 1995. Transgenic canola and soybean seeds with increased lysine. *Bio/Technology* 13:577–582.

Faus, I. 2000. Recent developments in the characterization and biotechnological production of sweet-tasting proteins. *Appl. Microbiol. Biotechnol.* 53:145–151.

Fiedler, U., and U. Conrad. 1995. High-level production and long-term

storage of engineered antibodies in transgenic tobacco seeds. *Bio/Technology* 13:1090–1093.

Giddings, G., G. Allison, D. Brooks, and A. Carter. 2000. Transgenic plants as factories for biopharmaceuticals. *Nat. Biotechnol.* 18:1151–1155.

Giritch, A., S. Marillonet, C. Engler, G. van Eldik, J. Botterman, V. Klimyuk, and Y. Gleba. 2006. Rapid high-yield expression of full-size IgG antibodies in plants coinfected with noncompeting viral vectors. *Proc. Natl. Acad. Sci. USA* 103:14701–14706.

Goldstein, D. A., and J. A. Thomas. 2004. Biopharmaceuticals derived from genetically modified plants. *Q. J. Med.* 97:705–716.

Goto, F., T. Yoshihara, N. Shigemoto, S. Toki, and F. Takaiwa. 1999. Iron fortification of rice seed by the soybean ferritin gene. *Nat. Biotechnol.* 17:282–286.

Gray, J. E., S. Picton, J. J. Giovannoni, and D. Grierson. 1994. The use of transgenic and naturally occurring mutants to understand and manipulate tomato fruit ripening. *Plant Cell Environ.* 17:557–571.

Holmberg, N., G. Lilius, J. E. Bailey, and L. Bülow. 1997. Transgenic tobacco expressing *Vitreoscilla* hemoglobin exhibits enhanced growth and altered metabolite production. *Nat. Biotechnol.* 15:244–247.

Holton, T. A., F. Brugliera, D. R. Lester, Y. Tanaka, C. D. Hyland, J. G. T. Menting, C.-Y. Liu, E. Farcy, T. W. Stevenson, and E. C. Cornish. 1993. Cloning and expression of cytochrome P450 genes controlling flower color. *Nature* 366:276–279.

Hu, W.-J., S. A. Harding, J. Lung, J. L. Popko, J. Ralph, D. D. Stokke, C.-J. Tsai, and V. L. Chiang. 1999. Repression of lignin biosynthesis promotes cellulose accumulation and growth in transgenic trees. *Nat. Biotechnol.* 17:808–812.

Jobling, S. A., R. J. Westcott, A. Tayal, R. Jeffcoat, and G. P. Schwall. 2002. Production of freeze-thaw-stable potato starch by antisense inhibition of three starch synthase genes. *Nat. Biotechnol.* 20:295–299.

Klee, H. J., M. B. Hayford, K. A. Kretzmer, G. F. Barry, and G. M.

Kishore. 1991. Control of ethylene synthesis by expression of a bacterial enzyme in transgenic tomato plants. *Plant Cell* 3:1187–1193.

Knutzon, D. S., G. A. Thompson, S. E. Radke, W. B. Johnson, V. C. Knauf, and J. C. Kridl. 1992. Modification of *Brassica* seed oil by antisense expression of a stearoyl-acyl carrier protein desaturase gene. *Proc. Natl. Acad. Sci. USA* 89:2624–2628.

Lucca, P., R. Hurrell, and I. Potrykus. 2001. Genetic engineering approaches to improve the bioavailability and the level of iron in rice grains. *Theor. Appl. Genet.* 102:392–397.

Ma, J. K.-C., and M. B. Hein. 1995. Immunotherapeutic potential of antibodies produced in plants. *Trends Biotechnol.* 13:522–527.

Mann, V., M. Harker, I. Pecker, and J. Hirschberg. 2000. Metabolic engineering of astaxanthin production in tobacco flowers. *Nat. Biotechnol.* 18:888–892.

Marillonnet, S., C. Thoeringer, R. Kandzia, V. Klimyuk and Y. Gleba. 2005. Systemic *Agrobacterium tumefaciens*-mediated transfection of viral replicons for efficient transient expression in plants. *Nat. Biotechnol.* 23:718–723.

Matzke, M. A., A. J. Matzke, G. J. Pruss, and V. B. Vance. 2001. RNA-based silencing strategies in plants. *Curr. Opin. Genet. Dev.* 11:221–227.

Meyer, P., I. Heidmann, G. Forkmann, and H. Saedler. 1987. A new petunia flower colour generated by transformation of a mutant with a maize gene. *Nature* 330:677–678.

Mol, J. N. M., T. A. Holton, and R. E. Koes. 1995. Floriculture: genetic engineering of commercial traits. *Trends Biotechnol.* 13:350–355.

Mol, J. N. M., A. R. van der Krol, A. J. van Tunen, R. van Blokland, P. de Lange, and A. R. Stuitje. 1990. Regulation of plant gene expression by antisense RNA. *FEBS Lett.* 268:427–430.

Molvig, L., L. M. Tabe, B. O. Eggum, A. E. Moore, S. Craig, D. Spencer, and T. J. V. Higgins. 1997. Enhanced methionine levels and increased nutritive value of seeds of transgenic lupins (*Lupinus angustifolius* L.) expressing a

sunflower seed albumin gene. *Proc. Natl. Acad. Sci. USA* **94**:8393–8398.

Murphy, D. J. 1996. Engineering oil production in rapeseed and other oil crops. *Trends Biotechnol.* **14**:206–213.

Nawrath, C., Y. Poirier, and C. Somerville. 1994. Targeting of polyhydroxybutyrate biosynthetic pathway to the plastids of *Arabidopsis thaliana* results in high levels of polymer accumulation. *Proc. Natl. Acad. Sci. USA* **91**:12760–12764.

Paine, J. A., C. A. Shipton, S. Chaggar, R. M. Howells, M. J. Kennedy, G. Vernon, S. Y. Wright, E. Hinchliffe, J. L. Adams, A. L. Silverstone, and R. Drake. 2005. Improving the nutritional value of Golden Rice through increased provitamin A content. *Nat. Biotechnol.* **23**:482–487.

Pilon-Smits, E. 2005. Phytoremediation. *Annu. Rev. Plant Biol.* **56**:15–39.

Qi, B., T. Fraser, S. Mugford, G. Dobson, O. Sayanova, J. Butler, J. A. Napier, A. K. Stobart, and C. M. Lazarus. 2004. Production of very long chain polyunsaturated omega-3 and omega-6 fatty acids in plants. *Nat. Biotechnol.* **22**:739–745.

Regierer, B., A. R. Fernie, F. Springer, A. Perez-Melis, A. Leisse, K. Koehl, L. Willmitzer, P. Geigenberger, and J. Kossmann. 2002. Starch content and yield increase as a result of altering adenylate pools in transgenic plants. *Nat. Biotechnol.* **20**:1256–1260.

Rooijen, G. J. H., and M. M. Moloney. 1995. Plant seed oil-bodies as carriers for foreign proteins. *Bio/Technology* **13**:72–77.

Roxas, V. P., R. K. Smith, Jr., E. R. Allen, and R. D. Allen. 1997. Overexpression of glutathione S-transferase/glutathione peroxidase

enhances the growth of transgenic tobacco seedlings during stress. *Nat. Biotechnol.* **15**:988–991.

Ruiz, O. N., H. S. Hussein, N. Terry, and H. Daniell. 2003. Phytoremediation of organomercurial compounds via chloroplast genetic engineering. *Plant Physiol.* **132**:1344–1352.

Sakamoto, T., Y. Morinaka, T. Ohnishi, H. Sunohara, S. Fujioka, M. Ueguchi-Tanaka, M. Mizutani, K. Sakata, S. Takatsuto, S. Yoshida, H. Tanaka, H. Kitano, and M. Matsuoka. 2006. Erect leaves caused by brassinosteroid deficiency increase biomass production and grain yield in rice. *Nat. Biotechnol.* **24**:105–109.

Sévenier, R., R. D. Hall, I. M. van der Meer, H. J. C. Hakkert, A. J. van Tunen, and A. J. Koops. 1998. High level fructan accumulation in a transgenic sugar beet. *Nat. Biotechnol.* **16**:843–846.

Shi, J., H. Wang, K. Schellin, B. Li, M. Faller, J. M. Stoop, R. B. Meeley, D. S. Ertl, J. P. Ranch, and K. Glassman. 2007. Embryo-specific silencing of a transporter reduces phytic acid content of maize and soybean seeds. *Nat. Biotechnol.* **25**:930–937.

Shintani, D., and D. DellaPenna. 1998. Elevating the vitamin E content of plants through metabolic engineering. *Science* **282**:2098–2100.

Song, W.-Y., E. J. Sohn, E. Martinoia, Y. J. Lee, Y.-Y. Yang, M. Jasinski, C. Forestier, I. Hwang, and Y. Lee. 2003. Engineering tolerance and accumulation of lead and cadmium in transgenic plants. *Nat. Biotechnol.* **21**:914–919.

Storozhenko, S., V. De Brouwer, M. Volckaert, O. Navarrete, D. Blancquaert, G.-F. Zhang, W. Lambert, and D. Van Der Straeten. 2007. Folate fortification of rice by

metabolic engineering. *Nat. Biotechnol.* **25**:1277–1279.

Takahashi, M., H. Nakanishi, S. Kawasaki, N. K. Nishizawa, and S. Mori. 2001. Enhanced tolerance of rice to low iron availability in alkaline soils using barley nicotianamine aminotransferase genes. *Nat. Biotechnol.* **19**:466–469.

Töpfer, R., N. Martini, and J. Schell. 1995. Modification of plant lipid synthesis. *Science* **268**:681–686.

Van Breusegem, F., L. Slooten, J.-M. Stassart, J. Botterman, T. Moens, M. Van Montagu, and D. Inzé. 1999. Effect of overproduction of MnSOD in maize chloroplasts on foliar tolerance to cold and oxidative stress. *J. Exp. Bot.* **50**:71–78.

Van Camp, W., H. Willekens, C. Bowler, M. Van Montagu, D. Inzé, P. Reupold-Popp, H. Sandermann, Jr., and C. Langebartels. 1994. Elevated levels of superoxide dismutase protect transgenic plants against ozone damage. *Bio/Technology* **12**:165–168.

Wen, S. X., L. D. Teel, N. A. Judge, and A. D. O'Brien. 2006. A plant-based oral vaccine to protect against systemic intoxication by Shiga toxin type 2. *Proc. Natl. Acad. Sci. USA* **103**:7082–7087.

Ye, X., S. Al-Babili, A. Klöti, J. Zhang, P. Lucca, P. Beyer, and I. Potrykus. 2000. Engineering the provitamin A (β-carotene) biosynthetic pathway into (carotenoid-free) rice endosperm. *Science* **287**:303–305.

Yu, J., and H. R. Langridge. 2001. A plant-based multicomponent vaccine protects mice from enteric disease. *Nat. Biotechnol.* **19**:548–552.

Zhang, H.-X., and E. Blumwald. 2001. Transgenic salt-tolerant tomato plants accumulate salt in foliage but not in fruit. *Nat. Biotechnol.* **19**:765–768.

REVIEW QUESTIONS

1. How can plants be genetically manipulated to produce flowers with unusual colors?

2. How can soybeans be genetically manipulated to increase their lysine content?

3. How can vitamins be overproduced in rice plants?

4. How would you engineer soybean plants to overproduce long-chain omega-3 and omega-6 fatty acids?

5. What is the effect of increasing the level of oxidized glutathione within a plant? How would you genetically manipulate a plant to do this?

6. How can the level of bioavailable iron in plants be increased?

7. How would you increase the amount of amylose compared to amylopectin in potato starch? How would you increase the amount of amylopectin compared to amylose? What is the advantage of performing these manipulations?

8. How does an antigen expressed in a transgenic plant act as an edible vaccine?

9. How would you engineer an edible vaccine directed against *V. cholerae*-caused diarrhea?

10. How can a plant's oxygen levels be manipulated? How does manipulation of a plant's oxygen levels affect the yield of that plant?

11. How would you engineer rice plants to overproduce tetrahydrofolate? Why would you do this?

12. Why is it necessary to genetically engineer soybean plants to have a small amount of phytate in their seeds when low-phytate mutants may be selected following conventional mutagenesis?

13. Briefly describe a vector system that may be used to engineer plants to produce large amounts of full-size IgG molecules.

14. Why are plants an attractive host system, compared to bacteria and animal cells in culture, for the production of human therapeutic proteins?

15. What is phytate? How can the levels of phytate in seeds be modulated? Why would you want to do this?

16. Describe a strategy for developing a plant vaccine against type 2 Shiga toxin.

17. How can the lignin content of trees be decreased? What is the benefit of this type of genetic manipulation?

18. How can manipulation of the level of brassinosteroids be used to increase plant yield?

19. How can plants be genetically modified to increase their effectiveness in the phytoremediation of certain metals?

Transgenic Animals

W HEN TRADITIONAL BREEDING METHODS ARE USED, many generations of selective matings are required to improve livestock and other domesticated animals genetically for traits such as milk yield, wool characteristics, rate of weight gain, and egg-laying frequency. At each successive generation, animals with superior performance characteristics are used as breeding stock. Eventually, high-production animals are developed as more or less pure breeding lines. This combination of mating and selection, although time-consuming and costly, has been exceptionally successful. Today, almost all aspects of the biological basis of livestock production can be attributed to this process. However, once an effective genetic line has been established, it becomes difficult to introduce new genetic traits by selective-breeding methods. For example, a strain with a newly discovered, valuable gene may also carry deleterious genes that, after crossing, would diminish the existing genetically determined production levels. Thus, a completely new program of multigenerational crosses with rigorous selection procedures has to be initiated to ensure that a new breeding line retains both its original attributes and the new trait.

Until recently, selective breeding was the only way to enhance the genetic features of domesticated animals. However, the combination of the successful transfer of genes into mammalian cells and the possibility of creating genetically identical animals by transplanting nuclei from somatic cells into enucleated eggs (nuclear transfer, or nuclear cloning) led researchers to consider putting single functional genes or gene clusters into the chromosomal DNA of higher organisms. Conceptually, the strategy used to achieve this end is simple. (1) A cloned gene is injected into the nucleus of a fertilized egg. (2) The inoculated fertilized eggs are implanted into a receptive female because successful completion of mammalian embryonic development is not possible outside of a female. (3) Some of the offspring derived from the implanted eggs carry the cloned gene in all of their cells. (4) Animals with the cloned gene integrated in their germ line cells are bred to establish new genetic lines.

TABLE 21.1 Protein compositions of milk from cattle and sheep

Protein	Concentration (g/liter) in milk from:	
	Cattle	Sheep
Caseins		
α$_{s1}$-Casein	10.0	12.0
α$_{s2}$-Casein	3.4	3.8
κ-Casein	3.9	4.6
β-Casein	10.0	16.0
Major whey proteins		
α-Lactalbumin	1.0	0.8
β-Lactalbumin	3.0	2.8
Other proteins		
Serum albumin	0.4	Unknown
Lysozyme	Trace	Unknown
Lactoferrin	0.1	Unknown
Immunoglobulins	0.7	Unknown

This approach has many practical applications. If, for example, the product of the injected gene stimulates growth, animals that acquire this gene should grow faster and require less feed. An enhancement of feed efficiency by a few percent would have a profound impact on lowering the cost of production of either beef or pork.

During the 1980s, with considerable effort, the idea of genetically manipulating animals by introducing genes into fertilized eggs was converted into reality. As with many new scientific enterprises, a set of terms was created to make communication easier. For example, an animal whose genetic composition has been altered by the addition of foreign (exogenous) DNA is said to be transgenic. The DNA that is introduced is called a transgene, and the overall process is called transgenic technology, or transgenesis.

The genetic improvement of animals by the introduction of relevant transgenes is only slowly being realized. In the meantime, however, transgenesis has become a powerful technique for studying fundamental problems of mammalian gene expression and development, for establishing animal model systems for studying human diseases, for producing foreign proteins in bird eggs, and for using the mammary gland to produce pharmaceutically important proteins in milk. With this last application in mind, the term "pharming" was coined to convey the idea that milk from transgenic farm ("pharm") animals can be a source of authentic human protein drugs or pharmaceuticals. There are a number of reasons why the mammary gland should be used in this way. Milk is a renewable, secreted body fluid that is produced in substantial quantities and can be collected frequently without harm to the animal. A novel drug protein that is confined to the mammary gland and secreted into milk should have no side effects on the normal physiological processes of the transgenic animal and should undergo posttranslational modifications that at least closely match those in humans. Finally, purification of a protein from milk, which contains only a small number of different proteins (Table 21.1), should be relatively straightforward.

FIGURE 21.1 Establishing transgenic mice with retroviral vectors. Cleavage stage embryos, usually at the eight-cell stage, are infected with a defective retrovirus carrying a transgene. Implanted females (foster mothers) give birth to transgenic pups. Matings are carried out to determine which pups have the transgene in their germ line cells. Transgenic lines can be established from these founder transgenic animals.

Transgenic Mice: Methodology

Transgenic technology has been developed and perfected in the laboratory mouse. Since the early 1980s, hundreds of different genes have been introduced into various mouse strains. These studies have contributed to an understanding of gene regulation, tumor development, immunological specificity, molecular genetics of development, and many other biological processes of fundamental interest. Transgenic mice have also played a role in examining the feasibility of the industrial production of human therapeutic drugs by domesticated animals and in the creation of transgenic

strains that act as biomedical models for various human genetic diseases. For transgenesis, DNA can be introduced into mice by (1) retroviral vectors that infect the cells of an early-stage embryo prior to implantation into a receptive female, (2) microinjection into the enlarged sperm nucleus (male pronucleus) of a fertilized egg, or (3) introduction of genetically engineered embryonic stem cells into an early-stage developing embryo before implantation into a receptive female.

The Retroviral Vector Method

Of the various gene transfer methods, the use of retroviral vectors (Fig. 21.1) has the advantage of being an effective means of integrating the transgene into the genome of a recipient cell. Retroviruses have RNA genomes that are used as templates for reverse transcriptase to synthesize a DNA copy that can be inserted into the host cell genome (see chapter 11). However, vectors derived from these viruses can transfer only small pieces (~8 kilobases [kb]) of DNA that, because of the size constraint, may lack essential adjacent sequences for regulating the expression of the transgene.

There is a further major drawback to the use of retroviral vectors. Although these vectors are designed to be replication defective, the genome of the retroviral strain (helper virus) that is needed to create large quantities of the vector DNA can be integrated into the same nucleus as the transgene. Despite special precautions, helper strain retroviruses could be produced by the transgenic organism. Consequently, for applications in which either a commercial product is to be synthesized by the transgenic organism or the transgenic organism is to be used as food, it is absolutely necessary that there be no retroviral contamination. In addition, transgenes introduced on some retroviral vectors are silenced in mouse embryos.

Transgenes carried on vectors derived from lentiviruses (Fig. 21.2)—a group of retroviruses that includes human immunodeficiency virus and similar viruses from other animal cells—however, are not silenced in embryos. Moreover, these vectors are capable of delivering large segments of DNA into the host genome, are stable for relatively long periods, have low immunogenicity, and can infect both dividing and nondividing cells.

FIGURE 21.2 A lentiviral transfer vector for introducing transgenes into animal cells. The transgene with an appropriate promoter sequence (*p*) is inserted into the lentiviral vector. The transfer vector is introduced into a packaging cell line that produces the viral proteins required for production of the viral RNA, including the transgene sequence, and for packaging the RNA into viral particles that will be used to deliver the transgene into animal cells. Long terminal repeats (LTR) at the 5' and 3' ends of the vector are required for production of lentiviral RNA, and the packaging signal (Ψ) is required for packaging the RNA into viral particles. Following infection of animal cells with lentivirus, lentiviral RNA is reverse transcribed, and the transgene is integrated into the animal cell genome via sequences in the LTRs. A polypurine tract sequence (PPT) and a woodchuck posttranscriptional regulatory element (WPRE) enhance the transduction of host cells and increase transgene expression in the animal cells. A regulatory element within the 3' LTR is deleted (indicated by a black dot) to prevent the production of vector RNA from a promoter contained within the LTR following introduction into host cells. Expression of the transgene is not affected by the deletion because it is expressed from its own promoter.

5' LTR Ψ PPT *p* Transgene WPRE 3' LTR

Superovulated
female

Female
pronucleus

Male
pronucleus

Fertilized egg

Holding
pipette

Injecting
pipette

Transgene

Fertilized egg

Implanted
female

Transgenic
founder

FIGURE 21.3 Establishing transgenic mice by DNA microinjection. Eggs are obtained from donor females that have been induced to superovulate and then mated with males. Purified samples of the transgene construct are microinjected into the male pronucleus of a fertilized egg. Implanted females (foster mothers) give birth to transgenic pups, from which transgenic lines can be established.

The last characteristic is an advantage for the expression of transgenes in neuronal, muscle, liver, and other nondividing cells. The lentivirus vector system is similar to other retroviral vector systems and is comprised of a transfer vector that carries the transgene and a packaging cell line that provides viral proteins for packaging the viral particles (Fig. 11.16). Lentiviral vectors have been used successfully to introduce a variety of transgenes into embryonic cells or early embryos of mice, pigs, cattle, and birds, and

these genes are highly expressed either ubiquitously or in a tissue-specific manner depending on the promoter used. Lentiviruses are also often used as delivery vehicles to introduce a construct to decrease gene expression in mice and other organisms by RNA interference (RNAi) (see below).

The DNA Microinjection Method

Because of the disadvantages of the retroviral vector method, microinjection of DNA is currently the preferred method for producing transgenic mice. This procedure is performed in the following way (Fig. 21.3). (1) The number of available fertilized eggs that are to be inoculated by microinjection is increased by stimulating donor females to superovulate. Female mice are given an initial injection of pregnant mare's serum and another injection, about 48 hours later, of human chorionic gonadotropin. A superovulated mouse produces about 35 eggs instead of the normal 5 to 10. (2) The superovulated females are mated so that eggs become fertilized, and then they are killed. The fertilized eggs are flushed from their oviducts. (3) Microinjection of the fertilized eggs usually occurs immediately after their collection. The microinjected transgene construct is often in a linear form and free of prokaryotic vector DNA sequences.

In mammals, after entry of the sperm into the egg, both the sperm nucleus (male pronucleus) and female nucleus are separate entities. After the female nucleus completes its meiotic division to become a female pronucleus, nuclear fusion (karyogamy) occurs. The male pronucleus, which tends to be larger than the female pronucleus, can be located by using a dissecting microscope. The egg can then be maneuvered, oriented, and held in place by micromanipulation while the DNA is microinjected. On a good day, several hundred male pronuclei can be inoculated.

After inoculation, 25 to 40 eggs are implanted microsurgically into a foster mother that has been made pseudopregnant by being mated to a vasectomized male. In mice, copulation is the only known way to prepare the uterus for implantation. In this case, because the male mate lacks sperm, none of the eggs of the foster mother are fertilized. The foster mother will deliver pups from the inoculated eggs about 3 weeks after implantation.

For identification of transgenic animals, DNA from a small piece of the tail can be assayed by either Southern blot hybridization or polymerase chain reaction (PCR) for the presence of the transgene. A transgenic mouse can be mated to another mouse to determine if the transgene is in the germ line of the founder animal. Subsequently, progeny can be bred with each other to form pure (homozygous) transgenic lines.

The procedure, although apparently simple, requires the coordination of a number of experimental steps. Even a highly trained practitioner can expect, at best, only 5% of the inoculated eggs to develop into live transgenic animals (Fig. 21.4). None of the steps in the procedure is 100% efficient; consequently, large numbers of microinjected fertilized eggs must be used. Furthermore, with this method, the injected DNA integrates at random sites within the genome, and often multiple copies of the injected DNA are incorporated at one site. Not all of the transgenic pups will have the appropriate characteristic. In some individuals, the transgene may not be expressed because of the site of integration, and in others, the copy number may be excessive and may lead to overexpression, which disrupts the normal physiology of the animal. Despite the overall inefficiency, it has

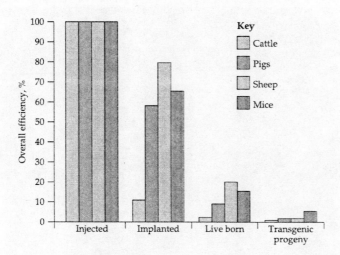

FIGURE 21.4 Overall efficiency of the transgenesis process after DNA microinjection. All the fertilized eggs (100%) of cattle, pigs, sheep, and mice are inoculated with a transgene, but the success of implantation and giving birth to offspring is much lower, and only 5% or fewer of the treated eggs become transgenic progeny.

become routine to use DNA microinjection of the male pronucleus to create lines of mice carrying functional transgenes.

The Engineered Embryonic Stem Cell Method

Cells from the early, blastocyst stage of a developing mouse embryo can proliferate in cell culture and still retain the capability to differentiate into all other cell types—including germ line cells—after they are reintroduced into another blastocyst embryo. Such cells are called pluripotent embryonic stem cells. When in culture, embryonic stem cells can be readily engineered genetically without altering their pluripotency. With this system, for example, a functional transgene can be integrated at a specific site within a dispensable region of the genome of embryonic stem cells. The genetically engineered cells can be selected, grown, and used to generate transgenic animals (Fig. 21.5). In this way, the randomness of integration that is inherent in the DNA microinjection and retroviral vector systems is avoided.

After transfection of embryonic stem cells in culture with a DNA vector that is designed to integrate within a specific chromosomal location, some cells will have DNA integrated at nontarget (spurious) sites, whereas in other cells, integration will occur at the target (correct) site. The target site should be located in a section of genomic DNA that encodes no essential products, so that after integration of the input DNA, there is no interference with any developmental or cellular functions. Moreover, it is essential that the transgene be integrated into a part of the genome that does not prevent it from being transcribed, for example, in euchromatin rather than heterochromatin (see chapter 7). In most of the embryonic stem cells, the input DNA will not be integrated at all. To enrich for the cells with DNA inte-

FIGURE 21.5 Establishing transgenic mice with genetically engineered embryonic stem (ES) cells. An embryonic stem cell culture is initiated from the inner cell mass of a mouse blastocyst. The embryonic stem cells are transfected with a transgene. After growth, the transfected cells are identified by either the positive-negative selection procedure or PCR analysis. Populations of transfected cells can be cultured and inserted into blastocysts, which are then implanted into foster mothers. Transgenic lines can be established by crosses from founder mice that carry the transgene in their germ lines.

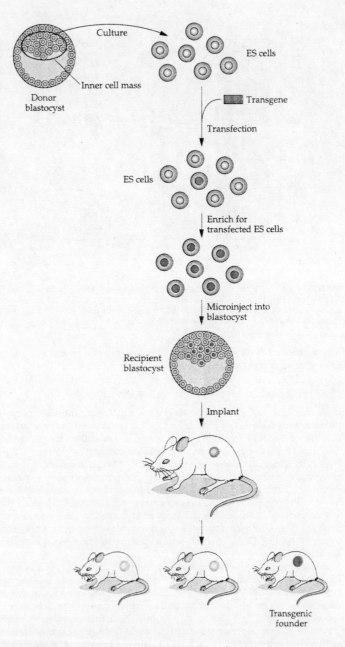

grated at the target site, a procedure called positive-negative selection is implemented. This strategy uses positive selection for cells that have vector DNA integrated anywhere in their genomes and negative selection against the vector DNA sequence that is integrated at spurious sites.

A targeting DNA vector for the positive-negative selection procedure usually contains (1) two blocks of DNA sequences (HB1 and HB2) that are homologous to separate regions of the target site; (2) the transgene, which will confer a new function on the recipient; (3) a DNA sequence that codes for resistance to the compound G-418 (Neor); and (4) two different genes for thymidine kinase *(tk1* and *tk2)* from herpes simplex virus types 1 and 2 (HSV-*tk1* and HSV-*tk2*) (Fig. 21.6A). The arrangement of these sequences is key to the positive-negative selection procedure. Between the two blocks of DNA that are homologous to the target site are the genes for the transgene and G-418 resistance (Neor gene). Outside of each of the homologous blocks are the genes HSV-*tk1* and HSV-*tk2*. If integration occurs at a spurious site, i.e., not at HB1 and HB2, either one or both of the HSV-*tk* genes have a high probability of being integrated along with the other sequences (Fig. 21.6A).

FIGURE 21.6 Positive–negative selection. **(A)** Result of nonspecific integration. Both genes for thymidine kinase *(tk1* and *tk2)*, the two DNA sequences that are homologous to a specific chromosomal region in the recipient cells (HB1 and HB2), a gene (Neor) that confers resistance to the cytotoxic compound G-418, and the transgene (TG) are incorporated into the chromosome. After transfection, cells are selected for resistance to both G-418 and the compound ganciclovir, which becomes cytotoxic to cells that synthesize thymidine kinase. Other nonhomologous integrations may occur and produce inserts with one or the other of the thymidine kinase genes. After treatment with G-418 and ganciclovir, all the cells with nonspecific integration of the input DNA that includes at least one of the thymidine kinase genes are killed. **(B)** Result of homologous recombination. The product of a double crossover between homologous blocks (HB1 and HB2) of DNA on the vector DNA and on chromosomal DNA does not contain either of the two thymidine kinase genes *(tk1* and *tk2)*. After treatment with G-418 and ganciclovir, only cells that have undergone homologous recombination survive.

A

B

Alternatively, if the integration event is due to homologous recombination by a double crossover at the target site, the HSV-*tk* genes are excluded and only the transgene and the Neo^r gene are incorporated into the genome (Fig. 21.6B). When transfected cells are grown in the presence of G-418, all the cells that lack the Neo^r gene are killed. Therefore, only cells with integrated DNA survive; i.e., these cells are positively selected. If the compound ganciclovir is added at the same time as G-418, the cells that express thymidine kinase are killed because thymidine kinase converts ganciclovir to toxic compounds that kill cells; i.e., these cells are negatively selected. The cells most likely to survive this dual-selection scheme are those that have DNA integrated at the target site. Although not foolproof, the positive-negative selection method enriches an embryonic stem cell population for cells that carry a transgene at a specific chromosomal location.

A more direct way to detect embryonic stem cells that carry a transgene at a targeted chromosomal site is to use PCR. The targeting DNA vector contains two blocks of DNA that are homologous to the target site, with one on either side of both the transgene and a cloned bacterial or synthetic (unique) DNA sequence that is not present in the mouse genome (Fig. 21.7). After the transfection of embryonic stem cells, the cells are pooled and samples are screened by PCR. One of the primers (P1) for PCR is complementary to a sequence within the cloned bacterial or synthetic (unique) DNA sequence of the integrating vector. The other primer (P2) is comple-

FIGURE 21.7 Testing for nonspecific integration and homologous recombination in transfected cells by PCR. **(A)** After nonspecific integration of the vector DNA, one of the primers (P2) is not able to hybridize to a chromosomal site that is a predetermined distance from the site of hybridization of P1, so a DNA fragment with a specific size is not amplified. P1 hybridizes to a unique segment (US) of the input DNA that does not occur in the chromosomal DNA of the recipient cells. TG, transgene; HB1 and HB2, homologous blocks. **(B)** Homologous recombination between DNA sequences (HB1 and HB2) of the input DNA that are complementary to chromosomal sites (CS1 and CS2) creates hybridization regions for both P1 and P2 that are a predetermined distance apart. Amplification by PCR generates a DNA fragment of a specific size that can be visualized by gel electrophoresis. In this case, the transgene (TG), which lies between the homologous blocks (HB1 and HB2), is integrated at a specific chromosomal location.

mentary to a DNA sequence that is part of the chromosome adjacent to the region of one of the homologous blocks of DNA. If integration is at a random site, the predicted amplified DNA product is not synthesized (Fig. 21.7A). However, if site-specific integration occurs, the PCR amplifies a DNA fragment of known size (Fig. 21.7B). In this way, pools of cells with embryonic stem cells containing the desired gene at the targeted site can be identified. By subculturing from these pools, cell lines carrying the site-specific integration can be established.

Embryonic stem cells carrying an integrated transgene can be cultured and inserted into blastocyst stage embryos, and these embryos can then be implanted into pseudopregnant foster mothers. Transgenic lines are established by mating the progeny that carry the transgene in their germ lines. Then, if required, littermates that carry a transgene in their germ lines are crossed to produce mice that are homozygous for the transgene.

Not only can a transgene be inserted into a specific chromosome site by homologous recombination in embryonic stem cells to provide a new function, but a specific mouse gene can also be targeted for disruption by the incorporation of a DNA sequence, usually a selectable marker gene, into its coding region (Fig. 21.8). One of the aims of targeted gene disruption (gene knockout) is to determine the developmental and physiological consequences of inactivating a particular gene. In addition, a transgenic line with a specific disabled gene can be used as a model system to study the molecular pathology of a human disease.

For example, inactivation of the mouse rhodopsin gene by targeted gene disruption leads to deterioration of the rod cells of the retina in transgenic mice that closely resembles the human disease retinitis pigmentosa. Thus, the progress of retinal degeneration and the effects of potential therapeutic agents that either delay or block the genetically induced retinopathy have been studied by using the rhodopsin knockout mouse. Hundreds of different types of knockout mice have been created as animal models for the study of various human abnormalities.

FIGURE 21.8 Gene disruption by targeted homologous recombination. The target vector carries a selectable marker gene (SMG) with flanking DNA sequences that are homologous to regions of the targeted gene. In this example, the targeted gene has five exons (1 to 5). Homologous recombination disrupts (i.e., knocks out) the targeted gene. *p*, promoter; *pa*, polyadenylation signal.

FIGURE 21.9 A *loxP* site with the repeats in the opposite (**A**) and same (**B**) orientation. The arrows indicate the directions of the repeat sequences.

Genetic Modification with the Cre–*loxP* Recombination System

Transgenic mice usually carry a transgene or gene modification (knockout gene) in all of their cells. However, it is helpful to have a process that selectively regulates the expression of a gene within a specific somatic tissue or cell type. The Cre–*loxP* recombination system, which is derived from genetic elements of bacteriophage P1, has been adapted for this purpose.

Bacteriophage P1 is one of several tailed viruses that infect *Escherichia coli*. It has a double-stranded DNA genome that is about 100 kb in length. After introduction into *E. coli*, the linear P1 genome forms a circle. The circularized P1 DNA acts as a template for replication, and depending on which set of genes is activated, the circular form is either maintained as a plasmid or used as a template for the production of viral genomes during the lytic cycle. On rare occasions, a circularized P1 genome integrates into the *E. coli* chromosome. Circularization and integration of the P1 genome are mediated by the product of the *cre* gene (circularization recombination [Cre recombinase] protein), which specifically cleaves and recombines the DNA of *loxP* (locus of crossing over [x] in P1) sites.

A *loxP* site consists of two 13-base-pair (bp) inverted repeats that are separated from each other by an 8-bp spacer sequence (Fig. 21.9). Briefly, Cre–*loxP* recombination entails the coming together of two remote *loxP* sites, each of which has two bound Cre recombinase molecules; cleavage by the Cre recombinase within the spacer regions between the repeat sequences; and the exchange and joining of DNA strands to form recombined DNA molecules. The outcome of the recombination event depends on the orientation of the repeats of the *loxP* sites (Fig. 21.10). If the repeats are in opposite directions, then the exchange inverts the DNA between the two *loxP* sites (Fig. 21.10A). If the repeats are in the same orientation, then the intervening sequence is excised (Fig. 21.10B). The repeat elements of bacteriophage P1 are naturally in opposite orientations. The Cre–*loxP* recombination system can function when the *loxP* sites are widely separated. For example, the two *loxP* sites that are essential for circularization of a P1 genome are about 100 kb apart. The specificity of the Cre–*loxP* system is absolute, because the Cre recombinase acts exclusively on *loxP* sites.

On the basis of these features, the Cre–*loxP* system was developed for producing cell-specific gene modifications in mouse cells. As a first step in the overall strategy, the *cre* gene is isolated and placed under the control of a cell-specific promoter. Transgenic mice with the *cre* gene construct are established, and the tissue specificity of the Cre activity is confirmed. Next, a *loxP* site with repeat sequences in the same direction is inserted on either

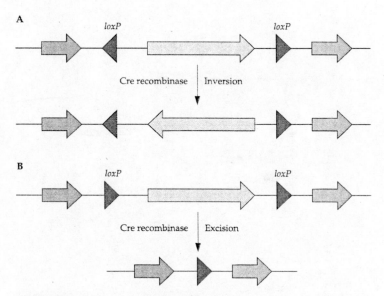

FIGURE 21.10 The outcome of Cre recombinase-mediated recombination depends on the relative orientation of the *loxP* sites. **(A)** Recombination between *loxP* sites in opposite orientations results in inversion of the DNA sequence between the two *loxP* sites. **(B)** Recombination between *loxP* sites in the same orientation results in deletion of the DNA sequence between the two *loxP* sites.

side of a cloned DNA sequence, such as a cloned exon (Fig. 21.11). The construct is integrated into a chromosome site of embryonic stem cells by homologous recombination. These cells are selected, cultured, and used to establish a transgenic mouse line. Then, a transgenic mouse with the tissue-specific *cre* transgene is mated with a transgenic mouse with the integrated *loxP*-flanked sequence. The DNA between the two *loxP* sites is deleted after the *cre* transgene is expressed in double-transgenic organisms (Fig. 21.11). In this way, the biological consequences of the loss of activity of a gene in a specific tissue can be monitored. The Cre–*loxP* recombination system can also be used to activate a transgene in a specific tissue. In this case, the sequence between the *loxP* sites prevents transcription. This construct is inserted between the promoter and the coding sequence of a transgene. When Cre is expressed in mice with the integrated construct, the DNA sequence that blocks transcription is excised, thereby enabling the expression of the transgene (Fig. 21.12). By controlling expression of Cre, for example, by adding an inducer that activates the *cre* promoter to the drinking water of mice, the expression of a transgene can be controlled.

The Cre–*loxP* technology has been used extensively to study the biological consequences of tissue-specific gene inactivation with the goal of establishing models for human diseases. For example, selective removal of the kinesin II gene, which is expressed exclusively in retinal photoreceptor cells, leads to an accumulation of opsin and arrestin and eventually to cell death. This result mimics aspects of inherited retinitis pigmentosa in humans and is used for detailed studies of the pathophysiological effects on the retina.

FIGURE 21.11 Cre–*loxP* recombination system for inactivating a gene in a specified cell type. (1) The *cre* gene is placed under the control of a cell-specific promoter (p^{cs}) and established as a transgene in a line of mice. (2) A *loxP* site is cloned on either side of an exon. The construct with the *loxP* sites is introduced into a chromosomal site of embryonic stem cells by homologous recombination, and a transgenic mouse line is established with these cells. The two transgenic lines are crossed. *p*, promoter. (3) In cells where both constructs are present, the Cre recombinase (beige circle) is synthesized, and two Cre molecules bind to each *loxP* site (dashed arrow). (4) The *loxP* sites undergo recombination (×), leading to the excision and circularization of a *loxP* site and an exon (Exon 2) that is eventually degraded and the formation of an inactivated gene that is retained in the chromosome. The right-angled arrow denotes transcription.

Large chromosomal aberrations, such as deletions, can also be created with the Cre–*loxP* system. In humans, a large deletion within chromosome 22 is associated with DiGeorge syndrome (DGS), which has cardiovascular dysfunction as a significant characteristic. It is not known whether DGS is due to the loss of a large number of genes or a few major ones. To determine the basis of DGS, a large deletion of the mouse chromosome that is comparable (syntenic) to human chromosome 22 was generated with the Cre–*loxP* excision strategy. The mice with this deletion had symptoms that resemble DGS. Moreover, when a transgene for a cardiovascular-specific transcription factor from this region was introduced into these mice, the DGS-like effects were partially overcome, which suggests that the loss of this gene in humans plays a key role in DGS.

FIGURE 21.12 Cre–*loxP* recombination system for activating a transgene in a specified cell type. (1) The *cre* gene is placed under the control of a cell-specific promoter (p^{cs}) and established as a transgene in a line of mice. (2) A piece of DNA with *loxP* sites that flank a transcription termination sequence (hatched box) is cloned between a promoter *(p)* and the first exon (Exon 1) of a gene. (3) The construct with the *loxP* sites is introduced into a chromosomal site of embryonic stem cells by homologous recombination, and a transgenic mouse line is established with these cells. The two transgenic lines are crossed. In cells where both constructs are present, the Cre recombinase (beige circle) is synthesized, and two Cre molecules bind to each *loxP* site (dashed arrow). (4) The *loxP* sites undergo recombination (×), leading to the excision and circularization of a *loxP* site and a transcription termination sequence that is eventually degraded and the formation of a transcriptionally active transgene that is retained in the chromosome. The right-angled arrows denote transcription, and the parallel vertical bars indicate termination of transcription.

RNA Interference

There are two main methods to silence gene expression in animal cells to study biological processes. One method abolishes expression of a gene by targeted disruption through homologous recombination in embryonic stem cells (knockout method), and the other decreases the expression of a target gene (knockdown method) by preventing messenger RNA (mRNA) translation using RNAi. The latter method exploits a natural mechanism for regulation of gene expression by endogenous RNA molecules in animals and plants and for protecting cells against exogenous RNA molecules

from invading viruses. In RNAi, double-stranded RNA is recognized by a ribonuclease (RNase) called Dicer that cleaves the RNA into smaller double-stranded RNA molecules known as small interfering RNA (siRNA). A large nuclease complex called RISC (RNA-induced silencing complex) separates the strands of siRNA, and the single-stranded RNA products, together with RISC, bind to homologous sequences on mRNA molecules (Fig. 11.13). The nuclease component of RISC then degrades the mRNA, which prevents the encoded protein from being synthesized. Short endogenous RNAs (micro-RNAs) transcribed from regions of the genomes of animals (and plants) are also recognized by Dicer and RISC and block translation of a target mRNA.

To create transgenic mice with reduced expression of a target gene, a small region of the target sequence is cloned into a vector as an inverted repeat separated by a short spacer region. The RNA transcript that is produced from this sequence forms a short (19- to 21-bp) hairpin RNA (small [or short] hairpin RNA [shRNA]) due to intramolecular basepairing (Fig. 21.13). Shorter sequences are used to avoid a general downregulation of translation that is often elicited with longer sequences (thought to occur as part of the viral defense response). The construct is introduced into mouse embryonic stem cells by pronuclear injection or on a lentiviral vector. Stable mouse lines have been generated that produce an shRNA that is processed by the animal's Dicer and RISC proteins into siRNA to reduce the expression of a target gene. This technique has been applied to a variety of animals, including cows, pigs, goats, frogs, and rats.

FIGURE 21.13 RNAi to knock down expression of a target gene in transgenic mice. A transgenic construct encoding an shRNA to target specific mRNA for degradation and a green fluorescent protein marker *(gfp)*, each under the control of its own promoter *(p)* (the direction of transcription is indicated by black arrows), is introduced into mouse embryonic stem cells by pronuclear injection or on a lentiviral vector. Transgenic mice are identified by production of green fluorescent protein (GFP). Transcription of the transgene encoding short inverted repeats (blue arrows) separated by a spacer sequence yields an shRNA that is processed by the host cell Dicer and RISC proteins to reduce expression of a target gene.

FIGURE 21.14 Conditional knockdown of target gene expression using RNAi. A blocking sequence, flanked by *loxP* sites in the same orientation, is inserted between the sequence encoding the shRNA and the promoter that controls expression of the hairpin RNA *(p)*. Cre recombinase-mediated recombination between *loxP* sites excises the blocking sequence and restores expression of the hairpin RNA.

In cases in which reduced expression of a target gene might impair the growth and development of the animal, the timing of expression of the shRNA can be controlled. For conditional knockdown, a blocking sequence is inserted into the vector between the sequence encoding the shRNA and the promoter that controls expression of the hairpin RNA. The blocking sequence carries a termination signal for RNA polymerase and can also contain a marker gene, such as *gfp*, encoding green fluorescent protein under the control of its own promoter. The blocking sequence is flanked by two *loxP* sites in the same orientation and therefore is excised following the induction of Cre recombinase. Excision of the blocking sequence restores expression of the hairpin RNA (Fig. 21.14) and downregulation of the target gene in the mouse genome.

Transgenesis with High-Capacity Vectors

Generally, transgenes are complementary DNAs (cDNAs), small genes (less than 20 kb), or parts of genes. Often, cDNAs are poorly expressed in mammalian cells. Also, when a segment of genomic DNA is used for transgenesis, important gene-specific regulatory sequences that lie either upstream or downstream of the gene are rarely retained as part of the insert. Moreover, complete genes and multigene complexes are too large

MILESTONE

Genetic Transformation of Mouse Embryos by Microinjection of Purified DNA
J. W. GORDON, G. A. SCANGOS, D. J. PLOTKIN, J. A. BARBOSA, and F. H. RUDDLE
Proc. Natl. Acad. Sci. USA 77:7380–7384, 1980

Somatic Expression of Herpes Thymidine Kinase in Mice following Injection of a Fusion Gene into Eggs
R. L. BRINSTER, H. Y. CHEN, M. TRUMBAUER, A. W. SENEAR, R. WARREN, and R. D. PALMITER
Cell 27:223–231, 1981

Gordon et al. were the first to show the feasibility of DNA transfer by microinjection into the pronucleus of the mouse egg. In their study, the procedure was tested by microinjecting several hundred eggs with a vector–gene construct that consisted of pBR322 carrying both the HSV thymidine kinase gene and a piece of the simian virus 40 genome. Of the 78 offspring that were obtained from the surrogate mothers, 2 retained some plasmid DNA. The authors concluded, "These data demonstrate that it is possible to use a recombinant plasmid as a vector to transfer foreign genes directly into mouse embryos,

and that these embryos can maintain the foreign genes throughout development." Unfortunately, the plasmid DNA was not intact, and the HSV thymidine kinase sequence did not become a transgene.

On the other hand, Brinster et al., who microinjected the pronuclei of a number of mouse eggs with a plasmid carrying the HSV thymidine kinase gene under the control of the promoter of the metallothionein I gene, found that one of their transgenic mice expressed HSV thymidine kinase at a high level in its liver and kidneys in comparison to three other transgenic mice that produced low levels of

this enzyme. Also, eight other transgenic animals carried the HSV thymidine kinase sequence but did not produce any active HSV thymidine kinase. Southern blot analysis showed that all of the transgenic mice contained multiple copies of the microinjected DNA.

These two studies laid the foundation for transgenesis of mice. Despite the technical complexity and relative inefficiency of the microinjection strategy, it has been exceptionally successful. Currently, scores of strains of mice with either foreign genes (transgenic mice) or endogenous genes that have been disrupted by the insertion of foreign DNA (knockout mice) are being used for studying gene regulation, mammalian development, viral pathogenesis, cancer, toxicology, and the mutagenicities of various agents, among other things. In addition, transgenic and knockout mice are of considerable biomedical importance as model systems for human diseases.

for conventional vectors. For these reasons, high-capacity vectors that carry genomic DNAs ranging in size from 100 to more than 1,000 kb have been developed for transgenesis. These vectors have been derived from bacterial, P1 bacteriophage-derived, mammalian, and yeast (YACs) artificial chromosomes. A number of transgenic mice have been produced by microinjection of the pronucleus of the fertilized egg or transfection of embryonic stem cells with YACs (described in chapter 7) that carry either an array of related genes or a single large gene. These organisms have been used to study developmental processes, as models for human disorders, and for the production of human therapeutic agents.

The production of mice that synthesize only human antibodies is another noteworthy example of YAC transgenesis. In theory, monoclonal antibodies can be effective agents for diminishing the proliferation of cancer cells and as a means of treating other human diseases. However, it is impossible to generate human monoclonal antibodies routinely. Also, unfortunately, rodent monoclonal antibodies are immunogenic to humans and elicit anti-mouse antibodies that result in destruction of the therapeutic antibody and sometimes allergic reactions. Recombinant DNA strategies have been devised to "humanize" existing rodent monoclonal antibodies.

An antibody is a tetrameric protein with two pairs of dissimilar chains. One of the chains is called the heavy chain, and the other is a light chain. The terms "heavy" and "light" refer to the difference in the molecular

masses of the antibody subunits. The genetic information for a specific heavy chain is created by rearrangement of several heavy-chain-specific DNA segments in a B cell (an antibody-producing cell). In addition, there are two different types of antibody light chains that are encoded after DNA rearrangements of other, light-chain-specific DNA segments. Each single B cell synthesizes only one kind of antibody molecule that has a unique set of rearranged segments for a heavy chain and a light chain.

The genetic repertoire for the formation of the vast numbers of different human antibodies consists of more than 100 heavy-chain DNA segments and a similar number of light-chain DNA segments. Each heavy- and light-chain gene locus is about 1 to 1.5 megabases in length. To create a transgenic mouse that is capable of synthesizing a full range of human antibodies against every antigen, the endogenous mouse heavy- and light-chain genes were inactivated, and YACs carrying most of the heavy- and light-chain DNA elements from each human immunoglobulin gene were inserted into the chromosomal DNA of the mouse (Fig. 10.28). A commercialized version of the human antibody-producing mouse has been designated the XenoMouse, and the first fully human monoclonal antibody produced in this mouse (panitumumab) has received regulatory approval for use as a treatment for advanced colorectal cancer. Clinical trials have shown that panitumumab is an effective control agent for colorectal cancer and does not elicit production of anti-panitumumab antibodies. The development of this cancer treatment took approximately 15 years to regulatory approval, including the development of the XenoMouse. Other therapeutic antibodies produced in the XenoMouse, including several for the treatment of various cancers and osteoporosis, are now in clinical trials.

Transgenic Mice: Applications

Transgenic mice can be used as model systems for determining the biological basis of human diseases and devising treatments for various conditions. In addition, transgenesis of mice is an exemplary system for proving whether the production of a potential therapeutic agent is feasible. Whole-animal models simulate both the onset and progression of a human disease. However, a mouse is not a human, even though it is a mammal, and so the information gathered from some transgenic models may not always be medically relevant. In other instances, however, critical insights into the etiology of a complex disease can be gained. With this in mind, mouse models for human genetic diseases, such as Alzheimer disease, amyotrophic lateral sclerosis, Huntington disease, arthritis, muscular dystrophy, tumorigenesis, hypertension, neurodegenerative disorders, endocrinological dysfunction, and coronary disease, as well as many others, have been developed.

Transgenic Disease Models: Alzheimer Disease

Alzheimer disease is a degenerative brain disorder that is characterized by the progressive loss of both abstract thinking and memory and is accompanied by personality change, language disturbances, and a slowing of physical capabilities. Clinical diagnosis of Alzheimer disease is poor, although 1% of the population between 60 and 65 years of age and 30% of the population over 80 years of age may develop it. Neurofibrillary tangles accumulate within the cell bodies of the neurons, dense extracellular aggregates called

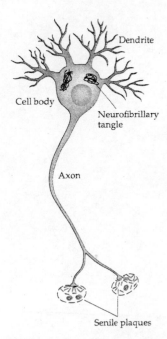

Dendrite

Cell body

Neurofibrillary
tangle

Axon

Senile plaques

FIGURE 21.15 Schematic representation of a neuron of the human cerebral cortex showing some of the histopathological features of Alzheimer disease. Senile plaques containing amyloid deposits and apparent cellular debris accumulate at the synaptic junction of a neuron. Within the cell body of a neuron, neurofibrillary tangles contain aggregated cytoskeletal and other proteins. Other changes that occur in affected neurons are not depicted.

senile plaques develop at the ends of inflamed nerves (neuritis), and brain cells (neurons) are lost in the neocortex and hippocampus of the brain in patients with Alzheimer disease (Fig. 21.15). The core of a senile plaque is composed of a closely packed, fibrillar structure that traditionally has been called an amyloid body. Originally, amyloid bodies were thought to be made up of carbohydrates, but more definitive analysis established that they are protein aggregates. However, despite the misnomer, the term "amyloid" has been retained.

The principal protein of Alzheimer disease amyloid bodies is a 4-kilodalton protein called Aβ (amyloid β, β-protein, β-amyloid protein, or β/A4). The Aβ protein ranges in length from 39 to 42 amino acid residues; the Aβ40 and Aβ42 forms are the main variants. All Aβ proteins are derived from an internal proteolytic cleavage of the β-amyloid precursor protein (APP). Faulty cleavage of the APP protein causes the production of Aβ40 and Aβ42, and inefficient clearance of the variants likely leads to their accumulation. A small number of families with a high incidence of Alzheimer disease have mutations in the *APP* gene, a finding that implicates this gene in the disorder. Unfortunately, for the most part, it is impossible to study the onset and pathogenesis of Alzheimer disease in human subjects. Accordingly, an animal model that mimics Alzheimer disease is an invaluable research tool.

Mouse models for Alzheimer disease were created with transgenes that contain mutations in the *APP* gene that occur in some families with a high incidence of early onset (before 50 years of age) of Alzheimer disease. In one set of these families, site 717 of APP (APP-717) contains phenylalanine instead of valine. In another group of families with Alzheimer disease, sites 670 and 671 of APP (APP-670/671) contain asparagine and leucine instead of lysine and methionine.

A transgene with the APP-717 mutation was constructed from an *APP* cDNA. Modified introns were added between exons 6 and 7, 7 and 8, and 8 and 9 of the *APP* cDNA. The introns were introduced into the *APP* cDNA because experiments have shown that transgenes with introns have an increased rate of transcription in comparison to constructs without them. The "*APP* cDNA–intron" construct is controlled by the platelet-derived growth factor β promoter that is expressed in brain tissue (Fig. 21.16). The complete construct is called the *PDAPP* minigene. Aging transgenic mice (more than 6 months old) with about 40 copies of the *PDAPP* minigene display amyloid plaques, neuronal cell death, and memory defects. An *APP-670/671* gene construct that is driven by a brain-specific promoter also produces transgenic mice with Alzheimer disease-like features, including an excess of Aβ42. Interestingly, neither aging *PDAPP* minigene mice nor *APP-670/671* transgenic mice have neurofibrillary tangles. Possibly, these structures are a secondary response to the overproduction of Aβ42 in humans.

The formation of amyloid plaques in humans has also been shown to be associated with increased production of the protein BACE1 (β-site APP-cleaving enzyme 1), one of the proteases that cleaves APP to produce Aβ. Transgenic mice that produce Aβ but also carry a knockout mutation in *BACE1* do not develop Aβ amyloid plaques. However, BACE1 knockout mice exhibit deleterious behavioral defects, which indicates that some BACE1 is required for normal development and/or normal adult brain activity. RNAi to reduce, but not abolish, production of BACE1 may therefore represent an attractive treatment to reduce or delay Alzheimer disease.

FIGURE 21.16 DNA construct for modeling Alzheimer disease in transgenic mice. The exons of the *APP* cDNA are marked by numbers (1 to 18), and the introduced introns are indicated by letters (A to C). The regulatory sequences are the platelet-derived growth factor β (PDGF-β) promoter and simian virus 40 poly(A) sequence. The dot marks the exon with the APP-717 mutation. The construct is called the *PDAPP* minigene.

This strategy is currently being tested in mouse models using mice that carry transgenes encoding mutant forms of APP that are genetically linked to familial Alzheimer disease in humans. shRNAs that target *BACE1* mRNA were carried on a lentiviral vector that was injected into the hippocampus (the region of the brain where amyloid plaques associated with Alzheimer disease are typically observed) in transgenic mice (Fig. 21.17). The mice injected with the RNAi construct showed a 38% reduction in the Aβ deposits and plaque formation within 1 month of injection. While there is much to learn about Alzheimer disease, the availability of animal models has helped to elucidate the molecular basis, and revealed some potential targets for treatment, of a disorder that affects about 4 million people in the United States at an annual cost of around $100 billion.

Using Transgenic Mice as Test Systems

The testing of RNAi in transgenic mice as a potential therapy to reduce levels of proteins that contribute to Alzheimer disease is one of many examples of the utility of transgenic laboratory animals in testing strategies to treat human genetic diseases. Transgenic mice have also been used to test the efficacy of strategies to protect animals against infectious diseases. One recent illustration is the development of transgenic mouse lines that express a soluble form of a porcine membrane receptor that could protect pigs against pseudorabies virus infection.

Pseudorabies virus is an alphaherpesvirus that infects pigs and causes major economic losses to pig producers. Viral infection can result in encephalitis and respiratory illness in young pigs and abortion and infertility in sows. Although vaccines are available and provide some protection, pseudorabies remains endemic in most regions of the world. An alternative approach has been proposed to produce transgenic pigs that resist pseudorabies virus infection or block replication of the pseudorabies

FIGURE 21.17 Lentiviral vector to knock down BACE1 expression in mouse models of Alzheimer disease. A sequence encoding the inverted repeats (blue arrows) of an shRNA targeting *BACE1* mRNA was inserted into the lentiviral vector downstream of the mouse RNA polymerase III promoter (p^{U6}). The gene for green fluorescent protein (*gfp*) under the control of the cytomegalovirus promoter (p^{CMV}) is used as a reporter gene to identify infected mouse cells. LTR, long terminal repeat (at the 5′ and 3′ ends of the vector); Ψ, viral packaging signal; PPT, polypurine tract sequence; WPRE, woodchuck posttranscriptional regulatory element for enhancing transduction and expression of the transgene in host cells.

virus genome. One proposed strategy is to block the entry of the virus into host cells by expressing a soluble form of the host cell receptor to which the virus normally attaches. It was hypothesized that expression of a soluble form of the receptor would prevent the virus from binding to the host membrane-bound receptor, the step that precedes viral penetration of the host cell. Several porcine alphaherpesvirus receptors were identified, and one promising receptor, nectin-1, provided protection to transformed cell lines challenged with the pseudorabies virus and exhibited broad specificity against alphaherpesviruses. Before the creation of transgenic farm animals, nectin-1 was tested for its ability to protect against pseudorabies infection in a mouse model.

The DNA sequence encoding the extracellular domain of the nectin-1 receptor was fused to the gene for the constant (Fc) region of human immunoglobulin G (IgG) and placed under the control of a promoter that enabled expression of the fusion protein in several cell types (Fig. 21.18). The fusion construct was designed to produce a secreted form of the nectin-1 receptor with enhanced stability and immunogenicity that would promote removal of the virus by the host immune system. When transgenic mice expressing the fusion protein were exposed to pseudorabies virus at 20 times the dose normally required to kill 50% of the animals, through intraperitoneal injection, 98% survived, in contrast to less than 10% of nontransgenic mice. Moreover, antibodies against the virus were not detected in the transgenic mice, which indicated that they were not infected. A similar level of protection was observed when the pseudorabies virus was inoculated through the nasal passage, which is the normal route of exposure in pigs; the epithelial cells lining the nasal passage and respiratory tract produced the nectin-1–IgG fusion protein. These results demonstrate that expression of a secreted form of the pseudorabies receptor in transgenic mice can protect the animals against viral infection. Nectin-1 is known to play a role in several important cell functions; however, transgenic mice expressing the protein appeared normal. Although expression of the porcine receptor in transgenic mice provided effective protection against the virus, it remains to be seen if the same level of protection is provided by expression of the soluble form of the receptor protein in pigs.

Conditional Regulation of Transgene Expression

Various protocols have been devised for turning on and off the expression of a transgene in a specific cell type at will. Of these methods, the tetracy-

FIGURE 21.18 Construct used to generate transgenic mice protected against pseudorabies virus infection. The extracellular domain of the porcine nectin-1 receptor was fused to the constant region of the human IgG protein (IgG-Fc) to create a stable, soluble form of the receptor that, when expressed in transgenic animals, would prevent entry of the pseudorabies virus into host cells. The cDNA sequence encoding this fusion protein was expressed under the control of the CAG promoter (p^{CAG}), which includes the chicken β-actin promoter and the cytomegalovirus enhancer sequence. The polyadenylation signal (pA) from the rabbit β-globin gene was also included at the 3′ end of the construct. The DNA fragment was microinjected into mouse eggs to generate transgenic founder mice. Adapted from Ono et al., *Proc. Natl. Acad. Sci.* **101:**16150-16155, 2004.

| p^{CAG} | Nectin-1 extracellular domain | IgG-Fc | pA |

cline-inducible system has been used extensively. This system is based on two transcription units in the same cell, with the product of one of the units determining the expression of a gene(s) of the other unit. In one form of the tetracycline-inducible system, the addition of doxycycline, a nontoxic analogue of tetracycline, turns off the expression of a transgene. Without doxycycline, the transgene is continuously expressed in a specific cell type. This "tet-off" system depends on the production of a chimeric (hybrid) protein composed of the tetracycline repressor and an amino acid sequence that activates the transcription process. The hybrid protein is called tetracycline-controlled transactivator (tetracycline transactivator, or tTA). The gene (*tTA*) that encodes tTA is under the control of a cell-specific promoter. The promoter that drives the transgene consists of a set of tetracycline operator (*tetO*) sequences upstream from a strong eukaryotic promoter. The tTA protein binds to the *tetO* region and activates the transcription of the transgene. The binding of the tTA protein to the *tetO*–promoter region is absolutely required for the initiation of transcription. On the other hand, when doxycycline is present, it binds to the tTA protein, and the doxycycline–tTA complex cannot bind to the *tetO*–promoter sequence, so transcription of the transgene does not occur. Thus, the presence or absence of doxycycline acts as a switch whenever and wherever the cell-specific promoter of the *tTA* gene is active (Fig. 21.19A).

A reverse system, called "tet-on," in which doxycycline must be present for transcription of the transgene, has also been devised. In this form, the nucleotide sequence for the tetracycline repressor carries mutations that prevent the combined repressor protein and transactivator from binding to the *tetO*–promoter sequence. This tetracycline repressor/transactivator protein is designated rtTA (reverse tetracycline-controlled transactivator). However, doxycycline binds to rtTA and changes its configuration, which allows the complex to attach to the *tetO*–promoter sequence and initiate transcription of the transgene (Fig. 21.19B).

Both transcription units of a tetracycline-regulatory system can be incorporated into a single plasmid; this reduces the number of steps that are required for the production of transgenic mice. Doxycycline is administered by adding it to the drinking water of the mice. The tet-off and tet-on systems have innumerable uses. For example, the biological consequences of the production of a defective protein or overexpression of a normal protein can be examined in detail, cell-specific disease conditions can be simulated, and gene-based treatments for diseases that affect a particular cell type can be tested.

A fascinating example of the utility of the tetracycline-regulatory system is the development of a mouse model for Huntington disease, a disease that normally occurs only in humans. This incurable, fatal neurological disorder affects about 1 in 10,000 people worldwide. The symptoms in most cases become evident when the patient is about 45 years old. Initially, muscle coordination is impaired. The disorder is progressive and unremitting. Eventually, both voluntary and involuntary movements become uncontrolled, speech is slurred, and severe psychiatric conditions appear. In the late stage of Huntington disease, the patients are mute, cognitively nonfunctional, and immobilized. The disease often lasts about 15 years from the time of onset. The neurological damage is confined to specific regions of the brain. At the genetic level, the alteration that is responsible for Huntington disease is the addition of CAG units to an existing sequential array of these trinucleotides in exon 1 of the *HD* gene, which

FIGURE 21.19 Schematic representation of tetracycline-regulated gene expression. **(A)** Tet-off system. The *tTA* gene is driven by a cell-specific promoter (*p*^cs^) and encodes a tetracycline repressor sequence (red) and a transcription activator (blue). The product of the *tTA* gene is a protein (tTA [purple circle]) that binds to a tetracycline operator (*tetO*)–eukaryotic promoter (*p*) sequence and, in the absence of doxycycline (– Dox), activates the transcription of the transgene. When doxycycline is present (+ Dox), it (yellow rectangle) binds to tTA, and the Dox–tTA complex cannot bind to the *tetO*–promoter region, so the transgene is not transcribed. **(B)** Tet-on system. The *rtTA* gene is driven by a cell-specific promoter (*p*^cs^) and encodes a mutated tetracycline repressor sequence (dark yellow) and a transcription activator (blue). The product of the *rtTA* gene is a protein (rtTA [pink circle]) that does not bind to a tetracycline operator (*tetO*)–eukaryotic promoter (*p*) sequence, and in the absence of doxycycline (– Dox), the transgene is not transcribed. When doxycycline is present (+ Dox), it (yellow rectangle) binds to rtTA, and the Dox–rtTA complex attaches to the *tetO*–promoter region and initiates the transcription of the transgene.

encodes the huntingtin protein. A CAG trinucleotide is the codon for glutamine, and during translation, a contiguous set of these codons produces a string of glutamine residues (polyglutamine) in the huntingtin protein. Symptoms of Huntington disease occur when the polyglutamine-coding segment has 38 or more CAG codons.

To create a mouse model for Huntington disease, the tet-off system was used with a variant of the *HD* gene that consists only of exon 1 with 94

FIGURE 21.20 A transgenic mouse model of Huntington disease carrying a mutant form of the *HD* gene encoding the huntingtin protein expressed under the control of the tet-off system. CAG$_{94}$ indicates a sequence of 94 CAG repeats in exon 1 of the mutant *HD* transgene that encode polyglutamine. p^{FB}, forebrain-specific promoter; tTA, tetracycline transactivator; *tetO*, tetracycline operator; *p*, promoter.

CAG repeats as the transgene (Fig. 21.20). The *tTA* gene was placed under the control of a promoter that is active in the cells of the forebrain. Loss of embryos was avoided during pregnancy by adding doxycycline to the drinking water, which turned off the expression of the mutant *HD* gene. At birth, doxycycline was not supplied to the transgenic mice, which allowed continuous expression of the mutant *HD* gene and the production of a protein with a long polyglutamine sequence. A neurological condition that was similar to Huntington disease in humans developed over time in these mice. Interestingly, the features of the disease disappeared when the expression of the mutant *HD* gene was prevented by the addition of doxycycline. Thus, at least in this model, continuous expression of a mutant *HD* gene is required for establishment of the disease, and brain cells can recover when this synthesis ceases.

While mouse models have contributed greatly to our understanding of human diseases, the short life span of the mouse may reduce its utility for the study of slow and progressive diseases, such as Huntington disease, that require observation over a longer time. Transgenic primate models, such as the rhesus macaque, may represent more accurate models for the study of human neurodegenerative diseases. Transgenic macaques were produced that expressed the mutant *HD* gene encoding the huntingtin protein with an expanded polyglutamine sequence. Rhesus oocytes were microinjected with a lentivirus vector containing the *HD* gene with 84 CAG repeats under the control of the human polyubiquitin C promoter. From 30 transplanted embryos, five live monkeys were delivered, and two of these died within 1 day of birth. Although the contribution of the *HD* gene to their deaths cannot be established, postmortem analysis confirmed the presence of multiple copies of the *HD* gene and expression of huntingtin with a polyglutamine sequence. One of the surviving monkeys carries a single copy of the *HD* transgene and at 6 months old showed features of Huntington disease that are found in humans with the disease, including involuntary, jerky body movements (chorea) and muscle contractions (dystonia). The macaques will be used to establish a transgenic line to study the

pathology of Huntington disease and to assess treatment and diagnostic strategies. Therapeutic strategies for Huntington disease will probably be directed toward either blocking the expression of the mutant *HD* gene in those people who test positive for more than 38 CAG repeats or clearing the abnormal protein from the neurons. In either case, the treatment must precisely target the mutant gene or protein, leaving the normal counterparts unaffected.

Conditional Control of Cell Death

The ability to induce cell death at different times and under defined conditions in a specific organ of a living organism is a helpful way to study organ failure caused by cell destruction and to determine how tissues and organs recover from various degrees of cell loss. Transgenic mice have been engineered for this purpose. For example, to examine the effects of liver cell damage, transgenic mice were created to express a receptor that is required for a bacterial toxin to cause cell death. The diphtheria toxin produced by the bacterial pathogen *Corynebacterium diphtheriae* binds to the human heparin-binding epidermal growth factor receptor, and the toxin–receptor complex is taken up into the cell, where it inactivates elongation factor 2 (EF-2). Protein synthesis requires functional EF-2 molecules, and cell death ensues in the absence of protein synthesis (Fig. 21.21). Mouse cells are not normally susceptible to diphtheria toxin because they do not have a receptor that recognizes the bacterial protein; therefore, transgenic mice were engineered to express the human heparin-binding epidermal growth factor receptor under the control of a liver-specific promoter. The transgenic mice were treated with high doses of diphtheria toxin, and severe

FIGURE 21.21 Genetically engineered cell death. **(A)** Cell membrane-localized human heparin-binding epidermal growth factor receptor (HB-EGFr) (brown rectangles) is synthesized in liver cells from an HB-EGFr cDNA transgene under the control of a liver cell-specific promoter (p^{liver}). **(B)** Diphtheria toxin (yellow and blue ovals) binds to HB-EGFr and is taken into the cell. A diphtheria toxin subunit (yellow oval) is released from an endosome and inactivates EF-2. Cell death follows the cessation of protein synthesis.

liver damage occurred; at lower concentrations of the toxin, the extent of liver damage was proportional to the dose of the toxin. There was no uptake of the diphtheria toxin in other mouse tissues. Also, the presence of human heparin-binding epidermal growth factor receptor in the cell membrane of the mouse liver cells had no obvious effects on liver cell functions or other processes in the absence of the diphtheria toxin. These mice are a convenient model for examining the consequences of moderate to severe liver damage due to cell loss. In addition, the effects of selective removal (ablation) of various cell types can be studied in mice by combining the human heparin-binding epidermal growth factor receptor coding sequence with different cell-specific promoters.

Cloning Livestock by Nuclear Transfer

In a highly publicized case, a sheep named Dolly was cloned by transfer of a nucleus from a mammary (udder) cell of an adult sheep into an egg cell. This was the first demonstration of pluripotency (totipotency) of a nucleus of a differentiated adult cell. Since the cloning of Dolly, somatic cell nuclei have been used to clone cattle, goats, sheep, and pigs. In these cases, the nuclear transfer procedures are similar (Fig. 21.22). Briefly, embryonic, fetal, or adult donor cells from a variety of cell types (e.g., mammary epithelial and ovarian cells, fibroblasts, and lymphocytes) are isolated, cultured, and genetically modified using methods described above. Although not always feasible with adult cells, prolonged culture is preferred, because experimenters have additional time to carry out successive genetic alterations, such as inactivating both alleles of a locus or creating multiple gene changes. After a cell line with a specific genetic modification(s) is established, individual donor cells are fused to an enucleated oocyte with short-duration electric pulses. For example, two 2.5-kilovolt/cm pulses for 10 microseconds each are used to fuse adult cattle fibroblasts with enucleated oocytes. The pulses simultaneously induce cell fusion and oocyte activation. Each fused cell is cultured to the blastocyst stage before being transferred into the uterus of a pseudopregnant female. At birth, genotype analysis is used to confirm the presence of the transgene.

Generally, the surviving animals produced by nuclear transfer are healthy. However, there is substantial loss of individuals before and after birth, and some of the cloned animals display abnormalities. Abnormalities, such as increased birth weight, are more prevalent in some livestock animals, for example, in cloned calves and lambs, than in others. One reason that has been postulated to explain this poor survival is the failure of the donor genome to undergo epigenetic reprogramming, that is, the pattern of DNA methylation and histone modification of the original donor cell is inappropriately maintained in the cells of the recipient animal. Because the epigenetic state of DNA controls gene expression, this could seriously impair cellular function. Despite the low efficiency, nuclear transfer has a number of advantages over pronuclear DNA microinjection. With nuclear transfer, site-specific genetic changes are possible; all offspring are transgenic, and small herds of the same sex can be produced within a short time. In contrast, with DNA microinjection, transgene integration occurs at random sites, expression is often constrained because of the chromosome location, unstable tandem arrays are formed, and the establishment of a transgenic line requires a number of generations. For these reasons, much

FIGURE 21.22 Cloning sheep by nuclear transfer. The nucleus of an ovum is removed (dashed arrow) with a pipette. Cells from the mammary epithelium of an adult are grown in culture, and the G_0 (quiescent, nondividing) state is induced by inhibiting cell growth. A G_0 cell and an enucleated ovum are fused, and the renucleated ovum is grown in culture or in ligated oviducts until an early embryonic stage before it is implanted into a foster mother, where development proceeds to term. In the experiment described by Wilmut et al. (1997), 277 enucleated ova were fused with G_0 mammary cells, and 1 of 29 transferred early-stage embryos produced a live lamb.

effort is being devoted to perfecting the cloning of livestock with nuclei from somatic cells.

Transgenic Livestock

There are several reasons for producing transgenic livestock. First, although mice have proven to be useful in biomedical research as models of human diseases and for testing of disease treatments, the physiology, anatomy, and life span of a mouse are different from those of humans. Thus, livestock are often better animals in which to model disease processes, gene regulation, and immune system development. Second, many livestock animals produce large amounts of milk and therefore can be used to produce and secrete large amounts of recombinant proteins and other molecules of pharmaceutical importance. Third, genetic engineering can be used to rapidly and specifically improve livestock traits, such as growth rate, disease resistance, and milk quality.

Conceptually, the methods used to generate transgenic cattle are similar to those used for transgenic mice. The essential steps in a modified mouse transgenesis DNA microinjection protocol (Fig. 21.23) entail (1) collecting oocytes, for example, from slaughterhouse-killed animals; (2) in vitro maturation of oocytes; (3) in vitro fertilization with bull semen; (4) centrifugation of the fertilized eggs to concentrate the yolk, which in normal eggs prevents the male pronuclei from being readily seen under a dissecting microscope; (5) microinjection of input DNA into male pronuclei; (6) in vitro development of embryos; (7) nonsurgical implantation of one embryo into one recipient foster mother in natural estrus; and (8) DNA screening of the offspring for the presence of the transgene.

When this nonsurgical procedure was put to the test for cattle, two transgenic calves were obtained from an initial pool of 2,470 oocytes. This result indicates that the methodology is feasible although inefficient. The poor yield of transgenic calves after DNA microinjection is likely due to the low probability of integration. In addition, time and effort are expended in rearing nontransgenic embryos. To spare this time and effort, small numbers of cells can be taken from a developing embryo prior to implantation and assayed for the transgene using PCR. The loss of these cells does not interfere with normal development. The test will ensure that only embryos carrying the transgene are implanted.

Production of Pharmaceuticals

Much of the research with transgenic livestock has been devoted to developing the mammary glands of these animals as bioreactors for the production of pharmaceutical proteins. This is likely due to the greater economic incentives, public acceptability, and ethical justification associated with using transgenic animals for the production of pharmaceuticals than with production of animals and animal products for human consumption. Recombinant proteins have been produced in the milk of a variety of transgenic mammals.

Transgenic mice are initially used to test whether a specified protein can be secreted into milk. For example, large quantities of the authentic cystic fibrosis transmembrane regulator (CFTR) protein are needed to

FIGURE 21.23 Steps in the development of transgenic cattle.

study its function and to formulate potential therapies for treating cystic fibrosis, a prevalent genetic disease. The primary effect of a faulty *CFTR* gene is an alteration of the protein that normally acts as a chloride channel. As a consequence of the disruption of the proper flow of chloride ions into and out of cells, mucus accumulates in the ducts of several organs, especially the lungs and pancreas. This mucus prevents normal organ function and becomes the site of a bacterial infection that is difficult to control with antibiotics.

The yields of CFTR with conventional in vitro cell expression systems have been low, possibly because of the biological consequences of the accumulation of CFTR in the cell membranes of transfected cells. The detrimental buildup of CFTR in the cell membranes of host cells could be avoided if the cell membranes were shed frequently. With such a system, not only would a heterologous transmembrane protein be associated with the released fragments of plasma membrane, but also, concentrating and purifying the recombinant protein would be relatively straightforward. In fact, during lactation, fat from within the mammary gland cell is encapsulated by plasma membrane, and together they are secreted into milk as a globule.

To test the feasibility of this concept, a full-length CFTR cDNA sequence was cloned into the middle of a defective goat β-casein gene that had a deletion extending from the end of exon 2 to the beginning of exon 7 (Fig. 21.24). The construct retained the promoter and termination sequences of the goat β-casein gene. The CFTR cDNA was cloned into a structural gene to provide introns for enhancing transcription of the transgene. The β-casein gene is actively expressed in mammary glands during lactation, and β-casein is a major milk protein. Transgenic mouse lines carrying the CFTR sequence under the control of the β-casein gene regulatory sequences were established. As predicted, the milk of transgenic females contained the CFTR protein bound to the membranes of fat globules. There were no negative effects on either CFTR-transgenic lactating mothers or pups that were fed milk that contained CFTR. The CFTR protein was glycosylated and readily extracted from the fat-rich fraction of the milk. Many other proteins that are potentially therapeutic for humans have also been synthesized by the mammary gland cells of lactating transgenic mice; however, to obtain large quantities of CFTR, other medically important transmembrane proteins, and various human therapeutic proteins, the transgenic constructs must be incorporated into the genome of a larger mammal, such as a cow, sheep, or goat.

With a method very similar to the one used for producing transgenic mice, and with transgene constructs that have mammary gland-specific

FIGURE 21.24 Goat β-casein gene–CFTR cDNA expression construct. The full-length cDNA for CFTR was cloned between exon 2 (EX2) and exon 7 (EX7) of the goat β-casein gene. The promoter (*p*) and transcription termination (*t*) sequences and exons 1, 8, and 9 (EX1, EX8, and EX9) of the β-casein gene were retained.

promoters driving human gene sequences, investigators have created transgenic sheep, goats, pigs, and rabbits for more than 100 different human proteins that are secreted into milk (Table 21.2). The transgene-derived proteins were glycosylated and had other posttranslational modifications. In many of these cases, the recombinant proteins had biological activities identical to those of proteins from human sources. If the mammary gland is to be used as a bioreactor, dairy cattle, which each annually produce approximately 10,000 liters of milk containing about 35 grams of protein per liter, are likely candidates for transgenesis. More specifically, if a recombinant protein were present at 1 gram per liter of milk and it could be purified with 50% efficiency, the yield from 20 transgenic cows would be about 100 kg per year. Coincidentally, the annual global requirement for protein C, which is used for the prevention of blood clots, is about 100 kg. On the other hand, one transgenic cow would be more than sufficient for the production of the annual world supply of factor IX (plasma thromboplastin component), which is used by hemophiliacs to facilitate blood clotting.

Although the quantity of milk produced by either a sheep or a goat is smaller than that produced by a cow, lactation in sheep and goats yields hundreds of liters of milk per year (Table 21.3). Goats can also be raised to produce milk more rapidly than cows. Recently the U.S. Food and Drug Administration approved the human protein antithrombin produced in goat's milk for use in individuals with a hereditary deficiency in the production of this protein and who are undergoing surgery or giving birth. Antithrombin is a protease inhibitor that acts as an anticlotting factor by inhibiting the activity of thrombin and other coagulation proteases and thereby prevents the excessive formation of blood clots and promotes the clearing of clotting factors. It is also has anti-inflammatory activity. Approximately 1 in 5,000 people is unable to produce this protein naturally, which puts them at risk for heart attacks and strokes. While antithrombin can be extracted from the plasma of donated blood, the supply is not sufficient to meet the needs of patients. Blood extraction is less efficient and more costly and has a higher risk of contamination with human pathogens than milk extraction, and the milk of transgenic goats is a significant source of human antithrombin, with yields of 2 to 10 grams per liter of milk. In cell cultures, yields on the order of 0.2 to 1 gram per liter of culture medium have been attained. It has been estimated that 75 transgenic goats are required to meet the annual worldwide demand for antithrombin. It is likely that several other human therapeutic proteins produced in transgenic goats will be available soon, including other blood proteinase inhibitors, such as antitrypsin; human clotting factors, such as factor IX for the treatment of hemophilia; and monoclonal antibodies.

Production of Donor Organs

Animals are a potential source of organs for transplantation into humans. Human-to-human organ transplants (allotransplantations, or allografts) of hearts, livers, and kidneys are 75 to 95% effective for the first year, and on average, transplant patients survive for 10 to 15 years. However, throughout the world, the demand for donated organs far exceeds the available supply. In the United States, for example, more than 80,000 kidney transplants were required in 2008, but only 15,000 were performed. With this in mind, animal-to-human transplants (xenotransplantations, or xenografts) have been proposed as a way to alleviate this disparity. In this context, swine

TABLE 21.2 Some human proteins that have been expressed in the mammary glands of transgenic animals

Antithrombin III
α_1-Antitrypsin
Calcitonin
Erythropoietin
Factor IX
Factor VIII
Fibrinogen
Glucagon-like peptide
α-Glucosidase
Granulocyte colony-stimulating factor
Growth hormone
Hemoglobin
Serum albumin
Insulin
Insulin-like growth factor 1
Interleukin 2
α-Lactalbumin
Lactoferrin
Lysozyme
Monclonal antibodies
Nerve growth factor
Protein C
Superoxide dismutase
Tissue plasminogen activator

TABLE 21.3 Milk production and estimated recombinant protein yields from organisms used for the expression of transgenes in mammary glands

Organism	Annual milk yield (liters)	Estimated recombinant protein per female (kg/year)
Rabbit	5	0.02
Pig	300	1.5
Sheep	500	2.5
Goat	900	4
Cow	10,000	60

have been considered the most likely source of organs for xenotransplantation because their organs are similar in size and physiological functions to those of humans, and because they are raised for food, it might be socially acceptable to use them as organ donors.

A major impediment to organ transplantation between species is hyperacute rejection of the animal organ. Hyperacute rejection entails the binding of preexisting antibodies of the host organism to a carbohydrate epitope (α-Gal) on the surfaces of the cells of the grafted organ. The bound antibodies elicit an inflammatory response (complement cascade) that destroys the antibody-coated cells and leads to the loss of the transplanted organ within hours. Under natural conditions, proteins on the surfaces of the cells lining the blood vessels protect the cells from the inflammatory response. These complement-inhibiting proteins are species specific. Therefore, it was reasoned that if the donor animal carried one or more of the genes for a human complement-inhibiting protein, a transplanted organ would be protected from the initial inflammatory response.

Transgenic pigs with different human complement inhibitor genes have been produced. Hyperacute rejection did not occur after kidneys from transgenic pigs were transplanted into a primate host, and survival times were 20 to 90 days, depending on the human complement inhibitor expressed. The survival times also depended on the levels of immunosuppressive drugs that were administered. Another strategy that shows some promise in pig-to-primate transplantation trials is the production of transgenic pigs with organs that do not produce the antigenic α-Gal epitope by deleting the gene encoding 1,3-α-galactosyltransferase.

The possibility that latent pig pathogens, such as porcine endogenous retrovirus (PERV), might become activated after xenotransplantation and cause infections in humans must also be addressed. Preliminary information indicates that PERV replicates in some established human cell lines, but not in newly established cell cultures or in human cells in vivo. Furthermore, there is no evidence that PERV produces adverse symptoms in humans. Certainly, all likely complications, as well as all of the ethical issues, must be resolved before xenografts are considered for clinical trials.

Disease-Resistant Livestock

Currently, infectious diseases of domestic animals are controlled by vaccination, drugs, physical isolation, and careful monitoring. The cost of disease prevention can be as much as 20% of the total production value. The development of transgenic animals with inherited resistance to bacterial, viral, and parasitic diseases would decrease the use of drugs used to treat

these problems, increase productivity, provide safer foods derived from these animals, and increase economic benefits. Genetic resistance to bacterial diseases, such as mastitis (mammary gland abscesses) in dairy cattle, bovine spongiform encephalopathy (BSE) (also called mad cow disease) in cattle, neonatal scours (dysentery) in swine, and fowl cholera, would be likely targets. If resistance in each case is genetically determined, it may be possible to create transgenic animals with specific protection against a bacterial disease after these genes have been isolated and characterized.

One approach that may be used to develop lines of animals that are resistant to infectious agents entails creating inherited immunological protection by transgenesis. The most favorable preliminary results to date have come from research in which the genes encoding the heavy and light chains of a monoclonal antibody have been transferred to mice, rabbits, goats, and pigs. The rationale behind this strategy is to provide a built-in, inherited biological protection mechanism for the transgenic animal that eliminates the need for immunization by vaccination.

The concept of introducing the transgenes for an antibody that binds to a specific antigen into a recipient animal is called in vivo immunization. Although the animal usually has an intact humoral immune system, expression of a monoclonal antibody against a specific pathogen would provide immediate protection without prior exposure to the pathogen. If the transgene encoding a monoclonal antibody was engineered to be secreted into milk, young suckling animals would acquire passive immunity against a pathogen.

Another strategy to protect livestock from infectious disease is to eliminate production of the host cell component that the infectious agent interacts with through genetic engineering. This strategy has been proposed for the prevention of prion diseases. Prion diseases are caused by aberrant forms of normal brain proteins. They are infectious in the sense that, once they are acquired by a cell, the aberrant proteins induce the normal versions of the brain proteins to misfold (Fig. 21.25). The misfolded proteins aggregate and disrupt normal brain function. One prion disease that is particularly problematic for the beef industry is BSE, caused by a mutant form of the protein known as prion protein BSE (PrP^{BSE}) to distinguish it from the normal protein, PrP^C. Scrapie is a similar prion disease found in sheep. BSE, often referred to as mad cow disease for the neuropathological symptoms in cows, has caused huge economic losses for cattle and dairy farmers and is the motivation for contentious barriers to the trade of livestock between countries. There is no known treatment for the disease, and therefore, many

FIGURE 21.25 Prion proteins that elicit BSE are aberrant forms (PrP^{BSE}) of a normal brain protein (PrP^C). Infection with PrP^{BSE} induces the normal versions of the brain proteins to misfold and aggregate, which disrupts normal brain function. Misfolded proteins can be transmitted to other animals and induce normal PrP^C proteins in those animals to misfold.

PrP^{BSE} PrP^C Misfolded PrP^C Aggregated PrP^C PrP^{BSE}

animals have to be destroyed, usually by incineration. Moreover, there is some evidence that prions can be transmitted to humans through consumption of prion-contaminated meat products to cause a variant form of encephalopathy, or Creutzfeldt-Jakob disease (in humans, the prion is referred to as PrPCJD). This insidious disease can be asymptomatic for very long periods but can eventually manifest as mental deterioration. Thus, it would be a relief for farmers, and indeed consumers of animal products, if livestock could be protected from prion protein infection.

The potential of engineering resistance by abolishing production of the normal version of the protein PrPC was tested first in mice and then in cattle, in which both alleles of the gene encoding PrPC were disrupted by the insertion of an antibiotic-resistant gene into the coding sequences (Fig. 21.26). The genetically modified animals were assessed for a variety of morphological and physiological features, in particular, for the presence of features that are used to diagnose spongiform encephalopathy, including mental status, sensory and motor functions, immune function, and brain tissue morphology. The brain tissue of infected animals becomes filled with holes that give the brain a characteristic sponge-like appearance. In all aspects, the transgenic cows were found to be normal and have remained normal for almost 2 years. Brain tissue homogenates were collected from wild-type and PrPC knockout cattle and incubated with brain homogenates of BSE-infected cattle carrying the abnormal version of the prion protein, PrPBSE (Fig. 21.26). Propagation of PrPBSE could not be detected in the homogenates of PrPC knockout animals while it was readily detected in the wild-type homogenates. These results indicate that loss of function of PrPC does not cause BSE and that the normal PrPC is required for propagation of the aberrant form of the prion protein and suggest that the genetically engineered PrPC knockout cattle could be resistant to BSE infection. Tests are now under way to determine if the PrPC knockout cattle are resistant to challenge with PrPBSE in vivo.

The bacterium *Staphylococcus aureus* is responsible for 25% of the cases of mammary gland infection (mastitis) in cows. These infections are contagious, recur frequently following termination of antibiotic treatment, and readily spread through an entire herd. Milk yields from infected cows are

FIGURE 21.26 Normal brain protein, PrPC, found in the brains of wild-type cattle, is required for propagation of the aberrant form of the protein, known as prion protein BSE (PrPBSE), that causes BSE.

significantly lowered. Currently, outbreaks of mastitis caused by *S. aureus* cannot be effectively controlled, with an annual cost of about $2 billion in the United States. Transgenic cows that secrete a staphylolytic agent into their milk to prevent the infections have been produced. *Staphylococcus simulans* produces lysostaphin, a peptidoglycan hydrolase that specifically attacks the cell wall of *S. aureus*. However, when cultured eukaryotic cells were initially transfected with the native lysostaphin gene, only inactive lysostaphin was produced because two asparagine residues were glycosylated. This problem was overcome by using in vitro mutagenesis to replace the codons for these two asparagine residues with those for glutamine (Fig. 21.27). The modified lysostaphin was nonglycosylated after synthesis in eukaryotic cells and was fully active against *S. aureus*.

The efficacy of this approach was first tested by engineering mice to express the altered lysostaphin gene under the control of the promoter of sheep β-lactoglobulin, which is secreted into milk. Based on the successful protection of the transgenic mice against large inocula of *S. aureus*, the approach has been extended to produce cows that express the lysostaphin transgene. The altered lysostaphin gene under the control of the ovine β-lactoglobulin promoter was introduced into cow fibroblasts, and the nuclei from these cells were then transferred to enucleated oocytes and activated. Blastocysts were implanted into the uterus of cows and several calves were subsequently born and used to establish transgenic lines. After nine infusions of *S. aureus* into the mammary glands of high-lysostaphin-expressing cows, no infections were observed. In contrast, 71% of the infused mammary glands of nontransgenic animals were infected. Moreover, even low levels of lysostaphin expression afforded a significant level of protection against the pathogen. While these results show promise for solving an important problem for the beef and dairy industries, the food safety issues associated with milk containing lysostaphin have yet to be addressed.

Improving Milk Quality

One of the goals of transgenesis of dairy cattle is to improve the nutritional value of milk for humans and for suckling animals. The major nutrients in milk are proteins, fat, and the carbohydrate lactose. Overexpression of proteins involved in the production of milk nutrients, for example, can

FIGURE 21.27 Native lysostaphin produced by *S. simulans* is a peptidoglycan hydrolase that cleaves the cell wall of the animal pathogen *S. aureus*. In animal cells transfected with the lysostaphin coding sequence from *S. simulans*, lysostaphin is glycosylated (yellow stars) and inactive against *S. aureus*. Alteration of the lysostaphin gene to replace the coding sequences for two asparagine residues in amino acid positions 125 and 232 (N^{125} and N^{232}) with glutamine residues (Q^{125} and Q^{232}) results in the production of nonglycosylated, active lysostaphin in animal cells.

improve the growth, health, and survival of suckling animals. Specific components of milk can also be altered to benefit human consumers. The amount of cheese produced from milk is directly proportional to the β-casein and κ-casein contents. An increase in β-casein content reduces the time required for protein coagulation and whey removal, with the desirable result of firmer curds. Increasing the production of these proteins in milk was achieved in cows engineered with additional copies of the β-casein and κ-casein genes. Other milk nutrients were largely unaffected by the presence of the casein transgenes: the vitamin, mineral, amino acid, fatty acid, and antibody contents were similar to those in nontransgenic milk. The cheese manufactured from the transgenic milk had a higher concentration of some amino acids, which increased its nutritional value, and a lower fat content.

Modification of the lactose content of milk would be welcomed by the many people who are lactose intolerant due to a deficiency in the production of the lactose-hydrolyzing enzyme lactase. Lactose-intolerant individuals experience severe indigestion after the consumption of milk or milk-containing foods. Expression of the mammalian lactase transgene in the mammary gland could decrease the lactose content of milk; however, the presence of some lactose is required for milk secretion. Although this has not yet been verified in cows, proof of principle was demonstrated in transgenic mice with a 50 to 85% reduction in milk lactose content. Similarly, many people who are allergic to bovine milk would benefit from the abolition of β-lactoglobulin, a major allergen in milk. Again, the feasibility of this approach has not yet been demonstrated in cows, mainly because the creation of knockout mutants by inserting a selectable marker in the protein-coding sequence is much more inefficient in livestock animals than it is in mice. This is due to the low frequency of homologous recombination in the cells of these animals.

Improving Animal Production Traits

Improving production traits, such as muscle mass in meat animals, is often more difficult than engineering animals to express a foreign gene in milk because multiple genes are involved in controlling growth and body composition and a detailed understanding of the genetic basis for the traits of interest is required. Initially, researchers sought to increase the body mass of livestock by introducing genes encoding growth hormones or insulin-like growth factor. Although these early efforts yielded animals with increased ability to convert feed into body weight, they were hampered by difficulties in controlling the expression of the transgenes. Overproduction of growth hormone was found to adversely affect the animals' health, which manifested as gastric ulceration, kidney dysfunction, lameness, inflammation of the lining of the heart, immobility of the joints, and susceptibility to pneumonia; the reasons for these symptoms are not known. To overcome this problem, inducible promoters were used, such as the metallothionein promoter, which can be activated by zinc administered in the animals' diet; however, expression was often poor because the transgene was incorporated into heterochromatin, transcriptionally silent regions of the genome.

Some cattle breeds, such as Belgian Blue, have larger and leaner muscle mass than other breeds because of naturally occurring mutations in the gene encoding myostatin, a growth factor that normally inhibits the growth

of skeletal muscle. Interestingly, humans with rare mutations that disrupt the function of myostatin are unusually muscular, and dogs of the whippet breed that have enhanced muscle mass, known as "double muscling," and increased racing speed carry mutations in both copies of the myostatin gene *(MSTN)*. These mutations result in production of a truncated, and therefore nonfunctional, myostatin protein. Some researchers have reasoned that a transgenesis approach could be used to disrupt myostatin function in other cattle breeds to increase meat production. Moreover, if disruption could be limited to male animals, then milk production in females would be unaffected. The feasibility of this approach has been demonstrated in mice, where a myostatin inactivator was targeted to the Y chromosome so that it would be expressed only in male animals. The myostatin inactivator consists of the N-terminal propeptide domain (latency-associated peptide [LAP]) of the myostatin protein. Following proteolytic cleavage, the N-terminal propeptide can hold the C-terminal portion of the protein, which is the biologically active component, in an inactive state (Fig. 21.28). This blocks myostatin activity that would normally lead to inhibition of muscle growth. A two-step strategy was used to target the gene encoding the myostatin inactivator to the mouse Y chromosome. In the first step, a cassette containing positive (Neor) and negative (HSV-*tk*) selectable markers flanked by *loxP* sites was inserted into a nonessential region of the Y chromosome of mouse embryonic stem cells by homologous recombination (Fig. 21.29A). Transformed cells were selected by resistance to the antibiotic G-418 conferred by the *neo* gene, and the integration site in the Y chromosome was confirmed by PCR. In the second step, a gene encoding the myostatin inactivator, under the control of a strong rat skeletal muscle promoter and enhancer and also flanked by *loxP* sites, was cloned into a plasmid and introduced by electroporation into the transfected embryonic stem cells carrying the selectable marker cassette (Fig. 21.29B). A second plasmid encoding Cre recombinase was also introduced into the transfected cells. Cre recombinase activity resulted in recombina-

FIGURE 21.28 Myostatin consists of an N-terminal propeptide domain (LAP) and an active C-terminal domain. Proteolytic cleavage and folding yield an active C-terminal dimer. Following proteolytic cleavage, the C-terminal dimer can form an inactive (latent) complex with the propeptide domain.

A

B

FIGURE 21.29 Strategy to generate transgenic mice with increased muscle mass. The gene encoding the myostatin inactivator, which consists of the N-terminal propeptide domain (LAP) of myostatin, was introduced into the Y chromosome of mouse embryonic stem cells using a two-step procedure. **(A)** In the first step, a cassette carrying genes encoding selectable markers *(neo and tk)* flanked by *loxP* sites was introduced into the Y chromosome by recombination between a nonessential sequence in the Y chromosome (Y) and a homologous sequence cloned into the vector. The positive selectable marker *(neo)* confers resistance to the antibiotic G-418, and the negative selectable marker *(tk)* confers sensitivity to ganciclovir. **(B)** In the second step, the selectable markers in the Y chromosome were replaced with a cassette carrying the myostatin inactivator *(lap)*, under the control of the rat skeletal muscle promoter *(p)* and enhancer *(e)*, by Cre recombinase-mediated exchange at the *loxP* sites. Adapted from Pirottin et al., *Proc. Natl. Acad. Sci. USA* **102:**6413–6418, 2005.

tion between *loxP* sites and integration of the myostatin inactivator gene into the Y chromosome (Fig. 21.29B). Exchange of the myostatin inactivator sequence for the selectable marker cassette was initially selected by resistance to ganciclovir, indicating loss of the *tk* gene, and then confirmed by

PCR. Transfected embryonic stem cells carrying the myostatin inactivator gene were cultured, inserted into blastocysts, and then implanted into pseudopregnant foster mothers. A single transgenic male founder mouse was obtained and then mated with nontransgenic females. As expected for a gene integrated into the Y chromosome, all male offspring carried the myostatin inactivator transgene whereas none of the female offspring were transgenic. In the transgenic males, the myostatin inactivator was expressed in skeletal muscle tissue and not in heart or liver tissue. Muscle mass was greater by 5 to 20% in transgenic males than in nontransgenic male control mice, suggesting that this may be a feasible approach to increase meat yields in livestock. Larger offspring often lead to birthing difficulties for female animals; therefore, it may be necessary to use promoters that can be controlled to delay expression of the transgene until after birth.

A diet rich in omega-3 fatty acids has been extolled as an aid in the prevention of cancer; autoimmune diseases, such as arthritis; and a variety of other diseases. Omega-3 fatty acids are long-chain polyunsaturated fatty acids found mainly in fish. Humans cannot produce these fatty acids, nor can livestock animals whose tissues are consumed in human diets; rather, they are acquired from a diet containing fish meal, fish oils, and flaxseed. The tissues of livestock animals contain high levels of omega-6 fatty acids, largely because they are fed a grain diet rich in these fatty acids (Fig. 21.30). Livestock lack the enzymes to convert omega-6 fatty acids to omega-3 fatty acids. Diets with high omega-6 content relative to omega-3 content contribute to a variety of diseases, including cancer, heart disease,

FIGURE 21.30 Some omega-3 and omega-6 fatty acids. Omega-3 fatty acids have long hydrocarbon chains with double bonds between several carbon atoms. In all omega-3 fatty acids, the first double bond is found at the third carbon from the methyl (-CH$_3$) end. Omega-6 fatty acids are also long-chain polyunsaturated fatty acids; however, the first double bond is found at the sixth carbon from the methyl end. In parentheses, the first number refers to the number of carbon atoms in the hydrocarbon chain, and the second number refers to the number of double bonds; for example, α-linolenic acid (C$_{18:3}$) has 18 carbons and three double bonds.

Omega-3 fatty acids

α-Linolenic acid (C$_{18:3}$)

Eicosapentaenoic acid (C$_{20:5}$)

Docosahexaenoic acid (C$_{22:6}$)

Omega-6 fatty acids

Linoleic acid (C$_{18:2}$)

Arachidonic acid (C$_{20:4}$)

and diabetes. One strategy to increase the omega-3 fatty acid content in the human diet is to produce pigs that synthesize omega-3 fatty acids. The roundworm *Caenorhabditis elegans* produces a desaturase that can convert omega-6 fatty acids to omega-3 fatty acids by introducing a double bond into the hydrocarbon chain. When this gene was transferred to mice, they gained the ability to synthesize omega-3 fatty acids. An optimized version of the *fat-1* gene (modified codon usage) was cloned into an expression vector under the control of the chicken β-actin promoter and the cytomegalovirus enhancer and was used to transfect fetal pig fibroblasts. Cultured cells that produced higher levels of omega-3 fatty acids and lower levels of omega-6 fatty acids were used to produce *fat-1* transgenic pigs by nuclear transfer. The transgenic pigs showed threefold-higher levels of omega-3 fatty acids and 23% lower levels of omega-6 fatty acids than their nontransgenic counterparts, indicating that they produced the Fat-1 desaturase and converted omega-6 to omega-3 fatty acids.

Transgenesis is also being used to address certain environmental concerns. For example, a major ecological problem with the mass rearing of pigs and poultry, i.e., monogastric organisms, is the overabundance of phosphorus in their fecal material. Phosphorus from pig or poultry manure that is stored outdoors or used as fertilizer can run off into water systems and cause excessive growth of cyanobacterial and algal populations (algal blooms) that in turn deplete the oxygen supply and subsequently kill fish and other aquatic organisms. In addition, large amounts of phosphorus in the environment are implicated in the production of gases that enhance the greenhouse effect and contribute to global warming.

Pigs and poultry excrete large amounts of phosphorus because, unlike ruminants, they are unable to digest and utilize phytate (*myo*-inositol 1,2,3,4,5,6-hexakisdihydrogen orthophosphate, or phytic acid) (Fig. 21.31A), the predominant storage form of phosphorus in plant-based animal feeds. For instance, the main food source for pigs is soybean meal, which has about 50% or more of its phosphate as phytate. The inability to catabolize phytate is due to the absence of the enzyme phytase, which is found in plants and microorganisms. Most phytases remove successive phosphates from phytate to produce inositol 2-monophosphate (Fig. 21.31B) or inositol

FIGURE 21.31 Molecular structures of phytic acid (**A**), inositol 2-monophosphate (**B**), and inositol (**C**).

(Fig. 21.31C). Phytase has been added to animal feed to facilitate the dietary uptake of phosphorus and to lower the phosphorus content of the excreta. However, this supplement is costly and inefficient because much of the enzyme activity is lost during the preparation and storage of the feed.

As an alternative strategy, it was reasoned that transgenic pigs expressing a phytase gene in their salivary glands could overcome the nutritional and pollution consequences of phytate in the diet. To this end, pronuclear embryo microinjection was used to introduce into pigs a transgene construct consisting of the phytase gene *appA* from *E. coli* under the control of the parotid secretory protein promoter that constitutively drives the transcription of a salivary-specific protein in mice. Established phytase-producing transgenic porcine lines were tested for growth and phosphorus excretion using soybean meal with 53% of its total phosphorus as phytate. Under these conditions, the soybean phytate was almost totally digested and the fecal phosphorus content was reduced 75% in comparison to non-transgenic controls. No adverse effects were noted among the phytase transgenic pigs. Tissues from the pigs that are utilized as meat for human consumption contain only trace amounts of the recombinant protein and have essentially the same composition as meat from nontransgenic pigs. "Enviropig," as it is aptly called, is currently under evaluation by the U.S. Food and Drug Administration for approval for commercialization.

Transgenic Poultry

Several features that are unique to avian reproduction and development make the production of transgenic strains by microinjection of DNA into fertilized eggs extremely inefficient. For example, during fertilization in birds, several sperm penetrate the ovum instead of one, as usually occurs in mammals. As a result, it is impossible to identify the male pronucleus that will fuse with the female pronucleus. Also, DNA injected into the cytoplasm of the fertilized egg does not integrate into genomic DNA. Finally, even if nuclear DNA microinjection were practicable, the technique would be difficult to implement because the avian ovum after fertilization becomes, in rapid succession, enveloped in a tough membrane, surrounded by large quantities of albumin, and enclosed in inner and outer shell membranes.

Despite these disadvantages, it is possible to inject a transgene into the region (germinal disc) on the yolk that contains the female and male pronuclei. The germinal disc is present before the eggshell is formed. After the administration of DNA to a germinal disc, each egg is cultured in vitro, and when an embryo forms, it is placed in a surrogate egg to produce a hatchling. Despite the technical difficulties, some transgenic lines of chickens have been established by this method.

By the time an avian egg outer shell membrane has hardened, the developing embryo (blastoderm stage) has two layers consisting of 30,000 to 60,000 cells. In trial experiments, inoculation of the blastoderm stage with replication-defective retrovirus vectors containing bacterial marker genes resulted in a few chickens and quail carrying these DNA sequences in their germ lines. Although some of these transgenic organisms did not produce virus, the use of retrovirus vectors to deliver genes for a product that is to be used as food would ultimately raise questions about its safety, whether real or imagined. Moreover, the size of the transgene that can be introduced into the recipient organism by retrovirus vectors is limited to

~8 kb, and occasionally, integration at the initial site is not permanent. Consequently, other methods of transgenesis have been examined.

The preferred vehicle for transgenesis is pluripotent cells that can be maintained continuously in culture and genetically modified by standard methods. To date, only blastoderm cells and primordial germ cells, which have limited growth in vitro, and stage X (the stage of the embryo in a newly laid egg) chicken embryonic stem cells, which survive for 21 days in culture, are available for this purpose. Briefly, primordial germ, stage X embryonic stem, or blastoderm cells (Fig. 21.32) are removed from a donor chick, transfected with a transgene construct, and implanted into the sub-germinal space of recipient embryos of freshly laid eggs. At hatching, some of the progeny consist of a mixture of cells. An organism with nonidentical cells from two or more individuals is called a chimera. In some of the chicken chimeras, cells that were descended from transfected cells become part of the germ line tissue and form germ cells. Transgenic lines can then be established from these chimeras by rounds of matings. Generally, the cells of the recipient far outnumber the cells with the transgene. However, the proportion of donor cells can be increased to enhance the probability of obtaining germ line chimeras. One strategy entails gamma-irradiation of the recipient embryos with a dose of 540 to 660 rads for 1 hour before the introduction of the transfected cells. The radiation treatment destroys some, but not all, of the blastoderm cells, thereby increasing the final ratio of donor to recipient cells in the chimeric chicken. Despite its inefficiency, this procedure has often been used to produce transgenic chickens.

Transgenesis could be used to improve the genetic makeup of existing chickens with respect to built-in (in vivo) resistance to viral, bacterial, and coccidial diseases; better feed efficiency; lower fat and cholesterol levels in eggs; and better meat quality. Avian researchers have also suggested that the egg, with its high protein content, could be used as a source for pharmaceutical proteins. By analogy to the mammary gland of livestock, the expression of a transgene in the cells of the reproductive tract of a hen that normally secretes large amounts of ovalbumin could lead to the accumulation of a transgene-derived protein that becomes encased in the eggshell. Ovalbumin constitutes more than 50% of the protein of egg white; therefore, expression of a transgene under the control of the ovalbumin promoter and regulatory elements can yield high levels of recombinant protein. Yields of up to 1 g of recombinant protein have been achieved per egg, and considering that a single hen lays more than 300 eggs per year, the productivity of these animal bioreactors could be substantial. The recombinant protein could either be fractionated from the sterile egg packages or consumed as a nutraceutical. Currently, as "proof-of-principle" experiments, transgenic chickens that synthesize monoclonal antibodies, growth hormone, insulin, human serum albumin, and alpha interferon have been created. Regulatory approval of therapeutic proteins produced in eggs may be more straightforward, as chicken eggs are already used to produce vaccines for injection into humans.

Transgenic Fish

As natural fisheries become depleted, production of this worldwide food resource has come to depend more heavily on aquaculture. In this context, enhanced growth rates, tolerance of environmental stress, and resistance to diseases are some of the features that may be created by transgenesis. To

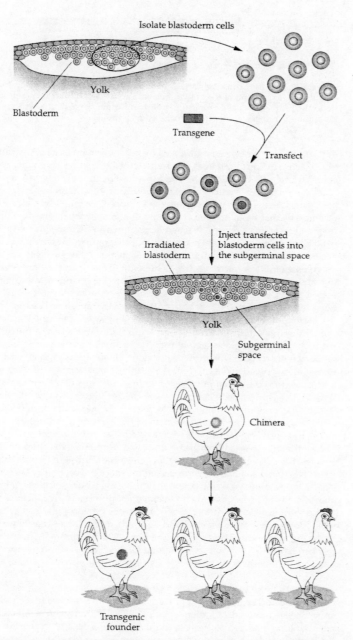

Isolate blastoderm cells

Yolk

Blastoderm

Transgene

Transfect

Inject transfected
blastoderm cells into
the subgerminal space

Irradiated
blastoderm

Yolk

Subgerminal
space

Chimera

Transgenic
founder

FIGURE 21.32 Establishing transgenic chickens by transfection of isolated blastoderm cells. Cells from blastoderm donors are removed, transfected with a transgene, and inserted into the subgerminal space of an irradiated recipient blastoderm. Some of the resulting chickens may be chimeric. The chimeras that have the transgene in germ line cells are bred to establish transgenic lines.

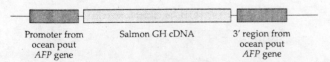

Promoter from Salmon GH cDNA 3' region from
ocean pout ocean pout
AFP gene *AFP* gene

FIGURE 21.33 "All-fish" construct used to generate Atlantic salmon with an enhanced growth rate. Expression of the growth hormone (GH) cDNA from salmon is controlled by the promoter and terminator–polyadenylation signals from the 3' end of the antifreeze protein *(AFP)* gene from the ocean pout fish.

date, transgenes have been introduced by microinjection or electroporation of DNA into the fertilized eggs of a number of fish species, including carp, catfish, trout, salmon, Arctic char, and tilapia. The pronuclei of fish are not readily seen under a microscope after fertilization; therefore, linearized transgene DNA is microinjected into the cytoplasm of either fertilized eggs or embryos that have reached the four-cell stage of development. Unlike mammalian embryogenesis, fish egg development is external; hence, there is no need for an implantation procedure. Development of transgenic fish occurs in temperature-regulated holding tanks. The survival of fish embryos after DNA microinjection is high (35 to 80%), and the production of transgenic fish ranges from 10 to 70%. The presence of a transgene is scored by PCR analysis of either nucleated erythrocytes or scale DNA. Founder fish are mated to establish true-breeding transgenic lines.

Many of the studies with transgenic fish have examined the effect of a growth hormone transgene on the growth rate. In one study, a transgene consisting of the promoter region from the antifreeze protein gene of a fish called the ocean pout, the growth hormone cDNA from salmon, and the termination–polyadenylation signals from the 3' end of the antifreeze protein gene from the ocean pout was injected into eggs of Atlantic salmon (Fig. 21.33). This expression system was chosen to enhance the transcription of the growth hormone in cold waters. In general, the transgenic salmon were larger and grew faster than the nontransgenic controls. An "all-fish" construct was assembled to avoid possible biological incompatibilities that might arise from using a growth hormone gene from nonfish sources. For even greater specificity, an "all-salmon" growth hormone construct was formulated and microinjected into sockeye salmon eggs. Young transgenic salmon grow much more rapidly than nontransgenic salmon and become adult fish that are on average about three to five times larger than nontransgenic fish. Theoretically, the faster growth of farmed salmon would lower the cost of the feed and lessen the pollution of coastal waters in the vicinity of the site of the holding pens. Aquaculture with transgenic fish can be carried out within contained facilities; however, the impact of the accidental release of transgenic fish on natural populations must be considered.

In addition to enhancing traits that aid the production of fish for food, transgenesis can be used to generate systems for monitoring aquatic pollutants. One such biosensor system entails the use of transgenic medaka fish genetically engineered to express red or green fluorescent protein under the control of pollutant-responsive promoters. The medaka, also known as the Japanese killfish, has been a popular aquarium pet for many years and is currently gaining rapid acceptance as a model organism in which to study biological processes due to its small size, which enables growth in small aquariums; hardiness; rapid development; and transparent body,

Estrogenic compounds

FIGURE 21.34 Transgenic medaka fish as biosensors of environmental pollutants. The promoter from the medaka vitellogenin gene (p^{vit}) was cloned upstream of the *gfp* reporter gene encoding green fluorescent protein, and the construct was introduced into medaka fish. The transgenic fish can be used to detect natural and synthetic estrogenic compounds because the vitellogenin promoter is activated in the presence of these compounds and green fluorescent protein is produced. Green fluorescent protein can be readily visualized in living fish.

which facilitates visualization of internal tissues and expression of reporter genes, such as those encoding fluorescent proteins. Transgenic medaka have been developed as biosensors to detect estrogenic compounds in aquatic environments. Estrogens are sex steroid hormones that stimulate the development and maintenance of the female reproductive system and secondary sex characteristics and also regulate some reproductive functions in males. Synthetic derivatives of natural estrogens are used in most oral contraceptives, as a therapy for postmenopausal disorders in women, to treat infertility and endometriosis, and to develop female-only fish populations in aquaculture. A wide variety of industrial chemicals, such as bisphenol A and polychlorinated biphenyls (PCBs), also have estrogenic activity in animals and are used in the manufacture of pharmaceuticals, plastics, paints, detergents, and insecticides. Thus, large amounts of estrogenic chemicals are flushed into aquatic ecosystems with domestic, agricultural, and industrial wastewater and sewage and can have a toxic effect on aquatic organisms. Indeed, one study has implicated high estrogen levels in wastewater effluent in the feminization of wild male fish that can lead to severe reductions in fish populations. To develop transgenic medaka to monitor levels of natural and synthetic estrogens in water, the estrogen-responsive promoter from the medaka vitellogenin gene was cloned upstream of the gene encoding green fluorescent protein and then injected into medaka eggs (Fig. 21.34). Vitellogenins are normally synthesized in females in response to endogenous estrogens, such as 17β-estradiol, and in

males in response to synthetic estrogenic compounds. Exposure of transgenic fish to 17β-estradiol and other natural and synthetic estrogenic compounds activates the vitellogenin promoter and production of green fluorescent protein that can be rapidly and directly visualized as emission of green fluorescence under normal light in living fish without additional reagents. This system can be expanded to include promoters responsive to other environmental toxins, such as heavy metals, that control the expression of red and green fluorescent proteins, in some cases in the same fish. Each color would indicate the presence of a different pollutant.

SUMMARY

Genetic modification of animals by recombinant DNA technology (transgenesis) entails introducing a cloned gene(s) into the genome of a cell that might, after proliferation and embryonic development in a receptive female, be present in the germ lines of some of the progeny. These founder animals are then used to establish true-breeding transgenic lineages. The cloned gene can be introduced into the male pronucleus of a fertilized egg by microinjection, delivered into a fertilized egg by using retroviral vectors, or transfected into embryonic stem cells.

Various strategies have been devised for regulating transgene expression, modifying transgenes, and inducing cell death at specific times in particular tissues of a transgenic organism. The Cre–loxP recombination system activates transgenes by selectively removing DNA elements that block transcription or inactivates transgenes by excising part of the coding sequence. The tet-on and tet-off protocols use the tetracycline analogue doxycycline to either turn on or turn off the transcription of a transgene. RNAi is often used to decrease (knock down) expression of a target gene. These systems have advanced our understanding of gene activity during development and the consequences of either gene overexpression or loss of gene function within a particular tissue.

Transgenic mice provide good models for many human diseases, such as Alzheimer disease, and are useful as test systems to evaluate potential therapies for human and animal diseases. They provide important information about the consequences of defective gene products, the course of the disease, and the effectiveness of different therapies. Transgenic mice have also been used to produce recombinant therapeutic proteins. The XenoMouse, which synthesizes completely human antibodies, was created by transgenesis with a high-capacity YAC carrying almost all of the genes for human heavy and light antibody chains.

Genetic manipulation can lead to improved livestock with enhanced growth rates and muscle mass, increased resistance to common diseases, and improved nutritional content of milk and meat products. A major application for transgenic livestock is to use the mammary gland as a bioreactor for the production of protein pharmaceuticals in milk. Transgenic animals have been created by DNA microinjection or nuclear cloning. The latter method entails transferring the nuclei from cells that have been genetically manipulated in culture to enucleated oocytes and obtaining among the progeny some animals that carry the transgene in all their cells.

Transgenesis of birds, especially chickens, can be used to improve strain attributes. In addition, eggs may be a repository for pharmaceuticals synthesized by transgenic chickens or for delivering recombinant-derived medication when an egg is consumed. Genetic augmentation of fish has been directed primarily to improving growth rates and conferring resistance to disease. In addition, transgenic fish are being considered as biosensors of environmental pollutants. Transgenes encoding fluorescent proteins under the control of promoters that are activated when particular contaminants, such as estrogenic compounds, are present have been incorporated into fish for determining the presence of pollutants in water.

REFERENCES

Baguisi, A., E. Behboodi, D. T. Melican, J. S. Pollock, M. M. Destrempes, C. Cammuso, J. L. Williams, S. D. Nims, C. A. Porter, P. Midura, M. J. Palacios, S. L. Ayres, R. S. Denniston, M. L. Hayes, C. A. Ziomek, H. M. Meade, R. A. Godke, W. G. Gavin, E. W. Overström, and Y. Echelard. 1999. Production of goats by somatic cell nuclear transfer. *Nat. Biotechnol.* 17:456–461.

Baron, U., D. Schnappinger, V. Helbl, M. Gossen, W. Hillen, and H. Bujard. 1999. Generation of conditional mutants in higher eukaryotes by switching between the expression of two genes. *Proc. Natl. Acad. Sci. USA* 96:1013–1018.

Betthauser, J., E. Forsberg, M. Augenstein, L. Childs, K. Eilertsen, J. Enos, T. Forsythe, P. Golueke, G. Jurgella, R. Koppang, T. Lesmeister, K. Mallon, G. Mell, P. Misica, M. Pace, M. Pfister-Genskow, N. Strelchenko, G. Voelker, S. Watt, S. Thompson, and M. Bishop. 2000. Production of cloned pigs from in vitro systems. *Nat. Biotechnol.* 18:1055–1059.

Brink, M. F., M. D. Bishop, and F. R. Pieper. 2000. Developing efficient strategies for the generation of transgenic cattle which produce biophar-

maceuticals in milk. *Theriogenology* 53:139–148.

Brinster, R. L., H. Y. Chen, M. Trumbauer, A. W. Senear, R. Warren, and R. D. Palmiter. 1981. Somatic expression of herpes thymidine kinase in mice following injection of a fusion gene into eggs. *Cell* 27:223–231.

Cibelli, J. B., S. L. Stice, P. J. Golueke, J. J. Kane, J. Jerry, C. Blackwell, F. A. Ponce de León, and J. M. Robl. 1998. Cloned transgenic calves produced from nonquiescent fetal fibroblasts. *Science* 280:1256–1258.

Clark, A. J. 1998. The mammary gland as a bioreactor: expression, processing and production of recombinant proteins. *J. Mammary Gland Biol. Neoplasia* 3:337–349.

Co, D. O., A. H. Borowski, J. D. Leung, J. van der Kaa, S. Hengst, G. J. Platenburg, F. R. Pieper, C. F. Perez, F. R. Jirik, and J. I. Drayer. 2000. Generation of transgenic mice and germline transmission of a mammalian artificial chromosome introduced into embryos by pronuclear microinjection. *Chromosome Res.* 8:183–191.

Cowan, P. J., A. Aminian, H. Barlow, A. A. Brown, C. G. Chen, N. Fisicaro, D. M. Francis, D. J. Goodman, W. Han, M. Kurek, M. B. Nottle, M. J. Pearse, E. Salvaris, T. A. Shinkel, G. V. Stainsby, A. B. Stewart, and A. J. d'Apice. 2000. Renal xenografts from triple-transgenic pigs are not hyperacutely rejected but cause coagulopathy in non-immunosuppressed baboons. *Transplantation* 69:2504–2515.

Devlin, R. H., T. Y. Yesaki, C. A. Biagi, E. M. Donaldson, P. Swanson, and W.-K. Chan. 1994. Extraordinary salmon growth. *Nature* 371:209–210.

Dewachter, I., J. Van Dorpe, L. Smeijers, M. Gilis, C. Kuiperi, I. Laenen, N. Caluwaerts, D. Moechars, F. Checler, H. Vanderstichele, and F. Van Leuven. 2000. Aging increased amyloid peptide and caused amyloid plaques in brain of old APP/V717I transgenic mice by a different mechanism than mutant presenilin1. *J. Neurosci.* 20:6452–6458.

Dewachter, I., J. van Dorpe, K. Spittaels, I. Tesseur, C. Van Den Haute, D. Moechars, and F. Van Leuven. 2000. Modeling Alzheimer's disease in transgenic mice: effect of age and of presenilin1 on amyloid bio-

chemistry and pathology in APP/London mice. *Exp. Gerontol.* 35:831–841.

DiTullio, P., S. H. Cheng, J. Marshall, R. J. Gregory, K. Ebert, H. M. Meade, and A. E. Smith. 1992. Production of cystic fibrosis transmembrane conductance regulator in the milk of transgenic mice. *Bio/Technology* 10:74–77.

Farah, M. H. 2007. RNAi silencing in mouse models of neurodegenerative diseases. *Curr. Drug. Deliv.* 4:161–167.

Galili, U. 2001. The α-Gal epitope (Galα1-3Galβ1-4GlcNAc-R) in xenotransplantation. *Biochimie* 83:557–563.

Gao, X., and P. Zhang. 2007. Transgenic RNA interference in mice. *Physiology* 22:161–166.

Giraldo, P., and L. Montoliu. 2001. Size matters: use of YACs, BACs and PACs in transgenic animals. *Transgenic Res.* 10:83–103.

Golovan, S. P., M. A. Hayes, J. P. Phillips, and C. W. Forsberg. 2001. Transgenic mice expressing bacterial phytase as a model for phosphorus pollution control. *Nat. Biotechnol.* 19:429–433.

Golovan, S. P., R. G. Meidinger, A. Ajakaiye, M. Cottrill, M. Z. Wiederkehr, D. J. Barney, C. Plante, J. W. Pollard, M. Z. Fan, M. A. Hayes, J. Laursen, J. P. Hjorth, R. R. Hacker, J. P. Phillips, and C. W. Forsberg. 2001. Pigs expressing salivary phytase produce low-phosphorus manure. *Nat. Biotechnol.* 19:741–745.

Gordon, J. W., G. A. Scangos, D. J. Plotkin, J. A. Barbosa, and F. H. Ruddle. 1980. Genetic transformation of mouse embryos by microinjection of purified DNA. *Proc. Natl. Acad. Sci. USA* 77:7380–7384.

Green, L. L. 1999. Antibody engineering via genetic engineering of the mouse: XenoMouse strains are a vehicle for the facile generation of therapeutic human monoclonal antibodies. *J. Immunol. Methods* 231:11–23.

Hadjantonakis, A. K., M. Pirity, and A. Nagy. 1999. Cre recombinase mediated alterations of the mouse genome using embryonic stem cells. *Methods Mol. Biol.* 97:101–122.

Imaizumi, T., K. L. Lankford, W. V. Burton, W. L. Fodor, and J. D. Kocsis. 2000. Xenotransplantation of transgenic pig olfactory ensheathing cells

promotes axonal regeneration in rat spinal cord. *Nat. Biotechnol.* 18:949–953.

Ivarie, R. 2006. Competitive bioreactor hens on the horizon. *Trends Biotechnol.* 24:99–101.

Jakobovits, A., R. G. Amado, X. Yang, L. Roskos, and G. Schwab. 2007. From Xenomouse technology to panitumumab, the first fully human antibody product from transgenic mice. *Nat. Biotechnol.* 25:1134–1143.

Kato, Y., T. Tani, Y. Sotomaru, K. Kurokawa, J. Kato, H. Doguchi, H. Yasue, and Y. Tsunoda. 1998. Eight calves cloned from somatic cells of a single adult. *Science* 282:2095–2098.

Kerr, D. E., K. Plaut, A. J. Bramley, C. M. Williamson, A. J. Lax, K. Moore, K. D. Wells, and R. J. Wall. 2001. Lysostaphin expression in mammary glands confers protection against staphylococcal infection in transgenic mice. *Nat. Biotechnol.* 19:66–70.

Krimpenfort, P., A. Rademakers, W. Eyestone, A. van der Schans, S. van den Broek, P. Kooiman, E. Kootwijk, G. Platenburg, F. Pieper, R. Strijker, and H. de Boer. 1991. Generation of transgenic dairy cattle using "in vitro" embryo production. *Bio/Technology* 9:844–847.

Kubota, C., H. Yamakuchi, J. Todoroki, K. Mizoshita, N. Tabara, M. Barber, and X. Yang. 2000. Six cloned calves produced from adult fibroblast cells after long-term culture. *Proc. Natl. Acad. Sci. USA* 97:990–995.

Kues, A. W., and H. Niemann. 2004. The contribution of farm animals to human health. *Trends Biotechnol.* 22:286–294.

Lai, L., J. X. Kang, R. Li, J. Wang, W. T. Witt, H. Y. Yong, Y. Hao, D. M. Wax, C. N. Murphy, A. Rieke, M. Samuel, M. L. Linville, S. W. Korte, R. W. Evans, T. E. Starzl, R. S. Prather, and Y. Dai. 2006. Generation of cloned transgenic pigs rich in omega-3 fatty acids. *Nat. Biotechnol.* 24:435–436.

Laible, G. 2009. Enhancing livestock through genetic engineering—recent advances and future prospects. *Comp. Immunol. Microbiol. Infect. Dis.* 32:123–137.

Laird, F. M., H. Cai, A. V. Savonenko, M. H. Farah, K. He, T. Melnikova, H. Wen, H.-C. Chiang, G. Xu, V. E. Koliatsos, D. R. Borchelt, D. L. Price,

H.-K. Lee, and P. C. Wong. 2005. BACE1, a major determinant of selective vulnerability of the brain to amyloid—cognitive, emotional, and synaptic functions. *Neurobiol. Dis.* 25:11693–11709

Loring, J. F. 1999. Designing animal models of Alzheimer's disease with amyloid precursor protein (APP) transgenes. *Methods Mol. Med.* 32:249–270.

Mansuy, I. M., and H. Bujard. 2000. Tetracycline-regulated gene expression in the brain. *Curr. Opin. Neurobiol.* 10:593–596.

McGowan, E., S. Sanders, T. Iwatsubo, A. Takeuchi, T. Saido, C. Zehr, X. Yu, S. Uljon, R. Wang, D. Mann, D. Dickson, and K. Duff. 1999. Amyloid phenotype characterization of transgenic mice overexpressing both mutant amyloid precursor protein and mutant presenilin 1 transgenes. *Neurobiol. Dis.* 6:231–244.

Mendez, M. J., L. L. Green, J. R. F. Corvalan, X.-C. Jia, C. E. Maynard-Currie, X. Yang, M. L. Gallo, D. M. Louie, D. V. Lee, K. L. Erickson, J. Luna, C. M.-N. Roy, H. Abderrahim, F. Kirschenbaum, M. Noguchi, D. H. Smith, A. Fukushima, J. F. Hales, M. H. Finer, C. G. Davis, K. M. Zsebo, and A. Jakobovits. 1997. Functional transplant of megabase human immunoglobulin loci recapitulates human antibody response in mice. *Nat. Genet.* 15:146–156.

Michie, C. 2001. Xenotransplantation, endogenous pig retroviruses and the precautionary principle. *Trends Mol. Med.* 7:62–63.

Mills, A. A., and A. Bradley. 2001. From mouse to man: generating megabase chromosome rearrangements. *Trends Genet.* 17:331–339.

Onishi, A., M. Iwamoto, T. Akita, S. Mikawa, K. Takeda, T. Awata, H. Hanada, and A. C. Perry. 2000. Pig cloning by microinjection of fetal fibroblast nuclei. *Science* 289:1188–1190.

Ono, E., K. Amagai, S. Taharaguchi, Y. Tomioka, S. Yoshino, Y. Watanabe, P. Cherel, L. M. Houdebine, M. Adam, M. Eloit, M. Inobe, and T. Uede. 2004. Transgenic mice expressing a soluble form of porcine nectin-1/herpesvirus entry mediator C as a model for pseudorabies-resistant livestock. *Proc. Natl. Acad. Sci. USA* 101:16150–16155.

Petitte, J. N., M. E. Clark, G. Liu, A. M. Verrinder Gibbins, and R. J. Etches. 1990. Production of somatic and germline chimeras in the chicken by transfer of early blastodermal cells. *Development* 108:185–189.

Pfeifer, A. 2006. Lentiviral transgenesis—a versatile tool for basic research and gene therapy. *Curr. Gene Ther.* 6:535–542.

Pirottin, D., L. Grobet, A. Adamantidis, F. Farnir, C. Herens, H. D. Schröder, and M. Georges. 2005. Transgenic engineering of male-specific muscular hypertrophy. *Proc. Natl. Acad. Sci. USA* 102:6413–6418.

Richt, J. A., P. Kasinathan, A. N. Hamir, J. Castilla, T. Sathiyaseelan, F. Vargas, J. Sathiyaseelan, H. Wu, H. Matsushita, J. Koster, S. Kato, I. Ishida, C. Soto, J. M. Robl, and Y. Kuroiwa. 2007. Production of cattle lacking prion protein. *Nat. Biotechnol.* 25:132–138.

Saito, M., T. Iwawaki, C. Taya, H. Yonekawa, M. Noda, Y. Inui, E. Mekada, Y. Kimata, A. Tsuru, and K. Kohno. 2001. Diphtheria toxin receptor-mediated conditional and targeted cell ablation in transgenic mice. *Nat. Biotechnol.* 19:746–750.

Sims, M., and N. L. First. 1993. Production of calves by transfer of nuclei from cultured inner cell mass cells. *Proc. Natl. Acad. Sci. USA* 90:6143–6147.

Tomizuka, K., T. Shinohara, H. Yoshida, H. Uejima, A. Ohguma, S. Tanaka, K. Sato, M. Oshimura, and I. Ishida. 2000. Double trans-chromosomic mice: maintenance of two individual human chromosome fragments containing Ig heavy and κ loci and expression of fully human antibodies. *Proc. Natl. Acad. Sci. USA* 97:722–727.

Urlinger, S., U. Baron, M. Thellmann, M. T. Hasan, H. Bujard, and W. Hillen. 2000. Exploring the sequence space for tetracycline-dependent transcriptional activators: novel mutations yield expanded range and sensitivity. *Proc. Natl. Acad. Sci. USA* 97:7963–7968.

Van Dorpe, J., L. Smeijers, I. Dewachter, D. Nuyens, K. Spittaels, C. Van Den Haute, M. Mercken, D. Moechars, I. Laenen, C. Kuiperi, K. Bruynseels, I. Tesseur, R. Loos, H. Vanderstichele, F. Checler, R. Sciot, and F. Van Leuven. 2000. Prominent cerebral amyloid angiopathy in transgenic mice overexpressing the London mutant of human APP in neurons. *Am. J. Pathol.* 157:1283–1298.

Wall, R. J., A. M. Powell, M. J. Paape, D. E. Kerr, D. D. Bannerman, V. G. Pursel, K. D. Wells, N. Talbot, and H. W. Hawk. 2005. Genetically enhanced cows resist intramammary *Staphylococcus aureus* infection. *Nat. Biotechnol.* 23:445–451.

Wilmut, I., A. E. Schnieke, J. McWhir, A. J. Kind, and K. H. S. Campbell. 1997. Viable offspring derived from fetal and adult mammalian cells. *Nature* 385:810–813.

Xu, X., K. U. Wagner, D. Larson, Z. Weaver, C. Li, T. Ried, L. Hennighausen, A. Wynshaw-Boris, and C.-X. Deng. 1999. Conditional mutation of *Brca1* in mammary epithelial cells results in blunted ductal morphogenesis and tumour formation. *Nat. Genet.* 22:37–43.

Yamamoto, A., J. J. Lucas, and R. Hen. 2000. Reversal of neuropathology and motor dysfunction in a conditional model of Huntington's disease. *Cell* 101:57–66.

Yang, S. H., P. H. Cheng, H. Banta, K. Piotrowska-Nitsche, J. J. Yang, E. C. Cheng, B. Snyder, K. Larkin, J. Liu, J. Orkin, Z. H. Fang, Y. Smith, J. Bachevalier, S. M. Zola, S. H. Li, X. J. Li, and A. W. Chan. 2008. Towards a transgenic model of Huntington's disease in a non-human primate. *Nature* 453:921–924.

Yang, X. D., X. C. Jia, J. R. Corvalan, P. Wang, and C. G. Davis. 2001. Development of ABX-EGF, a fully human anti-EGF receptor monoclonal antibody, for cancer therapy. *Crit. Rev. Oncol. Hematol.* 38:17–23.

1. How are transgenic mice created?

2. What is positive-negative selection, and how does it work?

3. What are knockout mice? How and why are they established?

4. What are knockdown mice? How are they generated?

5. Describe how the Cre–*loxP* recombination system is used to regulate the expression of a transgene.

6. What are the advantages and disadvantages of using transgenic mice as model systems for human diseases?

7. Describe an example of a transgenic mouse that was developed as a model system for a human disease.

8. What is nuclear cloning?

9. Discuss some ways in which transgenic livestock could contribute to human health.

10. Discuss how the mammary gland could be used as a bioreactor for the production of commercial products.

11. Discuss how transgenesis could be used to improve organ transplantation.

12. Describe a strategy to develop transgenic animals that are protected from infectious disease.

13. Why are pigs carrying a phytase transgene considered to be environmentally friendly?

14. What approaches have been developed to produce transgenic chickens?

15. Discuss how transgenesis might improve fish aquaculture.

This page intentionally left blank

IV MOLECULAR BIOTECHNOLOGY AND SOCIETY

INEVITABLY, NEW TECHNOLOGIES, especially when they are as widespread and pervasive as molecular biotechnology, affect society in diverse ways. There can be economic, social, and ethical consequences that result from both the implementation of a new way of doing something and the displacement of traditional processes. Moreover, because molecular biotechnology deals with the genetic engineering of life forms, it impinges on a number of socially sensitive issues. As a result, many questions have been raised about its propriety, safety, and acceptability to society. In part IV, we examine several of the controversial social, regulatory, political, and ethical aspects of molecular biotechnology.

This page intentionally left blank

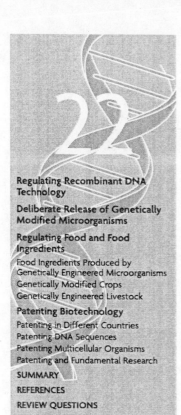

Regulating the Use of Biotechnology

MAJOR TECHNOLOGICAL ADVANCES, such as molecular biotechnology, are seldom implemented without controversy. Because molecular biotechnology can potentially affect many aspects of modern society, including food production and medical treatment, there are significant ethical, legal, economic, and social issues that need to be considered. For example, since its inception in 1973, serious doubts have been voiced by some individuals about the safety of recombinant DNA technology. These concerns prompted scientists to declare a self-imposed moratorium on certain types of recombinant DNA experiments until the adoption of official regulatory guidelines designed to ensure that recombinant microorganisms were unable to proliferate outside the laboratory and that laboratory workers were protected from any potential hazard. The formulation of these regulations took place in 1974 and 1975 in open meetings under the scrutiny of the press. Thus, the public became aware of the possibilities, both negative and positive, of genetically manipulating organisms. Nevertheless, in the late 1970s, apprehension persisted about the safety of this new technology. In particular, there was concern about the release, either accidental or deliberate, of genetically modified organisms into the environment and fear that they would become uncontrolled biological marauders of vulnerable ecosystems. Additional specific guidelines seemed to be necessary to ensure that such rare possibilities would be even less likely to occur.

In 1998, a vociferous and aggressive campaign was launched against planting genetically modified crops and marketing products derived from them. The reasons for this response are complex and encompass multiple concerns that range from human health and safety to environmental protection, corporate control of the food industry, world trade monopolies, trustworthiness of public institutions, integrity of regulatory agencies, and loss of individual choice.

Moreover, there has been much discussion about the ethics of genetic manipulation of animals. The objective of these discussions has been to distinguish between inappropriate and acceptable procedures. There are no easy answers to the ethical, legal, and social questions raised by the

various applications of molecular biotechnology. However, because the stakes are so high, many of these issues have been examined extensively.

Regulating Recombinant DNA Technology

In 1974, when it was realized that recombinant DNA technology could be used to engineer organisms with novel genes, concerns about safety, ethics, and unforeseen consequences were raised by scientists, the public, and government officials. Phrases such as "playing God," "manipulation of life," "the most threatening scientific research ever undertaken," and "man-made evolution" were often used by the popular press when describing recombinant DNA technology. The major apprehension was that, either inadvertently or possibly deliberately for the purposes of warfare, unique microorganisms that had never previously existed would be developed and would cause epidemics or environmental catastrophes. In response to a certain amount of public anxiety about these "doomsday bugs," a group of prominent molecular biologists called for a moratorium on several kinds of recombinant DNA research, especially experiments that involved pathogenic microorganisms.

Subsequently, in 1976, the U.S. National Institutes of Health (NIH), the primary U.S. research grant agency in the medical and health sciences, issued *Guidelines for Research Involving Recombinant DNA Molecules (NIH Guidelines)*. These rules and regulations rigorously defined physical (laboratory) containment levels for the conduct of recombinant DNA experiments. They also required that biological containment be a component of any recombinant DNA experiment, i.e., the preferred hosts for foreign DNA would be those microorganisms considered least likely to proliferate outside the laboratory or to transfer their DNA to other microorganisms. For research with known pathogenic organisms, elaborate negative-pressure, controlled, self-contained rooms were recommended. Research that was perceived to be less dangerous could be conducted in enclosed contained units equipped with high-quality filter systems. Although the *NIH Guidelines* did not have legal status, most researchers, including those who did not receive NIH funding and private companies that were starting recombinant DNA technology research programs, voluntarily complied. In addition, other countries, using the *NIH Guidelines* as a model, adopted their own sets of restrictions for the conduct of recombinant DNA research.

The initial *NIH Guidelines* were very stringent, and many scientists thought that they were excessive. For example, the costs of the containment facilities required by the guidelines effectively prevented smaller companies and researchers with modest grant support from initiating programs using recombinant DNA technology. In anticipation of the need to modify the original guidelines, the NIH Recombinant DNA Molecule Program Advisory Committee (RAC) was created. This committee was charged with overseeing the developments in recombinant DNA research and, if necessary, refining the regulations. The RAC had to hold open meetings to discuss its decisions, it had to publish and distribute the minutes of its meetings, and it had to allow any nonmember the opportunity to address the committee on any issue pertaining to recombinant DNA research. The membership of the RAC was broad and included both ethicists and members of the general public, although it consisted mostly of scientists.

As part of the original *NIH Guidelines*, one specific class of experiments that was "not to be initiated at the present time" under any circumstances

MILESTONE

Potential Biohazards of Recombinant DNA Molecules

P. BERG, D. BALTIMORE, H. W. BOYER, S. N. COHEN, R. W. DAVIS, D. S. HOGNESS, R. ROBLIN, J. D. WATSON, S. WEISSMAN, and N. D. ZINDER
Science 185:303, 1974

After Cohen et al. (*Proc. Natl. Acad. Sci. USA* **70**:3240–3244, 1973) described the basic strategy for inserting a DNA molecule from any source into a plasmid, the safety and ethical implications of recombinant DNA technology were discussed at length in the scientific community. These informal discussions led to the formation of a temporary committee (Ad Hoc Committee on Recombinant Nucleic Acids) that was composed of leading molecular biologists who were charged with examining the concerns in more detail. In 1974, this group published a brief note, which was dubbed the "Berg letter," simultaneously in three major scientific journals: *Science, Nature,* and the *Proceedings of the National Academy of Sciences of the United States of America.* In this communication, Berg et al. recommended that researchers defer creating microorganisms with novel genes for drug resistance and toxin production and cloning cancer-causing genes from viruses into bacterial host cells. Moreover, they suggested that a government body, which would represent the interests of the public, should prepare guidelines and regulations for recombinant DNA technology and that an international meeting of scientists should be convened to "discuss appropriate ways to deal with the potential biohazards of recombinant DNA molecules." This letter had a significant impact. It led to a scientific meeting at the Asilomar Conference Center in California that attempted to define various recombinant DNA experiments in terms of their relative risks and suggested which laboratory safeguards should be implemented for experiments that were considered to have a minimal, low, moderate, or high risk. In turn, the Asilomar recommendations (Berg et al., *Science* **188**:991–994, 1975) contributed to the development of the 1976 *NIH Guidelines* that established stringent regulations for all types of recombinant DNA experiments. The Berg letter was responsible for the formulation of the regulatory framework for recombinant DNA technology. It focused public attention on the potential risks and benefits of recombinant DNA technology and ignited a heated public debate about the technology. Historically, it represents an interesting example of scientists trying to anticipate the possible risks of a new technology before there was any substantial evidence that there were any hazards.

was the "deliberate release into the environment of any organism containing a recombinant DNA molecule." However, it was inevitable that genetically modified organisms that could function in natural settings would be developed.

By 1980, the original *NIH Guidelines* were relaxed considerably by the RAC as a result of experience and specific experimental data from studies that the committee and NIH had sponsored. For example, it was established that the host organism *Escherichia coli* K-12, which was most commonly used in recombinant DNA experiments, was unable to proliferate to any significant extent outside the laboratory. In addition, microbiologists convinced molecular biologists and others that existing safety procedures for work with pathogenic organisms were of a high standard and that more stringent rules were not required. Finally, it was conceded that it was extremely unlikely that a pathogenic organism would be created if the cloned gene had nothing to do with pathogenesis in the original organism. Most observers were satisfied that the safety of laboratory workers was ensured if good laboratory techniques were used. However, specific regulations were added to the guidelines to safeguard against accidental spills during large-scale fermentations with genetically modified organisms.

As a result of the easing of the containment requirements for more routine experiments, the use of recombinant DNA technology became more prevalent and flourished. The RAC and the *NIH Guidelines* had effectively quelled, to some extent, the original concern about the potential dangers of recombinant DNA research. However, two significant problems

remained. First, what kind of regulation was needed for foods that contained either genetically modified organisms or products that were derived from genetically modified organisms? Second, how were deliberate releases of genetically modified organisms into the environment to be managed?

A third potential problem area was avoided when pharmaceuticals that were made by recombinant DNA technology were deemed by regulatory authorities to be similar to pharmaceuticals produced by traditional means. In most countries, there was a strong consensus that existing regulations for the approval of pharmaceuticals for commercial use were sufficient to ensure both worker safety and public safety and that the process (i.e., recombinant DNA technology) by which a product was made was irrelevant. The axiom that the product alone should be evaluated for its safety and efficacy led to the approval of a range of recombinant DNA products, including human drugs, vaccines, and diagnostic devices.

Deliberate Release of Genetically Modified Microorganisms

Despite its initial prohibition, by 1982 it became clear that the RAC would have to cope with requests for open-field testing of genetically modified organisms, i.e., for their deliberate release into the environment. Uncharacteristically, neither guidelines nor protocols that advised applicants what information should be included in their submissions had been prepared. This initial reluctance to establish definitive regulations was due to a widely held belief among many molecular biologists that genetically modified organisms were not significantly different from their nonengineered progenitors, and if a difference was present, it was thought that it would be readily detected by conventional biological testing.

Three applications for field trials of genetically modified organisms were received by the RAC in 1982. Two dealt with genetically modified plants (corn [maize] and tobacco). The third proposal was concerned with testing a genetically modified strain of the microorganism *Pseudomonas syringae* to determine if it could limit the extent of frost damage to plants. This particular submission became part of the landmark case for the development of regulatory procedures for the release of genetically modified organisms into the environment.

The genetic engineering portion of the *P. syringae* proposal involved removing a gene that coded for an ice nucleation protein from the organism and then testing whether the modified "ice-minus" strain, when sprayed onto the leaves of plants, could prevent frost damage. Under natural conditions, wild-type "ice-plus" *P. syringae,* which is usually found on the surfaces of plant leaves, secretes a protein that at low temperatures causes the formation of ice crystals, which, in turn, causes frost damage to the plant. The rationale for the deletion of the gene encoding the ice nucleation protein was that if a strain that lacked this protein were sprayed onto leaves before they became colonized with the wild-type strain, it might lower the temperature at which ice formation would occur, thereby preventing the leaves from being damaged by bacterially induced ice crystals. There is a significant economic incentive for such a novel treatment, because in the United States, crop losses due to frost damage cost farmers billions of dollars each year.

In response to each of the requests for field testing of a genetically modified organism, the RAC followed, more or less, the procedures it had

established for handling the regulation of recombinant DNA experimentation in the laboratory.

1. The submissions were announced in the U.S. *Federal Register.*
2. Information was sent to 3,000 interested persons.
3. A panel of experts reviewed the proposals.
4. A public meeting was called for discussion of each proposal.
5. At the same time as the RAC was reviewing the proposals, the U.S. Department of Agriculture (USDA) also reviewed them.

After careful consideration, both the USDA and the RAC approved the "ice nucleation gene deletion" proposal. In 1983, the director of NIH gave final endorsement to the RAC decision. On the same day that permission was granted to proceed with the field trial, a lawsuit to block the test was filed by an organization called the Foundation on Economic Trends, which is headed by Jeremy Rifkin, who strongly opposes all forms of genetic engineering. The lawsuit was upheld, with the judge noting that the RAC had not carried out a proper hearing in accordance with U.S. statutes and, more importantly, that it had failed to request an environmental impact statement.

This legal decision dramatically demonstrated that, despite the scientific opinion of the RAC and its experts, the existing regulatory system for field testing of genetically modified organisms was inadequate. A prevalent opinion outside the confines of the RAC was that the release of a genetically modified organism into the environment could have far-reaching effects because living microorganisms proliferate, persist, disperse, and sometimes transfer their DNA to other microorganisms. Some critics of the release of genetically modified organisms into the environment believed that, after its introduction into the environment, an engineered organism could displace an existing important species from its ecological niche and as a result cause severe environmental damage. In addition, some opponents of release believed that genes could be transferred from an introduced genetically modified organism to indigenous strains, thereby creating, albeit inadvertently, an ecologically dangerous organism. Although these points of view presented worst-case adverse-effect scenarios that might be exceedingly unlikely, it was essential that the regulatory protocol for field testing include a thorough assessment of the potential risk that an introduced organism might pose for the environment.

The responsibility for assessing the initial submissions for the deliberate release of genetically modified organisms in the United States resides with the U.S. Environmental Protection Agency (EPA) and the USDA. The NIH drew up an initial set of criteria for field tests with genetically modified organisms, but it relinquished its authority in this area to these other agencies. The EPA decided to use two applications, both dealing with ice nucleation-defective bacteria, as prototype cases for developing an assessment process for the field testing of genetically modified organisms. Each proposal went through a series of reviews, which included appraisals of the environmental fate, ecological effects, and human health consequences of the test, as well as product analysis, by the following groups:

- The Office of Pesticide Program Review of the EPA
- The Toxic Substances, Research and Development Policy Planning, and Evaluation Committees of the EPA

- The General Counsel of the EPA
- The USDA, Food and Drug Administration (FDA), and NIH
- A Science Advisory Panel that consisted of a microbiologist, a plant pathologist, and a community ecologist
- Open public meetings
- Various state agencies, which in this instance included the California Department of Agriculture

It was not envisioned that this elaborate, time-consuming, and often redundant process would become the routine mechanism for approving field testing of genetically modified organisms; rather, it was assumed that, with experience, the system would be trimmed without loss of effective assessment of the potential hazards of each trial. After what was thought to be a very thorough set of analyses, permission was granted for both of the field trials with ice nucleation-negative bacteria. However, in both instances, although the circumstances were different, local residents who were worried about the release of a genetically modified organism in their neighborhoods obtained court orders that temporarily blocked each of the field trials. As a consequence of this delay, both the EPA and the USDA implemented better methodologies for determining the risks of introducing genetically modified organisms into the environment. In a short time, the staffs at these agencies became more proficient at handling and analyzing the data submitted by the applicants. The scientific community, including ecologists, helped the process by initiating research programs that were designed to examine the consequences of the release of organisms into model environments, and scientific organizations formulated frameworks for deciding whether a particular genetically modified organism would have an adverse effect on the environment.

Eventually, in 1987, the field trials with ice nucleation-negative bacteria were conducted at sites in California. The results indicated that these genetically modified organisms were not dispersed to off-site locations, nor did they persist at the site of application. At one site, the freezing temperature of the test plants was lowered by 1°C. However, for a number of reasons, genetically engineered ice-minus bacteria have not been developed commercially to protect crop plants from frost damage.

Since the first trials of ice-minus bacteria, open-field tests of genetically modified microorganisms have become commonplace. Overall, these studies have found that introduced microorganisms tend to remain confined to the test area, do not persist for more than a few months, do not transfer genes to indigenous microorganisms, and have similar basic biological functions in natural and laboratory settings. Generally, because there can be many different possible adverse effects for each genetically modified organism, a case-by-case approach has been adopted for granting permission to conduct a field test. These kinds of tests have been carried out in the United States, the United Kingdom, Australia, and other countries. However, biotechnology companies have been reluctant to develop genetically modified organisms that can be used in the environment because the cost of field testing is high and because final approval may be denied despite successful test results. Nevertheless, there is a growing consensus that the environmental release of genetically modified organisms after the appropriate laboratory and field tests will not be ecologically deleterious.

Regulating Food and Food Ingredients

In the United States, the FDA is responsible for regulating the introduction of foods, drugs, pharmaceuticals, and medical devices into the marketplace. The safety of both crop foods and food ingredients that include flavors and additives must be thoroughly assessed before they can be licensed for human consumption. The FDA has had a well-established, although not foolproof, system for the approval of new foods and food products for some time. Critics of the FDA, however, have argued that it tends to favor the interests of industry and is too lenient in enforcing its own regulations. Both the FDA and the food industry, which is represented by the International Food Biotechnology Council, have argued, somewhat convincingly, that new regulations are not required for foods and foodstuffs that are developed by recombinant DNA technology because any unlicensed food or food ingredient, regardless of how it is produced, must be assessed for safety by toxicity, allergenicity, and impurity testing. The approach in the United States has been that food products produced through recombinant DNA technology are not considered to be inherently riskier than those derived through traditional forms of genetic improvement, such as selective breeding or cross-pollination. In other words, new food products arising from genetic improvement, regardless of the method used, should be evaluated for risks, not the method by which the product was generated. Commercially available food products derived from genetically modified organisms are deemed as safe as those derived from their nonengineered counterparts.

Food Ingredients Produced by Genetically Engineered Microorganisms

Chymosin. A new food product is usually subjected to a large battery of tests. However, in order to streamline the process and lower the costs of developing a food product, the similarity of the new product to the one that it is designed to replace is taken into consideration. For example, the FDA approved the enzyme chymosin, an agent produced by recombinant DNA technology for use in cheese making, without demanding a full range of tests. Chymosin, one of the key components of rennet, is a milk-clotting proteolytic enzyme that hydrolyzes the κ-casein protein of milk. This enzymatic cleavage creates curds, which in turn are processed into cheese. Traditionally, the milk-clotting agent for cheese making is derived from the fourth stomach of calves and consists of a mixture of substances that collectively is called rennet.

To ensure a reliable, convenient, and possibly cheaper industrial supply of chymosin, one of the chymosin genes was cloned and expressed, and the product was harvested from *E. coli* K-12. When a petition requesting permission to use recombinant chymosin for the commercial production of cheese was presented to the FDA, it was necessary to decide what criteria should be required for the approval process. Because there has been a long history of using rennet containing chymosin in the cheese-making industry, the FDA reasoned that, if the recombinant chymosin was identical to the naturally occurring chymosin, then excessive testing was not necessary. In essence, the petitioner had to show that the recombinant chymosin was identical to the chymosin of rennet. To substantiate this, restriction mapping, DNA hybridization, and DNA sequencing were used to establish that

A

B

FIGURE 22.1 Preparations of L-tryptophan (A) produced in genetically engineered *E. coli* were found to be contaminated with EBT (B).

the cloned and native DNA sequences of the chymosin gene were identical. Moreover, the recombinant chymosin had the same molecular weight as purified calf chymosin, and the biological activities of the two forms of the enzyme were the same.

Next, it was essential to establish that the recombinant chymosin preparation was safe. The company showed that, as part of its purification process, recombinant chymosin is extracted from inclusion bodies and that the final preparation is free of whole bacterial cells, significant cell debris, and other impurities, including nucleic acids. Although the presence of minute amounts of *E. coli* K-12 cells in the final preparation of chymosin is undesirable, numerous studies have established that this strain is nontoxigenic and nonpathogenic to humans. To ensure that the recombinant chymosin preparations did not contain an unexpected toxin, animal testing was performed, and the results showed no adverse effects. After compiling all the information, the FDA concluded that the recombinant chymosin could be licensed for commercial use. Currently, about 85% of all cheeses in the United States are produced with recombinant chymosin.

Tryptophan. For the most part, agencies in various countries that are responsible for regulating food and foodstuffs derived from recombinant DNA technology have adopted a case-by-case approach. Each submission is considered separately, and depending on the judgment of the regulatory body, a series of tests is specified to ensure that the product is safe. Although the industry prefers and urges that government agencies create a single set of standards for all products derived by genetic engineering, there is considerable reluctance to go in that direction. Currently, the introduction of recombinant foodstuffs for human consumption is being handled with a degree of caution, especially since a false assumption that seems logical initially can cause unexpected and perhaps tragic results.

During 1989 and 1990 in the United States, an unusually high number of cases of the disease eosinophilia-myalgia syndrome (EMS) were reported. This generally rare disease causes severe, debilitating muscle pain and can be fatal as a result of respiratory arrest. A consistent feature among the occurrences of EMS was that the patients had been consuming large doses of the amino acid tryptophan as a food supplement. In each case, the source of the tryptophan was traced back to a single chemical company. The possible correlation between tryptophan and EMS was puzzling, because there had been no history of significant negative effects when tryptophan extracted from *E. coli* had previously been used as a dietary agent. Further investigation revealed that all of the suspected batches of the "tainted" tryptophan had been produced by a genetically engineered *E. coli* strain that had been designed to overproduce tryptophan. The company had assumed that the enhanced strain was identical to the previous one; therefore, no additional product safety tests were thought to be necessary. At the same time, what was thought to be a minor step in the purification process was changed, while the previous quality control measures that had been used to assay the purity of the final preparations were retained.

Chemical analyses of the commercial preparations that had been produced by the genetically engineered strain revealed that they contained novel metabolic derivatives of tryptophan, including 1,1'-ethylidenebis[L-tryptophan] (EBT) (Fig. 22.1). Initially, the presence of EBT was considered to be due to some metabolic quirk in the new strain. While research focused

on determining whether EBT caused EMS, other studies showed that EBT was produced by wild-type strains, as well. Toxicity studies established that EBT induced pathological changes in rats that are similar to EMS and, surprisingly, that even tryptophan, to a lesser extent, produced some EMS symptoms. Consequently, L-tryptophan, even without impurities, was banned for human consumption in the United States. It is not clear what actually caused EBT to appear in a product that had previously been safe. Most observers believe that the change in the purification process allowed EBT to contaminate the tryptophan. Presumably, although the company was unaware of it, the old method effectively removed it.

One of the lessons of this episode, even though genetic engineering may not have been the problem, is that biological equivalence between a strain and its genetically altered counterpart should not be assumed. This is as true for a strain produced by traditional methods as it is for one that has been genetically engineered. Furthermore, manufacturers are now more aware that a minor technical change in the purification phase can alter the nature of a product. However, what they do with this knowledge may be problematic; many companies do not want to run a complete battery of toxicity tests for a product that they believe has already been thoroughly tested. However, despite economic costs, many manufacturers are opting for a "better safe than sorry" approach.

Bovine somatotropin. The bovine somatotropin (also called BST, bST, bovine somatotrophin, or bovine growth hormone) controversy illustrates the constellation of issues that can arise from implementing a recombinant DNA product. In this case, Monsanto sought and won approval to market recombinant bovine somatotropin (Posilac). Concerns about animal health and welfare, human food safety, and the socioeconomic impact on small dairy farmers all came into play. Also, governmental agencies from different countries disagreed with some of the conclusions of the FDA.

In the 1930s, it was shown that injection of bovine somatotropin into a dairy cow increases its milk yield significantly. Because natural bovine somatotropin is both difficult and costly to accumulate in large quantities, it has not been used routinely as an augmenting agent by the dairy industry. However, with recombinant DNA technology, the gene for bovine somatotropin was cloned into *E. coli* and expressed. Recombinant bovine somatotropin was harvested, purified, and tested. Under trial conditions, milk production in dairy cows was increased by 20 to 25% after injection of recombinant bovine somatotropin.

The safety of natural bovine somatotropin in milk has been studied exhaustively. In treated cows, the levels of bovine somatotropin in milk are not higher than those in control cows. Moreover, bovine somatotropin is not active in humans, and all toxicity trials have shown that there are no adverse effects on test organisms. The FDA, using all the research results that it could assemble, concluded that both the meat and milk of recombinant bovine somatotropin-treated cows are safe for human consumption. This conclusion was supported by the U.S. Office of Technology Assessment after its independent analysis of many of the bovine somatotropin studies. On 5 November 1993, Monsanto's application to use recombinant bovine somatotropin as a milk production enhancer was granted.

An effective and powerful lobby group had been assembled to block governmental approval of recombinant bovine somatotropin. The principal reason for this opposition was based on the presumed economic conse-

quences that recombinant bovine somatotropin would have on the dairy industry. The fear was that many small dairy farms would become unprofitable because fewer cows would be required to maintain current levels of milk production. In addition to the attrition of small dairy farmers, opponents of recombinant bovine somatotropin thought that the industry would become dominated by large corporate interests at the expense of independent producers. At the time, these economic arguments may have been justified, and certainly any group is entitled to protect itself against what it perceives to be a threat to its livelihood. However, the main issue in the advertising campaign waged against recombinant bovine somatotropin was that "genetically engineered hormones" in "hormone-laced milk" would be harmful and cause cancer in humans. Using recombinant DNA technology as a bogeyman probably made this campaign emotionally effective.

In addition to economic concerns, the opponents of recombinant bovine somatotropin contended that its use would increase the incidence of bacterial infection of milk glands (mastitis) in dairy cattle. It was further argued that larger-than-normal amounts of antibiotics would have to be used to maintain the health of recombinant bovine somatotropin-treated animals, thereby resulting in increased levels of antibiotics in the cows' milk that might trigger allergic responses in some consumers. Moreover, increased antibiotic use could heighten the selection pressure for drug-resistant pathogens. The Veterinary Medicine Advisory Committee of the FDA and others have studied this issue and concluded that the frequencies of mastitis in treated and untreated cows are no different. On this basis, there is no reason to believe that the amounts of antibiotics in milk from recombinant bovine somatotropin-treated cows would be any greater than those from untreated cows. Moreover, by law, after any cow is treated with antibiotics, it is not milked for a specified period of time to enable the medication to be cleared from its system.

The concern about an increased risk of cancer was based on the presumed increased concentration of insulin-like growth factor I in the milk of treated cows. The FDA maintains that the amount of insulin-like growth factor I in recombinant bovine somatotropin-stimulated milk falls within the normal range observed for untreated milk. Moreover, any additional insulin-like growth factor I would add only a small amount to the existing pool of insulin-like growth factor I in human plasma. Taking into consideration these and other matters, the FDA reviewed the complete recombinant bovine somatotropin file in 1999 and found no reason to rescind its original decision.

Notwithstanding the certainty of both the FDA and the Joint Food and Agricultural/World Health Organization Expert Committee on Food Additives that recombinant bovine somatotropin poses no hazards for treated animals, the Canadian equivalent of the FDA (Health Canada) and the European Union both refused to approve recombinant bovine somatotropin on the grounds that it is detrimental to treated animals. In these instances, appointed committees concluded that recombinant bovine somatotropin supplementation increases the risk of mastitis, causes leg and foot disorders, decreases reproductive capabilities, and induces severe reactions at the site of injection. FDA analyses and more recent studies do not support these assertions. Clearly, the biological consequences of recombinant bovine somatotropin remain controversial. Currently, in the United States, about 15% of dairy producers use Posilac. There have been no

TABLE 22.1 Land area under cultivation with transgenic crops in countries that cultivated more than 1 million hectares in 2008

Country	Area (million hectares)	Transgenic crop(s)
United States	62.5	Soybean, corn, cotton, canola, squash, papaya, alfalfa, sugar beet
Argentina	21.0	Soybean, corn, cotton
Brazil	15.8	Soybean, corn, cotton
India	7.6	Cotton
Canada	7.6	Canola, corn, soybean, sugar beet
China	3.8	Cotton, tomato, poplar, petunia, papaya, sweet pepper
Paraguay	2.7	Soybean
South Africa	1.8	Corn, soybean, cotton

Adapted from James, *Global Status of Commercialized Biotech/GM Crops: 2008*, International Service for the Acquisition of Agri-Biotech Applications (ISAAA) brief no. 39 (ISAAA, Ithaca, NY, 2008).

reports since the onset of its commercial use that recombinant bovine somatotropin has had debilitating effects on treated cows. Studies also indicate that recombinant bovine somatotropin treatment has neither had an apparent impact on consumer prices nor led to extensive consolidation of small dairy farms. Moreover, a new market niche has been created. In many food stores, the consumer is given a choice of milk and milk products from either recombinant bovine somatotropin-treated or untreated cows.

By 1996, many of the initial apprehensions about regulating foodstuffs that were developed with recombinant DNA technologies appeared to have subsided in the United States as the FDA implemented traditional risk assessment procedures. The food industry preferred a minimal set of regulations to speed up the transition from the developmental phase to the marketplace. In this context, governmental agencies, as representatives of the public, have a dual responsibility. They are entrusted with protecting public health and ensuring that new developments are not needlessly curtailed. Presumably, any changes to the regulations will not be made for the sake of expediency at the expense of safety.

Genetically Modified Crops

While there is still polarization on the issue of genetically modified crops, many national governments have approved the commercialization of transgenic plants (Table 22.1). The United States cultivates more than 62 million hectares, which represents about 50% of the total global area planted with transgenic crops. In total, 25 countries now grow transgenic crops, with developing countries beginning to outpace industrial countries in the rate of increase. Four crops, soybean, corn, cotton, and canola, represent about 99% of the genetically engineered crops, with squash, papaya, alfalfa, sugar beet, tomato, sweet pepper, petunia, and carnation making up the balance. Most have been engineered to increase productivity by incorporating genes that confer tolerance for herbicides and resistance to insect predation. Other traits that have been approved but are marketed to a lesser extent include resistance to viral infection (especially in papaya) and altered plant quality (e.g., flower color in carnations).

While recognizing the need to increase agricultural production, the overarching purpose of regulating the commercialization of transgenic

crops, as for any crop, is to ensure that the crops are safe for humans and livestock to eat and safe to grow. Not only must the products be nontoxic for consumption, there must also be consideration of their potential impact on other organisms and on environments outside the area of cultivation, because the plants are usually grown in an open-field environment. For example, there is potential for plants carrying insecticidal toxins to adversely affect nontarget insects or to crossbreed with wild plants, which could enhance their invasiveness. In many countries, regulations governing transgenic crops are still being developed and are evolving.

In establishing regulations, the general consensus among national regulatory agencies has been to consider the characteristics of a transgenic plant rather than the process by which it was created. The prevalent view of transgenic plants has been that they are not different from traditional plant strains (cultivars) that are derived from traditional breeding experiments. In the United States, three agencies are responsible for assessing and approving applications for the development and release of genetically modified crops. The USDA is responsible for protecting agriculture and the environment from pests, the FDA is responsible for the safety of human food and animal feed, and the EPA is responsible for regulating pesticides, including plants that are engineered to produce pesticides. The same testing and licensing procedures are applied to all plants that carry genetic modifications, regardless of how these changes were introduced.

Many other countries have taken a similar approach when adopting legislation and follow general guidelines provided by the Organisation for Economic Co-operation and Development and the Cartagena Protocol on Biosafety, which was established to develop international standards for biosafety. The regulatory system in the European Union differs somewhat from that in the United States in placing greater emphasis on the process by which the crops have been developed. There is also a requirement for additional information that is used for labeling and to enable tracking of the origin of the plant.

In general, each new transgenic plant is considered on a case-by-case basis. Even when a previously approved transgene is introduced into a different plant variety or into the same plant genotype, each transgenesis event is assessed in a new application because the site of insertion into the plant genome is random and therefore the potential for disruption of the function or regulation of endogenous or introduced genes must be considered. Other traits that are assessed include the rate and method of reproduction, the potential for transfer of genetic material to other organisms, toxicity to other organisms, and sexual compatibility with wild relatives. For plants engineered with insecticidal proteins, strategies to manage insect resistance must also be in place (Table 22.2).

To date, in the United States, 12,000 field trials for genetically modified plants have been authorized. Over 100 transgenic crops have been approved for commercialization. Some argue that the lengthy and costly pre- and postcommercialization regulatory process is prohibitive to the development of new transgenic crops with traits other than herbicide and pest resistance, which would be produced on a smaller scale. They also argue that the high cost of meeting regulatory requirements, estimated to be $20 million to $30 million per product, precludes development by anyone other than large multinational companies. Proponents maintain that after 20 years of scrutiny and incorporation of many of the safeguards

TABLE 22.2 Some of the studies submitted to the U.S. EPA as part of the approval process for a variety of Bt corn

Molecular characterization of insect protected from transgenic corn

Evaluation of transgenic corn line in U.S. field trials

Assessment of the equivalence of *B. thuringiensis* subsp. *kurstaki* protein with commercial Bt corn varieties and microorganisms

Dietary toxicity study with Bt corn meal in the northern bobwhite

Aerobic soil degradation study of Bt protein

Acute oral toxicity study of Bt corn tryptic protein in albino mice

Assessment of the in vitro digestive fate of Bt protein

Stability of Bt protein in sucrose and honey solutions under nonrefrigerated temperature conditions

Evaluation of the dietary effects of purified Bt proteins on honeybee larvae

Evaluation of the dietary effects of purified Bt proteins on honeybee adults

Dietary toxicity study of activated Bt protein with green lacewing larvae

Dietary toxicity study of activated Bt protein with the parasitic hymenopteran *Brachymeria intermedia*

Dietary toxicity study of activated Bt protein with ladybird beetles

Evaluation of Bt corn feed as ingredient for catfish

Acute toxicity study of Bt protein with the earthworm in an artificial soil substrate

Effects of Bt protein on *Folsomia candida* and *Xenylla grisea* (Insecta: Collembola)

Expression of Bt protein in Bt corn

Tissue expression and corn earworm efficacy of Bt protein in Bt corn

Chronic exposure of *F. candida* to corn tissue expressing Bt protein

Corn pollen containing Bt protein: 48-h static-renewal test with *Daphnia magna* (Cladocera)

Adapted from National Research Council, *Genetically Modified Pest-Protected Plants: Science and Regulation*, p. 245 (National Academies Press, Washington, DC, 2000), with permission.

Bt corn, corn treated with the genetcially engineered *Bacillus thuringiensis cry* gene to make it resistant to pests.

to ensure that transgenic crops are safe for consumption and release into the environment, the regulatory process could be streamlined.

Despite the successful history of transgenic crops, recent legal cases in the United States may indicate that regulatory scrutiny will increase, rather than be relaxed as some producers had hoped. In three separate cases, it was ruled that field trials—for genetically engineered turf grass in Oregon, corn and sugarcane in Hawaii, and commercial cultivation of genetically engineered alfalfa in California—were approved by the USDA without adequate consideration of the environmental impact of the release.

Somewhat more challenging is the regulation of transgenic plants that produce pharmaceutical proteins. Frequently, these are agricultural crop plants, such as corn, tobacco, potato, rice, and safflower, although so far they have mainly been developed for production in contained facilities, for example, in cell cultures. Pharmaceutical plants grown in greenhouses, cell culture systems, and other contained facilities are regulated as drugs. The plants are genetically manipulated, often with several different genes, to maximize yields of proteins that are intended to be biologically active in humans or other animals. Thus, the plants potentially pose a greater risk to human health and the environment when grown in the field and therefore are given special consideration by regulators. For example, there are concerns that material derived from the plants could inadvertently end up in

the food chain, perhaps through seed dispersal. Prevention of such problems may require special confinement measures, such as dedicated farm machinery or containment netting, to separate pharmaceutical crops from food crops. Employing nonfood crops, such as tobacco, to produce pharmaceutical proteins would circumvent some of these problems and also provide tobacco farmers, who are facing income losses due to a decline in tobacco consumption, with an alternate market.

Genetically Engineered Livestock

The regulation of genetically engineered livestock is not fundamentally different from that of genetically modified crops. Generally, the same agencies in the United States are responsible for regulatory oversight of both. As with cultivation of plants, the goal for the commercial production of animals, regardless of the method of production, is to ensure that the animal products are safe for use and that the impact of the animals on the environment is as low as possible. In addition, the well-being of the animals must be protected. For new, rapidly developing, and expanding technologies, regulators are challenged with ensuring that these goals are met while recognizing the power of the technologies to solve important problems in agriculture and medicine. Moreover, for acceptance of the products of these animals and for commercial viability, society must be confident that safety issues have been addressed.

The regulatory issues for cloned livestock that have not undergone modification of their genomes are separated from those for transgenic animals. In the United States, the Center for Veterinary Medicine of the FDA considers that the cloning of livestock through somatic cell nuclear transfer is not different from other assisted reproductive technologies that have been practiced for many years and does not pose greater risks. Many cloned animals are unhealthy, most likely because the genome transferred from a differentiated somatic cell fails to undergo epigenetic reprogramming. This normally returns the genomes of differentiated egg and sperm cells to a nascent state in an early embryo, which is required for normal development. However, sick animals are generally destroyed, and their tissues are not consumed as food by humans or other animals. Healthy cloned animals are used primarily as breeding stock. Their offspring, which are consumed as food, are produced through sexual reproduction and therefore develop normally (i.e., undergo proper epigenetic programming) and are generally born healthy. The FDA takes the position that healthy animals produce safe foods. After extensive assessment of meat and milk composition, it was found that meat and milk derived from cloned animals is not different and is as safe to eat as that from animals produced using conventional agricultural practices. Additional regulations specific for cloned animals were determined to be unnecessary because any problems associated with the products from cloned animals can be identified through food inspections in current practice.

All genetically modified animals must be approved before they are commercialized, and to date, no animals that enter the food chain have received regulatory approval. In the United States, genetically engineered animals, whether containing heritable or nonheritable recombinant DNA and regardless of their intended use, are considered to be "new animal drugs" by the FDA. Each time a gene is introduced into an animal, approval must be obtained, even when the same gene is introduced into different

animals. As for transgenic plants, it is generally recognized that the site of insertion into the animal's genome is difficult to control and may affect the level of expression of the transgene or the animal's native genes and therefore could affect the health of the animal. All animals containing a recombinant DNA construct are regulated, including subsequent generations of animals that contain the construct that were derived from the original manipulated parent animals by breeding with a nontransgenic animal.

A distinction may be made between transgenic animals that are to be used for food production and nonfood transgenic animals. Transgenic animals that are used for nonfood research purposes (e.g., laboratory mice) or to produce human therapeutic proteins are contained within controlled environments and may not be as strictly regulated as those that are grown in open environments for food production unless safety issues are raised. Laboratory animals and animals raised in contained facilities for production of pharmaceuticals pose a low risk for unintended release into the environment. A transgenic goat that was engineered to produce human antithrombin protein was approved by the FDA in 2009 and was the first transgenic animal to receive regulatory approval for commercialization. Antithrombin is extracted from goats' milk and is used to prevent blood clots from developing during surgery and childbirth in humans who are unable to produce sufficient amounts of the protein. Genetically engineered animals, such as insects, that have been developed for nonfood uses, like biocontrol of pests, and that may be released into uncontrolled environments are evaluated by the EPA.

To gain approval, a genetically engineered food animal must be demonstrated to be safe for production and consumption, and the introduced characteristic must be shown to be effective as intended. The risk assessment by the FDA and the regulatory agencies of many other countries is consistent with those of the international standards still under development by the Codex Alimentarius Commission of the Food and Agriculture Organization and World Health Organization. The FDA considers several characteristics, including the method of introduction and detection and the nature of the introduced DNA (e.g., expression, stability, and potential for the construct to recombine with pathogens); the traits conferred by the introduction of the transgene(s) and any alterations from the normal phenotype of the corresponding nontransgenic animal, especially where it may impact the composition of the animal product (e.g., production of allergens, toxins, and novel metabolites and potential for unintended cell disregulation); and methods for production, processing, and disposal of transgenic animals and their tissues. Regulations also take into consideration the risk associated with the release of a genetically modified animal into the environment, whether intentional or accidental. Measures to prevent the escape of farm animals, and their products, from barns and pastures are required. Transgenic animals must be prevented from mating with nontransgenic relatives, which could spread the transgene, disrupt an ecosystem, or reduce biological diversity. Aquaculture facilities that raise transgenic fish, for example, must ensure that the fish cannot escape and poachers cannot get in.

Patenting Biotechnology

The principal objective of biotechnology is to produce commercial products for economic gain. However, no company will initiate high-risk, long-term projects without knowing that the results of its research efforts can be

legally protected from competitors. At the same time, society at large has a stake in encouraging industrial innovation. A strategy that meets both of these objectives is for the government to grant inventors exclusive rights to the novel products or processes that they develop. Collectively, these sanctioned privileges are called intellectual property rights and include trade secrets, copyrights, trademarks, and patents. Trade secrets comprise private information about specific technical procedures and formulations that a company wishes to protect from others. Copyrights protect the authorship of published works from unauthorized use. Trademarks can be either words or symbols that identify a particular product or process of one company. For example, the term FailSafe is the legally recognized designation for a polymerase chain reaction (PCR) procedure marketed by Epicentre Technologies. Other companies that sell similar PCR kits have created their own protected names.

For biotechnology, patents are the most important form of intellectual property. A patent is a legal document that gives the patent holder exclusive rights to implement the described invention commercially. Moreover, on the basis of the extent of the claims of the patent, the patent holder can develop other products that are directly derived from the original invention, while competitors would have to license the right to use the invention in order to develop a product based on it. On the other hand, a patent is a public document that must contain a detailed description of the invention, so it informs others about the nature and limits of the invention, allowing them to decide whether they should continue working in a particular direction or try to use the patented invention as a springboard to other possible innovations.

Patent decisions and laws vary from country to country, although there are ongoing attempts to develop international standards. The duration of the exclusive rights of a patent is 20 years from the date that the application is filed in all countries. However, in the United States, if there is a dispute about priority, the applicant who was first awarded the patent has the rights for 20 years (first-to-invent principle). In almost all other countries, the patent is given to the applicant who filed first (first-to-file principle). Usually it takes 2 to 5 years following the filing of the initial patent application before a patent is granted. In every jurisdiction, the holding of a patent can be of considerable economic value, and it is not a trivial matter to receive one. For this reason, both the patent application and the invention must meet a very strict set of criteria.

Generally, for either a product or a process to be patentable, it must satisfy four fundamental requirements:

1. The invention, after having been shown to work ("reduced to practice") must be "novel," meaning that the invention does not exist as another patent that is held by someone else in another country; is not an existing product or process; and, outside the United States, has not appeared in some published form before the submission of the patent application. In the United States, an inventor has 1 year following publication in which to apply for a patent.

2. A patent cannot be granted for something that was merely previously unknown, i.e., a discovery; rather, the invention must contain, as judged by the patent office, an inventive step that was "not obvious" to other workers in the field.

3. The invention must be "useful" in some way, whether it is a process, an instrument, a compound, a microorganism, or a multicellular organism.

4. Every patent application must contain a description of the invention that is sufficiently thorough that a person knowledgeable in the same field can implement it.

A patent cannot be granted for anything that is "a product of nature." The notion here is that it is not appropriate for society to give a monopoly to someone for something that occurs naturally, has merely been discovered, and therefore belongs to the public. Often companies and individuals skirt this constraint by applying for a patent that covers the process of purification of a product, thereby avoiding the direct question of ownership of either a natural substance or an organism that produces the product. In some countries, such as the United States, according to the Supreme Court in a landmark decision, virtually "anything under the sun that is made by man" is patentable; however, in other countries, including members of the European Union, therapeutic and diagnostic procedures are not patentable.

There is no simple, immediate system for the granting of a patent. The application must be prepared by an expert, normally a patent lawyer, and is organized in a defined pattern. In the United States, the application must have a title; an abstract describing succinctly the nature of the application; a section on the background of the invention that includes a full and open description of the current "state of the art" in the field of the invention; a comprehensive summary of the invention with, if considered helpful, figures and schematic representations; sections that explain the nature of the invention and describe how the invention works; and, finally, a list of claims about the invention and how the invention may be used. The application is sent to the U.S. Patent and Trademark Office (PTO), where it is reviewed by an examiner for novelty, nonobviousness, utility, feasibility, and general acceptability as a patentable invention.

If an examiner agrees that the invention meets all the criteria for patentability, then a patent is awarded. However, the receipt of a patent is not a license to produce and sell the invention. All statutory regulations must be met before any product can be marketed. For example, if a patent is granted for a genetically engineered microorganism, the manufacturer must satisfy the recombinant DNA regulations for its production, distribution, and release. Protection of patent rights is the responsibility of the patent holder, and generally that means bringing a lawsuit(s) against those who are presumed to be infringing on the patent. These disputes are decided by the courts and not the patent office. Similarly, if a person or company feels that an awarded patent is inappropriate, the legitimacy of the patent can be challenged by a lawsuit.

If a patent application is rejected by an examiner, then the applicant can appeal the decision to a Patent Appeals Board. If this appeal is turned down, then the decision can be challenged legally. For some applicants, patenting can be a frustrating experience. There are a number of cases in which the stakes are considered to be so high that costly court battles go on for years. Thomas Edison, who held more than a thousand patents in his lifetime, once described a patent as "an invitation to a lawsuit."

Product patents and process patents make up the two major categories of patents. Products include homogeneous substances, complex mixtures, and various devices; processes include preparative procedures, method-

TABLE 22.3 Common types of patent categories with examples of biotechnology inventions

Category	Examples
Product patents	
Substance	Cloned genes, recombinant proteins, monoclonal antibodies, plasmids, promoters, vectors, cDNA sequences, antigens, peptides, RNA constructs, antisense oligonucleotides, peptide nucleic acids, ribozymes, and fusion proteins
Composition of matter	Multivalent vaccines, biofertilizers, bioinsecticides, host cells, microorganisms, transformed cell lines, and transgenic organisms
Devices	Pulsed-field gel electrophoresis apparatus, DNA-sequencing units, and microprojectile gene transfer machine
Process patents	
Process of preparation	DNA isolation, synthesizing double-stranded DNA, vector–insert construction, PCR applications, and purification of recombinant proteins
Method of working	Nucleic acid hybridization assays, diagnostic procedures, and mutation detection systems using PCR
Use	Applying biofertilizers and bioinsecticides, fermentation of genetically modified microorganisms, and nontherapeutic animal treatment systems

ologies, or actual uses (Table 22.3). The patenting of biotechnology innovations has been based on the historical experience of patenting inventions by the agricultural, fermentation, pharmaceutical, and medical industries. For example, in 1873, Louis Pasteur received two patents (U.S. patents 135,245 and 141,072) for a process for fermenting beer that included the living organism (yeast) used in the process. Today, most but not all biotechnology patent applications are straightforward, and patents are granted without any significant problems. However, the first time a scientist attempted to patent a genetically modified microorganism that was engineered by the introduction of different plasmids, each of which carried the genes for a separate hydrocarbon degradative pathway, the case was highly controversial. This genetically modified bacterium, which was capable of breaking down many of the components of crude oil, was developed by A. Chakrabarty, who at the time worked for the General Electric Corporation. However, despite its potential usefulness in cleaning up oil spills, the patent application for the bacterium was rejected by the U.S. PTO on the grounds that microorganisms are products of nature and, as living things, are not patentable. In 1980, in a landmark decision, the U.S. Supreme Court decided that this organism was patentable according to the U.S. Patent Statute, arguing that "a live, human-made microorganism is patentable subject matter...as a manufacture or composition of matter."

The argument against patenting this genetically engineered microorganism tended to center on how the organism was developed. In the past, induced mutation followed by selection for novel properties was an acceptable way to create a patentable living organism. However, genetic engi-

neering was considered by some to be "tampering with nature." Consequently, it was argued that no inventor should benefit from manipulating "products of nature." This position was not upheld. Thus, in the United States from 1980 onward and later in other countries, organisms, regardless of the means that were used to develop them, must be judged by the standard criteria of novelty, nonobviousness, and utility to determine if they are patentable.

Patenting in Different Countries

The rights given by a patent extend only throughout the country in which the application was filed. Therefore, to protect an invention, a patent application must be filed separately in each country, and although the World Intellectual Property Organization is attempting to develop international standards, patent offices in different countries often reach quite different conclusions about the same patent application. For example, in 1989 the biotechnology company Genentech applied for a patent in the United Kingdom for, among other things, the production of human tissue plasminogen activator (tPA) by recombinant DNA processes. This protein exists in small amounts in the human body and converts plasminogen to plasmin. Plasmin is an active enzyme that degrades the fibrin of a blood clot. Consequently, human tPA has been considered as a possible therapeutic agent for the prevention and treatment of coronary thrombosis. Genentech, after considerable effort, assembled a complete version of a human tPA complementary DNA (cDNA) and cloned this cDNA into *E. coli* for the production of large amounts of pure tPA. In its patent application, Genentech claimed rights to human tPA as a product based on certain procedures of recombinant DNA technology that they developed, the cloning vector system, and the transformed microorganism. As a part of the "process" category, protection for the use of human tPA as a pharmaceutical agent was also sought by Genentech. A total of 20 claims were presented in the original patent application. Some of these were broad and others were narrow in scope. The patent was rejected by the United Kingdom's patent office. Genentech then appealed to the United Kingdom's Court of Appeals, which, after considerable deliberation, invalidated all of the claims for a variety of reasons. The judgment concluded that the patent was novel, but some of the judges argued that the submission was obvious; therefore, it could not be patented.

In contrast, Genentech was readily awarded a patent for human tPA in the United States. The U.S. patent not only protects the form of human tPA that was to be marketed by Genentech but also gives Genentech exclusive rights to all similar, but not identical, active forms of human tPA. Genentech won a lawsuit against two other biotechnology companies that were found to be infringing on its tPA patent, although they were selling nonidentical forms of tPA.

The Japanese version of Genentech's tPA patent is limited to the amino acid sequence of the human tPA that was cloned and patented by Genentech. In Japan, other companies can sell variant forms of human tPA. Thus, basically the same patent application was rejected, approved and given a broad interpretation, and approved and given a narrow interpretation by three different patent offices. For the present, at least, there are divergent views about what is or is not a patentable invention.

Patenting DNA Sequences

Currently, isolated nucleic acid sequences, whether DNA, RNA, or cDNA derived from RNA, and proteins are patentable. Although gene sequences and the mRNA and proteins encoded in these sequences are found naturally in organisms, purification from their natural state is considered sufficient to render them patentable. Since 1980, thousands of patent applications for whole genes have been approved by patent offices throughout the world. In the United States, more than 40,000 DNA-related patents have been issued, at a rate of 3,000 annually since 1998, and almost 20% of human genes have been patented. Some of these are used to make therapeutic proteins such as recombinant erythropoietin. Erythropoietin stimulates the formation of red blood cells and is used to prevent anemia in patients with kidney failure who require dialysis. Many of the other patented gene sequences are used as diagnostic probes. One example results from the discovery that particular mutations in the human gene *BRCA1* are linked to breast cancer. A patent, issued to Myriad Genetics Inc., claims methods to detect these mutations in *BRCA1* to diagnose a predisposition to breast cancer.

With the rapid accumulation of genetic sequences from genome sequencing projects and the undertaking of the partial sequencing of thousands of cDNA molecules from different organisms, tissues, and organs, the patenting of nucleic acid sequences became extremely contentious. In 1991, the issue of patenting gene fragments was broached when scientists from the U.S. National Institutes of Health filed for the patent rights for 315 partially sequenced human cDNAs (expressed sequence tags [ESTs]). Two additional filings brought the total number of partial sequences to 6,869. In 1994, in a preliminary ruling, the U.S. PTO notified the National Institutes of Health that it would reject the patent application on the grounds that the functions of the sequences were not known. In other words, partial sequences by themselves did not fulfill the requirement of utility and were not patentable. However, by 1997, over 350 patent applications for more than 500,000 partial DNA sequences had been filed, mostly by private companies, which purportedly met the standard for usefulness. One of these patent proposals sought protection for about 18,500 ESTs. Consequently, serious concerns were raised about granting patents for large numbers of sequenced genes and partially sequenced DNA fragments with broadly based applications.

Individuals who opposed the patenting of DNA fragments with unknown or loosely defined functions contended that genes and partial DNA sequences are discoveries or, more likely, products of nature and definitely not inventions. Others conceded that, although eventually some of these sequences might be useful, it was premature and speculative to award patents without additional information about the functions of the sequences. In this context, the thousands of ESTs are considered to be "means to ends" and not the actual end points. On the other side, those who favored patenting ESTs maintained that these collections were novel because they defined the normal messenger RNA (mRNA) complements of various tissues and organs and consequently had utility because each collection could be used as a diagnostic assay to determine the extent to which a disease alters the normal complement of mRNAs in various organs.

After developing some ad hoc rules, the U.S. PTO examined in more detail a full range of issues and concluded that genes and partial DNA sequences were patentable. On January 5, 2001, a set of guidelines for gene

patenting was released. The key requirement for this type of application was that each DNA sequence must have "specific and substantial credible utility." Moreover, the written specifications and claims for each sequence must be thorough and demonstrate the actual use of each sequence and not merely a potential function. These guidelines have established the criteria for patenting incomplete DNA sequences in the United States, although the granting of patents for any human DNA sequence remains controversial.

Also controversial is the increased scope of the DNA patent claims in recent years. Often included in the claims to DNA sequences and the proteins they encode are antibodies against the protein, even when the antibody has not actually been produced. Antibodies against human proteins are important from a commercial perspective because they are used for diagnostic purposes and as therapeutic agents, and therefore, there is considerable incentive to include them in patent applications. However, some argue that they do not meet the criteria for patentability because in many cases the antibodies have not been produced and therefore their characteristics are not specifically described and working examples are not provided.

Patenting Multicellular Organisms

The patenting of multicellular organisms continues to raise ethical and social concerns. However, there is nothing intrinsically new about the exclusive ownership of living material. In the past, microorganisms were routinely patented, and specific laws were promulgated to give plant

MILESTONE

Transgenic Non-Human Mammals

INVENTORS: P. LEDER and T. A. STEWART
Assignee: President and Fellows of Harvard College, Cambridge, MA
U.S. patent 4,736,866, 12 April 1988

In 1980, the U.S. Supreme Court defined a patentable invention as one that included "anything under the sun that is made by man." In 1988, a transgenic mouse was the first genetically engineered animal to be patented. In this case, the transgene consisted of a cancer-causing gene (oncogene) driven by a promoter in the long terminal repeat of the mouse mammary tumor virus (MMTV LTR). The oncogene was the *myc* gene from the chicken myelocytomatosis OK10 virus. The invention entailed cloning an MMTV LTR-*myc* fusion gene into a plasmid, injecting linearized plasmid DNA into the male pronuclei of fertilized one-celled mouse eggs, identifying offspring that expressed the *myc* gene, and establishing transgenic mouse lines. In some of these lines, the *myc* gene was expressed in several

different tissues, and in other lines, it was limited to one or a few tissues. The integration of the MMTV LTR-*myc* gene construct, according to Leder and Stewart, "increases the probability of the development of neoplasms (particularly malignant tumors) in the animal." These transgenic organisms can be used to test whether a compound either causes or prevents cancer and as a source of cell lines from cells of various tissues, such as the heart, that are difficult to culture. Since 1989, Du Pont has been selling one of these lines of transgenic mice under the trade name OncoMouse. More generically, others prefer to call this mouse line the "Harvard oncomouse" or, for short, just "oncomouse."

The granting of U.S. patent 4,736,866 was contentious, with much

of the concern directed at the ethical implications of such patents. Those who oppose the patenting of transgenic animals argue that this type of patent violates the sanctity of life, threatens the integrity of species, and fosters inhumane treatment of animals. Despite these allegations, since 1988, hundreds of patents have been granted in the United States for various transgenic organisms. For example, there are now patents for transgenic animals that act as models for benign prostatic disease, inflammatory disease, altered fat tissue metabolism, and thrombocytopenia, to name a few. To date, neither the U.S. courts nor the U.S. government has suggested that, in principle, any of these patents is inappropriate. The patenting of transgenic organisms is no longer an issue in the United States, and after much discussion and litigation, transgenic animals are now patentable in most jurisdictions throughout the world.

breeders the right to own various plant varieties. The transgenic mouse ("OncoMouse") that carries an activatable gene that makes it susceptible to tumor formation has been the precedent-setting case in many jurisdictions to determine whether genetically modified animals are patentable. Currently, patenting of genetically modified animals is sanctioned in most developed countries, including the United States, members of the European Union, Japan, Australia, and New Zealand. However, in other countries such as Canada, it is still not possible to patent a multicellular organism such as the OncoMouse.

Vigorous challenges to patenting transgenic animals have been put forward on moral grounds. In other words, the issue is whether society considers this form of patenting acceptable. From a historical perspective, it is unlikely that a position based on ethical considerations will be completely successful in preventing the patenting of all transgenic animals. For example, if an invention purports to facilitate a new treatment for human disease, the currently prevalent view in most countries is that human rights and needs supersede those of animals. However, patenting is not an absolute right, and governments, by passing specific laws, can determine what can or cannot be patented. If an invention is considered by various special interest groups to have a potentially negative economic impact on an existing agricultural practice, for example, then it is quite possible that a law preventing the implementation of the new technology could be passed.

Patenting and Fundamental Research

Not everyone believes that patenting is worthwhile. Some opponents argue that awarding a monopoly restricts competition, leads to higher prices, curtails new inventions, and favors large corporations at the expense of individual inventors or small companies. Despite these concerns, the patent system is well established and is here to stay. Moreover, patent ownership does not appear to prevent significant research and development by other researchers and companies. Indeed, it might be argued that if patents were serious impediments to innovation, then U.S. patent 4,237,224, which was granted to Stanley Cohen and Herbert Boyer in 1980 for recombinant DNA technology for both the use of viral and plasmid vectors and the cloning of foreign genes, should have seriously constrained the development of recombinant DNA technology (Fig. 22.2). Obviously, no such hindrance has occurred.

In the past, patenting and patent enforcement were rarely of interest to academic researchers working in the biological sciences. Now, however, there is a view within the academic scientific community that patents and the consequences of patenting may be detrimental to established scientific values. Traditionally, science, especially university-based research, has been an open system with a free exchange of ideas and materials through publications and personal communications. The ideas of others have been respected, and contribution to the technical development of an area of study has, in many instances, been a shared enterprise. However, more recently, some scientists have begun to feel that the integrity of traditional scientific inquiry has become secondary to self-interest, in that public recognition and financial gain from innovations are the prime motivations for conducting scientific research. It is argued that research is often carried out secretly and has created elite, noncooperating research groups. In the past,

A method for replicating a biologically functional DNA, which comprises: transforming under transforming conditions compatible unicellular organisms with biologically functional DNA to form transformants; said biologically functional DNA prepared in vitro by the method of: (a) cleaving a viral or circular plasmid DNA compatible with said unicellular organism to provide a first linear segment having an intact replicon and termini of a predetermined character; (b) combining said first linear segment with a second linear DNA segment, having at least one intact gene and foreign to said unicellular organism and having termini ligatable to said termini of said first linear segment, wherein at least one of said first and second linear DNA segments has a gene for a phenotypical trait, under joining conditions where the termini of said first and second segments join to provide a functional DNA capable of replication and transcription in said unicellular organism; growing said unicellular organisms under appropriate nutrient conditions; and isolating said transformants from parent unicellular organisms by means of said phenotypical trait imparted by said biologically functional DNA.

FIGURE 22.2 The first claim of U.S. patent 4,237,224, granted to S. Cohen and H. Boyer on 2 December 1980 and entitled "Process for producing biologically functional molecular chimeras."

there was a tendency to avoid secrecy in basic research. The belief was that scientific knowledge would grow if research results were published as articles in journals that could be read by anyone, thereby enabling researchers to direct their studies in appropriate directions and to benefit from the discoveries of others. With secrecy, time and effort may be wasted on repeating experiments that, unbeknownst to the researcher, have already been done. Now, scientists are advised by patent lawyers to keep their work secret until a patent is filed. Consequently, the lure of patenting has made a large number of scientists reluctant to talk about their work, at least until after the patent application has been filed.

Furthermore, because of chronic financial constraints, nonprofit institutions, and especially universities, have sought additional forms of revenue. Licensing fees and royalties from patents can be sources of new income. One example is the Cohen-Boyer patent for recombinant DNA, which, during its lifetime from 1980 to 1997, earned about $45 million for Stanford University and the University of California. Also, the Massachusetts Institute of Technology files more than 100 patents annually in all research fields and generates about $5.5 million per year from licensing patent rights. Most universities have established patent policies and offices that facilitate both patenting and the transfer of technology, at a price, to industry. Faculty members usually receive a portion of the income from their inventions. Clearly, entrepreneurial activity is a fact of life at many universities. The challenge is to prevent this legitimate function from dominating all aspects of academia.

In sum, the enthusiasm for patenting and patent protection has elicited the perception that traditional science may become hostage to patent holders and that research will become less fruitful. Others feel that the traditional way of doing science is an outmoded, inefficient, and indulgent exercise and that patent ownership and the drive for ownership will spur new discoveries. This controversy will not be readily resolved. It is clear that the emergence of molecular biotechnology has raised far-reaching considerations, even including how scientific inquiries ought to be conducted.

SUMMARY

Significant technological advances, such as molecular biotechnology, are seldom implemented without controversy. The issues and concerns raised by the ability of scientists to genetically engineer organisms have had far-reaching implications and have resulted in the establishment of official guidelines to ensure that the introduction of recombinant DNA products into the marketplace does not adversely affect human or animal health or the environment. In this chapter, various aspects of the regulation of recombinant DNA technology, food products from genetically modified organisms, and the release of genetically modified organisms into the environment are discussed.

Guidelines for the proper conduct of recombinant DNA technology experiments were established by the NIH in the late 1970s and were fine-tuned in the early 1980s, but two unresolved issues remained. First, how was the commercialization of genetically engineered products to be regulated? Second, how was the deliberate release of genetically modified organisms into the environment to be managed? Industry, believing that no special regulations should be implemented for genetically engineered products, has taken the view that the nature of the product and its properties, not the process that was used to manufacture the product, are what matter. This view was adopted in the United States for pharmaceutical products. On the other hand, there has been more concern about genetically engineered products that are consumed by humans and animals, including the food ingredients produced by genetically engineered organisms and transgenic crops and livestock. Generally, the FDA, which is responsible for ensuring the safety of pharmaceuticals and food products, has taken a case-by-case approach to the problem of accepting genetically engineered products as safe to eat and produce. Depending on the product, a specific set of criteria must be met before it can be released for human consumption.

Guidelines have also been developed for the release of genetically modified organisms into the environment. For transgenic plants grown in open fields, the potential for unintended impacts on other organisms in the cultivation area, such as insects, or in adjacent fields, such as weed plants, must be evaluated. This is also the case for genetically engineered animals that may escape from contained facilities, such as pastures or aquaculture pens.

Companies that produce biotechnology products often invest a great deal of time and resources to develop the products to the commercialization stage. Patents are a means to protect their investment by giving the patent holder exclusive rights to make, use, or sell the product for a specific period of time. These rights are a reward for developing a procedure, compound, or apparatus and are intended to spur innovation. The public also benefits from the disclosure of the details of an invention, knowledge that will both prevent loss of time and energy in the pursuit of something that has already been invented and stimulate further research. For a patent to be granted, an invention must be novel, not obvious, and useful. In addition, the invention should not be a "product of nature."

The key case that established that genetically engineered microorganisms were patentable was brought forward by A. Chakrabarty. In 1980, the U.S. Supreme Court ruled that a bacterium that had been created by a form of genetic manipulation could be patented. As a result of this landmark decision, U.S. patents have been granted for genetically modified plants and animals. Moreover, after considerable debate, transgenic animals and plants are also patentable in most countries in the world.

With the development of molecular biotechnology, questions about whether private industries should be allowed to own or patent genetically engineered organisms have been raised. On one hand, it has been argued that without such proprietary rights, biotechnology companies would not have the incentive to develop and market novel products. On the other hand, some critics find this type of privilege to be morally unacceptable, and they contend that patents of this sort inhibit research and constrain innovation. For a variety of reasons, patenting has also had an impact on how university-based biotechnology research is conducted.

REFERENCES

Adler, R. 1984. Biotechnology as an intellectual property. *Science* 224:357–363.

Berg, P., D. Baltimore, S. Brenner, R. O. Roblin III, and M. F. Singer. 1975. Asilomar conference on recombinant DNA molecules. *Science* 188:991–994.

Berg, P., D. Baltimore, H. W. Boyer, S. N. Cohen, R. W. Davis, D. S. Hogness, R. Roblin, J. D. Watson, S. Weissman, and N. D. Zinder. 1974. Potential biohazards of recombinant DNA molecules. *Science* 185:303.

Bradford, K. J., A. Van Deynze, N. Gutterson, W. Parrott, and S. H. Strauss. 2005. Regulating transgenic crops sensibly: lessons from plant breeding, biotechnology and genomics. *Nat. Biotechnol.* 23:439–444.

Carmen, I. 1992. Debates, divisions, and decisions: recombinant DNA Advisory Committee (RAC) authorization of the first human gene transfer experiments. *Am. J. Hum. Genet.* 50:245–260.

Caulfield, T., R. M. Cook-Deegan, F. S. Kieff, and J. P. Walsh. 2006. Evidence and anecdotes: an analysis of human gene patenting controversies. *Nat. Biotechnol.* 24:1091–1095.

Cohen, S. N., A. C. Chang, H. W. Boyer, and R. B. Helling. 1973. Construction of biologically functional bacterial plasmids in vitro. *Proc. Natl. Acad. Sci. USA* 70:3240–3244.

Eckenswiller, C., and J. Morrow. 1996. Why patent life forms? *Policy Options* 17:11–15.

Evans, P. 2001. Impact of U.S. PTO guidelines on gene patents. *Genet. Eng. News* 21:6, 44.

Flattmann, G. J., and J. M. Kaplan. 2001. Patenting expressed sequence tags and single nucleotide polymorphisms. *Nat. Biotechnol.* 19:777–779.

Flattmann, G. J., and J. M. Kaplan. 2001. Patenting expressed sequence tags and single nucleotide polymorphisms. *Nat. Biotechnol.* 19:683–684.

Gordon, J. 1999. Intellectual property, p. 309–320. In A. L. Demain et al. (ed.), *Manual of Industrial Microbiology and Biotechnology*, 2nd ed. ASM Press, Washington, DC.

Hashimoto, K. and T. Aida. 2008. Antibody patenting without antibodies: a global trend. *Nat. Biotechnol.* 26:1341–1343.

Holman, C. M. 2007. Patent border wars: defining the boundary between scientific discoveries and patentable inventions. *Trends Biotechnol.* 25:539–543.

Howard, T., and J. Rifkin. 1977. *Who Should Play God? The Artificial Creation of Life and What It Means to the Human Race.* Dell Publishing Co., New York, NY.

James, C. 2008. *Global Status of Commercialized Biotech/GM Crops: 2008.* International Service for the Acquisition of Agri-Biotech Applications (ISAAA) brief no. 39. ISAAA, Ithaca, NY.

Johnson, E. 1996. A benchside guide to patents and patenting. *Nat. Biotechnol.* 14:288–291.

Juskevich, J. C., and C. G. Guyer. 1990. Bovine growth hormone: human food safety evaluation. *Science* 249:875–884.

Kamb, M. L., J. J. Murphy, J. L. Jones, J. C. Caston, K. Nederlof, L. F.

Horney, L. A. Swygert, H. Falk, and E. M. Kilbourne. 1992. Eosinophilia-myalgia syndrome in L-tryptophan-exposed patients. *JAMA* 267:77–82.

Kochhar, H. P. S., and B. R. Evans. 2007. Current status of regulating biotechnology-derived animals in Canada—animal health and food safety consideration. *Theriogenology* 67:188–197.

Marshall, E. 1997. Companies rush to patent DNA. *Science* 275:780–781.

Mayeno, A. N., and G. J. Gleich. 1994. Eosinophilia-myalgia syndrome and tryptophan production: a cautionary tale. *Trends Biotechnol.* 12:346–352.

McHughen, A., and S. Smyth. 2008. US regulatory system for genetically modified [genetically modified organism (GMO), rDNA or transgenic] crop cultivars. *Plant Biotechnol. J.* 6:2–12.

National Institutes of Health. 2001. *Guidelines for Research Involving Recombinant DNA Molecules (NIH Guidelines).* Department of Health and Human Services. National Institutes of Health, Washington, DC. http://oba.od.nih.gov/rdna/nih_guidelines_oba.html.

Poste, G. 1995. The case for genomic patenting. *Nature* 378:534–536.

National Research Council. 2000. *Genetically Modified Pest-Protected Plants: Science and Regulation,* p. 245. National Academies Press, Washington, DC.

Royal College of Physicians and Surgeons of Canada. 1999. *Report of the rBST Safety Panel.* Health Canada, Ottawa, Ontario, Canada. http://www.hc-sc.gc.ca/dhp-mps/vet/issues-enjeux/rbst-stbr/rep_rcpsc-rap_crmcc_final-a-eng.php.

Rudenko, L. and J. C. Matheson. 2007. The US FDA and animal cloning:

risk and regulatory approach. *Theriogenology* 67:198–206.

Smyth, S., and A. McHughen. 2008. Regulating innovative crop technologies in Canada: the case of regulating genetically modified crops. *Plant Biotechnol. J.* 6:213–225.

Spök, A. 2006. Molecular farming on the rise—GMO regulators still walking a tightrope. *Trends Biotechnol.* 25:74–82.

Spök, A., R. M. Twyman, R. Fischer, J. K. C. Ma, and P. A. C. Sparrow. 2008. Evolution of a regulatory framework for pharmaceuticals derived from genetically modified plants. *Trends Biotechnol.* 26:506–517.

Tiedje, J. M., R. K. Colwell, Y. L. Grossman, R. E. Hodson, R. E. Lenski, R. N. Mack, and P. J. Regal. 1989. The planned introduction of genetically engineered organisms: ecological considerations and recommendations. *Ecology* 70:298–315.

U.S. Food and Drug Administration. 15 January 2009. Guidance for industry no. 187—regulation of genetically engineered animals containing heritable recombinant DNA constructs. http://www.fda.gov/cvm.

U.S. Patent and Trademark Office. 2001. Utility examination guidelines. *Fed. Regist.* 66:1092–1099.

Williamson, A. R. 2001. Gene patents: socially acceptable monopolies or an unnecessary hindrance to research? *Trends Genet.* 17:670–673.

Wilson, M., and S. E. Lindow. 1993. Release of recombinant organisms. *Annu. Rev. Microbiol.* 47:913–944.

Yablonsky, M. D., and W. J. Hone. 1995. Patenting DNA sequences. *Bio/Technology* 13:656–657.

REVIEW QUESTIONS

1. What is the RAC? What was its role in regulating recombinant DNA research?

2. What criteria are used by the FDA to determine if a recombinant protein is acceptable as a food or food additive?

3. Why are genetically engineered microorganisms that are designed to be released into the environment regulated?

4. Present an argument for or against the ban on production of L-tryptophan in a genetically engineered bacterium for human consumption.

5. Discuss the positive and negative aspects of licensing recombinant bovine somatotropin.

6. What are some of the criteria that regulatory agencies consider in approving transgenic crops?

7. Why is it important to evaluate transgenic livestock on a case-by-case basis?

8. What are the essential requirements for patenting an invention?

9. What are process patents? Product patents? Give examples.

10. What information must be present in a patent application?

11. Why is a patent helpful to researchers who do not hold the patent?

12. What is the purpose of a patent?

13. Prepare arguments for both sides of the following debate: "Resolved: patenting of genetically engineered multicellular organisms should be banned."

14. Go to the U.S. PTO website (http://patents.uspto.gov/) and conduct a search for biotechnology patents. Use various combinations of search words, such as transgenic AND mouse or DNA AND diagnostic. Summarize the inventions in the five most recent patents.

Societal Issues in Biotechnology

N O TECHNOLOGY IS without risks. However, it is important to weigh the benefits of a technological development against the risks and to manage the risks in a responsible and informed manner. Over the last 30 years, recombinant DNA technology has provided many commercial products, described throughout this book, that benefit society, and after much scientific scrutiny, most have proven to be safe. For the most part, society has accepted the technology. Vaccines and other medicines developed using recombinant DNA technology are generally accepted by the public and considered to be necessary and at least as safe as nonrecombinant medicines. On the other hand, food products derived from transgenic plants and animals make some people uneasy. They question whether the introduction of a transgene may make the food toxic, allergenic, or less nutritious or whether the transgenes can be transferred to other gut organisms, or perhaps even to the consumer, during digestion. Furthermore, some worry that once a transgene is released from the laboratory environment, in a cultivated plant or a farmed animal, it will have unintended, harmful consequences that cannot be foreseen or controlled. Some opponents of molecular biotechnology will never be convinced that the products are safe. For them, the transfer of genes among unrelated organisms is unnatural and therefore inherently wrong. Others want assurance that the risks are minimal and are justified because the products are necessary and that society in general, rather than a few select interest groups, will benefit from their availability.

Concerns about the Safety of Consuming Genetically Modified Foods

All foods produced today are derived from plants and animals that have been genetically manipulated to enhance desirable characteristics through either selective breeding or recombinant DNA technology. The genetic changes introduced through recombinant DNA technology are vastly smaller and better understood than those from traditional breeding, as only a few well-characterized genes are introduced. Also, because known

regulatory elements are included on the introduced genetic constructs, the spatial and temporal expression of recombinant genes can be controlled. Despite these advantages, some consumers are concerned that manipulating the genomes of food plants and animals through recombinant DNA technology can lead to the production of foods that are unsafe for human consumption. This fear has had a powerful effect on the food industry. For example, consumer concern over the safety of transgenic foods led major baby food producers to stop using them in their products, and several fast food chains have removed them from their menus. On the other hand, proponents of genetic engineering argue that by rejecting transgenic ingredients producers are marketing foods that are less safe. Conventional food is more likely to be contaminated with potent mycotoxins produced by molds, which could be prevented by growing crops that are engineered to be mold resistant. Allergens, naturally present in many foods, could be removed through genetic manipulation.

Alteration of the Nutritional Content of Food

All genetically engineered foods derived from plants and animals are tested on a case-by-case basis for "substantial equivalence" before approval for commercialization by regulatory agencies. This means that the safety and nutritional content of genetically engineered food must be substan-

TABLE 23.1 Comparison of nutritional content of glyphosate-tolerant transgenic corn grain (Roundup Ready corn line GA21) with that of the nontransgenic parental control line

Nutrient	Transgenic corn	Nontransgenic corn	Range (avg) for conventional corn
Proximates (% dry weight)			
Protein	11.05	10.54	6.67–14.69 (10.18)
Fat	3.90	3.98	2.03–4.90 (3.48)
Carbohydrates	83.7	83.8	77.4–89.5 (84.8)
Fatty acids (% total fatty acids)			
Palmitic (16:0)	10.70	10.72	8.57–17.46 (11.87)
Stearic (18:0)	1.68	1.67	1.02–2.86 (1.94)
Oleic (18:1)	24.2	24.1	17.4–38.5 (25.6)
Linoleic (18:2)	61.4	61.5	47.7–64.2 (57.5)
Minerals (% dry weight)			
Phosphorus	0.326	0.326	0.160–0.533 (0.321)
Calcium	0.0039	0.0043	0.0022–0.0163 (0.0043)
Amino acids (% total amino acids)			
Methionine	2.16	2.17	(2.05)
Cysteine	2.22	2.28	(2.12)
Lysine	3.11	3.02	(3.09)
Leucine	12.98	12.87	(12.91)
Tryptophan	0.61	0.61	(0.62)
Phenylalanine	5.31	5.33	(5.10)

Adapted from Chassy et al., *Comp. Rev. Food Sci. Food Saf.* 3:35–104, 2004.

Only some of the nutrients measured are listed. Also shown are the ranges of nutrient values found in conventional corn grains in the United States. The values in the rightmost column were provided by the International Life Sciences Institute Crop Composition database (http://www.cropcomposition.org). Note: the ranges for individual amino acids could not be calculated from available data.

tially the same as those of the corresponding conventional food. The nutrients that are measured include carbohydrates, proteins, fats, amino acids, fatty acids, vitamins, and minerals (Table 23.1). The natural variation in nutritional content among the conventional varieties of the food product due to varietal, developmental, or environmental factors is taken into consideration, and therefore, there is usually a range of levels that are considered acceptable for a given food. Also considered are any changes in antinutritional factors that occur naturally in foods. These include chelators, such as phytic acid, which effectively remove calcium, iron, zinc, and magnesium; protease inhibitors, which prevent protein digestion; and lectins, which reduce the bioavailability of carbohydrates. The measurements are used to determine whether undesirable changes in nutrient content have occurred as a consequence of genetic manipulation, that is, whether levels of important nutrients are reduced or levels of potentially harmful compounds have increased.

Numerous feeding trials in which insect-resistant or herbicide-tolerant transgenic corn (maize), rice, potatoes, soybeans, or tomatoes were fed to laboratory animals or livestock for prolonged periods, and often for several generations, have found no adverse effects related to nutrient deficiencies. There were no significant differences in the composition, quality, or digestibility of the food or in the development, health, or performance of animals fed genetically engineered and conventional plants. For example, more than 20 studies have shown that the yield and quality (fat, lactose, and protein content) of milk produced by lactating dairy cows fed corn genetically engineered to be insect resistant or corn, soybeans, or beets genetically modified to be tolerant of the herbicide glyphosate are the same as those of milk from cows fed a nontransgenic diet.

Detailed analyses of the compositions of products derived from cloned animals has led the U.S. Food and Drug Administration (FDA) Center for Veterinary Medicine to conclude that there is no difference between the nutritional contents of meat or milk from clones and conventionally bred animals. These studies measured milk yields and milk and meat fat, protein, and carbohydrate contents. The amounts of amino acids, fatty acids, and important vitamins and minerals were also determined. It is acknowledged that an exhaustive analysis of tissue composition is impossible due to the complexity of the molecules present and that composition is impacted appreciably by the diet of the animal and its environment.

Several plants have been engineered to improve the nutritional value of food (Table 23.2). In these cases, the nutritional content of the genetically engineered food is intentionally made different from that of the conventionally bred plant and in this regard does not meet the criteria for substantial equivalence. An important example of a nutritionally enhanced food is "golden rice," which was created to address dietary deficiencies of vitamin A. Insufficient consumption of vitamin A is a significant problem in developing nations, where each year hundreds of thousands of children are blinded due to retinal and corneal damage, suffer from infectious diseases, or die as a consequence of this nutritional deficiency. Carrots, tomatoes, meat, and milk are good dietary sources of vitamin A; however, in developing countries, they are not always readily available. Rather, rice grains, which do not contain vitamin A, are a primary food source. In 2000, after 7 years of research, scientists successfully engineered rice to produce β-carotene, a biosynthetic precursor of vitamin A, by introducing genes from daffodil and the bacterium *Erwinia uredovora*. In the initial strain, the levels of

TABLE 23.2 Some genetically modified plants with enhanced nutritional value

Plant	Enhanced trait	Transgene product
Canola	Increased vitamin E	γ-Tocopherol methyl transferase
Canola	Increased γ-linolenic acid (omega-6 fatty acid)	Δ^6 and Δ^{12} desaturases
Canola	Added β-carotene (vitamin A precursor)	Phytoene synthase, phytoene desaturase, lycopene cyclase
Cassava	Decreased cyanogenic toxins	Hydroxynitrile lyase
Coffee	Decreased caffeine	Antisense xanthosine-N-7-methyltransferase
Corn	Increased vitamin C	Dehydroascorbate reductase
Corn	Increased iron	Ferritin, phytase
Potato	Decreased solanine (glycoalkaloid toxin)	Antisense sterol glycotransferase
Rice	Added β-carotene	Phytoene synthase, phytoene desaturase, lycopene cyclase
Rice	Increased iron	Ferritin, metallothionein, phytase
Tomato	Increased β-carotene and lycopene	Lycopene cyclase, phytoene desaturase
Tomato	Increased flavonoids (antioxidants)	Chalcone isomerase

Adapted from EFSA GMO Panel Working Group on Animal Feeding Traits, *Food Chem. Toxicol.* 46:S2–S70, 2008.

β-carotene were too low to provide the recommended amounts through diet, a problem highlighted by opponents of the genetically engineered rice. However, a subsequent version, announced in 2004, produced 20 times more β-carotene, thereby reducing the amount of rice that would need to be eaten in order to obtain sufficient vitamin A to stave off malnutrition.

Despite the promise of this nutritionally enhanced food to solve vitamin A malnutrition, almost a decade after it was first developed, golden rice is not yet available commercially. Among other extensive environmental and biosafety analyses, golden rice, as for other nutritionally enhanced foods, must be assessed for substantial equivalence in nutritional composition to nontransgenic rice, except for the compound that is intentionally altered (i.e., β-carotene). Where all other compositional qualities are similar to those of a nonengineered comparator plant, the safety of the altered nutrient levels is evaluated against well-established nutritional guidelines. The large amounts of golden rice required for a complete safety assessment have been difficult to obtain in the greenhouse and in the limited field trials approved so far. Lack of financial support for a product that is being developed for low-income consumers and aggressive opposition to nutritionally enhanced food developed through genetic engineering have delayed completion of the requirements for regulatory approval. Opponents argue that rice containing the vitamin A precursor is unnecessarily risky because other methods to deliver vitamin A are available, including vitamin tablets and vitamin-fortified foods, such as sugar, and growing vegetables rich in vitamin A. However, these methods are often costly and difficult to sustain. Despite the obstacles, holders of the various patented technologies that contributed to the development of golden rice have provided licenses to developing countries at no charge in anticipation of its eventual commercialization (expected in 2011) as a humanitarian gesture to improve the health of billions of people.

Potential for Introducing Toxins or Allergens into Food

It is important to bear in mind that no foods can be guaranteed to be 100% safe. Many foods contain trace amounts of natural toxins that are harmless when consumed at low levels. For example, two common food plants, the potato and tomato, are members of the nightshade (Solanaceae) family that produce glycoalkaloids that can cause serious illness when consumed in relatively large quantities. Also, many foods naturally contain proteins that elicit an allergic response in some consumers. Extensive health safety tests of animals that compare genetically engineered foods to their nonengineered counterparts have concluded that the process of creating genetically engineered foods does not make the food different in digestibility or detrimental to the health of the consuming animal. However, it is necessary to ensure that the introduction of a specific transgene into a food product does not increase the risk of producing a toxin or allergen (Table 23.3). The regulatory agencies consider each food product derived from a transgenic plant or animal on a case-by-case basis and assess the risks against those associated with consuming the corresponding nontransgenic product.

There have been some highly publicized reports of adverse effects that have propagated unease among some consumers about eating genetically engineered foods. Often, the reports in the popular press have focused on particular aspects of the story that have led to confusion or have failed to mention that the data do not hold up to scientific scrutiny. For example, in August 1998, Arpad Pusztai, a scientist at the Rowett Research Institute in Aberdeen, Scotland, announced on a British television program that rats fed transgenic potatoes for 110 days were stunted and had suppressed immune function. He did not mention that the transgene encoded a plant lectin, a carbohydrate-binding protein. He also failed to emphasize that the experiments were preliminary and were being conducted to determine if this particular genetically modified plant was actually safe. Pusztai's revelation became instant news with the focus of attention on transgenic plants in general and not the specific gene that had been introduced into potatoes in this instance. The incident was further complicated when Pusztai's data were found by the director of his institute to be deficient scientifically. Eventually, after much controversy, Pusztai and an associate published a study suggesting that rats fed a diet consisting solely of transgenic potatoes engineered to express a plant lectin gene had compromised immune systems. Independent analysis of this report by a committee of the Royal Society in Britain and the National Institute for Quality Control of Agricultural Products in the Netherlands found serious scientific shortcomings that brought into question the validity of the results. Despite these expert assessments, this transgenic-potato saga was used by the critics of biotechnology as proof that transgenic plants are inherently dangerous to humans.

A transgene that is commonly introduced into crops encodes the crystal (Cry) protein, an insecticidal toxin, from the bacterium *Bacillus thuringiensis* (Bt toxin). When ingested by target insect larvae, the toxin interacts with specific receptors in the epithelium of the larval gut. The protein inserts into the epithelium, forming a pore through which gut contents leak, leading to the death of the insect. The Bt toxin has been used safely for over 40 years to protect crops from a variety of insect pests, either as an agricultural spray or produced by transgenic plants. The Cry protein is produced by *B. thuringiensis* in an inactive form as a full-length protein. Proteases

TABLE 23.3 Some examples of animal feeding studies conducted to assess the potential toxicity of genetically modified (GM) foods

GM food	Transgene	Test animal	Duration of feeding	Health effects
Corn	*epsps*	Rat	13 weeks	No adverse effects; animals were similar in overall health, body weight, food consumption, organ weights, blood and urine chemistry, and tissue appearance
Corn	*cry1Ab*	Chicken	38 days	No significant difference in survival and body weight
Corn	*cry1Ab*	Pig	91 days	No difference in nutrient digestibility and energy content
Soybean	*epsps*	Rat	13 weeks	No difference in animal activity, body weight, blood chemistry, and urine chemistry; no gross abnormalities
Soybean	*epsps*	Mouse	Gestation and lactation	No difference in litter size, body weight of pups, and testicular development
Potato	*bar*	Rat	10 weeks	No significant difference in body or organ weights, food consumption, sperm motility, litter size, survival and body weight of pups; significant reduction in male and female fertility

Adapted from Domingo, *Crit. Rev. Food Sci. Nutr.* **47**:721–733, 2007.

The health effects are compared to those in animals fed non-genetically modified food. *epsps* confers tolerance for glyphosate herbicide, *cry1Ab* confers resistance to lepidopteran insects, and *bar* confers tolerance for glyfosinate herbicide.

produced specifically by the insect cleave the protein, which actives the toxin. The proteases are active in the slightly alkaline environment of the insect gut. The protein is safe for human consumption because humans do not produce the specific protease required to activate the toxin or the epithelial receptors that bind the toxin, and the toxin is rapidly degraded under the acidic conditions found in the mammalian digestive system. Nonetheless, some consumers have questioned whether the Cry protein may be a potential allergen. This concern is fueled in part by reports that are often based on misinterpreted scientific studies. For example, in a 2005 campaign against Bt rice, Greenpeace stated that rice genetically engineered to produce the Cry1Ac protein "could cause an allergic reaction, as it did when tested on mice." Several scientific studies were cited to support the claim that the protein elicited an allergic reaction in mice. However, it was not explained that the purpose of the cited studies was to test the Cry1Ac protein as an adjuvant to increase the efficacy of a vaccine or that the Cry1Ac protein was chosen because it was known to have low toxicity in vertebrates. While anti-Cry1Ac antibodies typical of an immune response were produced in the immunized mice, they were not immunoglobulin E antibodies involved in the allergic response, nor was evidence of an allergic reaction presented. It was also not mentioned that Cry1Ac was already widely produced in crops consumed by humans and other animals without harmful effects. Interestingly, there has been almost no objection to the spraying of the Bt toxin over the last 4 decades; opposition seems only to be voiced against its production in transgenic plants.

To further support the allergenicity of Cry1Ac, opponents made reference to concerns among regulators regarding the potential allergenicity of another Bt product known as StarLink corn, an unfortunate association due to a regulatory breach by StarLink. The *B. thuringiensis* gene used to gen-

erate StarLink corn encodes the Cry9C protein, which differs from Cry1Ac and other Bt toxins. Although Cry9C is not similar to known protein allergens and is not derived from an organism known to produce allergenic proteins, it has greater heat stability and is not as readily digested, which are characteristics of some allergenic proteins. For these reasons, the FDA did not approve StarLink for human use but did allow it to be sold as animal feed and used for industrial purposes. However, in July 2000, Larry Bohlen, director of the Community, Health, and Environment Program for the U.S. affiliate of the international environmental organization Friends of the Earth, went grocery shopping and bought a large number of products that contained corn flour, including taco shells, corn flakes, and muffin mixes. He had these tested for the StarLink Cry9C gene using the polymerase chain reaction (PCR) test, and evidence of the gene was found in some of the taco shells. Clearly, food safety regulations had been broken. It was estimated that StarLink contaminated, at most, about 0.125% of all corn-based foods. The source of the contamination has never been traced. Aventis, the company that developed StarLink, has assumed that some farmers, probably inadvertently, mixed it with other varieties of corn despite written agreements that committed them to keep their harvested Bt crops segregated. The seed is no longer sold.

The StarLink episode had a number of ramifications. The critics of biotechnology pointed out that the regulatory system was seriously flawed and stressed that consumers should be aware of the hazards of genetically modified organisms. The biotechnology industry representatives noted there was no public health concern but that the regulatory issue had to be corrected. The FDA declared that it would no longer allow a product to be approved only for animal feed. A number of scientific advisory panels were convened to study in detail the consequences of Cry9C in human food, the possibility of consumer maladies due to eating products that may have been derived from StarLink, and how to improve the regulation and surveillance of transgenic crops. By 2001, there were no definitive cases of allergic reactions to Cry9C, but individuals who had symptoms compatible with a possible newly acquired allergy were monitored. No serious illness has been documented as a result of eating food contaminated with StarLink.

The potential for introduction of allergenic proteins into a food product that does not otherwise elicit an allergic response is a major concern. The FDA requires labeling to indicate genetically engineered foods containing proteins from organisms known to produce proteins that are allergens to humans. Major allergens are proteins from eggs, milk, shellfish, fish, tree nuts, soybeans, wheat, and peanuts. In most cases, such transgenic food products are not commercialized. For example, soybeans engineered to express a protein from Brazil nuts that was intended to increase the methionine content of the soybeans were found to react with sera from individuals known to be allergic to Brazil nuts. As a consequence, further development of the transgenic soybeans was voluntarily terminated by the developer.

Food allergies are a significant problem in developed countries. In the United States, about 5 to 8% of children and 1 to 2% of adults have food allergies, some of which can be fatal. Molecular biotechnology has the potential to reduce the allergenicity of some foods by preventing the synthesis of the allergenic protein (Table 23.4). A hypoallergenic variety of peanut is currently under development using RNA interference to reduce

levels of the seed storage protein Ara h 2, the most potent peanut allergen to which most hypersensitive individuals respond, often fatally.

Potential for Transferring Transgenes from Food to Humans or Intestinal Microorganisms

We consume a large amount of DNA, and the encoded protein products, in the plant and animal tissues that make up our daily diet. Indeed, these supply part of the nutrition from food. It has been estimated that an average adult consumes approximately 0.1 to 1 g of DNA per day. The DNA is partially degraded during food processing at high temperature or low pH and is further degraded into small fragments through chewing and the activities of nucleases in saliva and the gastrointestinal tract. Only a very small amount of the total DNA consumed remains in fragments that are capable of carrying an intact gene as the digested DNA passes into the small intestine. This was shown in patients who had an ileostomy, an operation in which the upper portion of the intestinal tract, the ileum, is severed from the lower portion of the small intestine, which allowed researchers to collect digestion products before they completed passage through the small intestine and colon. After eating soybeans genetically engineered with the *epsps* gene (encoding 5-enolpyruvylshikimate-3-phosphate synthase, which confers tolerance of the herbicide glyphosate), up to 3.7% of the consumed transgene was detected by PCR as a 180-base-pair fragment in the digestion products of the ileostomists. The full-length *epsps* gene (2.27 kilobase pairs) was detected in many of the collected samples. However, the *epsps* gene fragments were not detected in the feces of healthy volunteers with intact intestinal tracts and therefore were completely digested in the small and large intestines.

If the genes that are present in the food we eat remain intact in our intestinal tracts, can they be incorporated into our genomes, where they could disrupt the function of a gene or where they could be expressed, resulting in the production of a foreign protein? Several studies have shown that neither transgenic DNA nor the recombinant proteins encoded by the transgenes present in food are found in the tissues of humans and livestock that consume the food. PCR and Southern hybridization failed to detect recombinant DNA in the milk, eggs, skin, muscle, and other tissues of several livestock animals fed genetically engineered crops. Nonrecombinant chloroplast DNA, which is naturally present in multiple copies in plant cells, was detected in some tissues. This may have implications for transgenes that are incorporated into the chloroplast genome.

TABLE 23.4 Some foods containing allergenic proteins that may be reduced through genetic engineering

Food plant	Allergenic protein	Strategy to reduce allergenic protein
Rice	14–16-kilodalton allergen	Antisense RA17 gene silencing
Soybean	Gly m bd 30 K (P34; cysteine protease)	P34 sense cosuppression
Apple	Mal d 1	Mal d 1 RNA interference
Tomato	Lyc e 1 (profillin)	Lyc e 1 RNA interference
Tomato	Lyc e 3 (lipid transfer protein [LTP])	LTP RNA interference
Peanut	Ara h 2 (conglutin 7)	Ara h 2 RNA interference

Even when present in tissues, integration of functional genes from food DNA, transgenic or otherwise, into the genome of the consuming animal has never been found and is likely restricted by (1) the small fragment sizes of the DNA remaining in the gastrointestinal tract following food digestion, (2) the presence of cytosolic nucleases that further digest foreign DNA that is taken up by intestinal epithelial cells, (3) insufficient sequence homology for integration by homologous recombination, and (4) the requirement for appropriate transcription and translation signals for expression of an integrated gene.

The possibility that antibiotic resistance genes used as selectable markers during the process of creating transgenic plants could be transferred to microorganisms in the intestinal tract has also been investigated. Because most of the DNA derived from food that reaches the intestines, and particularly the colon, where most gut microorganisms reside, has been digested into small fragments, the risk of an intestinal microbe taking up and expressing a functional antibiotic resistance gene is extremely low. For example, an antibiotic resistance gene in transgenic corn was undetectable after 1 minute in sheep rumen fluid and in the intestines of chickens. Although there is no evidence from long-term studies of a variety of animals that antibiotic resistance genes consumed in transgenic food have been transferred to intestinal bacteria, to alleviate public concerns, alternate selection methods that avoid antibiotic resistance genes have been developed.

Controversy about the Labeling of Genetically Modified Foods

The labeling of biotechnology-derived foods is a contentious issue. In the United States, the composition of the product, not the process by which the product is produced, determines whether specific information should be added to a label. For example, corn syrup derived from Bt corn is identical to that from conventional corn. Consequently, in the United States, this type of product does not require a special label. In other words, the FDA policy follows the dictum, "If it quacks like a duck, walks like a duck, and looks like a duck, then it must be a duck." Labeling is required if the nutrient content of a genetically modified food is substantially different from that of the traditional product; if the food is novel, i.e., it never has been produced before; if it is likely to contain a potential allergen; or if it has an increased level of a toxic agent. In Europe, in contrast, the process has precedence over the product. Accordingly, it is mandatory for all European Union countries to label any food as "genetically modified" if more than 0.9% is from a genetically modified organism. The genetically modified food must also be traceable from its source on the farm through all stages of processing, storage, and transportation. This is to facilitate removal of the product should it be found to have adverse effects. Australia and New Zealand require the same designation if "novel DNA and/or protein is present in the final product," but not if the food is highly refined or there are no genetically modified ingredients in the final product. In most cases, the stringency of the labeling is not solely dependent on health concerns; often, economic and philosophical issues are also important considerations.

Historically, the food industry in the United States has argued against labeling genetically modified foods because it will be perceived as a warning and will unnecessarily stigmatize the product. On the other hand, as a mar-

keting strategy, some food companies and retail outlets are specifically labeling products that do not have any genetically modified ingredients. Since a label cannot be misleading or untruthful, the FDA has objected to descriptions such as "no genetically modified organisms" or "genetically modified free," because in the former case the product does not contain a viable organism and in the latter case there is no guarantee that some contamination has not occurred. Terms such as "genetically engineered" and "made through biotechnology" are acceptable to the FDA when there is no need to specify nutritional or health requirements. Consumer advocate groups in the United States have argued that the consumer has a right to know if a product comes from a genetically modified organism regardless of an equivalence of properties. Although legislation supporting this principle has been drafted by members of the U.S. Senate and House of Representatives, none of these proposals have had much success.

Concerns about the Impact of Genetically Modified Organisms on the Environment

There are currently more than 6.7 billion people on Earth, and the population is projected to grow to 9 billion in about 30 years. This is an enormous number of people to feed with an agricultural system that is already burdened by crop reductions due to disease, pests, adverse weather (drought, flooding, and hurricanes), competition with nonfood crops, and soil quality deterioration due to overuse of agricultural chemicals. Production of transgenic crops can offer solutions to some of these environmental problems by increasing the resistance of important crop plants to infectious disease, insect predation, and climate change and reducing applications of pesticides. However, some critics believe that our increasing dependence on genetically engineered crops is adversely affecting the environment by decreasing biodiversity and harming unintended organisms.

Impact on Biodiversity

In general, agriculture has decreased biodiversity. Crop plants are selected for high yields of their edible parts, hardiness, and other traits at the cost of loss of richness, not only of cultivated species, but also of wild plants as cultivation has expanded over a greater area. Newer, higher-yielding varieties have tended to replace traditional crops. The diversity of insects, birds, and other animals has also decreased as more land is dedicated to agriculture and host and food plants are lost. Application of agricultural chemicals to eradicate weeds and pests is a contributing factor. There is some concern that the trend toward extensive cultivation of crops that have been genetically engineered to resist environmental factors that normally limit plant growth, i.e., herbicide tolerance and insect resistance, could further decrease biodiversity. This concern stems mainly from the possibility that the transgenic plants could become weedy or invasive of natural habitats or that the transgenes can be transferred from genetically engineered crops to wild relatives or to non-genetically engineered crops and could confer on them a selective advantage. Enhanced growth of the unintentionally engineered plants could cause them to be invasive or to outcompete plants without the transgene.

Several species of weeds have been found to be resistant to the herbicide glyphosate. For the most part, this is due to overuse of the herbicide,

which selects for natural mutations that increase resistance in weeds, rather than to the transfer of the transgene through cross-breeding (hybridization), although the latter has been shown to occur at a low frequency. Pollination of wild relatives by genetically engineered crops can occur when they are within range of pollen distribution by wind, insects, etc., and when pollen production by the genetically engineered crop and flower production by the wild relative occur at the same time. Transfer of genes among plants that mainly self-pollinate (pollination of a flower by its own pollen), such as rice and soybeans, occurs at a low frequency. For example, transfer of a herbicide resistance gene from genetically engineered rice to wild red rice was found to occur at a frequency of less than 1%. The frequency of transfer is higher for plants that cross-pollinate (the pollen from one plant fertilizes the ovule of another plant). The glyphosate resistance gene from transgenic canola *(Brassica napus)*, an important oilseed crop, was transferred to a wild relative *(Brassica rapa,* or field mustard) at a frequency ranging from 7 to 14% depending on the *B. rapa* population. This was determined by collecting seeds from herbicide-sensitive *B. rapa* plants that had been interplanted with herbicide-tolerant transgenic *B. napus* and then assessing herbicide tolerance and production of the specific protein encoded by the transgene in the plants that developed from the *B. rapa* seeds. While cross-pollination occurred at a relatively high frequency between *B. napus* and *B. rapa,* hybridization between *B. napus* and three other wild relatives was extremely rare.

The spread of herbicide resistance genes reduces the ability of farmers to control weeds, and the weedy plants have the potential to become invasive, as they can proliferate in areas where the herbicides are used. Herbicide-resistant plants are unlikely to have an advantage in nonagricultural areas where herbicides are not applied. Moreover, hybridization does not always confer an advantage on the hybrid progeny. Hybrids resulting from cross-pollination by transgenic rice resistant to glyfosinate (a herbicide that disrupts glutamine biosynthesis) were less fit than their wild-type parents because flowering occurred too late to produce seed, which prevented proliferation of the hybrids. Hybrids that express a Bt toxin transgene may have a significant advantage when insect pressure is high.

The potential for gene flow to nontransgenic cultivars and wild relatives and its consequences are included in risk assessments required by regulatory agencies before a genetically engineered crop is commercialized, and strategies to manage the risks must be in place prior to cultivation. The assessment considers the mechanism by which the plant reproduces and pollen is disseminated, the nature of the transgene and any selective advantage it may impose, and the geographic context in which the crop will be grown, which includes the identification of sexually compatible wild relatives. Management strategies can include avoiding cultivation of a transgenic crop in areas where indigenous wild varieties are found and controlling embryo and/or seed viability through genetic engineering.

Impact of the Bt Toxin on Nontarget Insects

In May 1999, a report entitled "Transgenic pollen harms monarch larvae" by Losey et al. was published in the scientific journal *Nature*. In this study, pollen from Bt corn was sprinkled on milkweed leaves, the sole source of food for the larvae of the monarch butterfly, and extremely high mortality

was observed after monarch butterfly larvae fed on the treated leaves. The authors concluded that extensive Bt crop acreage could have "profound implications for the conservation of monarch butterflies." The study, which was conducted in the laboratory rather than under natural field conditions, incited much criticism. Scientists pointed out that appropriate controls were not used, the amount of pollen on the leaves was not calculated, and there was no indication whether the time of pollen shedding coincided with a feeding period of monarch butterfly larvae. These technical concerns were largely ignored because the monarch butterfly has iconic and aesthetic status in North America. Consequently, the study was widely reported and the threat to the monarch butterfly formed the cornerstone of the campaign against biotechnology in general. However, after 2 years of detailed studies, the initial skepticism of most entomologists was confirmed when it was proved that the risk of Bt toxin toxicity to the larvae of the monarch butterfly was negligible. Antibiotechnology factions have been reluctant to accept these findings. Much of their literature continues to stress that Bt crops are a threat to the survival of the monarch butterfly.

More recently, reports in the popular media have emerged suggesting that pollen containing the Bt toxin was responsible for severe reductions in the honeybee population in North America and Europe. Declines in the honeybee population, a phenomenon known as colony collapse disorder, were occurring at an alarming rate, and the consequences would be very serious if pollinators were not available to produce fruits. However, an analysis of 25 independent studies concluded that pollen containing the Cry proteins that are present in transgenic crops currently under cultivation and that are effective against coleopteran and lepidopteran predators are not toxic to honeybees, a hymenopteran insect. After a great deal of investigation, the general consensus among researchers is that because the Bt toxins are highly specific for target insects and are confined to plant tissues, the impact on nontarget insects is minimal. Several studies have shown that insect diversity and abundance have actually increased with the cultivation of Bt crops compared to application of chemical insecticide sprays that have a broader target range.

Environmental Benefits of Genetically Modified Organisms

Cultivation of plants that produce heterologous proteins that provide protection from pests has led to a global reduction in the application of agricultural chemicals, many of which have toxic effects on the environment. Spraying of insecticides was reduced by 94.5 million kg, or 19.4%, from 1996 to 2005 due to the cultivation of insect-resistant cotton alone. Insect-resistant corn accounted for a further 4.6% reduction. For example, the western corn rootworm is a devastating and pervasive insect pest of corn and causes huge economic losses in the United States and elsewhere. Because the predator is difficult to control, farmers routinely apply insecticides to their cornfields before infestation by the worm is apparent. The cultivation of genetically engineered varieties of corn that produce the Cry3Bb1 toxin, which is effective against the western corn rootworm, have obviated the spraying of insecticides against that insect.

Although some would argue that the widespread cultivation of herbicide-tolerant crops has increased our dependence on herbicides, it has actually resulted in a 25 to 30% reduction in herbicide applications to transgenic crops compared to conventional crops. While the use of glyphosate, the

herbicide to which most crops are engineered to be tolerant, has increased sharply over the last decade, the use of other herbicides has decreased. The herbicides that are applied are generally at lower strength and are less toxic. In addition, the herbicides can be applied to fields containing tolerant crops later in the season, after the crops have grown. This has dramatically reduced (and on many farms eliminated) soil tilling, the practice of turning the soil to remove weeds, and has thereby increased soil quality by reducing erosion and organic carbon loss and has decreased fuel consumption by farm machinery. The latter benefit is not trivial in its impact on the environment, as the estimated reduction in emissions of carbon dioxide, a greenhouse gas, as a consequence of growing herbicide-tolerant soybeans and canola is the equivalent of removing 400,000 cars from the road for 1 year.

Because different agricultural chemicals have different environmental toxicities, a better measure of their impact on the environment takes into consideration not only the amount of active ingredient applied, but also the toxicity of the chemical to farm workers, the consumer, and other organisms, such as birds and insects; its persistence in the soil; and its potential to leach into groundwater. These parameters are used to determine the relative environmental impact of each pesticide. Using these values, the global reduction in environmental impact resulting from changes in herbicide and pesticide applications to genetically modified crops was determined to be 15.3% over a 10-year period (1996 to 2005).

Many other examples have been presented throughout this book that illustrate the potential of genetic engineering to reduce damage to the environment. Pigs engineered with the phytase gene from bacteria utilize phosphorus in feed more efficiently and thereby reduce the phosphate content in their feces by up to 75%. Phosphate is a major environmental pollutant from pork production. Plants and bacteria can be genetically engineered to more effectively remove toxic compounds, such as heavy metals, from contaminated soils. Moreover, plants and animals can be engineered to more efficiently utilize nutrients and to grow under nonoptimal conditions. These features could enable cultivation of crops on less land or on land that would otherwise not be usable, thereby meeting the food demands of an increasing global population with reduced impact on resources.

Economic Issues

Who Benefits from Molecular Biotechnology?

Developers of biotechnology products that have applications in health care, agriculture, and industry have benefited financially from recombinant DNA technology. Global sales of all biotechnology goods and services by biotechnology companies exceed $70 billion annually, with firms in the United States accounting for more than half of the sales. Most of these companies develop pharmaceuticals. For example, in the United States and China, sales from health products account for 87 and 77% of total sales, respectively. Recombinant pharmaceutical products that are highly successful include the therapeutic proteins erythropoietin and human insulin, which respectively have sales of more than $8.8 billion and $5.3 billion annually.

Many smaller developers complain that the high cost of developing and commercializing a genetically engineered product prevents all but large multinational companies from profiting. For example, in the agricultural

biotechnology sector, where the cost of developing a genetically engineered product can exceed $20 million, due in part to stringent regulatory requirements, four companies own or co-own about 80% of the genetically engineered products that have received commercial approval: DuPont (United States), Monsanto (United States), Bayer Cropscience (Germany), and Syngenta (Switzerland). Moreover, high research and development costs have prohibited the commercialization of products that are not marketable on a large, profitable scale. This means that recombinant drugs that could target rare diseases or diseases that are found predominantly in low-income populations and transgenic crops other than herbicide-tolerant and insect-resistant crops and those that are not widely planted do not provide the revenues that are necessary to justify the high cost of product development. Improved varieties of crops that are important for resource-poor nations, such as rice, cassava, and millet, have not been developed as extensively. In addition, product development has been limited by antibiotechnology markets, such as the European Union, which in turn influence development in countries that rely on export to these markets.

Farmers in both developed and developing nations have perhaps been the greatest beneficiaries of recombinant DNA crop technology, not only due to increased yields from genetically engineered crops, but also from cost savings due to fewer applications of agricultural chemicals and to reduced labor and machinery costs. Profits are generally higher even after the higher cost of the transgenic seed is taken into consideration. Statistics for 2005 indicate that the global increase in farm income as a consequence of growing genetically modified crops was $5 billion. Most of the economic benefit (55%) was derived by farmers in developing countries. In particular, farmers in developing countries profited from cultivation of herbicide-tolerant soybeans and insect-resistant cotton. For example, a multiyear comparison of the productivity and profitability of small, resource-poor farms in South Africa growing nontransgenic cotton or bollworm-resistant Bt cotton found consistent yield increases of 156 to 185% for those growing Bt cotton. Although the Bt seed costs were roughly twice those of the conventional cotton, profits from the insect-resistant cotton were at least double due to higher yields, reduced pesticide costs, and reduced labor costs to spray the pesticide. For most insect-resistant crops, the greatest economic benefits are reaped in seasons when insect infestation is high. Because damage from insect predation is lower for the Bt crops, fungal infestations, which are often facilitated by insect damage to plant tissues, are also reduced. Cereals, oilseeds, and nuts contaminated with fungi are not suitable for sale due to increased risk of contamination with mycotoxins, such as aflatoxin, a carcinogenic toxin produced by *Aspergillus*. The economic benefits due to reduced mycotoxin contamination are significant at $30 million.

How Do Views about Genetically Engineered Food Affect Trade?

Exports of agricultural products from the United States to the European Union were valued at over $10 billion in 2008. However, differences in consumer acceptance and regulatory views have often made trade between the two regions difficult. In 1998, the European Union placed a moratorium on the importation of genetically modified corn, cotton, and soybean products. This prompted a complaint in 2003 by the United States, Canada, and Argentina to the World Trade Organization, which ruled in 2008 that the additional risk assessments and approvals required by the European Union

for some of the genetically engineered products were not based on scientific evidence and unfairly delayed trade. In contrast to the United States, only a few genetically engineered crops have been approved for cultivation and importation in the European Union, and to avoid labeling foods in which more than 0.9% is derived from an approved genetically engineered ingredient(s), exporters to the European Union have been forced to separate genetically modified crops from conventional crops, which is costly. Despite the view in many other countries that genetically modified foods are safe, Europeans are strongly opposed to the products. This is due in part to previous food scares, such as mad cow disease (bovine spongiform encephalopathy) in the 1990s, which left Europeans wary of food safety authorities who claimed that controversial foods were safe for human consumption. There is, however, concern among some farmers in the European Union that if new varieties of genetically engineered crops are not approved for importation from major feed producers in North and South America, where they are grown extensively, then there will be serious shortages of feed for livestock.

The resistance of the European Union to transgenic products has forced many developing countries to forgo the benefits of planting genetically engineered crops for fear that trade with the European Union will be jeopardized. In an extreme example, thousands of tons of food aid received by Zambia from the United States during the famine of 2001 were rejected. This was because the donation was believed to contain genetically modified corn. Subsequent to this, from 2002 to 2004, several other African countries refused food aid containing genetically modified organisms, putting 15 million Africans at risk for starvation. Many suspect that the decision to reject the aid was made to preserve trade relationships with countries that disfavor genetically modified food products. If donated seeds are planted, even inadvertently, then African crops may not be exported to markets such as the European Union. On the other hand, the United States has been accused of using food aid to introduce genetically modified food to developing countries.

SUMMARY

When assessing the acceptability of products of molecular biotechnology, people generally want to know what the benefits are compared to similar products derived from a conventional technology, who benefits from the biotechnology products, and the risks associated with the products. In particular, consumers are concerned about the safety of foods from genetically engineered microbes, plants, and animals and the impact of farming genetically engineered crops and livestock on the environment. The attitudes of consumers and the rigorous regulatory requirements for commercialization have greatly influenced the development and availability of biotechnology products.

Many countries, including the United States, have adopted the principle of "substantial equivalence" when evaluating the safety of genetically engineered foods. This means that a genetically modified plant or animal food product must be similar in composition to the corresponding conventional food. Levels of nutrients, anti-nutrients and natural toxins must not be different, and animal-feeding trials must not show differences in the development, health, or performance of the animals that would indicate reduced nutrition or increased toxicity or allergenicity of the genetically modified food. If the genetically engineered product is not substantially different from the conventional product, then labeling it as genetically engineered is not required. Labeling is required if the food contains a potential allergen or higher levels of a toxin, although it is unlikely that such products would be commercialized due to lack of consumer acceptance. The European Union, in response to strong consumer opposition to genetically modified foods, has adopted a precautionary approach and requires that all foods in which more than 0.9% is derived from a genetically engineered organism(s) be labeled. This has made trade difficult among countries with opposing views of biotechnology.

Cultivation of genetically modified crops or farming of transgenic livestock necessarily requires the release of the organism into the environment. Some people are concerned that this may increase the risk for unintended harm to natural

organisms in an environment or for transfer of the transgene to non-genetically engineered organisms, which could render them weedy or invasive. The vast majority of the transgenic crops currently grown have been engineered to resist predation by specific insects or to tolerate herbicides. They have resulted in substantial reductions in applications of agricultural chemicals and have reduced the agricultural footprint on the environment. Because the Bt insecticidal toxins are highly specific for their target insects and are confined to plant tissues, the impact on nontarget insects is very low. While the transgenes have been shown to be transferred to non-genetically engineered crops and wild relatives through cross-pollination, the herbicide-tolerant hybrids do not have an advantage in areas where the herbicides are not applied and insect-resistant hybrids have an advantage only when predation by

the specific insect is high. To prevent the spread of the transgene, cultivation of genetically engineered crops should be avoided in areas where sexually compatible nontransgenic crops and wild varieties are found.

Biotechnology products and services have enjoyed huge commercial success. Not only have the developers of the technology and products reaped the financial rewards, so have some of the downstream users of the biotechnology products. In particular, farmers in both developed and developing nations who plant genetically modified crops have benefited from increased profits due to higher yields and fewer pesticide applications. However, opponents point out that the cost of biotechnology products is high, for both the developer and the users, and this limits the products that are available.

REFERENCES

Brookes, G., and P. Barfoot. 2006. Global impact of biotech crops: socio-economic and environmental effects in the first ten years of commercial use. *AgBioForum* 9:139–151.

Chassy, B., J. J. Hlywka, G. A. Kleter, E. J. Kok, H. A. Kuiper, M. McGloughlin, I. C. Munro, R. H Phipps, and J. E. Reid. 2004. Nutritional and safety assessments of foods and feeds nutritionally improved through biotechnology. *Comp. Rev. Food Sci. Food Saf.* 3:35–104.

Davis, L. C. 2006. Genetic engineering, ecosystem change, and agriculture: an update. *Biotechnol. Mol. Biol. Rev.* 1:87–102.

Domingo, J. L. 2007. Toxicity studies of genetically modified plants: a review of the published literature. *Crit. Rev. Food Sci. Nutr.* 47:721–733.

Enserink, M. 2008. Tough lessons from golden rice. *Science* 320:468–471.

European Food Safety Authority. 2007. EFSA statement of the fate of recombinant DNA or proteins in meat milk and eggs from animals. http://www.efsa.europa.eu/EFSA/efsa_locale-1178620753812_1211902604524.htm.

European Food Safety Authority Working Group on Animal Feeding Trials. 2008. Safety and nutritional assessment of GM plants and derived food and feed: the role of animal

feeding trials. *Food Chem. Toxicol.* 46:S2–S70.

Flachowsky, G., K. Aulrich, H. Böhme, and I. Halle. 2007. Studies on feeds from genetically modified plants (GMP)—contributions to nutritional and safety assessment. *Anim. Feed Sci. Technol.* 133:2–30.

Leiberman, S., and T. Gray. 2008. GMOs and the developing world: a precautionary interpretation of biotechnology. *Br. J. Polit. Int. Relat.* 10:395–411.

Lemaux, P. G. 2008. Genetically engineered plants and foods: a scientist's analysis of the issues. Part I. *Annu. Rev. Plant Biol.* 59:771–812.

Lemaux, P. G. 2009. Genetically engineered plants and foods: a scientist's analysis of the issues. Part II. *Annu. Rev. Plant Biol.* 60:511–559.

Moreno-Fierros, L., N. García, R. Gutiérrez, R. López-Revilla, and R. I. Vázquez-Padrón. 2000. Intranasal, rectal and intraperitoneal immunization with protoxin Cry1Ac from *Bacillus thuringiensis* induces compartmentalized serum, intestinal, vaginal and pulmonary immune responses in Balb/c mice. *Microbes Infect.* 2:885–890.

Netherwood, T., S. M. Martín-Orúe, A. G. O'Donnell, S. Gockling, J. Graham, J. C. Mathers, and H. J. Gilbert. 2004. Assessing the survival of transgenic plant DNA in the human

gastrointestinal tract. *Nat. Biotechnol.* 22:204–209.

Pew Initiative on Food and Biotechnology. 2005. U.S. vs. E.U. An examination of the trade issues surrounding genetically modified food. http://www.pewtrusts.org/our-work_report_detail.aspx?id=24138.

Pray, C. E., and A. Naseem. 2007. Supplying crop biotechnology to the poor: opportunities and constraints. *J. Dev. Stud.* 43:192–217.

Singh, M. B., and P. L. Bhalla. 2008. Genetic engineering for removing food allergens from plants. *Trends Plant Sci.* 13:257–260.

Vázquez-Padrón, R. I., L. Moreno-Fierros, L. Neri-Bazán, G. A. de la Riva, and R. López-Revilla. 1999. Intragastric and intraperitoneal administration of Cry1Ac protoxin from *Bacillus thuringiensis* induces systemic and mucosal antibody responses in mice. *Life Sci.* 64:1897–1912.

Warwick, S I., M.-J. Simard, A. Légère, H. J. Beckie, L. Braun, B. Zhu, P. Mason, G. Séguin-Swartz, and C. N. Stewart. 2003. Hybridization between transgenic *Brassica napus* L. and its wild relatives: *Brassica rapa* L., *Raphanus raphanistrum* L., *Sinapis arvensis* L., and *Erucastrum gallicum* (Willd.) O.E. Schulz. *Theor. Appl. Genet.* 107:528–539.

REVIEW QUESTIONS

1. Discuss some of the reasons why foods derived from genetically engineered organisms might be safer for consumption than those developed through selective breeding. Discuss some of the reasons why genetically modified foods might be less safe.

2. What is meant by the term "substantial equivalence," and how is it used to assess food derived from genetically engineered organisms?

3. Why are animal-feeding trials important in the evaluation of the safety of genetically modified foods?

4. What are some of the benefits of golden rice? Why has commercialization been delayed?

5. How have some reports in the popular media contributed to the opposition to genetically engineered foods among consumers?

6. What is StarLink corn, and why is it no longer marketed?

7. When is a genetically engineered food required to be labeled in the United States and in the European Union? Why are the requirements different in the two regions?

8. Explain why the risk of incorporation of a transgene in genetically modified food into the genome of the consumer or intestinal bacterium is low.

9. Discuss the potential for cultivation of genetically engineered crops to decrease biodiversity.

10. Why is the risk of harm to nontarget insects lower for insect-resistant transgenic crops than for insecticide sprays?

11. Describe some ways in which genetically modified organisms can benefit the environment.

12. How have farmers benefited economically from growing insect-resistant transgenic crops?

13. How have consumer attitudes toward genetic engineering and stringent regulatory requirements limited the development of biotechnology products? How do they impact trade among nations?

This page intentionally left blank

Amino Acids of Proteins and Their Designations

Amino acid	Three-letter designation	Single-letter designation
Alanine	Ala	A
Arginine	Arg	R
Asparagine	Asn	N
Aspartic acid	Asp	D
Cysteine	Cys	C
Glutamic acid	Glu	E
Glutamine	Gln	Q
Glycine	Gly	G
Histidine	His	H
Isoleucine	Ile	I
Leucine	Leu	L
Lysine	Lys	K
Methionine	Met	M
Phenylalanine	Phe	F
Proline	Pro	P
Serine	Ser	S
Threonine	Thr	T
Tryptophan	Trp	W
Tyrosine	Tyr	Y
Valine	Val	V

This page intentionally left blank

Glossary

A An adenine residue in either DNA or RNA.

Ab *See* Antibody.

Absolute linkage *See* Complete linkage.

ACC 1-Aminocyclopropane-1-carboxylate. In plants, ACC is the immediate precursor of ethylene.

ACC deaminase A microbial enzyme that can cleave ACC to ammonia and α-ketobutyrate.

ACC oxidase A plant enzyme that catalyzes the oxidation of ACC to ethylene. Formerly called ethylene-forming enzyme.

ACC synthase A plant enzyme that catalyzes the synthesis of ACC from *S*-adenosylmethionine. Its activity is stimulated by indoleacetic acid.

Acetylation Addition of an acetyl group (CH_3COO^-) to a protein or other molecule.

Actin A major protein component of skeletal muscle. A contractile protein present within eukaryotic cells.

Activation Enhancement of the rate of transcription.

Activator (1) A substance or physical agent that stimulates transcription of a specific gene or operon. (2) A protein that binds to an operator and enhances the rate of transcription. Also called activator protein.

Activator site A DNA sequence to which an activator protein binds. Also called activating site.

Acyl carrier protein A low-molecular-weight protein that forms part of a larger complex for either fatty acid or polyketide biosynthesis.

Acylation Addition of an acyl group (RCO^-) to a molecule.

Adaptor (1) A synthetic double-stranded oligonucleotide that is blunt ended at one end and at the other has a nucleotide extension that can base pair with a cohesive end created by cleavage of a DNA molecule with a specific type II restriction endonuclease. After blunt-end ligation of the adaptor to the ends of a target DNA molecule, the construct can be cloned into a vector by using the cohesive ends of the adaptor. (2) A synthetic single-stranded oligonucleotide that, after self-hybridization, produces a molecule with cohesive ends and an internal restriction endonuclease site. When the adaptor is inserted into a cloning vector by means of the cohesive ends, the internal sequence provides a new restriction endonuclease site.

Adenine One of the organic bases found in either DNA or RNA.

Adjuvant A substance added to an immunogen (antigen) to increase the immunological response.

Aerobe A microorganism that requires oxygen for growth (respiration).

Affinity purification Selective isolation of a tagged molecule due to the specific binding of the tag (e.g., biotin) to another molecule (e.g., avidin or streptavidin).

Affinity tag A short sequence of amino acids that is engineered as part of a recombinant protein and binds to a specific element, compound, or macromolecule, which facilitates the identification or purification of the recombinant protein. Also called peptide tag, protein tag.

Ag *See* Antigen.

Airlift fermenter A cylindrical fermentation vessel in which the cells are mixed by air that is introduced at the base of the vessel and rises through the column of culture medium. The cell suspension circulates around the column as a consequence of the gradient of air bubbles in different parts of the reactor.

Alginate A polysaccharide polymer produced by different seaweeds and bacteria that is composed of β-D-mannuronate and α-L-guluronate.

Algorithm A precise procedure for solving a problem that is usually implemented by a computer program. Bioinformatics algorithms are developed to process, store, analyze, and visualize biological data.

Alignment Positioning of nucleotides or amino acids in two or more DNA, RNA, or protein sequences to line up regions of the sequences that are identical or similar.

Alkaloid One of a group of nitrogenous organic compounds derived from plants and having pharmacological properties.

Allele An alternative form of a gene.

Allelic frequency The ratio of the occurrence of one particular allele at a locus to the occurrence of all the alleles of the locus in a large number of individuals of a population.

Allelochemical A biologically synthesized chemical produced by one organism (usually a plant) and toxic or inhibitory to another. For example, many plant metabolites are toxic to insects or to some fungi.

Allergen A substance that stimulates an allergic reaction in sensitive individuals. Antibodies (immunoglobin E) are produced inappropriately by the immune system in response to the allergen, leading to a hypersensitivity response.

Allogeneic Having different antigens (an attribute of cell types). Also called allogenic.

Allolactose An isomer of D-lactose that is the actual inducer of the *Escherichia coli lac* operon. The enzyme β-galactosidase converts lactose to allolactose.

Allosteric control *See* Allosteric regulation.

Allosteric regulation A catalysis-regulating process in which the binding of a small effector molecule to one site on an enzyme affects the catalytic activity at another site on the enzyme.

Alternative splicing Cell-specific removal of an exon(s) during processing of a primary transcript that leads to a functional mRNA.

Amber mutation An alteration of the DNA resulting in the change of a codon specifying an amino acid to the nucleotide triplet TAG, which encodes UAG, a nonsense or stop codon.

Amino acid A building block of a protein.

Aminoacyl site The portion of a ribosome where the anticodon–codon interaction takes place during translation. Also called an A site.

Aminoacyl-tRNA A charged tRNA; a tRNA with its specific amino acid attached to its 3′ end.

1-Aminocyclopropane-1-carboxylate *See* ACC.

Amplicon (1) A herpes simplex virus type 1 plasmid vector. Also called amplicon plasmid. (2) A specific DNA fragment produced by a polymerase chain reaction.

Amylolytic Capable of breaking down starch into sugars (e.g., agents).

Anaerobe A microorganism that grows (respires) in the absence of oxygen.

Analytical protein microarray A high-density array of antibodies that captures proteins or other compounds or a protein array that captures antibodies.

Annealing The process of heating (denaturing step) and slowly cooling (renaturing step) double-stranded DNA to allow the formation of hybrid DNA or DNA–RNA molecules.

Annotated database Computer-stored data that are supplemented with additional information, such as detailed descriptions, comments, and references.

Antibiosis The prevention of growth or development of an organism by a substance or another organism.

Antibiotic A biological substance that is produced by one organism and that can inhibit the growth of, or kill, another organism.

Antibody A protein (immunoglobulin) that is synthesized by a B lymphocyte and that recognizes a specific site on an antigen. The basic immunoglobulin molecule consists of two identical heavy and two identical light chains.

Anticodon A set of three contiguous nucleotides in a tRNA molecule that are complementary to a set of three contiguous nucleotides (codon) in an mRNA.

Antifreeze protein A type of protein that binds to ice crystals and depresses the freezing temperature of the crystal below its melting temperature. Antifreeze proteins have been found in fish, insects, plants, fungi, and bacteria and protect cells from being damaged by ice crystals.

Antigen A compound that induces the production of antibodies.

Antigenic determinant *See* Epitope.

Anti-idiotype antibody An antibody that has the properties of an antigen.

Antiparallel orientation The arrangement of the two strands of a duplex DNA molecule, which are oriented in opposite directions, so that the 5′ phosphate end of one strand is aligned with the 3′ hydroxyl end of the complementary strand.

Antisense DNA (1) The sequence of chromosomal DNA that is transcribed. (2) A DNA sequence that is complementary to all or part of a functional RNA (mRNA).

Antisense RNA An RNA sequence that is complementary to all or part of a functional RNA.

Antisense therapy The in vivo treatment of a genetic disease by blocking translation of a protein with a DNA or an RNA sequence that is complementary to a specific mRNA.

Antiserum The fluid portion of the blood that contains the antibodies of an immunized organism.

Aphid A plant-sucking insect of the family Aphididae.

Apoplast The set of intercellular spaces that are inside a plant but outside the plant cells.

Apoptosis A controlled process leading to the death of the cell that occurs normally during the development of a multicellular organism or in response to cell damage or infection. Also known as programmed cell death.

Aptamer A synthetic nucleic acid, typically 15 to 40 nucleotides long, that has highly organized secondary and tertiary structures and binds with high affinity to a protein that normally does not bind to a nucleic acid.

Aquaculture Farming of fish or other marine or freshwater organisms under controlled conditions to produce food.

Arabidopsis thaliana A plant with a very small genome that is used as a model organism for the study of plant growth and development.

ARS *See* Autonomous replicating sequence.

Arthropod An invertebrate animal, such as an insect, spider, or crustacean, that has jointed limbs and an exoskeleton.

Articular cartilage Tough, rubbery, translucent, elastic tissue that forms the surfaces of bones within joints.

Atelocollagen Collagen from calf dermis digested under acidic conditions with the proteolytic enzyme pepsin to form positively charged subunits of approximately 300 kilodaltons each.

Atherogenic Causing the formation of lipid-containing plaques on the innermost layer of the wall of an artery.

Attenuated vaccine A virulent organism that has been modified to produce a less virulent form but nevertheless retains the ability to elicit antibodies against the virulent form.

Authentic protein A recombinant protein that has all the properties, including any posttranslational modifications, of its naturally occurring counterpart.

Autoantibody An antibody against one of one's own proteins.

Autologous cells Cells that are taken from an individual, cultured (or stored), and possibly genetically manipulated before being infused back into the original donor.

Autonomous replicating sequence Any cloned DNA sequence that initiates and supports extrachromosomal replication of a DNA molecule in a host cell; often used in yeast cells. Also called autonomously replicating sequence, autonomous(ly) replicating segment.

Autoradiography A technique that captures the image formed in a photographic emulsion as a result of the emission of either light or radioactivity from a labeled component that is placed next to unexposed film.

Autosomal Encoded on chromosomes other than the sex chromosomes.

Auxin *See* IAA.

Auxotroph A mutant that is unable to synthesize an essential metabolite, and therefore, the metabolite must be provided as a nutritional supplement for growth.

Avidin A glycoprotein component of egg white that binds strongly to biotin.

B cells Lymphocytes that produce antibodies and that are derived from bone marrow cells.

BAC *See* Bacterial artificial chromosome.

Bacmid A shuttle vector based on the *Autographa californica* multiple nucleopolyhedrosis virus genome that can be propagated in both *Escherichia coli* and insect cells.

Bacterial artificial chromosome A vector system based on the *Escherichia coli* F factor plasmid that is used for cloning large (100- to 300-kb) DNA inserts. Abbreviated BAC.

Bacteriocin A compound produced by one bacterium that can kill cells of another bacterial species.

Bacteriophage A virus that infects bacteria. Also called phage.

Bacteroid A modified bacterial cell formed following infection of a legume root hair and subsequent formation of a root nodule by a rhizobial strain when the bacteria inside the nodule shed their cell walls, thereby facilitating exchanges of nutrients between the bacteria and the plant.

Baculovirus A virus that infects insects.

Bank *See* Gene bank.

Base pair A term representing complementary nucleotides; in DNA, adenine (A) is hydrogen bonded with the base thymine (T), and guanine (G) is hydrogen bonded with cytosine (C). A thousand base pairs is often called a kilobase pair (kb).

Base pair substitution Permanent replacement in chromosomal DNA of a nucleotide pair with another nucleotide pair.

Batch culture *See* Batch fermentation.

Batch fermentation A process in which cells or microorganisms are grown for a limited time. At the beginning of the fermentation, an inoculum is introduced into fresh medium, and no medium is added or removed for the duration of the process.

β-1,3-Glucanase A plant enzyme, produced in response to infection by fungal pathogens, that hydrolyzes some components of fungal cell walls. Some bacteria can produce β-1,3-glucanase.

β-Ketoreductase An enzyme involved in the synthesis of polyketide antibiotics.

Betaine A low-molecular-weight compound that acts as a methyl group donor for methionine biosynthesis.

Bifunctional vector *See* Shuttle vector.

Binary fission Asexual cell division that produces equal-size daughter cells.

Binary vector system A two-plasmid system in *Agrobacterium* spp. for transferring a T-DNA region that carries cloned genes into plant cells. The virulence genes are on one plasmid, and the engineered T-DNA region is on the other plasmid.

Bioaccumulation Concentration of a chemical agent (e.g., DDT) in increasing quantities in the organisms of a food chain.

Biocontrol Any process using living organisms to restrain the growth and development of pathogenic organisms.

Biodegradation The breakdown of a compound into its chemical constituents by living organisms.

Bioinformatics Research into and development and application of computational tools to acquire, store, organize, analyze, and visualize data for biological, medical, behavioral, and health sciences.

Biolistics Delivery of DNA to plant and animal cells and organelles by means of DNA-coated pellets that are fired under pressure at high speed. Also called microprojectile bombardment.

Biological aging *See* Senescence.

Bioluminescence The production of light by biological organisms, such as insects and bacteria; usually catalyzed by the enzyme luciferase.

Biomarker A biological feature that is used to measure either the progress of a disease or the effect of a treatment.

Biomass (1) The cell mass produced by a population of living organisms. (2) The organic mass that can be used either as a source of energy or for its chemical components.

Biomass concentration The amount of biological material in a specific volume.

Biopolymer Any large polymeric molecule (protein, nucleic acid, polysaccharide, or lipid) produced by a living organism.

Bioreactor A vessel in which cells, cell extracts, or enzymes carry out a biological reaction. Often refers to a growth chamber (fermenter or fermentation vessel) for cells or microorganisms.

Bioremediation A process that uses living organisms to remove contaminants, pollutants, or unwanted substances from soil or water.

Biosensor A biological molecule or organism that is able to detect a particular molecule in the environment.

Biotechnology The application of scientific and engineering principles to the processing of material by biological agents to provide goods and services.

Biotin A B vitamin that is often used in biological research as a molecular tag because it has very high affinity for the proteins streptavidin and avidin.

Biotin labeling (1) The attachment of biotin to another molecule. (2) The incorporation of a biotin-containing nucleotide into a DNA molecule.

Biotransformation Conversion of a substance into a product by an organism or an enzyme.

BLAST Basic local alignment search tool. A computer program for determining a match between a query sequence and a sequence(s) in a database. BLASTn compares a DNA query sequence to a DNA database, and BLASTp compares an amino acid query sequence to a protein database.

Blastocyst A structure formed early in mammalian embryonic development that consists of a sphere of cells, which will later form the placenta, surrounding a fluid-filled cavity and a cluster of cells that will become the embryo.

Blot *See* Northern blotting; Southern blotting.

Blotting Transfer of a macromolecule by capillary action from a gel to a membrane.

Blunt end The end of a DNA duplex molecule in which neither strand extends beyond the other. Also called flush end.

Blunt-end cut To cleave phosphodiester bonds in the backbone of duplex DNA between the corresponding nucleotide pairs on opposite strands. This cleavage process produces no nucleotide extensions on either strand. Also called flush-end cut.

Blunt-end ligation Joining (ligation) of the nucleotides that are at the ends of two DNA duplex molecules, neither of which has an extension.

Boll weevil An insect pest of cotton plants.

Bovine spongiform encephalopathy An infectious disease of the central nervous system of cattle caused by prions that is characterized by lesions in the brain tissues. Also known as mad cow disease or BSE.

Box A short DNA sequence that plays a role in regulating, facilitating, enhancing, or silencing transcription.

bp *See* Base pair.

Brewer's yeast Strains of yeast, often *Saccharomyces cerevisiae*, that are used in the production of beer.

Broad-host-range plasmid A plasmid that can replicate in a number of different bacterial species.

Brush border membrane The microvillus-covered surface of pseudostratified and simple columnar epithelium cells.

Bubble column fermenter A fermentation vessel, or bioreactor, in which the cells or microorganisms are kept suspended in a tall cylinder by rising air that is introduced at the base of the column.

Bystander effect The death of an unmodified cell caused by a cytotoxic metabolite that is produced by a genetically modified cell and acquired by cell-to-cell contact.

C A cytosine residue in either DNA or RNA.

C terminus The last amino acid of a protein. Sometimes denotes the final amino acids of a protein. Also called carboxy(l) terminus, carboxy(l)-terminal end.

Calibrator lane The lane of a gel that contains electrophoretically separated size markers.

Callus A mass of undifferentiated plant tissue, from tissue cuttings or from individual plant cells, grown in culture on defined medium.

cAMP *See* Cyclic AMP.

Cancer Uncontrolled growth of the cells of a tissue or an organ in a multicellular organism.

Candidate gene A coding sequence that has some characteristics that make it likely that it could be responsible for a specific genetic disorder.

Candidate gene cloning A strategy for isolating a disease gene that is based on an informed guess about the possible gene product.

Canola A plant whose seed is used to produce high-quality cooking oil. Formerly called rapeseed. Canola is Canada's most economically important crop.

Cap *See* G cap.

Caprolactam An organic compound ($C_6H_{11}NO$) that is a lactam of 6-aminohexanoic acid. The primary industrial use of caprolactam is as a monomer in the production of nylon.

Capsid A structure that is composed of the coat protein(s) of a virus and is external to the viral nucleic acids. The capsid often determines the shape of the virus.

Carrier In genetics, an individual who has one mutant allele and one normal allele of a gene and whose phenotype is normal.

Cassette A combination of DNA elements that performs a specific function and that is maintained as a clonable unit.

Catalase An enzyme that catalyzes the decomposition of hydrogen peroxide into water and oxygen.

CD molecules Designation for surface molecules on various cells of the immune system, e.g., CD4 is present on the surfaces of helper T cells.

cDNA Complementary DNA. A double-stranded DNA complement of an mRNA sequence; synthesized in vitro by reverse transcriptase and DNA polymerase.

cDNA clone A double-stranded DNA molecule that is carried in a vector and that was synthesized in vitro from an mRNA sequence by using reverse transcriptase and DNA polymerase.

cDNA library A collection of cDNA clones that were generated in vitro from the mRNA sequences of a single tissue or cell population.

CDR *See* Complementarity-determining region.

Cecropin A A 35-amino-acid peptide with antimicrobial activity from the giant silk moth, *Hyalophora cecropia*.

Cell line A cell lineage that can be maintained in culture.

Cell-free protein synthesis *See* In vitro translation.

Cell-mediated immune response The activation of T cells of the immune system in response to the presence of a foreign antigen.

Cellulose A high-molecular-weight polysaccharide of unbranched chains of (1,4)-linked β-D-glucose units that, as part of lignocellulose, contributes to the structural framework of plant cell walls.

Cellulosome A multiprotein aggregate that is present in some cellulolytic microorganisms and that contains multiple copies of all the enzymes required to completely break down cellulose. This complex is often found on the outer surfaces of cellulolytic microorganisms.

Centromere The part of the chromosome that attaches to the spindle during cell division.

Cephem-type antibiotic An antibiotic that shares the basic chemical structure of cephalosporin.

Chagas disease A parasitic disease caused by the protozoan *Trypanosoma cruzi*.

Chaperone A protein complex that aids in the correct folding of nascent or misfolded proteins.

Charged tRNA A transfer RNA molecule that is coupled to its specific amino acid. Also called aminoacylated tRNA, aminoacyl tRNA.

Chemiluminescence The emission of light from a chemical reaction.

Chimera Usually, a plant or animal that has populations of cells with different genotypes. Sometimes it refers to a recombinant DNA molecule that contains sequences from different organisms.

Chimeric protein *See* Fusion protein.

Chitinase An enzyme that hydrolyzes the chitin components in fungal cell walls and insect exoskeletons. Produced by plants in response to infection by fungal pathogens. Some bacteria can produce chitinase.

Cholesterol A sterol that occurs widely in animal tissues. A precursor of various steroids. Often found in membranes.

Chromatin DNA and associated proteins that are compacted into chromosomes.

Chromatin immunoprecipitation A technique that uses specific antibodies to identify regions of a genome that are bound by a particular DNA-binding protein of interest in living cells.

Chromogenic substrate A compound or substance that contains a color-forming group.

Chromosomal integration site A chromosomal location where foreign DNA can be integrated, often without impairing any essential function in the host organism.

Chromosome A physically distinct unit of the genome.

Cistron A sequence of DNA that encodes a polypeptide chain.

Claims A section of a patent that states, in detail, the uses and possible applications of the invention described in the patent.

Cleave To break phosphodiester bonds of duplex DNA, usually with a type II restriction endonuclease. Also called cut, digest.

Clone (1) A population of cells or organisms that are genetically identical as a result of asexual reproduction, breeding of purebred (isogenic) organisms, or forming genetically identical organisms by nuclear transplantation. (2) A population of cells that all carry a cloning vehicle with the same insert

DNA molecule. (3) To insert a DNA segment into a vector or host chromosome.

Clone bank *See* Gene bank.

Cloning Incorporating a DNA molecule into a chromosomal site or a cloning vector.

Cloning site A location on a cloning vector into which DNA can be inserted.

Cloning vector A DNA molecule that can carry inserted DNA and can be perpetuated in a host cell. Also called cloning vehicle, vector, vehicle.

Cloning vehicle *See* Cloning vector.

Coding triplet A set of three contiguous nucleotides of the nontranscribed DNA strand of the coding region of a structural gene that is complementary to a transcribed triplet.

Codon A set of 3 nucleotides in mRNA that specifies a tRNA carrying a specific amino acid that is incorporated into a polypeptide chain during protein synthesis.

Codon optimization An experimental strategy in which codons within a cloned gene that are not the ones generally used by the host cell translation system are changed to the preferred codons without changing the amino acids of the synthesized protein.

Codon usage The mean frequency of occurrence of each codon determined from a large sample of structural genes of an organism.

Cofactor A low-molecular-weight compound that is a required component in an enzymatic reaction.

Cofermentation The simultaneous growth of two microorganisms in one bioreactor.

Cohesive ends Complementary single-strand extensions on the ends of duplex DNA molecules. Also called sticky ends. *See also* cos ends.

Cointegrate vector system A two-plasmid system for transferring cloned genes to plant cells. The cloning vector has a T-DNA segment that contains cloned genes. After introduction into *Agrobacterium tumefaciens*, the cloning vector DNA undergoes homologous recombination with a resident disarmed Ti plasmid to form a single plasmid carrying the genetic information for transferring the genetically engineered T-DNA region to plant cells.

Coleoptile A protective organ that covers the youngest leaves of a plant.

Collagen An insoluble fibrous protein commonly found in connective tissue. Collagen accounts for over 30% of the total protein in mammals.

Colon The large intestine.

Colony hybridization A technique that uses a nucleic acid probe to identify a bacterial colony with a vector carrying a specific cloned gene(s).

Combinatorial library During the ligation reaction with cDNAs of light and heavy antibody chains into a bacterio-

phage λ or M13 vector, many novel combinations consisting of one heavy and one light chain coding region are formed. The library comprises these combinations, each in a separate vector.

Competence The ability of bacterial cells to take up (usually plasmid) DNA molecules.

Complement A group of serum proteins that is activated by an antibody–antigen complex and has enzymatic and other biological activities, such as degrading antibody–antigen complexes, lysing cells, modulating antibody production, stimulating immune cells to migrate to a site of complement activity, and inducing the release of histamine.

Complement cascade The series of sequential activations and enzymatic reactions by serum proteins that is launched in response to the formation of an antibody–antigen complex.

Complementarity (1) A condition in which one of a pair of nucleotide bases forms hydrogen bonds with each other. Adenine (A) pairs with thymine (T) (or with uracil [U] in RNA), and guanine (G) pairs with cytosine (C). (2) A condition in which one of a pair of segments or strands of nucleic acid hybridizes (joins by hydrogen bonding) with the other.

Complementarity-determining region A part of the variable (V) regions of light and heavy antibody chains that makes contact with the antigen. The amino acid sequences of complementarity-determining regions are highly variable from one antibody of the same class to another. Abbreviated CDR.

Complementary base pairs Pairs of nucleotide bases that form hydrogen bonds with each other. In double-stranded DNA, adenine forms hydrogen bonds with thymine, and cytosine forms hydrogen bonds with guanine. In double-stranded regions of RNA molecules, and in both RNA–RNA and DNA–RNA strand interactions, adenine forms hydrogen bonds with uracil, and cytosine forms hydrogen bonds with guanine.

Complementary DNA *See* cDNA.

Complementary homopolymeric tailing The process of adding complementary nucleotide extensions to different DNA molecules, e.g., to the 3′ hydroxyl ends of one DNA molecule in dG (deoxyguanosine) and to the 3′ hydroxyl ends of another DNA molecule in dC (deoxycytidine), to facilitate the joining, after they are mixed, of the two DNA molecules by base pairing between the complementary extensions. Also called dG·dC tailing, dA·dT tailing.

Complementation *See* Genetic complementation.

Complete linkage Two or more adjacent gene loci on the same chromosome that are always inherited together. Also called absolute linkage.

Complete penetrance A situation in which all the individuals with a mutant allele(s) at a gene locus show the same abnormal (mutant) phenotype.

Computational biology Development and application of data analysis, modeling, and simulation techniques to study biological, behavioral, and social systems.

Concatemer A tandem array of repeating unit-length DNA elements.

Conformation The shape of a molecule or any other object.

Conifer An evergreen or softwood tree, such as pine, fir, or spruce.

Conjugation The unidirectional transfer of DNA from one bacterium to another, involving cell-to-cell contact.

Conjugative functions Plasmid-based genes and their products that facilitate the transfer of a plasmid from one bacterium to another.

Constant domains Regions of antibody chains that have the same amino acid sequence in different members of a particular class of antibody molecules.

Constitutive synthesis Continual production of RNA or protein by an organism.

Contig A set of overlapping contiguous clones that cover a chromosome region or a whole chromosome.

Continuous fermentation A process in which cells or microorganisms are maintained in culture in the exponential growth phase by the continuous addition of fresh medium that is exactly balanced by the removal of cell suspension from the bioreactor.

Copy number The average number of a specific type of plasmid molecules in a cell.

Corepressor A low-molecular-weight compound that combines with an inactive repressor protein to form a complex that binds to an operator region and prevents transcription.

cos ends The 12-base, single-strand, complementary extensions of bacteriophage λ DNA. Also called cos sites.

Cosegregation Two genetic conditions appearing to be inherited together.

Cosmid A vector that uses the cos end sequences of bacteriophage λ and in vitro bacteriophage packaging to form, after injection of the vector into a host cell, a plasmid that can carry as much as 45 kb of insert DNA.

Cosuppression The transformation of a plant with a gene, in the sense orientation, that the plant already possesses. This results in the downregulation of both the endogenous and introduced genes. Also called sense suppression.

Cotransfection The introduction of two different DNA molecules into a eukaryotic cell. In baculovirus expression systems, the procedure by which the baculovirus and the transfer vector are simultaneously introduced into insect cells in culture.

Coupling The phase state in which either two dominant or two recessive versions of two different genes occur on the same chromosome. Also called *cis* configuration. *See also* Repulsion.

CpG islands Clusters of GC-rich regions that precede many transcribed vertebrate genes.

Cross In genetic studies, the mating of two individuals. Also called mating.

Crossbreeding The mating of two different species or varieties to form a hybrid. Also known as hybridization.

Crossover (1) The site of recombination. A single crossover represents one reciprocal breakage-and-reunion event. A double crossover requires two simultaneous reciprocal breakage-and-reunion events. (2) The reciprocal exchange of DNA between two chromosomes or DNA molecules by a breakage-and-reunion process. Also called recombination, recombination event.

Crown gall A bulbous growth that occurs at the bases of certain plants and that is due to infection of the plant by a member of the bacterial genus *Agrobacterium*. Also called crown gall tumor.

Crown gall tumor *See* Crown gall.

Crucifer A plant, such as cabbage, that is a member of the family *Cruciferae*.

Cryptic site A functional macromolecular sequence in an unlikely location. Also used, in some instances, to denote a macromolecular sequence whose function is unknown.

Cultivar A variety of plant that is (1) below the level of a subspecies taxonomically and (2) found only under cultivation.

Culture A population of cells or microorganisms that are grown under controlled conditions.

Culture medium A solid or liquid mixture that is used to grow microorganisms, organisms, or cells.

Cut *See* Cleave.

Cyclic AMP Adenosine 3′,5′-cyclic phosphoric acid, an important regulatory molecule. Also called cAMP.

Cyclic-array sequencing A large-scale method for simultaneously determining the nucleotide sequences of millions of DNA fragments immobilized in a dense array.

Cytokine Any of several regulatory proteins, such as the interleukins and lymphokines, that are released by cells of the immune system and that act as intercellular mediators in the generation of an immune response.

Cytokinin A plant hormone that stimulates cell division.

Cytoplasm The contents of a cell enclosed by the cytoplasmic membrane (outside of the nucleus of a eukaryotic cell).

Cytosine One of the organic bases found in either DNA or RNA.

Cytosol The semifluid soluble portion of the cytoplasm of cells.

dA·dT tailing *See* Complementary homopolymeric tailing.

Damping off A disease of plant roots, generally caused by a pathogenic fungus.

Database A file system of formatted information that can be readily accessed, retrieved, and updated.

Dehalogenation The removal of halogen atoms (chlorine, iodine, bromine, or fluorine) from molecules, usually during biodegradation.

Deletion Loss of an internal portion of chromosomal DNA.

Denaturation (1) Separation of duplex nucleic acid molecules into single strands. (2) Disruption of the conformation of a macromolecule without breaking covalent bonds.

Denatured DNA Duplex DNA that has been converted to single strands by breaking the hydrogen bonds of complementary nucleotide pairs.

Deoxyribonuclease I *See* DNase I.

Deoxyribonucleic acid *See* DNA.

Deoxyribose The five-carbon sugar component of DNA.

Deoxyribozyme A DNA molecule that has catalytic activity.

Derepression Displacement of a repressor protein from a promoter or operator region of DNA; the "turning on" of a gene. When attached to the DNA, the repressor protein prevents RNA polymerase from initiating transcription.

Dermis The thicker, outermost layer of skin in vertebrates.

dG·dC tailing *See* Complementary homopolymeric tailing.

Diagnosis Determination of the cause of a disorder.

Diagnostic procedure A test or assay used to determine the presence of an organism, substance, or nucleic acid sequence alteration that represents a disease or pathogenic condition.

Diaminopimelic acid The immediate precursor to L-lysine in bacteria and plants and a component of some bacterial cell walls.

Diazotroph An organism that can fix nitrogen.

Dicistronic vector A mammalian cloning vector that is specially designed to carry two functional genes.

Dicotyledon A class of plants that has two seed leaves. Also called dicot.

Dideoxynucleotide A nucleoside triphosphate that lacks hydroxyl groups on both the 2′ and 3′ carbons of the pentose sugar. Also called ddNTP.

Digest *See* Cleave.

Dihydrofolate reductase An enzyme that catalyzes the formation of tetrahydrofolic acid.

Diploid A cell or organism that has a set of all pairs of its chromosomes.

Directed mutagenesis The process of generating nucleotide changes in cloned genes by any one of several procedures, including site-specific and random mutagenesis. Also called in vitro mutagenesis.

Disarm To delete from a plasmid or virus those genes that are cytotoxic or that induce crown gall formation.

Dithiothreitol A low-molecular-weight thiol-containing reducing agent. It is added to buffers in low concentrations to prevent protein sulfhydryl groups from being oxidized. At higher concentrations, it is used to reduce disulfide linkages in proteins.

DNA Deoxyribonucleic acid; the genetic material of living things.

DNA codon A set of three contiguous deoxyribonucleotide pairs of the coding region of a structural gene where the bases of one strand are transcribed into a codon.

DNA construct A cloning vector with a DNA insert.

DNA delivery system A generic term for any procedure that facilitates the uptake of DNA by a recipient cell.

DNA fingerprint A set of DNA fragments that are characteristic of a particular source of DNA, such as an insert of a clone. In some cases, restriction endonuclease DNA fragments are visualized by hybridization after gel electrophoresis. In other instances, the polymerase chain reaction (PCR) is used to generate a distinctive pattern of DNA bands that are evident after gel electrophoresis.

DNA fingerprinting A comparative diagnostic technique that characterizes the DNA of an organism or a sample.

DNA hybridization The pairing of two DNA molecules, often from different sources, by hydrogen bonding between complementary nucleotides. This technique is frequently used to detect the presence of a specific nucleotide sequence in a DNA sample.

DNA microarray An array of thousands of gene sequences or oligonucleotide probes bound to a solid support. Also called DNA chip, gene array.

DNA polymerase An enzyme that links an incoming deoxyribonucleotide, which is determined by complementarity to a deoxyribonucleotide in a template DNA strand, with a phosphodiester bond to the 3′ hydroxyl group of the last incorporated nucleotide of the growing strand during replication.

DNA probe A segment of DNA that is labeled (tagged) so that, after a DNA hybridization reaction, any base pairing between the probe and a complementary base sequence in a DNA sample can be detected.

DNA transformation *See* Transfection; Transformation.

DNA typing *See* Genotyping.

DNase I An enzyme that degrades DNA. It is used to remove DNA from RNA preparations and from cell-free extracts. Also called deoxyribonuclease I.

Domain A segment of a protein that has a discrete function or conformation. At the protein level, a domain can be as small as a few amino acid residues and as large as half of the entire protein.

Dominant (1) When heterozygous and homozygous genotypes determine the same phenotype, the gene is said to be

dominant. (2) An allele that produces the same phenotype whether the genotype is heterozygous or homozygous.

Dominant gene One of a pair of alleles that is sufficient to produce a phenotype in a heterozygote.

Dominant marker selection Selection in which a gene encodes a product that enables only the cells that carry the gene to grow under certain conditions. For example, plant and animal cells that express the introduced Neor gene are resistant to the compound G-418, and cells that do not carry the Neor gene are killed by G-418. Also called positive selection, positive selectable marker.

Double crossover Two simultaneous reciprocal breakage-and-reunion events between two DNA molecules.

Double heterozygote Two different gene loci, each with two different alleles.

Doubling time *See* Generation time.

Downstream (1) In molecular biology, the stretch of nucleotides of DNA that lie in the 3' direction from the site of initiation of transcription, which is designated +1. Downstream nucleotides are marked with plus signs, e.g., +2 and +10. The term also refers to the 3' side of a particular gene or sequence of nucleotides. (2) In chemical engineering, those phases of a manufacturing process that follow the biotransformation stage. Refers to recovery and purification of the product of a fermentation process. Also called downstream processing.

Downstream processing *See* Downstream.

Drug *See* Therapeutic agent.

Dry weight The weight of a sample of biological material that has been dried in an oven to remove the water.

Duplex DNA Double-stranded DNA.

E value Expectation value for a BLAST analysis; the lower the E value, the more significant the alignment score. The number of alternate alignments with a score equal to or better than the similarity score for a given alignment that can be expected to occur simply by chance.

Effector A low-molecular-weight compound that modifies the function of a regulatory protein.

Effector cells Cells of the immune system that degrade antigens.

Electrophoresis A technique that separates molecules (often DNA, RNA, or protein) on the basis of relative migration in a strong electric field.

Electroporation Electrical treatment of cells that induces transient pores, through which DNA is taken into the cell.

Electrotransfer Transfer of a macromolecule by an electric field from a gel to a membrane.

ELISA *See* Enzyme-linked immunosorbent assay.

Elongation Sequential addition of one monomer at a time to a polymer.

Embryonic stem cells Cells of an early embryo that can give rise to all differentiated cells, including germ line cells.

Emulsion PCR A technique that uses the polymerase chain reaction to produce tens of thousands of copies of a DNA template that is bound to a bead within a water-in-oil emulsion.

Encode To specify, after decoding by transcription and translation, the sequence of amino acids in a protein.

End-product inhibition The inhibition of the activity of an enzyme by a metabolite. The enzyme is often the first enzyme in a biosynthetic pathway, and the metabolite is generally the product of the last step in the pathway.

Endemic With respect to disease, prevalent in a particular geographic location.

Endocytosis Entrance of foreign material into the cell without passing through the cell membrane. The membrane folds around the material, resulting in the formation of a saclike vesicle into which the material is incorporated.

Endoplasmic reticulum A membrane-enclosed structure in a eukaryotic cell that is continuous with the nucleus and whose functions include the synthesis, processing, and transport of proteins (rough endoplasmic reticulum) and the synthesis of lipids (smooth endoplasmic reticulum).

Endoprotease An enzyme that cleaves the peptide bonds between amino acids within a protein. Cleavage is usually at one or more specific sites.

Endosperm A nutritive tissue in flowering plants that surrounds the developing embryo in a seed.

Endothelial cell A platelike cell that lines the inner surfaces of blood and lymph vessels.

Endotoxin A component of the cell wall of gram-negative bacteria that elicits an inflammatory response and fever in humans.

Enhancer A DNA sequence that increases the transcription of a eukaryotic gene when they are both on the same DNA molecule. Also called enhancer element, enhancer sequence.

Enolase An enzyme that catalyzes the conversion of 2-phosphoglycerate to phosphoenolpyruvate.

Enoylreductase An enzyme involved in the synthesis of polyketide antibiotics.

Enterobacter cloacae A free-living gram-negative soil bacterium that can act as a plant growth-promoting bacterium.

Enterotoxin A bacterial protein that, after its release into the intestine, causes cramps, diarrhea, and nausea.

Enzyme A protein or complex of proteins that acts as a catalyst to increase the rate of a chemical reaction.

Enzyme-linked immunosorbent assay A technique for detecting specific molecules in a mixed sample. An antibody (primary) is bound to the target molecule; another antibody (secondary), which binds to the primary antibody, is added later. The secondary antibody has attached to it an enzyme that can convert a colorless substrate into a colored product.

If the target molecule is not present in the sample, washing steps will remove both antibodies, and no colored product will be produced. Also called ELISA.

Enzyme replacement therapy Treatment of an inherited metabolic defect with a protein that facilitates a specific chemical reaction.

Epidermal growth factor A protein with kinase (phosphorylation) activity that is involved in triggering cell division in animal cells.

Epidermis The outermost layer of cells of an animal.

Epigenetic reprogramming Changes in epigenetic modifications during normal germ cell and embryonic development.

Epithelial cells Cells covering a surface or lining a cavity, e.g., gut epithelial cells.

Epitope A specific chemical domain on an antigen that is recognized by an antibody. Each epitope on a molecule, such as a protein, elicits the synthesis of a different antibody. Also called antigenic determinant.

Epitope tag An affinity tag that is recognized by an antibody.

Error-prone PCR Use of the polymerase chain reaction under conditions that promote the insertion of an incorrect nucleotide at every few hundred or so nucleotides of the template. Used as a method of random mutagenesis.

ES cells *See* Embryonic stem cells.

EST *See* Expressed sequence tag.

Established cell line A population of cells that is grown in vitro and that can be subcultured indefinitely.

Estrogenic compounds Natural and synthetic chemicals that act in a manner similar to that of the steroid hormone estrogen, which is responsible for the development of female sex characteristics.

Ethylene A gaseous compound that acts as a plant hormone. It is important in fruit ripening, flower senescence, seed germination, rooting of cuttings, root elongation, and the response of the plant to environmental stress.

Euchromatin The form of chromatin that is less compacted and is often more actively transcribed.

Eukaryotes Organisms, including animals, plants, fungi, and some algae, that have (1) chromosomes enclosed within a membrane-bounded nucleus and (2) functional organelles, such as mitochondria and chloroplasts, in the cytoplasm of their cells.

Excision The natural or in vitro enzymatic release (removal) of a DNA segment from a chromosome or cloning vector.

Excrete *See* Export.

Exogenous Derived externally, or foreign.

Exogenous DNA DNA that has been derived from a source organism and has been cloned into a vector and introduced into a host cell. Also referred to as foreign or heterologous DNA.

Exon A segment of a gene that is transcribed as part of the primary transcript and is retained, after being processed, with other exons to form a functional mRNA molecule.

Exonuclease III An *Escherichia coli* enzyme that removes nucleotides from the 3′ hydroxyl ends of double-stranded DNA. Also called ExoIII, exodeoxyribonuclease III.

Exopolysaccharide A high-molecular-weight polymer that is composed of sugar residues and is secreted by a microorganism into the surrounding environment.

ExoIII *See* Exonuclease III.

Export To transport a protein out of a cell. Also to secrete or to excrete.

Expressed sequence tag A partially sequenced cDNA clone for which a PCR assay exists. Also called EST, expressed-sequence-tagged site, eSTS.

Expression Transcription and translation of a gene.

Expression library A population of different DNA molecules cloned into an expression vector.

Expression profile Determination of the members of a transcriptome or proteome in a cell, tissue, or organism.

Extension A single-stranded DNA region consisting of one or more nucleotides at the end of a strand of duplex DNA. Also called protruding end, sticky end, overhang, cohesive end.

Extracellular matrix The organized carbohydrate and protein structure that is secreted by animal cells when they are part of a tissue.

Extrachromosomal DNA A replicatable DNA element that is not part of a chromosome.

Exudate A low-molecular-weight compound (sugar, amino acid, etc.) that leaks out of plant tissues, including seeds, roots, and leaves.

False negative A test result that does not recognize a target when it is present in a sample.

False positive A test result that indicates the presence of a target when it is not in a sample.

Fed-batch fermentation Growth of cells or microorganisms during which nutrients are added periodically to the bioreactor.

Feedback inhibition *See* End-product inhibition.

Fermentation (1) In chemical engineering, the growth of cells or microorganisms in specialized vessels (fermenters or bioreactors). (2) In biochemistry, the breakdown of carbon compounds by cells or organisms to synthesize ATP without using molecular oxygen.

Fermenter *See* Bioreactor.

Ferredoxin An iron–sulfur protein that acts as an electron carrier.

Ferritin A family of iron storage proteins found in animals, plants, fungi, and bacteria.

Fertile Capable of breeding and reproduction.

Fibroblast A spindle-shaped cell found in connective tissue.

5′ extension A short single-stranded nucleotide sequence on the 5′ phosphate end of a double-stranded DNA molecule. Also called 5′ protruding end, 5′ sticky end, 5′ overhang.

5′ phosphate end The phosphate group that is attached to the 5′ carbon atom of the sugar (ribose or deoxyribose) of the terminal nucleotide of a nucleic acid molecule.

Flavonoid A member of a class of plant phenolic compounds containing two aromatic rings connected by a three-carbon bridge.

Fluorescein A fluorescent dye often used to label antibodies so that they may be visualized after they have reacted with antigens in cells.

Fluorescence-activated cell sorting A technique used to separate cells based on the amount of fluorescence they emit. Also called FACS.

Fluorography Detection of the emission of light from a labeled source on X-ray film.

Fluorophore That portion of a molecule that can fluoresce.

Flush end *See* Blunt end.

Flush-end cut *See* Blunt-end cut.

Foliar Consisting of or pertaining to leaves.

Foreign DNA A DNA molecule that is incorporated into either a cloning vector or a chromosomal site.

Fosmid A cloning vector based on the F plasmid of *Escherichia coli* that can carry large segments of cloned DNA.

Fouling The coating or plugging of equipment by materials or microorganisms that prevents it from functioning properly.

Founder animal In transgenesis research, an organism that carries a transgene in its germ line and that can be used in matings to establish a pure-breeding transgenic line or one that acts as a breeding stock for transgenic animals.

Four-cutter A type II restriction endonuclease that binds and cleaves DNA at sites that contain four nucleotide pairs.

Frameshift mutation In chromosomal DNA, an insertion or deletion of base pairs that changes the reading frame of a gene.

Fructans Polymers of fructose that are not degraded in the human digestive tract.

Functional gene cloning A strategy for isolating a gene that depends on information about its product.

Functional genomics The large-scale study of gene expression.

Functional protein microarray An array, composed of as many members of a proteome as possible, that is used to study the activities of a proteome.

Fusion protein The product of two or more coding sequences from different genes that have been cloned together and that, after translation, form a single polypeptide sequence. Also called hybrid protein, chimeric protein.

G A guanine residue in either DNA or RNA.

G cap The 5′-terminal methylated guanine nucleotide that is present on many eukaryotic mRNAs; it is joined, after transcription, to the mRNA in a 5′-to-5′ linkage.

Gamete A cell with a haploid chromosome content. In animals, a sperm or egg; in plants, pollen or ovum.

Gametocyte A eukaryotic germ cell that divides by mitosis to form additional gametocytes or by meiosis to form gametids. Male gametids are spermatids, while female gametids are ootids.

Gap A missing internal segment of one strand of duplex DNA.

Gapped DNA A duplex DNA molecule with one or more internal single-stranded regions.

Gateway cloning technology A system that utilizes the attachment sites used by bacteriophage λ for integration and excision into and out of the *Escherichia coli* chromosome for cloning DNA, especially coding sequences into expression vectors.

Gel matrix A semisolid macromolecular lattice that is used for the electrophoretic fractionation of macromolecules.

Gelatinization Steam cooking of milled grain, a process that increases the surface area of the starch and converts the original mash into a material with a gel-like consistency.

Gene A segment of nucleic acid that encodes a functional protein or RNA. The unit of inheritance.

Gene bank A population of organisms, each of which carries a DNA molecule that was inserted into a cloning vector. Ideally, all of the cloned DNA molecules represent the entire genome of another organism. Also called gene library, clone bank, bank, library. This term is sometimes also used to denote all of the vector molecules, each carrying a piece of the chromosomal DNA of an organism, before the insertion of these molecules into a population of host cells.

Gene cloning Insertion of a gene into a DNA vector (often a plasmid) to form a new DNA molecule that can be perpetuated in a host cell. Also called recombinant DNA technology, genetic engineering, gene splicing, gene transplantation, molecular cloning, cloning.

Gene expression Synthesis of RNA, and often protein, directed by the nucleotide sequence in a specific segment of DNA (gene).

Gene flow The transfer of genes from one population to another through interbreeding.

Gene library *See* Gene bank.

Gene map The linear array of genes of a chromosome.

Gene therapy Use of a gene or cDNA to treat a disease.

Generally regarded as safe In the United States, a designation given to foods, drugs, and other materials that have been used for a considerable period and that have a history of not causing illness in humans, even though extensive toxicity testing has not been conducted. More recently, certain host organisms for recombinant DNA experimentation have been given this status.

Generation time The time that it takes for a population of single-celled organisms to double its cell number. Also called doubling time.

Genetic code The complete set of 64 codons that code for all 20 amino acids and 3 termination codons.

Genetic complementation When two genomes or DNA molecules that are in the same cell produce a function that neither genome or DNA molecule can supply on its own. Also called complementation.

Genetic engineering *See* Gene cloning.

Genetic heterogeneity The condition or state of a population in which different mutant genes produce the same phenotype. Also called heterogeneity.

Genetic immunization Delivery of a cloned gene that encodes an antigen to a host organism. After the cloned gene is expressed, it elicits an antibody response that protects the organism from infection by a virus, bacterium, or other disease-causing organism.

Genetic linkage *See* Linkage.

Genetic map The linear array of genes on a chromosome based on recombination frequencies. Also called linkage map.

Genetic mapping Determining the linear order of marker sites along a chromosome. Also called mapping.

Genetic polymorphism A situation in which two or more alleles of a locus in a population of individuals occur at a frequency of 1% or greater. Often, in the appropriate context, it is simply called polymorphism.

Genetic test An assay that determines whether the cause of a disorder is at the DNA level.

Genome (1) The entire complement of genetic material of an organism, virus, or organelle. (2) The haploid set of chromosomes (DNA) of a eukaryotic organism.

Genomics The study and development of genetic and physical maps, large-scale DNA sequencing, gene discovery, and computer-based systems for managing and analyzing the genome of an organism.

Genotype (1) The genetic constitution of an organism. (2) The alleles at a genetic locus.

Genotyping The determination of the alleles of a chromosome of an individual. Also called DNA typing, haplotyping.

Germ line cells Cells that produce gametes.

Germ line gene therapy The delivery of a gene(s) to a fertilized egg or an early embryonic cell. The transferred gene(s) is present in all nuclei of the cells of the mature individual, including the reproductive cells, and alters the phenotype of the developed individual.

Germinal disc A layer of cells on the surface of an egg yolk that will form the embryo.

Gluconeogenesis The synthesis of glucose from noncarbohydrates, such as fat or protein.

Glutathione A tripeptide comprising the amino acids glutamic acid, cysteine, and glycine that acts as an antioxidant.

Glycation The nonenzymatic covalent addition of sugar or sugar-related molecules to proteins.

Glycoalkaloids A group of toxic compounds found in some plants.

Glycogen synthase An enzyme that catalyzes one of the steps in the biosynthesis of glycogen from glucose.

Glycosylation The enzymatic covalent addition of sugar or sugar-related molecules to proteins or polynucleotides.

Glyphosate A broad-spectrum herbicide that inhibits the synthesis of aromatic amino acids in plants.

Golden rice Rice that has been genetically engineered to express three foreign genes and thereby to synthesize the vitamin A precursor β-carotene, imparting a yellow or golden color to the rice grains.

Golgi apparatus Flattened stacks of membranous sacs that process and sort proteins and other macromolecules, especially those that are secreted by the cell.

Gram-negative organism Any prokaryotic organism that does not retain the first stain (crystal violet) used in the Gram technique. It does retain the second stain (safranin O) and therefore has a pink color when viewed under a light microscope. Retention of the stain is due to the structure of the cell wall.

Gram-positive organism Any prokaryotic organism that retains the first stain (crystal violet) used in the Gram technique, which gives a purple-black color when viewed under a light microscope. Retention of the stain is due to the structure of the cell wall.

Gratuitous inducer A substance that can induce transcription of a gene(s) but that is not a substrate for the induced enzyme(s).

Green fluorescent protein A protein that emits green fluorescence after excitation by light of a specific wavelength. It is produced naturally by the jellyfish *Aequorea victoria* and other marine organisms and has a variety of applications in molecular biotechnology.

Guanine One of the organic bases found in either DNA or RNA.

GUS The bacterial enzyme β-glucuronidase, which is commonly used as a marker in the production of transgenic plants.

HAC *See* Human artificial chromosome.

Hairpin loop A segment of single-stranded DNA or RNA that is folded back upon itself and held together by base pairing in a structure that is locally double stranded; it may be represented on paper as having the appearance of a traditional lady's hairpin.

Haploid Having one copy of each autosome and one sex chromosome.

Haplotype The alleles of the loci of a chromosome. A set of closely linked genetic markers present on one chromosome that tend to be inherited together. The word is derived by combining "haplo" from haploid and "type" from genotype.

Haplotyping *See* Genotyping.

Heat shock proteins The proteins synthesized in the nearly universal response of organisms to environmental stress, such as high temperature.

Helper cells T cells that assist other cell types to respond immunologically to the presence of an antigen. Also called helper T lymphocytes.

Helper plasmid A plasmid that provides a function(s) to another plasmid in the same cell. Some helper plasmids are used to mobilize nonconjugative plasmids from a donor cell into a recipient cell.

Helper virus A virus that provides a function(s) to another virus or viral genome in the same cell.

Hemocoel Spaces between the organs of organisms with open circulatory systems, like most arthropods and mollusks.

Hemorrhagic colitis A type of gastroenteritis in which certain strains of the bacterium *Escherichia coli* infect the large intestine and produce a toxin (Shiga toxin) that causes bloody diarrhea and other serious complications. Hemorrhagic colitis occurs in people of all ages but is most common among children and older people.

Hepatocyte A cell that makes up the major mass of the liver and that is involved in synthesis of cholesterol, bile salts, and phospholipids as well as detoxification, modification, and excretion of various substances.

Heterochromatin Tightly compacted regions of chromatin that are usually transcriptionally silent.

Heterogeneity *See* Genetic heterogeneity.

Heterologous From a different source, as in heterologous DNA.

Heterologous probe A DNA probe that is derived from one organism and used to screen for a similar DNA sequence in a clone bank derived from another organism.

Heterologous protein *See* Recombinant protein.

Heteromer A protein with two or more different protein chains. Also called heteromeric polypeptide, heteromeric protein.

Heterozygote An individual that has different alleles at the same locus in its two homologous chromosomes.

HGP *See* Human Genome Project.

High-resolution map A genetic or physical map with closely spaced sites throughout.

Histone A protein that binds to DNA and aids in the compaction of chromosomes in the nucleus.

Holoenzyme A catalytically active enzyme containing all of the necessary cofactors and subunits.

Homodimer A protein with two identical polypeptide chains.

Homologous From the same source or having the same evolutionary function or structure.

Homology Similarity due to a common origin.

Homomer A protein with two or more identical protein chains. Also called homomeric polypeptide, homomeric protein.

Homopolymer A nucleic acid strand that is composed of one kind of nucleotide.

Homopolymeric tailing *See* Tailing.

Homozygote An individual that has identical alleles at the same locus in its two homologous chromosomes.

Hormone A chemical secreted by specialized cells that signal specific functions in target cells.

Host A microorganism, organism, or cell that maintains a cloning vector.

Human artificial chromosome A chromosome that is assembled from telomere, centromere, and human genomic DNA sequences. Also called HAC, microchromosome.

Human cytomegalovirus A virus belonging to the herpesvirus group.

Human Genome Project An international research effort dedicated to developing high-resolution human genetic and physical maps and the complete genomic DNA sequences of humans and other organisms. Also called HGP.

Human minisatellite DNA Human DNA that is noncoding and generally G+C rich and that contains tandem repeats of short (9- to 40-base-pair) stretches of DNA.

Humanized Having segments of a cloned (antibody) gene, usually from mice, replaced by comparable regions of human DNA. Such a recombinant protein is less likely to be recognized as a foreign protein when it is used as a human therapeutic agent.

Humoral immune response The production of antibody by B cells of the immune system in response to the presence of a foreign antigen.

Hybrid gene The combination of two genes or parts of two genes in the correct reading frame that encodes a single protein that has amino acid sequences from both genes.

Hybrid selection A protocol for determining which genomic clones hybridize to a cDNA or mRNA molecule.

Hybridization The pairing of two polynucleotide strands, often from different sources, by hydrogen bonding between complementary nucleotides.

Hybridoma The product of the fusion of a myeloma cell with an antibody-producing lymphocyte. This cell combination (hybridoma) can continue to divide in cell culture and secrete a single type of antibody.

Hydrogen bond A weak chemical bond that is formed when a hydrogen atom of a polar molecule that has a partial positive charge is attracted to an atom of another polar molecule that has a partial negative charge.

Hydrogen uptake positive A term describing a microorganism that is capable of assimilating (taking up) hydrogen gas. Also called Hup⁺.

Hydromechanical stress *See* Shear.

Hydroponics The growth of plants in liquid medium rather than in soil.

Hydroxyl group A functional group consisting of an oxygen atom and a hydrogen atom (–OH).

Hyperaccumulator A plant that can naturally accumulate large amounts of metal from the environment. These plants are often used for the phytoremediation of metals.

Hypervariable region The parts of both the heavy and light chains of an antibody molecule that enable it to bind to a specific site on an antigen.

Hypervariable segment A region of a protein that varies considerably between strains or individuals.

Hyphae Filamentous cells of some fungi.

IAA *See* Indole-3-acetic acid.

Ice nucleation protein A protein around which ice crystals form.

Ice-minus bacteria Bacteria that do not synthesize ice nucleation proteins.

I/E region *See* Integration–excision region.

Ileum The lower region of the small intestine just before the large intestine.

Immediate-early gene A viral gene that is expressed promptly after infection.

Immune response The processes, including the synthesis of antibodies, that are used by vertebrates to respond to the presence of a foreign antigen.

Immunoaffinity chromatography A purification technique in which an antibody is bound to a matrix and is subsequently used to bind a specific protein and separate it from a complex mixture.

Immunoassay A protocol that uses antibody specificity to detect the presence of a particular compound in a biological sample.

Immunogen A substance that induces an antibody response. Also called antigen.

Immunoglobulin *See* Antibody.

Immunosuppression Prevention or diminishment of the immune response by a substance, agent, or condition.

Immunotherapeutic procedure The use of an antibody or a fusion protein containing the antigen-binding site of an antibody to treat a disease and enhance the well-being of a patient.

Immunotoxin A fusion protein that has separate domains with antibody and toxin activities. The antibody portion of the molecule facilitates binding to a target molecule or cell, and the toxin inactivates the target molecule or kills the cell.

Impeller An agitator that is used for mixing the contents of a bioreactor.

In vitro mutagenesis *See* Directed mutagenesis.

In vitro translation Protein synthesis that is directed by either purified DNA with bacterial extracts or mRNA with wheat germ or rabbit reticulocyte extracts that provide ribosomes, tRNAs, and protein synthesis factors. The reaction mixture is often supplemented with ATP, GTP, and amino acids.

In vivo gene therapy The delivery of a gene(s) to a tissue or an organ of an individual to alleviate a genetic disorder.

Inactivated agent A virus, bacterium, or other organism that has been treated to prevent it from causing a disease.

Inclusion body A protein that is overproduced in a recombinant bacterium and forms a crystalline array of mostly inactive protein inside the bacterial cell.

Incompatibility group A classification scheme indicating which plasmids can coexist within a single cell. Plasmids must belong to different incompatibility groups to coexist within the same cell. Plasmids that belong to the same incompatibility group are unstable when placed into the same cell. A plasmid cloning vector should always belong to an incompatibility group different from that of the host bacterium's endogenous plasmids.

Independent assortment The formation of all possible gene combinations in gametes with genes on different chromosomes, followed by the random joining of male and female gametes. Also called Mendel's second law of inheritance.

Indole-3-acetic acid A plant hormone which stimulates both rapid responses, such as increases in cell elongation, and long-term effects, such as increases in cell division and differentiation. Abbreviated IAA.

Inducer A low-molecular-weight compound or a physical agent that interacts with or alters a repressor protein and prevents it from blocking transcription.

Induction Turning on the transcription of a specific gene or operon. The consequences of the action of an inducer.

Infectious agent Often, a proliferating virus, bacterium, or parasite that causes a disease in plants or animals.

Informatics *See* Bioinformatics.

Initiation The start of the biosynthesis of a polymeric macromolecule.

Initiation codon The codon AUG, which specifies the first amino acid (methionine [*N*-formylmethionine in prokaryotes]) of a protein. Also called initiator, translational start codon, translational initiation signal.

Initiation complex The fMet-tRNAfMet–mRNA–small ribosomal subunit–large ribosomal subunit combination in prokaryotes or the Met-tRNAMet–mRNA–small ribosomal subunit–large ribosomal subunit combination in eukaryotes that is ready for the elongation phase of translation.

Initiator *See* Initiation codon.

Initiator element *See* Response element.

Initiator tRNA The fMet-tRNAfMet in prokaryotes or Met-tRNAMet in eukaryotes that starts translation.

Insecticide A substance or living organism that kills insects.

Insert A DNA molecule that is incorporated into a cloning vector.

Insulin A small peptide hormone secreted by the pancreas that regulates glucose uptake by cells and other aspects of carbohydrate metabolism.

Integrating vector A vector that is designed to integrate cloned DNA into the host cell chromosomal DNA.

Integration Insertion of a DNA molecule (usually by homologous recombination) into a chromosomal site.

Integration–excision region The portion of bacteriophage λ DNA that enables bacteriophage λ DNA to be inserted into a specific site in the *Escherichia coli* chromosome and excised from this site.

Intein An internal segment of a protein that catalyzes its own excision from a protein precursor. Used in the construction of self-cleaving fusion proteins.

Interactome An extensive set of interacting proteins.

Interleukin-2 A lymphokine secreted by certain T lymphocytes that stimulates T-cell proliferation.

Internal ribosomal entry site A nontranslated sequence following a coding region of a polycistronic RNA that binds to a small ribosomal subunit and forms an initiation-of-translation complex.

Intervening sequence *See* Intron.

Intron A segment of a gene that is transcribed but is then excised from the primary transcript during processing into a functional RNA molecule. Also called intervening sequence.

Ion channel An integral protein within a cell membrane that facilitates selective ion transport.

IPTG Isopropyl-β-D-thiogalactopyranoside, an inducer of the *lac* (lactose) operon. In recombinant DNA technology, IPTG is often used to induce cloned genes that are under the control of the *lac* repressor–*lac* promoter system.

IRES *See* Internal ribosomal entry site.

Ischemia Inadequate blood supply to a local area due to blockage of the blood vessels to that area.

Isoelectric point The pH at which the net charge on a protein or other molecule is zero.

Isoschizomers Restriction enzymes that recognize and bind to the same nucleotide sequence in DNA and cut at the same site.

Isopropyl-β-D-thiogalactopyranoside *See* IPTG.

Jejunum The portion of the mammalian small intestine between the duodenum and the ileum. The jejunum is lined with small outgrowths called villi that facilitate the absorption of digested material.

kb *See* Kilobase pair.

k_{cat} The catalytic rate constant that characterizes an enzyme-catalyzed reaction. The higher the k_{cat}, the faster the conversion of substrate into product.

k_{cat}/K_m The catalytic efficiency of an enzyme-catalyzed reaction. The higher the value of k_{cat}/K_m, the more rapidly and efficiently the substrate is converted into product.

Ketosynthase A low-molecular-weight enzyme involved as part of a larger complex in polyketide biosynthesis.

Kilobase pair One thousand base pairs; a unit of length of DNA. Abbreviated kb.

Kindred A group of individuals who are related to each other either genetically or by marriage. Also called kinship.

Klenow fragment A product of proteolytic digestion of the DNA polymerase I from *Escherichia coli* that retains both polymerase and 3′ exonuclease activities but not 5′ exonuclease activity.

Kluyvera ascorbata A free-living gram-negative soil bacterium that can act as a plant growth-promoting bacterium.

K_m A dissociation constant that characterizes the binding of an enzyme to a substrate. The lower the K_m, the tighter the binding of the enzyme to the substrate. Also called Michaelis constant.

Knockout The targeted disruption of a gene by homologous recombination. Also called gene knockout.

Kozak sequence A specific sequence of nucleotides surrounding the start codon in higher eukaryotic organisms.

Label A compound or atom that is either attached to or incorporated into a macromolecule and is used to detect the

presence of a compound, substance, or macromolecule in a sample. Also called tag.

Large ribosomal subunit The larger component of a ribosome.

Latent agent Usually a virus that is present in a host organism but does not produce any symptoms.

Leader peptide *See* Signal sequence.

Leader sequence A sequence of nucleotides at the 5' end of an mRNA that is not translated into protein.

Lectin One of a group of plant proteins that can bind to specific oligosaccharides on the surface of a cell. Lectins are often found in seeds, where they act as a toxin against certain pathogenic agents.

Lentiviral vector A retroviral vector, derived from the lentivirus, that can be used to deliver a gene of interest into the genomes of dividing and nondividing host cells.

Library *See* Gene bank.

Ligand A molecule that specifically binds to a larger molecule.

Ligase chain reaction A technique for determining the presence or absence of a specific nucleotide pair within a target gene.

Ligation Joining of two DNA molecules by the formation of phosphodiester bonds. In vitro, this reaction is usually catalyzed by the enzyme T4 DNA ligase.

Lignocellulose The combination of lignin, hemicellulose, and cellulose that forms the structural framework of plant cell walls.

Linkage The occurrence of two or more genes on the same chromosome.

Linkage map *See* Genetic map.

Linker A synthetic double-stranded oligonucleotide that carries the sequence for one or more restriction endonuclease sites.

Lipase An enzyme that degrades lipids.

Lipofection Delivery into eukaryotic cells of DNA, RNA, or other compounds that have been encapsulated in an artificial phospholipid vesicle.

Lipopolysaccharide A compound containing lipid bound to a polysaccharide; often a component of microbial cell walls. Also called LPS.

Lipoprotein A compound containing both lipid and protein; the main structural material of cell membranes.

Liposome A spherical particle of lipid molecules in which the hydrophobic portions of the molecule are facing inward; a lipid vesicle with an aqueous interior that can carry nucleic acids, drugs, or other therapeutic agents.

Liquefaction Enzymatic digestion (often by α-amylase) of gelatinized starch to form lower-molecular-weight polysaccharides.

Liquid chromatography A technique used to separate molecules that are dissolved in a solution. Separation occurs as the molecules in the solution (the mobile phase) pass through a column containing a second solution (the stationary phase) because the molecules interact with the second solution to different extents and therefore pass through the column at different rates.

Live vaccine (1) A living, nonvirulent form of a microorganism or virus that is used to elicit an antibody response that protects the inoculated organism against infection by a virulent form of the microorganism or virus. (2) A living, nonvirulent microorganism or virus that expresses a foreign antigenic protein and is used to inoculate a human or animal. The latter type of organism is also called a live recombinant vaccine.

Locus The site on the chromosome where a specific gene is located.

Long template A DNA strand that is synthesized during the polymerase chain reaction, has a primer sequence at one end, and is extended beyond the site that is complementary to the second primer at the other end.

Long terminal repeats Similar blocks of genetic information that are found at the ends of the genomes of retroviruses. Also called LTRs.

LTRs *See* Long terminal repeats.

Luciferase In fireflies, the enzyme, encoded by the *luc* gene, that catalyzes the oxidation of luciferin and subsequent emission of light in a bioluminescence reaction. In bacteria, the enzyme, encoded by *luxA* to *luxE*, that catalyzes the production of light.

Luciferin In fireflies, the compound 4,5-dihydro-2-(-6-hydroxy-2-benzothiazolyl)-4-thiazole carboxylic acid, which is oxidized in the reaction used to produce light.

Lupine A grain legume that is grown extensively in Australia and New Zealand.

Lycopene A carotene photosynthetic pigment. Lycopene from tomatoes is thought to act as an antioxidant.

Lymphoma Cancer originating in the lymph nodes, spleen, and other lymphoreticular sites.

Lysis The destruction or breakage of cells by (1) viruses or (2) chemical or physical treatment.

Lysogeny A condition in which a bacteriophage genome (prophage) survives within the host chromosome and lytic functions are repressed.

Lytic cycle The process of viral production that usually leads to cell lysis.

MAb *See* Monoclonal antibody.

Macromolecule A molecule with a high molecular mass, such as a nucleic acid, protein, or polysaccharide.

Macrophage A large phagocytic white blood cell.

Macula Part of the retina of the vertebrate eye.

Maltose-binding protein An abundant bacterial protein located within the periplasmic space and involved in the uptake of maltose.

Marker An identifiable DNA sequence on a chromosome. Also called marker site, marker locus, genetic marker.

Marker peptide A portion of a fusion protein that facilitates its identification or purification.

Mass spectrometry Measurement of the mass-to-charge ratio of ions.

Matrix-assisted laser desorption ionization (MALDI) A mass spectrometry technique often used to determine the masses of peptides. The peptides are mixed with a matrix consisting of an organic acid and then ionized with a laser. The ions are accelerated through a tube by using a high-voltage current, and the time required for them to reach the ion detector is used to determine their molecular mass; lower-mass ions reach the detector first.

Mb *See* Megabase pair.

MCS *See* Polylinker.

Medaka The small freshwater teleost (bony fish) *Oryzias latipes*.

Megabase pair 1,000,000 base pairs; a unit of length of DNA. Abbreviated Mb.

Melittin A 26-amino-acid peptide with antimicrobial and hemolytic activities that is the major component of bee venom.

Meristematic tissue Plant tissue that is actively dividing. In young plants, it is usually found at the tips of the stem and the roots.

Merozoite A daughter cell of a protozoan parasite. It is the result of asexual reproduction.

Mesophile A microorganism that is able to grow within the temperature range of 20 to 50°C; optimal growth often occurs at about 37°C.

Messenger RNA An RNA molecule carrying the information that, during translation, specifies the amino acid sequence of a protein molecule. Also called mRNA.

Metabolite (1) A low-molecular-weight biological compound that is usually synthesized by an enzyme. (2) A compound that is essential for a metabolic process.

Metabolome The complete repertoire of metabolites of a cell, tissue, or organism.

Metagenomics The study of the collective genomes in an environmental sample.

Methylation The addition of a methyl group(s) to a macromolecule; for example, the addition of a methyl group to specific cytosine and, occasionally, adenine residues in DNA.

Michaelis constant *See* K_m.

Microchromosome *See* Human artificial chromosome.

Microinjection The introduction of DNA or other compounds into a single eukaryotic cell with a fine microscopic needle.

Microprojectile bombardment *See* Biolistics.

Minitransposon A smaller version of a transposon containing only a portion of the DNA carried by the transposon.

Mismatch The lack of base pairing between one or more nucleotides of two hybridized nucleic acid strands.

Missense mutation A genetic mutation that changes a codon for one amino acid into a codon specifying another amino acid.

Mobilizing functions The genes on a plasmid that facilitate the transfer of either a nonconjugative or a conjugative plasmid from one bacterium to another.

Modification (1) Enzymatic methylation of a restriction enzyme DNA recognition site. (2) A specific nucleotide change in a DNA or RNA molecule.

Molecular mass The sum of the masses of all the atoms in a molecule, usually expressed in daltons or kilodaltons.

Monochromosomal Referring to the presence of a single human chromosome in a somatic cell hybrid line.

Monoclonal antibody A single type of antibody that is directed against a specific epitope (antigenic determinant) and is produced by a hybridoma cell line, which is formed by the fusion of a lymphocyte with a myeloma cell. Some myeloma cells synthesize single antibodies naturally. Also called MAb.

Monocotyledon A class of plants that have one seed leaf. Also called monocot.

Monomer A unit of a polymer.

mRNA *See* Messenger RNA.

M13 + strand The single-stranded DNA molecule that is present in the infective bacteriophage M13.

Mucosal immunity Protection from the pathogenic effects of foreign microorganisms or antigenic substances as a result of antibody secretions of the mucous membranes. Mucosal epithelia in the gastrointestinal, respiratory, and reproductive tracts produce a form of immunoglobulin A that protects these ports of entry into the body.

Multigene RNA An RNA transcript of an operon.

Multiple cloning site *See* Polylinker.

Multiplex assay Simultaneous determination of a large number of different targets in one reaction vessel or by one analytical procedure.

Multipoint linkage analysis The determination of the order and map distances of many loci on a chromosome at one time. Also called multilocus mapping, multipoint mapping, multilocus linkage analysis.

Multivalent vaccine A single vaccine that is designed to elicit an immune response either to more than one infectious agent or to several different epitopes of a molecule.

Must The juice from crushed grapes before fermentation; used in wine making.

Mutagenesis Chemical or physical treatment that changes the nucleotides of the DNA of an organism.

Mutant An organism that differs from the wild type because it carries one or more genetic changes in its DNA. Also called a variant.

Mutant complementation *See* Genetic complementation.

Mutation A change of one or more nucleotide pairs of a DNA molecule.

Mutation detection assay A protocol that identifies the difference of one or a few nucleotide pairs between the same DNA molecules from different sources.

Mycelium A mass of interwoven threadlike filaments of a fungus or bacterium.

Myeloma A plasma cell cancer.

Mycotoxin A toxin produced by a fungus.

N terminus The first amino acid(s) of a protein. Also called amino terminus, amino-terminal end.

Narrow-host-range plasmid A plasmid that can replicate in one, or at most a few, different bacterial species.

Native protein The naturally occurring form of a protein.

Nebulization A process in which genomic DNA is fragmented by forcing it through a small pore, thereby creating a fine spray.

Negative control A system of regulation of transcription that requires the removal of a repressor from an operator.

Neomycin phosphotransferase An enzyme that inactivates the antibiotics neomycin and kanamycin. This enzyme is often used as a selective marker for transgenic plants.

Neonate A newborn.

Neoschizomers Restriction enzymes that recognize and bind to the same nucleotide sequence in DNA and cut at different sites.

Neutralizing antibody An antibody that reacts with an infectious agent (e.g., a virus) and destroys or inhibits its infectivity or virulence.

Neutrophil A type of white blood cell that fights infection. A form of granulocyte, filled with neutrally staining granules, which are tiny sacs of enzymes that help the cell to kill and digest microorganisms.

Nick (1) To break a phosphodiester bond in the backbone of one of the strands of a duplex DNA molecule. (2) A break in the backbone of one of the strands of duplex DNA.

Nicotine A colorless, poisonous alkaloid found in tobacco that is sometimes used as an insecticide.

Nitrilase An enzyme that catalyzes the hydrolysis of nitriles to carboxylic acids and ammonia.

Nitrogen fixation The conversion of atmospheric nitrogen to ammonia. Biological nitrogen fixation is catalyzed by the enzyme nitrogenase, which is found only in prokaryotes.

Nod box A DNA sequence that controls the transcriptional regulation of *Rhizobium* nodulation genes.

Nodulation The formation of nodules by symbiotic bacteria on the roots of plants.

Nonautologous From a different species or individual.

Nonreducing end The end of a cellulose strand that cannot act as a reducing agent; it does not contain an aldehyde moiety.

Nonvirulent agent *See* Attenuated vaccine.

Northern blotting Similar to Southern blotting, except that RNA which has been separated by gel electrophoresis is transferred from a gel onto a matrix, such as a nitrocellulose or nylon membrane, and the presence of a specific RNA molecule is detected by DNA–RNA hybridization.

Nuclear cloning Production of an organism by placing a nucleus from a somatic cell into an enucleated fertilized egg. Also called nuclear transfer.

Nucleocapsid The nucleic acid genome and surrounding protein coat of a virus.

Nucleoside A base (purine or pyrimidine) that is covalently linked to a five-carbon (pentose) sugar. When the sugar is ribose, the nucleoside is a ribonucleoside; when it is deoxyribose, the nucleoside is a deoxyribonucleoside.

Nucleotide A nucleoside with one or more phosphate groups linked to the 5′ carbon of the pentose sugar. Ribose-containing nucleosides are often called ribonucleoside monophosphate (NMP), ribonucleoside diphosphate (NDP), or ribonucleoside triphosphate (NTP). When the nucleoside contains the sugar deoxyribose, the nucleotides are called deoxyribonucleoside mono-, di-, or triphosphates (dNMP, dNDP, or dNTP).

Nucleus The membrane-enclosed structure in eukaryotic cells that contains the genetic material.

Off state A state in which a gene is not being transcribed.

OLA *See* Oligonucleotide ligation assay.

Oleosins Hydrophobic oil body proteins associated with plant seeds.

Oligonucleotide A short molecule (usually 6 to 100 nucleotides) of single-stranded DNA. Oligonucleotides are sometimes called oligodeoxyribonucleotides or oligomers and are usually synthesized chemically.

Oligonucleotide ligation assay A diagnostic technique for determining the presence or absence of a specific nucleotide pair within a target gene, which indicates whether a gene is wild type (normal) or mutant (defective). Abbreviated OLA.

Oligonucleotide-directed mutagenesis *See* Site-specific mutagenesis.

On state A state in which a gene is being transcribed.

Oncogene A gene that plays a role in the cell division cycle. Often, mutated forms of oncogenes cause a cell to grow in an uncontrolled manner.

Oncomouse A transgenic mouse that carries an activatable gene that makes it susceptible to tumor formation.

Oocyte An egg produced by female ovaries.

Open reading frame A sequence of nucleotides in a DNA molecule that encodes a peptide or protein. This term is often used when, after the sequence of a DNA fragment has been determined, the function of the encoded protein is not known. Abbreviated ORF.

Operator The region of DNA that is upstream from a prokaryotic gene(s) and to which a repressor or activator binds.

Operon A cluster of genes that are coordinately regulated.

Opine The condensation product of an amino acid with either a keto acid or a sugar.

ORF *See* Open reading frame.

ORFeome A large collection of cloned open reading frames of a proteome.

ori *See* Origin.

Origin The nucleotide sequence at which DNA synthesis is initiated. Also called origin of replication, *ori*.

Origin of replication *See* Origin.

Orthologues Sequences in different species that have a common origin.

Osmolyte A compound that regulates the osmotic pressure within a cell.

Outflow The volume of growing cells that is removed from a bioreactor during a continuous fermentation process.

Overhang *See* Extension.

Ovule The structure in seed plants that contains the female reproductive cells and develops into a seed after fertilization.

Oxidative phosphorylation A series of enzyme-catalyzed reactions in which the acetyl moiety of acetyl coenzyme A is converted to carbon dioxide and water with the concomitant synthesis of ATP.

Ozone A gaseous form of oxygen, O_3. Used for sterilizing water, purifying air, and bleaching.

P site *See* Peptidyl site.

PAC *See* P1 artificial chromosome.

Packaging cell line A cell line that is designed to produce viral particles that do not contain infective nucleic acid. This process has been described as "putting a sheep in wolf's clothing."

Palindromic sequences Complementary DNA sequences that are the same when each strand is read in the same direction (e.g., 5′ to 3′). These types of sequences serve as recognition sites for type II restriction endonucleases.

Panicle A pyramidal, loosely branched flower cluster.

Pantoea agglomerans A gram-negative bacterium typically found on plant surfaces. It is also an opportunistic human pathogen.

Parallelization Performing a large number of reactions, such as sequencing reactions, simultaneously.

Paralogue A sequence that arose by duplication within a species.

Parasporal crystal Tightly packaged insect protoxin molecules that are produced by strains of *Bacillus thuringiensis* during the formation of resting spores.

Partial digest Treatment of a DNA sample with a type II restriction endonuclease under conditions that result in a limited number of cuts in each DNA molecule to yield many possible combinations of cleaved pieces in the final sample.

Passaging Subculturing cells that are growing in vitro.

Passive immunity (1) Natural acquisition of antibodies by the fetus or newborn from the mother. (2) The artificial introduction of specific antibodies by the injection of serum from an immune animal. In both cases, it confers temporary protection on the recipient.

Patatin A storage protein commonly found in potatoes.

Patent A government-issued document that allows the holder the exclusive right to manufacture, use, or sell an invention for a defined period, usually 20 years.

Pathogenesis-related promoter The promoter for a plant gene whose transcription is activated upon infection of the plant by pathogens.

PCR *See* Polymerase chain reaction.

Pedigree A diagrammatic representation of the history of a trait in a multigeneration family.

Peptide A short chain of amino acids that are linked with peptide bonds.

Peptide bond The covalent bond between the α-carboxyl group of one amino acid and the α-amino group of an adjacent amino acid in a peptide or protein.

Peptide vaccine A short chain of amino acids that can induce antibodies against a specific infectious agent.

Peptidyl site The portion of a ribosome where the tRNA with the peptide chain participates in peptide bond formation with the aminoacyl–tRNA during translation. Also called P site.

Peptidyl-tRNA The tRNA that has a growing peptide chain attached to it during translation.

Periplasm The space (periplasmic space) between the cell (cytoplasmic) membrane of a bacterium or fungus and the outer membrane or cell wall.

Peritrophic membrane A semipermeable chitinous matrix lining the gut of most insects that is thought to be important in the maintenance of insect gut structure, facilitation of digestion, and protection from invasion by microorganisms and parasites.

Permeate In cross-flow filtration, the solution that passes through the membrane.

Peroxidase Enzymes that, together with hydrogen peroxide, catalyze the oxidation of certain organic compounds.

Pesticide A chemical or biological agent that is used to kill pests. Pesticides are often applied to crops to control weeds and to reduce predation by insects or pathogenic microorganisms.

Phage See Bacteriophage.

Pharmaceutical agent See Therapeutic agent.

Phase state The coupling or repulsion of two linked genes.

Phenotype An observable feature or set of traits that is determined by a gene or combination of genes of an organism.

Phenylalanine ammonia lyase An enzyme that converts phenylalanine to cinnamic acid and tyrosine to *p*-coumaric acid. This enzyme is central to the synthesis of phenylpropanoids, precursors of a range of phenolic compounds, including lignin, in plants.

Phenylketonuria An autosomal recessive disorder in humans that is due to the lack of the liver enzyme phenylalanine hydroxylase and that causes phenylalanine to accumulate. Abbreviated PKU.

Phosphate An inorganic ion that contains a central phosphorus atom linked to four oxygen atoms (PO_4^{3-}).

Phosphodiester bond The linkage of a phosphate group to the 3′ carbon of one nucleotide and the 5′ carbon of another nucleotide; the linkage between nucleotides of the same nucleic acid strand.

Phosphoramidite A chemically modified nucleoside used in the synthesis of short oligonucleotides.

Phosphorothioate linkage The linkage between nucleotides after a sulfur group replaces an available oxygen of a phosphodiester linkage.

Phosphorylation The addition of a phosphate group to a molecule.

Photolithography A manufacturing process that uses light. In the manufacture of some microarrays, the oligonucleotide probes are synthesized directly on a solid surface using multiple rounds of addition of modified nucleotides followed by exposure to light to stimulate joining of the nucleotide to a growing oligonucleotide chain. Nucleotide addition is prevented in some positions by shielding them from the light.

Photosynthetic Able to convert atmospheric carbon dioxide into organic compounds by using energy from sunlight.

Nearly all plants, most algae, and some bacteria are photosynthetic.

Phylogeny A prediction of evolutionary relationships among organisms that is determined from the comparison of molecular sequences and/or morphological characteristics.

Physical map A map of the positions of chromosome sites, such as restriction endonuclease recognition or sequence-tagged sites, on a chromosome. The distance between sites is measured in base pairs.

Phytase An enzyme able to break down phytate (phytic acid), a complex compound (inositol hexaphosphate) that is the major (60 to 80%) chemical form of phosphorus within cereal grains, oilseeds, and their byproducts. Many animals cannot digest and utilize the phosphorus within phytate, because they lack phytase in their digestive systems. The free inositol that is released upon digestion of phytate can chelate minerals such as iron, thereby facilitating its uptake.

Phytoextraction The absorption and concentration of metals from the soil into the roots and shoots of plants.

Phytohormone A substance that stimulates growth or other processes in plants; a plant hormone, e.g., auxin, cytokinin, gibberellin, ethylene, or abscisic acid.

Phytopathogen An organism, such as a fungus, bacterium, or virus, that causes disease in plants.

Phytoremediation The use of plants to remove or detoxify environmental contaminants, metals, or organic compounds.

Phytostabilization The use of plants to reduce the spread of metals in the environment.

Phytostimulation The stimulation of microbial biodegradation of organic compounds in the rhizosphere, the area around the roots of plants.

Phytotransformation The absorption and degradation of organic compounds by a plant.

Phytovolatilization The uptake by a plant of compounds from the environment and subsequent release into the atmosphere of volatile materials, such as mercury- or arsenic-containing compounds.

PKU See Phenylketonuria.

Plaque A clear area that is visible in a bacterial lawn on an agar plate and is due to lysis of the bacterial cells by bacteriophage.

Plasmid An autonomous, self-replicating extrachromosomal DNA molecule.

Plastid In plants, a double-membrane-bound organelle, such as a chloroplast.

Pluripotent See Totipotent.

Pneumatic reactor See Airlift fermenter.

Pollen Microspores of plants that carry male gametes.

Pollination The transfer of pollen to the female reproductive organ of a plant, enabling fertilization to take place.

Poly(A) tail *See* Polyadenylation.

Polyadenylation The addition of adenine residues to the 3′ ends of eukaryotic mRNAs. Also called poly(A) tailing. The adenine-rich 3′-terminal segment is called a poly(A) tail.

Polyadenylation signal A sequence that terminates transcription and provides a recognition site at the end of an mRNA for the enzymatic addition of adenine residues.

Polycistronic RNA An mRNA that encodes two or more proteins.

Polyclonal antibody A serum sample that contains antibodies that bind to different antigenic determinants of one antigen.

Polyhedron The combination of baculovirus nucleocapsids embedded in a matrix protein (polyhedrin).

Polyhydroxyalkanoate Biodegradable polymers produced by microorganisms as a carbon and energy storage material.

Polyketide A class of antibiotics.

Polyketide synthase An enzyme involved in the biosynthesis of polyketide antibiotics.

Polylinker A synthetic DNA sequence that contains a number of different restriction endonuclease sites. Also called multiple cloning site (MCS).

Polymer A macromolecule made up of a series of covalently linked monomers.

Polymerase chain reaction A technique for amplifying a specific segment of DNA by using a thermostable DNA polymerase, deoxyribonucleotides, and primer sequences in multiple cycles of denaturation, renaturation, and DNA synthesis. Also called PCR.

Polymorphic probe An assay system that identifies a chromosome site with two or more allelic DNA sequences that each occur with a frequency of 1% (0.01) or greater in a large population.

Polymorphic site A chromosome location that has two or more identifiable allelic DNA sequences that each occur with a frequency of 1% (0.01) or greater in a large population. Also called polymorphic locus.

Polymorphism Variation in phenotypic or genetic characteristics among individuals in a population.

Polynucleotide A linear series of 20 or more nucleotides linked by phosphodiester bonds.

Polypeptide A linear series of amino acids linked together with peptide bonds. Also called protein, protein chain.

Poly(3-hydroxybutyric acid) The best studied and best characterized of the polyhydroxyalkanoates.

P1 artificial chromosome A plasmid vector system based on bacteriophage P1 that uses electroporation for introducing a vector with a large DNA insert (100 to 300 kb) into *Escherichia coli*. Also called PAC.

P1 cloning system A plasmid vector system based on bacteriophage P1 that uses in vitro bacteriophage P1 packaging for introducing a vector with a large DNA insert (80 to 100 kb) into *Escherichia coli*.

Positional gene cloning A strategy for isolating an unknown disease gene. The disease gene is mapped to a chromosome site. A contig or genomic clone that covers the site of the disease gene is tested for exons. Examination of exons and mutation detection assays establish which gene is the disease gene.

Positive control A system of regulation of transcription that requires the addition of a protein activator to an activator site on the DNA.

Positive selectable marker *See* Dominant marker selection.

Positive selection *See* Dominant marker selection.

Positive-negative selection A protocol that both selects for cells that carry a DNA insert integrated at a specific targeted chromosomal location (positive selection) and selects against cells that carry a DNA insert integrated at a nontargeted chromosomal site (negative selection).

Posttranslational modification The specific addition of phosphate groups, sugars (glycosylation), or other molecules to a protein after it has been synthesized.

PR protein A pathogenesis-related protein synthesized in some plants in response to stress.

Preventive immunization Injection of an antigen to elicit an antibody response that will protect the organism against future infections. Also called vaccination.

Pribnow box A sequence of six nucleotides (TATAAT) in the promoter region of a prokaryotic gene that is recognized and bound by the sigma factor of RNA polymerase to initiate transcription.

Primary antibody The antibody that binds to the target molecule in an ELISA or other immunological assay.

Primary cell culture A population of growing cells that is started directly from a tissue or cells of an organism.

Primary transcript Unprocessed RNA that is transcribed from a eukaryotic structural gene that has exons and introns.

Primer A short oligonucleotide that hybridizes with a template strand and provides a 3′ hydroxyl end for the initiation of nucleic acid synthesis.

Primer walking A method for sequencing long (>1-kb) cloned pieces of DNA. The initial sequencing reaction reveals the sequence of the first few hundred nucleotides of the cloned DNA. On the basis of these data, a primer that contains about 20 nucleotides and is complementary to a sequence near the end of the sequenced DNA is synthesized and used for sequencing of the next few hundred nucleotides of the cloned DNA. This procedure is repeated until the complete nucleotide sequence of the cloned DNA is determined.

Prion An infectious agent consisting of an abnormal variant of a brain protein that induces the normal brain protein to misfold. Prions have been implicated in several neurodegen-

erative diseases, including bovine spongiform encephalopathy (mad cow disease) in cattle, scrapie in sheep, and Creutzfeldt-Jakob disease in humans.

Probe (1) For diagnostic tests, the agent that is used to detect the presence of a molecule in a sample. (2) A DNA sequence that is used to detect the presence of a complementary sequence by hybridization with a nucleic acid sample.

Probiotic A bacterium (or several bacteria) often used as a dietary supplement. Thought to improve the intestinal microbial balance and/or alleviate various intestinal ailments.

Prodrug An inactive compound that is converted into a pharmacological agent by an in vivo metabolic process.

Productivity The amount of product that is produced in a bioreactor within a given period of time.

Progeny The offspring of a mating.

Prokaryotes Organisms, usually bacteria, that have neither a membrane-bound nucleus enclosing their chromosomes nor functional organelles, such as mitochondria and chloroplasts.

Promoter A segment of DNA to which RNA polymerase attaches. It usually lies upstream of (5' to) a gene. A promoter sequence aligns the RNA polymerase so that transcription will initiate at a specific nucleotide.

Pronucleus The nucleus of an egg or sperm after fertilization but before the egg and sperm have fused.

Prophage A repressed or inactive state of a bacteriophage genome that is maintained in a bacterial host cell as part of the chromosomal DNA.

Protease An enzyme that hydrolyzes peptide bond linkages and cleaves proteins into smaller peptides. Also called proteinase, proteolytic enzyme.

Protease inhibitor A protein that can form a tight complex with a protease and block its activity.

Protein *See* Polypeptide.

Protein chain *See* Polypeptide.

Protein drug *See* Therapeutic agent.

Protein microarray An array of a large number of different proteins for massively parallel analyses.

Protein replacement therapy Treatment of an inherited disorder with a structural protein that restores normal function.

Proteolysis Enzymatic degradation of a protein.

Proteome The complete repertoire of proteins of a cell, tissue, or organism.

Proteomics The study of the structure, function, and interactions of the members of a proteome.

Protocorm The precursor form of a corm, an underground plant propagule.

Protoplast A bacterial, yeast, or plant cell that has had its cell wall removed either chemically or enzymatically.

Protoxin A latent, nonactive precursor form of a toxin.

Provirus A stage in the life cycle of a retrovirus in which the single-stranded RNA is converted into double-stranded DNA, which may then be integrated into the genome of a mammalian host cell.

Pseudomonas A genus of common gram-negative bacteria that are widely distributed. Many of the soil forms produce a pigment that fluoresces under ultraviolet light, hence the descriptive term fluorescent pseudomonads.

Pseudotype formation The packaging of the genome of one virus in the envelope or capsid protein of another virus. Also called phenotypic mixing.

Psoriasis A chronic skin disease characterized by red patches covered with white scales.

Psychrophile A microorganism that can grow at temperatures as low as 0 to 5°C.

Purine Fusion of a pyrimidine and an imidazole ring, e.g., adenine or guanine.

Pyrimidine A heterocyclic ring, e.g., thymine, cytosine, or uracil.

Pyrogen A bacterial substance that causes fever in humans.

Pyrophosphate Two covalently linked phosphate groups that are released during hydrolysis of a nucleoside triphosphate to a nucleoside monophosphate. Pyrophosphate is released following the formation of a phosphodiester bond between nucleotides during DNA synthesis.

Pyrosequencing A sequencing method that detects the release of pyrophosphate when a known nucleotide is added to a growing DNA strand in a template-dependent manner, that is, when DNA polymerase catalyzes the addition of the complementary nucleotide.

Pythium ultimum A pathogenic soil fungus that causes root diseases in a variety of plants.

Quencher The portion of a molecule that can quench fluorescence.

Query The input sequence for computer analysis, usually for similarity searches.

Random amplified polymorphic DNA A diagnostic procedure in which chromosomal DNA (usually from plants but sometimes from microorganisms or animals) is characterized by the DNA fragments that are synthesized when PCR is initiated after the addition of a single primer to the reaction mixture. Abbreviated RAPD.

Random mutagenesis A nondirected change of a nucleotide pair(s) in a DNA molecule.

Random-primer method A protocol for labeling DNA in vitro. A sample of random oligonucleotides containing all possible combinations of nucleotide sequences is hybridized to a DNA probe. Then, in the presence of a DNA polymerase and the four deoxyribonucleotides (one of which is labeled),

the 3′ hydroxyl ends of the hybridized oligonucleotides provide initiation sites for DNA synthesis that uses the separated strands of the probe DNA as a template. This reaction produces labeled copies of portions of the probe DNA.

RAPD *See* Random amplified polymorphic DNA.

Reading frame A series of codons that code for amino acids in a nucleotide sequence.

Read-through Transcription or translation that proceeds beyond the normal stopping point because the transcription or translation termination signal of a gene is absent or mutated.

RecA A protein, found in most bacteria, that is essential for DNA repair and DNA recombination.

Recessive gene An allele that does not demonstrably contribute to the phenotype in a heterozygote.

Recognition site *See* Restriction site.

Recombinant An individual with two or more linked genes that are a consequence of one or more crossover events.

Recombinant DNA technology *See* Gene cloning.

Recombinant protein A protein whose amino acid sequence is encoded by a cloned gene.

Recombinant toxin A single multifunctional toxic protein that has been created by combining the coding regions of various genes.

Recombinant vaccine *See* Subunit vaccine.

Recombination *See* Crossover.

Reducing end The end of a cellulose strand that can act as a reducing agent; it typically contains an aldehyde moiety.

Refugium A small tract of land where a crop that is otherwise treated with the microbial insecticide *Bacillus thuringiensis* is left untreated.

Regulatory protein A protein that plays a role in either turning on or turning off transcription.

Remedial *See* Therapeutic.

Renaturation The reassociation of two nucleic acid strands after denaturation.

Replacement therapy The administration of metabolites, cofactors, or hormones that are deficient as the result of a genetic disease.

Replica plating The transfer of cells from bacterial colonies on one petri plate to another petri plate; the locations of the colonies that grow on the second plate correspond to those on the original (master) petri plate.

Replicatable biological unit Any biological entity that is capable of being reproduced.

Replication The process of DNA synthesis.

Replicative form The molecular configuration of viral nucleic acid that is the template for replication in a host cell. Also called RF.

Reporter gene A gene that encodes a product that can readily be assayed. For example, reporter genes are used to determine whether a particular DNA construct has been successfully introduced into a cell, organ, or tissue.

Repression Inhibition of transcription by preventing RNA polymerase from binding to the transcription initiation site; a repressed gene is "turned off."

Repressor A protein that binds to the operator or promoter region of a gene and prevents transcription by blocking the binding of RNA polymerase.

Repulsion The phase state in which a dominant version and a recessive version of two different genes occur on the same chromosome. Also called *trans* configuration. *See also* Coupling.

Response element A sequence of deoxyribonucleotides of a gene that acts as a binding site for a protein (transcription factor) that regulates transcription. Also called initiator element, signal region.

Restenosis Recurring narrowing of a biological opening, tube, or canal.

Restriction endonuclease (type II) An enzyme that recognizes a specific duplex DNA sequence and cleaves phosphodiester bonds on both strands between definite nucleotides.

Restriction map The linear array of restriction endonuclease sites on a DNA molecule.

Restriction site The sequence of nucleotide pairs in duplex DNA that is recognized by a type II restriction endonuclease. Sometimes called restriction enzyme site, restriction endonuclease site, or recognition site.

Retentate The liquid retained after passages of a solution across an ultrafiltration membrane.

Retrotransposon A genetic element that reproduces by first synthesizing an RNA intermediate, which is then copied back into DNA by reverse transcriptase before inserting randomly into a genome.

Retrovirus A class of eukaryotic RNA viruses that can form double-stranded DNA copies of their genomes; the double-stranded forms can integrate into chromosomal sites of an infected cell.

Reverse-phase microarray An array of multiprotein complexes of cell lysates or tissue specimens.

Reverse transcriptase An RNA-dependent DNA polymerase that uses an RNA molecule as a template for the synthesis of a complementary DNA strand.

Reverse transcription–polymerase chain reaction A two-step protocol for synthesizing cDNA molecules. First, cDNA strands are synthesized in vitro by reverse transcriptase with oligo(dT) as a primer and mRNA as the template. Second, a specific cDNA strand is amplified by the polymerase chain reaction (PCR), with one primer directed to a sequence of the first cDNA strand and the other to a sequence of the complementary cDNA strand (second strand) that is synthesized during the first PCR cycle. Also called RT–PCR.

Reversible chain terminator A nucleotide that has a blocking group at the 3′ carbon of the deoxyribose sugar to prevent subsequent addition of nucleotides to a growing DNA strand. In DNA sequencing by single-nucleotide addition, the modified nucleotides are used to ensure that the DNA strand is extended by only a single nucleotide during each cycle. After the incorporated nucleotide is identified by detection of a unique fluorophore, the blocking group is removed to restore the 3′ hydroxyl group for the next cycle of nucleotide addition.

Rhizobacterium A microorganism whose natural habitat is near, on, or in plant roots.

Rhizofiltration The use of plant roots to remove metals from contaminated effluents.

Rhizosecretion Secretion of molecules from the roots of plants.

Rhizosphere The zone in the immediate vicinity of growing plant roots.

Ribonuclease An enzyme that cleaves RNA. Also called RNase.

Ribonucleic acid *See* RNA.

Ribose The five-carbon sugar component of RNA.

Ribosomal RNA The RNA molecules that form part of the large and small ribosomal subunits. Also called rRNA.

Ribosome The subcellular structure that contains both RNA and protein molecules and mediates the translation of mRNA into protein. Ribosomes contain both large and small subunits.

Ribosome-binding site A sequence of nucleotides near the 5′ phosphate end of a bacterial mRNA that facilitates the binding of the mRNA to the small ribosomal subunit. Also called Shine-Dalgarno sequence.

Ribozyme An RNA molecule that has catalytic activity.

Ribulose bisphosphate carboxylase The most abundant enzyme in the world, found in all green plants and responsible for the fixation of carbon dioxide in photosynthesis. Sometimes called RuBisCO.

RNA Ribonucleic acid; a polynucleotide that has ribose as its pentose sugar and uracil as one of its pyrimidines.

RNA interference A method to inhibit expression of a target gene. A small RNA binds to a complementary region of the mRNA of the target gene and prevents its translation into protein.

RNA polymerase An enzyme that links an incoming ribonucleotide, which is determined by complementarity to a base in a template DNA strand, with a phosphodiester bond to the 3′ hydroxyl group of the last incorporated ribonucleotide of the growing RNA strand during transcription.

RNase *See* Ribonuclease.

Rolling circle A mode of DNA replication that produces concatemeric duplex DNA.

Root nodule A small round mass of cells that is located on the roots of plants and contains nitrogen-fixing bacteria.

rRNA *See* Ribosomal RNA.

RT-PCR *See* Reverse transcription–polymerase chain reaction.

Rumen A compartment of the stomach of cows and other ruminants where ingested food is initially digested.

Saccharification Hydrolysis of polysaccharides, after liquefaction, by glucoamylase to maltose and glucose.

Scaffolding Assembly of sequence contigs in the correct order and orientation to reconstruct the sequence of a genome.

Scale-up Conversion of a process, such as fermentation of a microorganism, from a small scale to a larger scale.

SCP *See* Single-cell protein.

SDS *See* Sodium dodecyl sulfate.

SDS-PAGE *See* Sodium dodecyl sulfate–polyacrylamide gel electrophoresis.

Secondary antibody In an ELISA or other immunological assay system, the antibody that binds to the primary antibody. The secondary antibody is often conjugated with an enzyme, such as alkaline phosphatase.

Secondary metabolite A compound that is not necessary for growth or maintenance of cellular functions but is synthesized, generally for the protection of a cell or microorganism, during the stationary phase of the growth cycle.

Secrete *See* Export.

Secretion The passage of a molecule from the inside of a cell through a membrane into the periplasmic space or the extracellular medium.

Secretion complex A complex of proteins in the cytoplasmic membrane of bacterial cells for transporting proteins across the membrane.

Secretory proteins Any protein that is secreted by a cell.

Selectable Having a gene product that, when present, enables a researcher to identify and preferentially propagate a particular cell type.

Selection (1) A system for either isolating or identifying specific organisms in a mixed culture. (2) Survival of a more reproductively fit organism.

Selective breeding The deliberate mating of plants or animals with selected traits to develop offspring with desired characteristics. Also known as conventional breeding or traditional breeding.

Self-incompatibility In plants, the inability of the pollen to fertilize ovules (female gametes) of the same plant. Also called self-sterility.

Self-replicating elements Extrachromosomal DNA elements that have origins of replication for the initiation of their own DNA synthesis.

Self-sterility *See* Self-incompatibility.

Senescence The last stage in the postembryonic development of multicellular organisms, during which loss of functions and degradation of biological components occur. Also called biological aging.

Sensitivity The ratio of all true-positive test results to all positive test results, i.e., true positives plus false negatives.

Sequence-tagged site A short (200- to 500-bp) DNA sequence that occurs once in the genome and is identified by PCR amplification. Abbreviated STS.

Sequence-tagged-site content mapping Determination of shared sites among clones of a library by using markers that are based on unique polymerase chain reaction primers. This facilitates the assembly of a contig.

Serial analysis of gene expression A technique that identifies and quantifies short sequence tags to measure the expression levels of all of the genes that are transcribed in a cell, tissue, or organism under a set of conditions. Also called SAGE.

Serotype Classification of an organism or protein on the basis of its interaction with antibodies.

Shear The sliding of one layer across another, with deformation and fracturing in the direction parallel to the movement. This term usually refers to the forces that cells are subjected to in a bioreactor or a mechanical device used for cell breakage.

Shine-Dalgarno sequence *See* Ribosome-binding site.

Short template A DNA strand that is synthesized during the polymerase chain reaction and has a primer sequence at one end and a sequence complementary to the second primer at the other end.

Shotgun cloning Construction of a library of small, overlapping fragments of genomic DNA to sequence the fragments. The overlapping sequences are then assembled to obtain the sequence of the entire genome.

Shuttle vector A plasmid-cloning vehicle, usually a plasmid, that can replicate in two different organisms because it carries two different origins of replication. Also called bifunctional vector.

Siderophore A low-molecular-weight substance that binds very tightly to iron. Siderophores are synthesized by a variety of soil microorganisms and plants to ensure that the organisms can obtain sufficient amounts of iron from the environment.

Sigma factor An accessory bacterial protein(s) that directs the binding of RNA polymerase to specific promoters.

Signal peptide *See* Signal sequence.

Signal recognition complex A group of proteins that binds to the signal peptide of a newly synthesized protein and targets the protein for secretion across the cytoplasmic membrane through the secretion complex.

Signal region *See* Response element.

Signal sequence A segment of about 15 to 30 amino acids at the N terminus of a protein that enables the protein to be secreted (pass through a cell membrane). The signal sequence is removed as the protein is secreted. Also called signal peptide, leader peptide.

Signal-to-noise ratio The ratio of the extent of the response to an assay when the target entity is present (signal) in a sample to the extent when it is absent (noise) from the sample.

Silage Cattle feed that has been allowed to ferment.

Similarity Degree of relationship between two sequences.

Simplicity For diagnostic tests, the ease with which an assay can be implemented.

Single-cell protein A dried mass of a pure sample of a protein-rich microorganism, which may be used either as feed (for animals) or as food (for humans). Abbreviated SCP.

Single-site mutation A change in one base pair in DNA. Also called point mutation.

Single-strand conformation analysis A mutation detection assay that is based on the conformation of single strands of DNA. If there is a nucleotide difference between the DNA molecules from two different sources, then following denaturation and gel electrophoresis, the locations of the single strands in the two lanes of the gel will be different. Also called single-strand conformational analysis, single-strand conformation(al) polymorphism (SSCP), SSCA.

Site-specific mutagenesis A technique to change one or more specific nucleotides in a cloned gene in order to create an altered form of a protein with a specific amino acid change(s). Also called oligonucleotide-directed mutagenesis.

Six-cutter A type II restriction endonuclease that binds and cleaves DNA at sites that contain six nucleotide pairs.

Size markers A set of macromolecules with known molecular masses that are used to calculate the molecular masses of electrophoretically fractionated macromolecules.

Small ribosomal subunit The smaller component of a ribosome.

Sodium dodecyl sulfate An anionic detergent that denatures proteins.

Sodium dodecyl sulfate–polyacrylamide gel electrophoresis A technique for separating and then visualizing protein samples. Also called SDS-PAGE.

Somatic cell Any cell of a multicellular organism that does not produce gametes.

Somatic cell gene therapy The delivery of a gene(s) to a tissue other than reproductive cells of an individual with the aim of correcting a genetic defect.

Somatic cell hybrid panel A set of derived chromosome-specific hybrid cell lines that each carry a different portion of a particular chromosome. The members of such a panel have chromosomal deletions and, in some cases, carry translocated chromosomes that retain a segment of a particular chromo-

some. Ideally, the retained portions of the cell lines of a panel cover the entire chromosome. Also called somatic cell hybrid mapping panel, somatic cell deletion panel.

S1 nuclease An enzyme that specifically degrades single-stranded DNA.

Sonication Disruption of cells or DNA molecules by high-frequency sound waves. Also called ultrasonication.

Source DNA The DNA from an organism that contains a target gene; this DNA is used as starting material in a cloning experiment.

Source organism An organism (e.g., a bacterium, plant, or animal) from which DNA is purified and used in a cloning experiment.

Southern blotting A technique for transferring denatured DNA molecules that have been separated electrophoretically from a gel to a matrix (such as a nitrocellulose or nylon membrane) on which a hybridization assay can be performed.

Sparger A device that introduces air into a bioreactor in the form of separate, fine streams.

Specificity The ratio of all true-negative test results to all negative test results, i.e., true negatives plus false positives.

Splice site The nucleotides at (1) the end of an exon and the beginning of an intron and (2) the end of an intron and the beginning of the next exon that are required for the joining of two exons and the removal of an intron during the processing of a primary transcript into a functional mRNA.

Splice site mutation Loss or gain of a functional splice site that affects the proper removal of introns during mRNA processing.

Spore A small, protected reproductive form of a microorganism, often produced when nutrient levels are low.

Sporozoite A cell of a malaria parasite that develops in the mosquito's salivary glands, leaves the mosquito during a blood meal, and enters the liver, where it multiplies.

Sporulation Formation of spores or resting structures, usually after the near depletion of nutrients from the growth medium, by some bacteria or fungi.

SSCA *See* Single-strand conformation analysis.

Staggered cuts Symmetrically cleaved phosphodiester bonds that lie on both strands of duplex DNA but are not opposite one another.

Start codon *See* Initiation codon.

Steady state In a continuous fermentation process, the condition where the number of cells that are removed with the outflow is exactly balanced by the number of newly divided cells.

Stem cell A precursor cell that undergoes division and gives rise to lineages of differentiated cells.

Stenosis Narrowing of a biological opening, tube, or canal.

Sticky ends *See* Cohesive ends.

Stirred-tank fermenter A growth vessel in which cells or microorganisms are mixed by mechanically driven impellers.

Strain A microorganism or multicellular organism that is a genetic variant of a standard parental stock.

Strand A linear series of nucleotides that are linked to each other by phosphodiester bonds.

Streptavidin A protein from *Streptomyces* spp. that has a very high affinity for biotin and is often used for purification or detection of biotin-tagged molecules.

Streptokinase A bacterial enzyme that catalyzes the conversion of plasminogen to plasmin, thereby helping to dissolve blood clots.

Stress ethylene Ethylene that is synthesized in response to some form of environmental stress.

Structural gene A sequence of DNA that encodes a protein.

STS *See* Sequence-tagged site.

Subcloning Splicing part of a cloned DNA molecule into a different cloning vector.

Subcutaneous Lying beneath the dermis layer of the skin.

Subspecies A population(s) of organisms sharing certain characteristics that are not present in other populations of the same species.

Substantial equivalence A term used by many national regulatory agencies to describe genetically engineered products that are similar in composition and safety to their non-genetically engineered counterparts.

Substitutive therapy Treatment of an inherited disorder with a cofactor that restores enzyme function.

Substrate (1) A compound that is altered by an enzyme. (2) A food source for growing cells or microorganisms.

Substrate-induced gene expression A method used to identify catabolic genes that are expressed when a particular substrate is present. Also called SIGEX.

Subtilisin A proteolytic enzyme usually found in *Bacillus subtilis*.

Subunit vaccine An immunogenic protein(s) either purified from the disease-causing organism or produced from a cloned gene.

Sucrose density gradient centrifugation A procedure used to fractionate mRNAs or DNA fragments according to size.

Suicide gene A plasmid-borne, inducible sequence that produces a protein that directly or indirectly kills the host cell.

Superbug Jargon for the bacterial strain of *Pseudomonas* developed by A. Chakrabarty, who combined hydrocarbon-degrading genes carried on different plasmids into one organism. Although this genetically engineered microorganism is neither "super" nor a "bug," it is a landmark example, because it showed how genetically modified microbial strains could be used in a novel way and because it was the basis for the precedent-setting legal decision that, in the

United States, genetically engineered organisms are patentable.

Suppressor tRNA An abnormal tRNA that inserts an amino acid where a mutant mRNA specifies a stop codon in the middle of the coding portion of a gene. Insertion of this amino acid allows a normal-size rather than a shortened protein to be synthesized.

Symbiosis A close biological relationship between two organisms in which neither organism is extremely harmful to the other. In some cases, the relationship is mutually beneficial.

Syndrome A constellation of features that together make up the symptoms of a disorder or disease.

Systemic acquired resistance Resistance, in plants, to pathogenic agents that occur following an initial exposure to the same or another pathogenic agent. This resistance extends to plant tissues that are far from the site of the initial infection and may last for weeks to months.

Systemic immunity Immunity that affects the body as a whole; all-body immunity.

T A thymine residue in DNA.

T cells Lymphocytes that pass through the thymus gland during maturation. Different kinds of T cells play important roles in the immune response.

Tag *See* Label.

Tailing The in vitro addition of the same nucleotide by the enzyme terminal transferase to the 3′ hydroxyl ends of a duplex DNA molecule. Also called homopolymeric tailing.

Tandem array Usually, a DNA molecule that contains two or more identical nucleotide sequences in series.

Tandem mass spectrometry Initial mass analysis of ions (precursor ions) followed by a second mass analysis of the daughter ions of a selected precursor ion. Also called MS/MS, tandem MS.

Target For diagnostic tests, the molecule or nucleic acid sequence that is being sought in a sample.

Target gene A descriptive term for a gene that is to be either cloned or specifically mutated.

Targeting vector A cloning vector carrying a DNA sequence capable of participating in a crossover event at a specified chromosomal location in the host cell.

TATA box The DNA sequence to which RNA polymerase binds and that lies upstream from the site of initiation of transcription and ensures that transcription starts at a specified nucleotide. Also called a Pribnow box in prokaryotes and a Hogness box in eukaryotes, after the researchers who discovered the function of the TATA box in prokaryotes and eukaryotes, respectively.

T-DNA The segment of a Ti plasmid that is transferred and integrated into chromosomal sites in the nuclei of plant cells.

Telomere The defined end of a chromosome containing specific DNA sequences.

Temperature-sensitive protein A protein that is functional at one temperature but loses function at another (usually higher) temperature.

Template strand The polynucleotide strand that a polymerase uses for determining the sequence of nucleotides during the synthesis of a new nucleic acid strand.

Termination The cessation of the biosynthesis of a polymeric macromolecule.

Termination codon A naturally occurring codon that does not base pair with the anticodon of any tRNA. Generally, the three codons in this class (UAA, UAG, and UGA) are used to terminate translation, although in some rare instances one of these codons does code for an amino acid. Also called translational stop signal.

Termination factor A protein that enters the A site of a ribosome when a stop codon in the mRNA is present and terminates protein synthesis by stimulating cleavage of the polypeptide from the tRNA in the P site. Also known as a release factor.

Terminator A sequence of DNA at the 3′ end of a gene that stops transcription. Also called transcription terminator.

Tetanus An infectious disease marked by spasms of voluntary muscles and caused by the toxin from the bacterium *Clostridium tetani*.

T4 DNA ligase An enzyme from bacteriophage T4-infected cells that catalyzes the joining of duplex DNA molecules and repairs nicks in DNA molecules. The enzyme joins a 5′ phosphate group to a 3′ hydroxyl group.

T4 DNA polymerase end labeling A process in which DNA that has been cut with a restriction endonuclease(s) is mixed with T4 DNA polymerase and one labeled deoxyribonucleotide. The 3′ exonuclease activity of the T4 DNA polymerase removes deoxyribonucleotides from the 3′ ends of the DNA fragments. Immediately after a deoxyribonucleotide that is the same as the deoxyribonucleotide in the reaction mixture is cleaved off, the T4 DNA polymerase activity incorporates a labeled deoxyribonucleotide from the reaction mixture. No further incorporation of deoxyribonucleotides occurs because there is only one kind of deoxyribonucleotide in the reaction mixture.

Thaumatin A plant protein that has a sweet taste. It is also synthesized in some plants in response to infection by pathogens.

Therapeutic Referring to treatment of a disease.

Therapeutic agent A compound that is used for the treatment of a disease and for improving the well-being of an organism. Also called pharmaceutical agent, drug, protein drug.

Thermophile A microorganism that grows optimally at high temperatures, usually above 50°C. Some thermophiles can grow at temperatures of 90 to 100°C.

Thermosensitivity Loss of activity of a protein at high temperature.

Thermostability Retention of activity at high temperature.

Thioredoxin A small protein that acts as an electron carrier.

3' extension A short, single-stranded nucleotide sequence on the 3' hydroxyl end of a double-stranded DNA molecule. Also called 3' protruding end, 3' sticky end, 3' overhang.

3' hydroxyl end The hydroxyl group that is attached to the 3' carbon atom of the sugar (ribose or deoxyribose) of the terminal nucleotide of a nucleic acid molecule.

Thrombin A blood protein that plays a role in blood clotting.

Thrombus A blood clot.

Thymidylate synthase An enzyme that catalyzes the methylation of the uracil moiety in dUMP to convert it to dTMP.

Thymine One of the organic bases found in DNA.

Ti plasmid A large extrachromosomal element that is found in strains of *Agrobacterium* and is responsible for crown gall formation.

Tissue plasminogen activator A protein involved in dissolving blood clots. Abbreviated tPA.

Totipotent Generally, the state in which a cell is able to respond to any one of a number of different stimuli and, subsequently, to develop into any one of a number of differentiated cell types. Also called pluripotent.

Toxoid A toxin that has been treated to destroy its toxicity but is left capable of inducing antibodies.

tPA *See* Tissue plasminogen activator.

Tracking dye A low-molecular-weight, visible, colored compound that moves with the ion front during gel electrophoresis.

Transcribed triplet A set of three contiguous nucleotides of the transcribed DNA strand of the coding region of a structural gene that determines a codon in the mRNA.

Transcript An RNA molecule that has been synthesized from a specific DNA template.

Transcription The process of RNA synthesis that is catalyzed by RNA polymerase; it uses a DNA strand as a template.

Transcription factor A protein that facilitates RNA synthesis by binding to a specific DNA sequence or another transcription factor that is bound to a specific DNA sequence.

Transcription mapping Assigning gene transcripts, in the form of cDNA clones or expressed sequence tags, to specific chromosome regions by fluorescence in situ hybridization, hybridization, polymerase chain reaction, analysis of somatic cell hybrid mapping panels, or other strategies. Also called transcript mapping, transcriptional mapping.

Transcriptome The complete repertoire of RNA molecules of a cell, tissue, or organism.

Transduction The transfer of nonviral DNA by a virus to a cell.

Transfection The transfer of DNA to a eukaryotic cell.

Transfer RNA The RNA molecules that decode the sequence information contained in an mRNA molecule during the translation process. Also called tRNA.

Transformation (1) The uptake and establishment of DNA in a bacterium or yeast cell in which the introduced DNA often changes the phenotype of the recipient organism. (2) Conversion, by various means, of animal cells in tissue culture from controlled to uncontrolled cell growth.

Transformation efficiency The number of cells that take up foreign DNA as a function of the amount of added DNA; expressed as transformants per microgram of added DNA.

Transformation frequency The fraction of a cell population that takes up foreign DNA; expressed as the number of transformed cells divided by the total number of cells in a population.

Transgene A gene from one source that has been incorporated into the genome of another organism. Often refers to a gene that has been introduced into a multicellular organism.

Transgenesis The introduction of a gene(s) into animal or plant cells that leads to the transmission of the input gene (transgene) to successive generations.

Transgenic animal A fertile animal that carries an introduced gene(s) in its germ line.

Transgenic plant A fertile plant that carries an introduced gene(s) in its germ line.

Transient Of short duration.

Translation The process of protein (polypeptide) synthesis in which the amino acid sequence of a protein is determined by mRNA mediated by tRNA molecules and carried out on ribosomes.

Translational initiation signal *See* Initiation codon.

Translational start codon *See* Initiation codon.

Translational stop signal *See* Termination codon.

Translocation (1) The movement of peptidyl-tRNA and mRNA from the aminoacyl site to the peptidyl site on the ribosome during the elongation phase of translation; this movement opens the aminoacyl site for the next codon. (2) The transfer of chromosome material from one chromosome to another. (3) The movement of compounds through a plant.

Transposable element *See* Transposon.

Transposase An enzyme that is encoded by a transposon gene and that facilitates the insertion of the transposon into a new chromosomal site and excision from a site.

Transposon A DNA sequence (mobile genetic element) that can insert randomly into a chromosome, exit the site, and relocate at another chromosomal site. For example, Tn5 is a bacterial transposon that carries the genes for resistance to the antibiotics neomycin and kanamycin and the genetic information for its insertion and excision. Also called transposable element.

Trichloroethylene An organic compound, used as a solvent and degreasing agent, that often persists in the environment.

Tripartite mating A process in which conjugation is used to transfer a plasmid vector to a target cell when the plasmid vector is not self-mobilizable. When (1) cells that have a plasmid with conjugative and mobilizing functions are mixed with (2) cells that carry the plasmid vector and (3) target cells, mobilizing plasmids enter the cells with the plasmid vector and mobilize the plasmid vector to enter the target cells. Following tripartite mating, the target cells with the plasmid vector are separated from the other cell types in the mixture by various selection procedures.

tRNA *See* Transfer RNA.

True negative A test result that does not indicate the presence of a target when it is not in a sample.

True positive A test result that always recognizes a target when it is present in a sample.

Two-dimensional polyacrylamide gel electrophoresis A technique to separate different proteins in a complex mixture first based on differences in their net charges (first dimension) and then on differences in their molecular weights (second dimension).

Two-hybrid system An assay for identifying pairwise protein-protein interactions.

2μm plasmid A naturally occurring, double-stranded, circular DNA plasmid (6,318 bp) found in the nuclei of *Saccharomyces cerevisiae*. Many yeast plasmid vectors are derived from the 2μm plasmid. Also called 2μm circle, 2μ plasmid, 2-micron plasmid.

U A uracil residue in RNA.

Upstream (1) In molecular biology, the stretch of DNA base pairs that lie in the 5′ direction from the site of initiation of transcription. Usually, the first transcribed base is designated +1 and the upstream nucleotides are indicated with minus signs, e.g., −1 and −10. Also, to the 5′ side of a particular gene or sequence of nucleotides. (2) In chemical engineering, those phases of a manufacturing process that precede the biotransformation step; the preparation of raw materials for a fermentation process. Also called upstream processing.

Upstream processing *See* Upstream.

Uracil One of the organic bases found in RNA.

Vaccination *See* Preventive immunization.

Variable domains Regions of antibody chains that have different amino acid sequences in different antibody molecules. These regions are responsible for the antigen-binding specificity of the antibody molecule.

Variant An organism that is genetically different from the wild-type organism. Also called mutant.

Vascularization The formation of blood vessels.

Vector *See* Cloning vector.

Vegetative Referring to the normal growth cycle of a microorganism.

Vehicle *See* Cloning vector.

***vir* genes** A set of genes on a Ti plasmid that prepare the T-DNA segment for transfer into a plant cell.

Virion An infectious virus particle.

Viroid A circular single-stranded RNA that forms a highly base-paired (to itself) double-stranded-like structure and acts as a disease-causing agent. Viroids do not encode any proteins.

Virulence The degree of pathogenicity of an organism.

V_{max} The maximal rate of an enzyme-catalyzed reaction. V_{max} is the product of E_0 (the total amount of enzyme) and the value of k_{cat} (the catalytic rate constant).

Washout The loss of the slower-growing microorganism when two organisms are being grown together.

Western blotting Transfer of protein from a gel to a membrane.

Whey A liquid by-product of cheese making, containing mostly lactose and some milk proteins and minerals.

Wild type A genetic term that denotes the most commonly observed phenotype, or the normal state, in contrast to a mutant condition.

X linkage The presence of a gene on the X chromosome.

X-ray diffraction A technique to determine the three-dimensional structure of a molecule based on the diffraction pattern of X rays by the atoms of the molecule.

Xenobiotic A chemical compound that is not produced by living organisms; a manufactured chemical compound.

Xenogeneic From a different species or individual (an attribute of cells or tissue). Also called xenogenic.

Xenomouse A transgenic mouse that has been engineered to produce a full range of human antibodies against every antigen.

Xenotransplantation A procedure for transferring cells, tissues, or organs from one species to another species.

Xylem A tissue that transports water and dissolved minerals in plants. Xylem contributes significantly to the mechanical strength of the plant.

Xylose A five-carbon sugar that is a major constituent of hemicellulose.

YAC *See* Yeast artificial chromosome.

Yeast A single-celled fungus.

Yeast artificial chromosome A yeast-based vector system for cloning large (>100-kb) DNA inserts. Abbreviated YAC.

Yeast episomal vector A cloning vector for the yeast *Saccharomyces cerevisiae* that uses the 2μm plasmid origin of replication and is maintained as an extrachromosomal nuclear DNA molecule.

Zinc finger proteins Sequence-specific DNA-binding proteins that contain domains that bind Zn^{2+}.

Index